Current Practice of Medicine

Volume 1

Current Practice of Medicine

Series Editor
ROGER C. BONE, MD
President
The Medical College of Ohio
Toledo, Ohio

I GENERAL INTERNAL MEDICINE
Joseph D. Sapira, MD
Past Professor of Medicine
University of Alabama Birmingham
University of South Alabama
University of Maryland
St. Louis University;
Olivette, Missouri

II CARDIOLOGY
Joseph S. Alpert, MD
Professor and Chairman
Department of Medicine
University of Arizona
Health Sciences Center
Tucson, Arizona

III PULMONARY AND CRITICAL CARE MEDICINE
Roger C. Bone, MD
President
The Medical College of Ohio
Toledo, Ohio

IV ENDOCRINOLOGY AND METABOLIC DISEASE
Stanley G. Korenman, MD
Chief of Endocrinology
Department of Medicine
University of California, Los Angeles School of Medicine
Center for the Health Sciences
Los Angeles, California

CHURCHILL LIVINGSTONE, INC. • CURRENT MEDICINE, INC.

Distributed Worldwide by
CHURCHILL LIVINGSTONE, INC.
650 Avenue of the Americas
New York, NY 10003

DEVELOPED BY CURRENT MEDICINE, INC.
PHILADELPHIA

MANAGING EDITOR	Lori J. Bainbridge
PROJECT EDITOR	Peter Stevenson
DEVELOPMENTAL EDITORS	Jim Slade, Karen Nevers, Barbara Cohen-Kligerman
EDITORIAL ASSISTANTS	Charlene French, Danielle Shaw
INDEXER	Maria Coughlin
ART DIRECTOR	Paul Fennessy
LAYOUT	Jerilyn Bockorick, Lisa Caro, Robert LeBrun, Patrick Whelan
COVER DESIGN	Jerilyn Bockorick
ILLUSTRATION DIRECTOR	Ann Saydlowski
ILLUSTRATOR	Gary Welch
PRODUCTION MANAGER	David Myers
ASSISTANT PRODUCTION MANAGER	Lori Holland
TYPESETTING MANAGER	Colleen Ward

Printed in Hong Kong by Paramount Printing Group Limited.

ISBN: 0-443-07894-7 (*series*)
ISBN: 0-443-07889-0 (*volume*)
ISSN: 1079-980X
5 4 3 2 1

Although every effort has been made to ensure that drug doses and other information are presented accurately in this publication, the ultimate responsibility rests with the prescribing physician. Neither the publishers nor the authors can be held responsible for errors or for any consequences arising from the use of information contained herein. Products mentioned in this publication should be used in accordance with the prescribing information prepared by the manufacturers. No claims or endorsements are made for any drug or compound at present under clinical investigation.

© Copyright 1996 by Current Medicine, 400 Market Street, Suite 700, Philadelphia, PA 19106. All rights reserved. No part of this publication may be reproduced, stored in a retrieval system, or transmitted in any form or by any means electronic, mechanical, photocopying, recording, or otherwise, without prior written permission of the publisher.

Contributors

I. GENERAL INTERNAL MEDICINE

SECTION EDITOR

JOSEPH D. SAPIRA, MD
Past Professor of Medicine
University of Alabama Birmingham
University of South Alabama
University of Maryland
St. Louis University;
Olivette, Missouri

DALE BERG, MD
Assistant Professor of Medicine
Department of Medicine
Medical College of Wisconsin
Milwaukee, Wisconsin

JULIUS J. CHOSY, MD
Professor of Medicine
Department of Medicine
University of Wisconsin School of Medicine
Madison, Wisconsin

WILLIAM M. CONNELLY, BS, JD
Adjunct Professor
Department of Psychiatry;
Board of Trustees
Medical College of Ohio;
Connelly, Soutar and Jackson
Attorneys at Law
Toledo, Ohio

ROBERT M. HEANEY, MD
Associate Professor
Department of Internal Medicine;
Associate Dean, Graduate Medical Education
St. Louis University School of Medicine
St. Louis, Missouri

JEFFEREY D. LANG, MD
Fellow in General Medicine
Department of Medicine
McMaster University School of Medicine
Hamilton, Ontario, Canada

MACK LIPKIN, MD
Associate Professor of Clinical Medicine
Department of Medicine
New York University School of Medicine;
Director, Primary Care
New York University/Bellevue Medical Centers
New York, New York

THOMAS G. MACKIN, MD
Connelly, Soutar and Jackson
Attorneys at Law
Toledo, Ohio

ANDREW H. MELCZER, PHD
Assistant Vice President
Health Care Finance;
Director, Health Policy Research
Illinois State Medical Society
Chicago, Illinois

KEVIN O'ROURKE, OP, JCD, STM
Professor
Department of Internal Medicine
St. Louis University School of Medicine;
Director, Center for Health Care Ethics
St. Louis University Health Sciences Center
St. Louis, Missouri

CHARLES B. RODNING, MD, PHD
Professor and Vice Chairman
Department of Surgery and Structural and Cellular Biology
University of South Alabama College of Medicine
Mobile, Alabama

DAVID L. SACKETT, FRSC, MD, FRCP
Professor
Department of Clinical Medicine
University of Oxford
Oxford, England

WILLIAM SALAZAR, MD
Division of Primary Care
New York University Medical Center;
Governor Hospital
Department of Medicine
New York, New York

JAMES SEBASTIAN, MD
Associate Professor of Medicine
Department of Medicine
Medical College of Wisconsin
Milwaukee, Wisconsin

WILLIAM G. TROYER, JR., MD
Chief of Staff;
Professor of Medicine
Department of General Internal Medicine
University of Illinois Hospital
Chicago, Illinois

MARK D. WILLIAMS, MD
Assistant Professor
Department of Surgery
University of South Alabama College of Medicine
Mobile, Alabama

II. CARDIOLOGY

SECTION EDITOR

JOSEPH S. ALPERT, MD
Professor and Chairman
Department of Medicine
University of Arizona
Health Sciences Center
Tucson, Arizona

RICHARD C. BECKER, MD
Associate Professor of Medicine
University of Massachusetts Medical School;
Director, Coronary Care Unit;
Director, Thrombosis Research Center
University of Massachusetts Medical Center
Worcester, Massachusetts

CHARLES M. BLATT, MD
Instructor in Medicine
Harvard Medical School;
Associate Physician
Brigham and Women's Hospital
Boston, Massachusetts

BRAD S. BURLEW, MD
Associate Professor
University of Tennessee School of Medicine;
Director, Cardiac Catheterization Laboratory
University of Tennessee Bowld Hospital
Memphis, Tennessee

SEEMANT CHATURVEDI, MD
Assistant Professor
Department of Neurology
Wayne State University;
Staff Neurologist
Detroit Medical Center
Detroit, Michigan

MELVIN D. CHEITLIN, MD
Professor of Medicine
Division of Cardiology
Department of Medicine
University of California, San Francisco, School of Medicine;
San Francisco General Hospital
San Francisco, California

JOHN S. CHILD, MD, FACC
Co-Chief for Clinical Cardiology;
Professor of Medicine
Division of Cardiology
Department of Medicine
University of California, Los Angeles,
 School of Medicine
Los Angeles, California

JACK W. COBURN, MD
Professor of Medicine
Department of Medicine
University of California, Los Angeles,
 School of Medicine;
Staff Physician
West Los Angeles Veterans Affairs Medical
 Center
Los Angeles, California

PETER F. COHN, MD
Professor of Medicine
Division of Cardiology
Department of Medicine
State University of New York at Stony
 Brook Health Sciences Center
Stony Brook, New York

DEBORAH M. DEMARCO, MD
Assistant Professor of Medicine
Division of Rheumatology
Department of Medicine
University of Massachusetts Medical School
Worcester, Massachusetts

RICHARD B. DEVEREUX, MD
Professor of Medicine
Cornell University Medical College;
Director, Echocardiography Laboratory
The New York Hospital
New York, New York

GORDON A. EWY, MD
Professor and Chief of Cardiology
Department of Medicine
University of Arizona College of Medicine;
Director, Department of Cardiology
University of Arizona Medical Center
Tucson, Arizona

MARK N. FIENGO, DO
Eastern Connecticut Cardiology Group
New London, Connecticut;
Clinical Instructor of Medicine
Hahnemann University Hospital
Philadelphia, Pennsylvania

MICHAEL A. FIFER, MD
Director, Coronary Care Unit
Assistant Professor of Medicine
Department of Medicine
Harvard Medical School
Boston, Massachusetts

EDWARD A. FISHER, MD
Clinical Associate Professor
Department of Medicine;
Assistant Director of Echocardiography
Mt. Sinai Hospital
New York, New York

MARC FISHER, MD
Professor of Neurology and Radiology
Department of Medicine
University of Massachusetts School of
 Medicine;
Chief of Neurology
Medical Center of Central Massachusetts
Worcester, Massachusetts

DAVID F. GIANSIRACUSA, MD
Professor of Medicine;
Associate Chair
Department of Medicine
University of Massachusetts Medical School
Worcester, Massachusetts

D. BRENT GLAMANN, MD
Assistant Professor
Department of Internal Medicine
University of Texas Southwestern Medical
 Center
Dallas, Texas

MARTIN E. GOLDMAN, MD
Associate Professor
Department of Medicine
Mt. Sinai Medical School;
Director, Non-Invasive Cardiology
Mt. Sinai Hospital
New York, New York

THOMAS B. GRABOYS, MD
Associate Clinical Professor of Medicine
Harvard Medical School;
Director, Lown Cardiovascular Center;
Physician, Brigham and Women's Hospital
Boston, Massachusetts

HAIM HAMMERMAN, MD
Director, Coronary Care Unit
Department of Cardiology
Rambam Medical Center
Haifa, Israel

L. DAVID HILLIS, MD
Professor
Department of Internal Medicine
University of Texas Southwestern Medical
 Center
Dallas, Texas

HOWARD R. HORN, MD
The LW Diggs Alumni Professor of
 Medicine and Chair of Excellence in
 Medical Education

Department of Medicine
University of Tennessee, Memphis, College
 of Medicine;
Senior Physician
University of Tennessee Bowld Hospital
Memphis, Tennessee

**RUSSELL D. HULL, MBBS, MSC,
FRCP(C), FACP, FCCP**
Professor of Medicine
Department of Medicine
University of Calgary
Calgary, Alberta, Canada

WILLIAM B. KANNEL, MD, MPH, FACC
Professor of Medicine and Public Health
Department of Medicine
Boston University School of Medicine
Boston, Massachusetts

ROBERT A. KLONER, MD
Director of Research
Hospital of the Good Samaritan
The Heart Institute
Los Angeles, California

CARL V. LEIER, MD
Professor of Medicine and Pharmacology
Division of Cardiology
Department of Internal Medicine
Ohio State University College of Medicine
Columbus, Ohio

MARTIN M. LEWINTER, MD
Director of Cardiology;
Professor of Medicine
University of Vermont College of Medicine
Burlington, Vermont

A. JAMES LIEDTKE, MD
Professor of Medicine
Department of Medicine
University of Wisconsin Medical School
Madison, Wisconsin

ERIC L. MICHELSON, MD
Professor of Medicine
Medical College of Pennsylvania and
 Hahnemann University
Philadelphia, Pennsylvania

CHARLES K. MOORE, MD
Assistant Professor of Medicine
Department of Medicine
University of Mississippi Medical Center
Jackson, Mississippi

NAVIN C. NANDA, MD
Professor of Medicine
Division of Cardiology
Department of Medicine
University of Alabama School of Medicine
Birmingham, Alabama

J.V. Nixon, MD
Professor of Medicine
Medical College of Virginia
Virginia Commonwealth University
Richmond, Virginia

John B. O'Connell, MD
Professor and Chairman of Medicine
Department of Medicine
University of Mississippi Medical School
Jackson, Mississippi

Elizabeth O. Ofili, MD, MPH
Chief, Section of Cardiology;
Associate Professor of Medicine
Department of Internal Medicine
Morehouse School of Medicine
Atlanta, Georgia

John A. Paraskos, MD
Professor of Medicine
Department of Cardiovascular Medicine
University of Massachusetts Medical School
Worcester, Massachusetts

Mark J. Pirwitz, MD
Fellow
Department of Internal Medicine
University of Texas Southwestern Medical Center
Dallas, Texas

Eric N. Prystowsky, MD
Consulting Professor of Medicine
Department of Medicine
Duke University Medical Center
Durham, North Carolina;
Director, Clinical Electrophysiology Laboratory
St. Vincent Hospital
Indianapolis, Indiana

Timothy J. Regan, MD
Professor of Medicine
Department of Medicine
University of Medicine and Dentistry of New Jersey
Newark, New Jersey

Stuart Rich, MD
Chief, Section of Cardiology;
Professor of Medicine
Department of Medicine
University of Illinois at Chicago
Chicago, Illinois

John Speer Schroeder, MD
Professor of Medicine
Department of Medicine
Stanford University School of Medicine
Stanford, California

Susan Simandl, MD
Assistant Professor of Medicine
Division of Cardiology
Department of Medicine
State University of New York at Stony Brook Health Sciences Center
Stony Brook, New York

Sidney C. Smith, Jr., MD
Chief, Division of Cardiology
Professor of Medicine
University of North Carolina at Chapel Hill School of Medicine
Chapel Hill, North Carolina

Sanjiv Sobti, MD
Fellow
Department of Medicine
University of Medicine and Dentistry of New Jersey
Newark, New Jersey

John A. Spittell, Jr., MD, MACP, FACC
Professor (Emeritus) of Medicine
Cardiovascular Department
Mayo Medical School;
Consultant, Cardiovascular Disease
Mayo Clinic
Rochester, Minnesota

Peter C. Spittell, MD, FACC
Assistant Professor of Medicine
Division of Cardiovascular Diseases
Department of Internal Medicine
Mayo Medical School
Rochester, Minnesota

Paul D. Stein, MD
Professor of Medicine
Department of Medicine
Case Western Reserve University School of Medicine
Cleveland, Ohio;
Medical Director, LeVine Health Enhancement Center
Henry Ford Hospital
Detroit, Michigan

Neil J. Stone, MD
Associate Professor of Medicine
Division of Cardiology
Department of Medicine
Northwestern University Medical School
Chicago, Illinois

Jay M. Sullivan, MD
Chief, Division of Cardiology;
Professor of Medicine
Department of Medicine
University of Tennessee, Memphis, College of Medicine;
Senior Physician
University of Tennessee Bowld Hospital
Memphis, Tennessee

Paul T. Vaitkus, MD
Head, Cardiac Catheterization Laboratory
Assistant Professor
University of Vermont College of Medicine
Burlington, Vermont

Pantel S. Vokonas, MD
Professor of Medicine
Department of Medicine and Public Health
Boston University School of Medicine;
Director, Department of Veterans Affairs Normative Aging Study
Boston, Massachusetts

Park W. Willis IV, MD
Associate Professor
Division of Cardiology
Department of Medicine
University of North Carolina at Chapel Hill School of Medicine
Chapel Hill, North Carolina

Gregg M. Yamada, MD
Instructor
Department of Medicine
University of Arizona College of Medicine
Tucson, Arizona

III. PULMONARY AND CRITICAL CARE MEDICINE

Section Editor
Roger C. Bone, MD
President
The Medical College of Ohio
Toledo, Ohio

Guillermo A. do Pico, MD, FCCP
Professor of Medicine
Department of Medicine
University of Wisconsin Medical School
Madison, Wisconsin

Takateru Izumi, MD
Professor of Medicine
Chest Research Institute
Kyoto University
Kyoto, Japan

Glen A. Lillington, MD, FRCPC, FACP
Clinical Professor of Medicine
Pulmonary/Critical Care Division
Stanford University School of Medicine;
Stanford Chest Clinic
Stanford University Medical Center
Stanford, California;
Professor Emeritus of Medicine
University of California, Davis, School of Medicine
Davis, California

SAMUEL LOUIE, MD
Associate Professor of Medicine
University of California, Davis, School of Medicine;
Pulmonary/Critical Care Division
University of California, Davis, Medical Center
Davis, California

KEITH C. MEYER, MD, FACP, FCCP
Assistant Professor of Medicine
Department of Internal Medicine
University of Wisconsin Medical School
Madison, Wisconsin

MICHAEL S. NIEDERMAN, MD
Associate Professor of Medicine
State University of New York at Stony Brook Health Sciences Center
Stony Brook, New York;
Director, Critical Care Subsection
Winthrop-University Hospital
Mineola, New York

GREGORY R. OWENS, MD
Professor of Medicine and Anesthesiology
Department of Medicine
University of Pittsburgh School of Medicine;
Chief, Pulmonary and Critical Care Medicine
Montefiore University Hospital
Pittsburgh, Pennsylvania

SUSAN K. PINGLETON, MD
Professor of Medicine
Director, Division of Pulmonary and Critical Care Medicine
University of Kansas Medical Center
Kansas City, Kansas

ROBERT L. ROSEN, MD
Associate Professor
Department of Internal Medicine
Rush Medical College of Rush University
Chicago, Illinois

LEWIS J. RUBIN, MD
Head, Division of Pulmonary and Critical Care Medicine;
Professor of Medicine and Physiology
University of Maryland School of Medicine
Baltimore, Maryland

STEVEN A. SAHN, MD
Professor of Medicine
Division of Pulmonary and Critical Care Medicine
Department of Medicine
Medical University of South Carolina
Charleston, South Carolina

OM P. SHARMA, MD
Professor of Medicine
Department of Medicine
University of Southern California School of Medicine
Los Angeles, California

NEIL V. WARAVDEKAR, MD
Grissom, Halvorson and Gilson (private practice)
Frederick, Maryland

CLIFFORD W. ZWILLICH, MD
Vice Chairman
Department of Medicine;
Chief, Pulmonary/Critical Care Division
The Milton S. Hershey Medical Center
Hershey, Pennsylvania

IV. ENDOCRINOLOGY AND METABOLIC DISEASE

SECTION EDITOR
STANLEY G. KORENMAN, MD
Chief of Endocrinology
Department of Medicine
University of California, Los Angeles School of Medicine
Center for the Health Sciences
Los Angeles, California

MARTIN J. ABRAHAMSON, MD
Assistant Professor
Department of Medicine
Harvard Medical School;
Clinical Director, Diabetes Care Center
Beth Israel Hospital
Boston, Massachusetts

ITAMAR B. ABRASS, MD
Professor and Head
Division of Gerontology and Geriatric Medicine
Department of Medicine
University of Washington School of Medicine
Seattle, Washington

STEPHEN B. BAYLIN, MD
Professor of Oncology and Medicine
Oncology Center Laboratories
Johns Hopkins University School of Medicine
Baltimore, Maryland

SHALENDER BHASIN, MD
Professor of Medicine
Harbor-University of California, Los Angeles, Medical Center
Department of Medicine
Torrance, California

GEORGE P. CHROUSOS, MD, ScD
Professor of Medicine
Department of Pediatrics
Georgetown University School of Medicine
Washington, DC;
Chief, Pediatric Endocrinology Section
National Institutes of Health Clinical Center
Bethesda, Maryland

ANDRÉE C. DE BUSTROS, MD, MPH
Section Head, Endocrinology
Christ Hospital and Medical Center
Oak Lawn, Illinois

LESLIE J. DEGROOT, MD
Professor of Medicine
Department of Medicine
University of Chicago Pritzker School of Medicine
Chicago, Illinois

VINCENT DEQUATTRO, MD
Professor of Medicine
Department of Medicine
University of Southern California School of Medicine;
Chief, Hypertension Service
Los Angeles County University of Southern California Medical Center
Los Angeles, California

ROBERT G. DLUHY, MD
Associate Professor
Endocrine-Hypertension Division
Department of Medicine
Harvard Medical School
Boston, Massachusetts

DAVID A. EHRMANN, MD
Associate Professor of Medicine
Department of Medicine
University of Chicago Pritzker School of Medicine;
Bernard Mitchell Hospital
Chicago, Illinois

DAVID FELDMAN, MD
Professor of Medicine
Division of Endocrinology, Gerontology, and Metabolism
Department of Medicine
Stanford University School of Medicine
Stanford, California

J. FRANCISCO FIERRO-RENOY, MD
Research Fellow
Department of Medicine
University of Chicago Pritzker School of Medicine
Chicago, Illinois

JEFFREY S. FLIER, MD
Professor of Medicine
Department of Medicine
Harvard Medical School;
Beth Israel Hospital
Boston, Massachusetts

JACK GELLER, MD
Adjunct Professor of Medicine
Department of Internal Medicine
University of California, San Diego, School
 of Medicine;
Mercy Hospital Medical Center
San Diego, California

DAVID HEBER, MD, PhD
Professor of Medicine
University of California, Los Angeles,
 School of Medicine
Los Angeles, California

JEROME M. HERSHMAN, MD
Chief, Endocrinology and Metabolism
 Division
West Los Angeles Veterans Affairs Medical
 Center;
Professor of Medicine
University of California, Los Angeles,
 School of Medicine
Los Angeles, California

L. MICHAEL KETTEL, MD
Associate Professor of Medicine
Department of Reproductive Medicine
University of California, San Diego,
 Medical Center
San Diego, California

LYNN KOHLMEIER, MD
Fellow
Division of Endocrinology
Department of Medicine
Stanford University School of Medicine
Stanford California;
Brigham and Women's Hospital
Boston, Massachusetts

FREDRIC B. KRAEMER, MD
Associate Professor of Medicine
Division of Endocrinology
Department of Medicine
Stanford University School of Medicine
Stanford, California;
Department of Veterans Affairs
Palo Alto, California

DEPING LEE, MD
Assistant Professor
Department of Research Medicine;
Associate Director
Hypertension Diagnostic Laboratory
University of Southern California School of
 Medicine
Los Angeles, California

MARIA ALEXANDRA MAGIAKOU, MD
Guest Researcher
Developmental Endocrinology Branch
National Institute of Child Health and
 Human Development
National Institutes of Health
Bethesda, Maryland

ROBERT MARCUS, MD
Professor of Medicine
Department of Medicine
Stanford University School of Medicine
Stanford, California;
Director, Aging Study Unit
Veterans Affairs Medical Center
Palo Alto, California

SHLOMO MELMED, MD
Professor of Medicine
Department of Medicine
University of California, Los Angeles,
 School of Medicine;
Director, Division of Endocrinology and
 Metabolism
Cedars-Sinai Medical Center
Los Angeles, California

MYRON MILLER, MD
Professor and Vice Chairman
Department of Geriatrics and Adult
 Development;
Professor and Chief
Division of Clinical Geriatrics
Department of Medicine
Mt. Sinai School of Medicine of the City
 University of New York
New York, New York

VALERY T. MILLER, MD
Research Professor
Department of Medicine
George Washington University School of
 Medicine and Health Sciences
Washington, DC

STEPHEN R. PLYMATE, MD
Research Associate Professor
Department of Medicine;
Geriatric Research Education and Clinical
 Center
University of Washington School of
 Medicine
Tacoma, Washington

JANE E-B. REUSCH, MD
Assistant Professor of Medicine
Department of Medicine
University of Colorado School of Medicine;
Denver Veterans Affairs Medical Center
Denver, Colorado

ROBERT L. ROSENFIELD, MD
Professor of Medicine
Departments of Medicine and Pediatrics
University of Chicago Pritzker School of
 Medicine;
Wyler Children's Hospital
Chicago, Illinois

ROBERT S. SCHWARTZ, MD
Professor of Medicine
Division of Gerontology and Geriatric
 Medicine
Department of Medicine
University of Washington School of
 Medicine
Seattle, Washington

KARL E. SUSSMAN, MD
Professor of Medicine
Department of Endocrinology
Veterans Affairs Medical Center
Denver, Colorado

GORDON H. WILLIAMS, MD
Professor of Medicine
Department of Medicine
Harvard Medical School;
Endocrine-Hypertension Division
Brigham and Women's Hospital
Boston, Massachusetts

Foreword

During the past few decades, the practice of medicine has evolved from an "art form" applied at a leisurely pace to a "science" demanding rapid and accurate diagnosis with quick and effective therapies. This textbook, *Current Practice of Medicine*, is designed to offer the primary care physician a ready reference for the practice of such a science. Its chapters are condensed but comprehensive, and are greatly enhanced by the liberal application of figures and tables. Key concepts are presented in a form that can be assimilated and applied directly to the management of a patient. Perhaps the most remarkable advancement in clinical practice has been the ever-increasing armamentarium of methods for imaging the organs of pathology, either directly by endoscopy, or indirectly by computed tomography or magnetic resonance imaging. The images obtained from such tools are represented plentifully in this textbook. In this era of rapid scientific developments, it is essential for a textbook to be up to date. To circumvent the lead time required to produce a work of this magnitude, each of the four volumes of *Current Practice of Medicine* will be updated regularly. For ease of use, a companion CD-ROM version is planned, allowing the text to be linked to MEDLINE for extensive evaluation of cited references. *Current Practice of Medicine* is a modern textbook well suited for the practicing internist of today. No doubt it will serve its purpose well.

Tadataka Yamada, MD
Ann Arbor, Michigan

Series Preface

Medical knowledge is said to double approximately every five years. Complicated diagnostic tools, emerging pharmaceuticals, and innovative treatment protocols continually challenge today's physician. To provide the highest quality health care to patients, the general practitioner must keep pace with the burgeoning medical literature.

Today's physicians have access to many good sources of information, including continuing education courses, journals and textbooks, and interactive computer software. However, until now, a complete medical information source that is always within an arm's reach has been lacking. As Editor of the *Current Practice of Medicine* series, I am proud to introduce a comprehensive medical reference source that will satisfy the substantial informational needs of the general practitioner. The series is designed to provide the general practitioner with easily accessible, in-depth commentary on contemporary medicine.

Four bound volumes, each filled with hundreds of photographs, tables, and detailed medical illustrations, cover every aspect of internal medicine:

- Allergy and Immunology
- Cardiology
- Dermatology
- Endocrinology and Metabolic Disease
- Gastroenterology
- General Internal Medicine
- Hematology
- Hepatology
- Infectious Diseases
- Nephrology
- Neurology
- Oncology
- Psychiatry
- Pulmonary and Critical Care Medicine
- Rheumatology

The Section Editors have asked the premier specialists of their respective fields to contribute up-to-date and reliable chapters specifically intended for the general practitioner.

Current Practice of Medicine is an ambitious series. It is a valuable addition to the reference libraries of all physicians who deal with the complicated mysteries presented by patients. I am proud to oversee the important and essential information that these volumes contribute to medical knowledge.

I would like to thank all of the contributing authors and the Section Editors, whose efforts are central to the great success of this series. I also offer my sincere thanks to Abe Krieger, President of Current Medicine; Lori J. Bainbridge, Managing Editor; Pete Stevenson and Jim Slade, Developmental Editors; and everyone on the staff of Current Medicine who helped to make this project possible.

Roger C. Bone, MD
Toledo, Ohio

Series Contents

VOLUME 1

Section I. General Internal Medicine
Joseph D. Sapira, Section Editor

Section II. Cardiology
Joseph S. Alpert, Section Editor

Section III. Pulmonary and Critical Care Medicine
Roger C. Bone, Section Editor

Section IV. Endocrinology and Metabolic Disease
Stanley G. Korenman, Section Editor

VOLUME 2

Section V. Dermatology
Jeffrey P. Callen, Section Editor

Section VI. Rheumatology
Daniel J. McCarty, Section Editor

Section VII. Allergy and Immunology
Phillip L. Lieberman, Section Editor

Section VIII. Infectious Diseases
Harold C. Neu and Robert H. Rubin, Section Editors

VOLUME 3

Section IX. Neurology
William C. Koller, Section Editor

Section X. Psychiatry
Jan Fawcett, Section Editor

Section XI. Hematology
Jiri Palek, Section Editor

Section XII. Oncology
David S. Ettinger, Section Editor

VOLUME 4

Section XIII. Gastroenterology
David Y. Graham and Atilla Ertan, Section Editors

Section XIV. Hepatology
Willis C. Maddrey, Section Editor

Section XV. Nephrology
Richard J. Glassock, Section Editor

Volume Contents

SECTION I. GENERAL INTERNAL MEDICINE
Joseph D. Sapira, Section Editor

CHAPTER 1
The Medical Interview
Mack Lipkin and William Salazar

CHAPTER 2
Screening
Robert M. Heaney

CHAPTER 3
Physical Diagnosis in Medicine
Dale Berg and James Sebastian

CHAPTER 4
Diagnostic Tests
Jefferey D. Lang and David L. Sackett

CHAPTER 5
Referrals
Julius J. Chosy

CHAPTER 6
Medical Economics
Andrew H. Melczer

CHAPTER 7
Health Policy
William G. Troyer

CHAPTER 8
Health Care Ethics
Kevin O'Rourke

CHAPTER 9
The Humanities in Medicine
Mark D. Williams and Charles B. Rodning

CHAPTER 10
Malpractice
William M. Connelly and Thomas G. Mackin

SECTION II. CARDIOLOGY
Joseph S. Alpert, Section Editor

CHAPTER 1
Evaluation of the Patient with Chest Pain
John A. Paraskos

CHAPTER 2
Evaluation of the Patient with Heart Failure
Carl V. Leier

CHAPTER 3
Evaluation of the Patient with Hypotension and Shock
Richard C. Becker

CHAPTER 4
Evaluation of the Patient with Palpitations and Non–Life-Threatening Cardiac Arrhythmias
Mark N. Fiengo and Eric L. Michelson

CHAPTER 5
Evaluation of the Patient with Syncope
Charles M. Blatt and Thomas B. Graboys

CHAPTER 6
Evaluation of the Patient Resuscitated from Cardiac Arrest
Eric N. Prystowsky

CHAPTER 7
Risk Factors for and Prevention of Atherosclerotic Cardiovascular Disease
Pantel S. Vokonas and William B. Kannel

CHAPTER 8
Approach to the Patient with Hyperlipidemia
Neil J. Stone

CHAPTER 9
Chronic Ischemic Heart Disease
Susan Simandl and Peter F. Cohn

CHAPTER 10
Unstable Angina and Non–Q Wave Myocardial Infarction
John Speer Schroeder

CHAPTER 11
Q-Wave Myocardial Infarction
Haim Hammerman and Robert A. Kloner

CHAPTER 12
Mitral Stenosis and Regurgitation
Sidney C. Smith, Jr., and Park W. Willis IV

CHAPTER 13
Mitral Valve Prolapse
Richard B. Devereux

CHAPTER 14
Aortic Stenosis and Regurgitation
Michael A. Fifer

CHAPTER 15
Tricuspid and Pulmonic Valve Disease
D. Brent Glamann, Mark J. Pirwitz, and L. David Hillis

CHAPTER 16
Hypertrophic Cardiomyopathy
Gregg M. Yamada and Joseph S. Alpert

CHAPTER 17
Congestive Cardiomyopathy
Sanjiv Sobti and Timothy J. Regan

CHAPTER 18
Restrictive Cardiomyopathy
Martin E. Goldman and Edward A. Fisher

CHAPTER 19
Infectious Myocarditis
Martin E. Goldman

CHAPTER 20
Infectious Endocarditis
Gordon A. Ewy

CHAPTER 21
Pericardial Disease
Paul T. Vaitkus and Martin M. LeWinter

CHAPTER 22
Congenital Heart Disease, Including Unrepaired Lesions in the Adult
Melvin D. Cheitlin

CHAPTER 23
Congenital Heart Disease in the Adult Postoperative Patient
John S. Child

CHAPTER 24
Pulmonary Hypertension
Stuart Rich

CHAPTER 25
Pulmonary Embolism
Paul D. Stein and Russell D. Hull

CHAPTER 26
Cardiac Tumors
Elizabeth O. Ofili and Navin C. Nanda

CHAPTER 27
Nonpenetrating Cardiac Trauma
A. James Liedtke

CHAPTER 28
Diseases of the Aorta
Gregg M. Yamada and Joseph S. Alpert

CHAPTER 29
Diseases of Peripheral Arteries and Veins
John A. Spittell, Jr., and Peter C. Spittell

CHAPTER 30
Cerebrovascular Complications of Cardiac Disorders
Seemant Chaturvedi and Marc Fisher

CHAPTER 31
Rheumatic Diseases and the Heart
Deborah M. DeMarco and David F. Giansiracusa

CHAPTER 32
The Aging Heart
J.V. Nixon

CHAPTER 33
Pregnancy and the Heart
Brad S. Burlew, Howard R. Horn, and Jay M. Sullivan

CHAPTER 34
The Transplanted Heart
Charles K. Moore and John B. O'Connell

SECTION III. PULMONARY AND CRITICAL CARE MEDICINE

ROGER C. BONE, SECTION EDITOR

CHAPTER 1
Pulmonary Diagnostic Studies
Robert L. Rosen

CHAPTER 2
Obstructive Diseases
Gregory R. Owens

CHAPTER 3
Neoplasms of the Lung
Samuel Louie and Glen Lillington

CHAPTER 4
Infectious Lung Diseases
Michael S. Niederman

CHAPTER 5
Disorders of the Pulmonary Circulation
Lewis J. Rubin

CHAPTER 6
Interstitial Lung Disease
Om P. Sharma and Takateru Izumi

CHAPTER 7
Occupational and Environmental Lung Diseases
Guillermo A. do Pico and Keith C. Meyer

CHAPTER 8
Diseases of the Pleura
  Steven A. Sahn

CHAPTER 9
Disorders of the Control of Breathing
  Neil V. Waravdekar and Clifford W. Zwillich

CHAPTER 10
Critical Care
  Susan K. Pingleton

SECTION IV. ENDOCRINOLOGY AND METABOLIC DISEASE
STANLEY G. KORENMAN, SECTION EDITOR

CHAPTER 1
Neuroendocrinology
  Myron Miller

CHAPTER 2
Anterior Pituitary
  Shlomo Melmed

CHAPTER 3
Thyroid Dysfunction
  Jerome M. Hershman

CHAPTER 4
Thyroid Masses
  J. Francisco Fierro-Renoy and Leslie J. DeGroot

CHAPTER 5
Adrenal Cortex Glucocorticoids
  Lynn Kohlmeier and David Feldman

CHAPTER 6
Glucocorticoid Therapy and Withdrawal
  George P. Chrousos and Maria Alexandra Magiakou

CHAPTER 7
Pheochromocytoma
  Vincent DeQuattro and Deping Lee

CHAPTER 8
Aldosteronism and Endocrine Blood Pressure Syndromes
  Robert G. Dluhy and Gordon H. Williams

CHAPTER 9
Abnormal Uterine Bleeding
  L. Michael Kettel

CHAPTER 10
Secondary Amenorrhea
  Robert L. Rosenfield and David A. Ehrmann

CHAPTER 11
Male Hypogonadism
  Stephen R. Plymate

CHAPTER 12
Male Reproductive Problems
  Shalender Bhasin

CHAPTER 13
Disorders of Serum Calcium Concentration
  Robert Marcus

CHAPTER 14
Diabetes Mellitus and Hypoglycemia
  Martin J. Abrahamson and Jeffrey S. Flier

CHAPTER 15
Management of Hyperglycemic Emergencies and Other Hyperglycemic States
  Jane E-B. Reusch and Karl E. Sussman

CHAPTER 16
Complications of Diabetes
  Fredric B. Kraemer

CHAPTER 17
Breast Disease
  David Heber

CHAPTER 18
Nutrition and Lipids
  David Heber

CHAPTER 19
Endocrine Manifestations of Cancer
  Andrée C. de Bustros and Stephen B. Baylin

CHAPTER 20
Aging: Prostatic Disease, Benign Prostatic Hyperplasia, and Carcinoma
  Jack Geller

CHAPTER 21
Special Presentation of Endocrine Disease in the Elderly
  Itamar B. Abrass and Robert S. Schwartz

CHAPTER 22
Menopause and the Postmenopausal State
  Valery T. Miller

VOLUME INDEX

GENERAL INTERNAL MEDICINE

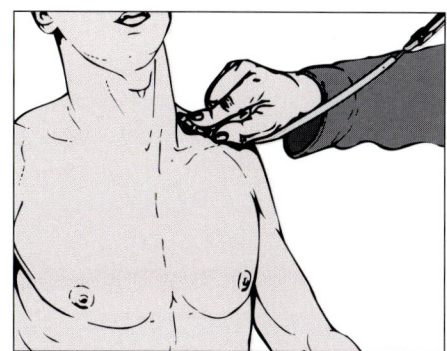

Section Editor

Joseph D. Sapira

This section of *Current Practice of Medicine* differs from the others in that it is less concerned with the content and more with the *process* of medicine. Thus, it should be of interest to all physicians.

The chapter on interviewing will enhance the physician's effectiveness, regardless of his or her specialty. Analyses of diagnostic tests in general, and of screening tests in particular, provide both theoretical and practical suggestions. A chapter on physical diagnosis uniquely combines discussions of common problems and specific useful maneuvers. This contrasts with the chapter on the humanities in medicine, which is of the genre that Osler called "night-table reading." The chapter on medical economics is a rare opportunity to read a discussion based on data by an impartial writer. Chapters concerning referrals, health policy, and medical ethics are succinct articulations of what most physicians have felt, in terms they do not normally use.

Hopefully, after absorbing the wisdom provided in the first nine chapters, the reader will not have to apply lessons learned from the final chapter on medical malpractice, except for the tips on providing expert testimony.

I thank the contributors for their efforts, and we look forward to comments from our readers.

The Medical Interview

Mack Lipkin
William Salazar

> **Key Points**
> - The medical interview is the clinical skill that most determines efficiency, diagnostic accuracy and completeness, patient and physician satisfaction, and freedom from malpractice suits.
> - The average generalist will conduct 160,000 to 200,000 interviews in a career, yet will never work to improve on this skill in a systematic, data-based way.
> - Work on interview skills, knowledge, and attitudes leads to lasting improvement, efficiency, and increased satisfaction.
> - The interview has ten structural elements and three functions. Each of these elements has specific associated behaviors that correlate with improved outcomes of care and satisfaction.
> - Dealing with difficult patients, obtaining sexual history, breaking bad news, and working with patients from other cultures and no common language are situations that physicians find particularly vexing and that lead to poor care.
> - The generalist practitioner should work on his or her interview skills regularly through self-taping, use of a tutor or peers, and attending courses.

The medical interview is the most important tool of the physician [1••]. On a personal level, it occupies more time and is done more often than anything else in the physician's professional life. Because the average primary care physician will perform 160,000 to 200,000 interviews in a 40-year career, it behooves physicians to maximize their efficiency (a 10% increase in efficiency per interview would save more than 2 years) and their satisfaction. A good deal of the dissatisfaction in modern medicine is dissatisfaction with the interview and the relationships that it produces.

The good news is that helpful knowledge is available to guide skill enhancement in interviewing. This chapter summarizes this knowledge and guides physicians to resources for working on skills. Since the time when most current physicians were trained, there has been an explosion of new research about what is important, what works, and what pleases physician and patient. Some of this research is done on the micro level, such as looking at the form and sequence of questions. Some explores important new constructs regarding the structure and function of the interview. By studying this new knowledge, taking it to heart, and practicing the skills involved, physicians can expect significantly improved efficiency, accuracy, and completeness of data collection; improved doctor-patient relationships; and greater satisfaction. The central modern construct concerning the interview is that it has structure and functions.

THE THREE FUNCTIONS OF THE INTERVIEW

One way to improve skills in medical interviewing is through better execution of the three functions of the interview [2]: 1) gathering information (Table 1); 2) developing and maintaining a therapeutic relationship (Table 2); and 3) communicating information (Table 3).

TABLE 1 GATHERING INFORMATION AND DETERMINING THE NATURE OF THE PROBLEM	
Skills	Examples
Open-ended questions	"Tell me about your concerns."
Facilitation	"Uh, uh, tell me more about that."
Direction	"This is important, and I would like to hear more about it later; for now, would you tell me about your chest pain?"
Summarizing and checking the continuous worries	"You have talked about your chest pain, about your family, and about the problems that you have taking the medication. Is there anything else that concerns you?"

TABLE 2 DEVELOPING AND MAINTAINING A THERAPEUTIC RELATIONSHIP	
Skills	Examples
Reflection	"You seem to be very upset about this issue."
Legitimation	"I can certainly understand why taking medications is so difficult for you."
Support	"I want you to know that I am here to help you through this difficult decision."
Partnership	"Then how would you like to be helped now?"
Respect	"It is really nice to see you coming to the clinic on your own, despite how difficult it is for you."
Nonverbal skills	Touch; positive eye contact
Empathy	"I understand your suffering."
Unconditional positive regard	"I admire how you keep trying."
Avoid shame and humiliation	"How could you forget that?"

Each function has specific associated behaviors which, if done well, will improve the physician's work. Each function has a separate set of skills that are specific, learnable, and focused [3]. However, overlap and interrelation exist among them. To use these skills and to fulfill the three functions of the interview efficiently, the interviewer needs to integrate them with the structural elements (*see* later discussion).

Collecting information is considered by most physicians to be the core function of the medical interview. Whether this information is psychological or biological, appropriate data collection skills can increase the efficiency and accuracy of the information that is collected.

The second function of the interview is critical to all interviews and has a major impact on the other functions. "Therapeutic" here means a relationship that promotes care, cooperation, and healing. The interaction between patient and physician gives the patient freedom to talk more openly and in more detail about the feelings he or she is experiencing. Use of the interviewing techniques in Table 2 contributes to interview efficiency and to rapport. To maintain rapport, the physician needs to handle the patient's emotions appropriately. Throughout the interview, the physician should remain aware of and responsive to emotions when they become apparent and when they ought to be present but are not. Part of history taking involves sharing control and decision making. This "activates" the patient as an agent of his or her own care and has been shown to improve biologic outcome [4]. Patients who feel understood by their physicians are generally more satisfied and feel better, which in turn brings more physician satisfaction.

Use of the simple skills listed in Table 3 influences adherence to treatment recommendations. Patients will better understand the nature of their illness, the suggested diagnostic procedures, and the treatment possibilities. Unless physician and patient negotiate agreement regarding the nature of the problem, the patient will not comply. After the patient fully understands the disease process, the physician and patient can achieve an alliance for the patient's care. Issues of informed consent, coping mechanisms, and lifestyle change can be managed more effectively. The information provided to the patient should be brief. It is important to remember that anxiety interferes with the ability to understand the illness, and most patients are quite anxious when they are first told about an illness. Initially, the physician should stick to a few key points.

Motivational Skills

Motivational skills are important in helping patients adhere to the recommendations of their physicians (Table 4).

THE STRUCTURAL ELEMENTS OF THE INTERVIEW

Careful structuring of the interview is central to effectiveness. Each of the 10 structural elements must be used. Each influences the quality of data, of the process, and of the ensuing doctor–patient relationship. Each element has specific behaviors associated which, if done well, improve, and if done poorly, detract from the effectiveness of the interview [5•].

Optimizing the environment includes removing barriers, handing off the beeper, eliminating distractions, ensuring privacy, and making eye contact on the same level. It also includes making the office accessible, having pleasant and polite receptionists and phone operators, and having as attractive a setting as feels adequate to the physician.

The *opening* includes preparing oneself to listen and, using the initial observation of the patient, to gather preliminary data and generate hypotheses. We use the first observation of the patient in the waiting room as a preliminary evaluation: Is she thin or jaundiced? Is he disheveled? Does she slump over? Is the family there, and if so, who? This rapid look also prepares us for engaging with *this* person.

Table 3. Educating patients and implementing a treatment plan

Skills	Examples
Establishing baseline knowledge and attributions	"Would you tell me your understanding of diabetes and its causes?"
Avoiding complex medical terminology	"You have a positive PPD: this means that the `germs' entered your body, went to your lungs, and fell asleep. You do not have tuberculosis."
Checking	"Just to make sure that I have made myself clear, can you tell me how you will be taking the medications at home?"

PPD—purified protein derivative.

Table 4. Motivational skills

Skills	Examples
Establish a baseline	"What is your understanding of this medication that I prescribed for you?"
Explore obstacles to adherence	"Many patients have problems taking medications every day. What is your experience?"
Elicit and negotiate goals	"Would you tell me what will make it easier for you to follow the diet?"
Elicit and negotiate problems	"I think the idea of cutting down your fat intake is good. Explain to me how you would do it."
Elicit and negotiate solutions	"How about starting with red meat?"
Offer help	"I am really eager to help you with this. Call anytime with questions or to talk."

Preparing to listen involves focusing, leaving behind other worries and thoughts, and getting centered. Some physicians do this through imaging, through self-hypnosis, or through sheer intentional concentration. This step markedly improves the physician's data-gathering effectiveness.

Greeting the patient appropriately sets the stage for a positive interaction. From the greeting, the patient can ascertain who the physician is, that the physician knows him or her, and what tone and type of exchange the physician practices (*ie*, authoritarian, person to person, or informal). It may indicate whether the physician can perceive and adapt to the patient's style. Overall, the greeting sets the initial tone for the interview.

In the *introduction* phase, physician and patient each discuss why they are there, what their expectations are, and what the limits to this or all interactions are. Social talk may occur. Most valuable is the physician's act of showing (in contrast to merely feeling or intending) care for the patient. Today, many patients have bad experiences with doctors. Patients may be fearful or angry and may be inclined to project these feelings, and they may hurt physically or psychologically. "I see you are in pain. May I help make you more comfortable or get you something?" is a remarkably powerful way of engaging the patient's belief that you care and are interested in the patient's needs.

Every new interview raises the probability of *barriers to communication*. Unless the physician detects them and corrects for them, the interview tool is as worthless as an uncalibrated meter. Some barriers are physical—delirium, deafness, and severe pain—some are cognitive—delirium, dementia, attention deficits, and hyperactivity. Other barriers are psychological, such as depression, grief, rage, and delusions or hallucinations. Many are cultural, such as language differences, health belief model differences, and fears of deportation or ridicule. Some are status differences. Unless these (and other) barriers are identified and overcome, the physician is wasting time and effort and is probably obtaining bad data as well [6•].

Once the stage has been set, the usual practice is to elicit a "chief complaint." In reality, the average patient coming to a generalist has three complaints in mind [7]. The first complaint presented may not be what is really important to the patient or to the doctor. Therefore, it is wisest to *survey all the problems* before choosing which to pursue first. The physician might ask something like "What brings you in today?" After the patient responds with, "I have terrible allergies" or whatever, the doctor can say something like, "So what else?" "Well, I have been having real trouble sleeping." "What else?" "Sometimes I cough up some phlegm with some red spots in it." "Anything else?" "Not really."

Obviously, the most significant problem to the physician came up third. If the physician had not surveyed problems, information about the blood-tinged sputum might not have been elicited or gotten to. This is realistic. Patients often leave the complaint that frightens or embarrasses them the most to last, especially chest pain, shortness of breath, bleeding, and alcoholism. Once as complete a list as possible has been obtained, the physician can *negotiate a priority problem* with the patient. This is necessary because the patient's priority may be back pain or insomnia, whereas the physician's may be blood-tinged sputum. Unless the physician explicitly acknowledges and deals with the value and importance of the patient's issues (the acknowledgment may be as simple as, "I definitely want to get to your back pain—if not today, then next time"), the patient's cooperation, likelihood of return, and willingness to comply may be compromised. How does the physician negotiate the priority complaint [8•]? The physician states his or her reasons and has the patient do likewise; then, patient and physician decide together.

The best way to proceed on the negotiated priority is to ask the patient to tell the story of X from the beginning. This establishes a *narrative thread* that organizes the flow of talk. To the extent possible, allowing the patient to tell his or her own story in his or her own words is most efficient and produces the most accurate information. Of course, the physician may have to focus a rambler, someone with mental status deficits, and so forth. With the narrative thread in place, the physician can digress to elaborate (*eg,* "Tell me about your family," or "What was happening then?") and then come back to the thread with "And what happened next?"

The narrative thread is particularly helpful in *developing the life context of the patient and illness*. The physician can ask, "Who is at home?" or, "What is your work?", and so forth and then return to the story after obtaining the needed information.

Certain techniques facilitate learning about the patient as a person efficiently. One is to show interest, at the first opportunity, about the personal issues and feelings of the patient. A second is to demonstrate respect, sensitivity, gentleness, and concern about these issues as soon as possible and often. A third is to listen actively, which means hearing not only the cognitive content of what the patient is saying, but also the matters not spoken of explicitly. For example, the physician may hear the feelings expressed; what is omitted; how what is said reflects what the patient thinks or feels about the subject; when the patient changes the subject; when the patient's eyes fill; and much more.

The end of the visit is very important. The physician generally educates and negotiates with the patient at this point about diagnostic plans and therapeutic options. To educate effectively includes assessing where the patient is and what he or she knows, using simple language, omitting all but the crucial information, and reviewing and revising with the patient. The physician lets the patient know what to do between visits if the patient needs the doctor. Most importantly, however, the physician should allow the patient to review in his or her own words what has happened and what will happen.

DEALING WITH UNUSUAL OR DIFFICULT SITUATIONS

Taking the Sexual History

The sexual history is increasingly important to the medical interview in the era of AIDS. Despite the increasing incidence of sexual issues, physicians often experience obstacles and discomfort in asking about sex, and the majority rarely take sexual histories. In primary care settings, the prevalence of sexual problems and concerns is approximately 50%. The goals of taking the sexual history are outlined in Table 5. Unlike most situations, in which starting with an open-ended question and then coning down is best, in taking the sexual history, it is good to start with direct questions. An open-ended approach is not useful initially because patients do not usually volunteer information about sexual problems when asked a general question [9].

Working with Interpreters

When practitioner and patient do not share a language, using an interpreter becomes essential for accurate communication. The most important barriers are health belief model and language. Kleinman [10] has formulated a set of questions that is useful in eliciting the patient's belief system (Table 6). The physician should always use a trained medical interpreter when it is feasible and practical. Interpreter-dependent interviews take more time. In working with interpreters, questions should be short and simple. Language that the interpreter can handle should be used, with brief comments and explanations for the interpreter added as needed. Ambiguous statements and questions, as well as abstractions, idiomatic expressions, and metaphors, are risky and create confusion (Table 7).

TABLE 5 QUESTIONS FOR THE SEXUAL HISTORY TAKING

"Have you ever had sex?"
"Are you having sex these days?"
"Are there any problems related to sex that you would like to discuss with me?"
"Have you had sex with men, with women, or with both?"

TABLE 6 QUESTIONS TO ELICIT PATIENTS' EXPLANATORY MODELS OF ILLNESS

"What do you call your problem? What name does it have?"
"What do you think has caused your problem?"
"Why do you think it started when it did?"
"What does your sickness do to you? How does it work?"
"How severe is it? Will it have a short or long course?"
"What do you fear most about your sickness?"
"What are the chief problems your sickness has caused you?"
"What kind of treatment do you think you should receive?"
"What are the most important results you hope to receive from your treatment?"

TABLE 7 GENERAL GUIDELINES FOR WORKING WITH INTERPRETERS

Learn about the patient's background
Clarify with the interpreter before the session how you are going to work together
Meet regularly with your interpreters (if any)
Become familiar with special terminology the patient uses
If possible, maintain interpreter–patient pairing
Be patient
Use short questions without complicated clauses
Use language that the interpreter can handle
Be brief
Make allowances for terms and concepts that do not exist in the target language
Avoid ambiguous statements and questions
Use family only as a last resort (as confidentiality is compromised)

(*From* New York Task Force on Immigrant Health, Division of Primary Care Internal Medicine, New York University Medical Center, Bellevue Hospital Center, New York, NY.)

Table 8. Strategies for physicians to cope with negative emotional responses

Physician's reaction	Coping strategies
Avoidance	Attempt to understand and master feelings that lead to avoidance; stay with the patient; discuss the situation with colleagues
Identification with the patient	Recognize the reaction; avoid tendency to deny seriousness of the disease or to give way to despair
Hostility or rejection	Acknowledge and analyze the reaction; do not attempt to like the unlikable patient; use behavioral approaches; if the situation is intolerable, transfer the patient to another physician
Feelings of impotence or inadequacy	Discover areas in which physical and emotional help and comfort can be rendered; be realistic about limitations
Feelings of loss of control or threatened authority	Acknowledge and analyze the reaction; be realistic about personal limitations and actual range of influence and authority; be aware that the patient's need for control over his or her own body may conflict with the physician's urge to control the situation
Uncertainty about dealing with the patient; coping strategies have not been effective	Request a consultation or referral (psychiatric, psychosocial, or both)

Interviewing Difficult Patients

Patients that are difficult have been labeled "crocks," "gomers," "obnoxious," "hateful," and so forth. These patients usually evoke very strong responses in primary care providers. The early recognition of emotional reactions to these patients will make the doctor-patient interaction and communication more manageable. A given physician may personally find a particular patient difficult to work with for some reason. What is difficult for one physician may be easy for another. There are some predictable responses to regular types of patients with so-called maladaptive personality styles. These are well discussed by Putnam and coworkers [11••]. Table 8 presents some simple strategies for coping with difficult patients.

Breaking Bad News

Physicians must break bad news all too often—"You have cancer," "You have AIDS," "Your child isn't going to be normal." Table 9 shows the essential steps involved [12•]. In addition to these steps it has been shown unequivocally that taping such encounters and giving the tape to the patient at the end of the session helps to improve understanding, retention, and quality of remaining life [13].

How to Improve Interviewing Skills

Most practitioners have had little useful formal work on interviewing skills. More physicians have taken lessons in a sport than in this most important clinical skill! However, in our work we have yet to find a practitioner (among more than 3000) who could not benefit from explicit work on his or her interviewing skills, including us. For this work involves a lifetime of learning. How can physicians, then, work on these skills? The simplest way is to audio- or videotape oneself, say for an afternoon, and review the tape. The reviewer will encounter much to improve. Doing the review with one or more colleagues adds objectivity and perspective. Finding a skilled mentor is not easy, but having one makes a difference. Undertaking to teach residents about these issues can help.

Table 9. Points to be considered when breaking bad news to a patient

Make preparations as fully as possible (*eg*, check notes, test results, and time arranged for follow-up investigations or admission)

Break bad news in a suitable room, perhaps with a staff member present. Arrange furniture appropriately and ensure privacy with no interruptions

Allow enough time

Make sure that patients and/or relatives know who you are and understand the purpose of the consultation

Remember that what is hopeful news for you might still be bad news for the patient, and vice versa, depending on the circumstances

Do not assume that someone else has handled important parts of giving the information; check patient's understanding

Do not be falsely reassuring, but give as much positive, practical support and information as possible

Ensure that the patient has enough time to let news sink in; check understanding before he or she leaves

Offer a follow-up appointment, a number to call, or addresses of helpful agencies

Check your own feelings before seeing another patient

From Fallowfield and Lipkin [12•]; with permission.

The American Academy on Physician and Patient (New York University Medical Center, New York, NY) offers courses of proven benefit. Reading some of the key articles, if available, can help, and annotated bibliographies are also available from the American Academy on Physician and Patient.

References and Recommended Reading

Recently published papers of particular interest have been highlighted as:
- Of interest
- •• Of outstanding interest

1. •• Lipkin M, Frankel R, Beckman H, *et al.*: Performing the interview. In *The Medical Interview: Clinical Care, Education, and Research.* Edited by Lipkin M, Putnam SA, Lazare A. New York: Springer-Verlag; 1995.
2. Cohen-Cole SA: Interviewing the cardiac patient: I, II, III. *Qual Life Cardiac Care* 1986, 2:101–112.
3. Lazare A, Putnam SA, Lipkin M: The three function model of the medical interview. In *The Medical Interview: Clinical Care, Education, and Research.* Edited by Lipkin M, Putnam SA, Lazare A. New York: Springer-Verlag; 1995.
4. Kaplan SH, Greenfield S, Ware JE: Assessing the effects of physician patient interactions on the outcomes of chronic disease. *Med Care* 1989, 27:5110–5127.
5. •• Lipkin M: The medical interview and related skills. In *The Office Practice of Medicine.* Edited by Branch WT. Philadelphia: WB Saunders; 1994.
6. • Quill TE: Barriers to communication. In *The Medical Interview: Clinical Care, Education, and Research.* Edited by Lipkin M, Putnam SA, Lazare A. New York: Springer-Verlag; 1995.
7. Beckman HB, Frankel RM: The effect of physician behavior on the collection of data. *Ann Intern Med* 1984, 101:692–696.
8. • Lazare A: Negotiation. In *The Medical Interview Clinical Care, Education, and Research.* Edited by Lipkin M, Putnam SA, Lazare A. New York: Springer-Verlag; 1994.
9. Williams S: The sexual history. In *The Medical Interview: Clinical Care, Education, and Research.* Edited by Lipkin M, Putnam SA, Lazare A. New York: Springer-Verlag; 1995.
10. Kleinman AM, Eisenberg L, Good B: Culture, illness and care: clinical lessons from anthropologic and cross-cultural research. *Ann Intern Med* 1978, 88:251–258.
11. •• Putnam SA, Lipkin M, Drossman DD, *et al.*: Personality styles. In *The Medical Interview: Clinical Care, Education, and Research.* Edited by Lipkin M, Putnam SA, Lazare A. New York: Springer-Verlag; 1995.
12. • Fallowfield LJ, Lipkin M: Breaking sad or bad news. In *The Medical Interview: Clinical Care, Education, and Research.* Edited by Lipkin M, Putnam SA, Lazare A. New York: Springer-Verlag; 1994.
13. Hogbin B, Fallowfield LJ: Getting it taped: the "bad news" consultation with cancer patients. *Br J Hosp Med* 1989, 41:330–333.

Screening
Robert M. Heaney

> **Key Points**
> - Significant mortality of patients younger than 65 years of age is preventable; screening is the prototype secondary preventive intervention.
> - When deciding whether or not to subject a patient to preventative screening, the physician must make several considerations, including the importance and treatability of the screening target, and the safety, effectiveness, and cost of the screening test.
> - Numerous institutions, including the American Cancer Society, the American College of Physicians, the National Academy of Sciences, and other groups, have issued screening recommendations for preventative care.
> - Advances in molecular biology will open up new opportunities for future screening.

ROLE OF SCREENING IN PREVENTIVE MEDICINE

Prevention is central to the practice of medicine. The opportunity to prevent disease, suffering, disability, and death presents itself in every patient encounter, regardless of the setting. Abundant evidence shows that much of the mortality of populations under 65 years of age is preventable [1].

Definitions

Preventive medical care can be thought of as primary, secondary, or tertiary [2], depending on where in the spectrum of a disease the patient and the physician intervene (Fig. 1). Primary prevention takes place before the onset of the disease process. Prototypes of primary prevention include public health measures, such as water treatment and immunization against infectious diseases. By extension, identification and modification of risk factors, such as smoking, are also considered to be primary prevention.

Tertiary prevention occurs at the other end of the disease spectrum. Interventions to prevent progressive or catastrophic worsening of an already established disease process, such as aspirin or warfarin therapy in patients with ischemic congestive cardiomyopathies, are tertiary. In a sense, rehabilitative services are tertiary prevention against progressive disability and early death for patients who have arthritis or have had a stroke.

Secondary preventive interventions occur after a disease has started but before symptoms occur. For secondary prevention to be of value, the disease process must be detectable early, and it should be measurably better to treat the disease on detection rather than to wait for symptoms. Screening is the prototype secondary preventive intervention.

"Screening is the application of a test to detect a potential disease or condition in a person who has no known signs or symptoms of that disease or…risk factor" [3•]. The decision to use a screening test can be difficult because most of the patients in whom it is used will not have the disease; will not benefit from the test; and will

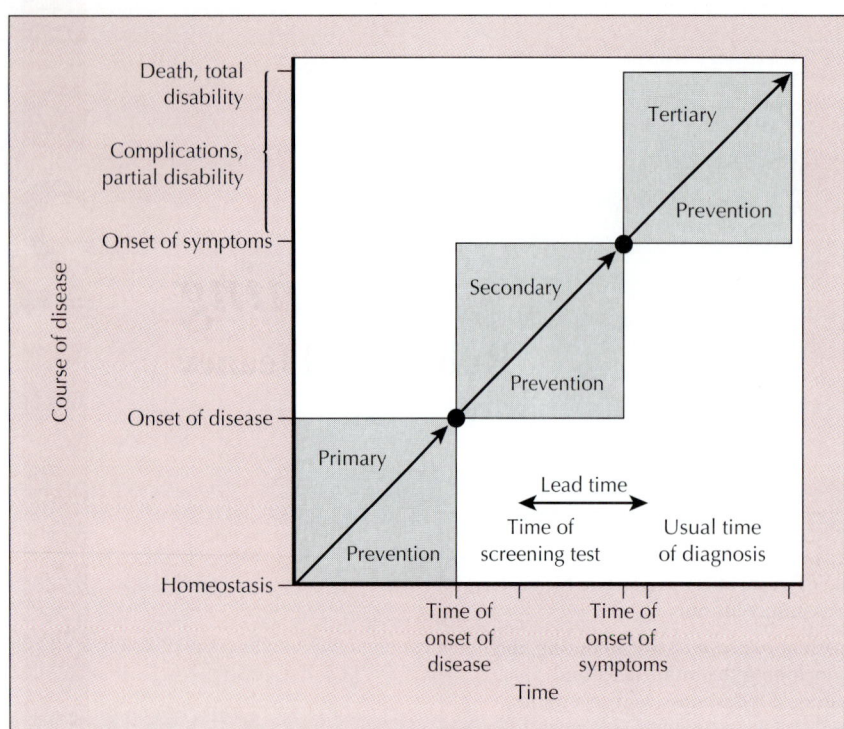

FIGURE 1 Primary, secondary, and tertiary prevention in the spectrum of disease. (*From* Kern [2]; with permission.)

suffer risk, anxiety, cost, and discomfort. This places a special burden on physicians and groups recommending a screening test. They must understand the performance characteristics of the test, the populations and patients most at risk for the disease, and the real benefits that outweigh the harm and justify the costs of the screening test.

Types of Screening

Many terms are used to describe screening [3•]. *Mass screening* is used to describe screening done in public settings, or anywhere that a patient's individual circumstances are not determined. *General screening* refers to screening applied individually to patients who fit very broad criteria, such as age and sex. Use of the term *routine screening* has been discouraged because of the connotation of automatic, unthinking repetition. *Selective screening* refers to screening that is only for patients with specific risk factors, such as a family history of a condition [4]. Most patients come to physicians for specific medical problems, not for preventive care. *Case finding* describes a medical practice strategy that seeks opportunities to perform preventive interventions, including general and selective screening, when the patient presents for other problems [2].

TABLE 1 EFFECT OF MORTALITY RATE ON TOTAL DEATHS PREVENTED ANNUALLY		
Reduction in mortality with intervention, %	Deaths per year from target condition, n	Total deaths prevented with intervention, n
50	10	5
1	100,000	1000

From US Preventive Services Task Force [1]; with permission.

CRITERIA FOR SCREENING RECOMMENDATIONS

Various criteria for screening recommendations have been developed [5,6]. Their current application seeks to ensure clinical efficacy: that is, that more benefit results than harm is done to those to whom the screening test is offered.

Importance of the Screening Target

The first consideration is the importance of the screening target itself. Does the disease or condition have a prevalence, an incidence, or both that warrants screening? What is the attributable morbidity or mortality? Recommendations have been developed for extremely common conditions (coronary artery disease, 1.5 million myocardial infarctions and 500,000 deaths each year [7]) and quite uncommon conditions (testicular cancer, annual incidence of < 1 per 10,000 and 350 deaths per year [8]). An intervention with a small mortality reduction in a common condition will have a greater impact than an intervention with a dramatic mortality reduction in an uncommon condition (Table 1) [1].

Effectiveness of the Preventive Intervention

Once found, the screening target must be treatable. Although lung cancer is far more common than testicular cancer, there are no current recommendations to screen for lung cancer [1]. Several large, well-designed studies, such as the Memorial Sloan-Kettering project [9], failed to find any mortality benefit in the screened groups, despite the fact that more lung cancers were detected at lower, earlier stages. Screening for lung cancer must await the development of better treatments for local and metastatic disease.

A preventive intervention should be safe, and it should be comfortable enough that a reasonable compliance rate can be

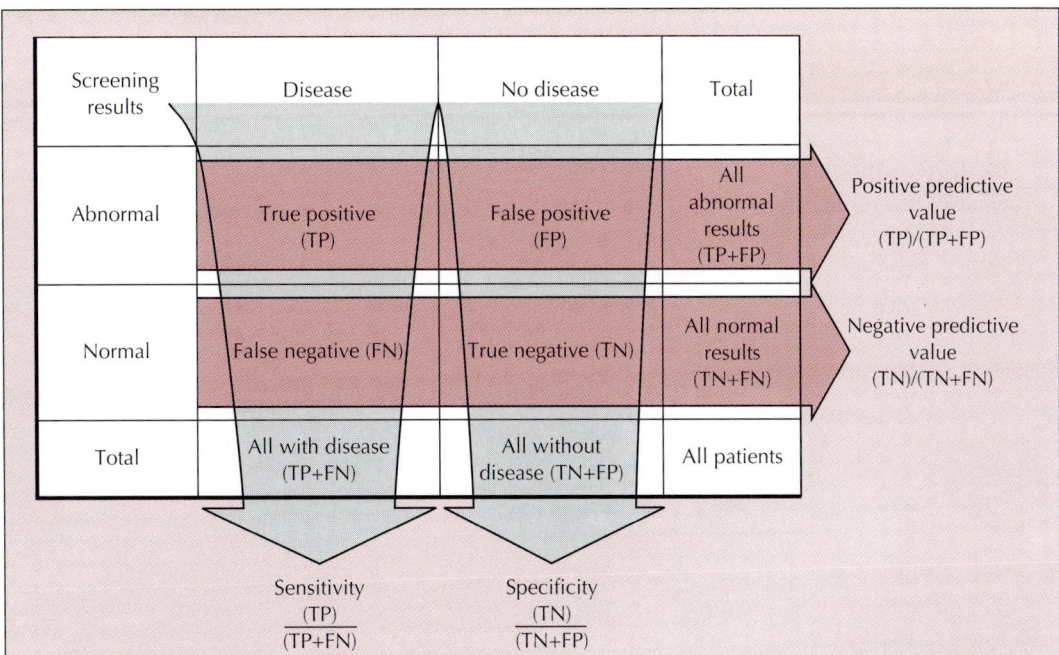

FIGURE 2 Sensitivity, specificity, and predictive values of a screening test.

expected. In a large study conducted by the Kaiser Foundation Health Plan [10], the use of rigid sigmoidoscopy was associated with a lower colorectal cancer death rate. However, only approximately one third of the patients in the study group actually received sigmoidoscopy even once. Perforation rates have been estimated at 0.01% to 0.2%. Perforation usually requires surgery and has a 5% to 10% mortality rate.

Effectiveness of the Screening Test

For a screening intervention to be effective, the test used must be effective. It should be reliable: the test should produce the same result when repeated, whether by different observers or in different settings. The Papanicolaou smear used in cervical cancer screening has shown a significant variation in results in as many as 57% of 20,000 smears compared in two laboratories [11].

A screening test should be accurate. It should have an acceptable sensitivity and specificity. Sensitivity is a measure of the test's ability to find the disease in question; specificity, conversely, is the ability of the test to find health (the absence of the disease in question). A simple two-by-two table (Fig. 2) can show the calculation of sensitivity and specificity.

Sensitivity and specificity are properties of the test, not the patient. What a patient needs to know after getting a screening test result is, Do I have the disease, or am I healthy? Both patients and physicians need to know the predictive value of the test. Figure 2 also demonstrates the calculation of predictive values.

Even tests with good reliability, sensitivity, and specificity can perform relatively poorly. The results of the first large study on prostate-specific antigen screening for prostate cancer [12] are shown in Table 2. In this referral practice, the prostate-specific antigen findings had excellent sensitivity and specificity in the pooled patients, but a prostate-specific antigen value greater than 4.0 had only a 33% chance of representing prostate cancer. In the subgroup of patients between 50 and 59 years of age, the positive predictive value of the test fell to 20%.

TABLE 2 SENSITIVITY, SPECIFICITY, PREVALENCE, POSITIVE PREDICTIVE VALUE, AND NEGATIVE PREDICTIVE VALUE FOR PROSTATE-SPECIFIC ANTIGEN SCREENING FOR PROSTATE CANCER

	Patients, n		
PSA findings	Biopsy-proven prostate cancer	Prostate cancer negative (biopsy or clinical)	Total
PSA ≥ 4.0	85	171	256
PSA < 4.0	13	1619	1632
All PSA values	98	1790	1888
	Sensitivity = 87%	Specificity = 94%	Positive predictive value = 33%
			Negative predictive value = 99%
			Prevalence of prostate cancer = 5%

PSA—prostate-specific antigen.
From Catalona et al. [12]; with permission.

TABLE 3 EFFECT OF PREVALENCE ON THE PREDICTIVE VALUE OF AN EXCELLENT SIGN, SYMPTOM, OR LABORATORY TEST*

Prevalence, %[†]	Predictive value of a positive test result, %[‡]	Predictive value of a negative test result, %	
		No disease[§]	Disease[¶]
99	99.9	16	84
95	99.7	50	50
90	99.4	68	32
80	99	83	17
70	98	89	11
60	97	93	7
50	95	95	5
40	93	97	3
30	89	98	2
20	83	99	1
10	68	99.4	0.6
5	50	99.7	0.3
1	16	99.9	0.1
0.5	9	99.97	0.03
0.1	2	99.99	0.01

*Both sensitivity and specificity equal 95% in every case.
[†]Pretest likelihood or prior probability of disease.
[‡]Posterior probability of disease following a positive test result.
[§]Posterior probability of no disease following a negative test result.
[¶]Posterior probability of disease following a negative test result.
From Sackett et al. [19]; with permission.

The low positive predictive values are due to the low prevalence of prostate cancer in the study and comparison groups. This effect of prevalence on the predictive values of an excellent test are shown in Table 3. A screening test has its greatest utility when the likelihood that the patient has the target disease is relatively high, a condition not likely to be met in a routine office practice. The positive predictive values of many other screening tests are less than 20%, even in research settings. In this situation, not only are most of the patients who receive the screening test free of the disease, but most of those with positive test results do *not* have it either.

EVALUATING SCREENING RECOMMENDATIONS

Quality of the Evidence

Groups recommending a screening intervention should explicitly rate the quality of the evidence on which they make their recommendation. Table 4 lists grading criteria for evidence [1] that place the greatest weight on controlled and cohort or case-control studies but takes into account historical evidence and the opinions of experts.

Introduction of Bias

Even controlled studies can present problems. Dilution of the intervention group (when patients offered screening do not receive it) and contamination of the control group by inadvertent personal screening lead to underestimates of the true effect of screening. Both occurred in the Kaiser Permanente Multiphasic Evaluation Study [10]. Case-control and uncontrolled studies are also subject to serious patient-selection bias.

Uncontrolled studies may have to deal with several other biases peculiar to screening [3•]. Lead time bias is illustrated in Figure 1. This lead time will increase the time between diagnosis and death, even if no treatment is given or the treatment has no effect. It took several decades to be reasonably certain that lead-time bias was not the primary effect of mammographic screening for breast cancer (Fig. 3), and there is still significant disagreement on this issue for younger women [13]. Length bias occurs when lesions discovered by screening programs have different, less aggressive natural histories than lesions that present with symptoms, as probably happens in colorectal cancer screening with colonoscopy [14]. Some conditions discovered by screening would spontaneously remit and would never come to clinical attention without the screening, confusing the interpretation of the data by overdiagnosis [3•].

Threshold for Screening

Lastly, in making a decision about a screening test, some consideration must be given to cost. Ideally, comparisons of the benefits, harms, and costs should be made from explicit data, with informed patient input given before the decision is made to screen [15]. The following formula is useful: The threshold for screening is low when the costs are low (*eg*, testicular self-examination) and the benefits are substantial [1]. The threshold for screening for colorectal cancer with colonoscopy is much higher because the benefits of screening are more nearly balanced by the costs and harms of the procedure [1]. When the benefits of screening are not known, for instance in screening for prostate cancer, it is not yet possible to set a threshold or make a definite recommendation [1].

SOURCES OF SCREENING RECOMMENDATIONS

Since the American Medical Association first proposed the routine annual physical examination of asymptomatic patients in 1922, there has been a growing stream of recommendations for preventive medical care from many sources. All major sources of recommendations now advocate selective rather than "routine" screening and have steadily expanded the scope of their recommendations. Increasingly, recommendations are based on sound scientific information from well-designed patient outcome studies.

The Canadian Task Force [6] first issued a series of recommendations for their periodic health examination in 1979, and these were most recently updated in 1993. Their recommendations are conservative, are explicitly tied to the Canadian population and health care system, and are updated regularly.

The American College of Physicians, Medical Practice Committee advised in 1981 that annual checkups for healthy adults be abandoned. Since then, they have regularly issued comparisons between different sets of guidelines, with suggestions for implementing screening in office practice. Through its Clinical Efficacy Assessment Project, the American College of Physicians, in conjunction with Blue Cross/Blue Shield, has developed and is expanding a set of practice guidelines [4].

The American Cancer Society [16] has created an aggressive set of cancer-related screens and has regularly challenged other groups to justify making the decision not to screen.

The US Preventive Services Task Force began work in 1984, following the model developed by the Canadians. They developed 169 recommendations for 60 target conditions affecting patients from infancy to old age. They stress the importance of patients' personal health practices, the utility of counseling and patient education (not traditionally considered part of a physician's role), and the necessity for selective use of their recommendations.

Other groups with selective recommendations include the National Academy of Sciences, the Institute of Medicine, the American College of Obstetricians and Gynecologists, other specialty societies, and Frame and Carlson [5].

SCREENING RECOMMENDATIONS FOR SPECIFIC CONDITIONS

The screening recommendations that follow—for vascular diseases (Table 5), neoplastic diseases (Table 6), metabolic diseases (Table 7), and other diseases (Table 8)—are drawn largely from the US Preventive Services Task Force's guide [1] and are expanded on in that report. They should be considered as guidelines for *healthy, asymptomatic* patients. Appropriate detection strategies should be followed for ill or symptomatic patients.

COMPARATIVE RECOMMENDATIONS

As mentioned previously, recommendations may vary between authors and advisory groups. Differing interpretation of data, assessment of outcome and values, and focus on benefits versus harm lead to these differences. On some recommendations, however, there is broad agreement. Hayward and coworkers [4] compared the recommendations from major sources for seven screening tests, three immunizations, and counseling. These recommendations, like all screening recommendations, should be used as guidelines for an individual's medical care.

	TABLE 4 GRADE QUALITY OF EVIDENCE
	Description
I	Evidence obtained from at least one properly designed randomized, controlled trial
II1	Evidence obtained from well-designed controlled trials without randomization
II2	Evidence obtained from well-designed cohort or case-control analytic studies, preferably from more than one center or research group
II3	Evidence obtained from multiple time series with or without the intervention; dramatic results in uncontrolled experiments (*eg*, the results of the introduction of penicillin treatment in the 1940s) could also be regarded as this type of evidence
III	Opinions of respected authorities, based on clinical experience, descriptive studies, or reports of expert committees

From US Preventive Service Task Force [1]; with permission.

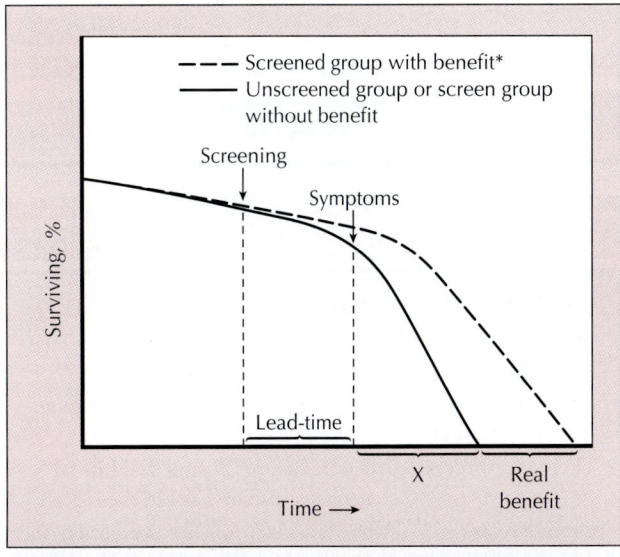

FIGURE 3 Survivorship with lead-time bias versus a real intervention effect.

Table 5 Screening for Vascular Diseases and Risk Factors

Condition	Intervention	Interval	Selective screening
Hypertension	Sphygmomanometry	Yearly over age 3 y	None
Hypercholesterolemia	Total cholesterol measurement and dietary counseling	Every 5 y (upper age limit unknown)	More frequently for individuals with a family history or other vascular risk factors
Asymptomatic coronary artery disease	None (emphasize primary prevention)	None	Resting ECG for high-risk individuals; exercise ECG for sedentary or high-risk individuals before exercise programs or high risk jobs (eg, pilots)
Cerebrovascular disease	None (emphasize primary prevention)	None	Cervical auscultation in high-risk individuals
Peripheral vascular disease	None (emphasize primary prevention)	None	Auscultation, palpation of abdominal aorta in high-risk individuals

ECG—electrocardiogram.

Table 6 Screening for Neoplastic Diseases

Condition	Intervention	Interval	Selective screening
Lung cancer	None (emphasize primary prevention)	None	None
Breast cancer	Clinical breast examination	Yearly for age >40	Mammography earlier for women at high risk; continued past age 75 if pathology is present
	Mammography	Every 1–2 y for ages 50–75	
	Breast self-examination	Unknown	
Colorectal cancer	Occult fecal blood	Yearly for age >50	Colonoscopy for individuals who are at high risk, are known to have polyps, or have chronically heme-positive stools
	sigmoidoscopy	Initial at age 50, every 2–3 y to follow	
Prostate cancer	Digital rectal examination	Yearly for age >50	
	Prostate-specific antigen measurement	Unknown	
Cervical cancer	Papanicolaou smear	Every 3 y from menarche to age 65	Yearly for high-risk individuals
Skin cancer	None (skin protection)	None	Yearly clinical examination for high-risk individuals age >40
	Skin self-examination	Unknown	
Gonadal cancer	Testicular self-examination	Unknown	
	Adnexal examination	At the time of Papanicolaou smear	Yearly adnexal examinations in women at high risk
Pancreatic cancer	None	None	—
Oral cancer	None (emphasize primary prevention)	—	Dental and physician oral examinations yearly in high-risk individuals

Table 7 Screening for Metabolic Diseases

Condition	Intervention	Interval	Selective screening
Obesity	Weight and height measurement, dietary counseling	Yearly	None
Diabetes mellitus	Oral glucose tolerance test in pregnancy	Between 24 and 28 wk	Random blood glucose or urine glucose testing in high-risk individuals
Thyroid disorders	Measurement of T_4 and TSH in neonates and of TSH in the elderly	Unknown	Clinical examination in patients with known radiation exposure
Osteoporosis	None (consider primary prevention and post menopausal estrogen replacement)	None	Consider skeletal radiography, densitometry, or quantitative computed tomography for high-risk individuals

T_4—thyroxine; TSH—thyroid-stimulating hormone.

Table 8 Screening for other diseases

Condition	Intervention	Interval	Selective screening
Infectious diseases			
Hepatitis B	Hepatitis B surface antigen testing	Pregnancy	On diagnosis of a sexually transmitted disease in high-risk individuals
Syphilis	RPR, VDRL	Pregnancy	As above
Chlamydia infection	Antigen screen	Pregnancy	As above, and yearly in women with multiple STDs
Genital herpes simplex	Culture	Pregnancy	
Gonorrhea	Culture	Pregnancy	As above
HIV infection	ELISA for the human immunodefiency virus antibody		As above, and yearly in patients with multiple STDs
Tuberculosis	Skin testing with purified protein derivative	Every 1–5 y	In patients with a likelihood of exposure
Asymptomatic bacteriuria	Combined "dipstick" testing	Unknown	Urine culture in pregnancy; "dipstick" testing possibly in patients with diabetes mellitus or age >65
Hematologic diseases			
Anemia	Measurement of hemoglobin level	Once in childhood and again in pregnancy	None
Hemoglobinopathy			Electrophoresis for patients with a family history
Lead poisoning			Erythrocyte protoporphyrin measurement yearly for children at high risk
Loss of visual acuity			Consider an eye screen in the elderly
Glaucoma	Intraocular pressure measurement	Unknown	Consider yearly evaluation in the elderly
Loss of hearing	Hand-held audiometry	Unknown	Periodically in the elderly
Alcoholism	History, screening, questionnaire (*eg*, CAGE [17])	Unknown	None
Other drug abuse	History	Unknown	None
Mental disorders			
Dementia	None	None	
Depression	None	None	Consider history or screening questionnaire around episodes of bereavement.

ELISA—enzyme-linked immunosorbent assay; RPR—rapid plasma reagin test; STDs—sexually transmitted diseases; VDRL—Venereal Disease Research Laboratory test.

Future Opportunities for Screening

The most promising role of prevention in future medical practice may lie in changing the few personal behaviors that are linked to the leading causes of death. Smoking, failure to use seat belts, drunken driving, sedentary lifestyle, poor diet, and indiscriminate sexual practices contribute tremendous excess mortality [1]. Smoking cessation alone could dramatically change disease patterns and screening recommendations. Alcoholism can be reliably detected, creating opportunities for intervention [17].

As new therapies for vascular diseases, cancers, and other conditions are developed, screening recommendations will change. The leading cancer killer—lung cancer—awaits improved treatment strategies before any screen can be recommended [1,3•].

Molecular biology offers exciting new opportunities for both screening and therapy. The finding that a small region on chromosome 5 was associated with the familial adenomatous polyposis syndrome and the development of an allele-specific assay for syndrome-producing mutations [18] will very likely revolutionize colorectal cancer screening for patients with a family history of this syndrome. Molecular intervention at the genome, expression, and differentiation levels may revolutionize cancer therapy.

References and Recommended Reading

Recently published papers of particular interest have been highlighted as:
- Of interest

1. US Preventive Services Task Force: *Guide to Clinical Preventive Services: An Assessment of the Effectiveness of 169 Interventions. Report of the US Preventive Services Task Force.* Baltimore: Williams & Wilkins; 1989.
2. Kern DE: Preventive medicine in ambulatory practice. In *Principles of Ambulatory Medicine*, edn 3. Edited by Barker RL, Burton JR, Zieve PD. Baltimore: Williams & Wilkins; 1991.
3. • Eddy RM: How to think about screening. In *Common Screening Tests.* Edited by Eddy DM. Philadelphia: American College of Physicians; 1991:1–21.
4. Hayward RAS, Steinberg EP, Ford DE, *et al.*: Preventive care guidelines, 1991. *Ann Intern Med* 1991, 114:758–783.
5. Frame PS, Carlson SJ: A critical review of periodic health screening using specific screening criteria: I. Selected diseases of respiratory, cardiovascular, and critical nervous systems. *J Fam Pract* 1975, 2:29–36.
6. Canadian Task Force on the Periodic Health Examination: The periodic health examination. *Can Med Assoc J* 1979, 121:1193–1254.
7. National Center for Health Statistics: Advance Report of Final Mortality Statistics, 1986. *Monthly Vital Stat Rep [Suppl]* 1988, 37:1–24
8. American Cancer Society: Cancer statistics, 1993. *CA Cancer J Clin* 1992, 43(1):7–26.
9. Melamud MR, Flehinger BT, Zaman MB, *et al.*: Screening for early lung cancer: Results of the Memorial Sloan Kettering study in New York. *Chest* 1984, 86:44–53.
10. Selby JV, Freedman GD, Collen MF: Sigmoidoscopy and mortality from colorectal cancer: The Kaiser Permanente Multiphasic Evaluation Study. *J Clin Epidemiol* 1988, 41:427–434.
11. Yobs AR, Platt AE, Hieklin MD: Retrospective evaluation of gynecologic cyto diagnosis: II. Interlaboratory reproducibility as shown in rescreening large consecutive samples of reported cases. *Acta Cytol* 1987, 31:900–910.
12. Catalona WJ, Smith DS, Ratliff TL, *et al.*: Measurement of prostate-specific antigen in serum as a screening test for prostate cancer. *N Engl J Med* 1991, 324:1156–1161.
13. Eddy DM: Screening for breast cancer. *Ann Intern Med* 1989, 111:389–399.
14. Eddy DM: Screening for colorectal cancer. *Ann Intern Med* 1990, 113:373–384.
15. Eisenberg JM: *Cost-Benefit and Cost-Effectiveness Analysis in Teaching Clinical Decision Making.* Edited by Cebul RD, Beck LH. New York: Praeger; 1985.
16. American Cancer Society: *Summary of Current Guidelines for the Cancer-Related Checkup: Recommendations.* Atlanta: American Cancer Society; 1992.
17. Ewing JA: Detecting alcoholism: the CAGE questionnaire. *JAMA* 1984, 252:1905–1907.
18. Powell SM, Petersen GM, Krusl AJ, *et al.* Molecular diagnosis of familial adenomatous polyposis. *N Engl J Med* 1993, 329:1982–1987.
19. Sackett DL, Haynes RB, Tugwell P: *Clinical Epidemiology: A Basic Science for Clinical Medicine*, edn 2. Toronto: Little Brown and Co.; 1985.

Physical Diagnosis in Medicine

Dale Berg
James Sebastian

> **Key Points**
> - Physical diagnosis plays a central role in making diagnostic and management decisions in the everyday practice of medicine.
> - Physical diagnostic techniques are most useful when the clinician approaches them with knowledge of the techniques, outcomes, and scientific characteristics (*ie*, knowledge of sensitivity and specificity of the tests).
> - With a thorough but succinct examination of various musculoskeletal structures (*eg*, shoulder, knees, back or hands), the clinician will be able to define the underlying diagnosis.
> - Knowledge of the techniques of cardiac palpation and auscultation provides the clinician tools for evaluating cardiac extrasounds, especially murmurs.
> - Knowledge of the techniques of percussion, tactile fremitus, and auscultation afford the clinician tools for evaluating pulmonary problems.

The past several decades have seen increasing use of the technologic aspects of medicine for making diagnostic and therapeutic decisions. These methods, which include computed tomography and magnetic resonance imaging, echocardiography, cardiac catheterization, and a veritable potpourri of laboratory tests, have provided new and exciting modalities to assist physicians in providing quality medical care. These techniques, via their emphasis in medical school and postgraduate training, have taken over as the central features of medical diagnosis and management at the expense of the techniques of physical examination and history taking.

Objective evidence that medical students and house staff are deficient in physical examination skills is provided in a 1992 study by St. Clair and coworkers [1], in which internal medicine house staff were asked to auscult classic cardiac findings under optimal auscultatory conditions. Only 37% of the house staff at this institution could detect incontrovertible mitral stenosis. Only a slight majority (52% and 54%, respectively) detected mitral regurgitation or aortic insufficiency.

Yet physical examination is indeed a first-line, pivotal, basic foundation on which the remainder of the evaluative and management schemes are based. This is self-evident to general internists and other primary care providers, and has been demonstrated by several studies, (for example, Peterson and coworkers [2]). When the examination is performed correctly and the result interpreted using scientific parameters of sensitivity, specificity, positive predictive values, negative predictive values, and likelihood ratios, as eloquently described by Sackett and coworkers [3••], it becomes integral to effective, appropriate, efficient, and economical patient care, thus precluding the need for expensive and invasive examinations. Even when a specific diagnosis cannot be established on the basis of the bedside history and physical examination, clinicians can construct a weighted differential diagnosis on which a logical and diagnostic approach can be formulated.

This chapter provides a brief overview of the most commonly used physical examination techniques for seven discrete and common medical problem areas.

Hand Pain, Stiffness, or Dysfunction

It is exceedingly common for patients to present with pain, stiffness, or dysfunction of one or both hands. The primary care physician can evaluate and diagnose most of these problems by performing a basic physical examination of the hands (Table 1). Various specific entities can be diagnosed by performing the previously described site-specific physical examination.

Felon

A felon is an exquisitely tender, swollen, erythematous nodule at the tip of a digit. This lesion is a type of "collar button abscess" that forms in the terminal pulp cavity of the distal phalanx, usually as the result of an antecedent puncture wound.

Heberden's and Bouchard's Nodes

Heberden's and Bouchard's nodes are nontender nodules on the distal interphalangeal (Heberden's) or proximal interphalangeal (Bouchard's) joints of the digits. They usually occur on the digits of the hands, the feet, or both in middle-aged or older patients and are consistent with degenerative joint disease.

Sclerodactyly

Sclerodactyly is characterized by a diffuse and quite painless decreased range of motion of the digits resulting from a palpable thickening of the skin and underlying connective tissue about the digits. The differential diagnosis of etiologies includes the autoimmune and rheumatologic disorders of mixed connective tissue disease, CREST syndrome (calcinosis, Raynaud's disease, esophageal dysmotility, sclerodactyly, and telangiectasia), rheumatoid arthritis, scleroderma, and Buerger's disease.

Swan Neck and Boutonnière Signs

Swan neck deformity is hyperextension contracture of the proximal interphalangeal and joint flexion contracture of the distal interphalangeal joint; the boutonnière deformity is the converse, in that the proximal interphalangeal joint has a significant flexion contracture and the distal interphalangeal joint has a contracture of hyperextension. These signs are found in severe chronic polyarticular arthritides.

Boxer's Fracture

The presence of tenderness and swelling over the medial aspect (ulnar side) of the hand that occurs after the patient forcibly hits an object with a closed fist is a simple fracture of the diaphysis of the fifth metacarpal bone.

Trigger Finger and Locked Finger

Triggering is the snapping sensation of the digit on flexion, extension, or both. Locking is the reversible inability to extend the affected finger or fingers, usually at the proximal interphalangeal joint. These conditions result from inflammation at the site where the long flexor tendons pass through the metacarpophalangeal joint pulley.

Ganglion

Ganglions are soft, fluctuant, nontender lesions that occur on the palmar or dorsal side of the hands, wrists, or both, each adjacent to a tendon or tendon sheath. They are well-defined benign cystic structures. The term *ganglion* or *ganglion cyst* can be misleading given the fact that these structures have nothing to do with the nervous system.

Dupuytren's Disease

Dupuytren's disease is the presence of a flexion contracture, usually in the fourth and fifth digits (*ie*, the affected digits cannot be actively or passively extended). Furthermore, palpable nodules are often present in the palmar fascia of the affected digits. The presence of this disease is correlated with ethanol abuse and hepatic diseases.

de Quervain's Disease

The presence of tenderness in and about the tendons that comprise the anatomic "snuff box" at the dorsal aspect of the base of the thumb characterizes de Quervain's disease. There is inflammation of the tendons of the abductor pollicis longus muscle, the extensor pollicis longus muscle, and the extensor pollicis brevis muscle. Examination reveals positive findings for Finklestein's sign (*ie*, pain is reproduced when the patient is instructed to grasp the thumb with adjacent digits while flexing the wrist ulnarly and palmarly).

Radial Nerve Dysfunction

If any evidence of radial nerve dysfunction is present, a screening examination should be performed (Table 2).

Table 1 Overall Physical Examination of the Hands

Perform active and then passive range-of-motion assessment of the wrist, metacarpophalangeal, proximal interphalangeal, and distal interphalangeal joints
- Wrist joints
  - Flexion: 80°
  - Extension (dorsiflexion): 70°
  - Abduction: 30°
  - Adduction: 30°
- Metacarpophalangeal joints
  - Flexion: 90°
  - Extension: 30°
- Proximal interphalangeal joints
  - Flexion: 120°
  - Extension: 0°
- Distal interphalangeal joints
  - Flexion: 80°
  - Extension: 0°

Immobilize the joint or joints if a fracture is suspected
Visually inspect and palpate the digits and hands
Screen for the function of the three nerves that innervate the hands: the ulnar, median, and radial nerves (*see* Table 2).

Table 2 Overall screening examination of nerves in the hands	
Procedure	Nerve
Fine touch on the palmar skin of digits 1, 2, and 3	Median
Fine touch on the dorsal skin of digits 1, 2, and 3	Radial
Fine touch on the ulnar aspect of the hand	Ulnar
Active apposition of the thumb	Median
Active abduction of the digits	Ulnar
Active dorsiflexion of the hand at the wrist	Radial

Table 3 Overall physical examination of the back

Perform passive and active range-of-motion assessment of the lower back
  Extension: 30°
  Flexion: 75° to 90°
  Lateral bending: 30°, left and right
  Rotation: 30°, left and right
Palpate the spinous processes of the back
Palpate the paraspinous musculature
Perform a screening neurologic examination of the S-1, L-5, and L-4 roots of the lower extremities (*see* Table 4)
Perform a rectal examination to determine sphincter tone
Perform the straight-leg-raising examination by placing the patient in a supine position and passively flexing each leg at the hip

Wristdrop hand

Wristdrop hand is the development of significant weakness in hand dorsiflexion at the wrist joint. The patient has a "limp" wrist that can be passively but not actively extended. This may be the result of damage to the radial nerve, possibly secondary to a Colles fracture of the radius or a spiral fracture of the humeral shaft.

Median Nerve Dysfunction

If any evidence of median nerve dysfunction is present, a screening examination should be performed (Table 2).

Carpal tunnel syndrome

The sensory manifestations of carpal tunnel syndrome, which is a very common entity, include the development of paresthesias and numbness of the volar (palmar) side of digits 1, 2, and 3. A further manifestation is the presence of thenar (thumb) muscular atrophy. In addition, Tinel's sign may be present. This is the development of paresthesias and dysthesias in the distribution of the median nerve while the examiner percusses gently over the midpoint of a line transversely placed at the base of the thenar and hypothenar eminences for more than 30 seconds. The site for percussing should be adjacent to the palmaris longus tendon immediately on the radial side. Finally, Phalen's sign should be performed. In this examination, the patient is directed to flex both hands at the wrist passively (reverse prayer position) for 60 seconds. The development of paresthesias and dysthesias in the distribution of the median nerve is consistent with carpal tunnel syndrome. In their review of carpal tunnel syndrome, Katz and coworkers [4•] reported the sensitivity of Tinel's and Phalen's signs to be in the range of 25% to 75%, whereas the specificity of these signs was 70% to 90%.

Low Back Pain or Stiffness

One of the most common problems with which patients present to primary care physicians is pain and stiffness in the back. Clearly, physical examination plays a central role [5] in the evaluation of back pain and dysfunction and effectively supersedes all other first-line techniques (Table 3). The specific entities that can be diagnosed by performing the previously described site-specific physical examination are discussed in the following sections.

Acute Musculoskeletal or Ligamentous Strain

With acute musculoskeletal or ligamentous strain, there is often spasm and tenderness of the involved back musculature but no radicular findings or neurologic deficits. The underlying pathology is the tearing of muscle and ligamentous structures from the lifting of a heavy object, with resultant pain and inflammation.

Herniated Disk

With sciatica or herniated disk [6•], weakness of the muscles innervated by the L-5 and S-1 nerve roots is manifest as by great toe weakness and an inability to perform a tiptoe walk for S-1, and by decreased ankle jerk with an inability to perform a heel walk for L-5 (Table 4). Concurrent posterolateral thigh and leg pain, paresthesias, and sensory deficits are invariably present. The underlying pathology is the posterior herniation of the disk annulus, the soft connective tissue bridge between two vertebral bodies. This herniation may result in entrapment or impingement of the nerve root (*ie*, the manifestations of sciata, unilaterally).

Compression Fracture

With compression fracture, there is significant tenderness over the affected vertebra, which is quite localized and can be severe. Concurrent findings are usually due to the underlying process. An example of this is a dowager's hump, which is an accentuated thoracic kyphosis in patients with past compression fractures, especially in osteoporosis. The compression can be trauma related or result from a loss of bone substance, thus weakening the individual vertebral body. Disorders predisposing to compression fractures include osteoporosis, neoplastic disease, and infectious diseases.

Facet Disease (Spondylolisthesis)

In facet disease, there is usually a paucity of specific findings, even when the patient presents with an acute exacerbation of

Physical Diagnosis in Medicine

Table 4 Neurologic screening examination of the lower extremities	
Procedure	Nerve
Instruct the patient to walk on tiptoes, *ie*, actively plantar flex at the ankle	S-1
Instruct the patient to walk on the heels, *ie*, actively dorsiflex at the ankle	L-5
Instruct the patient to actively extend the leg at the knee	L-4

the pain syndrome. The underlying pathogenesis is of acquired anterior subluxation, also referred to as spondylolisthesis, of a vertebral body on an adjacent vertebral body. This is, quite invariably, a result of degenerative joint disease of the facet joints.

Ankylosing Spondylitis

Ankylosing spondylitis is characterized by a marked abnormal straightening of the back, manifested specifically with a loss of the normal thoracic kyphosis and lumber lordosis. Furthermore, palpable tenderness exists over the sacroiliac joints, and the normal range of motion of the back is significantly decreased. The underlying pathogenesis is inflammatory arthritis affecting the central (*ie*, appendicular) skeleton.

Epidural Disease

On examination, the patient with epidural disease may have fever and quite often has pain over the affected vertebra. There can be weakness of the musculature innervated by L-4, L-5, and the sacral nerves (*see* Table 4). This weakness is manifest as great toe weakness; weakness of foot dorsiflexion and foot plantar flexion; and an inability to walk on the toes, the heels, or both. Furthermore, a weakened anal sphincter and the presence of an enlarged, fluid-filled urinary bladder are often demonstrable by percussion. This condition is a result of disease from an infectious source, either endocarditis or an adjacent osteomyelitis, or from a malignant neoplastic source.

KNEE PAIN OR DYSFUNCTION

As the members of our society become more active, more injuries of and problems with the knees occur. Therefore, the primary care physician must know the physical examination of the knee. This is especially true given the fact that the vast majority of knee problems are diagnosed by a thorough, site-specific physical examination [7,8•] (Table 5). A number of specific entities are diagnosed by physical examination.

Prepatellar Bursitis

Prepatellar bursitis is characterized by nontender swelling and fluctuance over the anterior and superior aspects of the patella. This results from an inflammation of the prepatellar bursa, a bursa that is located immediately anterior (superficial) and superior to the patella.

Infrapatellar Bursitis

Infrapatellar bursitis is characterized by moderately tender swelling on one side or both sides of the inferior aspect of the patellar ligament. The most marked manifestations are located immediately deep and inferior to the patella. This results from an inflammation of the infrapatellar bursa, a bursa that is located immediately deep and inferior to the patella itself.

Semimembranous Bursitis

Semimembranous bursitis is marked by a moderately tender mass in the superior medial aspect of the popliteal fossa. The mass becomes more palpable on extension, whereas it relaxes on knee flexion and thus becomes nonpalpable. This is the result of an inflammation of the semimembranous bursa, a bursa that is located deep in the superior medial popliteal fossa and immediately adjacent to the head of the gastrocnemius and the insertion of the semimembranous muscle.

Anterior Cruciate Ligament Tear

The presence of a moderate to large effusion and a marked decrease in range of motion characterize an anterior cruciate ligament tear. On further examination there are positive anterior drawer sign and positive Lachman's sign findings. These two signs can be difficult to demonstrate if the injury is acute because of the pain and swelling. The underlying pathogenesis is a partial or complete tear of the anterior cruciate ligament, usually resulting from a force applied to the tibia anteriorly (recall that this ligament connects the anterior tibia with the femur).

Posterior Cruciate Ligament Tear

The presence of a tender effusion in the affected knee and decreased range of motion characterize a posterior cruciate ligament tear. On further examination, there are positive posterior drawer sign findings. The underlying pathogenesis is a partial or complete tear of the posterior cruciate ligament. As one can recall, the posterior cruciate ligament attaches the posterior tibia to the femur. The tear is usually the result of a direct blow to the proximal tibia when the knee is flexed.

Medial Meniscus Tear

With a medial meniscus tear, minimal joint instability or effusion is present. On further examination, there are positive McMurray's test findings. The results of Childress' test, (*ie*, the "duck waddle test," in which the patient is unable to fully flex the affected knee while instructed to move in the duck waddle position) may also be positive. Positive results are indicative of a rupture of the posterior horn of the medial meniscus. The underlying pathogenesis is one of damage to the cartilage (meniscus) in the medial compartment of the knee. The damage occurs when the knee is twisted medially and flexed, with concurrent bearing of weight.

Lateral Meniscus Tear

With a lateral meniscus tear, minimal joint instability or effusion is present. On further examination, McMurray's test findings are positive. The underlying pathogenesis is one of damage to the cartilage (meniscus) in the lateral compartment of the knee. The damage occurs when the knee is twisted laterally and flexed, with concurrent bearing of weight.

Medial Collateral Ligament Tear

The knee with a medial collateral ligament tear often has mild to moderate medial mobility, which is even more prominent if there has been concurrent damage to the anterior cruciate ligament. Unless there has been concurrent damage to the menisci, the results of McMurray's test are negative. The underlying pathogenesis is partial or complete tear of the medial collateral ligament, usually a result of excessive valgus bending of the knee during activity.

Lateral Collateral Ligament Tear

On examination, the knee with a lateral collateral ligament tear often has mild to moderate lateral mobility, which is even more prominent if there has been concurrent damage to the anterior cruciate ligament. Unless there has been concurrent damage to the menisci, the results of McMurray's test are negative. The underlying pathogenesis of this is the partial or complete tear of the lateral collateral ligament, usually as a result of excessive varus bending of the knee during activity.

Degenerative Joint Disease

In degenerative joint disease, crepitus is quite often present in the affected knee or knees, as is decreased range of motion. Furthermore, a small effusion in the involved knee may be present. Often, a valgus or varus deformity exists, the lateral or medial compartments, respectively, are more significantly involved.

SHOULDER PROBLEMS

Physical examination is extremely important in the evaluation of the shoulder. Clearly the vast majority of problems can by diagnosed by a site-specific, thorough physical examination

---

TABLE 5 OVERALL EXAMINATION OF THE KNEE

Perform active and passive range-of-motion assessment of the knee:
  Flexion: 130°
  Extension: 5°
  Adduction and abduction: Minimal
  Internal and external rotation: Minimal

Ballot the patellas. With the patient in a supine position and the knee extended, gently press on the suprapatellar area with one hand and on the patella with the other hand, attempting to press the patella against the tibial condyles

Palpate the structures around the knee for areas of fluctuance, swelling, or both

With the patient in a supine position and the knee extended, gently press on the lateral side of the knee 1 cm inferior to the patella, visually inspecting the medial side of the knee. Repeat the procedure on the medial side, visually inspecting the lateral side, if there is a concavity before that remains concave after applying pressure. If a loss of the concavity or even a convex appearance to the side of the knee (a bulge), an effusion is present

Instruct the patient to assume and maintain a neutral anatomic stance. If the tibia is abnormally adducted on the femur, the patient has a varus deformity (*ie*, is bowlegged). If the tibia is abnormally abducted on the femur, the patient has a valgus deformity (*ie*, is knock-kneed)

Perform Lachman's manuever: With the patient in a supine position and the knee held by examiner and flexed at 30°, gently yet firmly pull on the tibia in an anterior direction so as to sublux it anteriorly. Perform with the knee in internal and external rotation positions to increase the sensitivity of the examination. If the tibia slides anteriorly over the femur (positive Lachman's sign) it is consistent with an anterior cruciate ligament tear.

Examine the patient for the perform posterior drawer sign. With the patient in a supine position and the knee held by the examiner and flexed at 90°, gently yet firmly push on the tibia in a posterior direction so as to sublux it posteriorly; use the contralateral knee as a control. If the tibia slides posteriorly under the femur (positive posterior drawer sign) it is consistent with a posterior cruciate ligament tear.

Perform McMurray's test. With the patient in a supine position, flex the hip and the knee until the heel touches the buttock. Steady the knee with one hand and grasp the heel with the other hand rotating the foot as far lateral (external rotation) as possible and the extend the knee to 90°. Return to the beginning and rotate the foot as far medial (internal rotation) as possible, and then passively extend the knee to 90°. Concurrently palpate the knee being tested. Repeat in the contralateral knee as a control. The presence of a click over the lateral aspect of the knee (a lateral McMurray sign) is consistent with a lateral meniscal tear, whereas, the presence of a click over the medial aspect of the knee (a medial McMurray sign) is consistent with a medial meniscal tear

Perform Apley's test. Instruct the patient to assume a prone position and then passively flex the leg at the knee to a right angle. Place the other hand immediately proximal to the knee to hold the femur down and concurrently flex the knee to a more acute angle. Query the patient regarding any sensations in the knee. Repeat in the contralateral knee as a control. Medial pain is consistent with medial collateral ligament dysfunction, whereas lateral pain is consistent with lateral collateral ligament dysfunction

From Daniel [7] and Rothenberg and Graf [8•]; with permission.

Table 6. Overall Physical Examination of the Shoulder

Perform active and passive range-of-motion assessment of the shoulder, at the glenohumeral joint. Stabilize the shoulder by placing a hand on the superior aspect of the acromion while the patient is abducting
  External rotation: 90°
  Internal rotation: 90°
  Extension: 50°
  Flexion: 180°
  Abduction: 180°
  Adduction: 50°
Inspect and palpate the sternoclavicular joint, the acromioclavicular joint, the humerus, and the musculature of the shoulder
Palpate the bicipital groove. This is the anatomic groove through which the long head of the biceps muscle passes on the proximal humerus, between the greater and lesser tubercles
Palpate over the lateral, superior aspect of the shoulder
If any suspicion of fracture or subluxation, check for any ipsilateral neurologic deficits (see Table 2)

From Smith and Campbell [9•]; with permission.

[9•] (Table 6). The specific entities that can be diagnosed by physical examination are described in the following sections.

Anterior Glenohumeral Dislocation

In anterior glenohumeral dislocation, the acromion is inappropriately prominent and the head of the humerus is anteriorly and medially displaced to a position beneath the coracoid process. The patient positions and holds the arm close to the body, with the elbow flexed. Finally, there is a complete loss of passive or active adduction of the arm at the shoulder. This dislocation usually results from arm hyperextension (*eg*, while pitching a baseball overhand or serving a tennis ball overhand).

Acromioclavicular Separation

In acromioclavicular separation, the distal clavicle is superiorly displaced from the acromion. Furthermore, the patient is unable to abduct or flex the ipsilateral arm actively. In most cases, the separation of the clavicle from the acromion can be detected via visual and tactile inspection. This separation is the result of trauma, specifically force being placed on the shoulder with an inferoposterior thrust.

Clavicular Fracture

The patient with a clavicular fracture is unable to abduct or elevate the entire upper extremity. On visual inspection and palpation, the fracture is quite evident. The underlying pathogenesis is one of direct trauma to the shoulder, the anterosuperior chest wall, or both, usually as the result of a fall.

Bicipital Tendinitis

The patient with bicipital tendinitis has tenderness over the anterior shoulder and positive findings for Yergason's sign (*ie*, reproduction of the pain on flexion of the elbow against force) and Speed's sign (*ie*, reproduction of the pain on curling the shoulders actively inward). This is the result of inflammation of the long head of the biceps in the bicipital groove.

Subacromial Bursitis

With subacromial bursitis, there is significant tenderness over the anterior and inferior aspects of the acromion and the development of signs of impingement, including both the presence of positive impingement test findings (*ie*, pain over the anterior acromion when the patient's arm is maximally passively flexed and the examiner presses on the shoulder girdle), and quite often the findings of bicipital tendinitis.

Supraspinatus Tendinitis

With supraspinatus tendinitis, there is significant tenderness over and adjacent to the greater tuberosity of the humerus and the acromion process and a marked decrease in active and passive abduction of the humerus at the glenohumeral joint over 90°. The underlying pathogenesis of this entity, which is also known as calcific tendinitis, is the noninfectious inflammation of the rotator cuff tendons in general, and of the supraspinatus tendon specifically.

Rotator Cuff Tears

Rotator cuff tears are characterized by tenderness over the greater tuberosity of the humerus and weakness of the motions of abduction and external rotation of the arm at the shoulder. The passive range of motion of the arm is normal, but active motion, especially abduction, is significantly limited. Furthermore, there is a marked limitation to active abduction from 0° to 30°. This is the result of a tear in one or more of the tendons or muscles that comprise the rotator cuff (*ie*, the supraspinatus, the infraspinatus, and the teres minor).

MURMURS

Cardiac murmurs are frequently noted during routine physical examination (Table 7). Although many murmurs are benign (innocent), others require further definition because they may be correlated with a malignant natural history. Furthermore, some lesions that these murmurs represent can be markers for other disease processes or may need antibiotic prophylaxis to prevent procedure-induced endocarditis (Table 8).

On the basis of the initial physical examination findings and the preliminary differential diagnosis, the examiner can then use other bedside maneuvers to assist in defining the underlying lesion. These specific maneuvers should not be performed blindly without having first defined the basic attributes of the murmur. Specific maneuvers are discussed in the following sections.

Systolic Murmurs Loudest at the Base

An attempt should be made to differentiate between aortic stenosis, a pathologic lesion that can result in malignant outcomes (including heart failure, left ventricular hypertrophy, syncope and sudden cardiac death) and that sometimes requires antibiotic prophylaxis; idiopathic hypertrophic subaortic steno-

TABLE 7 DIAGNOSTIC FEATURES OF A MURMUR

Place the patient in a supine position and auscult over the base and apex using the diaphragm with the patient breathing at baseline; note the following features of the murmur:
  Timing—when the murmur occurs in the cardiac cycle
    Systolic—between S_1 and S_2
    Diastolic—between S_2 and S_1
  Location—the location that is is easiest to auscult and/or palpate
    Base—deep to the manubrium sternum
    Apex—deep to the left fourth interspace
  Intensity[10•]
    Heard, but not immediately
    Faintest murmur is heard immediately after placing the stethoscope on the chest
    Loud, without a thrill
    Loud, with a thrill (*ie*, a palpable vibratory component to the murmur)
    Can be heard with the stethoscope at an angle
    Heard even with the stethoscope not touching the chest wall
  Radiation—locations where the murmur can be heard distant from the loudest point
  Associated manifestations—the company that the murmur keeps. Examples include the fixed split S_2 of atrial septal defect, the decreased intensity of S_2 in aortic stenosis, and the systolic click of mitral valve prolapse. Specifics are described in the text

S_1—first heart sound; S_2—second heart sound.

TABLE 8 DIFFERENTIAL DIAGNOSIS OF LESIONS FOR VARIOUS MURMURS
If systolic murmur is loudest at the base Aortic sclerosis Aortic stenosis Idiopathic hypertrophic subaortic stenosis Pulmonic stenosis, organic or functional **If diastolic murmur is loudest at the base** Aortic insufficiency Pulmonic insufficiency **If diastolic murmur is loudest at the apex** Austin Flint murmur of aortic insufficiency Mitral stenosis **If systolic murmur is loudest at the apex** Mitral insufficiency Tricuspid insufficiency Mitral valve prolapse Ventricular septal defect

sis (IHSS) another malignant lesion; and the benign entity aortic sclerosis, which does not require antibiotic prophylaxis.

To differentiate an aortic lesion from a subaortic lesion, such as IHSS, refer to Table 9. With the patient supine and breathing at baseline, auscultate using the diaphragm over the base, and then repeat the examination at this location 30 seconds after the patient has assumed a standing position. If the murmur intensity decreases or is unchanged after standing, it is aortic stenosis or sclerosis, whereas an increase on standing is consistent with IHSS. Furthermore, if the murmur increases in intensity or stays the same with squatting, it is aortic stenosis or sclerosis, whereas if it decreases with squatting, it is IHSS. Finally, if the carotid pulse decreases in intensity after an extrasystole, it is IHSS.

Severe aortic stenosis, unlike aortic sclerosis, results in a loss in the intensity of the second heart sound, a paradoxical splitting of the second heart tone (*ie*, P_2A_2 with inspiration, rather than the normal splitting of A_2P_2 with inspiration), or both; and has a decrease in the pulse pressure, with carotid upstrokes that are low and slow (*ie*, pulsus parvus et tardus) (Table 10).

Systolic Murmurs Loudest at the Apex

The four most common lesions that manifest with systolic murmurs best heard at the apex are tricuspid regurgitation, mitral regurgitation, mitral valve prolapse, and ventricular septal defect. Maneuvers to differentiate these lesions are extremely useful.

The first step is to differentiate tricuspid regurgitation from the other lesions. This is accomplished by several specific maneuvers. The first is the Rivero-Carvallo maneuver, which consists of auscultating over the apex with the diaphragm at the end of expiration and then during a deep, held inspiration. If the intensity of the murmur is increased with inspiration, it is mitral regurgitation, mitral valve prolapse, or a ventricular septal defect. There have been reports of 100% sensitivity and 88% specificity [13••]. Furthermore, if the examiner auscultates over the apex with the diaphragm before and during the placement of manual pressure on the liver for 15 to 20 seconds and the intensity of the murmur increases (Vitums' sign), it is consistent with tricuspid regurgitation. This sign has been reported to be 56% sensitive and virtually 100% specific [14]. Finally, if the examiner visually inspects the patient for jugular venous pulsations, these pulsations are often elevated, with

TABLE 9 MANEUVERS TO DIFFERENTIATE AORTIC VALVE LESIONS FROM IDIOPATHIC HYPERTROPHIC SUBAORTIC STENOSIS	
Procedure	**Outcome**
Change in the intensity of the murmur after attaining a standing from a supine position	Increased IHSS Decreased aortic valve
Change in the intensity of the murmur after attaining a squatting from a supine position	Decreased IHSS Increased aortic valve

IHSS—idiopathic hypertrophic subaortic stenosis.

Physical Diagnosis in Medicine

TABLE 10 MANEUVERS TO DIFFERENTIATE SEVERE AORTIC STENOSIS FROM AORTIC SCLEROSIS

Procedure	Aortic stenosis	Aortic sclerosis
Radiation of the murmur	Into the right carotid and right midclavicular areas	Minimal
Brachioradial delay [12]: with the patient supine or sitting, palpate the brachial and radial pulses simultaneously in one arm	The pulse in the radial site is delayed Sensitivity: 100% in severe aortic stenosis and 25% in mild aortic stenosis Specificity: 100%	Pulses are simultaneous
Second heart tone	Decreased intensity Paradoxical splitting (P_2A_2) with inspiration)	Discrete S_2 Physiological splitting (A_2P_2) with inspiration
Point of maximal impulse	Laterally displaced	Normal
Pulse wave contour	Pulsus parvus et tardus (low and slow)	Normal
Pulse pressure	<40 mm Hg	>40 mm Hg

S_2—second heart sound.

large V waves and great Y descents (Lancisi's sign), in tricuspid regurgitation [14].

Once tricuspid regurgitation has been diagnosed, no further maneuvers are necessary. However, if tricuspid regurgitation is unlikely based on these maneuvers, the next step is to differentiate mitral valve prolapse from mitral regurgitation. Mitral valve prolapse has a concurrent click before the murmur in systole, whereas none of the other lesions have a systolic click. Furthermore, the murmur and click of mitral valve prolapse increase in intensity after the patient assumes a standing position; if the murmur does not change, it is consistent with mitral regurgitation or another lesion.

ABDOMINAL PAIN

One of the most common problems with which patients present to physicians, and to primary care physicians specifically, is abdominal pain. Physical examination of the abdomen is pivotal in the evaluation of abdominal pain (Tables 11, 12, and 13). It will assist not only in making a diagnosis, but in an emergency (*ie*, an acute abdomen).

High-pitched bowel sounds heard on auscultation of the abdomen are called tinkles and are consistent with small bowel obstruction. Periods of markedly increased bowel sounds that are intermittent and few in nature are rushes; they are consistent with either normal findings, or early small bowel obstruction. Periods of markedly increased bowel sounds that are recurrent and heard without the assistance of a stethoscope are referred to as borborygmi and are consistent with a hyperdynamic small bowel. Finally, decreased or absent bowel sounds are consistent with ileus (*ie*, hypofunctioning of the small intestine).

To assess the liver, place the patient in a supine position and auscultate using the diaphragm of the stethoscope over the area inferior to the xiphoid process. Concurrently, scratch the skin lightly in the right midclavicular line, starting at the right nipple and moving inferiorly. This is used as a screening test to estimate the size and location of the liver. The scratching sound is accentuated over the liver itself. A scratching sound 10 to 12 cm in the right midclavicular line indicates a normal sized liver; if the hepar is greater than 12 cm, hepatomegaly is indicated; and, if it is less than 8 cm, a small liver is indicated. The upper border of the liver can be confirmed by percussion in the right midclavicular line, whereas the inferior border can be confirmed and described in further detail via palpation. If the edge is smooth and

TABLE 11 OVERALL PHYSICAL EXAMINATION OF THE PATIENT WITH ABDOMINAL PAIN

With the patient in a supine relaxed position, auscultate the abdomen using the diaphragm for 30 to 40 seconds.
  Perform this procedure before any other abdominal examination
Determine liver size and consistency by performing the scratch test and by performing percussion and palpation
Perform direct palpation using the dominant hand in the abdomen in all four quadrants and about the umbilicus. Always palpate the painful area last
Perform rebound palpation, using the dominant hand in the abdomen in all four quadrants and about the umbilicus. Always palpate the painful area last

Visually inspect the skin of the adbomen, with attention given to the periumbilical and flank areas
Attempt to localize the tenderness to one quadrant of the abdomen, and then perform quadrant-specific maneuvers to assist in divining the diagnosis (see Table 12)
If the abdomen appears to be distended, perform specific maneuvers to differentiate between adipose, gas, a gravid uterus, and ascites (*see* Table 13) [15•,16]
Perform a rectal examination
Perform a genitourinary examination in men and women. Palpate the penis and scrotum in men, and perform a pelvic examination in women

Table 12 Maneuvers to evaluate abdominal pain

Quadrant	Maneuver or procedure	Outcome and diagnosis

Right upper quadrant	With the patient supine and with the hips and knees flexed, deeply palpate the right upper quadrant as the patient is instructed to inhale deeply	If inspiration is inhibited by pain:
		  Cholecystitis
		  Ascending cholangitis

Right upper quadrant	Directly palpate the liver	If the liver is diffusely enlarged and tender:
		  Hepatitis
		  Distention from acute congestive failure

Right or left upper quadrant	With the patient sitting upright, percuss, using the second digit, over the right costophrenic angle, using the contralateral side as a control; a variant is to punch the costophrenic angle gently with the ulnar aspect of a closed fist	If tenderness is present over the costophrenic angle:
		  Pyelonephritis
		  Psoas abscess

Right lower quadrant	With the patient in supine and with the hips and knees flexed, perform deep and rebound palpation at McBurney's point (one third of the distance medial to the anterosuperior iliac spine on a line drawn from the anterosuperior iliac spine to the umbilicus)	If tenderness is present: Appendicitis
Right lower quadrant	With the patient supine and with the hips and knees flexed, perform deep and rebound palpation in the left lower quadrant	If rebound and deep tenderness are present in the right lower quadrant (Rovsing's sign): Appendicitis

Left or right lower quadrant (in women)	Perform a bimanual pelvic examination	If adnexal tenderness or an adnexal mass is present:
		  Ectopic pregnancy
		  Pelvic inflammatory disease

Table 13 Maneuvers to differentiate the etiology of abdominal distention

Procedure	Outcome	Sensitivity and specificity

With the patient supine, percuss the abdomen in an arc from the umbilicus inferolaterally; note the location of a change in percussion note from resonant to dull	Dull throughout:
	  Adipose
	Dull in flanks only:
	  Ascites
		Sensitivity: 80% [15•,16]
		Specificity: 69% [15•,16]
		Sensitivity: 94% [15•]
		Specificity: 29% [15•]

Examine the patient for shifting dullness: If there is a level of dullness perceived by percussion, note and mark that level, then roll the patient over 90° and repercuss in the same arc; note and mark the level of dullness	If no change in the level occurs:
	  Adipose
	  No significant ascites
	If a change in the level occurs:
	  Ascites
	  Severe mesenteric adiposity
		Sensitivity: 60% [15•,16]
		Specificity: 90% [15•,16]

With the patient in a supine position, percuss with a sharp staccato motion over a specific spot in the left or right inferolateral abdomen; concurrently, place the contralateral hand, palm to abdominal skin, on the contralateral side of the abdomen; if possible instruct an assistant to gently place the ulnar aspect of the hand longitudinally over the midline of the abdomen	If there is a wave, fast and seen in the skin:
	  Adipose
	If the presence of a wave sensation felt by the contralateral hand occurs after the adipose wave:
	  Fluid wave of ascites
		Sensitivity: 50% [15•]
		Specificity: 82% [15•]
		Sensitivity: 80% [15•,16]
		Specificity: 92% [15•,16]
		Sensitivity: 53% [15•]
		Specificity: 90% [15•]

nontender, it is normal; if nodules or masses are present, it is consistent with cirrhosis, primary hepatocellular carcinoma, or metastatic disease; and if the liver is diffusely tender and enlarged, it is consistent with hepatitis.

To discover any direct tenderness, instruct the patient to assume a supine position with the knees and hips flexed. Directly palpate, the abdomen in all four quadrants and about the umbilicus using the dominant hand with the palm adja-

TABLE 14 OVERALL EXAMINATION OF A PATIENT WITH SHORTNESS OF BREATH

Percuss the lung fields with the third digit of the dominant hand on the third digit of the nondominant hand applied to specific sites in the thorax. A tympanic note (*ie*, hyperresonance) is consistent with decreased lung tissue emphysema or pneumothorax. A dull note is consistent with a pleural effusion or consolidation

Instruct the patient to state the word "coin," "toy," or "boy" repetitively. Each time feel for the transmission of the sound using the palms of both hands as the sensor (tactile fremitus)

With the patient sitting up and leaning forward, auscult using the diaphragm and the lung fields

Visually inspect the mucous membranes and nail beds; use your own mucous membranes as a control

Auscultate the heart for any gallops or evidence of heart failure. S_3 is quite specific for systolic heart failure, whereas S_4 may indicate diastolic heart failure

Perform a sputum examination if the patient has a productive cough. Yellow-green (*ie*, purulent) sputa is correlated with an inflammatory (asthma) or infectious etiology. Pink frothy sputa is consistent with pulmonary edema, and hemoptysis may result from bronchitis, cancer, or mycobacterial diseases

S_3—third heart sound; S_4—fourth heart sound.

SHORTNESS OF BREATH

Another quite common problem with which patients present to primary care physicians is shortness of breath, with or without a cough. The many causes of this problem, including bronchitis, pneumonia, asthma, chronic obstructive pulmonary disease, pneumothorax, pleural effusions, and heart failure, can all be diagnosed via the techniques of physical diagnosis (Table 14).

Breath sounds are quite helpful in assessing the underlying etiology of shortness of breath. If the peripheral breath sounds have an expiratory phase that is longer than the inspiratory phase and are louder than those in control areas (*ie*, if they sound similar to those over the trachea [bronchial breath sounds]), they are consistent with consolidation or atelectasis. Table 15 provides information on differentiating pleural effusion from consolidation.

Adventitious sounds [17] include wheezes and rales. Wheezes indicate partial airway obstruction. Predominantly inspiratory wheezes suggest rigid stenosis of an airway, whereas predominantly expiratory wheezes suggest reversible airway disease. A high-pitched wheeze (*ie*, stridor) is consistent with high-grade stenosis of an airway, an emergent condition. If the stridor is predominantly inspiratory, it is consistent with upper airway obstruction, whereas if it is predominantly expiratory, it is consistent with lower airway obstruction. Crackles and rales will sound like the rubbing of hairs next to the ears, and may indicate interstitial inflammation, fibrosis, or fluid in the pulmonary parenchyma itself. Sounds that sound like secretions in tubes or something that needs to be coughed up, are rhonchi, which are suggestive of fluid or secretions in the airways themselves.

During the inspection of the mucous membranes and nail beds, the examiner can assess certain features of the severity and chronicity of the pulmonary dysfunction. The color of the mucous membranes and nail beds is important to note: pink is normal; a bright red discoloration is suggestive of carbon monoxide inhalation or ingestion of cyanide; a diffuse blue discoloration is consistent with cyanosis; and a pallor or white discoloration is consistent with anemia.

The nails should be carefully examined for clubbing through visual inspection of the nail plate, and attention given to the angle made by the nail plate and the proximal nail fold. This angle is normally 160°; an angle of greater than 160° is one criterion for clubbing. If this first criterion for clubbing is present, press on the proximal nail plate with finger, attempting to move the plate from the bed. If the plate cannot be moved on the bed, this is normal, whereas if the plate can be

cent to the skin. Always palpate the painful area last. If there is tenderness to deep palpation (*ie*, pain produced by direct pressure), it is quite nonspecific, except to localize the tenderness to a specific quadrant. Voluntary guarding (*ie*, the patient voluntarily contracts muscles to prevent palpation) is nonspecific, whereas in involuntary guarding the abdominal wall is rigid to palpation, which is indicative of peritoneal irritation. Although this is not specific for a diagnosis, it is a marker for an emergent or acute abdomen.

To discover any rebound tenderness, palpate the abdomen and rapidly withdraw the hand from the point of maximal deep palpation. Always palpate the painful area last. If no pain is present on withdrawal of the hand, there is no rebound tenderness, whereas if pain is present, this is rebound tenderness and indicates local or diffuse peritoneal irritation. If the rebound tenderness is localized, it is an aid in developing a quadrant-specific differential diagnosis and is a marker for an emergent or acute abdomen.

TABLE 15 MANEUVERS TO DIFFERENTIATE CONSOLIDATION FROM PLEURAL EFFUSION

Procedure	Consolidation	Pleural effusion
Percussion	Dull over site	Dull over site
Examination for tactile fremitus	Increased usually	Decreased
Auscultation	Increased breath sounds	Decreased breath sounds

TABLE 16 PHYSICAL EXAMINATION FINDINGS OF COMMON ETIOLOGIES OF SHORTNESS OF BREATH

Etiology	Percussion	Auscultation Breath sounds	Auscultation Adventitious sounds	Tactile fremitus	Heart	Sputum
Pleural effusion	Dull over effusion	Decreased over effusion	Minimal	Decreased over effusion	Tachycardia	Scant
Typical pneumonia	Dull over pneumonia	Increased over pneumonia	Diffuse rhonchi; crackles over pneumonia	Increased over pneumonia	Tachycardia	Green-yellow
Atypical pneumonia	Normal	Normal	Diffuse crackles	Normal	Tachycardia	Scant
Bronchitis	Normal	Normal	Diffuse wheezes; diffuse rhonchi	Normal	Tachycardia	Yellow-white
Asthma	Normal	Normal	Diffuse wheezes	Normal	Tachycardia	Yellow-white
Chronic bronchitis	Normal	Normal	Diffuse wheezes; diffuse rhonchi	Normal	Tachycardia; increased P_2; wide split S_2	Yellow-white
Emphysema	Tympanic	Diffusely decreased	A few wheezes	Normal	Tachycardia; increased P_2; wide split S_2	Scant
Heart failure	Normal, unless an effusion is present	Normal	Diffuse crackles	Normal	Tachycardia; S_3	Frothy, pink
Pneumothorax	Unilateral tympany	Unilateral decrease	Minimal	Unilateral decrease	Tachycardia	Scant

S_2—second heart sound; S_3—third heart sound (ventricular gallop).

moved on the bed (*ie*, if there is sponginess at the base), this is consistent with clubbing. Clubbing is a marker for chronic hypoxemia or a chronic neoplastic or inflammatory condition.

The specifics regarding examination for the diagnoses of pleural effusion, typical pneumonia, atypical pneumonia, bronchitis, asthma, chronic obstructive pulmonary disease, heart failure, and pneumothorax are listed in Table 16.

CONCLUSION

This brief overview of physical examination has hopefully served to reinforce the tools we as physicians have virtually at the tips of our fingers, at the focal point of our vision, at our threshold of hearing, and within the range of our olfactory senses. These techniques, when used and interpreted effectively are a time- and cost-effective set of tools for providing quality medical care. In addition, we hope that this overview has piqued interest in further developing skills in physical examination.

REFERENCES AND RECOMMENDED READING

Recently published papers of particular interest have been highlighted as:
- Of interest
- • Of outstanding interest

1. St. Clair EW, Oddone EZ, Waugh RA: Assessing housestaff diagnostic skills using a cardiology patient simulator. *Ann Intern Med* 1992, 117:751–756.
2. Peterson MC, Holbrook JH, Von Hales D, *et al.*: Contributions of the history, physical examination, and laboratory investigation in making a medical diagnosis. *West J Med* 1992, 156:163–165.
3.•• Sackett DL: The science and art of the clinical examination. *JAMA* 1992, 267:2650–2657.
4.• Katz JN: The carpal tunnel syndrome: diagnostic utility of the history and physical examination findings. *Ann Intern Med* 1990, 112:321–327.
5. Deyo RA, Rainville J, Kent DL: What can the history and physical examination tell us about low back pain? *JAMA* 1992, 268:760–766.
6.• Deyo RA, Loeser JD, Bigos SJ: Herniated lumber intervertebral disk. *Ann Intern Med* 1990, 112:598–603.
7. Daniel DM: Diagnosis of a ligament injury. In *Knee Ligaments: Structure, Function, Injury, and Repair*. Edited by Daniel DM, *et al*. New York: Raven Press; 1990:3–10.
8.• Rothenberg MH, Graf BK: Evaluation of acute knee injuries. *Postgrad Med* 1993, 93:75–86.
9.• Smith DL, Campbell SM: The painful shoulder. *J Gen Intern Med* 1992, 7:328–339.
10.• Freeman AR, Levine SA: Clinical significance of systolic murmurs. *Ann Intern Med* 1933, 6:1371–1379.
11.• Rothman A, Goldberger AL: Aids to cardiac auscultation. *Ann Intern Med* 1983, 99:346–353.
12. Leach RM, McBrien RM: Brachioradial delay in severe aortic stenosis. *Lancet* 1990, 335:1199–1201.
13.•• Lembo NJ, Dell'Italia LJ, Crawford MH, O'Rourke RA: Bedside diagnosis of systolic murmurs. *N Engl J Med* 1988, 318:1572–1578.
14. Cha SD, Gooch AS: Diagnosis of tricuspid regurgitation. *Arch Intern Med* 1983, 143:1763–1764.

15.• Williams JW, Simel DL: Does this patient have ascites? *JAMA* 1992, 267:2645–2648.

16. Simel DL: Quantitating bedside diagnosis: clinical evaluation of ascites. *J Gen Intern Med* 1988, 3:423–428.

17.• Bohadana AB: Breath sounds in the clinical assessment of airflow obstruction. *Thorax* 1978, 33:345–351.

SELECT BIBLIOGRAPHY

Sapira JD: *The Art and Science of Bedside Diagnosis*. Baltimore: Urban and Schwarzenberg; 1990.

Schneiderman H, Wilms J, eds: *Physical Diagnosis*. Baltimore: Williams and Wilkins; 1994.

Schneiderman H: *Bedside Diagnosis*. Philadelphia: American College of Physicians; 1992.

Diagnostic Tests

Jefferey D. Lang
David L. Sackett

Key Points
- Diagnostic tests must be managed properly to avoid useless or low-yield procedures, to minimize potentially dangerous or invasive tests, and to hasten the time to definitive diagnosis by skipping preliminary steps.
- The most common diagnostic strategy employs pattern recognition only for the purpose of generating a short list of diagnostic possibilities that is refined.
- Interpretation of diagnostic test results depends on sensitivity, specificity, and likelihood ratios, as well as pretest probability.
- Test threshold and treatment threshold help the physician to decide whether to test further, treat, or abandon a diagnosis.

There is a science to the art of diagnosis, and we are beginning to understand it. Although there is no substitute for clinical experience and judgment, there are several simple steps that all physicians can incorporate into their work-ups to make the diagnostic process more efficient and hasten selection of rapidly evolving diagnostic technologies.

DIAGNOSTIC STRATEGIES

The diagnosing clinician uses several strategies, but only two are discussed in this chapter. One method is both the simplest and the most complex because it involves the recognition of a constellation of clinical findings that conforms to a previously learned pattern of disease (*eg*, the joints of rheumatoid arthritis, the exophthalmos of Graves' disease, and much of dermatology). Pattern recognition is difficult to teach and is prone to error when employed casually, but can be particularly useful when recognizing diagnostic elements of high specificity (pathognomonic features). The more common and reliable diagnostic strategy employs pattern recognition only for the purpose of generating a short list of diagnostic possibilities based on the first few moments of the patient interview [1]. Clinicians subsequently refine this list with each ensuing piece of information carefully elicited from the history and physical examination. Subsequent testing (*eg*, laboratory tests or radiography) can complete this hypothetico-deductive process and confirm or refute initial hypotheses in a highly focused and logical manner. Each step in the diagnostic process is based on the results of the previous step and is dedicated to further developing and narrowing the short list of diagnostic possibilities for the individual patient. This chapter focuses on this latter diagnostic strategy.

DEFINITIONS OF NORMAL

Normal can be defined in many ways depending on the context (Table 1) [2]. For our purposes, we are most interested in separating patients with disease or at risk for disease from those without disease. We are especially interested in identifying

TABLE 1 DEFINITIONS OF 'NORMAL'

Term	Property	Consequences of clinical application
Gaussian	Normal distribution of test results about central mean	Limits of test result would extend toward infinity in both directions
Percentile	Result lies within a preset percentile of previous diagnostic test results	Prevalence of all disease would be 5%
Risk factor	Result carries no additional risk of morbidity or mortality	Assumes altering the risk factor alters risk
Culturally desirable	Socially or politically correct	Confusion over the role of medicine in society
Diagnostic	Test result that separates those with high probability of disease from those without	Need to know the predictive values of the test as they pertain to your practice
Therapeutic	Test result that identifies those likely to benefit from intervention	Need to keep up with new knowledge about therapy as therapy changes

Adapted from Sackett *et al.* [2]; with permission.

diseases in which treatment does more good than harm. The old medical school axiom "don't miss treatable disease" is more important today than ever, as treatments are developed, refined, and tested in experimental trials. The *diagnostic definition of normal* calls normal those patients without the thoughtfully arbitrary identifying features of the disease in question, separating those who are well from those who are ill: patients with fasting blood sugars greater than 7.8 mmol/L have diabetes, and those with both symptoms and greater than 10^5 colony-forming units of bacteria in their urine have a urinary tract infection. Patients without these defining features are considered "normal."

The *therapeutic definition of normal* calls only those patients with conditions that improve with therapy abnormal and requires constant updating as our ability to identify risk and effectively treat disease improves. This definition also is arbitrary and varies among different patients, cultures, and physicians. In addition, for some diseases there is no clearly identifiable cut-off between disease and no disease. For example, the risk of mortality increases steadily at all levels of systemic blood pressure and serum cholesterol. Even typical values connote some risk, and no values appear to be without risk. This therapeutic definition permits some flexibility in choosing who to treat and who to observe and allows us to avoid labeling those patients unlikely to benefit from intervention as sick. One might be prepared to accept a serum cholesterol level of 5.7 mmol/L in an otherwise healthy young person, but would aggressively treat this "abnormality" in a 50-year-old patient with hypertension or other coronary risk factors.

SELECTION

As technology evolves, we are confronted with an increasing arsenal of diagnostic tests, each touted as the latest and greatest. Some diagnostic tests have definite normal and abnormal results, but the majority have multiple potential results and are subject to interpretation (*eg*, a ventilation-perfusion scan for pulmonary embolus, a serum calcium determination, or even a chest radiograph with a solitary nodule). No dichotomy between normal and abnormal makes sense in these tests.

Moreover, diagnostic test results must always be interpreted in light of the patient's clinical circumstance and the results of previous testing. Several guides to selection of appropriate diagnostic tests have been published recently (Table 2), and these can help clinicians make decisions on the appropriateness of a given diagnostic test [3•].

As an example, an elderly gentleman presents with anemia and, because of the possibility of an underlying occult malignancy, you want to rule in or out iron deficiency as the cause accurately. The gold standard is, of course, bone marrow

TABLE 2 READERS' GUIDES FOR INTERPRETATION OF STUDIES OF DIAGNOSTIC TESTS

Are the results of the study valid?
Primary guides
    Has there been an independent "blind" comparison with a reference standard?
    Did the patient sample include an appropriate spectrum of patients to whom the diagnostic test will be applied in clinical practice?
Secondary guides
    Did the results of the test influence the decision to perform the reference standard?
    Were the methods for performing the test described in sufficient detail to permit their exact replication?

What are the results?
Are likelihood ratios for the test results presented, or are the data necessary for their calculation provided?

Will the results help me in caring for my patients?
Will the reproducibility of the test result and its interpretation be satisfactory in my setting?
Are the results applicable to my patient?
Will the results change my management?
Will the patient be better off as a result of the test?

Adapted from Jaeschke *et al.* [3•]; with permission.

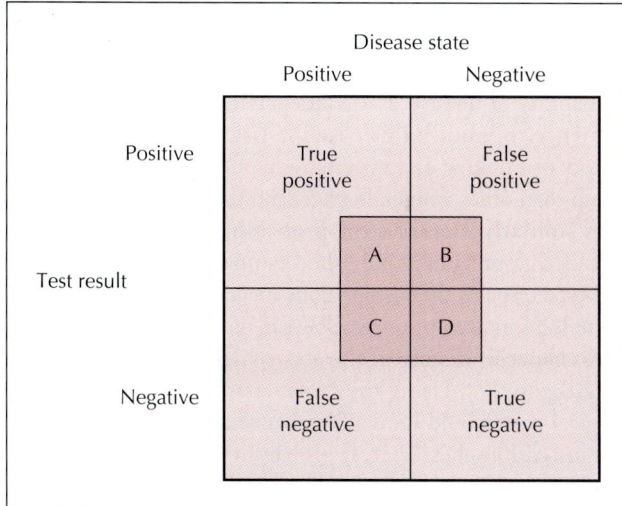

FIGURE 1 Two-by-two table for calculating test sensitivity.

biopsy with a stain for iron stores; however, this procedure is invasive, uncomfortable for the patient, and very likely unnecessary. You are aware of several laboratory tests that can help in the diagnosis, but you are unaware of the relative value of each test or whether they are all necessary. Because you are confronted by this type of problem frequently, you also believe that it is important to have a good knowledge of the recent literature. At this point you might pursue one of several options: 1) you can ask a colleague or expert in the field, but may get a biased interpretation of the literature [4•] or information based on a different type of practice than your own; 2) you can consult a text, but you know that texts are often years out of date even at the time of publication; or 3) you can search the current literature yourself to derive your answer. You choose the latter route, and your librarian helps with a computer-based search of the MEDLINE database at the National Library of Medicine using a simpler, user-friendly access method known as Grateful Med. You choose the search terms iron deficiency, likelihood ratios, diagnostic tests, and meta-analysis. An article by Guyatt *et al* [5•] appears promising, and you retrieve it. You then apply the readers' guide to see if you can base your clinical decisions on it. This meta-analysis pooled data from primary articles with independent blind comparisons to the reference standard of bone marrow biopsy and included a broad range of patients. The test results did not influence the application of the reference standard, and the details of the test were clear. Likelihood ratios were presented (*see* following), and the article provided evidence on reproducibility and applicability to your patient. Overall the article fulfills all the important criteria, and the results can help guide your diagnosis and management. The next step requires you to apply these results to your patient.

INTERPRETATION

Interpretation of diagnostic test results depends on several important properties of the test, including sensitivity, specificity, and likelihood ratios, as well as the probability of disease in the patient before the test, or pretest probability [6•]. These properties are described below.

Sensitivity and Specificity

The value of any given test is measured by how well it identifies patients with a target disorder. The proportion of people with the target disorder who have a positive test result is termed the *sensitivity* of the test and can be calculated from a simple two-by-two table as A/A+C (Fig. 1). A test's *specificity* is defined as the proportion of people without disease who have a negative test result and can be calculated as D/B+D. Sensitivity and specificity are intrinsic properties of the test, are calculated from only those with and without disease, respectively, and do not change with the prevalence of disease (the proportion of patients with true disease, calculated from a cohort sample as A+C/A+B+C+D). They may, however, change with severity of disease, such that patients with more advanced disease are more likely to have a positive test result, or a higher test value, as in the case of carcinoembryonic antigen for colon carcinoma. Prevalence, however, changes the positive and negative predictive values of the test (A/A+B and D/C+D, respectively), or the chances that a given test result is a true result. As prevalence decreases, even with a highly sensitive and specific test, the probability that a positive test result is true-positive decreases. Tables 3 and 4 are examples of a good test (sensitivity = 90%; specificity = 90%) and the impact of changing prevalence. In this example, the probability of a positive test result being true-positive is only 50% when prevalence of disease is 10% and increases to 85% when applied to a population with a prevalence of disease of 40%.

TABLE 3 EXAMPLE TEST		
	Disease	
Test result	**Positive**	**Negative**
Positive	90	90
Negative	10	810
Prevalence = 10%		
n = 1000		
Sensitivity = 90%; specificity = 90%		
Positive predictive value = 0.5		
Negative predictive value = 0.99		

TABLE 4 EXAMPLE TEST		
	Disease	
Test result	**Positive**	**Negative**
Positive	360	60
Negative	40	540
Prevalence = 40%		
n = 1000		
Sensitivity = 90%; specificity = 90%		
Positive predictive value = 0.85		
Negative predictive value = 0.93		

This example highlights the importance of applying diagnostic tests thoughtfully to appropriate patient populations, thus minimizing false-positive results and unnecessary further investigation.

A test with a high sensitivity is useful for ruling out disease (*Se*nsitive test when *N*egative rules *out* disease, or *SnNout*). Similarly, a test with high specificity is useful for ruling in disease (*Sp*ecific test when *P*ositive rules *in* disease, or *SpPin*). Calling a test result positive or negative may be useful when the test is a good *SpPin* or *SnNout*, but for most tests a great deal of information is lost by creating this dichotomy. A more useful measure of a test's value, which takes into account different baseline risks, is the likelihood ratio.

Pretest Probability

A baseline estimate of the probability of disease in a given patient before embarking on a series of diagnostic tests can help refine the order of tests and the aggressiveness of the investigation. For example, consider two patients who present with chest pain. One is a 55-year-old woman with a history of hypertension and heavy smoking who describes central heavy pain precipitated by exertion. The second is a 30-year-old anxious man who describes left-sided nonexertional chest pain of a transient nature associated with dyspnea. Intuitively, we can estimate that the probability of significant coronary artery disease is quite different in the two individuals—high in the middle-aged woman and low in the young man. As a result, one might make markedly different decisions as to the aggressiveness of the ensuing investigation and might treat results from tests in a different manner in the two patients.

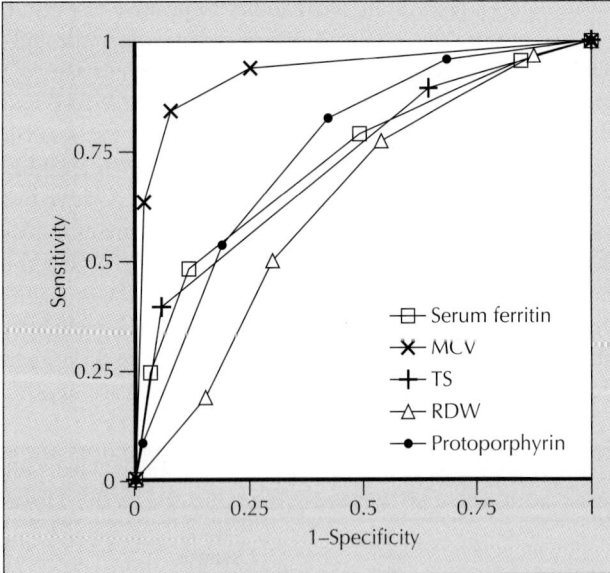

FIGURE 2 Receiver operating characteristic curves for serum ferritin radioimmunoassay, red cell protoporphyrin determination, transferrin saturation (TS), mean cell volume (MCV) determination, and red cell distribution width (RDW). For each value of each test, the y-axis represents the sensitivity of the test (the proportion of patients without iron deficiency who are falsely classified as having iron deficiency). (*From* Guyatt *et al.* [5•]; with permission.)

The logical conclusions are that most diagnostic tests do not definitely diagnose disease but rather modify our baseline estimate of risk (pretest probability), yielding a new (post-test) probability of disease. Each independent test can be used in sequence to modify this baseline risk. In the first patient, history of smoking and hypertension put her into a higher risk group than other women her age, and the typical nature of her pain similarly increases the probability of disease. In fact, considering previously published estimates based on age, sex, and type of pain, the history alone increases the risk of disease from 3.2% in asymptomatic 55-year-old women to almost an 80% chance of disease in the above-mentioned woman with typical pain [7]. Using the same data, the young man with atypical pain would have a 5% chance of disease, confirming our initial hunches. Pretest probabilities (also called prevalence) are available in the literature and some texts [8] or can be estimated from one's own practice. How then can we anticipate the effect of a test result on our patient's likelihood of disease once we are aware of the baseline risk for the target disorder?

Likelihood Ratios

For most tests, no one value is diagnostic for disease but instead alters the pretest probability of disease. For example, serum ferritin can be measured to help in the evaluation of iron deficiency anemia, and although a very low value for ferritin, *eg*, less than 15 µg/L, is extremely specific for iron deficiency (SpPin) and a high value, *eg*, greater than 100 µg/L, makes the disease very unlikely (SnNout), there are a range of values in between with intermediate sensitivity and specificity. A graphic plot of sensitivity (true-positive rate) versus 1 - specificity (false-positive rate) shows that there is a clear trade off (Fig. 2). The more sensitive a test, the more false-positive results are usually seen. This type of graph is called a receiver operating characteristic (ROC) curve and can be useful in evaluating the characteristics of a diagnostic test and in determining the most appropriate point to use for a cut-off. In general, the greater the area under the curve, the better the diagnostic test.

These ratios of true-positive findings to false-positive findings also can be calculated and expressed as *likelihood ratios*. Different likelihood ratios can be calculated for each test result or range of results. This technique uses all the available information from the testing procedure and is an expression of the *odds* of a patient with disease having a given test result compared with a person without disease having the same test result. These likelihood ratios can then be used to modify mathematically the pretest odds of disease to arrive at a post-test or posterior probability in a simplified application of Bayes' theorem.

For our example using serum ferritin level for the diagnosis of iron deficiency anemia, we can extract the likelihood ratios from the article from Guyatt *et al.* [5•] and apply them to our patient. The table summarizes the results of the overview. How likely is true iron deficiency anemia in a patient with serum ferritin level of less than 15 µg/L? Table 5 shows that 474 of 809 patients with iron deficiency had this test result (probability or sensitivity of 0.586). Only 20 of 1860 patients

Table 5. Sensitivity of test for iron deficiency

Serum ferritin, µg/L	Iron deficient patients, n	Non–iron-deficient patients, n	Likelihood ratio	95% Confidence interval
≥ 100	48	1320	0.08	0.07–0.09
45 < 100	76	398	0.54	0.48–0.60
35 < 45	36	43	1.83	1.47–2.19
25 < 35	58	50	2.54	2.11–2.97
15 < 25	117	29	8.83	7.22–10.44
≤ 15	474	20	51.85	41.53–62.27

Adapted from Guyatt *et al.* [5•]; with permission.

without iron deficiency (probability or 1 - specificity of 0.011) had this test result. The ratio of these two probabilities is the likelihood ratio of the test and is 51.85 in this case. Therefore, this test result is approximately 52 times more common among those with iron deficiency anemia than those without. Likelihood ratios can be calculated similarly for the different ranges of values for the test.

By estimating the pretest likelihood of disease, we can derive a post-test probability for the disease in question. In an otherwise healthy young woman with a history of heavy menses and anemia, our pretest probability for the disorder might be quite high, maybe 80% or more. Similarly, in an elderly man with a history of weight loss, change in bowel habits, and occult blood–positive stool, our pretest probability also would be high. These probabilities can be converted to odds by the formula:

Odds = Probability/1 – Probability

In this case, with a probability of 80%, the odds would be 0.8/0.2, or 4.0. This figure can be multiplied by the likelihood ratio (in the case of a ferritin level of <15 µg/L, 51.85) to come up with post-test odds (207.4) and converted back to probability by the formula:

Probability = Odds/1 + Odds

and a final probability of 99%. We have ruled in iron deficiency.

In general, likelihood ratios of greater than 10 or less than 0.1 make for convincing changes to pretest probabilities. Less extreme values cause moderate shifts. Tests with likelihood ratios of less than 10 or greater 0.1 are most useful when the pretest probability is in the midrange. For example, if the pretest probability was thought to be 10% (odds 0.11), a very low ferritin level results in a post-test probability of 85%, whereas if the pretest probability was thought to be 40%, a ferritin level of 30 µg/L (likelihood ratio 2.54) results in a post-test probability of only 63%. This process seems complicated, but it is learned rapidly and is easy to use. An alternative to this mathematical process is to use a nomogram (Fig. 3). This nomogram is simple to use, can be carried in the pocket of your coat, and involves only placing a straight edge linking the pretest probability and the likelihood ratio and reading the post-test probability from the card.

Unfortunately, few studies explicitly provide the values for likelihood ratios, but this is improving. They can be calculated easily if the sensitivity and specificity are known or from a simple two-by-two table using the following formula:

LR = Sensitivity/1 – Specificity

This is a valuable and quick way of approaching a diagnostic test. It takes into account the baseline risk (pretest probability) and allows multiple levels of test results to give the best estimate of likelihood of disease.

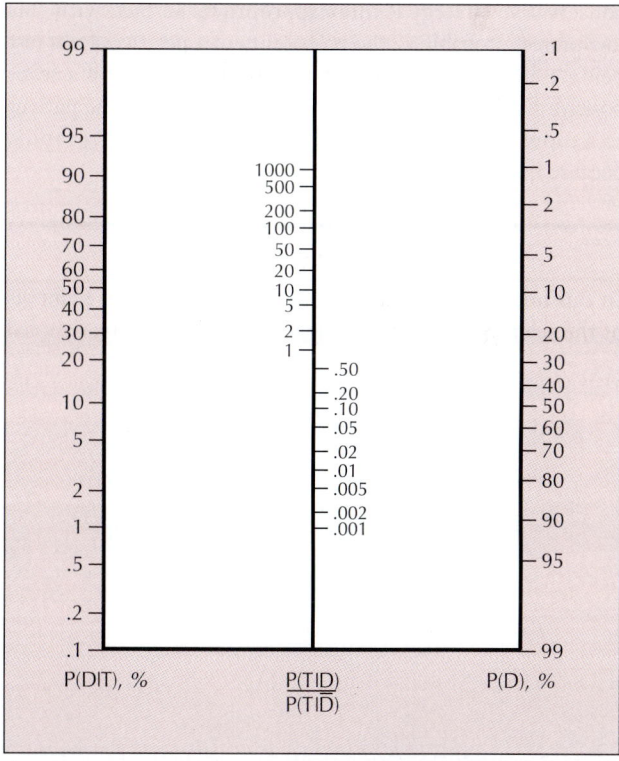

Figure 3 Nomogram for Bayes's Theorem. P(D) is the probability that the patient has the disease before the test. P(D|T) is the probability that the patient has the disease after the test result. P(T|D̄) is the probability of the test result if the patient has the disease, and P(T|D̄) is the probability of the test result if the patient does not have the disease. With this terminology the usefulness of both positive and negative test results can be assessed. A line drawn from P(D) on the right through the ratio of P(T|D̄) to P(T|D̄) in the yields P(D|T) on the left.

TEST AND TREATMENT THRESHOLD

At each point in the diagnostic process a decision must be made whether to test further, treat, or abandon a diagnosis. These thresholds can be thought of usefully as probabilities between 0 (the target disorder is ruled out) and 1 (it is ruled in). These thresholds vary among diseases and patients and have been described as the "test threshold" (below which no tests would be carried out because of their high rates of false-positive results) and the "treatment threshold" (above which further testing is unnecessary and treatment should begin). The "action" is in between these thresholds: it is where we test and guide our treatment by the test result. In the chest pain example, the two patients are at clearly different risks for having disease, and the diagnostic strategies applied should be accordingly different. With an 80% pretest probability of having disease, the woman with typical pain would be better treated by aggressive antianginal therapy (or by proceeding directly to the definitive diagnostic test—cardiac angiography rather than to an insensitive test such as graduated exercise testing). In this example, one could argue that the stress test is potentially dangerous because it may delay definitive investigation or treatment and may place the patient at undue risk.

In contrast, with a very low pretest probability of 5% to 10%, as seen in the male patient with atypical chest pain, a conservative strategy is more appropriate. In fact, with this low pretest probability, the probability of a positive stress test being a false-positive finding is greater than that of a true-positive finding. It also is not justifiable to subject the patient to a more definitive diagnostic test, such as angiography, because the risk outweighs any potential benefit.

CONCLUSION

In this brief chapter, we have described some of the elements of the science of the art of diagnosis. Their mastery, coupled with clinical experience, can speed the effective diagnosis of patients and ensure that they receive the best treatment (which often is no treatment).

REFERENCES AND RECOMMENDED READING

Recently published papers of particular interest have been highlighted as:
- Of interest

1. Barrow HS, Norman GR, Neufeld VR, Feightner JW: The clinical reasoning of randomly selected physicians in general medical practice. *Clin Invest Med* 1982, 5:49.
2. Sackett DL, Haynes RB, Guyatt GH, Tugwell P: *Clinical Epidemiology: A Basic Science for Clinical Medicine*, edn. 2. Boston: Little, Brown and Company; 1991.
3.• Jaeschke R, Guyatt GH, Sackett DL, and the Evidence-Based Medicine Working Group: Users' guides to the medical literature. Part III: how to use an article about a diagnostic test. Part A: are the results of the study valid? *JAMA* 1994, 271(9):703–707.
4.• Antman EM, Lau J, Kupelnick B, *et al.*: A comparison of results of meta-analyses of randomized control trials and recommendations of clinical experts. *JAMA* 1992, 268:240–248.
5.• Guyatt GH, Oxman AD, Ali M, *et al.*: Laboratory diagnosis of iron deficiency anemia: an overview. *J Gen Intern Med* 1992, 7:145–153.
6.• Jaeschke R, Guyatt GH, Sackett DL, and the Evidence-Based Medicine Working Group: Users' guides to the medical literature. Part III: how to use an article about a diagnostic test. Part B: what are the results and will they help me in caring for my patients? *JAMA* 1994, 271(9):703–707.
7. Diamond GA, Forrester JS: Analysis of probability as an aid in the clinical diagnosis of coronary artery disease. *N Engl J Med* 1979, 300:1350–1358.
8. Panzer RJ, Black ER, Griner PF: *Diagnostic Strategies for Common Medical Problems*. Philadelphia: American College of Physicians; 1991.

Referrals
Julius J. Chosy

> **Key Points**
> - Proper referral and consultation are important for optimum health care delivery, control of costs, and quality of care.
> - Accurate communication is essential; referring physicians should state clearly what it is they want to know and what they want the consultant to do.
> - Consultants must define the task, address the referring physician's concerns, and know what responsibility for care is to be assumed.
> - Consultants should use problem lists, make recommendations that are succinct, to the point, and specific, and then follow up if possible.
> - Consultants should transmit what is important to both the patient and the referring physician.

Referral and consultation among physicians and other health care providers facilitates optimum health care delivery. The primary physician as care coordinator matches patients' needs and preferences with the judicious use of medical services. Doing so protects patients from the possible adverse effects of unnecessary care and ensures the appropriate use of health care services [1••]. In this era of explosive growth in biomedical knowledge, technology, subspecialized care, and costs, referral and consultation decisions greatly affect the cost and quality of care [2••].

Physicians in training are exposed to a variety of consultation services, but few training programs offer formal instruction in the principles and the art of referral and consultation (seven leading medical textbooks do not cover the subject at all). In this chapter the principles of referral and consultation and the rules of behavior involved are discussed.

REFERRAL

Referrals may involve requests for a wide range of services, from a limited consultation (for example, to a nutrition service for diet assessment) to a complete transfer of patient care responsibility. The outcome of these arrangements among the primary physician, the patient, and the consultant is generally improved care for the patient; however, poor communication between the participants can lead to misunderstanding, duplication of care, or even lapses in care.

Consultation and referral patterns, their variability, and the clinical decision processes that govern them are not well understood. Patient characteristics, physician specialty, length of training, and reimbursement plan appear to be important [1••,3,4]. The results of two recent studies suggest that the greater a practitioner's diagnostic certainty or knowledge in a specialty area, the higher the referral rate to that specialty [5,6•].

The reasons for referral and consultation are varied and complex (Table 1) [2••,7•,8,9]. They mainly involve seeking advice or help in diagnosis or patient

TABLE 1 REASONS FOR REFERRAL
Diagnosis or confirmation of diagnosis
Recommendations for therapy or management
Implementation of therapy or management
Performance of a specialty procedure
Routine specialty examination
Prior care by subspecialty consultant
Reassurance for patient, relative, or physician
Request by patient
Education of patient or physician
Medical-legal reasons
Transfer of patient care

TABLE 2 THE FIVE STEPS OF REFERRAL AND CONSULTATION
1. Referring physician and patient recognize need for consultation
2. Referring physician communicates reason for consultation and clinical information about patient to consultant
3. Consultant evaluates patient's condition
4. Consultant communicates findings and recommendations to referring physician
5. Patient, referring physician, and consultant decide about continuing care

management, performing a procedure, reassurance, pleasing someone, patient education, and divestiture of responsibility for care.

The literature includes many articles regarding when to refer patients with a particular problem or disease. The chief plea of consultants is that patients be referred "soon enough." "Soon enough" depends on the problem in question, the condition of the patient, and the skills of the primary physician and consultant. Certainly, when a physician is feeling a certain level of discomfort, it is time to refer. When the patient's condition is at a plateau or getting worse and further improvement might be possible, it is time to refer. A physician should not wait until the patient has become resentful or is compelled to ask for a referral. Patients often know when they are being held back from a second opinion. Enough medical information is available through the media for patients to be familiar with their options. Physicians should not be afraid to seek a second opinion: to do so will either validate their care and thereby their reputation, or it will lead to patients' getting the care they need, or both.

A somewhat sensitive reason for referral is the wish to be free of a particularly troublesome or hypochondriacal patient. It is an appropriate reason to refer when the physician can no longer provide the attentive listening and objective responses good medical care requires. In fairness to both the patient and the consultant, it should be made clear to the consultant.

What should be done when a patient asks for a referral that is not indicated or a second opinion that is believed unnecessary? Unless the patient can be readily convinced otherwise, it is probably best to arrange it. What if the patient asks to see a specific consultant who the physician believes to be a poor one? Always, the physician's obligation is to do right by the patient so that the issue must be handled tactfully but honestly and an alternate consultant suggested.

Steps in Referral

The process of referral and consultation involves five essential steps (Table 2) [8]. Problems may occur at any point, usually because of failures in communication or discordant expectations [1••,7•,8–12]. The most important step is formulating the question being asked. The consultant can't provide what is wanted if physicians themselves don't know or have not asked for it clearly. The physician must ask, "What is it I want to know, and what is it I want the consultant to do?".

For example, in requesting a neurology consultation, rather than saying, "Diabetic patient with progressive lower extremity weakness," say, "Insulin-dependent diabetic with steroid-dependent COPD and three-month history of progressive lower extremity weakness. Considering diabetic plexopathy versus steroid myopathy. Would appreciate your opinion and suggestions for evaluating the cause of this problem."

In requesting a rehabilitation medicine consultation, it is less helpful to say, "Admitted for pneumonia, needs rehab" than to say "76-yo patient admitted for treatment of pneumonia who is now deconditioned because of extended bedrest. Wishes to be discharged home. Lives alone. Please evaluate for self care and mobility and intervene as necessary."

When choosing a consultant, the primary physician's responsibility is to ensure the best possible outcome for the patient. In these days of managed care, capitation, gatekeepers, and pressure to generate revenue and contain costs, there may be limitations on referral choices. In a system with referral limitations, the physician remains obliged to get the right consultant for the patient when needed, even if it means requesting approval from a medical director to go outside.

Physicians choose consultants based on reputation, the recommendations of colleagues, and their own personal experience. Consultants are sought who will give a skilled and thoughtful response, whose personality fits the patient well, and who will keep the referring physician informed.

The mode of contact with the consultant varies with circumstances and personal style. Commonly, contact is by telephone, which has the advantage of speed and the opportunity to clarify questions and expectations. In other instances formal letters or consultation forms are used. Some physicians use verbal instructions to their patients to convey the purpose of a consultation, but this carries a great risk for miscommunication.

It is important to provide the consultant with all relevant clinical information (Table 3), including results of diagnostic tests and procedures to avoid unnecessary duplication [13]. It is helpful for the consultant to know of any previous therapy that has failed so that the same therapy is not recommended again. Consultants must know what responsibility for care they are to assume. It is courting disaster, for example, for the consulting physician to write aminoglycoside orders while thinking, incorrectly, that the primary physician will monitor blood levels and renal function. The consultant needs to know if a request is an emergency, urgent, or routine, as emergency consults must be seen immediately and urgent ones urgently. It is helpful for the consultant to know what the referring physician has told the patient about the referral so that the patient's expectations can be anticipated. Similarly, it is helpful for the consultant to know about any special attitudes of the patient, such as inordinate fear, fixed opinions of tests or treatments, or unreasonable expectations of outcome.

CONSULTATION

Now we turn to the consultant's role and the rules of effective consultation (Table 4) [1••,6•,7•,8,10–12]. The consultant's first task is to define what the referring physician wants. That is not always evident in the written consultation request or referral letter. A quick phone call to the referring physician may be needed to ascertain what the questions are and what specifically the consultant is being asked to do and when.

Next, consultants should look for themselves. It may be that they will have more time for interviewing and examining the patient, reviewing old records, or tracking down information than did a time-pressured referring physician. Because of their expertise and special perspective they may recognize the significance of information overlooked by others. They can also give the patient another chance to provide answers. The problem of one patient referred to find the cause of chronic postcholecystectomy right upper quadrant pain was illuminated when the consultant, after listening to the patient, confirmed the presence of a tender mass just where the patient said it was; at laparotomy, a stitch abscess was removed. And a telephone call to another hospital's record room may easily answer the question of whether a lung nodule was there 2 years ago. Consultants who look at the radiographs themselves may see something important that the radiologist didn't see or report.

Recommendations should be succinct and directed to the questions that generated the consultation. Compliance with recommendations increases when recommendations are fewer than six, are specific, and are focused on issues central to current patient care, when drug doses are specific and when frequent follow-up visits are made by the consultant [7•,10–12]. Use problem lists in consultation note or letter. A group of British general practitioners overwhelmingly preferred a letter with a problem list over one containing the same information in the conventional narrative format (Fig. 1) [14]. Computerized mini-medical records containing problem lists are well received in multispecialty practices where interphysician communication is vital [15]. Unless it is certain that the referring physician will see the consultant's note in the chart in suitable time, the referring physician should be telephoned. There is no substitute for direct contact to discuss recommendations and plans.

Major interventions should not be undertaken that have not been mutually agreed upon beforehand. It is extremely disconcerting for a referring physician to learn that a patient referred for evaluation of an abnormal mammogram has had a radical mastectomy.

Finally, it is important to communicate with the patient as well as the referring physician. Most consultants report their conclusions and recommendations verbally to the patient. Others think the results of the consultation should be conveyed to the patient by the referring physician, who knows the patient better, particularly if there is bad news. A more controversial approach is to provide the patient with an individualized letter with a copy to the referring physician. This method was heavily favored by a group of Australian cancer consultants who believed that for initial cancer consultations, doctor–patient and doctor–doctor communications would be improved by this technique [16].

AWKWARD ISSUES

In the process of referral and consultation several awkward issues can be counted upon to arise. One is the problem of the referring physician or the consultant concluding that poor medical care has been given by the other. In this situation, as always, the patient's best interests come first, and an appropriate care plan should be recommended to the patient as gently and tactfully as possible. Another is the situation in which the patient wants the consultant to become the primary physician or to completely take over care when such was not intended by the referring physician. A sure way for a consulting physician's practice to suffer is to develop a reputation for "stealing"

TABLE 3 INFORMATION CONSULTANTS NEED FROM REFERRING PHYSICIAN
Specific reason for consultation
Current medical problems
Current medications
Diagnostic test and procedure results
Previous therapeutic failures
Specific responsibility for care consultant is to assume
How soon consultant needs to see patient
What patient has been told about referral
Any special patient attitude about the problem

TABLE 4 RULES FOR EFFECTIVE CONSULTATION
Define what referring physician wants
Establish urgency
Look for yourself
Address referring physician's concerns
Make specific and succinct recommendations
Limit number of recommendations to fewer than six, if possible
Include problem list
Call referring physician
Make follow-up visits

A

Re John Jones, Date of birth: 1/1/1985
456 Any Street, London N17 33X

Dear Dr Smith,

Thank you for referring this boy with frequent attacks of cough and wheeze. He misses a lot of school, sleeps badly, and is short of breath on exertion. I think he has poorly controlled asthma. I note that both his parents smoke and that their housing conditions are very poor. As you know, his younger brother has Down's syndrome.

I was very generally optimistic but emphasized the potential for serious attacks and the need for close family involvement in the management.

I prescribed sodium cromoglycate 10 mg (two puffs) three times a day. His relief drug is terbutaline 1 mg (four puffs) four hourly. Both are to be taken via a nebuhaler (he has excellent technique). I have advised his parents to stop smoking.

His peak flow was 180 today. I have issued a peak flow meter, and the parents will establish what his best peak flow is. I have given them a danger peak flow value of 100—if his peak flow falls to less than this they will bring him to casualty.

Review 1 month.

B

Re John Jones, Date of birth: 1/1/1985
456 Any Street, London N17 33X

Dear Dr Smith,
Problems:
 Poorly controlled asthma
 Passive smoker
 Poor housing
 Younger brother has Down's syndrome

Thank you for referring this boy with frequent attacks of cough and wheeze. He misses a lot of school, sleeps badly, and is short of breath on exertion.

I was generally optimistic but emphasized the potential for serious attacks and the need for close family involvement in the management.

I prescribed sodium cromoglycate 10 mg (two puffs) three times a day. His relief drug is terbutaline 1 mg (four puffs) four hourly. Both are to be taken via a nebuhaler (he has excellent technique). I have advised his parents to stop smoking.

His peak flow was 180 today. I have issued a peak flow meter, and the parents will establish what his best peak flow is. I have given them a danger peak flow value of 100—if his peak flow falls to less than this they will bring him to casualty.

Review 1 month.

FIGURE 1 Referral letters (**A**), without and (**B**), with a problem list. (*From* Lloyd and Barnett [14]; with permission.)

patients. The referral-consultant relationship should be explained to the patient, who should be urged to discuss concerns with the referring physician. Should the patient be unwilling to do so, however, it is not unethical to accept the patient in this circumstance.

To be a good consultant, make communication a priority, establish what the consultant's task is, be specific and to the point, follow up, and transmit what is important to the patient and to the referring physician.

REFERENCES AND RECOMMENDED READING

Recently published papers of particular interest have been highlighted as:
• Of interest
•• Of outstanding interest

1.•• Franks P, Clancy C, Nutting P: Gatekeeping revisited—protecting patients from overtreatment. *N Engl J Med* 1992, 327:424–429.

2.•• Nutting P, Franks P, Clancy C: Referral and consultation in primary care: do we understand what we're doing? *J Fam Pract* 1992, 35:21–23.

3. Kravitz R, Greenfield S, Rogers W: *et al.*: Differences in the mix of patients among medical specialties and systems of care: results from the medical outcomes study. *JAMA* 1992, 267:1617–1623.

4. Greenfield S, Nelson E, Zubkoff M:*et al.*: Variations in resource utilization among medical specialties and systems of care: results from the medical outcomes study. *JAMA* 1992, 267:1624–1630.

5. Reynolds G, Chitnis J, Roland M: General practitioner outpatient referrals: do good doctors refer more patients to hospital? *BMJ* 1991, 302:1250–1252.

6.• Calman N, Hyman R, Licht W: Variability in consultation rates and practitioner level of diagnostic certainty. *J Fam Pract* 1992, 35:31–38.

7.• Lee T, Pappius E, Goldman L: Impact of inter-physician communication on the effectiveness of medical consultations. *Am J Med* 1983, 74:106–112.

8. McPhee S, Lo B, Saika G, Meltzer R: How good is communication between primary care physicians and subspecialty consultants(?) *Arch Intern Med* 1984, 144:1265–1268.

9. Armstrong D, Fry J, Armstrong P: Doctors' perceptions of pressure from patients for referral. *BMJ* 1991, 302:1186–1188.

10. Goldman L, Lee T, Rudd P: Ten commandments for effective consultations. *Arch Intern Med* 1983, 143:1753–1755.

11. Sears C, Charlson M: The effectiveness of a consultation: compliance with initial recommendations. *Am J Med* 1983, 74:870–876.

12. Pupa L, Coventry J, Hanley J, Carpenter J: Factors affecting compliance for general medicine consultations to non-internists. *Am J Med* 1986, 81:508–514.

13. Barker L,: Distinctive characteristics of ambulatory medicine. In *Ambulatory Medicine*, edn 3. Edited by Barker L, Burton J, Zieve P. Baltimore: Williams and Wilkins 1991:3–13.

14. Lloyd B, Barnett P: Use of problem lists in letters between hospital doctors and general practitioners. *BMJ* 1993, 306:247.

15. Carey T, Thomas D, Woolsey A, Proctor R, Philbeck M, Bowen G, Blish C, Fletcher S: Half a loaf is better than waiting for the bread truck: a computerized mini-medical record for outpatient care. *Arch Intern Med* 1992, 152:1845–1849.

16. Stockler M, Butow P, Tattersall M: The take-home message: doctors' views on letters and tapes after a cancer consultation. *Ann Oncol* 1993, 4:549–552.

Medical Economics

Andrew H. Melczer

> **Key Points**
> - The health care marketplace is undergoing immense change.
> - Physicians are facing economic pressures resulting from concern over the high cost of health care.
> - The cost of health care is largely driven by general inflation, volume increases, and increased intensity resulting from new technologies.
> - The health care marketplace is consolidating, and payors are seeking to provide care to insureds through integrated systems, often using managed care and capitated approaches.
> - Given the complexities of the problem, it is unlikely that any "magic bullets" can be found to solve the health care cost crisis.

The health care system in the United States is undergoing immense change. This chapter explores what is currently occurring in the health care marketplace and focuses on the pressures facing physicians. Over the past several years a great deal of attention has been focused on the high costs of health care. There have been growing expressions of concern by government agencies, the business community, and more recently the news media that the cost of health care in the United States is very high—perhaps too high, given the benefit derived from it, especially in comparison with the funds expended and the health status of people in other countries. Concern has also increased regarding the 37 million uninsured Americans. There is a growing feeling that something must be done to ensure better access to medical care for all Americans.

In response, health care reform is moving ahead quickly in the absence of and perhaps in spite of any legislative or regulatory changes. The government and other purchasers have been changing the manner in which they do business. Payors increasingly are seeking to do business with systems and networks of providers. Payment incentives, utilization review, and external quality assurance are changing the manner in which providers render care. Providers (including physicians) are forming groups and cutting overhead costs while continuing to provide their patients with access to quality medical care.

THE COST "PROBLEM"

From 1965 to 1985 national health expenditures (NHEs) in the United States increased from $41.9 to $422.6 billion [1]. NHEs were $755.6 billion in 1991 and $884.2 billion for 1993 (Fig. 1). From 1980 to 1993 NHEs increased 252%, an annualized increase of 10.2%, which far exceeds the 4.5% annualized increase in the general inflation rate over the same period. The percentage of gross national product (GNP) spent on health care also has increased significantly from less than 6% of GNP in 1965 to 9.2% in 1980, and to 13.9% in 1993. It is anticipated that the percentage of GNP spent on health care will continue to increase and may reach 18% by the year 2000.

On a per capita basis NHEs have increased from $206 in 1965, to $1063 in 1980, to $1710 in 1985, to $3299 in 1993 (Fig. 2) [1]. This represents a 10.0% annualized increase from 1980 to 1985 and a 8.6% annualized increase from 1985 to 1993.

Government policy makers are concerned about the large amount of funds going to health care. Medicare, Medicaid, and other government programs spent $388 billion on health care in 1993 (up from $105.2 billion in 1980), an 10.6% annualized rate of increase at a time when governments are facing extreme budgetary pressures [1]. The private sector is also concerned. Over the past few years businesses have seen their costs for health insurance skyrocket. Increases have exceeded inflation consistently. Health insurance increases of 20% annually have not been unusual. For several years increases of only 20% were considered "good." Businesses continue to see an ever-increasing portion of their gross income go for health care—and not to the bottom line.

The public also has become alarmed. Most individuals do not buy health insurance directly; usually health insurance is an employee benefit. However, individuals have had to pay more and more for health care out-of-pocket as a result of the imposition of deductibles, increasing deductibles, coinsurance, and the increase in coinsurance rates. Consumers are also finding that more and more services are "not covered."

Health care providers, including physicians, are often blamed for the "uncontrollable" increases in health care expenditures. However, there are many factors that are responsible for the increases—principally inflation, volume increases, and increased intensity resulting from new technologies.

Health Care Price Inflation

The consumer price index (CPI) increased 70.3% from 1980 to 1992, a 4.5% annualized rate of increase [2]. Over the same period the CPI–medical care component increased 153.9%, an annualized increase of 8.1%. Over the same period the CPI–medical care component increased over twice as much as the overall CPI (Fig. 3). These rates have moderated over the past several years. However, they continue to run at a rate nearly twice that of the overall CPI. From 1965 to 1993, NHEs increased 2,010.3% compared with a 352.5% increase in the CPI. Stated differently, inflation accounts for about 18% of the increase in NHEs from 1965 to 1993.

Changes in Volume

Changes in volume are responsible for a large portion of the increase in NHEs over the past two decades.

Population changes

At the simplest level the general population of the United States increased 30.0% from 1965 to 1991 [3]. In addition, the distribution of the population has changed. Over this period the number of individuals aged 65 and over grew by 72.7%, and the number of individuals aged 75 and over grew by 103.6%. The elderly use a "disproportionate" share of health care: it is estimated that the age 65 and over population uses three to five times as much health care as the under age 65 population on a per capita basis and that the over age 75 population uses even more health care on a per capita basis. Adjusting population growth for age differences, ie, taking account of demographic changes, population growth alone

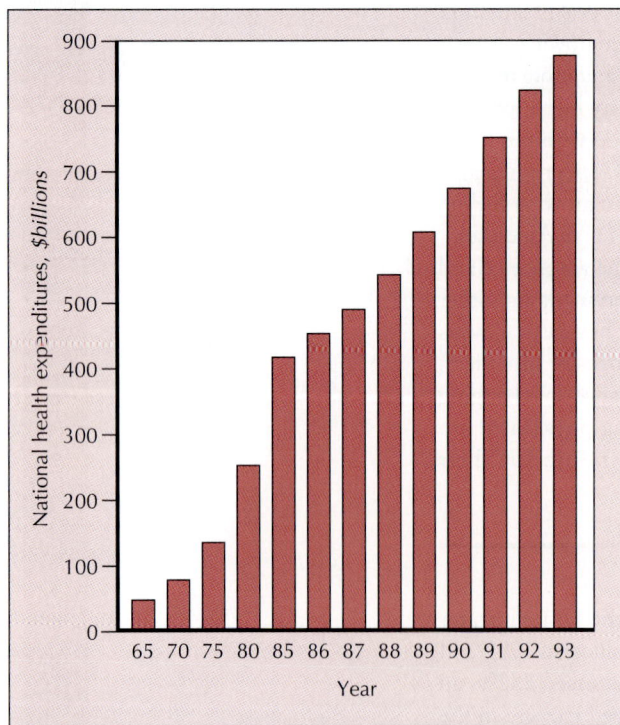

FIGURE 1 Total health care expenditures in the United States. (*Adapted from* Levit [1]; with permission.)

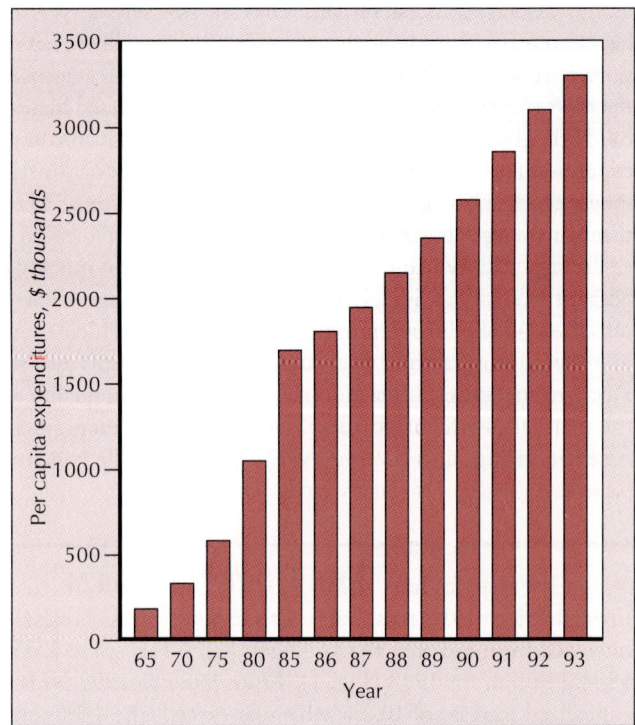

FIGURE 2 Per capita health care expenditures in the United States. (*Adapted from* Levit [1]; with permission.)

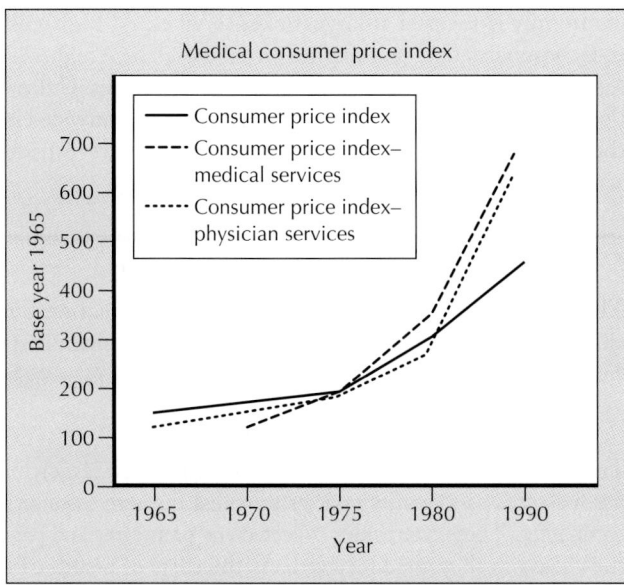

FIGURE 3 Medical inflation. (*Adapted from* Bureau of Labor Statistics [2].)

would have been expected to result in an 87% growth in NHEs from 1965 to 1991. Stated differently, population shifts account for approximately 5% of the increase in NHEs from 1965 to 1991.

Increases in access

Access to health care continues to be a serious concern. However, access has improved significantly over the past 25 years. Increased access to health care increases the use of health care services and NHEs.

Medicare and Medicaid increased access for a large number of previously uncovered elderly (age 65 and over), disabled, and poor individuals. Health insurance also has expanded for the working population, largely as a result of union actions that have set a pattern for many nonunionized companies and industries. Furthermore, health insurance has the effect of lowering the out-of-pocket price faced by patients. Lower prices lead to increased demand—and increased NHEs. Much of the increase is warranted because previously unmet needs are met. It appears that increased access to appropriate health care services is responsible for a substantial portion of NHE growth over the past 25 years, perhaps as much as 15% to 20% of the total increase in NHEs.

Changes in Intensity

Significant changes have occurred in the intensity of medical care provided to patients. This is principally because of new technology and the professional liability crisis.

New technology

Over the past 25 years much new technology has been developed and entered the mainstream of medical practice. New technologies range from neonatal intensive care units to organ transplants to renal dialysis to computed tomography, magnetic resonance imaging, and positron emission tomography scans to new drug therapies. New technologies have enhanced the quality of care and the quality of life. Diseases that in the past caused long-term pain, loss of function, or both, such as cataracts, can now be treated.

New technologies tend to be expensive. This is doubly true because they often stimulate demand for medical care. For example, a new technology may make a "terminal" or "untreatable" diagnosis "treatable" and, as such, can offer enormous societal benefits. However, it can also result in substantial increased costs of medical care, both the direct costs and the "out year" costs of patients kept alive by new technologies. It appears that at least 25% to 30% of the increase in NHEs over the past 25 years can be attributed to new technologies.

Defensive medicine

As a result of the professional liability situation, some physicians order more and different tests and procedures than may actually be needed to determine the appropriate diagnosis or treatment. These "extra" tests and procedures are ordered "for the record" in case of a professional liability suit. Physicians want to document that no stone was left unturned, regardless of the cost. For example, when a roentgenogram will suffice, a computed tomography scan is performed "to be doubly sure."

The costs of defensive medicine have been estimated by the American Medical Association and others. Estimates range from $25 to $65 billion for 1990 (from 3.8% to 9.8% of NHE) and account for between 4.1% and 10.5% of the overall increase in NHEs from 1965 to 1990.

Summary

The factors listed above account for 67% to 83% of the increase in NHEs over the past 25 years and perhaps significantly more. The other 17% to 33% of the increase is composed of inflation specific to the health care field (largely associated with specialized medical personnel and increased administrative costs).

Cost Containment

Many attempts are underway to contain costs, including utilization review and increasing deductibles and copayments. At the same time, attempts are being made to expand health care benefits for those currently insured, *eg*, to provide expanded coverage for nursing home care or drug benefits. Attempts are also being pursued to increase access to health care for the poor, indigent, and currently uninsured populations. These initiatives have the potential to increase NHEs significantly. Given the complexities, it is clear that there are no "magic bullets" to solve the cost "crisis." Nonetheless, payors continue to pursue approaches to health care cost containment.

The Insurance Market

Insurers have taken a number of steps to contain costs. The federal Medicare program covers approximately 36.5 million individuals, and Medicaid, a joint federal–state program, covers approximately 34.0 million individuals. Together these two programs cover over 25% of the US population. Private insurance covers approximately 150 million US citizens, just less than 60% of the total population. The remaining 37 million individuals are uninsured.

Managed care

Managed care has been on the rise for many years. Managed care insurance plans originally included only health maintenance organizations (HMOs). During the 1980s preferred provider organizations (PPOs), exclusive provider organizations (EPOs), and point-of-service (POS) plans were developed as hybrids between traditional fee-for-service medicine and restrictive HMOs. Preferred provider organizations, EPOs, and POS plans provide incentives for insured people to use cost-effective health care providers and for doctors to render cost-effective services.

Availability of insurance

Insurers do not want to accept too much risk. In order to limit risk, they employ three practices that have the effect of limiting the availability of insurance. First, preexisting condition limitations, periods during which the insurance company will not pay for conditions that existed prior to being covered by the plan, are imposed. Second, health screening is used to deny coverage to "unhealthy" people. Third, insurance companies risk-rate their policies, charging higher premiums to those more likely to use the insurance.

Price Controls

The first step in cost containment traditionally has been to limit the prices charged by and paid to providers. Medicare was a pioneer in this area, initially limiting physician payment rates based on an inflation index. In 1983 Medicare cut hospital payment rates under the Prospective Payment System, which is based on diagnosis-related groups (DRGs). Medicaid also has limited charges and payments. Medicaid rate schedules in many states were frozen for long periods of time.

Private payors also have attempted to control the prices they face. HMOs and PPOs were developed in part as a response to increasing prices. They usually pay providers based on some sort of negotiated rate structure that is commonly below the providers' usual charges. Doctors are willing to agree to a lower price in return for a higher volume of patients.

Price controls have not resulted in controlling costs. In fact, as a result of "cost shifting," providers must charge higher prices to full-paying patients to cover the ever larger number of patients who do not pay full charges and often do not even cover the direct costs of services; these may include Medicare, Medicaid, and indigent patients. Price controls have had the effect of distorting prices in the market.

Utilization Review and Rationing

The second step to cost containment traditionally has been to limit use, particularly use of high-cost services. This is done by eliminating "unnecessary" care and by ensuring services are provided in the most cost-effective setting. Utilization review commonly is focused at large-ticket services, *eg*, high-cost tests, hospitalization, and surgical procedures. These high-cost services present the greatest potential for cost savings. Utilization review also may focus on ensuring that care is provided in the most cost-effective setting. Utilization review restricts access to care and thus is a mechanism for rationing.

HEALTH SYSTEM RESPONSES

The health care system has been undergoing a great deal of change in response to the cost problem and the resultant cost-containment strategies.

Delivery Systems

Traditionally health care insurance has consisted largely of fee-for-service indemnity policies provided through insurance companies. These companies collected the premiums and paid the claims as they were received. As the costs of health care have increased, other insurance models have grown and become more prominent. These alternative delivery systems have been designed to contain costs.

Health maintenance organizations have been around since the 1940s. They seek to contain costs by providing all care to enrollees in a managed care environment by directly controlling access and negotiating favorable payment rates. At the end of 1980 there were 244 HMOs nationally. In 1976, 6 million individuals were enrolled in HMOs [4]. Currently there are 546 HMOs with 52.4 million enrollees, more than 25% of the total of those insured (Fig. 4).

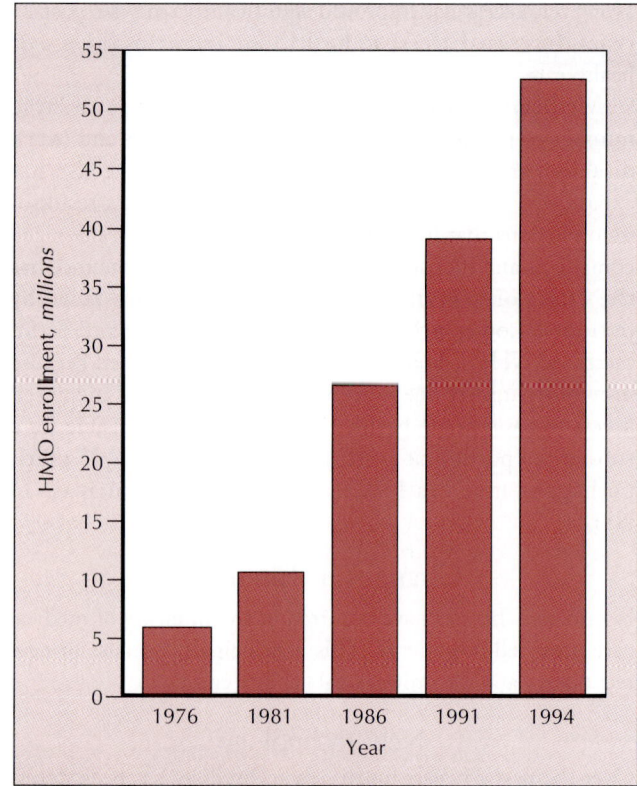

FIGURE 4 Enrollment in health maintenance organizations. (*Adapted from* Marion Merrill Dow [4]; with permission.)

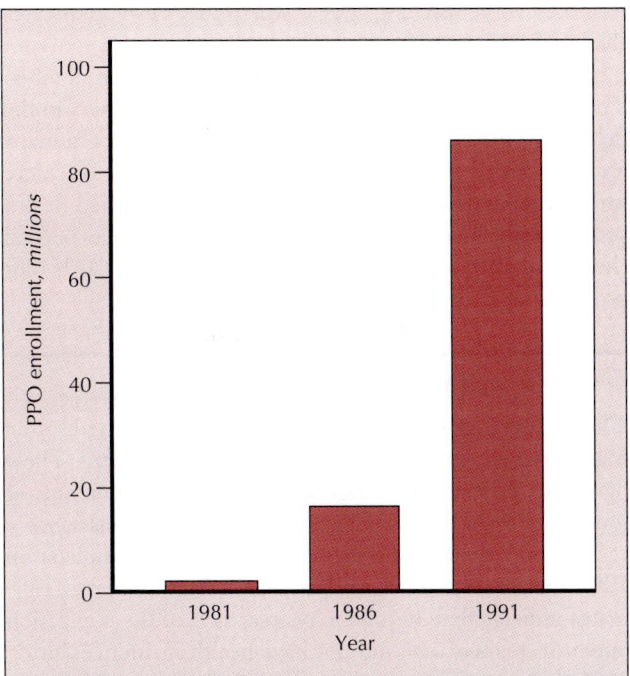

FIGURE 5 Enrollment in preferred provider organizations. (*Adapted from* Marion Merrill Dow [5]; with permission.)

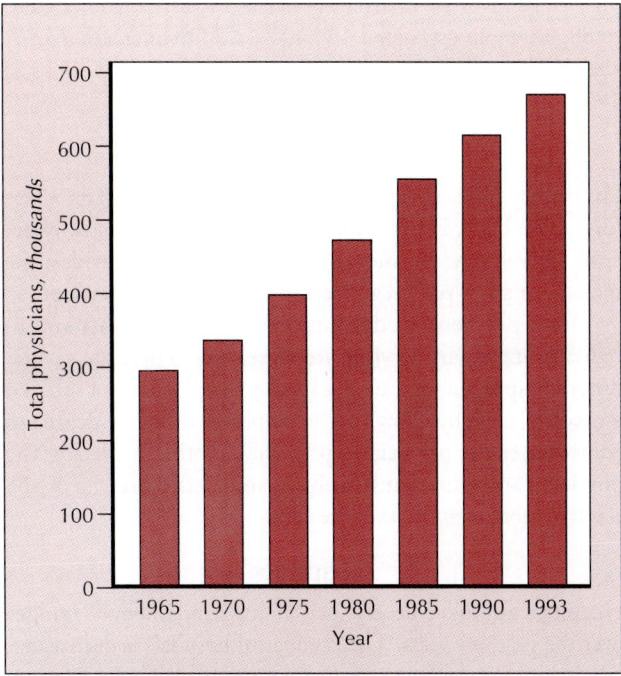

FIGURE 6 Total physicians in the United States. (*Adapted from* American Medical Association [6]; with permission.)

Preferred provider organizations are a relatively new phenomenon. They identify providers who give "cost-effective" care and agree to accept discounted payment rates in return for more patients. Preferred provider organizations usually require providers to adhere to strict utilization review. In 1986 there were 305 PPOs; by the end of 1991, there were 978 PPOs [5]. Approximately 13.5 million individuals were enrolled in PPOs in 1986, and by 1991 that figure had grown to over 85 million (Fig. 5). The average physician's fee discount was 20% nationally.

Physicians

The number of physicians in the United States has increased from 292,100 in 1965 to 670,300 in 1993—an 129% increase (Fig. 6) [6]. The number providing patient care was 259,400 in 1965 and 550,400 in 1993—a 112% increase. Over this same period the number of practicing physicians per 100,000 population increased from 132 to 212—a 61% increase.

Despite this growth, there is a shortage of physicians in many geographic areas and in many specialties, particularly primary care. Rural states tend to have lower physician–population ratios, as do rural areas of urban states. In many communities primary care is unavailable.

Physician expenses and income

Over the past 20 years physicians' incomes and expenses have increased dramatically, as has the cost of living. From 1975 to 1992 physicians' median total income before expenses increased 278% to $287,000 [7]. Practice expenses increased 348% over the same period, from 41% to 48% of gross income. Median physician income increased to $139,000. On average physicians worked nearly 60 hours per week and took off slightly more than 5 weeks, including vacations and holidays, during 1993.

Trends in practice setting

To remain competitive in an increasingly complex environment, physicians are forming group practices. More groups and larger groups have been forming over the past 25 years. The number of physician group practices has increased from 4300 in 1965, to 10,800 in 1980, to 16,600 in 1991—a 286% increase (Fig. 7) [8]. During this same period the number of

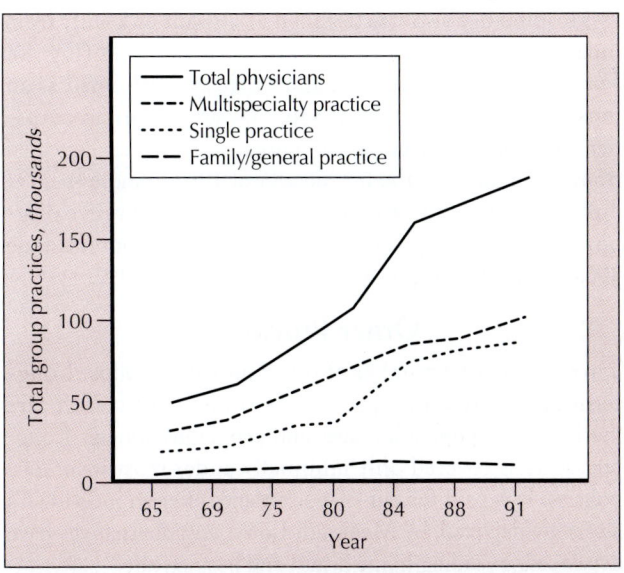

FIGURE 7 Total group practice physicians in the United States. (*Adapted from* American Medical Association [8]; with permission.)

physicians involved in group practices increased from 28,400 to 88,300 to an estimated 184,400—a 549% increase. *Nearly one third of all physicians were involved in a group practice in 1991*, up from approximately 10% in 1965.

Payment modalities

Historically physicians predominantly have been paid on a fee-for-service basis. It has been argued that this system is inherently inflationary: the more services a physician provides, the more he or she is paid, regardless of the need for the services.

Other payment modalities used to control costs and to reduce unnecessary services are increasing. There are several different approaches: one is to make the physician a salaried employee, thereby allowing the employer a certain degree of control over the physician's practice. Another is placing the physician at risk in that if a physician is "efficient," he or she receives more income, and vice versa.

Hospitals

Hospitals also have been experiencing fundamental changes over the past few years. The number of hospitals is decreasing, admissions are declining, outpatient use of services is soaring, and those who control reimbursement are less willing to pay what hospitals charge. In 1975 there were 7156 hospitals in the United States [9]. By 1992 the number of hospitals declined to 6539. There were 5292 nongovernmental community hospitals. Average hospital size was approximately 174 beds.

The total number of hospital beds in 1975 was 1.466 million, and by 1992 the figure had decreased to 921,000. Even with this decline, the occupancy rate declined from 75.3 in 1982 to 65.6 in 1992. There are several reasons for these declines, not the least of which is the shift from fee-for-service to set fees per discharge, which give hospitals an incentive to treat patients as efficiently as possible and discharge them quickly. Utilization review also has identified patients who stay in the hospital an extra day or 2 for "hotel" services. These patients are now sent home.

Hospital use also has declined as a result of a shift from inpatient to outpatient provision for many services (Fig. 8). For example, hernia repairs, almost always performed as an inpatient procedure 15 years ago, now are usually an outpatient procedure. The number of outpatient visits has increased from 54.5 million in the first quarter of 1982 to more than 94 million in the last quarter of 1992. Outpatient invasive diagnostic and surgical procedures have increased from less than 400,000 in 1983 to approximately 2.9 million in 1992.

Other Providers

There are a large number of other provider groups. Long-term care represents a growing portion of the health care market as the population ages and people live longer. Long-term care is covered only minimally under most insurance policies. It is paid for out-of-pocket and, after an individual's assets are depleted, by Medicaid. Lower cost alternatives have developed, including home health and hospice care.

Drugs represent a growing portion of health care expenditures. New drugs continue to prolong life and increase quality of life. Furthermore, the aging of the population has resulted in more people reaching ages at which they develop diseases that can be managed by expensive drug therapies.

Allied health professionals have been growing in number. These individuals usually assist physicians and others in the delivery of medical care. The shortage of physicians in many areas has fueled allied health professionals' attempts to achieve more independent practice. This is a concern: allied health professionals should not be allowed to provide services beyond their limited training. Quality-of-care concerns arise if they provide such services.

The Access Problem

Thirty-seven million people are uninsured in the United States, and another 30 to 40 million are underinsured. These figures are presented on a regular basis. There are a number of sources for these figures and a wide range of interpretations.

The primary source is a government survey completed in 1987 and updated on a regular basis. In fact, the latest estimates indicate that 36 million people, 17% of the population under 65 years of age, did not have health insurance during 1991. In fact, many more people were without health insurance for some portion of 1991. According to an Urban Institute study, half of the uninsured are without insurance for 4 months or less and 76% for less than 12 months. Only 15% are uninsured for greater than 24 months.

The poor access to care in the United States is demonstrated by the fact that the health status of people in the United States (as judged by traditional, but potentially confounded measures) is no better than many other countries that spend a considerably lower percentage of their GNP on health care. Life expectancy and infant mortality rates for the

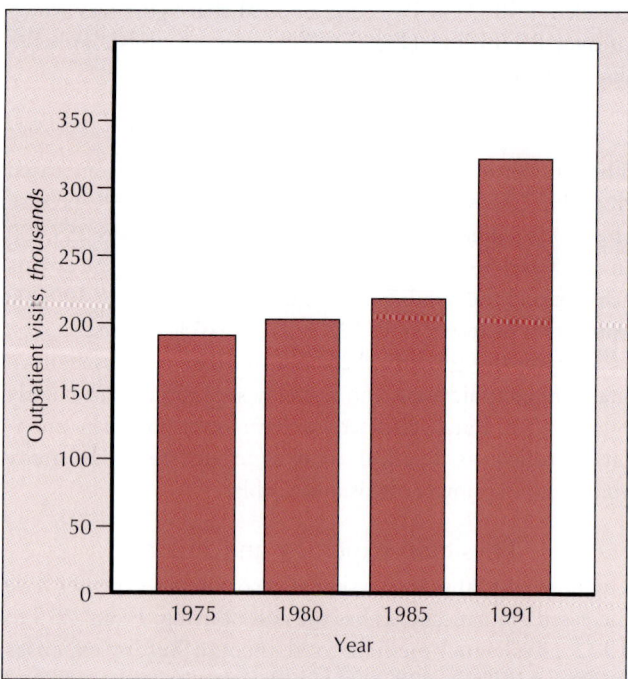

FIGURE 8 Total outpatient hospital visits in the United States. (*Adapted from* American Medical Association [9]; with permission.)

United States are considerably higher than those of many other countries. These figures, and many others, appear to confirm that the "expensive" health care of the United States does not have a positive impact on health status. However, these statistics do not indicate the underlying health habits and problems of the population. For example, the infant mortality rate in the United States is in part higher because of economic and cultural factors which impede access to care. Those who receive timely and adequate prenatal care appear to experience infant mortality rates similar to populations in other countries. Furthermore, life expectancy is lower because of the higher rate of homicides, AIDS, and drug abuse in the United States compared with other Western countries, and other lifestyle choices.

Conclusions

The medical care environment is shifting dramatically and rapidly. New health care delivery and payment systems continue to develop and evolve. Many attempts are underway to contain costs, including utilization review and increasing deductibles and copayments. At the same time, attempts are being made to expand health care benefits for those currently insured, eg, to provide expanded coverage for nursing home care and drugs. Attempts also are being pursued to increase access to health care for the poor, indigent, and currently uninsured populations. These initiatives and others have the potential to increase NHEs significantly and rapidly.

The increasing level of health care costs will remain a concern for government, businesses, the public, and especially providers. Given the complexities of the problem, it is unlikely any "magic bullets" can be found to solve the health care cost crisis. Nonetheless, it is likely that government and businesses will continue to pursue various approaches to health care system reform.

References and Recommended Reading

Recently published papers of particular interest have been highlighted as:
- Of interest
- • Of outstanding interest

1. Levi KR, Sensenig AL, Cowan CA, *et al.*: National health expenditures, 1993. *Health Care Financing Rev* 1994, 16:1–30.
2. Bureau of Labor Statistics, US Department of Labor: CPI detailed report. Data for December 1993, December 1992, December 1991, December 1990, December 1980, December 1975.
3. US Department of Commerce: Statistical abstract of the United States; 1992.
4. Marion Merrill Dow: Managed care digest, HMO edition. Kansas City: Marion Merrell Dow; 1994.
5. Marion Merrill Dow: Managed care digest, PPO edition. Kansas City: Merion Merrell Dow; 1994.
6. American Medical Association: Physician characteristics and distribution in the US. Chicago: American Medical Association; 1994.
7. American Medical Association: Socioeconomic characteristics of medical practice. Chicago: American Medical Association; 1993.
8. American Medical Association: Medical groups in the US. Chicago: American Medical Association; 1993.
9. American Hospital Association: Hospital statistics. Chicago: American Hospital Association; 1994.

Health Policy
William Troyer

> **Key Points**
> - Government intervenes periodically into health care with focused programs.
> - Funding medical research, building hospitals, increasing access to health care for poor and aged populations, health maintenance organization planning grants, and increasing medical school enrollment are examples.
> - Over time, some programs may produce unintended consequences such as rising costs.
> - For the past 25 years, cost control and universal access, which are mutually contradictory, have preoccupied policy makers.
> - Cost controls are threats to quality of care.
> - Current proposals to ensure quality of care, such as clinical guidelines and appropriateness of care studies, are experimental.
> - Preservation of quality will be the most pressing problem in the next phase of the evolution of health care in the United States.

In 1948 Congress created the modern National Institutes of Health (NIH) by merging the National Cancer Institute (NCI) with the newly created National Heart Institute. In 1945 the NCI budget was $180,000, by 1950 (as the NIH) it had grown to $46 million, and by 1994 it had increased to $12 billion. Even allowing for the depreciation of buying power of the 1948 dollar (about 80%), the results are staggering. Congress had set in motion an act of public policy that was to fuel a revolution in health care in the United States. A half century later, all levels of the private and public sectors of the economy are struggling with the consequences.

Before plunging into an analysis of the impact of health policy on medicine in the past five decades, it might be wise to tarry a moment and consider the nature of public policy, the anatomy of health care, and the significant events leading up to 1948. We shall learn that public policy, while often crafted to solve a public problem such as an inequity or a social need such as a program of medical research to combat the major diseases of the day, sows the seeds of another problem that may appear generations later.

FORCES OF CHANGE

The events leading up to 1948 began a half century before. Around the last half of the 19th century major universities were changing, in Harold Shapiro's words, from "centers of dogma to centers of inquiry" [1]. Universities began to create new knowledge and test new and old theories instead of just passing information on to another generation. This philosophy spread to medical education, but only sparingly, until the Flexner Report of 1910. Prepared by Abraham Flexner, a sociologist, this report advised sound training in the basic sciences for medical students. To meet this recommendation, which eventually became a requirement for accreditation, many freestanding medical schools sought to affiliate or merge with a university. The requirement that the university faculty engage in scholarly activity, *eg*, research, became the rule rather than the exception in medical schools. The advent of scientific research, the university's involvement, the celebration and success of the American inventor, and the public's interest in it provided the groundwork for the modern-day medical research establishment.

Other forces were at work creating public demand for more medical research that would in turn result in treatment for disease. Advances in surgery, notably neurosurgery pioneered by Harvey Cushing; pharmaceutical development, pioneered by Paul Erlich for syphilis; and Banting and Best's discovery of insulin for diabetes mellitus were only a few research-based treatments that found their way into practice to whet the public's appetite for more.

DISEASE INTEREST GROUPS

The American Heart Association, the American Cancer Society, and the National Foundation for Infantile Paralysis (polio), all founded in the 1920s and 1930s, were the forerunners of the single-disease advocacy groups that are so prevalent today. Franklin Delano Roosevelt, himself a victim of polio and later an organizer of a polio rehabilitation center in Warm Springs, Georgia, helped keep this issue in the public eye for years. These voluntary groups began as fundraisers for research and evolved into the educational, patient support, and research advocacy groups that we know today.

WORLD WAR II CONTRIBUTIONS

World War II was a pivotal event in the evolution of medical care. More than 12 million military personnel saw at firsthand the kinds of miracles American medicine could perform. The advances in blood banking, anesthesia, surgery, and antibiotic therapy were truly astonishing. Compared with World War I, the death rate from disease decreased twenty times in World War II. The war effort also developed technology that in later years would be adapted for use in medicine. The atomic bomb led to radioisotopes; Ultra, the allied project that broke the German secret military code, employed primitive computers that eventually became sophisticated enough for computed tomography scanners and magnetic resonance imaging; and radar and sonar eventually led to ultrasonography. Later the space exploration program would continue the development of technology, especially miniaturization.

World War II produced another legacy—employer sponsored and financed health insurance. To avoid inflation during World War II, wages were frozen except in unusual circumstances. Labor unions negotiated for fringe benefits, including health insurance, that were not regulated so severely by the government. By the end of the war the stage was set for increased demand for medical care, and a battle-tested research technology and establishment were available to fill those desires. Sufficient facilities and personnel to deliver health care to the general population and a financing mechanism to pay for health care of the retired and poor were still lacking. In the next decades public policy would be pressed to correct these deficiencies.

HEALTH CARE ACCESS, QUALITY, AND COST

One way to conceptualize the relationship of health care and money is to think of it as a three-legged stool, with one leg representing access to care, another quality of care, and a third cost. Assuming no change in quality or productivity (efficiency), any increase in access results in an increase in cost, a decrease in quality, or both. In the real world quality standards change constantly because of research advances and rising expectations of patients and their families. Both rising expectations and rising quality standards tend to increase cost.

TOO MANY HOSPITAL BEDS

Even before World War II, planning had started for increased hospital construction by a national commission organized by the American Hospital Association. In 1946 Congress passed the Hill-Burton Act, which authorized a program of hospital construction with federal participation in the financing. Nearly 13 billion dollars of hospital construction occurred over the next 25 years [2]. The act set a limit that became a standard, as maximums or minimums so often do, of 4.5 hospital beds per 1000 people. Assuming 80% occupancy of those beds, this calculates out to 1314 hospital days per year per 1000 covered enrollees, which is nearly three times the number of hospital days per year that a well-managed health maintenance organization (HMO) with a patient population representative of the general population including the poor and retirees requires today. This is the first but by no means the last example of government-sponsored health policy that was passed to correct a perceived short-term problem (which it did), but in so doing created a bigger problem for the longer term—in this case a hospital bed surplus and the attendant effects it had on practice patterns and patient expectations for the past four decades.

During the 1950s hospitals slowly expanded, biomedical research flourished from rising NIH budgets, and unions bargained for and obtained first-dollar health insurance coverage for their members. Congress occasionally debated, but rejected, the notion of universal national health insurance, but something had to be done for the elderly. The price of health care began to rise along with expectations of the wonders brought by biomedical research and the pharmaceutical companies. Polio was conquered by the Salk vaccine, tuberculosis was checked with streptomycin and isoniazid, and some heart defects became repairable thanks to skillful surgery and cardiac catheterization. But those treatments were not generally available to the unemployed or the retired unless they were so sick they could not be turned away from the emergency room. The very poor and the elderly in the era before Medicare/Medicaid were like the "self-pay" patients of today. Physicians usually treated these patients for little or no fee, and many hospitals had indigent care funds to cover much of the hospital costs.

INCREASING ACCESS

It took congress nearly 5 years of debate and a false start before Medicare Parts A and B and Medicaid were passed. Medicare Part A covers payment of hospital expenses for people over 65 years of age and is financed by the Social Security trust fund. Medicare Part B covers payment of physicians's fees and is financed by the contributions of those enrolled in Part A. Medicaid, contrary to common opinion, is not one homogenous program for the poor, *ie*, those with an income below or close to the poverty line ($14,000 for a family of four). It is a series of programs, jointly funded by federal and state governments and administered by the states for various subpopulations of the poor. The largest of these programs is Aid to Dependent Children and Their Mothers (AFDC). Another is Aid to the Blind and Disabled. At one time there were 16 programs, but many have been eliminated or consolidated as cost pressures have mounted.

The addition of the Medicare and Medicaid populations increased the rate of growth in cost of medical services from an average of 3.2% per year before Medicare and Medicaid to nearly 8% per year afterward. During the same period the service portion of the Consumer Price Index increased from 2.0% to 5.8% annually. In the 15 years before Medicare and Medicaid, hospital expenditures rose an average of 8% per year; after passage the rate of growth increased to 14% per year. Between 1965 and 1970 government, state, and federal expenditures increased from $10.8 billion to $27.8 billion. More ominous than the total amount of money spent was the widening gap of the rates of expenditures for medical and other services. In 1965 this was 1.2%; in 1970 it was 2.2%. In the 1980s this measure of cost inflation in medical service increased to 6% to 7% above the average consumer price increase.

These inflationary increases in the costs of medical care, if sustained, meant that the costs of medical care would double in 10 to 12 years relative to prices in general. This increase would be reflected in a larger percent of the gross national product (GNP) spent on health services. In the 1950s the percent of GNP spent on health services was 6%. In 1994 this is expected to be 14%. Other industrialized countries spend a smaller percentage of their GNP on health care than the United States. This marker can be misleading: first because a change in percent can be caused by changes in the numerator, the denominator, or both; and second, the health budgets of foreign countries do not necessarily cover the same components as those included in the United States'. For example, the budget of the National Health Service in the United Kingdom does not include money spent for long-term care as does the United States' budget. And finally, as Victor Fuch reminds us, health insurance, which is mostly employer provided, is another form of wages [3]. On the other hand government-funded health insurance is funded by taxes that many Americans view adversely.

INCREASING THE SUPPLY OF DOCTORS

To deal with the increased demand for medical services and the inflationary costs of medical services, governments began to increase the supply of doctors and support other cost-control measures. The number of medical schools slowly increased following World War II. In the 1950s there were approximately 65 schools, and by 1965 this number increased to 88. By 1980 there were nearly 40 more. The number of graduates rose as well. In 1955 there were approximately 6000 graduates. In the late 1980s this number increased to 17,000. Medical schools were induced to increase enrollments by government payments for each medical student and with bonuses for increased enrollment. This government program was successful in its intent to increase the physician supply, but more than doubled the aggregated cost of physicians' services. Individually physicians' incomes have increased slightly less than inflation during the past 15 years.

DISTORTING THE SPECIALTY MIX

Prior to the enactment of Medicare in 1965, graduate medical education, internships and residencies were financed from hospital patient care revenues or philanthropy. Subspecialty training programs' fellowships were different. These originally were developed out of research grants, with the goal of training future faculty for medical schools. In 1965 Medicare took over the funding of all house staff programs. Because specialists practiced, researched, and taught in hospitals, the house staff training programs were tilted, some would say lopsidedly, toward tertiary care and away from primary care. In retrospect Medicare funding of graduate medical education in the tertiary care environment contributed to today's perceived imbalance between generalists and specialists. In addition to Medicare funding, other variables affected this skill mix among physicians. The higher incomes of specialists, their shorter work week, and the greater certainty of their practice field were among those variables.

CONTROLLING COSTS

From 1970 on public policy has been directed at controlling the cost of health care and perversely toward increasing access. The list is long, and even a brief discussion of them is beyond the scope of this chapter. Among the cost-control measures tried were direct cost control on hospital charges and physicians' fees, which worked while in place but more than made up for the savings when they were lifted. These measures are analogous to patients' weight on a crash diet—it works while they are on it, but they gain it all back and more when they go off. Another cost-saving remedy has been utilization review, which started as a peer review program in the 1970s and has evolved into a $200 million commercial industry—an estimate that does not include hospital and physician costs.

Both the government and the insurance industry have tried to influence medical practice. Congress passed legislation nearly 20 years ago to encourage HMO planning grants and loan guarantees for HMO "start-ups," and the private sector developed preferred provider organizations, which negotiate for discounts on hospital charges and physicians' fees in a return for promises of patient volume.

DIAGNOSIS-RELATED GROUPS

Finally in 1982 Congress authorized a federal version of managed care for the Medicare population called diagnosis-related groups (DRGs). Even after 10 years of widespread use there is little evidence and agreement that DRGs have successfully contained cost.

FOOD AND DRUG ADMINISTRATION

Efforts to improve quality have been mediated largely through the judicial and regulatory system. Twenty-five years ago, following several near tragedies related to birth defects and severe side effects of new drugs, the Food and Drug Administration (FDA) was empowered by Congress to take a more active role in evaluating and regulating the introduction of new drugs to the general market. This program has very likely been successful, but at a price of delay and cost. New drugs are not usually first introduced into the United States without being used in foreign countries for several years. This is because of the safety and efficiency standard imposed by the FDA. The cost of development of a new drug can now be as high as several hundred million dollars.

LEGAL EFFECTS

The judicial system's effect on the cost-quality balance has been largely negative. Both the courts and the Federal Trade Commission consistently have weakened the ability of organized medicine, which I define here as anything in between a hospital medical staff and the American Medical Association (AMA) to discipline members. This has occurred as a result of a series of court rulings that have interpreted organized medicine's attempts at discipline as violations of the antitrust laws.

The number of professional liability actions has increased, and when it has not, the decrease in incidence has been accompanied by an increase in settlement costs. Malpractice premiums account for approximately $9 billion annually. The threat of a malpractice suit has given rise to what is known as "defensive medicine." This is defined as the cost of "unnecessary" additional laboratory tests, procedures, and consultations that are not needed for the prudent care of the patient but rather are to be used in anticipation of malpractice litigation to defend charges of negligence. The cost of defensive medicine is difficult to determine empirically; the AMA estimates it to be 5% to 10% of the costs of hospital and physician service, ie, $30 billion to $60 billion annually.

One other government action deserves mention—underfunding of Medicare and Medicaid and the Employee Retirement Income Security Act (ERISA). Both Medicare and Medicaid pay less than commercial insurance for hospital care. Medicare pays about 80% of cost (not charges). Medicaid payments vary from state to state but are usually less than Medicare. Because costs must be recovered from other payors, hospitals usually charge or negotiate higher payments from preferred provider organization, HMOs, and indemnity payors. This in turn drives up insurance premiums even higher than the general increase in health costs. Many employee groups are self-insured under ERISA. This act permits exemption from state insurance laws that typically both require community rating (charging all enrollees the same rate) and prohibit disqualification for preexisting conditions and concurrent adverse experiences. All of the foregoing practices result in seemingly higher costs for health care. Hospitals shift costs incurred by government-sponsored patients to the private sector; very large groups of healthy employees get favorable rates; smaller groups of employees get unfavorable rates; and employees with preexisting conditions or adverse experience can't get jobs or get terminated from the health plan, their jobs, or both.

APPROACHING CRISIS

Currently, we face a situation in which the cost of health care is rising at an unacceptable rate, and 15% of the population is uninsured. Political opinion appears to be unable to tolerate uncontrollable health costs and denial of access to health care for the uninsured. It seems likely that additional access along with some kind of cost controls will occur. In the past when additional access occurred, as in 1965 when Medicare and Medicaid were passed by Congress, additional funding was added to the system, and the physician and nursing supply as well as hospital facilities were expanded. The increase in demand occurred nearly all at once, whereas the expansion of provider supply occurred over a number of years. While these events were occurring the research establishment was steadily improving the quality of care, resulting in both high quality and high cost. It is probable that the outcome of present events will be increased access and cost controls. The results are likely to be an erosion of quality. Preservation of quality is likely to be the most pressing problem for the next phase of the evolution of health care in the United States.

The concept of quality health care seems like such a simple concept, but it resists definition and defies quantification. A suitable analogy of a Supreme Court justice's definition of another very subjective concept, pornography, is appropriate. Justice Byron White said, "I can't define it, but I know it when I see it." Most physicians could say the same thing about quality medical care. In 1986 Congress created the Agency for Health Care Policy and Research (AHCPR). Currently, AHCPR is creating clinical guidelines for the management of common conditions. These guidelines are created by panels of experts whose consensus decisions are based on the scientific literature. Many specialty organizations are engaged in developing guidelines of medical conditions seen by their members. The Editor of the *New England Journal of Medicine*, Jerome P.

Kassirer, MD, in a penetrating editorial on the quality of care [4••] asks many questions about clinical guidelines [5] and appropriateness [6•] of medical care studies. Suffice it to say that the methodologic foundations of guidelines and appropriateness studies need improvement.

What To Do: Some Suggestions

Other ways of reducing costs and thereby preserving quality should be considered. Tort reform has great potential for saving money, but the changes in behavior that will be required of health care providers and the legal and judiciary system will occur slowly. Productivity increases also may result from more frequent use of midlevel nurse practitioners and physician assistants. Both types of practitioners have been shown to function satisfactorily in primary care settings as well as in hospitals [7,8]. Increased use of such physician extenders could reduce the demand for physicians' services so significantly that along with expanded managed care, significant physician unemployment could result [9].

The future of health care in this country will depend on the delicate balance among access, quality, and cost of health care. The tasks of physicians, both collectively in their societies and individually, is to first educate themselves about health policy, the practice of appropriate, cost-effective medicine, and then educate their patients and public officials about the impact of various public policy initiatives on their patients. The shaping of public policy is largely an educational function of our elected officials. It is not easy to dispel old myths and prejudices even with facts, but it can be done. It is right both ethically and politically to put patients' long-term interests first. If we do that, physicians' interests will take care of themselves.

References and Recommended Reading

Recently published papers of particular interest have been highlighted as:
•• Of outstanding interest

1. Shapiro HT: The future of the kaleidoscope: medical education and the university. Presented at the Annual Meeting of the American Association of Medical Colleges, October 28, 1985; Washington, DC.
2. Starr P: *The Social Transformation of American Medicine*. New York: Basic Books; 1982:347–350.
3. Fuchs V: No pain, no gain: Perspectives on cost containment. *JAMA* 1993, 269:631–633.
4.•• Kassirer JP: The quality of care and the quality of measuring it. *N Engl J Med* 1993, 329:1263–1264.
5. Tannenbaum SJ: What physicians know. *N Engl J Med* 1993, 329:1268–1271.
6.•• Phelps CE: The methodologic foundations of studies of the appropriateness of medical care. *N Engl J Med* 1993, 329:1241–1245.
7. Safriet BJ: Health care dollars and regulatory sense: The role of advanced practice nursing. *Yale J Regulation* 1992, 9:419–487.
8. Mundinger MA: Advanced practice nursing—good medicine for physicians? *N Engl J Med* 1994, 330:211–214.
9. Jones FG: Study forum examines health care systems in Germany, Holland: Part II: The German system. *Physician Executive* 1993, 19:58–62.

Select Bibliography

Starr P: *The Social Transformation of American Medicine*. New York: Basic Books; 1982.

Health Care Ethics
Kevin O'Rourke

> ### Key Points
> - The most basic method of ethical theory is founded on human need.
> - Good human acts fulfill human needs in a balanced manner; bad actions do not.
> - Human acts may be subjectively good even if they are objectively bad.
> - Participants in medical decisions may have different needs or values in mind; medical decision making is a collaborative process.
> - Identifying medical facts is essential for ethical decision making in health care.

Ethics is the discipline or science by which we determine which human actions are good and which are bad. If we agree that some actions are good and some are bad, it implies that there is a norm or measure for judging human actions. That is, there must be standards to which good actions conform and bad actions do not conform. This essay discusses the standards or norms by which free human actions are judged to be good or bad.

Some ethical systems seek to weigh good and evil. This is shortsighted because it allows a person to do evil in order to achieve good. Some ethical systems use "principles" such as autonomy or beneficence. But these "principles" are not definite and are not grounded in human need. A more thorough and well-grounded theory of ethics is based on the purpose of human activity.

Humans act in order to fulfill their needs. What are our human needs? Although we can enumerate many human needs, some of which are very significant, such as food and water, and some of which are not so significant but make life more pleasant, such as ice cream and television. Four needs are most basic or fundamental: physiological, psychological, social, and creative or spiritual (Table 1).

FUNCTIONS TO FULFILL NEEDS

To fulfill our needs, we have powers or functions: biologic, emotional, social, and creative. All the needs and their corresponding human functions are important, but creative needs and functions are most important because they direct the attainment of all human needs. Nevertheless, creative functions are dependent to some degree on physiologic function. A person cannot think and love without a cerebral cortex. In sum, the functions by which we fulfill human needs are interdependent. The human functions that enable us to fulfill our needs are conceived most aptly as dimensions of a cube rather than floors of a building, because they cannot be separated one from another even though some needs and functions are more important than others.

Our needs, or drives as they are sometimes called, motivate us to pursue objects and activities that will satisfy our fundamental needs. We call the objects or activities that fulfill our needs "goods." When seeking goods that will fulfill the funda-

TABLE 1 FUNDAMENTAL HUMAN NEEDS
Physiological needs, satisfied through food and drink
Psychological needs, satisfied through sense, pleasure, rest, and relaxation
Social needs, satisfied through family, friends, and community
Creative or spiritual needs, satisfied through knowledge, truth, and love

mental human needs, we know from experience that a person must be careful to fulfill needs in a balanced manner. That is, when fulfilling a need, a person must make sure that fulfilling other needs is still possible. For example, eating appetizing food fulfills my physiologic and psychological needs, but if I eat too much, I may get sick and be unable to study for the chemistry examination I have tomorrow. By fulfilling my need for food in an unbalanced manner, I have made it impossible to fulfill my creative need (*ie*, passing the chemistry examination). Everyone has heard of people who study so intently that they harm their health. This is another example of fulfilling needs in an unbalanced manner. The significance of fulfilling human needs in a balanced manner is expressed in the distinction between people who live to eat and people who eat to live.

When a human act achieves the goal of fulfilling a human need in a balanced manner, we call such an action a good action. Moreover, the action is described as having value. If a human act does not fulfill a human need or if it fulfills a human need in an unbalanced manner, we call such an action a bad action. Thus, if one person steals food from another, he is performing a bad action because although he may be fulfilling his physiologic need, he is not fulfilling his social needs. Or if a person fulfills his physiologic and psychological needs by drinking beer but drinks so much that he impairs his ability to drive a car safely, he is unable to fulfill his social and creative needs and hence is performing a bad action, whether or not other people are injured as a result of his drunkenness.

DECISIONS OF CONSCIENCE

The free judgments by which a person chooses to fulfill his or her basic needs are known as ethical decisions, or decisions of conscience. In making decisions of conscience, difficulties arise most often in regard to social needs. Our desire to fulfill our physiologic, psychological, and creative needs usually involves our own well-being. But in order to fulfill our social needs, we must be concerned about the well-being of others; that is, we must respect their needs and rights. Experience teaches us how difficult it is to keep the needs and rights of others in mind as we seek to fulfill our own needs. That is why society devotes so much attention to establishing justice through laws, courts, and police forces. We also know, however, that respecting the rights and needs of others is vitally important because it is the basis for friendship and community, peace and progress.

As we affirm that the purpose of human acts is to fulfill human needs in a balanced manner, we also affirm that a person who fails to act in a balanced manner is still trying to do something that he or she considers to be good. To state it another way, if a person chooses to do something that does not fulfill his or her needs in a balanced manner, the person chooses an action that is subjectively good but objectively evil. The distinction between subjective and objective morality is most important in ethics. This distinction helps us understand the nature of good and evil. A human action that is both objectively and subjectively good is a human act that fulfills a person's needs in a balanced manner. However, an action may be objectively evil and only subjectively good. This happens when the act is only a partial or an apparent good. The error in judgment that leads a person to choose an apparent good rather than a true or balanced good may be due to an intellectual error or to moral weakness. Hence, a person may choose to take the property of another, thinking erroneously that it is his or her own property. If the person is not responsible for the ignorance that disposes him or her to act in this way, the action might be considered evil objectively, but subjectively good because the person taking the property is unaware that he or she is violating the property rights of another person. Moral weakness might cause a person to choose a partial or apparent good, such as when the opportunity to steal money without being caught causes a person to neglect fulfillment of his social needs. If a person determines to steal a large sum of money, he concentrates on the good that will come to him when he has more money and thinks little about the harm that will come to the people from whom he steals the money. If the thief thinks of his victims at all, he might excuse his violation of human rights by saying, "They won't miss it!" Conflicts regarding moral judgments arise when people, either because of ignorance or moral weakness, do not consider all their human needs when making ethical decisions.

DIFFERENT VALUES

When making ethical decisions regarding health care, patients and health care professionals may have different needs or values in mind. For example, the medical team is interested in prolonging life—a physiologic need or value. Patients, however, may have spiritual norms they wish to fulfill. Thus, a patient who is a Jehovah's Witness will seek to fulfill her religious beliefs, which prohibit blood transfusions, even though she may die as a result of her choice. Insofar as she is concerned, she is making a good ethical decision because fulfilling her spiritual need is more important than fulfilling her physiologic need. In the mind of the medical team, however, she is making a bad decision because she is thwarting her ability to live and prolong life, a physiologic good. Medical teams sometimes try to persuade Jehovah's Witnesses to have blood transfusions or, what is more problematic, give them transfusions if they are comatose. Ethical patient care requires that the medical team realize that fulfilling spiritual needs is more important than fulfilling physiologic needs because spiritual needs have the most important place in the levels of human needs.

Ethical Norms

To facilitate ethical decision making, ethical norms have been constructed that express which actions are good and which are bad. These ethical norms are an effort to codify or express the experience that people have had in making individual ethical decisions. Therefore, we have positive ethical norms, such as "tell the truth" and "honor your father and mother," and negative ethical norms, such as "do not steal" and "do not commit adultery." Thus, ethical behavior implies the observance of ethical norms not because they are norms, but because of the ethical wisdom that they express. In most cases, ethical norms can be followed simply without a great deal of discussion because their validity can easily be discerned. Sometimes, however, more investigation is needed to see if the norm has validity in a particular situation: that is, more investigation may be needed to discern whether the ethical norm is relevant in a particular case. Thus, the good protected by observing the ethical norm "do not steal" is the good of private property. However, should a person starve to death rather than steal money or food? Is the good of human life more important than the good of private property? Thus, some ethical norms are subject to evaluation when it seems the norm would impose irrational behavior. Another way of stating this is the following: the circumstances in which an act is performed may change the ethical evaluation of the act. Is this true of all ethical norms? For example, determining whether the removal of life support is ethical or unethical depends on the circumstances that relate to the patient's medical condition. Given the medical condition of the patient, will continued use of a respirator be beneficial for the patient? Are all ethical norms relative in the sense that circumstances may change the moral evaluation of every act? Are some human acts always wrong, no matter what the circumstances? This issue is highly debated in ethics. It seems that some ethical norms, such as respecting the worth of innocent human life, are so important that they oblige under all conditions and circumstances, and circumstances do not change the moral evaluation of the act.

Ethical Norms for Medicine

In the course of history, several general norms have been formulated to guide the ethical practice of medicine. These norms are derived from the experience of physicians and nurses seeking to fulfill the needs of patients and caregivers in a balanced manner. Because ethical medicine seeks to fulfill all the needs of the patient, an ethical physician or nurse seeks to do more than keep the patient alive. Some of the norms for the ethical practice of medicine are listed in Table 2.

Clearly, in applying these norms, there is often a need to resolve conflicts that arise between different norms. For example, do community needs ever modify the norm to observe confidentiality? It seems so, because cases of venereal disease must be reported to public authorities so that the community may take steps to limit the disease. More concretely, how far can we go in observing the last norm in Table 2 without impeding the effort to provide health care for those who are able to pay for their care? Most of the time, however, these aforementioned principles can be applied correctly, with little discussion about meaning or applicability.

Taking time to study carefully whether a particular action will fulfill the human needs of a particular person in a balanced manner is a time-consuming and difficult process. For this reason, the following process or medical decision making is suggested: 1) medical facts must be obtained; and 2) then, options for action regarding patient benefit must be analyzed. Thus, patient benefit becomes the central theme of ethical decision making. The determination of patient benefit requires an analysis of how well patient needs will be fulfilled. Unfortunately, uncertainty often makes ethical decisions in health care confusing or difficult. When life support is being removed, for example, the ethical decision is made more difficult if the effect of removing the life support is often unknown: will continuing the life support be a benefit for the patient or will it impose an excessive burden? If some degree of moral certitude cannot be obtained regarding the effect of continuing the life support, sound ethical decision making requires that the more cautious action, the action most likely to protect patient benefit, be followed.

Perfect options are seldom available. The best or better option, given the circumstances, must be selected. Often, the choice of the better option results from a comparison of human needs that will be fulfilled by the particular options. Thus, determination of patient benefit must take into consideration the four basic levels of human function mentioned previously. Finally, one option must be selected. The option chosen will not always be the perfect option theoretically, but it should be the best option under the circumstances. For example, two options for treating an illness are suggested, one may be too expensive or impose an excessive burden. Hence, the best treatment for emphysema may be to move to a warm and dry climate. However, many people have neither the money to relocate nor the inclination to leave friends and family. Thus, an option for treating the emphysema must be chosen that is in theory less effective but that is the best hope for cure or palliative care under the circumstances. The process of decision

Table 2 Norms for the Ethical Practice of Medicine

Do no harm to the patient
Obtain informed consent from the patient or the proxy
Respect human life and bodily integrity
Tell the truth
Maintain confidentiality, especially concerning harmful facts and information
Respect the faith of the patient
Do not use patients in research projects without their consent
Allow patients to die if life-prolonging therapy is ineffective or imposes an excessive burden
Offer health care because people are in need, not because they can pay for it

making described above is called reasoned analysis, or prudential personalism, because it endeavors to bring human reason to the center of ethical decision making and seeks to benefit persons in their quest for human fulfillment [1].

CONCLUSIONS

The following describes the collaborative process of reasoned analysis for making ethical decisions regarding matters of health care:

- Identify all the pertinent medical facts.
- Make a diagnosis and then formulate the various possible therapies. select a therapeutic plan that seems to fulfill the needs of the patient.
- Explain the diagnosis, the possible therapies, and the preferred therapeutic plan to the patient or to the proxy if the patient is incapacitated.
- Decide with the patient or proxy which therapy will fulfill the needs of the patient in the most effective manner.
- In case of conflict that cannot be resolved through discussion, use ethical consultation.

The physician should recommend a therapeutic plan because the patient has little ability to evaluate a therapy from the aspect of physiologic or psychological need. The patient, however, has the primary ability to evaluate therapy from the aspect of social and creative need. Thus, the choice of therapy (informed consent) is a collaborative process. The patient has the right to reject the proposed therapeutic plan.

REFERENCES AND RECOMMENDED READING

1. Ashley B, O'Rourke K: Health Care Ethics, edn 3. St. Louis: Catholic Health Association; 1989.

SELECT BIBLIOGRAPHY

Ashley B, O'Rourke K: *Ethics of Health Care.* Washington: Georgetown University Press; 1994.

Beauchamp J, Childress J: Ethical theories. In *Principles of Biomedical Ethics.* New York: Oxford University Press; 1993.

Brennan T: Informed consent. In *Just Doctoring: Medical Ethics in the Liberal State.* Berkeley: University of California Press; 1991.

Dunn E: Ethics and family practice: some modern dilemmas. *Canadian Fam Phys* 1990, 36:1785.

Jonsen A: Causistry as methodology in clinical ethics. *Theoretical Medicine* 1991, 12(4):295–307.

The Humanities in Medicine
Mark D. Williams
Charles B. Rodning

> **Key Points**
> - If *humanitas* denotes a way of life centered on human interests and values, then all endeavors and relationships of humankind are within its domain, including the arts and sciences.
> - The ascendancy of the sciences since the Renaissance has contributed to a "metaphorical split" of the biomedical sciences from the humanities.
> - Because the ideational environments of patients and physicians, ranging from objective to subjective and rational to irrational, will influence the therapeutic milieu created within the patient–physician relationship, a physician must be artistic, humanistic, and scientific to serve patients effectually.
> - As symbolized by *Vitruvian Man*, the goal of a physician must be to develop a balance between knowledge and wisdom by study of the arts and humanities, as well as the biomedical sciences.

Homo sum; humani nihil a me alienum puto.
(I am a man; and nothing human is foreign to me.)
Heautontimoroumenos I, Terence (Publius Terentius Afer)

Vitruvian Man (Man in Circle and Square), created by Leonardo da Vinci, epitomizes a perception of humankind that existed during the Renaissance (Fig. 1). The inherent harmony, measured proportions, and symmetry of a man are depicted, with the extended extremities subtending a circle and a square—the most divine and perfect of geometric figures. The circle is centered on the umbilicus and is interpreted as the generative or maternal symbol. The square is centered on the symphysis pubis and is interpreted as the masculine or paternal symbol ("foursquare"). The widened stance forms a third geometric figure, an equilateral triangle bounded by the lower extremities. The balance and stability of this configuration, with the feet resting naturally on the surfaces and the hands stretched easily to the boundaries, depicts the reality of a human being, not an abstraction. It also depicts a vision of the incarnation of humankind—harmoniously created in the image of the Divine, reaching to touch perfection [1].

HUMANITAS DEFINED

The domain of the humanities (from the Latin *humanus*, "man") is broad and deep because it involves all the endeavors and relationships of humankind. *Humanitas* denotes an attitude, a doctrine, or a way of life centered on human interests and values, especially a philosophy that asserts the dignity and worth of humankind and a capacity for self-realization by the application of reason and rationality [2,3]. This capacity for self-realization occurs within interdependent cultural spheres of influence and interests, including artistic, economic, ethical, moral, historical, legal, literary, medical, philosophical, political, psychological, recreational, religious, and sociological.

Semiotically, *humanitas* can be interpreted as an entity and as a methodology. As an entity, *humanitas* ("humanism," "humanity," and "humanitarian") connotes a reaction to, and an attempt to interpret and explain, the multifarious world and universe in which humans are born, live, and die and in which they experience love and hate, triumph and defeat, joy and despair, hope and loss, pleasure and pain, health and disease, honor and humiliation, common sense and insanity, and wisdom and stupidity. As a methodology, *humanitas* ("humanize," "humane," "humanly," and "humanistic") connotes a system of nurture, education, development, and maturation employing reason and rationality for the benefit of humankind. Predicated on the evolution of sentience and linguistics, humans are qualitatively aware of their *conditio humani* and, by analogy, of that of other humans [4]. These definitions and perspectives have substantial relevance to the relationships that form between patients and physicians *vis-à-vis* health and medical care.

The avowed goal of medical education is to develop a proper balance between the sciences and the humanities in preparing physicians to deliver that health and medical care. A study of the humanities enables physicians to develop what Clouser [5] has referred to as "qualities of mind" or an awareness relevant to the nuance and subtlety of the patient–physician relationship. These qualities include incredulity, critical analytic skills, flexibility of perspective, discernment of values, nondogmatism, empathy, and self-knowledge. These skills are evermore required because of contemporary multicultural interactions. The dichotomy that currently exists between the sciences and the humanities has occurred because the ascendancy of the sciences since the Middle Ages, and particularly during this century, has skewed this balance [3,6].

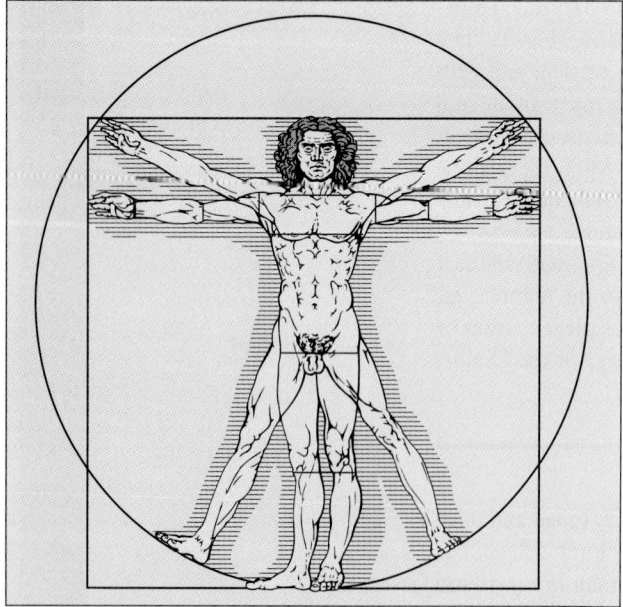

FIGURE 1 *Vitruvian Man*, Leonardo da Vinci, 1490. Gallerie dell' Academia, Venice.

IDEATIONAL ENVIRONMENT

Life is short, art long, opportunity fleeting, experiment treacherous, judgment difficult.
"Aphorisms," *Corpus Hippocraticum,* Hippocrates

The ideational environment [7] of contemporary physicians has been substantially influenced by the sciences. Physicians, unlike most persons, believe in science and that science can elucidate disease and illness. The fact that nonscientific variables may influence the content of the patient–physician relationship and may occasionally even supersede the ultimate therapeutic result poses a conundrum. This dilemma originates in and revolves around the distinction between the mechanistic reductionistic model of disease and the biopsychosocial model of illness [8].

What are the humanities if not the study of scientific and nonscientific ideational environments? The language of the humanities, unlike the language of the sciences, is intensely personal and appeals to sensibilities. Ideational environments may be as real and as consequential for patients and physicians as biological, physical, and social environments. Knowledge of patients' ideational environments enables physicians to develop compassion, empathy, rapport, and understanding, which are essential components of the therapeutic milieu.

Study of the humanities also enables physicians to understand their own ideational environments and the subjective and objective philosophical scales underlying their value judgments that are rendered daily. An objective approach to an analysis of values, perhaps encouraged by scientific methodologic principles, implies an external value structure and a moral order of the world that can be judged as right or wrong, as typified by the formal ethics and morals espoused by Immanuel Kant and Judeo-Christian tradition. Most caregivers, including clinical medical ethicists and philosophers [9•,10,11], prefer objectivity. In contrast, during this century, there has been a tremendous increase in the popularity of subjectivism, as expressed by the existentialist thought of Albert Camus and Jean-Paul Sartre. Values are perceived as idiosyncratic expressions of personal opinion and inner subjective feelings that cannot be evaluated as right or wrong. Cognizance, study, and discussion of these and other philosophical perspectives enable physicians to develop that attentiveness (from the Latin *attendere,* "to stretch toward") essential for the establishment of effective therapeutic relationships as they struggle intellectually with their attitudes regarding illness, the ill, scientific innovations, clinical productivity, and self-worth. Awareness and acknowledgment of these attitudes enable physicians to function with maturity and prudence.

ASCENDANCY OF SCIENCE

If we have our own *why* of life, we shall get along with almost any *how.*
Twilight of the Idols, Friedrich Wilhelm Nietzsche

Although the sciences and the humanities are linguistically and semiotically distinguished, the humanities actually encompass all human endeavors, including the sciences. The approach within each domain can be characterized as follows:

Scientia	Humanitas
Fact	Faith
Information	Wisdom
Experimental	Metaphorical
Reductionistic	Expansive
Quantitative	Qualitative
Observational	Analogical
Exoteric	Esoteric
Certainty	Uncertainty
Perceptive	Intuitive
Incredulity	Credulity
Linear	Nonlinear

The goal of any discovery is to balance the scientific methodologic approach to answer how (what, when, where, and who) with the humanistic methodologic approach to answer why. It is axiomatic that the accretion of knowledge in the scientific domain has substantially influenced humankind's perception of its situation and status in relationship to the biosphere. This has been exemplified by the rendering of human anatomy by da Vinci, Vesalius, and Harvey; the heliocentric interpretation of the universe by Copernicus and Kepler; the chemistry of van Helmont, Priestly, and Lavoisier; the physics of Galileo, Newton, Faraday, Gilbert, Bohr, Planck, and Einstein; the genetics of Mendel, Morgan, Watson, and Crick; the evolutionary theory of Darwin and Wallace; the introduction of vaccination by Jenner; the application of anesthesia by Long, Wells, and Morton; the concepts of asepsis and antisepsis by Semmelweis, Pasteur, and Koch; and the discovery of antibiotic medications by Ehrlich, Fleming and Waksman [12]. The point to be emphasized is that the relationship between the sciences and the humanities is bidirectional, dynamic, and evolving.

METAPHORICAL SPLIT

Where is the wisdom we have lost in knowledge?
The Rock, Chorus I, T.S. Eliot

The intellectual or metaphorical gap or split that has developed between the sciences and the humanities is a characteristic of Occidental society since the Enlightenment [3,6,13•,14]. The split was the consequence of a search for certainty and universality of knowledge as a basis for social order and as a reaction to the irreconcilable and unresolvable conflicts in religious and political life that characterized the Reformation. This untethering of the sciences from overt ecclesiastical and political control resulted in unprecedented growth in the understanding of human biology and in the application of this knowledge to medicine. However, this metaphorical split between the sciences and the humanities, what Snow [15] has referred to as a "two-cultures gap," has been detrimental to the relationship between patients and physicians, between scientists and clinicians, and between the medical profession and the public. A scientific world suffused with professional norms, procedures, priorities, and standards is discordant with a humanistic world suffused with fears, hopes, opinions, and values [10,11].

This perceived gap, the isolation and separation of the sciences from culture such that science is a value-neutral cognitive system that produces universal truths, is an illusion. The sciences are and must be subservient to human values, as philosophical and sociological observations and studies have repeatedly demonstrated. Can society justify spending billions of dollars to determine the sequence of the human genome while children are suffering from and dying of malnutrition and preventable diseases? Which endeavor has greater beneficence and value, or are they equivalent? A failure to understand and apply humanistic as well as scientific principles to articulate answers to these and other questions exposes the medical profession to criticism for being complacent and self-serving [13•,14,16••,17].

MEDICAL EDUCATION

Education, properly understood, is that which teaches discernment.
Meditations of a Parish Priest, Joseph Roux

Organized conventional medicine has been characterized as possessing an abundance of knowledge (sciences) and a paucity of wisdom (humanities); thus, it has been criticized for excessive reliance on scientific fact and insufficient emphasis on values, caring, personal relationships, and social skills [2,18,19]. In addition, no universally accepted curriculum incorporating the humanities currently exists. Both perspectives have contributed to a consensus that curricula must be re-oriented properly to serve current and future societal contingencies, constituencies, mandates, and requirements [2,18,20,21•–23•]. The Edinburgh Declaration of the World Council on Medical Education is exemplary of this re-orientation and evolving philosophy to heighten emphasis of the humanities (Table 1) [24].

Several authorities have recommended formal education in the humanities at the undergraduate, graduate, or postgraduate levels [16•,20,22•]. Bibliographies containing primary and secondary sources from our Occidental cultural heritage have been compiled that include science, economics, history, politics, literature, philosophy, religion, psychology, and sociology (Table 2). Systematic and thorough study of such a curriculum is a challenge that would require substantial commitment, conscientiousness, dedication, and will by students and physicians. However, the intellectual rewards and enhanced ability to serve patients are potentially great if physicians would but recall the Oslerian perspective of medical education as "a life-course, ending only with death" [25]. Physicians must also counteract the tendency of modern industrial society to trivialize the literary masterpieces of our predecessors. Although it is impossible to prove scientifically, common sense suggests that the intellectual and cultural heritage of Occidental society is a correlatively valid source of information and insight within the realm of medical education, health and medical care, and patient–physician relationships. Study of the humanities enables physicians to place scientific and nonscientific issues in appropriate and relevant contexts [26]. The literary masterpieces of our predecessors remain contextually meaningful and remind physicians that they do not function in a vacuum but rather serve as part of the cultural heritage and tradition of contemporary society.

A "COMPLEAT" PHYSICIAN

Medicine is the most humane of sciences, the most empiric of arts, and the most scientific of humanities.
Humanism and the Physician, E.D. Pellegrino

A section of the *Corpus Hippocraticum* entitled "Of the epidemics" records that the practice of medicine "consists in three things: the patient, the disease, and the physician. The physician is the servant of the art...it is the patient who must combat the disease along with the physician" [27]. According to this tradition, physicians vow "first to do good and to do no harm." This celebrated summary of the practice of medicine is indicative of the accumulated knowledge and wisdom that a "compleat" physician must possess to achieve empowerment, entitlement, and mastery of the discipline (Fig. 2) [28,29].

A physician must be scientific. A physician must know about diseases in general and be able to classify diseases according to their etiologies, symptoms and signs, pathophysiologies, and natural histories. Such knowledge underlies a physician's diagnosis of a patient's malady. This in turn facilitates assessment of the prognosis and the stages through which an illness will progress, from its onset, through various crises or turning points, to its sequelae or consequences. The accuracy of the diagnosis and the certainty of the prognosis influence the effectiveness of any remedy a physician prescribes to achieve cure or palliation.

However, a physician must also be humanistic. Patients are never identical. A physician must know a patient as an individual, and all the relevant circumstances of that individual's life, as well as the particular characteristics of the illness, must be discerned. The Hippocratic conception of a physician's work favors the practice of general medicine rather than divisive subspecialization. An individual, not the disease per se, is to be treated, and to treat that individual well, a physician must examine the patient as a whole, not merely the organ or system involved. The formula for obtaining a case history, for example, mandates an inquiry into the patient's life [27]:

> ...his antecedents, his occupation, his temperament, habits, regimen, and pursuits; his conversation, manners, taciturnity, thoughts, sleep, and sometimes his dreams, what they are and when they occur; his picking and scratching; his tears— from these, as well as from symptoms and signs, we form our judgment.

A physician must recognize and attend to the patient as a unique individual.

Finally, a physician must be artistic. The practice of medicine requires more than scientific and humanistic knowledge of health and disease. It requires the sort of experience that can be acquired only from actual practice—the art of medicine. Physicians are called on to apply all the knowledge and wisdom they have acquired as they focus on the care of an individual patient. This integrative process introduces an element of artistry, mystery, and subjectivity into the entire endeavor because knowledge of the human organism, as sophisticated as it may currently be, remains elementary. Decisions about patient care are often rendered on the basis of incomplete, and occasionally even incorrect, information. It is prudence acquired by experience that enables physicians to cope with this burden and to help their patients cope with this burden.

TABLE 1 EDINBURGH DECLARATION

The aim of medical education is to produce doctors who will promote the health of all people, and that aim is not being realized in many places, despite the enormous progress that has been made during this century in the biomedical sciences. The individual patient should be able to expect a doctor trained as an attentive listener, a careful observer, a sensitive communicator, and an effective clinician; but it is no longer enough only to treat some of the sick. Thousands suffer and die every day from diseases which are preventable, curable, or self-inflicted, and millions have no ready access to health care of any kind....

Scientific research continues to bring rich rewards; but man needs more than science alone, and it is the health needs of the human race as a whole, and of the whole person, that medical educators must affirm....

1. Enlarge the range of setting in which educational programs are conducted, to include all health resources of the community, not hospitals alone....

3. Ensure continuity of learning throughout life, shifting emphasis from the passive methods so widespread now to more active learning, including self-directed and independent study as well as tutorial methods.

4. Build both curriculum and examination systems to ensure the achievement of professional competence and social values, not merely the retention and recall of information.

5. Train teachers as educators, not solely experts in content, and reward educational excellence as fully as excellence in biomedical research or clinical practice....

Reform of medical education requires more than agreement; it requires a widespread commitment to action, vigorous leadership, and political will....

By this declaration we pledge ourselves and call on others to join us in a sustained and organized program to alter the character of medical education so that it truly meets the defined needs of the society in which it is situated. We also pledge ourselves to create the organizational framework required for these solemn words to be translated into sustained and effective action. The stage is set; the time for action is upon us.

From Warren [24]; with permission.

CONCLUSIONS

Unto whomsoever much is given, of him much be required.
Luke, The Physician, 12:48, *Bible* (King James Version)

Physicians can create a milieu for healing to occur, an incompletely understood physical and psychological biologic phenomenon; however, physicians cannot, no matter what their prowess, cause healing to occur. Physicians must recognize this distinction. *Scientia* can answer how something occurred, but it

Table 2 Occidental Literary Heritage

Science

Aristotle	*History of Animals*
Galen	*Natural Faculties*
Aulus Cornelius Celsus	*De Medicina*
Avicenna	*...Canon of Medicine....*
Maimonides	*Regimen Sanitatis*
Galileo Galilei	*...Concerning the Two New Sciences*
William Harvey	*Circulation of the Blood*
Sir Isaac Newton	*Mathematical Principles*
Claude Bernard	*...Study of Experimental Medicine*
Thomas Robert Malthus	*An Essay on Population*
Sir Charles Lyell	*Principles of Geology*
Walter Bradford Cannon	*Wisdom of the Body*
Rudolf Ludwig Karl Virchow	*Cellular Pathology....*
Max Karl Ernst Ludwig Planck	*Treatise on Thermodynamics*
Thomas Hunt Morgan	*Evolution and Genetics*
Alfred North Whitehead	*Process and Reality*
Norbert Weiner	*Cybernetics*
Albert Einstein	*Relativity....*

Medical history

Garrison FH	*...History of Medicine*
Bettmann OL	*Pictorial History of Medicine*
Lyons AS, Petrucelli RJ	*Medicine: An Illustrated History*

Psychology/Sociology

William James	*Principles of Psychology*
Sigmund Freud	*...Psycho-Analysis*
Max Weber	*Essays in Sociology*
John Dewey	*Experience and Education*

Religion

Saint Augustine	*City of God*
Saint Thomas Aquinas	*Summa Theologica*
Sir Thomas Browne	*Religio Medici*
Saint Thomas A'Kempis	*Imitation of Christ*
Martin Luther	*Treatise on Christian Liberty*
Saint Ignatius of Loyola	*Constitutions*
Martin Buber	*I and Thou*

Economics/History/Politics

Jean Jacques Rousseau	*Social Contract*
Adam Smith	*...The Wealth of Nations*
American State Papers	*Declaration of Independence, Articles of Confederation, Constitution*
John Stuart Mill	*Utilitarianism*
Thomas Jefferson	*Democracy*
Benjamin Franklin	*...Liberty and Necessity....*
Alexis Charles Henri Maurice Clérel de Tocqueville	*Democracy in America*

Literature

Homer	*Iliad, Odyssey*
Dante Alighieri	*Divine Comedy*
Goeffrey Chaucer	*Canterbury Tales*
William Shakespeare	*Tragadie et Comedia*
Miguel De Cervantes	*History of Don Quixote de la Mancha*
John Milton	*Paradise Lost*
Jonathan Swift	*Gulliver's Travels*
Johann Wolfgang von Goethe	*Faust*
Alexander Pope	*Essay on Criticism*
William Wordsworth	*Intimations of Immorality*
William Blake	*Songs of Innocence*
Charles Dickens	*Great Expectations*
Ralph Waldo Emerson	*Conduct of Life*
Victor Marie Hugo	*Les Misérables*
Henrik Ibsen	*Enemy of the People*
Charles Ludwidge Dodgson	*Alice's Adventures in Wonderland*
Anton Pavlovich Chekhov	*Ward No. 6*
Alexander Sergygyevich Pushkin	*The Captain's Daughter*
Walt Whitman	*Leaves of Grass*
Count Leo Tolstoy	*War and Peace*
Fyodor Mikhailovich Dostoevsky	*Brothers Karamazov*
William Carlos Williams	*In the American Grain*
Somerset Maugham	*Of Human Bondage*
Ernest Hemingway	*For Whom the Bell Tolls*

Philosophy

Plato	*Apology*
Marcus Aurelius	*Meditations*
William of Ockham	*Summa Totius Logicas*
Nicolò Machiavelli	*Prince*
John Locke	*Essay Concerning Human Understanding*
George Berkeley	*Principles of Human Knowledge*
David Hume	*...Concerning Human Understanding*
Sir Francis Bacon	*Advancement of Learning*
René Descartes	*Discourse on the Method*
Immanuel Kant	*...Metaphysic of Morals*
George Wilhelm Friedrich Hegel	*Philosophy of History*
Gottfried Wilhelm Leibnitz	*Characteristica*
Friedrich Wilhelm Nietzsche	*Will to Power....*
Sören Aabye Kierkegaard	*Either/Or....*
Arthur Schopenhauer	*World as Will and Idea*
Ludwig Wittgenstein	*Tractatus Logico-Philosophicus*
Bertrand Arthur William Russell	*Human Knowledge...*
George Santayana	*Reason in Science*

Adapted from Adler [28]; with permission.

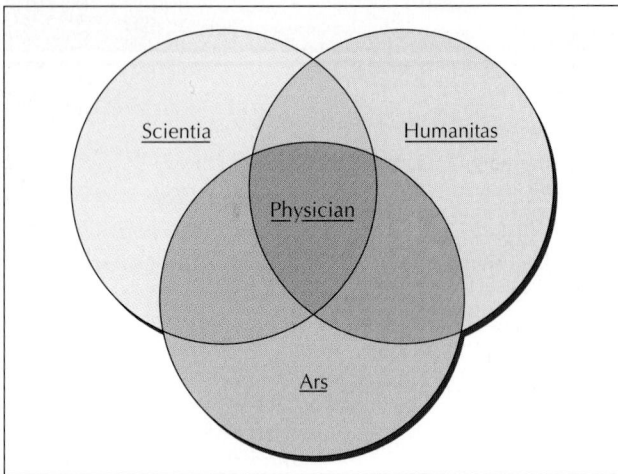

FIGURE 2 Interdependent attributes of a "compleat" physician.

cannot answer why something occurred or the moral value of the occurrence. For the latter, physicians must apply *humanitas*. Physicians must guard against using the sciences to answer why, just as they must guard against using the humanities to answer how. Doctors (from the Latin *docere*, "to teach") must educate their patients and their students to address and understand this eternal dichotomy [17]. In treating something as complex as the human organism, the sciences and the humanities serve bilateral, complementary, interdependent, and mutual roles.

Linkage between how and why and between the sciences and the humanities is needed. The art of medicine serves as this link. To speak of right action in medicine, to define disease and illness, or to enjoin the preservation of human health presupposes ideals of human well-being. Because medical therapies involve the manipulation of human nature, all the traditional philosophical questions about what one can know, what one ought to do, and how one should use technocratic power are raised in contexts intimately bound to human life, suffering, and death [2,18]. Comprehending and explaining the workings of the human organism must be commensurate and compatible with a realistic and achievable goal of maximal restoration of health for patients. The sciences and the humanities should ideally inhabit the intellectual milieu, the ideational environment, of every physician if physicians are to serve their patients with authority, excellence, expertise, and foresight—striving to achieve mastery, "reaching to touch perfection" [1].

Acknowledgment

The authors are grateful to Ms. Betty J. Young and Ms. Judy L. Northcutt for typing the manuscript.

References and Recommended Reading

Recently published papers of particular interest have been highlighted as:
• Of interest
•• Of outstanding interest

1. Creed JC: Vitruvian Man. *JAMA* 1986, 256:1541.
2. Pellegrino ED: *Humanism and the Physician* Knoxville, TN: University of Tennessee Press; 1979.
3. Durant W, Durant A: *The Story of Civilization*, vols I–XI. New York: Simon and Schuster; 1954–1975.
4. Diamond J: *The Third Chimpanzee: The Evolution and Future of the Human Animal*. New York: Harper Perennial; 1992.
5. Clouser KD: Humanities in medical education: some contributions. *J Med Philos* 1990, 15:289–301.
6. Manchester W: *A World Lit Only by Fire: The Medieval Mind and the Renaissance. Portrait of an Age*. Boston: Little Brown; 1992.
7. Murdock G: *Theories of Illness, A World Survey*. Pittsburgh: University of Pittsburgh Press; 1980.
8. Engel GL: The need for a new medical model: a challenge for biomedicine. *Science* 1977, 196:129–136.
9.• Self DJ, Skeel JD: A study of the foundations of ethical decision making of clinical medical ethicists. *Theor Med* 1991, 12:117–127.
10. Thomasma DC: Why philosophers should offer ethics consultations. *Theor Med* 1991, 12:129–140.
11. Barnard D: Reflections of a reluctant clinical ethicist: ethics consultation and the collapse of critical distance. *Theor Med* 1992, 13:15–22.
12. Garrison FH: *An Introduction to the History of Medicine With Medical Chronology, Suggestions for Study and Bibliographic Data*. Philadelphia: WB Saunders; 1929.
13.• Bellett AJD: Value issues in biomedical science: public concerns and professional complacency. *Immunol Cell Biol* 1992, 70:363–368.
14. Toulmin SE: *Cosmopolis: The Hidden Agenda of Modernity*. New York: Free Press; 1989.
15. Snow CP: *Two Cultures and a Second Look*. Cambridge, England: Cambridge University Press; 1964.
16.•• Almy TP, Colby KK, Zubkoff M, *et al.*: Health, society, and the physician: problem-based learning of the social sciences and humanities. *Ann Intern Med* 1992, 116:569–574.
17. Reiser SJ: The era of the patient: using the experience of illness in shaping the missions of health care. *JAMA* 1993, 269:1012–1017.
18. Engelhardt HT Jr: The birth of the medical humanities and the rebirth of the philosophy of medicine: the vision of Edmund D. Pellegrino. *J Med Philos* 1990, 15:237–241.
19. Epstein RM, Campbell TL, Cohen-Cole SA, *et al.*: Perspectives on patient-doctor communication. *J Fam Pract* 1993, 37:377–388.
20. Elstein M, Harris J: Teaching of medical ethics. *J Med Educ* 1990, 24:531–534.
21.• Andre J: Learning to see: moral growth during medical training. *J Med Ethics* 1992, 18:148–152.
22.• Menken M: Humanitas in medical education. *J Med Educ* 1992, 26:429–432.
23.• Spiro H: What is empathy and can it be taught? *Ann Intern Med* 1992, 116:843–846.
24. Warren K: World conference on medical education, Edinburgh. *Lancet* 1988, ii:462–463.
25. Osler W: *Aequanimitas: With Other Addresses to Medical Students, Nurses, and Practitioners of Medicine*. Philadelphia: P. Blakiston; 1905.
26. Bronowski J: *The Common Sense of Science*. Cambridge, MA: Harvard University Press; 1953.
27. Hippocrates: *Corpus Hippocraticum*, vol I and II. Translated by Jones WHS. London: William Heinemann; 1931.
28. Adler MJ: Medicine. *Great Ideas: A Synopticon of Great Books of the Western World*, vol II. Edited by Adler MJ. Chicago: Encyclopaedia Britannica; 1952:113–132.
29. Rodning CB: Gift of attention. *South Med J* 1992, 85:403–406.

Malpractice

William M. Connelly
Thomas G. Mackin

> ### Key Points
> - Negligence is broadly defined as conduct that falls below the standard established by law to protect people against unreasonable risks of harm.
> - Medical malpractice is defined as professional misconduct or unreasonable lack of care.
> - The elements of a claim of medical negligence are duty, breach of that duty, proximate cause, and damages.
> - A physician is held to the standard of care that a physician of ordinary skill, care, and diligence would provide to a patient in similar circumstances or conditions.
> - When a physician holds himself or herself out as a specialist in a particular field of medicine, that physician is held to the standard of care for that specialty in light of today's knowledge.

Malpractice is generally defined as professional misconduct or unreasonable lack of care [1]. The term *medical malpractice* is commonly used to describe the liability of a medical care provider arising from the rendering of professional medical services. This general description, however, encompasses several different theories of civil liability, including medical negligence (Table 1) [2••]. Of these theories of liability, medical negligence is predominant and most often reaches litigation, where it is often accompanied by one of the other theories of liability. Although the type of claim that can be made under the theory of medical negligence may vary from state to state, generally a medical negligence claim includes any claim asserted in a civil action that arises out of the medical diagnosis, care, or treatment of any person by a physician or any health care provider, including a hospital [3].

This chapter provides a brief overview of the elements of a claim for medical negligence as set forth through judicial decisions and statutory law. Although the legal principles discussed in this chapter are, for the most part, well established, the law in each state may vary according to the developed case law or the law as codified by the state's legislature. This chapter also considers several defenses to a claim for medical negligence.

STANDARDS FOR ESTABLISHING A CLAIM FOR MEDICAL NEGLIGENCE

Negligence is broadly defined as conduct that falls below the standard established by law to protect people against unreasonable risks of harm [4]. To prove a claim of negligence, the party bringing the claim, *ie*, the plaintiff, must prove by preponderance of the evidence [5] that the party from whom the plaintiff is seeking relief, *ie*, the defendant, owes the plaintiff a duty, that the defendant breached that duty, that the breach of that duty was the "proximate" cause of the harm, and that the plaintiff

TABLE 1 POTENTIAL CLAIMS AS PART OF MALPRACTICE LAWSUIT

Medical negligence
Wrongful death
Failure to obtain informed consent
Product liability
Assault
Battery
Breach of fiduciary duty

suffered damage compensable in the law as a result of the breach of that duty [6]. Each one of these elements is discussed below in the context of a claim for medical negligence.

Duty of Care

A physician does not owe a duty of care to the public at large, but a physician does owe an individual a duty when the physician–patient relationship exists. Such a relationship arises out of contract and imposes on a physician an obligation to use the appropriate degree of skill or care during the existence of the physician–patient relationship, but a physician is not, in the absence of an expressed promise, an insurer of the patient's recovery or a guarantor of results [7]. A physician–patient relationship is consensual and is created by either an expressed or implied agreement in which the physician agrees to provide service to a patient and that patient agrees to accept that service for the purpose of receiving medical treatment [8]. Although the relationship between a physician and a patient is considered to be contractual in nature, generally a patient cannot bring a claim of breach of contract on the grounds that the physician negligently performed under the terms of their agreement [9].

In most cases, the physician–patient relationship is established when the physician agrees to provide medical service in exchange for consideration. A physician–patient relationship may be created when a patient justifiably relies on a promise of care given to that patient by a physician [10]. A physician–patient relationship may exist even though there is no physical meeting between the medical professional and the patient. For example, a pathologist owes a duty to a patient to accurately interpret a tissue biopsy even though the pathologist has never met the patient. One court even found that the question of whether a physician–patient relationship exists should be determined by a jury: in that case a physician, a hospital insurance plan doctor, told a member of that plan to go home and return during business hours in a telephone discussion in which the individual complained of chest pain. After returning home and before the plan was open, the individual died [11].

Generally, a physician–patient relationship ends when a patient completes treatment. A physician may terminate the relationship only if the patient is afforded a reasonable notice and the opportunity to secure other medical attention if it is necessary [12]. If a physician does not provide a patient with an opportunity to find another physician, the physician may expose himself or herself to liability for abandoning a patient. It is not considered abandonment, however, when a specialist, after completing treatment of a patient, terminates the relationship by returning the patient to the original physician [13].

Breach of Duty of Care

At the start of a medical negligence case, the plaintiff must overcome the presumption that the medical services provided met the applicable standard of care [14]. Interestingly, evidence that a physician followed a recognized practice or procedure, although helpful to the judge or jury in determining whether the appropriate standard of care was followed, is not conclusive concerning the issue of negligence. The critical issue in determining whether a physician was negligent depends on whether the procedure used was reasonable under the circumstances.

Determining the appropriate standard of care

The physician being sued is held to the standard of care that a physician of ordinary skill, care, and diligence would provide to a patient in similar conditions or circumstances [13]. A physician is not required to possess the highest degree of knowledge or skill, but a physician must exercise the skill, care, or diligence that would be exercised by that physician's peers with similar education and training under the same or similar circumstances [15]. Because the issue of whether a physician has departed from the appropriate standard of care focuses on whether the physician's conduct was acceptable when compared with other physicians of similar training, the geographic location of the incidence does not control the standard of care owed to a patient by a physician [16].

Additionally, if a physician considers himself or herself to be specialist in a particular field of medicine, that physician is held to the standard of care for that specialty in light of the present day's knowledge. For instance, the standard of care for a surgeon, in the practice of a board-certified specialty, is that of a reasonable surgeon practicing in the same specialty and considering the state of scientific knowledge existing in the field when the malpractice is claimed to have occurred [13].

Proving a Breach of Care
Expert Testimony Required

In some states, such as Ohio, expert testimony is required in most cases on the issue of whether the treatment departed from the appropriate standard of care [17]. The expert must be qualified to express an opinion concerning the specific standard of care that prevails in the medical community in which the alleged malpractice took place [18]. The purpose of expert testimony is to aid the trier of fact, ie, the jury or judge, in determining whether the defendant committed malpractice (Table 2).

The courts that require expert testimony generally have established certain requirements that a person must satisfy to be considered an expert. For a person to be an expert in an Ohio medical negligence case, that person must be licensed to practice medicine by the state medical board and devote at least half of his or her time to active clinical practice in his or her field of licensure or to its instruction in an accredited school of medicine [17].

Whether an individual is qualified as an expert does not depend on whether the witness is the best witness on the subject or whether the proposed expert is within the same "school" if the fields of medicine overlap. If a given procedure may be performed by more than one type of specialist, a witness may testify as an expert in a malpractice case even though his or her practice is not in the same field of specialty as the defendant's. For example, a surgeon was found qualified as an expert in a case involving a podiatrist because that surgeon testified that he was familiar with the proper procedures and treatment rendered by a podiatrist and that foot surgery was part of his training and practice [19]. However, when an expert witness is not in the same field as the defendant, the jury may not find that expert as credible as an expert in the specialty area of the defendant.

Exceptions

The exception to this rule occurs when the nature of the departure from the standard of care is such that the lack of skill is so apparent as to be within the comprehension of a layman and requires only common knowledge and experience [20]. For instance, no expert testimony is necessary to show a breach of the appropriate standard of care when the evidence establishes that a needle was left in the patient after surgery [21].

Breach of the appropriate standard of care also may be established though the use of a legal doctrine called *res ipsa loquitur*, which means "the thing speaks for itself" [22]. *Res ipsa loquitur* applies only when the injury is one that could not have occurred in the absence of negligence; the instrumentality causing the injury was at the time of the injury under the exclusive control of the defendant; and there was no contributory negligence or assumption of the risk on the part of the patient [23]. This doctrine permits a jury to draw an inference, in the majority of states, that the treating physician was negligent, but it cannot be used when the claim of medical malpractice is based solely on the fact that treatment was unsuccessful or terminated with a poor or unfortunate result [24]. Use of this doctrine at a trial means that the plaintiff has proof to a reasonable degree of medical certainty. However, that proof may be rebutted by other evidence, leaving the issue of negligence for the jury or judge to decide.

Proximate Cause

The third element of a medical malpractice claim is causation. "Proximate," or legal cause, "is that which in a natural and continued sequence contributes to procedure the result, without which it would not have happened [25]." This means that the breach of the appropriate standard of care produces the injury as a result of the nature and the continuous consequence of events, unbroken by an superseding act of negligence [26].

In the context of a medical malpractice claim, to prove causation a plaintiff must establish through expert testimony that the injury was caused by the physician's negligence to a "reasonable degree of medical certainty." A reasonable degree of medical certainty means that an event is more than likely to occur, or is medically more probable to occur, as opposed to a mere possibility [27]. The reasonable degree of medical certainty standard is used to prevent speculation on the part of the jury as to whether there is evidence of negligence. However, use of this standard does not mean that all other possible causes for the injury must be eliminated.

This element of proving medical negligence is perhaps the most difficult for a plaintiff bringing a claim of malpractice because the mere fact that there was a bad result is not sufficient to establish causation. In one case, a patient presented with an advanced case of lung cancer. The cancer was observable on the patient's radiographs, but the patient was not properly treated or monitored after the cancer was discovered. The court found that there was no malpractice because the patient would have died as a result of the advanced condition of the cancer regardless of the treatment received [28]. In another case, a court found that the condition that most likely caused an infant's handicapped condition occurred prior to the infant's delivery. As a result, the court noted that a physician's failure to investigate the infant's low blood platelet count was not the proximate cause of the injury [29].

Causation may be established if there is evidence that the treating physician incorrectly diagnosed a patient, which thus led to incorrect treatment. Causation also may be established by evidence of failure by a physician to diagnose injury, resulting in a delay in treatment or a lack of treatment. To establish causation in a failure-to-diagnose case, the medical expert must testify that the lack or delay in treatment either diminished the chances of the patient's recovery, prolonged the patient's illness, or increased the patient's suffering. In other words, the failure to properly diagnose must have made the patient's condition worse than it would have been had the physician followed the appropriate standard of care [30].

TABLE 2 TIPS FOR THE PHYSICIAN WHO IS GOING TO TESTIFY AS AN EXPERT WITNESS

Commit to taking the time necessary to testify professionally
Become intimately familiar with the record of the case
Review the relevant literature on the subject at issue so that you are up-to-date
If possible, anticipate questions to be asked of you by opposing counsel
Remember, do not underestimate the medical knowledge that can be obtained on a very specific medical issue by the opposing attorney
Be aware of any opinions you have presented in a medical periodical relating to the topic on which you are going to testify

Finally, with regard to proximate cause, an issue may arise as to whether an act of negligence after an earlier breach of care breaks the causal chain and relieves the original negligent physician of liability. In general, the law does not relieve a wrongdoer, called a *tort-feasor*, from liability when subsequent or successive negligence occurs in the natural and ordinary course of things, or is foreseeable, and is reasonably probable as a result of the original negligence [31].

Damages

For the final element, to prove damages, a plaintiff must prove an injury considered to be compensable in law. Some damages are not compensable in the law. For instance, the Ohio Supreme Court has held that a woman was not entitled to recover the damages and expenses that she would incur to raise a baby after she gave birth to a healthy baby, although she had earlier undergone a tubal ligation [32]. In a medical negligence case, the most common forms of damages recoverable by a plaintiff are compensatory damages, which are intended to compensate an injured party for the actual loss that he or she suffered. Compensatory damages are designed to put the plaintiff in the position that the plaintiff would have been in had there been no malpractice [33].

In a medical malpractice case, the amount of compensatory damage that the plaintiff is entitled to recover includes economic loss, including expenditures for medical care and treatment; lost wages and other expenditures; and noneconomic loss, including pain and suffering, loss of companionship, and loss of enjoyment of life. Relief for noneconomic injury is more controversial because it is difficult to put a monetary value on the pain and suffering endured by a patient or the loss of the pleasure of doing something.

A plaintiff also may be entitled to recover for future damages if the injury is permanent. Future damages are those suffered as a result of the injury and that will arise after the determination of liability by the jury [34]. Derivative claims may also be available for family members, such as a wife or parents if the injury is to a minor.

Over the past several years there has been a question as to whether a limit should be placed on the amount of recoverable damages in a claim for medical negligence. In most of the jurisdictions where the issue has been addressed, the courts have overturned statutory language designed to limit damage awards on the ground that such limitations are unconstitutional and deny the right to a jury trial [34].

Defenses

In addition to defeating a medical negligence claim by establishing that the plaintiff has not proven one of the necessary elements identified above, a physician may be able to assert one or more affirmative defenses to defeat a claim of malpractice. Affirmative defenses include the possibility that the statute of limitation, the time within which a claim must be brought, has expired or that the plaintiff's own negligence was the cause of the injury.

Statute of Limitations

The time for filing a lawsuit claiming that injuries occurred as a result of medical negligence is generally governed by state statute, which limits the time for filing the lawsuit in court to, for example, 1 year from when the claim "accrues" [3]. A claim accrues when the physician–patient relationship is terminated or when the patient discovers the injury or should have discovered the injury though the exercise of reasonable care [35]. The fact that the patient misses an appointment is not sufficient to conclude that the physician–patient relationship has terminated when that patient is continuing to take medication prescribed by that physician [36–38].

The plaintiff may be permitted to extend the time for filing a claim for medical malpractice beyond the original statute of limitations (in Ohio, for an additional 180 days) when the party against whom the claim will be brought receives notice of the intent to bring a claim [39]. The deadline for filing a claim also may be extended if the injury is to a minor. In that situation, the action accrues, and the statute of limitations begins to run when the minor becomes an adult at the age of "majority," which is 18 years in most states.

Contributory Negligence

For a patient's negligence to bar recovery in a medical malpractice claim, that "contributory" negligence must have been an active and contributing cause of the injury, and it must have occurred simultaneously with the fault of the treating physician. It also must have entered into the creation of the claim and have been an element in the transaction that constituted the negligence [40]. This defense may apply, for example, when a patient fails to provide an accurate medical history to a treating physician [41].

If You Are the Subject of a Malpractice Suit

In addition to considering the legal requirements set forth above, if you are served with a complaint for medical negligence you should take some practical steps to protect yourself. First, immediately notify your malpractice insurance carrier. Second, consider retaining separate counsel from any other defendant. Third, in anticipation of your deposition being taken, prepare a chronology of events and arrange the file in chronological order. Fourth, keep in contact with your attorney and keep informed about the status of your case (Table 3).

Table 3 What to do if you are sued for malpractice
Notify your insurance carrier
Consider obtaining separate counsel from the other defendants
Organize your file chronologically
Keep informed

References and Recommended Reading

Recently published papers of particular interest have been highlighted as:
- Of interest
- •• Of outstanding interest

1. Black HC, ed.: *Black's Law Dictionary*, edn 5. St. Paul: West Publishing Co; 1979:864.
2. •• Ohio Rev Code Ann § 2317.54 (Anderson 1991).
3. Ohio Rev Code Ann § 2305.11(D)(3) (Anderson Supp 1992).
4. *Torts*, § 285 (1965).
5. Black HC, ed.: *Black's Law Dictionary*, edn 5. St. Paul: West Publishing Co.; 1979:864.
6. Prossor W: *Handbook on the Law of Torts*. St. Paul: West Publishing Co.; §143 (4th ed. 1977).
7. *Turner v Children's Hospital, Inc.*, 76 Ohio App3d 541, 547, 602 NE2d 423 (1991).
8. *United Calendar Manufacturing Corporation v Huang*, 94 AD2d 176, 179, 463 NYS2d 497 (1983).
9. *Robb v Community Mutual Insurance Company*, 63 Ohio App3d 308, 305, 580, NE2d 494 (1983).
10. *O'Neil v Montefiore Hospital*, 11 AD2d 132, 134, 202 NYS2d 436 (1960).
11. McCafferty MP, Meyer SM: *Medical Malpractice Bases of Liability*. McGraw-Hill; 1985:16–17.
12. *Hammonds v Aetna Casualty and Sur. Company*, 24 NE2d 793 (ND Ohio 1965).
13. *Bruni v Tatsumi*, 46 Ohio St2d 127, 127, 346 NE2d 673 (1976).
14. *Finley v United States*, 314 F Suppl 905 (SD Ohio 1970).
15. *Promen v Ward*, 70 Ohio App3d 560, 565, 591 NE2d 813 (1990).
16. *Bruni v Tatsumi*, 46 Ohio St2d 134–35.
17. Ohio Rev Code Ann § 2743.43 (Anderson 1992).
18. *Herring v Knab*, 458 F Suppl 359 (SD Ohio 1978).
19. *King v LaKamp*, 50 Ohio App3d 84, 85, 553 NE2d 71 (1986).
20. *Anderson v Motta*, 73 Ohio App3d 1, 595 NE2d 1029 (1991).
21. *Wright v Carter*, 604 NE2d 1236 (Ind Ct Appl 1992).
22. Black HC, ed.: *Black's Law Dictionary*, edn 5. St. Paul: West Publishing Co; 1979:1173.
23. *Morgan v Children's Hospital*, 18 Ohio St3d 185, 188–89, 480 NE2d 464 (1985).
24. *Johnson v Hammond*, 68 Ohio App3d 491, 494, 589 NE2d 65 (1990).
25. *Taylor v Webster*, 12 Ohio St2d 53, 56, 231 NE2d 870 (1987).
26. Black HC, ed.: *Black's Law Dictionary*, edn 5. St. Paul: West Publishing Co; 1979:1103.
27. *Cooper v Sisters of Charity, Inc.*, 27 Ohio St2d 242, 272 NE2d 97 (1971).
28. *Breining v United States*, 861 F2d 1342 (5th Cir 1988).
29. *Chupka v Rigsby*, 75 Ohio App3d 795, 799–801, 600 NE2d 832 (1991).
30. *Tomcak v Ohio Department of Rehabilitation and Corrections*, 62 Ohio Misc2d 324, 598 NE2d 900 (1991).
31. Black HC, ed.: *Black's Law Dictionary*, edn 5. St. Paul: West Publishing Co; 1979:1103.
32. *Johnson v University Hospital of Cleveland*, 44 Ohio St3d 49, 540 NE2d 1370 (1989).
33. Black HC, ed.: *Black's Law Dictionary*, edn 5. St. Paul: West Publishing Co; 1979:352.
34. Ohio Rev Code Ann § 2323.56 (Anderson 1992).
35. *Ishler v Miller*, 56 Ohio St2d 447, 449–451, 384 NE2d 296 (1978).
36. *Matter v Griffin Hospital*, 207 Conn 125, 240 A2d 666, 679 (1988).
37. *Willinger v Mercy Catholic Medical Center*, 398 A.2d 1188 (Pa 1978).
38. *Caldwell v Ohio Power Company*, 710 F Suppl 194 (ND Ohio 1989).
39. *Edens v Barberton Area Family Practice Center*, 43 Ohio St3d 176, 176, 539, NE2d 1124 (1989), syllabus.
40. *Seley v G.D. Searle & Company*, 67 Ohio St3d 192, 208–209, 423 NE2d 831 (1981).
41. *McKoy v Furlong*, 69 Ohio App3d 62, 65, 590 NE2d, 39 (1990).

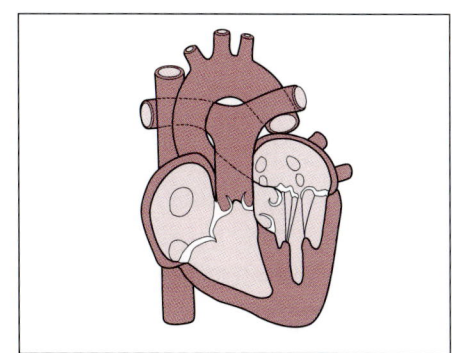

CARDIOLOGY

II

Section Editor
Joseph S. Alpert

Cardiovascular disease continues to be the most common cause of death in developed countries such as the United States. Despite remarkable advances in the understanding and management of cardiovascular diseases, with resultant marked declines in mortality for these conditions, cardiovascular problems still plague our patients.

The primary care physician often encounters patients with cardiovascular disease. Most of these patients suffer from hypertension, and/or the ravages of atherosclerosis: coronary artery disease, cerebrovascular disease, and peripheral vascular disease. In addition, the average primary care physician often confronts patients with valvular heart disease, atrial fibrillation, and various other arrhythmias, some benign and some malignant. Consequently, the primary care physician must have considerable familiarity with the presentation, diagnosis, and treatment of cardiovascular disease.

The Cardiology section of *Current Practice of Medicine* provides a thorough update of cardiovascular illness and the latest developments in cardiovascular treatment. I thank the many authors who labored to create this unique text.

Evaluation of the Patient with Chest Pain

John A. Paraskos

> **Key Points**
> - Much of the economic and medical resources used in evaluating patients with chest pain is unnecessary.
> - A carefully obtained history is crucial to assessing the likelihood of coronary disease before any testing is obtained (*ie*, the pretest likelihood for coronary disease).
> - The pretest likelihood is assessed from the patient's age, gender, character of the pain or discomfort, and associated risk factors.
> - Both the choice and interpretation of noninvasive tests to establish the diagnosis depend on the pretest likelihood and the perceived urgency or instability of the clinical scenario.
> - The choice and timing of coronary arteriography depend on the urgency of the clinical scenario and the inability of noninvasive tests to establish the diagnosis reliably.

Evaluation of chest pain consumes a tremendous amount of economic and medical resources. Identification of patients whose chest pain results from myocardial ischemia is a challenging and important problem in clinical medicine, considering the potentially lethal consequences of error. Many of the resources expended in cardiac evaluation, however, are unnecessary.

The most important evaluative tool in most cases is a careful history augmented by physical examination and simple laboratory procedures. Angina pectoris is a diagnosis of history; an effective physician can often allay the patient's anxiety and prevent unnecessary diagnostic procedures by a careful history and a thorough knowledge of the likelihood of coronary artery disease (CAD) in a given population. Whenever a patient presents with chest pain, it is important to assess rapidly the likelihood of coronary disease in that individual, the likelihood that the character of the pain is cardiac in origin, and the multiplicity of other conditions that can produce similar symptoms. This differentiation is complicated by the overlap of signs and symptoms of myocardial ischemia with several noncardiac causes of chest pain (Table 1). Any of the thoracic structures can be a source of chest pain, as can structures outside the thorax, particularly the gastrointestinal tract. Because the heart and esophagus share the same spinal cord sensory innervation, myocardial ischemia and esophageal pain are sometimes indistinguishable [1,2•]. A burning substernal discomfort typical of esophageal pyrosis is not uncommon in myocardial ischemia; conversely, substernal tightness or pressure or even crushing pain typical of angina pectoris, may be caused by esophageal disease. After a careful initial evaluation, many patients must be treated as if they have myocardial ischemia until the diagnostic dilemma is resolved by further observation, diagnostic studies, or response to therapy. If coronary disease is likely and the character of the pain is clearly or possibly ischemic, consultation with an internist or cardiologist is appropriate.

This chapter provides a useful method of determining the likelihood of coronary disease in any individual based on risk factors and pain characteristics. Physical findings associated with various causes of chest pain and procedures needed to confirm the diagnosis are also discussed.

CHEST PAIN AS A MANIFESTATION OF MYOCARDIAL ISCHEMIA

Angina pectoris is usually substernal and transient. It is often brought on by exercise and relieved by rest or nitrates. Angina may be provoked by a large meal and be mistaken for indigestion. If the coronary disease is stable, the pain episodes are usually short-lived (*ie*, 5 to 15 minutes) and provoked by exertion or meals.

Unstable angina is characterized by a less predictable prognosis, with a higher likelihood of acute myocardial infarction (MI) or sudden death. This instability is usually caused by a complication in the coronary artery (*eg*, plaque rupture, thrombosis, or spasm). Features that mark instability are new-onset angina, accelerating angina (occurring more frequently or at lower workloads), rest angina, angina that wakes the patient from sleep, prolonged anginal episodes, anginal episodes not responsive to nitrates, and angina associated with severe nausea, weakness, dyspnea, sweating, palpitations, syncope, or pulmonary edema.

The pain of MI usually includes a number of these features of instability. It is usually not triggered by exertion and is not relieved by rest, antacids, or nitrates. The pain of MI is more often accompanied by nausea and sweating, and patients are often immobilized by a sense of impending doom.

Patients suspected of having acute MI are admitted for intensive care monitoring, because short-term survival is enhanced by early intervention, especially for life-threatening ventricular arrhythmias. Patients with unstable angina also have a serious short-term prognosis and usually require hospitalization and consultation with a cardiologist so that therapeutic decisions can be made promptly.

When evaluating ischemic pain, the clinician should consider several questions. Is the chest pain typical for myocar-

TABLE 1 CAUSES OF CHEST PAIN

Cardiovascular
Coronary artery disease
   Obstructive, spastic, nonathero-
     sclerotic, and congenital
   Cocaine abuse
Severe aortic stenosis or aortic
   insufficiency
Hypertrophic cardiomyopathy
Aortic dissection
Pericarditis
Myocarditis
Dressler's syndrome
Pulmonary embolism
Pulmonary hypertension
Thoracic aneurysm
Hepatic engorgement
Mitral valve prolapse

Pulmonary
Pneumonitis
Pleurisy
Pulmonary infarction or hemorrhage
Pulmonary embolism or *in situ*
   thrombosis
Tracheitis and tracheobronchitis
Spontaneous pneumothorax
Intrathoracic tumor

Gastrointestinal
Hiatal hernia with reflux esophagitis
Esophageal spasm
Esophageal perforation
Esophagitis
Irritable esophagus
Mallory-Weiss syndrome
Peptic ulcer disease
Gastritis
Cholecystitis and biliary colic
Pancreatitis
Gas entrapment syndromes
   Gastric distention
   Hepatic or splenic flexure distention

Musculoskeletal
Costochondritis (Tietze's syndrome)
Costochondral or xiphisternal arthralgia
Sternoclavicular arthralgia
Manubriosternal arthralgia
Costovertebral arthritis
Epidemic myalgia
Fibromyalgia
Myositis
Thoracic outlet syndromes
Sternal or rib fractures
Slipping rib syndrome
Precordial catch syndrome (muscle spasm)
Muscle strain
Ostealgia from neoplasm, inflammation,
   or infarction
Sternal marrow pain (acute leukemia)
Trauma

Neurologic
Radicular syndrome
Thoracic disc disease
Brachial plexus syndrome
Intercostal neuritis
Reflex autonomic dysfunction
   (shoulder-hand syndrome)
Neurofibromatosis
Herpes zoster involving thoracic
   dermatome with postherpetic pain

Functional or psychiatric
Anxiety with periapical hyperesthesia
Hyperventilation with increased
   muscle tension
Panic attacks
Cardiac neurosis
Psychogenic regional pain syndrome
Malingering
Depression

Miscellaneous
Diaphragmatic spasm or flutter
Superficial thrombophlebitis
   (Mondor's syndrome)
Mediastinitis
Mediastinal emphysema
Mediastinal tumors

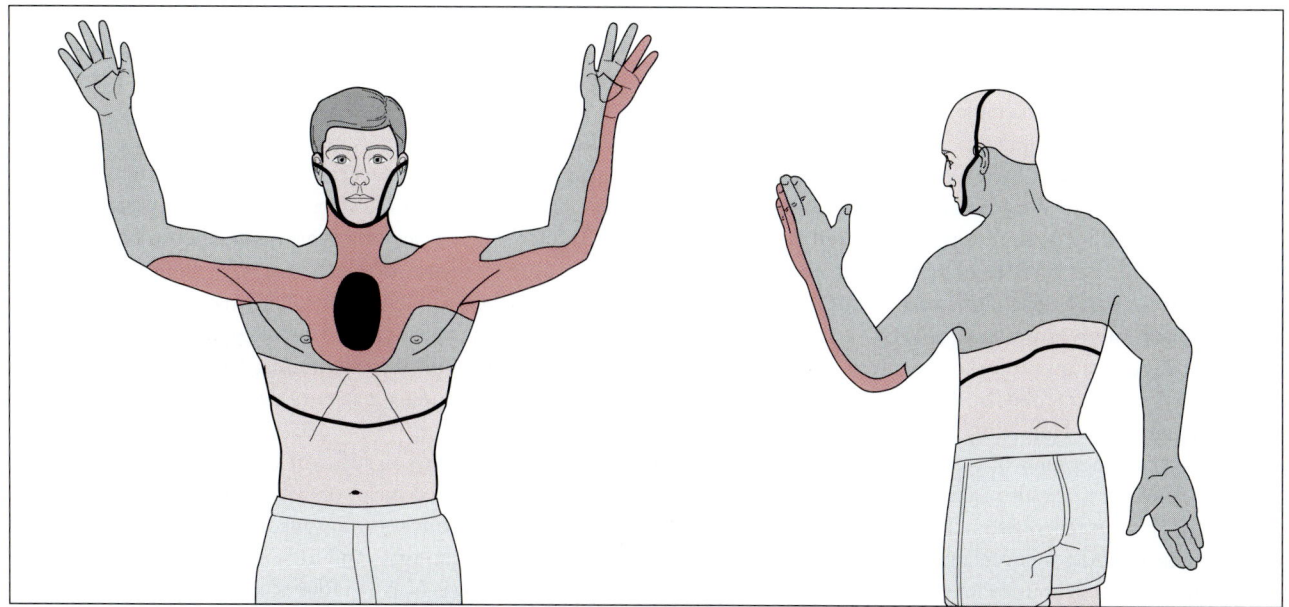

FIGURE 1 Location and radiation of ischemic pain. The black area represents the most frequent location of ischemic pain. Dark shading represents the most common sites of radiation, and light shading includes all but the rarest areas of sites of radiation (C3–T6). The heavy lines encompass the rarest sites of radiation (C2–T8). (From Rippee [17]; with permission.)

dial ischemic pain, atypical for but possibly caused by ischemic pain, or clearly unlikely to be ischemic in origin? Also, is the pain likely to be of a serious nature? Even typical angina pectoris does not always indicate serious coronary disease; rather, it may be associated with less threatening causes (*eg*, mitral valve prolapse, nonthreatening stable coronary disease). Alternatively, chest pain may be caused by other life-threatening conditions that require immediate attention (*eg*, aortic dissection, critical aortic stenosis, accelerating hypertension, pulmonary thromboembolism, pulmonary hypertension). After addressing these questions, the clinician can judge whether intensive care unit monitoring is warranted and what emergency procedures are required. In answering these questions, a careful history is the most important tool [3,4••].

Many episodes of myocardial ischemia and even MI are asymptomatic [5]. Others may be painless but provoke other symptoms such as profound weakness, severe diaphoresis, nausea, or malaise. These symptoms may be considered anginal equivalents and may alert the clinician to the correct diagnosis.

CHARACTERISTICS OF MYOCARDIAL ISCHEMIC PAIN

The location of myocardial ischemic pain is typically in the lower substernal area with radiation to either or both arms (more often the left than the right). Another typical site of radiation is to the anterior aspect of the neck or lower jaw. Ischemic pain rarely extends beyond the area from the pharynx and lower jaw to the epigastrium (C3–T6); the extreme possible limits are from the occiput to the epigastrium (C2–T8) (Fig. 1). In atypical presentations, myocardial ischemic pain may be localized in the jaw, teeth, mid or upper back, shoulder, elbow, or wrist, mimicking a dental or orthopedic problem. Ischemic pain is not so sharply localized, however, that its area can be covered by a fingertip. Sharply localized inframammary pain is particularly unlikely to be ischemic in origin. Chest pain that radiates from the sternum to the back or vice versa may indicate aortic dissection.

Ischemic pain is usually described as heavy or constricting (ranging from crushing to mild pressure). It may also be described as expansible or burning, but rarely as sharp or stabbing. The pain is "deep" and "visceral" and is commonly associated with sweating, dyspnea, nausea, and hiccupping.

Duration of ischemic pain is useful to distinguish it from pain of other causes. A single episode of transient myocardial ischemia (angina pectoris) usually lasts 2 to 20 minutes, with extremes of 30 seconds to over 1 hour. Lightening-like stabs are clearly nonischemic. Episodes of discomfort lasting over 20 to 30 minutes should raise suspicion of MI or unstable angina. Therefore, if a patient has suffered for months from multiple episodes of pain lasting hours at a time and fails to demonstrate electrocardiographic (ECG) evidence for recent or remote MI, the pain is unlikely to be ischemic in origin.

The time-intensity curve of the pain may give helpful information. Typically, angina pectoris builds in intensity for several to 30 minutes, then wanes and disappears over several additional minutes. The pain of acute MI also waxes over the course of minutes. Chest pain that abruptly reaches a maximum intensity is unusual in ischemic pain and should raise suspicion of aortic dissection.

Inciting factors of the pain are often important clues to the correct diagnosis. Physical effort is the usual inciting factor for a transient episode of myocardial ischemia caused by fixed coronary obstructive disease. Exertion is more likely to cause angina early in the morning and with use of the arms or isometric activity. For many patients, working with the arms above shoulder level is more likely to provoke angina than other activities. Emotional stress, exposure to cold, walking up

Evaluation of the Patient with Chest Pain

a grade or against the wind, and exertion after a large meal are other common initiating or contributing factors. Ischemic pain that develops at rest or wakes the patient from sleep is more suggestive of MI, unstable angina, or occasionally, coronary spasm (*ie*, variant angina).

Chest pain worsened by respiration is not ischemic. Such pain, brought on by a deep breath or cough, is usually sharp and either caused by pleural or pericardial inflammation or a chest-wall condition such as a fractured rib, costochondritis, or intercostal neuritis. Ischemic pain is not aggravated by a single motion of an arm, neck, or torso, and such a pattern strongly suggests a musculoskeletal cause. Pain that can be reproduced or worsened by local palpation is also not ischemic, although following MI, some patients may have local precordial tenderness of obscure cause.

Patterns of relief are also valuable in assessing the cause of chest pain. Prompt relief within 2 to 10 minutes of rest is most characteristic of effort-induced angina pectoris. A more gradual disappearance over 1 hour or longer is more typical of musculoskeletal pain. Occasionally, effort-induced ischemic pain disappears while the activity continues; this is known as *walk-through* or *second-wind angina*. Relief within several minutes of the administration of sublingual nitrates is characteristic of MI; however, the pain of spastic gastrointestinal disorders also has been noted occasionally to respond dramatically to nitrates. Prompt relief with induced bradycardia (as with a Valsalva's maneuver or carotid sinus pressure) is frequently described in angina pectoris. Relief with food or antacids suggests esophagitis or peptic disease. Partial relief by sitting forward is more typical of pericarditis or pancreatitis. Occasionally, pericarditis develops as a complication of MI, and these patients can have pericardial chest pain with both pleuritic and positional components.

ATYPICAL ANGINA PECTORIS AND NONISCHEMIC CHEST PAIN

Nonischemic chest pain syndromes include sharply localized pain, especially costochondral or inframammary; pain radiating outside the limits of C2 to T8; momentary "catches" or stabs of pain; pain incited by motion, respiratory effort, or local pressure; and recurrent, long-lasting, unabating pain (many hours to days) in the absence of ECG evidence of ischemia or infarction. A single convincing nonischemic feature should cancel several ischemic-like features if it is clearly part of the same chest-pain symptom complex.

Atypical angina pectoris is a phrase often used to refer to pain caused by myocardial ischemia with clinical features not typical of ischemic chest pain. Characteristics of a chest pain syndrome sometimes cannot be clearly classified as either nonischemic or typical for ischemia. Whether these patients are treated as coronary patients depends on the clinician's judgment.

The likelihood of significant coronary disease has been estimated at a pooled mean prevalence of 89% for all patients with chest pain typical for angina, 50% for those with chest pain atypical for angina, and 16% for all other subjects [6]. The prevalence was heavily influenced by age and gender (Fig. 2). The estimate of the prevalence of significant coronary disease has important implications for the interpretation of noninvasive tests for myocardial ischemia [7] (Figs. 3 and 4).

PHYSICAL EXAMINATION

The physical examination may be unremarkable during an episode of life-threatening myocardial ischemia or an evolving MI. More often, however, a careful physical examination provides useful clues to the diagnosis. For nonischemic causes of chest pain, it may help lead to the correct diagnosis. Cases of chest-wall tenderness, musculoskeletal disease, breast disease, thoracic outlet syndromes, or neurologic syndromes may be disclosed by abnormal physical findings. Disorders of the gastrointestinal tract often fail to provide characteristic findings; however, upper quadrant or epigastric tenderness or marked tympany suggests bowel distention or inflammation.

Cardiovascular examination may first call attention to a noncoronary cause for myocardial ischemia. The diagnosis of

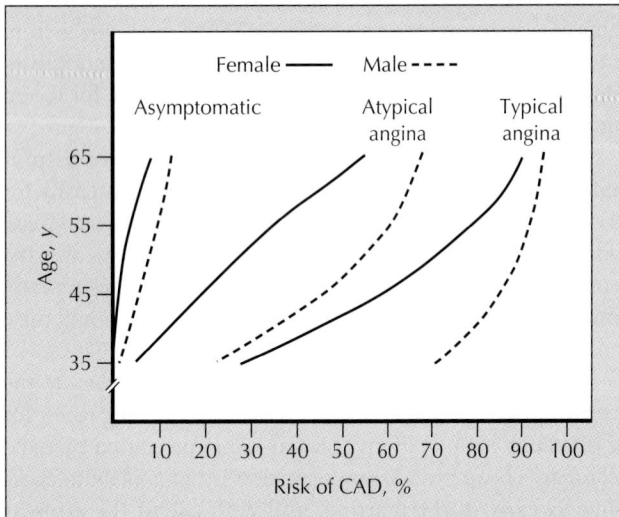

FIGURE 2 Influence of age, gender, and symptoms on risk of coronary artery disease (CAD). (*From* Epstein [7]; with permission.)

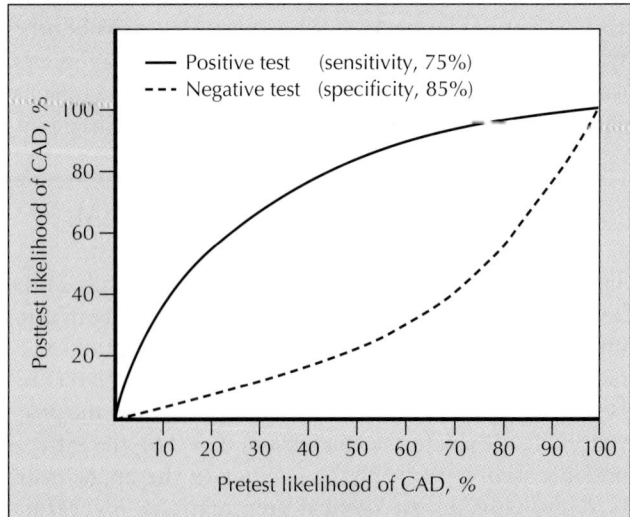

FIGURE 3 Influence of pretest likelihood of coronary artery disease (CAD) on the posttest likelihood of CAD for a test with 75% sensitivity and 85% specificity. (*From* Epstein [7]; with permission.)

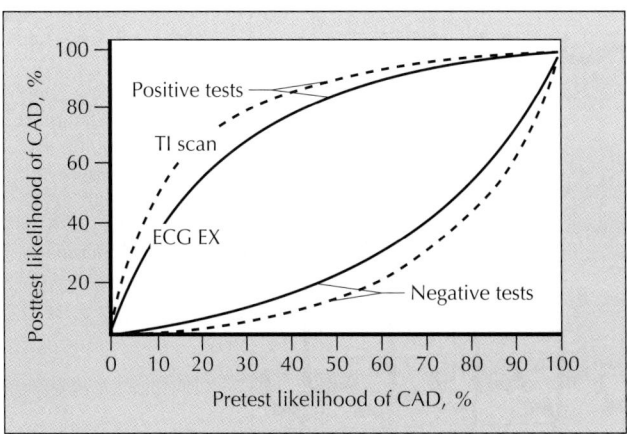

FIGURE 4 Influence of pretest likelihood of coronary artery disease (CAD) on the posttest likelihood of CAD for electrocardiographic exercise testing (ECG EX) and thallium perfusion scintigraphy (Tl scan). (*From* Epstein [7]; with permission.)

aortic dissection may be suggested by absent pulses or the inequality of blood pressure of the arms or legs. Suspicion of aortic dissection is heightened if aortic regurgitation or an enlarging pleural effusion exist. A late-peaking aortic systolic murmur associated with a diminished intensity of the second heart sound and a delayed carotid upstroke may provide the first clue to critical aortic stenosis. Hypertrophic cardiomyopathy also may be associated with angina pectoris in the absence of coronary occlusive disease and is likely to be manifested by a brisk carotid upstroke and a harsh systolic murmur at the left sternal edge, which typically increases with Valsalva's maneuver. The patient with mitral valve prolapse may be recognized by the characteristic nonejection click or mid to late systolic plateau or crescendo murmur at the apex or lower left sternal edge. Pericardial or pleural friction rubs may unmask underlying serosal inflammation. Friction rubs may occur with transmural MI or aortic dissection. Also, the presence of organic heart disease (*eg*, valvular lesion, hypertrophic cardiomyopathy) does not exclude concomitant CAD as a cause of the chest pain.

Although it is common for CAD to present without abnormal physical findings, it often gives evidence of ventricular dysfunction. The findings may present transiently during an episode of ischemia, or they may represent more prolonged changes caused by "stunned" myocardium or MI. Fourth heart sounds are ubiquitous in patients with significant symptomatic coronary disease, and they may become more prominent during ischemic episodes. Third heart sounds, paradoxically split second heart sounds, holosystolic murmurs, pulsus alternans, a fall in blood pressure, pulmonary congestion, pallor, as well as cold and clammy skin occasionally may be encountered during severe myocardial ischemia. Transient rises in blood pressure also may occur. Evidence for hypercholesterolemia (*eg*, xanthelasma, tuberous xanthoma) raises the suspicion of associated CAD, but does not confirm that the pain is ischemic. Femoral or carotid bruits or diminished peripheral pulses indicate the presence of atherosclerosis and, therefore, a higher likelihood of CAD. Arcus cornealis, earlobe creases, and hairy external auditory canals are nonspecific and of no diagnostic assistance.

Although tachycardia and tachypnea are nonspecific findings, they may be signs of left ventricular failure. Tachycardias may contribute to myocardial ischemia. Bradycardias often develop during the early stages of an inferior or posterior wall infarction.

During an acute ischemic episode, pulmonary congestion suggests a previously compromised left ventricle or severe ischemia involving a significant portion of the left ventricle. Severe ischemia may present dramatically as "flash" pulmonary edema in which the patient rapidly develops severe pulmonary congestion.

Dramatic presentations of ischemia with pulmonary edema, often with evidence of incipient shock, should alert the clinician to the possibility of a large MI or near-global ischemia. Left main coronary or very proximal left anterior descending obstruction, severe three-vessel disease, or severe aortic stenosis should be considered.

A rare physical finding of severe stenosis of the left main or left anterior descending coronary artery is an early to mid-diastolic high-pitched murmur; this is best heard along the left sternal border. It is produced by turbulent flow in the nearly obstructed coronary artery. The murmur is diastolic in timing, because flow in the left coronary system occurs predominantly in diastole. Because of its location and timing, this murmur is usually confused with that of aortic regurgitation.

ELECTROCARDIOGRAPHIC, RADIOLOGIC, AND ECHOCARDIOGRAPHIC STUDIES

Electrocardiography

Electrocardiography performed at rest and in the absence of stress or ongoing chest pain, is an insensitive test for the presence of CAD. Most patients with CAD have normal resting ECGs. The presence of Q waves may indicate previous MI but is not found in most patients with CAD. ST-T wave abnormalities, arrhythmias, and conduction abnormalities are nondiagnostic findings.

Aside from the history and physical examination, ECG is the most valuable tool for initial patient assessment during chest pain. Evidence for ischemia may be in the form of horizontal or downsloping ST-segment depression of at least 1 mm (Fig. 5), with or without abnormally inverted or peaked hyperkalemic-appearing T waves (Fig. 6). More subtle findings include nonspecific T-wave flattening or inversion, straightened ST segments, or inverted U waves (Fig. 7). These latter findings are nonspecific and only mildly support the diagnosis of possible myocardial ischemia.

Myocardial injury or MI usually causes ST-segment elevation with eventual development of abnormal Q waves. Reciprocal changes in the early to mid-precordial leads (V_1 through V_4) may represent true posterior-wall infarction. In all the multivariate analytic systems for the evaluation of chest pain, ECG plays a pivotal role. A normal ECG taken during an episode of chest pain is important testimony against ischemic disease, but it does not exclude ischemia or infarction. If the history and patient setting are suggestive, the diagnosis must be entertained despite a normal ECG.

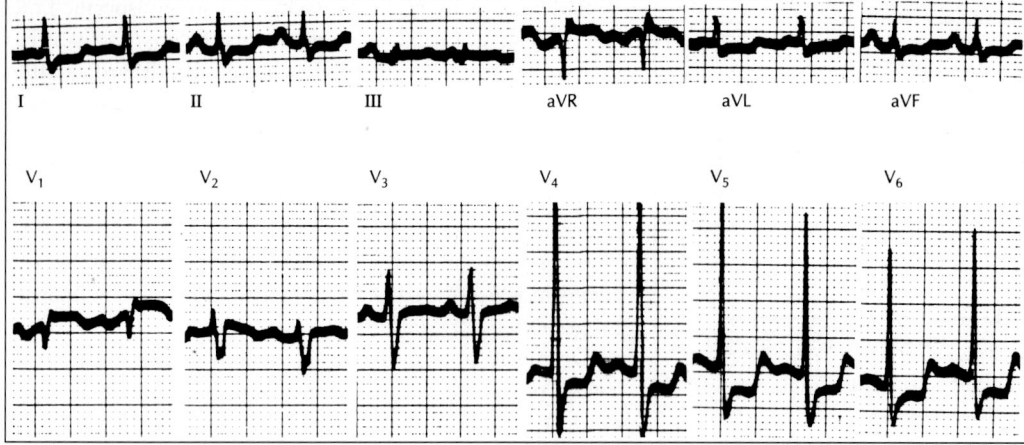

FIGURE 5 Exercise electrocardiogram demonstrating 2 to 3 mm of horizontal to downsloping ST segment depression in V_4 through V_6. (From Schamroth [18]; with permission.)

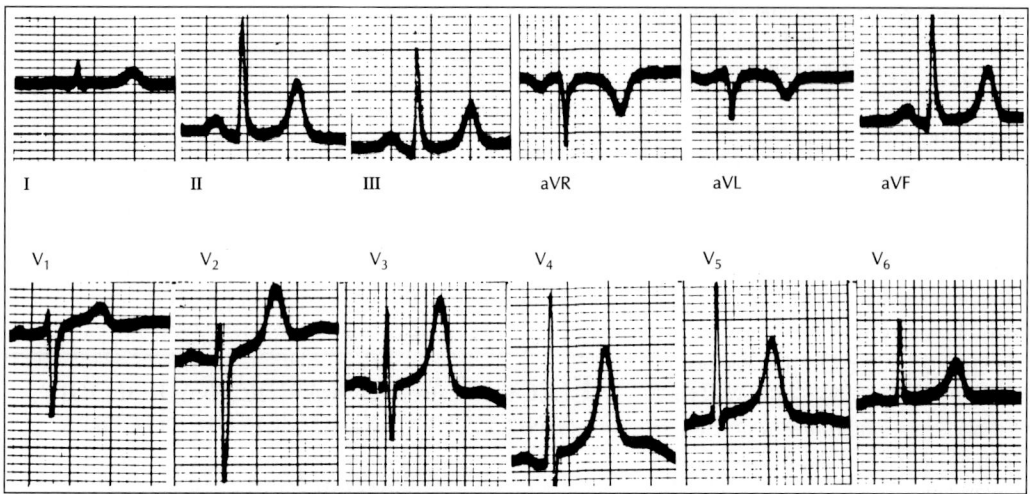

FIGURE 6 Electrocardiogram taken during ischemic chest pain demonstrates peaked T waves in II, III, aVF, and V_2 through V_6. (From Schamroth [18]; with permission.)

Electrocardiography may be helpful in supporting a diagnosis of acute pericarditis with diffuse ST elevations and possible PR-segment depression. Occasionally, the ECG suggests acute right ventricular strain, which in turn suggests a massive pulmonary embolism. In acute right ventricular strain, the QRS vector is often altered so that an S wave appears in lead I while a significant Q wave with T-wave inversion develops in lead III (S_1, Q_3, T_3 pattern of McGinn and White). T-wave inversion in leads II and aVF may also be present so that an inferior-wall MI is simulated. Inverted T waves in the right precordial leads (V_3 and V_4) may occur, but ST-segment deviations are absent or of small amplitude. Electrocardiography also may be valuable in the patient with chest pain by uncovering arrhythmias, conduction abnormalities, or hypertrophy patterns.

Chest Radiography

Chest radiographs are likely to be unremarkable during an acute ischemic episode or in an uncomplicated MI. Pulmonary vascular congestion, however, may occur in either. The heart shadow is usually normal. A large heart shadow during an ischemic episode or in the early stages of an infarct suggest antecedent myocardial damage, valvular disease, or pericardial effusion. Pulmonary infiltrates, pneumothorax, rib fractures, and metastatic lesions are other sources of chest pain that may be discovered by the chest film. A widened mediastinum on the posteroanterior view is nonspecific, but a normal mediastinal width makes aortic dissection much less likely.

Echocardiography

Echocardiography may be helpful in delineating the cause of

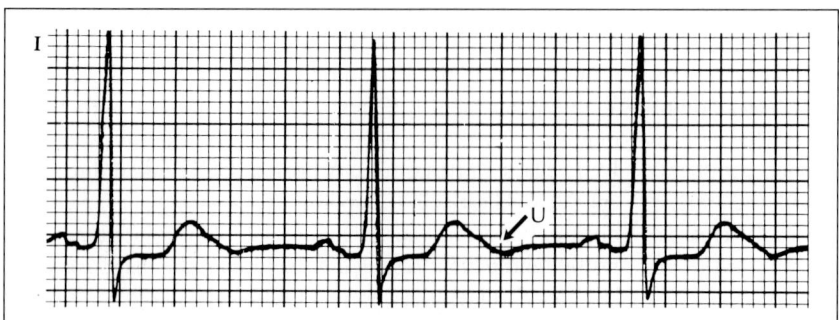

FIGURE 7 Electrocardiogram taken during ischemic chest pain demonstrates less than 1 mm horizontal ST depression associated with inverted U waves. (From Schamroth [18]; with permission.)

cardiac chest pain. A transthoracic echocardiogram may reveal wall-motion abnormalities during an episode of ischemic heart pain and in the early stages of MI, even when the ECG is still normal. Unsuspected valvular disease, pericardial effusion, widened aortic root, and occasionally, dissection of the ascending aorta may be demonstrated. A transesophageal echocardiogram is useful and accurate in the early diagnosis of aortic dissection [8].

LABORATORY STUDIES

Arterial blood gases or pulse oximetry are usually at normal levels in acute ischemic heart disease, unless significant left ventricular congestion or antecedent lung disease coexist. Hypoxia with associated hypocapnia are nonspecific findings common to pulmonary congestion, pulmonary embolism, and other acute respiratory problems.

A complete blood count may be valuable in the differential diagnosis of chest pain. Severe anemia is occasionally first manifested by angina. Acute MI and pulmonary embolism both may be associated with a modest granulocytosis; however, a markedly elevated leukocyte count (> 15,000/mL) with a shift to the left should raise suspicion of an infectious origin.

Evaluation of cardiac enzymes during the initial patient assessment may be helpful as well, but routine measurements of creatine kinase MB fraction are often normal in the early stages of an infarction. Use of a more sensitive immunochemical assay may allow the diagnosis or exclusion of infarction within 3 hours of presentation, when the initial creatine kinase MB is negative. Musculoskeletal causes of chest pain (*eg*, skeletal muscle injury, myositis, thoracic outlet syndrome) can be expected to raise the total creatine kinase level. The MB fraction of creatine kinase is often difficult to obtain in an emergency situation and is too often inaccurate.

EMERGENCY EVALUATION

In the initial diagnostic approach to the patient with recent or ongoing chest pain, emphasis is on rapid triage with simple but potent diagnostic tools. Central to the diagnostic effort is a careful, focused history with rapid determination of pertinent physical findings, ECG and monitoring, chest radiography when possible, and simple laboratory tests. Rapid determination is made of the presence of a true emergency. Even the possibility of a myocardial source for the pain makes the case a true medical emergency until proven otherwise. Administration of supplemental oxygen and placing of an intravenous line should be rapidly performed if myocardial ischemia or MI are reasonably possible causes. Rapid diagnosis of MI and exclusion of aortic dissection are even more important when considering thrombolytic therapy, rapid revascularization, or prompt surgical intervention.

If the patient presents in the absence of chest pain and with stable vital signs, the physician should first assess the likelihood of unstable and life-threatening coronary syndrome. The initial work-up is similar to that required in an emergency. Features of the pain that suggest instability should initiate a prompt and definitive evaluation in favor of hospitalization with monitoring and early coronary arteriography [9,10].

NONINVASIVE EVALUATION

If the patient's history of chest pain more likely represents stable angina pectoris or is less likely caused by serious coronary disease, the work-up can proceed on an outpatient basis with use of noninvasive procedures. Most of these procedures involve monitoring the ECG under either physiologic or pharmacologic stress. Simultaneous use of myocardial imaging techniques greatly improves the sensitivity, specificity, and predictive value of the tests. Selection of the most appropriate test depends on the patient's exercise capacity, ability to tolerate pharmacologic intervention, and especially the pretest likelihood of significant obstructive coronary disease.

The choice of a suitable noninvasive test for ischemic disease is decided by the predictive accuracy of the test for that patient. The predictive accuracy of the test is determined by the patient's pretest likelihood for coronary disease, which is determined by the patient's gender, age, chest-pain characteristics, family history, and other risk factors [7]. Angina pectoris is rare before 35 years of age, especially in women; however, its likelihood increases with each decade. Between ages 35 and 65 years, men have a higher likelihood of CAD; after age 65, it is distributed relatively equally among men and women. The presence and number of risk factors also increase the likelihood of disease. Combining these factors, the clinician can arrive at a level of suspicion (low, intermediate, or high) for CAD. Various tests for ischemia provide a degree of positive or negative confirmation of that pretest likelihood (*eg*, the posttest likelihood deviates to a greater degree from the pretest likelihood).

Exercise Treadmill Test

The exercise treadmill test (ETT) or simple exercise ECG with treadmill (or bicycle ergometry) has the lowest predictive accuracy [7] and the least ability to quantitate the severity of ischemia. ETT is more likely to be valuable in those with a normal resting ECG, because resting ST-T abnormalities or left bundle-branch block interferes with interpretation of the test. ETT is best reserved for those with a somewhat moderate or intermediate pretest likelihood of disease, in whom the probability of a false-negative result is also low. A positive test carries a chance of being falsely positive and may require further testing with myocardial imaging.

If a patient develops anginalike chest pain associated with horizontal or downsloping ST-segment depression of more than 1 mm, the likelihood of CAD is high. If the test is positive with marked ST depression at a low level of exercise, widespread ischemia is suggested. Other features of widespread ischemia are ischemic changes associated with a drop in blood pressure while exercise continues and prolonged postexercise ischemic changes. For such patients, cardiac catheterization is usually the next step.

A person with high pretest likelihood of CAD still has a moderate possibility of disease, even in the absence of ischemic changes on the ETT. If it is necessary to establish the diagnosis of CAD, this person will require more sensitive tests with myocardial imaging or even coronary arteriography.

Exercise Perfusion Scintigraphy

Exercise perfusion scintigraphy with thallium or sestamibi carries a better predictive accuracy than simple ETT. In the minute before termination of exercise, the radionuclide is injected into a peripheral vein. Myocardial imaging begins within minutes, either with standard planar scintigraphy or single-photon emission computed tomography. The initial images are compared with those taken 4 hours later when redistribution allows ischemic areas to take up the radionuclide. Scanning can be done 24 hours later with reinjection to improve sensitivity. This imaging method improves the image quality and allows improved quantitative analysis of perfusion defects [11]. A negative test, even in a patient with a high pretest likelihood of disease, decreases the possibility of myocardial ischemia considerably; other causes of chest pain should be strongly considered. Rarely is the pretest likelihood so compelling that other imaging techniques (eg, stress echocardiography, coronary arteriography) needed to exclude a false-negative nuclear test.

Dipyridamole Perfusion Scintigraphy

Dipyridamole perfusion scintigraphy is often useful in those patients who are unable to exercise adequately on a treadmill [12]. Dipyridamole causes maximum dilation of the coronary arteries. In the presence of significant CAD, coronary flow reserve is limited and disparities occur in the distribution of the thallium. Predictive accuracy is equivalent to an exercise scintigram. Patients with severe obstructive lung disease or asthma often cannot tolerate dipyridamole; in such patients, stress may be accomplished with dobutamine or adenosine.

Stress Echocardiography

Stress echocardiography can be accomplished with dipyridamole, dobutamine, or adenosine [13•]. Early results suggest excellent predictive accuracy. Treadmill or bicycle echocardiography also can be performed, but the exertion and hyperventilation involved may interfere with adequate transthoracic echocardiographic imaging.

Other Noninvasive Techniques

Other noninvasive techniques including positron-emission tomography [14] and 24-hour ambulatory ECG (Holter monitoring) [15] are occasionally useful in the evaluation of ischemic chest pain. Holter monitoring is too insensitive to be used routinely as a diagnostic test for ischemia, but it may be particularly valuable in patients who experience pain only at rest or are strongly suspected of having episodes of silent ischemia.

When the likelihood of a cardiac condition is excluded or considered unlikely, further work-up of recurrent chest pain of obscure origin depends on the special characteristics of the patient and the pain. Esophageal manometry with or without provocation, ambulatory 24-hour esophageal monitoring of pH, and psychologic testing may be in order for the few patients who continue to be uncomfortable and in whom simple measures to treat esophageal disease fail [16•].

Coronary Arteriography

The most reliable test for the diagnosis and quantitation of CAD is cardiac catheterization with selective coronary arteriography. Indications for coronary arteriography include chest pain suspicious for CAD undiagnosed by thorough noninvasive evaluation, chest pain thought to result from coronary disease but unresponsive to medical therapy, unstable angina, and postinfarction angina. The more unstable the angina, the more reasonable it is to use coronary arteriography early, even as one of the first diagnostic tests.

Coronary arteriography in at least two orthogonal views allows an excellent assessment of the extent of CAD as well as the potential for instability in the form of high-grade proximal stenoses, intraluminal thrombus, and ruptured or complicated plaques. Along with the patient's clinical course, this information is used to select medical therapy, angioplasty, or coronary artery bypass surgery in the management of the patient.

Conclusions

When a patient's chest pain has characteristics suspicious for myocardial ischemia and the patient's age, gender, and other risk factors make coronary disease possible, the clinician should exclude myocardial ischemia as a cause. If the characteristics suggest an unstable pattern of myocardial ischemia, the clinician should exclude acute or recent MI and assess the advisability of urgent antithrombotic therapy or the need for invasive diagnostic procedures. The patient's history, supported by simple physical examination and laboratory evaluation, is central to the process. The need for further consultation and more elaborate diagnostic procedures is determined by this initial evaluation. The more carefully the history is taken, the less likely it is that expensive procedures are ordered unnecessarily.

After the history, physical examination, and ECG, the choice of tests for diagnostic evaluation include ETT, ETT with imaging, and coronary arteriography. Imaging techniques with radionuclide or echocardiography greatly improve diagnostic accuracy. Although expensive, their use could limit the number of coronary arteriograms otherwise required.

References and Recommended Reading

Recently published papers of particular interest have been highlighted as:
- Of interest
- • Of outstanding interest

1. Richter JE, Bradley LA, Castell DO: Esophageal chest pain: current controversies in pathogenesis, diagnosis, and therapy. *Ann Intern Med* 1989, 110:66–78.
2.• Davies HA: Anginal pain of esophageal origin: clinical presentation, prevalence, and prognosis. *Am J Med* 1992, 92(suppl 5A):5S–10S.
3. Goldman L, Weinberg M, Weisberg M, *et al.*: A computer-derived protocol to aid in the diagnosis of emergency room patients with acute chest pain. *N Engl J Med* 1982, 307:588–596.
4.•• Lee TH, Juarez G, Cook EF, *et al.*: Ruling out acute myocardial infarction: a prospective multicenter validation of a 12-hour strategy for patients at low risk. *N Engl J Med* 1991, 324:1239–1246.
5. Cohn PF: Silent myocardial ischemia. *Ann Intern Med* 1988, 109:312–317.

6. Diamond GA, Forrester JS: Analysis of probability as an aid in the clinical diagnosis of coronary artery disease. *N Engl J Med* 1979, 300:1350–1358.

7. Epstein SE: Implications of probability analysis on the strategy used for noninvasive detection of coronary artery disease: role of single or combined use of exercise electrocardiographic testing, radionuclide cineangiography and myocardial perfusion imaging. *Am J Cardiol* 1980, 46:491–499.

8. Hashimoto S, Kumada T, Osakada G, *et al*.: Assessment of transesophageal Doppler echography in dissecting aortic aneurysm. *J Am Coll Cardiol* 1989, 14:1253–1262.

9. Pryor DB, Shaw L, Harrell FE Jr, *et al*.: Estimating the likelihood of severe coronary artery disease. *Am J Med* 1991, 90:553–562.

10. Lee TH, Ting HH, Shammash JB, *et al*.: Long-term survival of emergency department patients with acute chest pain. *Am J Cardiol* 1992, 69:145–151.

11. Mahmarian JJ, Boyce TM, Goldberg RK, *et al*.: Quantitative exercise thallium-201 single photon emission computed tomography for the enhanced diagnosis of ischemic heart disease. *J Am Coll Cardiol* 1990, 15:318–329.

12. Beller GA: Pharmacologic stress imaging. *JAMA* 1991, 265:633–638.

13.• Mazeika PK, Nadazdin A, Oakley CM: Dobutamine stress echocardiography for detection and assessment of coronary artery disease. *J Am Coll Cardiol* 1992, 19:1203–1211.

14. Demer L, Gould K, Goldstein R, *et al*.: Assessment of coronary artery disease severity by positron emission tomography: comparison with quantitative arteriography in 193 patients. *Circulation* 1989, 79:825–835.

15. Deanfield JE, Rubiero P, Oakley K, *et al*.: Analysis of ST segment changes in normal subjects: implications for ambulatory monitoring in angina pectoris. *Am J Cardiol* 1984, 54:1321–1325.

16.• Richter J: Overview of diagnostic testing for chest pain of unknown origin. *Am J Med* 1992, 92(suppl 5A):41S–45S.

17. *Intensive Care Medicine*, edn 2. Edited by Rippe JM. Boston: Little, Brown and Co.; 1992: 361.

18. *The Electrocardiology of Coronary Diseases*, edn 1. Edited by Schamroth L. Philadelphia: JB Lippincott; 1975.

SELECT BIBLIOGRAPHY

Constant J: The clinical diagnosis of non-anginal chest pain: the differentiation of angina from non-anginal chest pain by history. *Clin Cardiol* 1983, 6:11–16.

Rude RE, Pool WK, Muller JE, *et al*.: Electrocardiographic and clinical criteria for recognition of acute myocardial infarction based on analysis of 3697 patients. *Am J Cardiol* 1983, 52:936–942.

Sampson JJ, Cheitlin MD: Pathophysiology and differential diagnosis of cardiac pain. *Prog Cardiovasc Dis* 1971, 23:507–531.

Evaluation of the Patient with Heart Failure

Carl V. Leier

> **Key Points**
> - Heart failure is a clinical presentation of an underlying cardiovascular disorder or disease.
> - An effort should be made to diagnose the cause of heart failure, specifically to determine whether the heart failure is caused by a remedially reversible disorder or disease.
> - The medical history, a good cardiovascular examination, electrocardiogram, chest roentgenogram, and two-dimensional Doppler echocardiogram are the essential components of the initial evaluation of the heart failure patient.
> - Either cardiomegaly or a depressed ejection fraction alone is not indicative of inoperable underlying heart disease.
> - Unclear etiology, possible underlying reparable heart disease, symptomatic dysrhythmias and conduction disturbances, New York Heart Association (NYHA) functional class III and IV classification, unstable course, and the need for specialized cardiovascular testing should prompt cardiology consultation or referral to a heart failure–transplantation center.

Heart failure is one of the cardiovascular conditions that is not decreasing in frequency. As interventions for other cardiovascular disorders (*eg*, cardiac surgery and anesthesiology, antiarrhythmic approaches) have improved and as the mean age of the general population has risen, the overall prevalence of heart failure has increased.

This chapter discusses optimal care and management of the heart failure patient. Optimal patient care and cost-effective management are inseparable because proper evaluation and therapy for heart failure keep patients alive, employed, out of hospitals, and off transplant lists.

INITIAL EVALUATION

The patient with ventricular dysfunction can present in several ways. There may be no symptoms (*eg*, if the patient is referred for evaluation of an abnormal examination, chest roentgenogram, electrocardiogram [ECG], or echocardiogram) or there may be acute pulmonary edema or cardiogenic shock. A standard approach does not exist. Evaluation and therapy for each patient must be modified according to clinical presentation, acuity, and severity of heart failure; reversibility of the underlying disease process; and concomitant disease states. Nevertheless, general recommendations can be made to guide the optimal evaluation of the heart failure patient.

Medical History and Physical Findings

Important aspects of medical history

As in most conditions, the acuity and severity of symptoms determine the level of urgency in the evaluation and therapy for the patient with heart failure. A patient presenting with a 3-day history of orthopnea and 12 hours of resting dyspnea deserves more vigorous work-up and treatment than the patient with a 6-month history of steadily increasing pedal edema and easy fatigability, although both patients may ultimately undergo similar testing and often are placed on comparable long-term treatment.

Heart failure alone should never be considered a primary diagnosis. Heart failure is a symptom complex or syndrome; thus, it is always caused by some underlying cardiovascular disorder (*ie*, the primary diagnosis). On establishing the presence of heart failure by medical history and physical examination, the physician focuses on potential underlying causes, particularly reversible causes or those treatable with specific interventions (*eg*, coronary angioplasty-atherectomy and valvular repair or replacement). In general, intermittent symptoms of recent onset are more likely to be caused by reversible lesions (*eg*, occlusive coronary artery disease, ischemic papillary muscle dysfunction with episodic mitral regurgitation) than are long-standing symptoms. Although surgically treatable, chronic valvular stenosis or insufficiency often presents with long-standing symptoms. A history of major coronary risk factors (*eg*, smoking, diabetes mellitus, family history), concomitant angina pectoris, and intermittent or nocturnal symptoms should suggest occlusive atherosclerotic coronary artery disease and resultant disorders (*eg*, intermittent myocardial ischemia, diastolic or systolic dysfunction and papillary muscle dysfunction with mitral regurgitation). "Flash" pulmonary edema is usually caused by occlusive coronary artery disease, uncontrolled severe hypertension (often secondary to renal artery stenosis), periodic noncompliance to diet and drug therapy, or a combination of these factors.

Although a recent viral illness or influenza should raise the consideration of viral myocarditis in a patient with new onset heart failure, the symptoms of the viral event are often indistinguishable from those experienced during an episode of congestive heart failure. There is a paucity of evidence found through testing such as myocardial biopsy and serologic testing for a viral disease in most of these patients; however, the ability to diagnose postviral cardiomyopathy should improve as better diagnostic techniques are developed for viral infections and retrovirus alterations.

As many as 30% to 35% of patients with idiopathic dilated cardiomyopathy have a family history of cardiomegaly or heart failure [1], suggesting that some patients with dilated cardiomyopathy develop their illness by genetic transmission. However, until these defects are defined and biotechnologically correctable, the clinical approach to these patients is the same as that to other patients with dilated cardiomyopathy.

Increasing age, diabetes mellitus, and a history of systemic hypertension should suggest that diastolic dysfunction may play a pathophysiologic role, often the primary role, in the patient's heart failure.

Advancing age, clinical severity of heart failure, refractory response to optimal medical management, and a history of syncope or cardiac arrest are some of the major historical points that portend a less favorable prognosis [2••,3,4].

Key physical findings
The initial physical examination is generally directed at evaluating the extent and severity of heart failure and looking for clues for an underlying cause.

Indicators of extent and severity of heart failure
The severity and general character of a patient's heart failure are cumulatively assessed on physical examination by the presence and degree of a general appearance of well-being, anxiety or distress, pallor, cyanosis, tachypnea, Cheyne-Stokes respiratory pattern, tachycardia, pulsus alternans, pulsus paradoxus, narrow pulse pressure, systemic hypotension, hypokinetic and laterally displaced apical impulse, ventricular gallop sounds, murmurs, pulmonary rales, pleural effusion, elevated jugular venous pressure (if absent, hepatojugular reflux), hepatomegaly with or without tenderness and ascites, and pedal edema. It is important to record the initial (*ie*, baseline) positive and pertinent negative findings because they, along with symptoms, are the principal means of guiding therapy.

Clues for underlying cause of heart failure
Most patients with chronic congestive cardiac failure have evidence of both right and left heart failure. Patients with decompensated nonischemic dilated cardiomyopathy and patients with predominant right heart dysfunction (*eg*, cor pulmonale and right ventricular dysplasia) usually present with predominant signs of right heart failure, including jugular venous distention, hepatomegaly with or without ascites, or prominent peripheral edema. If the patient presents with predominant signs and symptoms of left heart failure, the primary considerations for differential diagnosis are systemic hypertension, occlusive coronary artery disease, and an aortic or mitral valvular disorder.

The presence of systemic atherosclerotic vascular disease suggests occlusive coronary artery disease as the cause of the patient's heart failure.

Systemic hypotension unrelated to drug therapy in the patient with adequate or high ventricular filling pressures suggests considerable cardiac dysfunction and an unfavorable prognosis; vasodilator and converting enzyme inhibitor therapy are often difficult to administer in such a patient. A recording of elevated blood pressure may be a consequence of the neurohormonal reaction to cardiac failure (particularly acute cardiac failure); however, long-standing or severe uncontrolled systemic hypertension is often a major contributor or is the predominant cause of cardiac decompensation. The patient with hypertensive heart failure usually responds favorably to proper antihypertensive, afterload-reducing therapy. Basically, hypertensive heart failure is easier to treat than hypotensive heart failure. The elevated systemic blood pressure of hypertensive heart failure gives the physician a wider range of blood pressure and afterload levels to work with during vasodilator or converting enzyme inhibitor therapy, and the elevated systemic blood pressure is treatable.

Several systemic illnesses are associated with cardiac disease and failure; a few include various neuromuscular disorders (*eg*, muscular dystrophy, myotonia dystrophia, Friedreich's ataxia) thyroid disease, acromegaly, and amyloidosis. The presence of a hyperdynamic precordium and circulation (tachycardia and bounding, full pulses) raises the possibility of high-output heart failure and the various causes, including anemia, hyperthyroidism, and arteriovenous malformations; most of these conditions are treatable.

Recording of body weight is an important guide to therapy.

Blood/Serum Studies

Every patient with heart failure should have a baseline complete blood count and measurement of serum electrolytes, urea nitrogen, creatinine, and magnesium. Hyponatremia, azotemia, and anemia of chronic disease are often indicative of a severe, advanced stage of heart failure. Other laboratory tests that may be indicated include sedimentation rate, C-reactive protein, and, occasionally, viral serology tests when myocarditis is suspected; coagulation studies (*ie*, prothrombin time, activated partial thromboplastin time, and platelet count) if anticoagulation therapy is anticipated; hepatic enzymes assessing the patient with severe heart failure and liver congestion; and arterial blood gas and pH in severe heart failure complicated by respiratory distress or problematic low cardiac output.

Chest Roentgenography

In addition to excluding unrelated but complicating conditions (*eg*, lung neoplasia) in a generally middle-aged to older population, the chest roentgenogram gives the physician a reasonable assessment of heart size, cardiac chamber enlargement, pulmonary congestion, and pleural effusion, and it can render clues regarding cause (Fig. 1). Along with the physical examination, the chest roentgenogram is the optimal (and least expensive) method of following heart size and pulmonary congestion during long-term management.

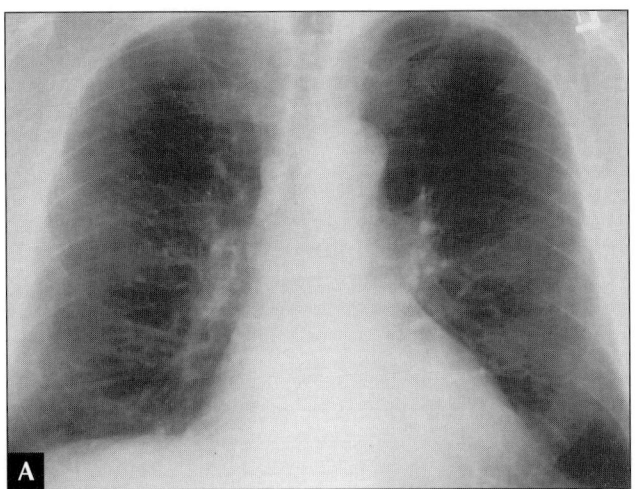
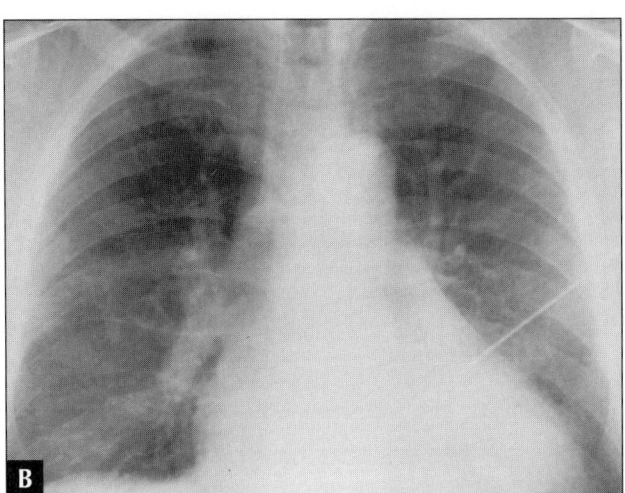
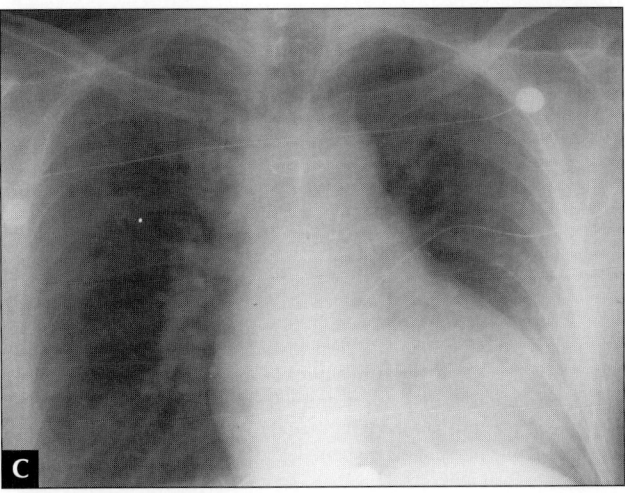
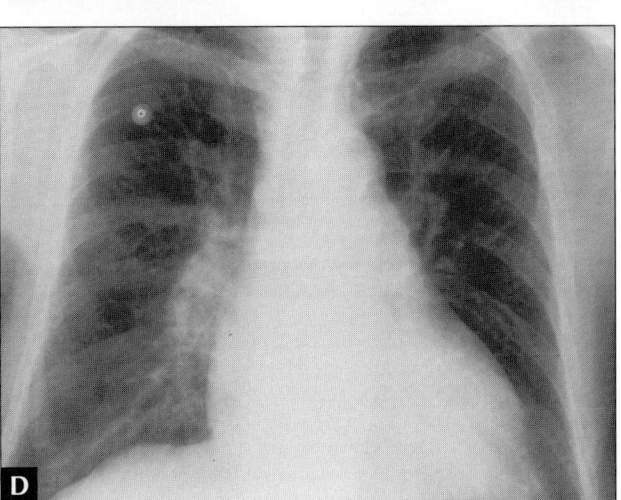

FIGURE 1 **A**, Relatively unremarkable chest roentgenogram of a 52-year-old tire dealer who presented at an emergency room 3 weeks earlier with acute "flash" pulmonary edema. At cardiac catheterization-angiography, high-grade obstructive lesions were noted along the proximal segments of the right coronary artery and left anterior descending coronary artery. **B**, Chest roentgenogram shows marked cardiomegaly, pulmonary venous engorgement, and pleural effusion of the base and minor fissure of the right chest; this 66-year-old salesman presented with decompensation of chronic heart failure secondary to nonischemic dilated cardiomyopathy. **C**, Moderate pulmonary edema on chest roentgenogram of a 49-year-old factory administrator who presented with a 9-month history of dyspnea on exertion, 4 hours of increasing dyspnea at rest, and chest "tightness." He had undergone coronary artery bypass surgery 8 years before this hospital admission. Electrocardiogram and cardiac enzyme analyses indicated an acute anterior myocardial infarction in the presence of a prior inferior wall infarction. **D**, Chest roentgenogram of a 78-year-old retired restaurant owner afflicted with 9 to 10 months of increasing dyspnea on exertion, orthopnea, and pedal edema. Mild to moderate left ventricular systolic dysfunction, marked biventricular diastolic dysfunction, and normal epicardial coronary arteries were noted at cardiac catheterization.

Electrocardiogram, Specialized Electrocardiographic Studies, and Electrophysiologic Testing

The ECG establishes the cardiac rhythm for the period of the test and provides clues regarding chamber enlargement and conduction disturbances (Fig. 2). Infarct patterns suggest occlusive coronary artery disease as the cause or contributing condition, although nonischemic cardiomyopathies are the most common disorders causing "pseudoinfarct" patterns. Some studies have found atrial fibrillation and left ventricular conduction defects to be some of the predictors of a poor outcome in heart failure [2••,3,4].

In the case of acute heart failure, an early ECG is invaluable in determining whether a patient might benefit from immediate thrombolytic therapy or urgent cardiac catheterization and angioplasty.

Although controversial, signal-averaged electrocardiography (SAE) appears to have little predictive power in nonischemic cardiomyopathy [2••,5]. The prognostic value in ischemic cardiomyopathy is probably better, but the information is of limited practical value because therapeutic interventions have not yet been shown to significantly alter the clinical course of the heart failure patient with an abnormal SAE [2••].

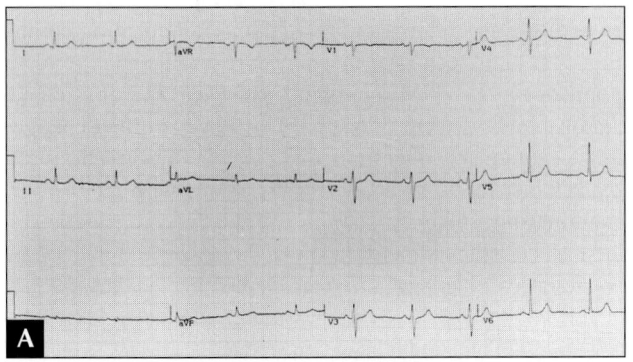

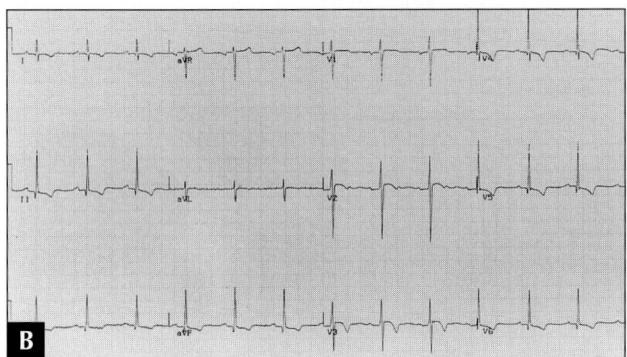

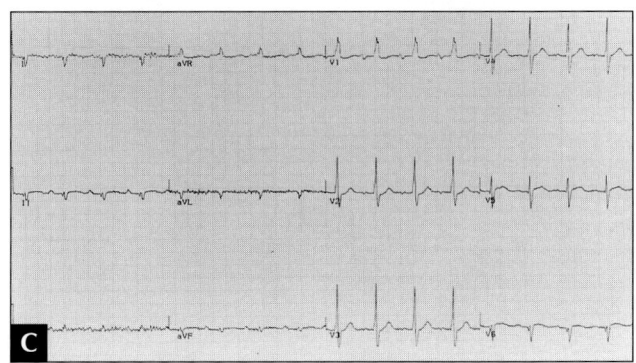

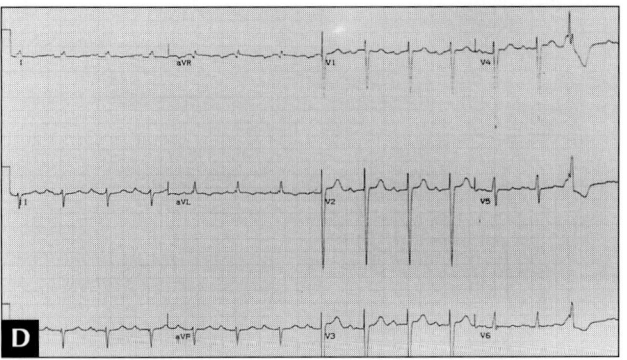

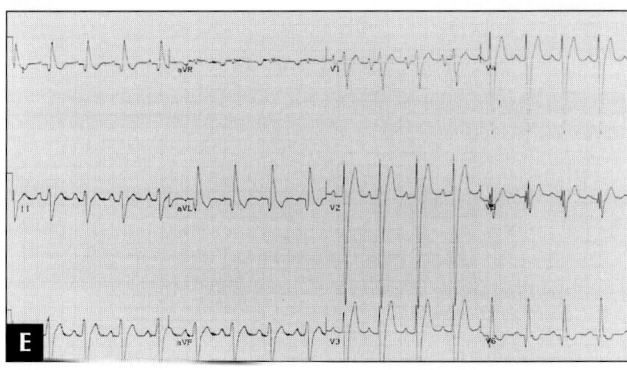

FIGURE 2 **A**, Normal electrocardiogram of a 68-year-old retired university professor who first presented with the sole complaint of 3 months of increasing dyspnea on exertion. Proximal high-grade obstructive coronary artery disease was noted at cardiac catheterization (see Fig. 4A). **B**, The electrocardiogram of a 52-year-old farmer with a 5-year history of increasing dyspnea on exertion, easy fatigability, and two episodes of severe decompensation (pulmonary edema). The left ventricular hypertrophy pattern noted on the electrocardiogram is a consequence of a 25- to 30-year history of inadequately controlled essential hypertension. **C**, Electrocardiogram of a 58-year-old laborer with a 3-week history of increasing weakness and pedal edema. Four weeks before admission, he experienced episodic severe chest pain and intermittent nausea and vomiting. The electrocardiogram shows an extensive posterolateral myocardial infarction, marked right axis deviation, and left posterior fascicular block. Physical examination, echocardiography, and cardiac catheterization further demonstrated moderate mitral regurgitation, elevated left and right ventricular end-diastolic and pulmonary artery pressures, depressed cardiac output, moderately increased left ventricular diastolic volume, and reduced ejection fraction (24%) secondary to a large akinetic zone involving the inferior, posterior, and lateral regions of the left ventricle. Complete occlusions of the proximal right coronary artery and left circumflex coronary artery were seen on coronary angiography. **D**, This electrocardiogram, showing biventricular enlargement, left axis deviation, a premature ventricular beat, abnormal P waves, and prolonged PR interval, was taken of a 42-year-old housewife with a 3-year history of progressively symptomatic dilated cardiomyopathy. She was referred for further treatment and transplantation evaluation. **E**, Myocardial dystrophy is the likely explanation for the electrocardiographic changes observed in this 20-year-old patient with Duchenne muscular dystrophy. Sinus tachycardia, abnormal P waves, left axis deviation, intraventricular conduction delay, lateral wall "pseudoinfarct" pattern, and biventricular enlargement are represented on the recording. In addition to musculoskeletal limitations, he had been afflicted with advancing symptoms and signs of heart failure for 3 to 4 years before this admission. He was dyspneic at rest and had orthopnea, hepatomegaly, and pedal edema on admission.

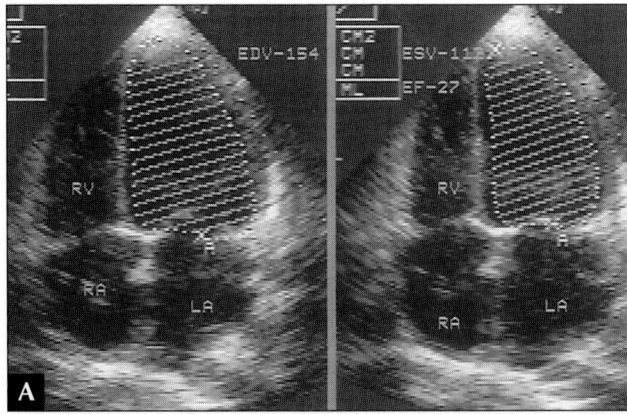
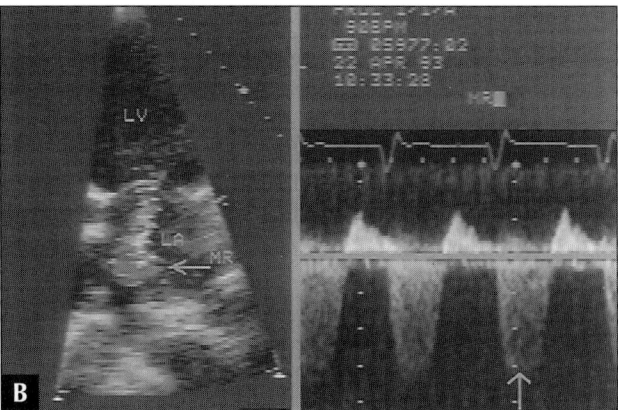
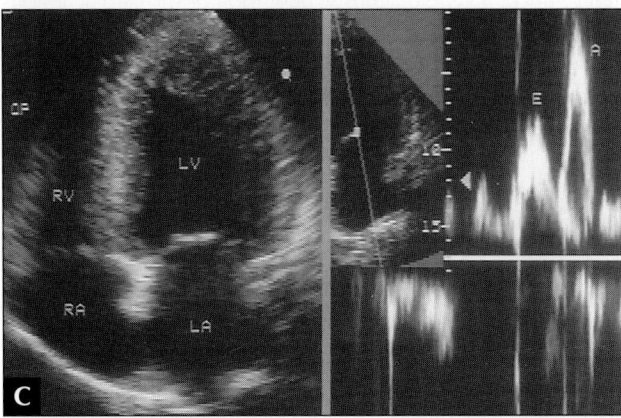

FIGURE 3 A, Two-dimensional echocardiographic apical four-chamber views in a 36-year-old patient who presented with congestive heart failure secondary to nonischemic dilated cardiomyopathy, demonstrating marked left ventricular (LV) enlargement and depressed systolic function with modest volume change from diastole (left) to systole (right). End-diastolic volume equals 154 cc; end-systolic volume, 111 cc; and ejection fraction (EF), 27%. **B**, Color Doppler (left) and continuous wave Doppler (right) images from a patient with dilated cardiomyopathy and considerable mitral regurgitation (arrows), which was barely audible on auscultation. (See Color Plate.) **C**, Two-dimensional apical four-chamber view of a 53-year-old patient with long-standing hypertension and heart failure demonstrating (left) marked concentric left ventricular hypertrophy (wall thickness, 1.5 cm; LV mass index, 154 g/m^2). Systolic function was normal (EF, 65%), but pulsed Doppler of mitral inflow (right) demonstrates markedly diminished early filling velocities (E) and enhanced atrial contribution to filling (A) consistent with considerable diastolic dysfunction. (See Color Plate.) (Courtesy of Anthony C. Pearson, Division of Cardiology, The Ohio State University.)

Continuous Holter ECG recordings are indicated in the heart failure patient with suspected symptomatic rhythm disturbances. These disturbances can manifest as periodic frequent ventricular ectopic beats with resultant drop in the effective ventricular rate, sustained ventricular tachycardia, torsades de pointes, bradycardia (sinus slowing or atrioventricular block), and atrial flutter or fibrillation. Holter recordings are not recommended as a routine component of the initial evaluation of the heart failure patient without arrhythmia-related symptoms, although several studies have shown that frequent ventricular ectopic beats portend a less favorable prognosis [2••,3–9]. Once again, therapies are not yet available to improve prognosis through the simple suppression of asymptomatic ventricular ectopy.

Electrocardiogram event recorders with memory (with or without transtelephonic link) are useful in assessing patients with infrequent, arrhythmia-induced symptoms.

Invasive electrophysiologic testing requires referral to a cardiologist (specifically, to a cardiac electrophysiologist) and is generally reserved for the heart failure patient troubled with sustained ventricular tachycardia [2••]. If the tachycardia is readily inducible during the electrophysiologic study, the procedure can then be used to determine (and follow) more selective antiarrhythmic intervention (*eg*, specific drug selection and antitachycardia or cardioverter-defibrillator device). An electrophysiologic study, often combined with upright-tilt testing, can be helpful in the evaluation of near-syncope or syncope when the cause for such has not been adequately defined by continuous ECG monitoring.

Echocardiography

Echocardiography is a pivotal diagnostic study in the initial evaluation of the heart failure patient. In addition to providing information on the size and function of the four heart chambers, echocardiography is the test of choice to determine whether mitral or tricuspid regurgitation (both can be inaudible on examination) and ventricular diastolic dysfunction play a role in the patient's presentation (Fig. 3).

Exercise Testing

For patients who can adequately relate their symptoms to the physician, exercise testing is not an essential component of the initial evaluation. However, exercise testing can be helpful in corroborating a patient's symptoms, following the patient's therapy, assessing a patient's candidacy for employment or cardiac transplantation, and prescribing an exercise conditioning program [4,10–15]. Expiratory gas analysis is also not essential, but this technique provides a more precise evaluation of exercise capacity and effort [13]. A maximal exercise oxygen consumption of more than 18 to 20 mL/kg/min suggests that the patient and therapy are doing reasonably well. Oxygen consumption of less than 14 mL/kg/min indicates severe impairment of exercise capacity and the need to consider a patient's candidacy for cardiac transplantation, particularly if the patient has been receiving optimal heart failure therapy [15].

Cardiac Catheterization-Angiography

Cardiac catheterization provides direct hemodynamic data (*ie*, right heart, pulmonary artery, and left ventricular filling pressures), an accurate assessment of ventricular diastolic function, and precise measurements required to derive certain hemodynamic parameters (*eg*, pulmonic and systemic vascular resistances and ventricular stroke work). Coronary angiography is used to define whether heart failure is secondary to occlusive coronary artery disease and to determine the potential for revascularization (Fig. 4). At most centers, cardiac catheterization-angiography requires referral to a cardiologist.

Most patients with heart failure deserve strong consideration for a diagnostic cardiac catheterization-angiography before their condition is declared irreparable. It is often impossible to distinguish nonischemic from ischemic forms of cardiac failure, and unless a reversible cause for heart failure is found, congestive heart failure has a grim long-term prognosis. An ejection fraction of 0.25 or less is no longer considered a contraindication to a revascularization procedure because revascularization can be effective in reversing such a patient's ventricular dysfunction and heart failure if reversible myocardial ischemia, rather than infarction, is causing the ventricular dysfunction (Fig. 4) [16••].

Patients with another end-stage illness limiting their overall clinical course and survival (*eg*, metastatic malignant neoplasia) and elderly patients who are not likely to survive a major surgical procedure may not benefit greatly from cardiac catheterization-angiography.

Patients who present with acute heart failure are more likely to have a remedially reparable cardiac lesion compared with patients with more chronic forms of heart failure. For patients presenting with acute pulmonary edema or cardiogenic shock, precise diagnostic definition of the cardiac lesions and urgent, specific intervention (*eg*, angioplasty and valvular repair or replacement) offer the optimal and, often, the only means of improving an otherwise dismal clinical course and reduced survival [17,18].

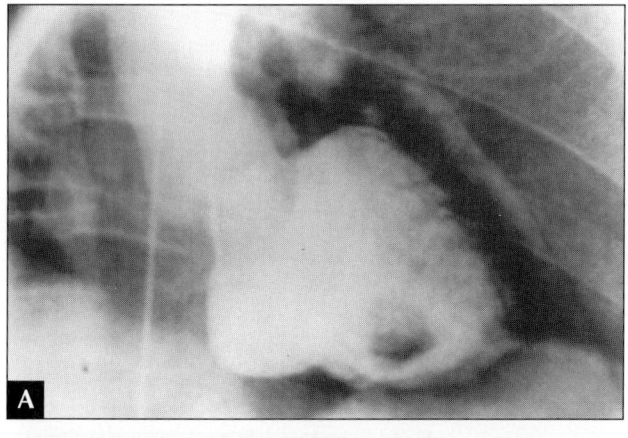
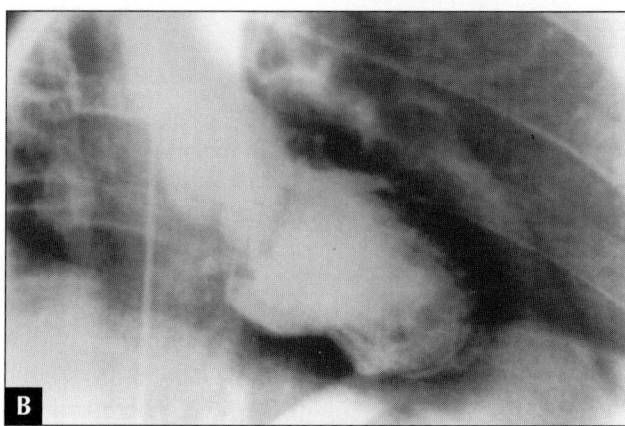
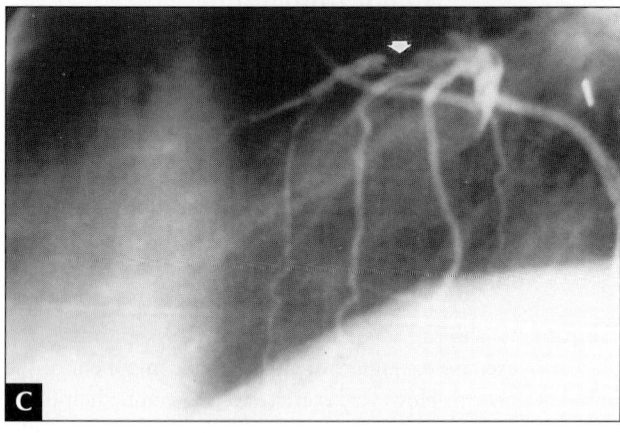
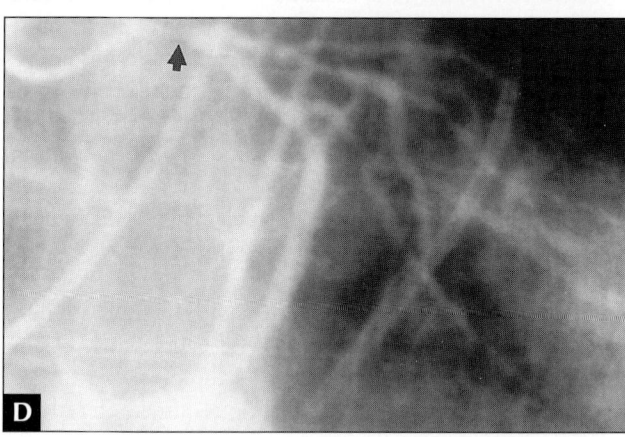

FIGURE 4 **A** through **C**, Angiographic frames of the patient presented in Figure 2A. Coronary artery bypass surgery was successful in bringing this patient from relative physical inactivity before surgery to a daily 2-mile run or 2000-yard swim within 9 months of his surgery. **A**, Contrast injection of left ventricle in diastole. Some chamber enlargement is present. **B**, Considerable anterior and apical hypokinesis are demonstrated in this end-systolic frame. The hypokinetic regions demonstrated thallium redistribution, indicating viable hibernating myocardium. The preoperative ejection fraction of 0.28 rose to 0.48 six months after surgery. **C**, Left lateral view of a left coronary artery injection demonstrating an occlusive lesion of the proximal left anterior descending coronary artery (arrow). Scattered plaques were noted along the proximal right coronary artery. The patient did not recall ever experiencing angina pectoris. **D**, Left coronary injection of a 76-year-old man who went to his local emergency room on two occasions with severe dyspnea, weakness, roentgenographic pulmonary edema, and transient electrocardiographic anterior ischemic changes. A high-grade obstructive lesion is present in the left main coronary artery (arrow) with additional obstructive disease in the proximal left anterior descending artery. A nondominant right coronary artery was completely occluded. He remains symptom-free (receiving only daily aspirin) with increased physical activity 18 months after coronary bypass surgery.

Myocardial Biopsy

Without specific, proven-effective therapy as an end point for obtaining a specific diagnosis, there are no absolute indications for performing an endomyocardial biopsy in heart failure. On the other hand, transvenous endomyocardial biopsy is the best way of diagnosing or confirming several pathogenic cardiac conditions, including myocarditis, Löffler's eosinophilic endocarditis, amyloidosis, and other inflammatory and infiltrative disorders [19]. If any of these conditions is suspected, referral to a cardiologist skilled in the management of heart failure and the performance of the endomyocardial biopsy should be considered. Corticosteroid or any immunosuppressive therapy is not empirically indicated (*ie*, without an endomyocardial biopsy) for a patient who presents with dilated cardiomyopathy and suspected myocarditis. Most of these patients do not have myocarditis, and the risk–benefit ratio of empiric corticosteroid or any other immunosuppressive therapy in cardiomyopathic heart failure likely exceeds that of an endomyocardial biopsy and directed therapy. The endomyocardial biopsy is an important tool in heart research and is the principal means of following cardiac rejection after transplantation.

Pharmacohemodynamic Evaluation

Patients with apparently refractory heart failure should generally undergo intense pharmacohemodynamic study before being placed on a cardiac transplant list or being declared to have terminal, refractory congestive heart failure [10,20,21•]. Such patients should be referred to a comprehensive heart failure center to take advantage of expertise in the use of standard heart failure medication, pharmacohemodynamic evaluation of standard and experimental agents, therapeutic application of experimental compounds, and assessment and treatment of transplant candidates.

General clinical indications for the application of pharmacohemodynamic testing in the initial evaluation of the advanced heart failure patient include the following:

- When the status of ventricular preload and afterload at rest and during exercise cannot be determined with certainty from clinical examination and other laboratory data
- When a potentially effective drug has a greater than average potential for adversely affecting hemodynamics and clinical status
- When determination of the most effective drug or its optimal dose is necessary to treat a patient with severely compromised congestive heart failure.

The pharmacohemodynamic approach and protocols vary by center [12,20,21•]. They must often be modified for each heart failure patient.

Other Testing Modalities

Radionuclide studies

Resting or exercise radionuclide perfusion studies (*eg*, thallium studies) can help in determining myocardial viability in patients who present with occlusive coronary artery disease complicated by congestive heart failure. A patient with operable occlusive coronary artery disease and a substantial amount of viable myocardium should be considered for a revascularization procedure. Magnetic resonance spectroscopy and positron-emission tomography scanning are being developed to enhance our ability to distinguish viable from nonviable myocardium in patients with heart failure [22•].

Although rest and exercise radionuclide angiography does not add much information to that obtained from rest and exercise echocardiography, the right and left ventricular ejection fraction values from radionuclide angiography are regarded as more accurate.

Pulmonary function studies

Dyspnea and related symptoms of many patients are secondary to combined cardiac and pulmonic disease. After a patient's heart failure is optimally treated, pulmonary function studies (*ie*, lung volumes, flow rates, maximal ventilation, and diffusing capacity) are indicated in patients with any clinical evidence (*eg*, history of smoking, findings on physical examination) of lung disease. For patients with reduced expiratory flow rates, bronchodilators should be tested to determine the reversibility of impaired flow rates and whether certain patients need bronchodilators as part of their overall therapeutic plan.

FOLLOW-UP EVALUATION

The outpatient care of the patient with heart failure is facilitated by patient (and spouse) participation in the day-to-day management of the condition by recording daily weights at home, promptly reporting new or worsening symptoms to the physician's office continually learning about the condition and treatment, and, if feasible, joining a support group of heart failure patients.

General Clinical Evaluation

An immense amount of information can be quickly attained by observing the patient and spouse (or close family member or friend) during the initial greeting. A favorable or steady course and an unfavorable course (*eg*, worsening or new symptoms) can be sensed by the physician, then verified by further questioning and cardiovascular examination. The clinical impression extracted from this initial brief contact generally guides the direction, activities, and intensity of the outpatient visit.

The standard clinical question, "How are you doing?" is a reasonable way to start a focused recent medical history. Further questioning is then directed at the patient's (or spouse's) response, the course of prior symptoms, activity and sleep patterns, outpatient body weight recordings, dietary issues, and medications.

The focused follow-up cardiovascular examination in heart failure includes assessment of body weight, supine and upright heart rate and blood pressure, estimation of jugular venous pressure (with or without hepatojugular reflux), palpation of carotid pulses and precordium, auscultation for the presence and intensity of gallop sounds and murmurs (particularly mitral and tricuspid regurgitation), palpation and measurement of the liver (vertical span along the right clavicular line), and palpation of the legs and ankles for edema and tenderness. General appearance and the respiratory rate pattern are gleaned from the patient during the examination. A careful lung examination for rales and pleural effusion follows a history of dyspnea at rest, increasing dyspnea, tachypnea, weight gain, and the finding of rales or effusion during a prior examination.

At this point, the clinician has most of the information needed to adjust the patient's activities, diet, and medication, order additional laboratory studies, and determine the timing of the subsequent visit. If the patient has recently experienced an unfavorable course, the decision is made to alter outpatient management or to admit the patient to the hospital.

Follow-up Laboratory Testing

A standard schedule of outpatient laboratory testing cannot satisfy the clinical needs of most patients with ventricular dysfunction and heart failure. Follow-up laboratory testing is best individualized to avoid inappropriate risk, expense, and use of laboratory time and resources for a low yield of useful information and clinical benefit. Common sense is the guiding principle. However, routine or common tests are necessary for patients receiving certain medications (eg, anticoagulation therapy) or are occasionally useful for patients with more symptomatic or advanced stages of heart failure.

Chronic stable mild heart failure (NYHA functional class I or II)

Patients in the NYHA class I or II category require fewer outpatient visits and less laboratory testing. After a stable course is achieved, an occasional (eg, every 6 to 12 months) serum potassium and urea nitrogen (or creatinine) determination is usually the maximal laboratory requirement. A chest roentgenogram to follow heart size or an echocardiogram to determine chamber size and function is reasonable at greater than 12-month intervals.

Chronic moderate to severe heart failure (NYHA functional class III or IV)

Patients with NYHA functional class III or IV heart failure require more frequent follow-up visits than patients with milder heart failure. As the severity of heart failure increases, symptoms and complications escalate in frequency and intensity, the overall clinical condition becomes more unstable, and the medication requirements and side effects increase. Functional class III or IV patients are generally seen in the outpatient setting at 2-week to 3-month intervals, with serum potassium and urea nitrogen (or creatinine) determinations made every 1 to 4 months. To avert hospitalization during a relatively unstable period, more frequent visits (as many as 1 to 2 per week) and laboratory testing may be required. Determining serum sodium and magnesium concentrations is informative in patients with advanced heart failure who are receiving vigorous diuretic therapy but is rarely required more than once every 2 to 3 months. Unless the patient enters an unstable decompensated phase, optimal outpatient management includes an annual echocardiogram to assess cardiac chamber size and function and the degree of mitral and tricuspid regurgitation and an annual chest roentgenogram to assess heart size.

With effective history taking, intermittent exercise testing is not essential for the optimal treatment of most patients with chronic heart failure. However, exercise testing can assist in the evaluation of symptoms, clinical course, and therapeutic plan of patients who do not convey meaningful, consistent, or interpretable information about their symptoms. An exercise study can also be useful for the following: assessing a patient with symptoms disparate from clinical or other laboratory findings, determining a prescription for or the effectiveness of a physical conditioning program, following a major change in therapy, and evaluating whether a patient should continue or seek employment, apply for employment disability, or undergo evaluation for cardiac transplantation [10–15].

The exercise protocol (eg, maximal treadmill, 6-minute walk) is less important than ensuring that sequential studies are performed similarly by the same laboratory and that the managing physician is in attendance if symptom corroboration and effort-motivation are issues of concern. Patients rarely perform maximal exercise in the home or work setting, but a maximal exercise performance study (treadmill or upright bicycle) is preferred. The study uses oxygen consumption, symptoms (Borg scale) and heart rate at set submaximal levels, and exercise duration with peak oxygen consumption at maximal exhaustive exercise as study end points. The respiratory quotient and anaerobic threshold are objective indicators of adequate effort. Treadmill and bicycle exercise are not appropriate surrogates for all the physical activities of a patient; therefore, the mode of exercise testing may have to be modified to recreate heart failure symptoms primarily associated with specific activity (eg, arm ergometry for a commercial painter who is symptomatic only while working).

Certain patients require other testing modalities to address specific complaints and problems. For example, Holter or event ECG recordings should be considered in the heart failure patient with palpitations and near-syncopal episodes, and ECG should be considered in a patient with a recent change in cardiac rhythm or a recent episode of prolonged angina, and a repeat cardiac catheterization or coronary angiography should be considered in a heart failure patient whose remote catheterization showed nonocclusive coronary lesions but now presents with angina or angina-equivalent symptoms.

Decompensation

The patient whose symptoms are escaping a previously effective therapeutic plan deserves special, more intense consideration and, often, referral to a cardiologist or heart failure center.

After review of the patient's symptoms, inquiries should be made into changes in personal and home situations. Family or marital difficulties, financial problems, dietary alterations or indiscretions, and intentional or inadvertent changes in medications or dosing schedule often provide clues for the mechanisms of the clinical deterioration. A focused cardiovascular examination is then performed to establish physical evidence of clinical deterioration (eg, body weight, level of jugular venous distention, liver size, rales, pedal edema) and to reveal complications of heart failure (eg, new onset atrial fibrillation, recent development of mitral regurgitation) that may explain or significantly contribute to the deteriorating course. Decompensation is not uncommonly precipitated by noncardiovascular conditions (*eg*, respiratory infection and recent addition of a nonsteroidal antiinflammatory drug).

If the explanation for the unfavorable course is not apparent from history and physical examination and to further assess the extent of decompression, laboratory testing is indicated and generally includes assessment of serum electrolytes, urea nitrogen, creatinine, complete blood count and, occasionally, hepatic enzymes; chest roentgenogram to evaluate heart size and degree of pulmonary congestion; and two-dimensional Doppler echocardiography to assess changes in chamber size and function and the presence and degree of mitral and tricuspid regurgitation.

If the patient's deteriorating clinical condition is threatening or does not respond in a reasonable time (1 to 3 days) to a rational change in therapy, the patient should be hospitalized for monitored observation, intravenous therapy directed at improving symptoms and the patient's cardiovascular status (*eg*, intravenously administered diuretics, vasodilators, or dobutamine), and possibly additional diagnostic studies.

If the decompensation was caused by development of refractoriness to apparently optimal therapy or by deterioration of the underlying cardiac disease process, the patient may benefit from pharmacohemodynamic assessment to 1) determine why a patient is not responding to therapy as well as expected (*eg*, tolerance, excessive or ineffective dosing), 2) evaluate the evolution of new cardiovascular symptoms that may be drug- or dose-related, 3) assess the status and course of the underlying cardiovascular condition, and 4) advance the medical management by optimizing drug and dose selection. A more effective therapeutic plan can usually be determined from pharmacohemodynamic evaluation [10,20,21•]. The failure to achieve such portends a poor prognosis and the need to consider cardiac transplantation.

EVALUATING THE CARDIAC TRANSPLANTATION CANDIDATE

The complete evaluation of the heart failure patient for cardiac transplantation is best done via referral to a heart failure or transplantation specialist. Nevertheless, the referring internist or cardiologist can greatly assist in the preliminary assessment of the transplantation candidate. Basically, the typical candidate approved as a transplant recipient is a person younger than 60 years of age (65 years or younger at some centers) with symptomatic advanced heart failure refractory to optimal therapy. The patient is in otherwise good health without a chronic infection, infectious source, major chronic disease, or terminal illness. Compliance to physician and nurse instructions, stable psychological make-up, and an intact familial and social support structure are other important favorable features of an acceptable transplant-recipient candidate.

REFERENCES AND RECOMMENDED READING

Recently published papers of particular interest have been highlighted as:
- Of interest
- •• Of outstanding interest

1. Unverferth DV, Wooley CF: Familial dilated cardiomyopathy. In *Dilated Cardiomyopathy*. Edited by Unverferth DV. Mt. Kisco, NY: Futura Publishing Co.; 1985:159–165.

2.•• Leier CV: The cardiomyopathies: mortality, sudden death, and ventricular arrhythmias. In *Cardiovascular Clinics: Contemporary Management of Ventricular Arrhythmias*. Edited by Greenspon AJ, Waxman HL. Philadelphia: FA Davis Co.; 1992:275–306.

3. Unverferth DV, Magorien RD, Moeschberger ML, *et al.*: Factors influencing the one-year mortality of dilated cardiomyopathy. *Am J Cardiol* 1984, 54:147–152.

4. Willens HJ, Blevins RD, Wrisley D, *et al.*: The prognostic value of functional capacity in patients with mild to moderate heart failure. *Am Heart J* 1987, 114:377–382.

5. Gonska B, Bethge K, Figulla H, *et al.*: Occurrence and clinical significance of endocardial late potentials and fractionations in idiopathic dilated cardiomyopathy. *Br Heart J* 1988, 59:39–46.

6. Meinertz T, Hofmann T, Kasper W, *et al.*: Significance of ventricular arrhythmias in idiopathic dilated cardiomyopathy. *Am J Cardiol* 1984, 53:902–907.

7. Holmes J, Kubo SH, Cody RJ, *et al.*: Arrhythmias in ischemic and nonischemic dilated cardiomyopathy: prediction of mortality by ambulatory electrocardiography. *Am J Cardiol* 1985, 55:146–151.

8. Hofmann T, Meinertz T, Kasper W, *et al.*: Mode of death in idiopathic dilated cardiomyopathy: a multivariate analysis of prognostic determinants. *Am Heart J* 1988, 116:1455–1463.

9. Stevenson LW, Fowler MB, Schroeder JS, *et al.*: Poor survival of patients with idiopathic cardiomyopathy considered too well for transplantation. *Am J Med* 1987, 83:871–876.

10. Leier CV: Cardiovascular testing procedures in the evaluation and management of chronic congestive heart failure. In *Diagnostic Procedures in Cardiology*. Edited by Warren JV, Lewis RP. Chicago: Year Book Medical Publishers; 1985:390–396.

11. Franciosa JA, Ziesche S, Wilen M: Functional capacity of patients with chronic left ventricular failure. *Am J Med* 1979, 67:460–466.

12. Leier CV, Huss P, Magorien RD, *et al.*: Improved exercise capacity and differing arterial and venous tolerance during chronic isosorbide dinitrate therapy for congestive heart failure. *Circulation* 1983, 67:817–822.

13. Weber KT, Kinasewitz GT, Janicki JS, *et al.*: Oxygen utilization and ventilation during exercise in patients with chronic cardiac failure. *Circulation* 1982, 65:1218–1223.

14. Meiler SEL, Ashton JJ, Moeschberger ML, *et al.*: An analysis of the determinants of exercise performance in congestive heart failure. *Am Heart J* 1987, 113:1207–1217.

15. Mancini DM, Eisen H, Kussmaul W, *et al.*: Value of peak exercise oxygen consumption for optimal timing of cardiac transplantation in ambulatory patients with heart failure. *Circulation* 1991, 83:778–786.

16.•• Louie HW, Laks H, Milgalter E, *et al.*: Ischemic cardiomyopathy criteria for coronary revascularization and cardiac transplantation. *Circulation* 1991, 84(suppl III):290–295.

17. Lee L, Bates ER, Pitt B, *et al.*: Percutaneous transluminal coronary angioplasty improves survival in acute myocardial infarction complicated by cardiogenic shock. *Circulation* 1988, 78:1345–1351.

18. Goldberger JJ, Peled HB, Stroh JA, *et al.*: Prognostic factors in acute pulmonary edema. *Arch Intern Med* 1986, 146:489–493.

19. Starling RC, Unverferth DV: Value of endomyocardial biopsy: indications and applications. In *Progress in Cardiology*. Edited by Zipes DP, Rowlands DJ. Philadelphia: Lea and Febiger; 1989:33–41.

20. Stevenson LW, Dracup KA, Tillisch JH: Efficacy of medical therapy tailored for severe congestive heart failure in patients transferred for urgent cardiac transplantation. *Am J Cardiol* 1989, 63:461–464.

21.• Haas GJ, Leier CV: Invasive cardiovascular testing in chronic congestive heart failure. *Crit Care Med* 1990, 18:51–54.

22.• Mody FV, Brunken RC, Stevenson LW, *et al.*: Differentiating cardiomyopathy of coronary artery disease from nonischemic dilated cardiomyopathy utilizing positron emission tomography. *J Am Coll Cardiol* 1991, 17:373–383.

SELECT BIBLIOGRAPHY

ACC/AHA Guidelines Committee: American College of Cardiology/American Heart Association Guidelines for the Management of Heart Failure. Dallas, TX: American Heart Association; 1994.

Braunwald E, Grossman W: Clinical aspects of heart failure. In *Heart Disease*. Edited by Braunwald E. Philadelphia: WB Saunders; 1992:444–463.

Cohn JN: Approach to the patient with heart failure. In *Textbook of Internal Medicine*, edn 2. Edited by Kelley WN. Philadelphia: JB Lippincott; 1992:340–347.

Leier CV: The cardiomyopathies: mortality, sudden death and ventricular arrhythmias. In *Contemporary Management of Ventricular Arrhythmias, Cardiovascular Clinics 22/1*. Edited by Greenspon AJ, Waxman HL. Series Editor-in-Chief, Brest AN. Philadelphia: FA Davis; 1992:275–306.

Evaluation of the Patient with Hypotension and Shock

Richard C. Becker

> **Key Points**
> - Cardiogenic shock is caused by a marked reduction in overall myocardial performance.
> - Cardiogenic shock developing in patients with myocardial infarction is associated with an in-hospital mortality rate approaching 80%.
> - The cardinal manifestations of cardiogenic shock are hypotension and hypoperfusion.
> - Prompt stabilization is an absolute prerequisite in the early management of cardiogenic shock.
> - Definitive treatment is determined by the underlying disorder or disease state.

Hypotension and shock are typically caused by a marked reduction in myocardial performance. The most common underlying condition, acute myocardial infarction, is associated with an in-hospital mortality rate approaching 80%. Rapid recognition, stabilization, diagnostic evaluation, and treatment are absolute prerequisites for patient survival.

DETERMINANTS OF A NORMAL SYSTEMIC BLOOD PRESSURE

Systemic blood pressure is determined by the volume of blood ejected into the systemic circulation (cardiac output) and by the peripheral vascular resistance. Therefore, disturbances in blood pressure are caused by either a reduced cardiac output (the hallmark of cardiogenic shock) or a reduced peripheral vascular resistance (the hallmark of septic shock).

Peripheral Vascular Resistance

Peripheral vascular resistance varies inversely with the fourth power of the arteriolar (resistance vessels) radius. Therefore, vascular resistance is determined by vascular tone, which is directly influenced by:

1. Metabolic and mechanical autoregulatory mechanisms (adenosine is the primary metabolic regulator),
2. Neurogenic constrictor influences operating through norepinephrine,
3. Neurogenic vasodilator influences operating through acetylcholine and histamine, and
4. Circulating and locally released vasoactive substances, including catecholamines, angiotensin II, bradykinin, and prostaglandins.

The autonomic nervous system plays a particularly prominent role in the maintenance of systemic blood pressure, because it directly influences both cardiac output and peripheral vascular resistance.

Blood Volume

An adequate intravascular volume is required to maintain systemic blood pressure. This is accomplished primarily through the renin-angiotensin-aldosterone system;

TABLE 1 DETERMINANTS OF CARDIAC PERFORMANCE

Preload (ventricular filling)
  Venous return
  Total blood volume
  Intrathoracic pressure
  Intrapericardial pressure
  Atrial contribution
Afterload (ventricular wall stress; impedance)
Contractility (intrinsic activity of myocardium)
  Sympathetic nervous system
  Circulating catecholamines
  Local environment (anoxia, ischemia, acidemia)
  Contractile mass
  Inotropic stimulation
Heart rate

other contributors include arginine vasopressin and atrial natriuretic polypeptide.

Cardiac Performance

The three primary determinants of cardiac performance are preload, afterload, and contractility. As cardiac output is the product of heart rate and stroke volume, the former is considered to be a fourth determinant of cardiac performance (Table 1).

SHOCK STATE

When systemic hypotension is prolonged and severe, a series of compensating mechanisms are initiated in an attempt to restore blood volume, increase peripheral vascular resistance, and improve cardiac performance. Marked stimulation of the autonomic and renin-angiotensin-aldosterone systems occurs in patients with cardiogenic shock. If adequate end-organ perfusion is not restored, endogenous mediators are released from monocytes, macrophages, and neutrophils. As in septic shock, these mediators may contribute directly to the perpetuation of the shock state and be responsible for end-organ damage (Fig. 1).

CLINICAL PRESENTATION

The two cardinal manifestations of cardiogenic shock are hypotension and hypoperfusion. Hypotension is defined as a systolic blood pressure less than 90 mm Hg or a mean arterial blood pressure less than 70 mm Hg. As some patients experience end-organ (tissue) hypoperfusion at a higher blood pressure, a working definition of mean arterial pressure of 30 mm Hg or more below the baseline blood pressure may be preferred.

The presence of hypoperfusion can be determined indirectly from several key clinical observations: 1) altered mental status (agitation, restlessness, obtundation); 2) pale or mottled, cool, clammy skin; and 3) reduced urine output (< 30 mL/h). Most patients with cardiogenic shock are tachycardic (> 100 bpm). The peripheral pulses are typically weak and thready and tachypnea (> 20 respirations/min) is also common.

The common laboratory abnormalities are:
- Hypoxia, hypocarbia, metabolic acidosis
- Elevated blood lactate
- Leukocytosis (mild to moderate), thrombocytopenia (disseminated intravascular coagulation)
- Sinus tachycardia
- Pulmonary edema, adult respiratory distress syndrome
- Arterial hypotension, decreased cardiac output

INITIAL STABILIZATION

Care of critically ill patients is unique in many ways. Unlike other clinical situations that permit a series of diagnostic tests to be performed before instituting treatment, cardiogenic shock is imminently life-threatening; therefore, prompt stabilization is required before a thorough diagnostic evaluation can be performed (Table 2).

TABLE 2 RECOMMENDATIONS FOR STABILIZING CRITICALLY ILL PATIENTS

Assure adequate oxygenation (low threshold for tracheal intubation)
Obtain intravenous access (central access preferred)
Restore arterial pressure (mean, > 70 mm Hg)
  Volume replacement
  Vasopressor agents (dopamine, norepinephrine)
Correct acid–base abnormalities
Correct rhythm disturbances and conduction abnormalities

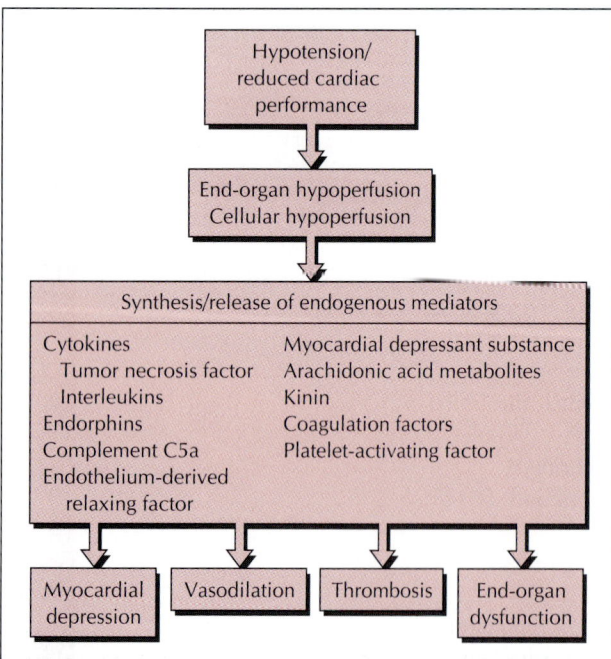

FIGURE 1 The shock state is initiated when tissue hypoperfusion initiates the release of endogenous mediators, which in turn are responsible for myocardial depression, vasodilation, thrombosis, and end-organ dysfunction.

TABLE 3 COMMON CAUSES OF CARDIOGENIC SHOCK
Acute myocardial infarction
Ventricular septal rupture
Acute mitral insufficiency
Right ventricular infarction
Myocarditis
Dilated cardiomyopathy
Advanced valvular heart disease
Aortic stenosis
Aortic insufficiency
Mitral stenosis
Mitral insufficiency
Tachy- and bradyarrhythmias
Cardiac tamponade
Pulmonary embolism
Hypertrophic cardiomyopathy
End-stage hypertensive heart disease

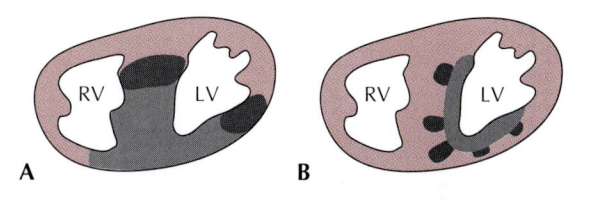

FIGURE 2 Patients with myocardial infarction complicated by cardiogenic shock demonstrate marginal extension at autopsy that can be either subepicardial (**A**) or lateral (**B**) in location. LV—left ventricle; RV—right ventricle.

DIFFERENTIAL DIAGNOSIS

A number of common diseases of the heart can cause hypotension and cardiogenic shock (Table 3). The most common is abnormal myocardial function caused by severe coronary artery disease, multiple myocardial infarctions (MIs) also known as ischemic cardiomyopathy, or acute massive MI.

The incidence of cardiogenic shock complicating MI ranges from 5% to 15%. The degree of left ventricular compromise correlates closely with the overall extent of ventricular damage. The Starling mechanism of functional compensation fails when the surface area of necrosis exceeds 30% [1,2]. Smaller infarctions may cause complications associated with shock, including ventricular septal rupture, free-wall rupture, and papillary muscle rupture.

A consistent pathologic observation among patients with fatal cardiogenic shock is progressive myocardial necrosis (Fig. 2). Persistent occlusion of the infarct-related coronary artery is also common. Severe multivessel coronary artery disease, prior infarction, or compromised collateral circulation may cause shock in the absence of a large infarction.

DIAGNOSTIC EVALUATION

Following initial stabilization of the patient, the clinician must promptly begin a thorough diagnostic evaluation. In many instances, a diagnosis can be secured through a careful physical examination, chest radiography, electrocardiography, and routine blood tests. At times, vital historical information can be provided by friends, family members, and medical records. Specialized testing, including echocardiography (transthoracic/transesophogeal), coronary angiography, computed tomography, magnetic resonance imaging, and pulmonary artery catheterization, may be required to confirm a diagnosis. The checklist in Table 4 should be helpful in making a diagnosis.

MANAGEMENT

Whenever possible, patients with cardiogenic shock should be managed in an intensive care unit. Close observation is an absolute prerequisite, and both intraarterial and hemodynamic monitoring should be considered strongly.

Intraarterial Monitoring

Direct blood pressure measurement is more accurate than noninvasive, indirect measurement in patients with hemodynamic instability and shock. Intraarterial monitoring allows careful titration of vasoactive drugs and provides immediate access for frequent blood sampling, including blood gas analysis. The preferred cannulation site is the radial artery; however, other sites (femoral artery, dorsalis pedis artery, brachial artery) also may be used. Potential complications of intraarterial monitoring include bleeding, thrombosis, embolism, limb ischemia, pseudoaneurysm formation, infection, and peripheral neuropathy.

Hemodynamic Monitoring

Pulmonary artery catheterization for hemodynamic monitoring has four primary objectives (Table 5):
1. To assess left ventricular and right ventricular function,
2. To assess changes in hemodynamic status,
3. To guide treatment with pharmacologic and nonpharmacologic agents, and
4. To gather prognostic information.

The hemodynamic information obtained from pulmonary arterial catheterization can be used directly in both patient management and diagnosis (Tables 6 and 7).

Potential complications of catheterization include balloon rupture, knotting, pulmonary infarction, arterial perforation, thromboembolism, heart block, arrhythmias, myocardial perforation with tamponade, and infection.

Pharmacologic Therapy

Dopamine is an immediate precursor of norepinephrine. It has both α- and β-adrenergic agonist properties as well as dopaminergic-receptor agonism within the mesenteric and renal vascular beds. At doses required to increase mean arterial pressure and cardiac output (5 to 8 μg/kg body weight/min), heart rate and myocardial oxygen demand may be increased [3]. In the presence of acidemia, higher doses (up to 15 μg/kg/min) may be required to produce a hemodynamic

Table 4. Diagnostic Benchmarks in Cardiogenic Shock

	General physical appearance	Signs or history	Jugular venous pressure	Heart sounds	Lung examination	Chest radiograph	Electrocardiography	Other diagnostic tests
Myocardial infarction	Apprehensive Cool, moist skin Agitation	Symptom onset at rest Chest pain Dyspnea Hypotension Tachycardia	↑, ↔	S₃, S₄ gallops ± Holosystolic murmur (papillary muscle dysfunction)	Rales in > 50% of both lung fields	Pulmonary edema	ST-segment elevation ± Q waves	Elevated creatine kinase Abnormal MB fraction (may not be elevated early) Focal wall motion abnormality on echocardiogram
Ventricular septal rupture	Anxious Diaphoretic	Recent MI (3–5 d)* Sudden change in clinical status Chest pain Dyspnea Tachycardia	↑	S₃, S₄ gallops Localized holosystolic murmur (new) Palpable systolic thrill (lower left sternal border)	Rales in > 50% of lung fields	Pulmonary edema	Persistent ST-segment elevation Pseudonormalization of T waves Prominent V waves	L→R shunt on echocardiogram O₂ saturation "step-up"
Mitral insufficiency (acute)	Anxious Diaphoretic	Sudden dyspnea Recent inferior/ inferoposterior MI or History of mitral valve prolapse or History of blunt/ penetrating trauma	↑, ↔	S₁ decreased S₃ gallop Holosystolic murmur obscuring S₂ (A₂ component)	Rales in > 50% of lung fields	Pulmonary edema	Recent MI Nonspecific ST-T wave abnormality	Mitral insufficiency ± flail mitral leaflet on echocardiogram
Right ventricular infarction	Apprehensive Diaphoretic	Chest pain Nausea	↑↑	S₂, S₃, S₄ gallops (right sided)	Clear or basilar rales	Clear	Inferior injury pattern with posterior extension ≥0.5 mm ST elevation in V₃R, V₄R Bradyarrhythmias Conduction abnormalities (2°, 3° heart block)	Inferoposterior hypokinesis and right ventricular hypokinesis on echocardiogram
Myocarditis	Apprehensive Cool, moist skin	Viral prodrome Progressive shortness of breath Low-grade temperature Narrow pulse pressure	↑	S₃, S₄ gallops	Rales in > 50% of lung fields	Pulmonary edema Heart size normal or enlarged	Sinus tachycardia Nonspecific ST/T changes Pseudoinfarction pattern Bundle-branch block	Chamber dilation Hypokinesis on echocardiogram
Dilated cardiomyopathy	Diaphoretic Cool Peripheral mottling	History of chronic heart failure Narrow pulse pressure Chronic venous stasis pigmentation-ulceration	↑↑	S₃, S₄ gallops Holosystolic murmur (mitral, tricuspid regurgitation)	Rales in > 50% of lung fields	Pulmonary edema Cardiomegaly	Sinus tachycardia/ tachyarrhythmias (atrial/ventricular) Low voltage Bundle-branch block Diffuse ST/T-wave changes	Four-chamber dilation on echocardiogram

*May occur earlier (24–48 hours) following thrombolytic therapy.

(Continued on next page)

Table 4 Diagnostic Benchmarks in Cardiogenic Shock (continued)

	General physical appearance	Signs or history	Jugular venous pressure	Heart sounds	Lung examination	Chest radiograph	Electrocardiography	Other diagnostic tests
Hypertrophic cardiomyopathy	Anxious Diaphoretic	History of chest pain, dyspnea, syncope Family history of sudden death Apical "triple" beat Rapid carotid upstroke	↑, ↔ (prominent A wave)	Prominent S_4 gallop Holosystolic blowing murmur at apex Holosystolic harsh murmur left sternal border (↑ Valsalva)	Rales in > 50% of lung fields	Pulmonary edema	Left ventricular hypertrophy Q waves inferolateral leads	Septal hypertrophy on echocardiogram Outflow tract obstruction on Doppler studies
Aortic stenosis	Pale Diaphoretic	Carotid shudder, delayed upstroke	↑	S_1 soft; single S_2 (P_2) S_3, S_4 gallops Harsh, late-peaking systolic murmur (radiation to carotid arteries)	Rales in > 50% of lung fields	Pulmonary edema	Left ventricular hypertrophy	Aortic valve thickening Reduced leaflet motion Pressure gradient across aortic valve
Aortic insufficiency	Diaphoretic	History of hypertension, endocarditis, or trauma Chest ± back pain Dyspnea Asymmetric blood pressure/pulses Paralysis/sensory deficits	↑, ↔	S_1 soft or absent S_2 (P_2) prominent S_3, S_4 gallops Early, low-pitch diastolic murmur	Rales in > 50% of lung fields	Pulmonary edema "Calcium" sign	Nonspecific ST/T-wave changes	Aortic dissection Aortic insufficiency Transesophogeal echocardiogram
Mitral stenosis	Diaphoretic Cyanotic	Progressive dyspnea Frothy blood-tinged sputum Prior thromboembolism	↑ (prominent A wave)	S_1 prominent or reduced (immobile valve leaflets) P_2 prominent Opening snap Diastolic rumbling murmur	Rales in > 50% of lung fields	Pulmonary edema Right ventricular prominence Left atrial enlargement	Tachyarrythmia (particularly atrial fibrillation) Right-axis deviation Right ventricular hypertrophy Atrial enlargement	Calcified, stenotic mitral valve
Pulmonary embolism	Anxious Cyanotic	Sudden pleuritic chest pain, dyspnea, cough, hemoptysis, or syncope Risk factors for pulmonary embolism Tachypnea (> 20 breaths/min)	↑ (prominent A wave)	S_2 (P_2) increased S_3, S_4 gallops (right sided) Holosystolic murmur (tricuspid regurgitation)	Clear	Oligemia Elevated hemidiaphragm Pleural effusion "Wedge-shaped" infiltrate Prominent hilar vessel	S_1, Q_3, T_3 pattern Nonspecific ST/T-wave changes Right bundle-branch block	V/Q mismatch Abnormal pulmonary angiography Right ventricular prominence on echocardiogram
Cardiac tamponade	Pale Anxious Apprehensive	Hypotension Narrow pulse pressure Distended neck veins Pulsus paradoxus	↑↑ (absent Y descent)	Distant (rapid pericardial fluid accumulation) ± Friction rub	Clear	Normal or enlarged cardiac silhouette	Low voltage T-wave flattening	Pericardial effusion Right atrial, right ventricular collapse on echocardiogram Abnormal Doppler flow patterns

L→R—left to right; MI—myocardial infarction; P_2—pulmonic second heart sound; S_1—first heart sound; S_2—second heart sound; S_3—third heart sound; S_4—fourth heart sound; ↔—normal; ↑—increased; ↑↑—markedly increased.

TABLE 5 KEY HEMODYNAMIC REFERENCE POINTS FOR PATIENTS WITH PULMONARY ARTERY CATHETERS	
Cardiac chamber catheter site	**Normal pressures, mm Hg**
Right atrium	
Range	0–6
Mean	3
Right ventricle	
Systolic	15–30
Diastolic	0–6
Pulmonary artery	
Systolic	15–30
Diastolic	5–13
Mean	10–18
Pulmonary capillary bed	
Mean	2–12

improvement; at this dose, atrial and ventricular tachyarrhythmias may occur.

Dobutamine is a synthetic derivative of isoproterenol. It increases cardiac output at doses between 2.5 and 5.0 µg/kg/min without significantly increasing either heart rate or myocardial oxygen demand [4]. Therefore, in the setting of MI complicated by cardiogenic shock, dobutamine is considered the inotropic agent of choice.

Norepinephrine is a potent α-receptor agonist (increases peripheral vascular resistance). It exhibits some myocardial $β_1$-receptor agonism as well. Norepinephrine should be used in patients with hypotension refractory to other inotropic agents.

The efficacy of dopamine and dobutamine may decline with long-term administration. Tachyphylaxis may represent a downregulation of myocardial adrenergic receptors. Phosphodiesterase inhibitors increase cyclic AMP concentrations without relying directly on adrenergic receptors. Amrinone and milrinone have been used successfully in the treatment of cardiogenic shock [5].

Patients with increased left ventricular mass and diastolic dysfunction, hypertensive heart disease, or hypertrophic cardiomyopathy have unique requirements. In fact, inotropic agents may worsen their clinical condition. Calcium channel blockers (verapamil, diltiazem) or β-blockers (esmolol [Brevibloc, Du Pont Pharmaceuticals, Wilmington, DE]) given as a continuous intravenous infusion may improve ventricular distensibility and diastolic filling. In refractory congestive heart failure accompanied by hypotension, a pure α-agonist such as phenylephrine hydrochloride (Neo-Synephrine, Winthrop Pharmaceuticals, New York, NY), used in combination with supportive care, may be beneficial.

Thrombolytic therapy is useful in the treatment of massive pulmonary embolism. Intravenous tissue-plasminogen activator appears to be the agent of choice; however, urokinase has shown promise as well [6•]. Unfortunately, while reducing the incidence of congestive heart failure and cardiogenic shock among patients with MI, thrombolytic therapy has not been shown to improve survival when administered in the presence of cardiogenic shock [7•].

Antiarrhythmics (procainamide, lidocaine) or electrical cardioversion should be used as needed for patients with hemodynamically compromising supraventricular and ventricular tachyarrhythmias. Occasionally, intravenous amiodarone is required in the care of patients with cardiogenic shock and incessant ventricular tachycardia.

Mechanical Intervention

Intraaortic balloon counterpulsation (IABP) can rapidly stabilize many patients with cardiogenic shock, particularly

TABLE 6 HEMODYNAMIC PARAMETERS IN PATIENTS WITH HYPOTENSION AND SHOCK (GUIDELINES FOR DIAGNOSIS)							
	RA, mm Hg	RV, mm Hg*	PA, mm Hg*	PWP, mm Hg	AO, mm Hg	CI L/min/m²	SVR, dyne/sec/cm⁻⁵
Normal	0–6	25/0–6	25/6–12	6–12	120/80	≥2.5	1200–1500
Hypovolemia	0–2	15/0–2	15/2–6	2–6	≥ 90/60	< 2.0	> 1500
Cardiogenic shock	8	50/8	50/35	35	< 90/60	< 2.0	> 1500
Septic shock							
Early	0–2	25/0–2	25/0–6	0–6	< 90/60	< 2.5	< 1000
Late	0–4	25/4–10	25/4–10	4–10	< 90/60	< 2.0	> 1000
Massive PE	8–12	50/12	50/12	<12	< 90/60	< 2.0	> 1200
Tamponade	12–18	30/12–18	30/12–18	12–18	< 90/60	< 2.0	> 1200
Right ventricular infarction	12–20	30/12–20	30/12	<12	< 90/60	< 2.0	> 1200
Ventricular septal rupture	6	60/6–8	60/35	30	< 90/60	< 2.0	> 1500

*The first value represents the mean value; the second is the range.
AO—aortic pressure; CI—cardiac index; PA pulmonary artery; PE—pulmonary embolism; PWP—pulmonary wedge pressure; RA—right atrium; RV—right ventricle; SVR—systemic vascular resistance.

those with global myocardial ischemia or MI complicated by papillary muscle rupture or ventricular septal rupture. It is contraindicated in patients with severe aortic insufficiency. The observed hemodynamic changes following IABP insertion include:

1. A 10% to 20% increase in cardiac output,
2. A reduction in systolic and an increase in diastolic blood pressure,
3. A diminution in heart rate, and
4. An increase in urine output.

In some patients, combined IABP and inotropic therapy is required to achieve and maintain an acceptable blood pressure (systolic, > 90 mm Hg systolic; mean, > 70 mm Hg) and cardiac index (> 2.2 L/min/m²).

Recently, more powerful circulatory assist devices, such as the Hemopump (Johnson and Johnson Interventional Systems, Rancho Cordova, CA) and the percutaneous cardiopulmonary support system, have been used in the care of patients with cardiogenic shock caused by left heart failure [8,9]. As with IABP, these devices are designed for rapid clinical stabilization while preparations are made for definitive, corrective intervention.

Coronary angiography and urgent coronary angioplasty may improve survival for patients with MI complicated by cardiogenic shock [10–12]. Although randomized trials have not been conducted, restoration of coronary arterial patency in retrospective studies and pooled series has been associated with a nearly 50% reduction in the mortality rate.

Alternative mechanical interventions include:
1. Pericardiocentesis for patients with cardiac tamponade,
2. Balloon valvuloplasty for those with critical aortic or mitral stenosis when surgical correction is not feasible, and
3. Pacemaker placement for patients with severe brady-arrhythmias, conduction disturbances, or right ventricular infarction refractory to fluid administration and inotropic support.

Surgical Intervention

Corrective surgery is most beneficial in patients with mechanical defects (papillary muscle rupture, ventricular septal rupture), critical valvular heart disease (aortic stenosis, aortic insufficiency, mitral stenosis), and severe coronary artery disease (three-vessel disease, left main disease). In a majority of cases, initial stabilization is achieved by inotropic support with or without a circulatory assist device. Overall, the best results are achieved when surgical intervention is undertaken promptly [13,14].

Cardiac transplantation is a therapeutic alternative for a small and highly selective group of individuals with cardiogenic shock. Mechanical circulatory support as a "bridge" to cardiac transplantation includes a total artificial heart and ventricular assist devices [15,16] (Table 8).

TABLE 7 MEASURES CALCULABLE FROM HEMODYNAMIC DATA

$$\text{Cardiac index} = \frac{\text{Cardiac output (L/min)}}{\text{Body surface area (m}^2\text{)}}$$

Normal: 2.5–4.5 L/min/m²

$$\text{Mean arterial pressure} = \frac{(2 \times \text{Diastolic}) + \text{Systolic}}{3}$$

Normal: 70–95 mm Hg

$$\text{Systemic vascular resistance} = \frac{\text{MAP-RA}}{\text{CO}} \times 80$$

Normal: 1200–1500 dyne/sec/cm⁻⁵

CO—cardiac output; MAP—mean arterial pressure; RA—right atrial pressure.

TABLE 8 TREATMENT OPTIONS IN CARDIOGENIC SHOCK

Pharmacologic	Mechanisms of action
Dobutamine	Inotropic support
Dopamine	Inotropic support
Norepinephrine	Inotropic support, vasopressor
Phenylephrine	Vasopressor
Tissue-plasminogen activator	Thrombolysis (pulmonary embolism ± MI)
Urokinase	Thrombolysis (pulmonary embolism ± MI)
Lidocaine, procainamide, amiodarone	Antiarrhythmic
Mechanical	
Intraaortic balloon pump	Improve cardiac output, Increase coronary artery perfusion
Hemopump	Improve cardiac output
Percutaneous cardio-pulmonary support	Improve cardiac output, Improve tissue perfusion
Pacemaker	Restore heart rate, Restore atrioventricular synchrony
Coronary angioplasty	Improve myocardial perfusion
Pericardiocentesis	Improve preload, ventricular filling
Surgery	Correct mechanical defects

References and Recommended Reading

Recently published papers of particular interest have been highlighted as:
• Of interest
•• Of outstanding interest

1. Klein MD, Herman MV, Gorlin R: A hemodynamic study of left ventricular aneurysm. *Circulation* 1967, 35:614–630.

2. Page DL, Caulfield JB, Kastor JA, *et al.*: Myocardial changes associated with cardiogenic shock. *N Engl J Med* 1971, 285:133–137.

3. Meuller HS, Evans R, Ayres SM: Effect of dopamine on hemodynamics and myocardial metabolism in shock following acute myocardial infarction in man. *Circulation* 1978, 57:361–365.

4. Francis GS, Sharma B, Hodges M: Comparative hemodynamic effects of dopamine and dobutamine in patients with acute cardiogenic circulatory collapse. *Am Heart J* 1982, 103:995–1000.

5. Klocke RK, Mager G, Kux A, *et al.*: Effects of a 24-hour milrinone infusion in patients with severe heart failure and cardiogenic shock as a function of the hemodynamic initial condition. *Am Heart J* 1991, 121:1965–1973.

6.• Goldhaber SZ, Kessler CM, Heit JA, *et al.*: Recombinant tissue-type plasminogen activator versus a novel dosing regimen of urokinase in acute pulmonary embolism: a randomized controlled multicenter trial. *J Am Coll Cardiol* 1992, 20:24–31.

7.• Becker RC: Hemodynamic, mechanical and metabolic determinants of thrombolytic efficacy: a theoretic framework for assessing the limitations of thrombolysis in patients with cardiogenic shock. *Am Heart J* 1993, 125:919–929.

8. Smalling RW, Sweeney M, Lachterman B, *et al.*: Transvalvular left ventricular assistance in cardiogenic shock secondary to acute myocardial infarction. *J Am Coll Cardiol* 1994, 23:637–644.

9. Phillips SJ, Zeff RH, Kongtahworn C, *et al.*: Percutaneous cardiopulmonary bypass: application and indication for use. *Ann Thorac Surg* 1989, 47:121–123.

10. Abbottsmith CW, Topol EJ, George BS, *et al.*: Fate of patients with acute myocardial infarction with patency of the infarct-related vessel achieved with successful thrombolysis versus rescue angiography. *J Am Coll Cardiol* 1990, 16:770–778.

11. Lee L, Bates ER, Pitt B, *et al.*: Percutaneous transluminal coronary angioplasty improves survival in acute myocardial infarction complicated by cardiogenic shock. *Circulation* 1988, 78:1345–1351.

12. Lee L, Erbel R, Brown TM, *et al.*: Multicenter registry of angioplasty therapy of cardiogenic shock: initial and long-term survival. *J Am Coll Cardiol* 1991, 17:599–603.

13. Phillips SJ, Kongtahworn C, Slanner JR, Zeff MT: Emergency coronary artery reperfusion: a choice therapy for evolving myocardial infarction: results in 339 patients. *J Thorac Cardiovasc Surg* 1983, 86:679–688.

14. DeWood MA, Notske RN, Hensley GR, *et al.*: Intra-aortic balloon counterpulsation with or without reperfusion for myocardial shock. *Circulation* 1980, 61:1105–1112.

15. Joyce LD, Johnson KE, Pierce WS: Summary of the work experience with clinical use of total artificial hearts as heart support devices. *J Heart Transplant* 1986, 5:229–235.

16. Fortin DF, Califf RM: Long term survival from acute myocardial infarction: salutary effect of an open coronary vessel. *Am J Med* 1990, 88:9N–15N.

Selected Bibliography

Hibbard MD, Holmes DR, Bailey KR, *et al.*: Percutaneous transluminal coronary angioplasty in patients with cardiogenic shock. *J Am Coll Cardiol* 1992, 19:639–646.

Kleiman NS, Terrin M, Meuller HS, *et al.* for the TIMI Investigators: Mechanisms of early death despite thrombolytic therapy: experience from the TIMI II study. *J Am Coll Cardiol* 1992, 19:1129–1135.

McCallister BD, Christian TF, Gersh BJ, Gibbons RJ: Prognosis of myocardial infarctions involving more than 40% of the left ventricle after reperfusion therapy. *Circulation* 1993, 88(part 1):1470–1475.

Evaluation of the Patient with Palpitations and Non–Life-Threatening Cardiac Arrhythmias

Mark N. Fiengo
Eric L. Michelson

Key Points
- Palpitations are a frequent but relatively nonspecific cardiac symptom.
- Palpitations are not a reliable indicator of any particular cardiovascular finding or arrhythmia.
- Palpitations are clinically important when there is associated functional incapacity or concern of the patient, when they cause severe hemodynamic sequelae, or serve as harbingers of life-threatening cardiac arrhythmias in selected patients.
- A thorough history, physical examination, and judicious use of laboratory testing usually guides management.
- Management must encompass the nature and severity of the palpitations, the patient's general medical and cardiac conditions, the mechanism of the arrhythmia, and an algorithm for risk stratification.

Palpitations are a common symptom and frequent cause of outpatient visits to generalists and cardiovascular subspecialists. This chapter emphasizes a holistic yet focused, practical, and cost-effective approach to evaluating patients with palpitations. It is a reference for initiating management strategies in most patients with palpitations and non–life-threatening cardiac arrhythmias.

PALPITATIONS

Definitions

In this discussion, *palpitation* is defined broadly as an uncomfortable or abnormal awareness of the heart beating. Symptoms vary and may be described as heavy beating of the heart, fluttering in the chest, skipped beats, rapid heart beating, irregular heart beating, pounding in the neck, or some other unpleasant sensation depending on the underlying cardiac rhythm and the patient. Palpitations are a relatively nonspecific symptom and are not a reliable indicator of any particular cardiovascular finding or arrhythmia.

Symptomatic Manifestations of Arrhythmias

Cardiac symptoms as a manifestation of arrhythmias can be very nonspecific. Patients may present with a variety of complaints. Among individuals with documented cardiac arrhythmias, some are completely asymptomatic, some have palpitations, and some have symptoms that may suggest angina, dyspnea, fatigue, effort intolerance, near-syncope or syncope, or even noncardiac symptoms such as gastrointestinal upset [1,2].

Mechanisms

Arrhythmias can produce palpitations through multiple mechanisms. Arrhythmias can cause symptoms related to disorders of rhythm, disorders of rate, alterations in patterns of cardiac contractility, or alterations in cardiovascular hemodynamics. Intermittent disorders of rhythm such as paroxysmal supraventricular tachycardias, paroxysmal atrial fibrillation, atrial premature beats, and ventricular premature beats are frequent causes of palpitations. Disorders of rate also can be perceived as palpitations, and even sinus tachy- or bradycardia can cause symptoms (Fig. 1). In many cases, only normal sinus rhythm is found when using ambulatory electrocardiographic (ECG) recording techniques. This finding may suggest either a noncardiac origin or an awareness of increased contractility secondary to a surge in catecholamines (*eg*, before an interview, examination, or appearance on stage).

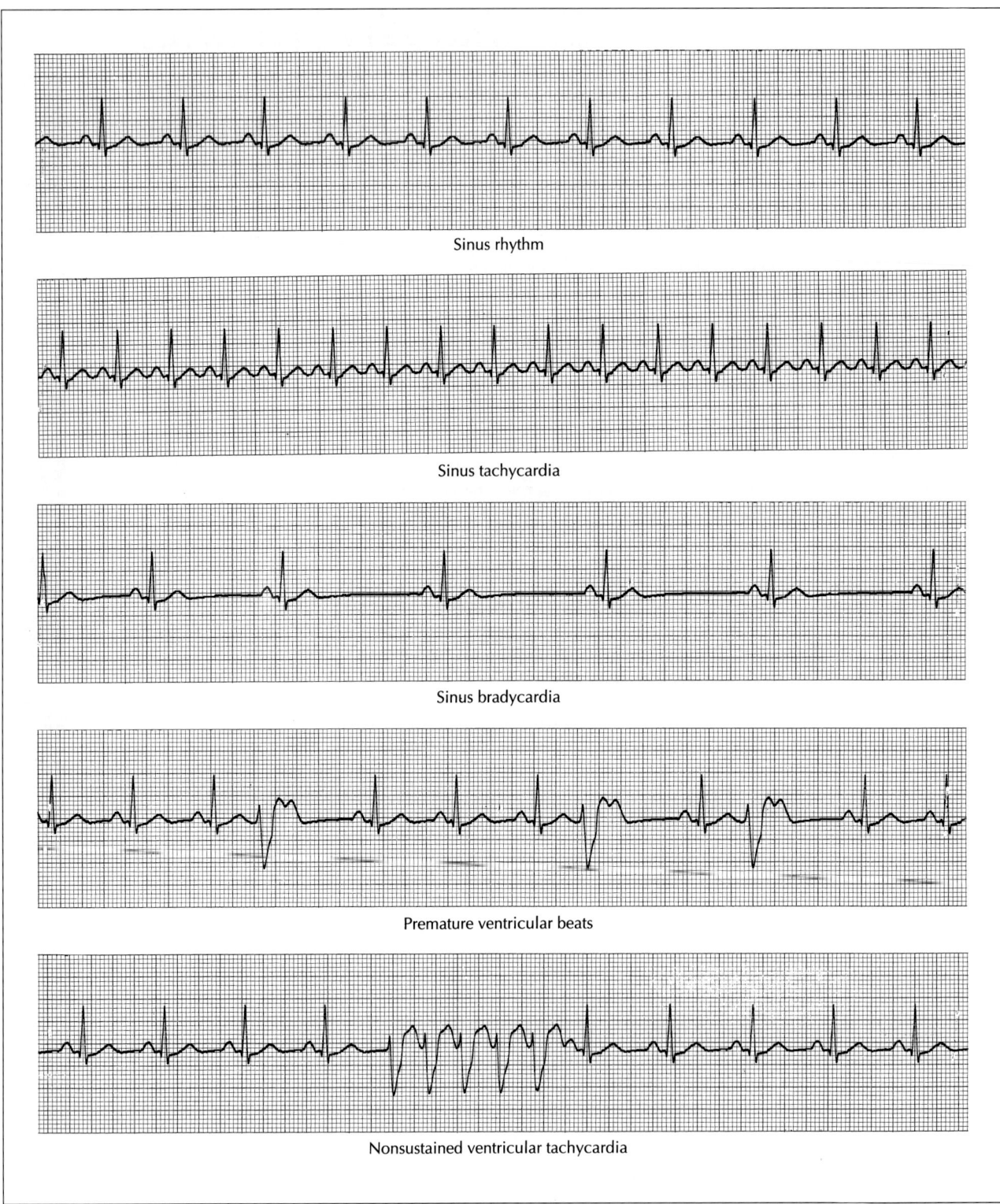

FIGURE 1 Electrocardiographic rhythms typically associated with palpitations.

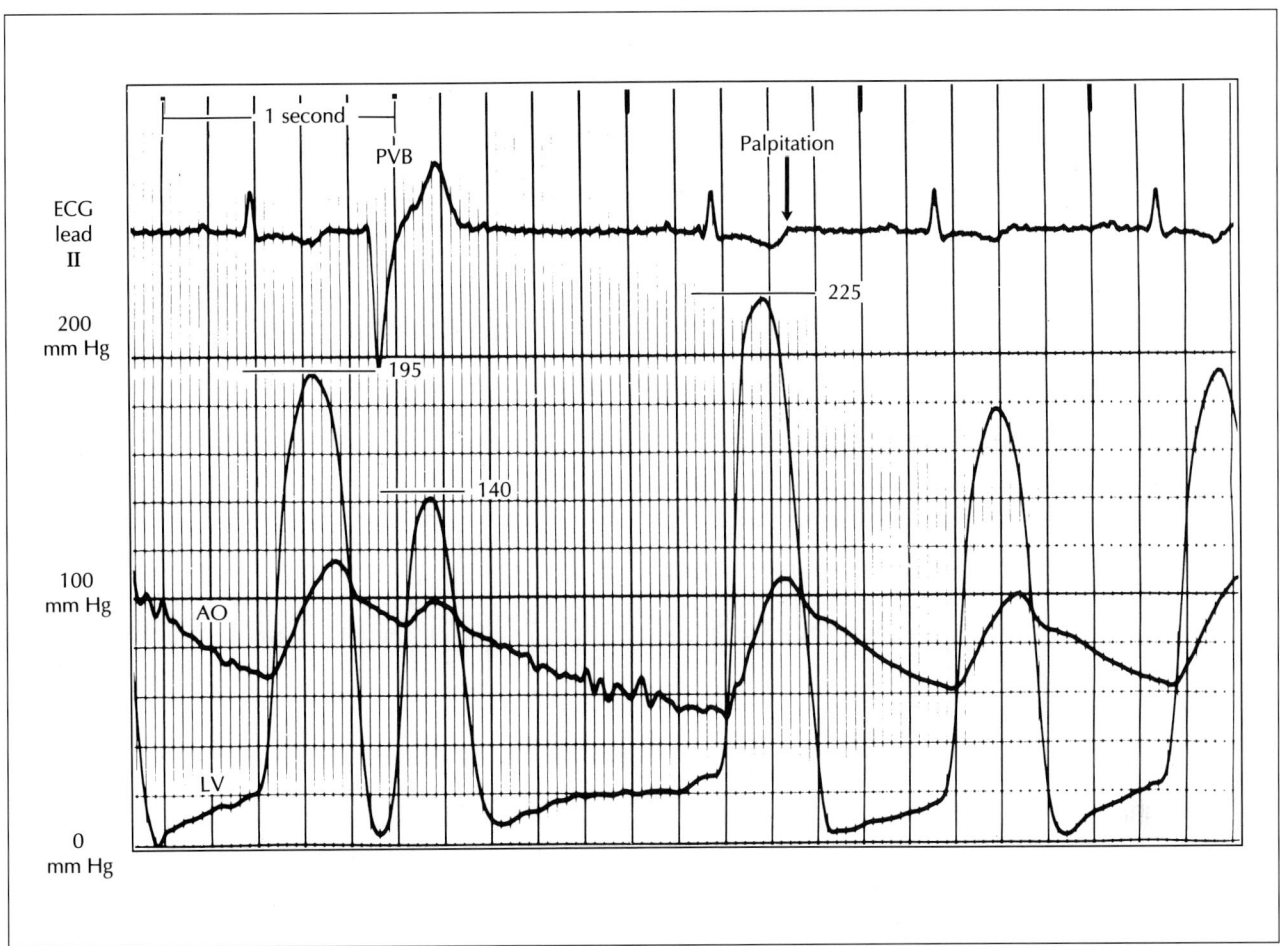

FIGURE 2 Increased left ventricular pressure (LV) after premature ventricular beat (PVB) in a patient with severe aortic stenosis and palpitations (arrow). AO—aortic pressure; ECG—electrocardiogram.

The alterations in cardiac contractility and increased stroke volume that occur after premature ventricular beats also may be interpreted as palpitations (Fig. 2). Any arrhythmia associated with atrioventricular (AV) dissociation or varying patterns of AV conduction may cause symptoms related to a variety of mechanisms including altered atrial contribution to ventricular filling, which affects cardiac output, or atrial contraction against closed AV valves, which causes engorgement and regurgitation of blood into the pulmonary veins and venae cavae (Fig. 3). Characteristically, AV nodal reentrant tachycardia causes a regular, rapid "pounding in the neck" related to (right) atrial contraction against the closed (tricuspid) AV valve with each heartbeat [3].

Patient Evaluation

Initial Evaluation and Medical History

The ideal initial evaluation of the patient with palpitations is a thorough history and physical examination [4••,5••]. Most important to the general medical history is to determine the presence of common conditions (*eg*, hypertension or thyroid disease) that affect the cardiovascular system and possibly potentiate arrhythmias as well as to identify less common systemic disorders (*eg*, sarcoidosis) (Table 1). Any history of cardiovascular disease should be reviewed. Common disorders such as coronary artery disease and mitral valve prolapse, as well as less common disorders such as Wolff-Parkinson-White syndrome, congenital long-QT syndrome, and hypertrophic cardiomyopathy should be considered. A thorough social history must be reviewed, and patients should be asked if they use tobacco, alcohol, caffeine or illicit drugs. Family history should be reviewed regarding parents, siblings, and other family members with a history of cardiovascular disease, sudden cardiac death, or arrhythmias. As part of the initial history, it is also essential to determine the use of concomitant medications, whether prescription or over-the-counter drugs, that may affect the cardiovascular system (Table 2). It is similarly important to determine the patient's overall sense of well-being, because palpitations may be a manifestation of depression or anxiety or may reflect stress.

Characteristics of Palpitations

Once a detailed, general medical history is obtained, the physician should characterize the patient's symptoms of palpitations qualitatively and quantitatively [6,7]. This

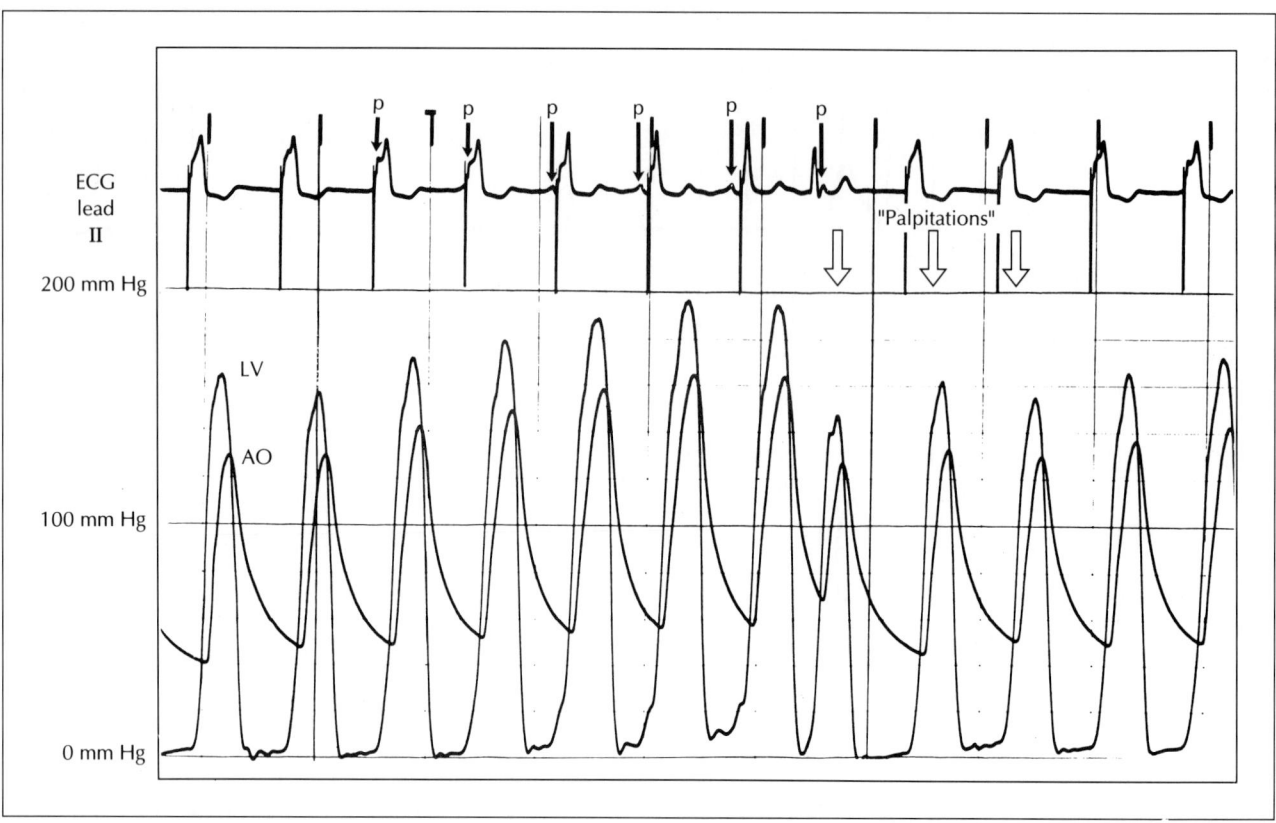

FIGURE 3 Pacemaker syndrome—the effects of atrioventricular dissociation on cardiac hemodynamics. There is a drop of 40 mm Hg in systemic blood pressure with atrioventricular asynchrony associated with palpitations (open arrows). Arrows indicate P waves. AO—aortic pressure; LV—left ventricular pressure.

includes establishing the frequency and duration of symptoms, the temporal pattern of symptoms, and the situations or circumstances that provoke or relieve symptoms (Table 3). The onset and termination of palpitations may help to identify the responsible arrhythmia. Symptoms that begin and terminate abruptly favor a reentrant or reciprocating tachycardia, such as AV reciprocating tachycardia or AV nodal reentrant tachycardia, whereas symptoms that begin abruptly but persist for days favor a diagnosis of paroxysmal atrial fibrillation [8•]. The rate and regularity, or irregularity, are also important characteristics. Exacerbating or ameliorating factors, associated symptoms (*eg*, dyspnea, lightheadedness, and angina), and response to prophylaxis, avoidance of potentiating factors, or interventions all may provide clues to an effective arrhythmia evaluation and management strategy.

Physical Examination

The physical examination should focus on the stigmata of structural heart disease. It should also focus on recognition of noncardiac disorders and the systemic manifestations of diseases (*eg*, thyroid disorder) known to affect the heart and predispose patients to arrhythmias.

Laboratory Testing

Initial routine laboratory testing should be limited to those tests likely to lead to a diagnosis or guide a management strategy. These may include a serum potassium or hemoglobin determination or an evaluation of thyroid function.

Electrocardiography is the cornerstone in the evaluation of patients with palpitations and is often useful in determining the mechanism of the responsible arrhythmia as well as the presence of underlying cardiac disease. The ECG can make the diagnosis of preexcitation syndrome, long-QT syndrome, Mobitz type I or type II heart block, or other conduction system disease. Supraventricular or ventricular premature beats also may be identified, but the modern, computerized, multilead ECG often records only 12 to 15 seconds of rhythm, which is usually insufficient to diagnose rhythms that are not clearly present clinically when the recording begins. If a diagnosis is not made, ambulatory ECG monitoring is usually the next step. If symptoms are frequent (*ie*, daily), testing is by ambulatory ECG recording; if symptoms are intermittent, testing is by event monitoring. In either case, correlation of symptoms with ECG findings is essential [1]. Figure 1 shows single-lead ECG strips of various rhythms typically documented by ambulatory ECG recording or event monitoring. Often, at least two leads are recorded simultaneously to facilitate interpretation.

The initial thorough history, physical examination, and routine laboratory testing are usually within the purview of

Table 1 Patient History

General medical history
Hypertension
Thyroid disease
Electrolyte disorder
Neuropsychiatric disorder
Sarcoidosis
Amyloidosis
Hemochromatosis

Cardiovascular history
Ischemic heart disease
Hypertrophic heart disease
Mitral valve prolapse
Valvular heart disease
Preexcitation/Wolff-Parkinson-White Syndrome
Long-QT syndrome
Rheumatic heart disease
Heart failure/cardiomyopathy

Social history
Ethanol use
Caffeine use
Tobacco use
Illicit drug use
Stress

Family history
Cardiovascular disease
Sudden cardiac death
Arrhythmias

Table 2 Noncardiac Drugs Associated with Palpitations*

α-Adrenergic agonist Phenylpropanolamine Phenylephrine	**Endocrine** Thyroxine
β-Adrenergic agonist Terbutaline Isoproterenol Albuterol	**Anticholinesterase** Physostigmine Neostigmine
Methylxanthine Theophylline	**Antimuscarinic** Atropine Scopolamine
Psychoactive Phenothiazines Tricyclics	**Illicit** Amphetamine Cocaine

*Partial listing of more commonly associated drugs.

Table 3 Characteristics of Palpitations

Frequency	Rhythm regularity/irregularity
Temporal pattern	Exacerbating factors
Situations/circumstances	Ameliorating factors
Onset/termination	Associated symptoms
Duration	Response to prophylaxis or interventions
Heart rate	

the generalist in the evaluation of patients with palpitations. Exceptions may include patients known to have more advanced or specific cardiovascular disorders or those having palpitations associated with more severe or potentially life-threatening sequelae.

Risk Stratification

Risk stratification is critical to the evaluation of patients who present with palpitations. The physician must stratify patients as to those with symptomatic but benign arrhythmias, those with prognostically important arrhythmias, and those with potentially life-threatening or hemodynamically important tachy- or bradyarrhythmia.

In patients with unremarkable history, physical examination, ECG, and routine laboratory results and who experience minor symptoms without significant arrhythmia on ambulatory monitoring, no further cardiovascular evaluation is usually necessary. Reassurance for the patient is appropriate. Conversely, in patients whose findings are more remarkable and symptoms more incapacitating, or for whom an increased risk of sudden death is clearly suspected, more aggressive diagnostic evaluation is warranted, in some cases including cardiac catheterization or electrophysiologic studies (Table 4). These cases are usually referred to a cardiovascular specialist, and some highly specialized invasive tests (*eg*, electrophysiologic studies) are done by subspecialists. The challenge to the clinician is to identify those individuals at increased risk for lethal or hemodynamically important arrhythmias from among those patients with intermediate findings and to choose the most appropriate diagnostic modality. In Table 5, low-risk patients are stratified as those who often require minimal evaluation, and high-risk patients are those who may require a more extensive work-up. Table 6 elaborates on several common rhythm abnormalities within these patient profiles, and based on this patient risk profile, Figure 4 presents an algorithm for the evaluation of patients with palpitations.

In managing patients with palpitations, cost-effectiveness of the evaluation must encompass several factors in addition to the direct cost of diagnostic testing. These include the adverse effect of palpitations on the patient's quality of life and productivity at work as well as the consequences of not recognizing a potentially lethal underlying cardiovascular problem.

Conclusion

Palpitations are a common symptom that can be frustrating for both the patient and physician. An optimal approach to evaluating the patient with palpitations is holistic; systematic with respect to the history, physical examination, and laboratory testing; and must include risk stratification. The evaluation strategy must be practical, cost-effective, and relevant to a well-defined algorithm for patient management.

TABLE 4 DIAGNOSTIC MODALITIES

Test	Clinical indication
Electrocardiography*	Initial test for patients with palpitations or suspected arrhythmia
24-hour electrocardiographic monitoring*	Frequent symptoms of palpitations or near-syncope
Ambulatory event recording*	Less frequent symptoms of prolonged palpitations or near-syncope
Echocardiography	Assessment of known or suspected structural heart disease and for evaluation of cardiac function or ischemic heart disease
Radionuclide studies	Assessment of known or suspected ischemic heart disease and less commonly for evaluation of cardiac function
Exercise stress testing*	Evaluation of exercise-induced arrhythmia or screening for ischemic heart disease
Head-up tilt testing	Evaluation of vasodepressor/vasovagal syncope
Signal-averaged electrocardiography	Risk stratification of patients with previous myocardial infarction
Invasive†	
Cardiac catheterization	Evaluation of cardiac/coronary anatomy and cardiac function in high-risk patients with known or suspected ischemic/ structural or valvular heart disease
Electrophysiologic testing	Evaluation of patients with life-threatening or hemodynamically important arrhythmias

*Initial testing modalities usually available to generalists
†Invasive diagnostic modalities done by cardiovascular specialists and subspecialists

TABLE 5 RISK STRATIFICATION OF PATIENTS WITH PALPITATIONS FOR LETHAL OR HEMODYNAMICALLY IMPORTANT ARRHYTHMIAS

Low risk
Patients without structural heart disease
Patients without a history of near-syncope or syncope
Patients without evidence of myocardial ischemia
Patients with preserved left ventricular function

High risk
Patients with structural heart disease
Patients with history of syncope
Patients with left ventricular ejection fraction < 40% or symptomatic heart failure
Patients with known coronary artery disease or myocardial infarction
Patients with conduction system disease
Patients with long-QT syndrome
Patients with Wolff-Parkinson-White syndrome

TABLE 6 EVALUATION OF ARRHYTHMIAS IN PATIENTS WITH PALPITATIONS

Benign arrhythmias that generally do not require extensive evaluation
Sinus bradycardia
Sinus arrhythmia
Isolated atrial premature beats
Isolated ventricular premature beats

Arrhythmias that may require more extensive evaluation
Tachy-brady syndrome
Atrioventricular nodal reentrant tachycardias
Atrioventricular reciprocating tachycardias
Nonsustained ventricular tachycardia
Prognostically important ventricular premature beats (couplets, triplets, multiform, R-on-T beats, very frequent beats)

Arrhythmias that generally require further evaluation
Persistent atrial or sinus tachycardia
Preexcitation/Wolff-Parkinson-White syndrome
Atrial fibrillation/atrial flutter
Sustained ventricular tachycardia

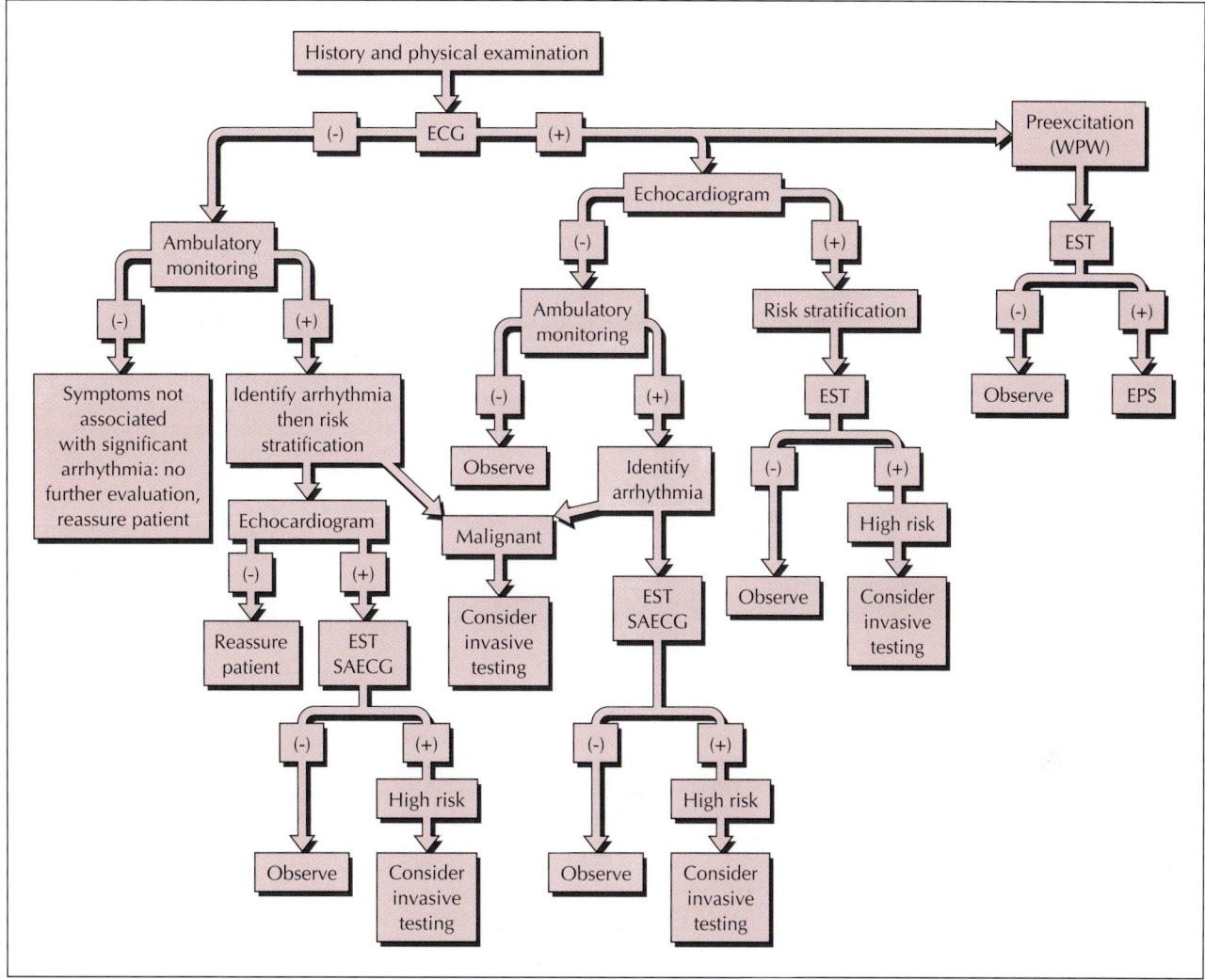

FIGURE 4 Diagnostic evaluation of palpitations. ECG—electrocardiography; EPS—electrophysiologic study; EST—exercise stress test; SAECG—signal-averaged ECG; WPW—Wolff-Parkinson-White syndrome.

References and Recommended Reading

Recently published papers of particular interest have been highlighted as:
- Of interest
- Of outstanding interest

1. Zeldis SM, Levine BJ, Michelson EL, Morganroth J: Cardiovascular complaints: correlation with cardiac arrhythmias on 24-hour electrocardiographic monitoring. *Chest* 1980, 78:456–462.
2. Page RL, Wilkinson WE, Clair WK, *et al.*: Asymptomatic arrhythmia in patients with symptomatic paroxysmal atrial fibrillation and paroxysmal supraventricular tachycardia. *Circulation* 1994, 89:224–227.
3. Gursoy S, Steurer G, Brugada J, *et al.*: The hemodynamic mechanism of pounding in the neck in atrioventricular nodal reentrant tachycardia. *N Engl J Med* 1992, 327:772–774.
4.•• Goldman L, Braunwald E: Chest discomfort and palpitation. In *Harrison's Principles of Internal Medicine*, edn 13. New York: McGraw-Hill; 1994:60–61.
5.•• Braunwald E: The history. In *Heart Disease: A Textbook of Cardiovascular Medicine*. Philadelphia: WB Saunders; 1992:1–12.
6. Pritchett ELC, MaCarthy EA, Lee KL, Wildinson WE: The clinical presentation of paroxysmal supraventricular tachycardia in untreated patients. In *Cardiac Electrophysiology*. Edited by Zipes DP, Jalife J. Philadelphia: WB Saunders; 1990:703–707.
7. Kastor JA: Atrial fibrillation. In *Arrhythmias*. Philadelphia: WB Saunders; 1994:25–34.
8.• Kannel WB, Wolf PA: Epidemiology of atrial fibrillation. In *Atrial Fibrillation: Mechanisms and Management*. Edited by Falk FH, Podrid PJ. New York: Raven Press; 1992:81–93.

Evaluation of the Patient with Syncope

Charles M. Blatt
Thomas B. Graboys

> **Key Points**
> - Five percent to 10% of emergency visits and hospitalizations involve investigation and management of patients with syncope.
> - Patient history is key in defining the cause of the syncopal event; a witness is often a critical historian.
> - Patient history must focus on a detailed setting for the syncopal event and should define any situational relationships.
> - The physical examination must assess orthostatic potential and focus on potential cardiac and carotid obstructive lesions.
> - Multiple unwitnessed syncopal events under curious circumstances should be suspected as factitious.
> - Over-the-counter medications may interact with prescribed medications, especially in the elderly, and must be considered as a cause of syncope.
> - Referral to a specialist is warranted when either neurologic or cardiac brady- or tachyarrhythmic causes are suggested by preliminary testing.

Syncope accounts for 5% to 10% of emergency room visits and hospitalizations. Traditionally, syncope is viewed as either cardiac or neurologic in origin. These processes overlap, however, because of the dominant role of the vagus nerve and myocardial mechanoreceptors in the generation of neurocardiogenic syncope. Intense peripheral vasodilation followed by bradycardia is mediated by inhibition of sympathetic efferents and enhancement of parasympathetic efferent activity. Psychogenic syncope bridges the gap between cardiac and neurogenic syncope by many inadequately defined mechanisms. Causes of syncope are listed in Table 1; a diagnostic approach is shown in Figure 1.

HISTORY

Patient history is the key to determining the origin of the syncopal event. Physical examination and laboratory tests are important in a minority of events. The clinician should establish a clinical description of the syncopal event with questions such as the following:

    Was the syncope witnessed or unwitnessed?
    Does the patient have a memory of the event?
    Was the event prodromal?
    Was it a singular or recurrent episode?
    Were injuries associated with the syncopal event?
    Can a situational relationship be established?
        Did the patient rise abruptly [1]?
        Did the patient urinate (postmicturition) [2]?
        Did the patient defecate [3]?
        Did the patient eat a meal (postprandial) [4]?

Did the patient cough?
Did the patient swallow?
Was the patient exposed to intense pain?
Was the patient exposed to the sight of blood?
Has the patient recently started a new drug regimen?

The physician must first exclude potential polypharmaceutic drug–drug interactions that might induce either a brady- or tachycardiac event. For the elderly patient, β-adrenergic and calcium-blocking agents may induce sinoatrial block, and benign drugs (*eg*, the popular antihistamines astemizole and terfenadine) may induce ventricular tachyarrhythmia. Aggravation of ventricular arrhythmia or "proarrhythmia" by antiarrhythmic drugs, a concept introduced by our group a decade ago [5], should also be excluded among patients with syncope who are receiving these agents.

Witnesses

The witness to the syncopal event fills in the history that the patient cannot provide. If episodes of syncope are multiple and all unwitnessed with curious circumstances in which a witness could not be present, factitious syncope must be considered. Witnesses should be located and interviewed to focus the inquiry and lead to a more cost-effective diagnostic approach. Panic attacks, anxiety episodes, and conversion reactions may be diagnosed with the aid of a witness, thus eliminating the need for further testing that would delay introduction of therapy [6].

Patient Memory

How the patient remembers the syncopal event may be helpful, and the patient should be asked to recreate in detail the circumstances leading to the event. A postictal confusion, with or without evidence of urinary or fecal incontinence, clearly points to a neurologic cause, whereas clearheadedness immediately after the event points away from seizure as a cause. A completely prodromal event, independent of body position or activity, may focus diagnostic events to uncovering complete heart block, especially for the older patient in whom a sclero-

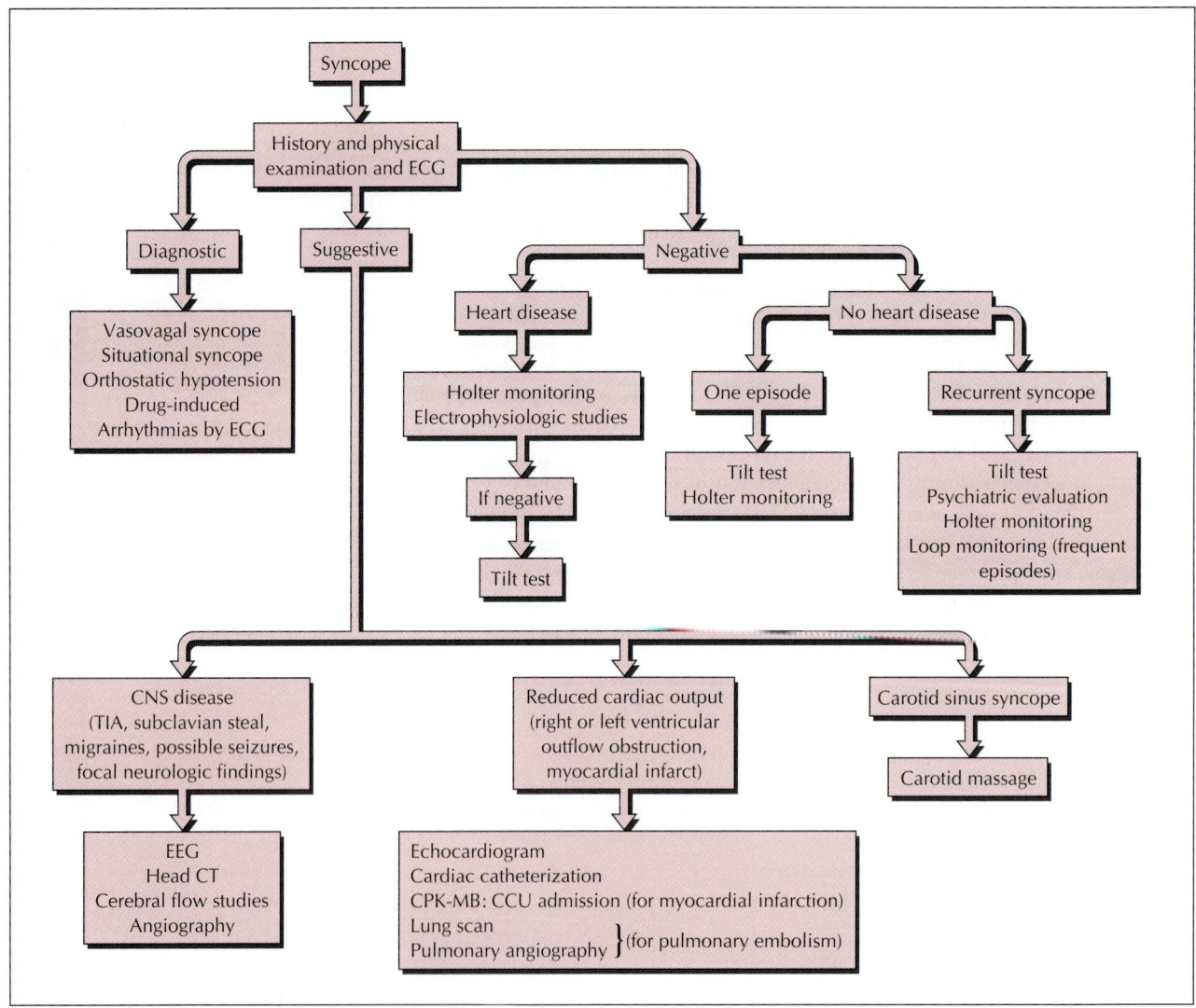

FIGURE 1 Diagnostic approach to syncope. CCU—coronary care unit; CNS—central nervous system; CPK-MB—creatine phosphokinase-muscle brain units; CT—computed tomography; ECG—electrocardiography; EEG—electroencephalography; TIA—transient ischemic attack. (From Kapoor [8••]; with permission.)

TABLE 1 CAUSES OF SYNCOPE	
Arrhythmia	Situational
Bradyarrhythmia	Coughing
Tachyarrhythmia	Defecation
Supraventricular	Eating
Ventricular	Micturition
Carotid sinus sensitivity	Swallowing
Cerebrovascular disease	Valvular
Drug induced	Aortic stenosis
Vasodilation	Pulmonic stenosis
Arrhythmogenic	Miscellaneous
Neurocardiogenic	Idiopathic hypertrophic subaortic stenosis
Orthostatic	
Pulmonary embolism	Atrial myxoma (right or left)
Psychogenic	
Anxiety	
Conversion	
Panic	

TABLE 2 PHYSICAL EXAMINATION FINDINGS
Orthostatic vital signs
Blood pressure
Supine, sitting, standing after 30 and 60 seconds
Heart rate
Appropriate rise
Persistent decline with standing
Cardiac bruits
Cardiac obstructive murmurs
Aortic stenosis
Mitral stenosis
Hypertrophic cardiomyopathy
Ectopy
Neurologic examination

calcific process may affect the cardiac conduction system. The nature of the prodrome, if witnessed or recalled, is likely to help define a vagally mediated event, including pallor, diaphoresis, nausea, and suggestive historical details.

Multiple Events

Multiple syncopal episodes may define a patient with a benign process or point to a psychogenic cause [7•]. In general, the clinical history tends to be more valuable in distinguishing vasodepressor syncope from syncope caused by either atrioventricular block or ventricular tachycardia [8••].

Setting the Stage

The history obtained from the patient and any witnesses should set the stage of the syncopal event in detail, with precise definition of the time of day; altitude; relation to meals; events of the preceding 24 hours; change in routine patterns of sleep, bowel movement, and food intake; coincident medication, including novel combinations of prescription and over-the-counter medication; and preceding breathlessness, palpitations, and chest discomfort. The witness must be questioned for evidence of seizure activity; was the patient postictal or incontinent? In addition to the obvious tonic-clonic grand mal activity, evidence of petit mal must be sought. Pulmonary embolism is often overlooked as a cause of syncope, and a conducive historical setting for this problem must be considered. This history includes recent inactivity, travel, or surgery.

PHYSICAL FINDINGS

Although a meticulous history is the cornerstone of defining the cause of syncope, physical findings also may contribute to the correct diagnosis (Table 2). Foremost is the demonstration of any abnormalities in orthostasis. Blood pressure readings should be taken in both arms while the patient is supine, sitting, and standing. A normal response is a slight decrease in pressure when assuming the upright posture, but blood pressure is maintained within 30 to 60 seconds and a slight increase in heart rate occurs. Among older patients complaining of postural dizziness or near loss of consciousness, orthostatic hypotension induced by antihypertensive drugs is a frequent cause of postural dizziness of frank syncope. Potent antihypertensive drugs may induce a decrease of 20 to 30 mm Hg in blood pressure when assuming an upright posture.

Autonomic Dysfunction

While standing, patients with idiopathic orthostatic hypotension experience a gradual decrease in blood pressure without a commensurate increase in heart rate. This type of autonomic dysfunction also may be a sign of Shy-Drager's disease. Individuals with high vagal tone not only may demonstrate changes in heart rate while obtaining postural blood pressures but also profound sinus bradycardia. Slow heart rates as a manifestation of vagotonia may indicate the patient's predisposition to vasodepressor or vasovagal syncope.

Auscultation of the Carotid Vessels and Heart

Careful examination of the carotid vessels for bruits and auscultation of the heart determine the presence of aortic stenosis or obstructive cardiomyopathy. The presence of a high density of ectopic beats also may help to define arrhythmia as a potential cause of syncope. Central nervous system examination can exclude evidence for focal neurologic deficit. In most patients, however, physical findings are not helpful and not nearly as critical to the diagnosis as a proper history.

LABORATORY EVALUATION

Ambulatory and Transtelephonic Electrocardiographic Monitoring

Laboratory evaluation of a patient with syncope (Table 3) should focus on where the diagnosis will most likely be found.

Any historical suggestion of cardiac arrhythmia, either tachycardia or bradycardia, demands 48 to 72 hours of ambulatory monitoring. A transtelephonic device with loop memory capacity may be the only practical means of documenting cardiac rhythm when events are infrequent [9]. Also, the exercise tolerance test may provide invaluable information regarding the ability to provoke ventricular tachycardia of hemodynamic significance as well as bradycardia or advanced atrioventricular block [10].

Carotid Sinus Massage

The coincidence of coronary artery disease may be demonstrated by an exercise test, and the application of carotid sinus massage during the routine 12-lead electrocardiogram may provide information regarding carotid bulb sensitivity. A sensitive carotid may be stimulated by a tight collar when the neck is rotated, thus generating a syncopal event [11].

Signal-Averaged Electrocardiogram

The signal-averaged electrocardiogram [12] is used to demonstrate the presence of high-frequency, low-amplitude electrical activity at the terminal portion of the QRS complex and may indicate susceptibility to ventricular arrhythmia. Electrophysiologic provocation studies [13] may provide further clues regarding the ease of stimulating a brady- or tachyarrhythmia and help to define the sinoatrial recovery time, which may be helpful under well-defined circumstances [14]. The tachybrady syndrome, wherein the abrupt termination of rapid supraventricular tachycardia (including atrial fibrillation) produces a prolonged sinus pause, may give rise to prolonged asystole and near or complete syncope. Whether to pursue invasive studies depends on exclusion of the more obvious causes of syncope. Our practice is to defer electrophysiologic study until a full noninvasive evaluation is completed [15].

Autonomic Testing

Autonomic testing using head-up tilt and an isoproterenol infusion has been studied in detail [16,17•,18••]. The appearance of intense bradycardia and hypotension during head-up tilt, with or without the infusion of isoproterenol, and the induction of near syncope or syncope suggestive of the clinical scenario are diagnostic of neurocardiogenic syncope. An increase in myocardial contractility and a coincidental decline in left ventricular end diastolic dimension precede the onset of syncope [19]. A vagus-mediated slowing of the heart rate appears to play a secondary role to vasodepression in inducing a hypotensive syncopal episode. This appears to explain the inefficacy of cardiac pacing in the management of patients with neurocardiogenic syncope [20•].

Echocardiography

Echocardiography occasionally supplements and clarifies issues raised on physical examination. Systolic murmurs may require further clarification regarding the potential for hemodynamically critical aortic stenosis, pulmonary stenosis, idiopathic hypertrophic subaortic stenosis (IHSS), or atrial myxoma to be the source of syncope. The patient with unsuspected IHSS receiving a diuretic may experience a syncopal episode; with rehydration the patient may have no further symptoms. Ventricular or atrial tachyarrhythmia in the setting of IHSS also may cause syncope.

MANAGEMENT

Single Event

Typically, the first episode of lost consciousness is based on a vasovagal event; however, this diagnosis is one of exclusion. Patient history is typical, with an absence of neurologic prodrome or sequelae and a spontaneous resumption of consciousness without the need for resuscitation. These features define the diagnosis and determine further management. In many cases, a solitary episode of lost consciousness suggests either cardiac or neurologic syncope and requires further evaluation.

Multiple Episodes

There is more concern if the patient experiences two or more syncopal episodes, particularly if they share historical characteristics. At times, several days of hospitalization are needed to define the syncope as neurologic, which may only be disclosed through a sleep-deprived electroencephalogram, for example, or a cardiac rhythm disorder that may either have been a brady- or tachycardiac event. Evaluation of the patient with syncope depends on the unique nature and frequency of the event and the clinical condition of the patient.

WHEN TO REFER

The generalist should maintain responsibility for the overall care of the patient and integration of the evaluation and therapy for syncope with the patient's preexisting medical and social problems. It is often the valued role of the generalist to maintain a critical perspective on results of the general and specialized testing. If one test does not fit a scenario that the bulk of the other diagnostic tests support, it may need to be

TABLE 3 LABORATORY EVALUATION

By the generalist
Carotid sinus massage
Electrocardiography
Ambulatory electrocardiographic monitor
Transtelephonic "loop memory"
Exercise tolerance test
Electroencephalography
If indicated by physical examination:
  Echocardiography
  Carotid arterial noninvasive tests

By the specialist
Signal-averaged electrocardiography
Cardiac electrophysiologic study
Tilt-table autonomic testing

discarded. One test result should not countermand the weight of clinical sensibility if the other objective tests lean away from the diagnosis supported by that single test.

Under most circumstances, the generalist proceeds with a thorough history and physical examination, including carotid sinus massage, an electrocardiogram and a 24-hour ambulatory monitor. If the physical examination suggests an obstructive lesion of the carotid arteries, referral for carotid noninvasive testing is indicated. If the vascular obstruction is reported as significant, referral to a neurologist or vascular surgeon is warranted. The neurologist also should be consulted when the history suggests a seizure disorder.

Cardiac murmurs suggestive of valvular obstructive disease or hypertrophic obstructive cardiomyopathy require prompt referral. Consultation with a cardiologist is indicated if pathology is defined or the murmur remains enigmatic and the history suggests a cardiac source of syncope.

Referral to the cardiologist also is advised when the 24-hour ambulatory monitor provides various types of data. An unambiguous, complete atrioventricular block requires pacemaker implantation. Tachyarrhythmia, particularly ventricular, requires referral to the cardiologist to determine the need for further assessment with electrocardiographic signal averaging or arrhythmia provocation (electrophysiologic studies).

References and Recommended Reading

Recently published papers of particular interest have been highlighted as:
- Of interest
- • Of outstanding interest

1. Lipsitz LA: Orthostatic hypotension in the elderly. *N Engl J Med* 1989, 321:952–956.
2. Kapoor WN, Peterson JR, Karpf M: Micturition syncope. *JAMA* 1985, 253:796–798.
3. Kapoor WN, Peterson J, Karpf M: Defecation syncopes: a symptom with multiple etiologies. *Ann Intern Med* 1986, 146:2377–2423.
4. Lipsitz LA, Pluchino FC, Wei JY, *et al.*: Cardiovascular and norepinephrine responses after meal consumption in elderly (older than 75 years) persons with postprandial hypotension and syncope. *Am J Cardiol* 1986, 58:810–815.
5. Velebit V, Podrid PJ, Lown B, *et al.*: Aggravation and provocation of ventricular arrhythmias by antiarrhythmic drugs. *Circulation* 1982, 65:886–894.
6. Linzer M, Pontinen M, Gold DT, *et al.*: Impairment of physical and psychosocial health in recurrent syncope. *J Clin Epidemiol* 1991, 44:1037–1044.
7.• Linzer M, Felder A, Hackel A, *et al.*: Psychiatric syncope: a new look at an old disease. *Psychosomatics* 1990, 31:181–188.
8.•• Kapoor WN: Diagnostic evaluation of syncope. *Am J Med* 1991, 90:91–106.
9. Cumbee SR, Pryor RE, Linzer M: Cardiac loop ECG recording: a new noninvasive diagnostic test in recurrent syncope. *South Med J* 1990, 83:39–43.
10. Podrid PJ, Graboys TB, Lampert S, Blatt CM: Exercise stress testing for exposure of arrhythmia. *Circulation* 1987, 75:60–65.
11. Lewis T: A lecture on vasovagal syncope and the carotid sinus mechanism. *BMJ* 1932, 1:873–876.
12. Kuchar DL, Thorburn CW, Sammel NL: Signal-averaged electrocardiogram for evaluation of recurrent syncope. *Am J Cardiol* 1986, 58:949–953.
13. Krol RB, Morady F, Flaker CG, *et al.*: Electrophysiologic testing in patients with unexplained syncope: clinical and noninvasive predictors of outcome. *J Am Coll Cardiol* 1987, 10:358–363.
14. Linzer M, Prystowsky EN, Divine GW, *et al.*: Predicting the outcome of electrophysiologic studies in syncope: validation of a derived model. *J Gen Intern Med* 1991, 6:113–120.
15. Lown B: Management of patients at high risk of sudden death. *Am Heart J* 1982, 103:689–697.
16. Almquist A, Goldenberg IF, Milstein S, *et al.*: Provocation of bradycardia and hypotension by isoproterenol and upright posture in patients with unexplained syncope. *N Engl J Med* 1989, 320:346–351.
17.• Grubb BP, Temesy-Armos P, Han H, Elliot L: Utility of upright tilt-table testing in the evaluation and management of syncope of unknown origin. *Am J Med* 1991, 90:6–10.
18.•• Kapoor WN, Brant N: Evaluation of syncope by upright tilt testing with isoproterenol: a nonspecific test. *Ann Intern Med* 1992, 116:358–363.
19. Shalev Y, Gal R, Tchou PJ, *et al.*: Echocardiographic demonstration of decreased left ventricular dimensions and vigorous myocardial contraction during syncope induced by head-up tilt. *J Am Coll Cardiol* 1991, 18:746–751.
20.• Sra JS, Jazayeri MR, Avitall B, *et al.*: Comparison of cardiac pacing with drug therapy in the treatment of neurocardiogenic (vasovagal) syncope with bradycardia or asystole. *N Engl J Med* 1993, 328:1085–1090.

Evaluation of the Patient Resuscitated from Cardiac Arrest

Eric N. Prystowsky

> ### Key Points
> - Sudden cardiac death is the most common cause of mortality in adults less than age 65 years of age.
> - Coronary artery disease is the most common cause of cardiac arrest.
> - Survivors of cardiac arrest should undergo a complete history and physical examination as well as cardiac catheterization and electrophysiologic testing.
> - An implantable cardioverter defibrillator (ICD) is often necessary to prevent sudden cardiac death.
> - Antiarrhythmic drug therapy, alone or with the ICD, is often useful.
> - Survivors of cardiac arrest are at a high risk for a recurrent episode if not treated properly, so referral to a clinical electrophysiologist is suggested.

Sudden cardiac death is the most common cause of mortality in adults less than 65 years of age [1•]. It is estimated that sudden cardiac death claims a patient approximately every 1 to 2 minutes [2]. There are various cardiac causes for sudden death (Table 1). In a relatively small percentage of patients, bradycardia may be the first arrhythmia identified in the cardiac arrest victim, but ventricular fibrillation or rapid sustained ventricular tachycardia (VT-S) is more common (Fig. 1) [3–7].

Cobb and coworkers [8••] are pioneers in establishing community-based intervention for cardiac arrest victims. They have developed a rapid response system for emergency services in Seattle using the Seattle Fire Department. Approximately 60% of Seattle residents 12 years of age and older have had some training in cardiopulmonary resuscitation. Even in such an emergency care system, only approximately 30% of cardiac arrest victims are discharged from the hospital alive. Most communities, especially in more rural areas of the United States, have far fewer successful resuscitations. In Memphis, approximately 10% to 13% of patients with cardiac arrest and out-of-hospital ventricular tachycardia or ventricular fibrillation who are given emergency care are discharged from the hospital alive [9]. Because survival rates are so poor in patients with out-of-hospital cardiac arrest caused by ventricular fibrillation or VT-S, physicians should determine who is at greatest risk for these arrhythmias to prevent the first episode and decrease sudden death.

Causes of Sudden Cardiac Death

Heart Disease

Sudden cardiac death because of ventricular fibrillation occurs most commonly in patients with heart disease. By far, coronary artery disease is the most common condition associated with sudden cardiac death [10,11], and it is important to identify whether cardiac arrest occurred at the time of acute myocardial infarction (MI) (Fig. 2). Cobb and coworkers [12] reported a 1-year mortality rate of 2% in patients with an acute MI at the time of cardiac arrest compared with 22% in patients without acute MI. Coronary artery spasm can cause ventricular fibrillation, but it has been documented as the cause of cardiac arrest in only a small percentage of patients [13•].

Some patients with hypertrophic or dilated cardiomyopathy as well as those with certain forms of congenital heart disease, (*eg*, postoperative tetralogy of Fallot) also can be at risk for sudden cardiac death [14]. There is sometimes a familial pattern of sudden cardiac death, especially in certain idiopathic dilated cardiomyopathies or in hypertrophic cardiomyopathy.

Electrophysiologic Abnormalities

Patients with the Wolff-Parkinson-White syndrome rarely have cardiac arrest [15]. The most common form of tachycardia in this syndrome is paroxysmal supraventricular tachycardia, which is usually a regular, narrow QRS-complex tachycardia. In some patients, atrial fibrillation may cause a rapid ventricular rate because of conduction from the atrium to the ventricle over the accessory pathway; this can subsequently degenerate into ventricular fibrillation (Fig. 3) [15].

Patients with the idiopathic long-QT syndrome are at risk for syncope and cardiac arrest [16•]. Typically, these patients have torsade de pointes, a polymorphic ventricular tachycardia, which can degenerate into ventricular fibrillation. Long-QT syndrome has a strong familial pattern, with autosomal dominant and recessive modes of inheritance. The hallmark is a prolonged QT interval, although this is not present in every electrocardiogram. Therapy can usually prevent cardiac arrest. It is important to make an accurate diagnosis and to evaluate other family members who may be at risk.

Infrequently, patients with no evidence of structural heart disease can have ventricular fibrillation. In a recent series of 19 patients with idiopathic ventricular fibrillation, six had a history of syncope and two had presyncope before cardiac arrest [17]. However, ventricular tachyarrhythmias are an uncommon cause for syncope in patients with no identifiable structural heart disease. Thus, it is not advisable to pursue aggressively this cause for syncope in most patients, unless a strong suspicion exists for the presence of ventricular tachycardia.

Iatrogenic Causes

Aggressive diuresis with subsequent marked hypokalemia can lead to cardiac arrest because of ventricular fibrillation. A more common iatrogenic cause of cardiac arrest is proarrhythmia resulting from drug use, especially antiarrhythmic drugs. Several types of ventricular proarrhythmias exist, including drug-associated ventricular fibrillation, new-onset VT-S, incessant ventricular tachycardia, and torsade de pointes. Patients with depressed left ventricular function and those with a history of VT-S are more likely to develop proarrhythmia during antiarrhythmic drug treatment.

An example of torsade de pointes ventricular proarrhythmia is shown in Figure 4. This patient had heart disease and atrial fibrillation. Intravenous procainamide failed to terminate atrial fibrillation, and electrical cardioversion restored sinus rhythm. The QT interval was markedly prolonged immediately after cardioversion. Approximately 10 minutes later, the patient developed torsade de pointes and required resuscitative efforts. Because ventricular proarrhythmia often occurs during the first few days of therapy, we recommend starting antiarrhythmic drugs in-hospital for patients with heart disease.

APPROACH TO SURVIVORS OF CARDIAC ARREST

Evaluation

Survivors of cardiac arrest should undergo a complete history and physical examination. The history may reveal data suggesting a long-term problem with cardiac dysfunction, such as exertional shortness of breath. Alternatively, the patient may relate a history of chest pain that has increased in severity over several weeks before cardiac arrest. In our experience, patients almost always have some degree of retrograde amnesia when they awake after cardiac arrest. This usually precludes any useful information regarding events that immediately preceded the cardiac arrest, unless an observer can provide these data. It should be ascertained whether the patient took any new prescription or over the counter drugs. Some aggressive diets,

TABLE 1 COMMON CAUSES OF CARDIAC ARREST

Heart disease
Coronary artery disease
Cardiomyopathy
Congenital heart disease
Electrophysiologic abnormalities
Wolff-Parkinson-White syndrome
Long-QT syndrome
Idiopathic ventricular fibrillation
Iatrogenic
Proarrhythmia with drugs
Electrolyte derangements

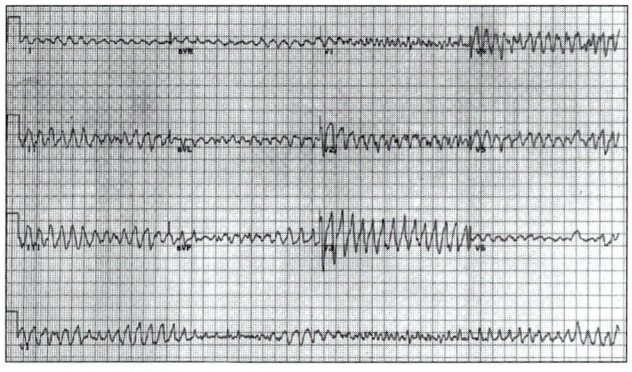

FIGURE 1 Twelve-lead electrocardiogram of ventricular fibrillation recorded during electrophysiologic study of a patient in whom arrhythmia was induced with programmed ventricular stimulation.

(*eg*, liquid protein diets) can lead to marked abnormalities in electrolytes and development of ventricular tachyarrhythmias. When appropriate, one should investigate and screen for use of illicit drugs, especially cocaine.

Physical examination may reveal the presence of atherosclerosis, detected by findings of peripheral vascular disease such as a decreased arterial pulse or the presence of xanthomas or xanthelasma. Cardiac examination may disclose a ventricular

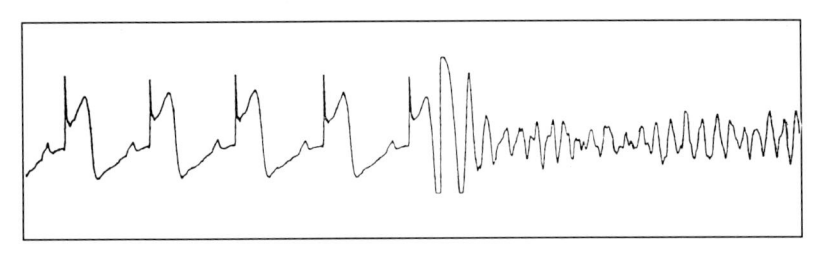

FIGURE 2 Emergence of ventricular fibrillation during the first hour of acute myocardial infarction. (From Prystowsky [23]; with permission.)

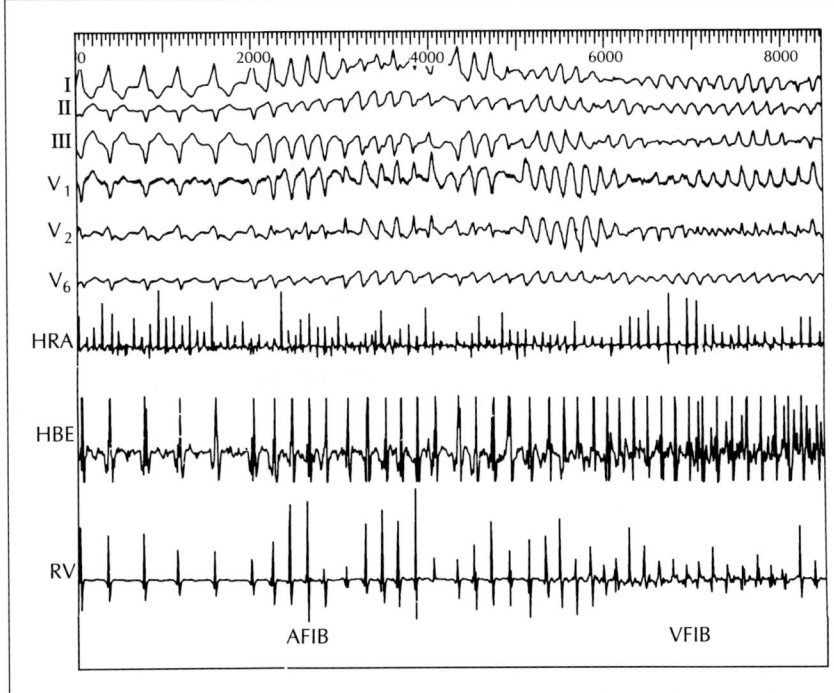

FIGURE 3 Atrial fibrillation (AFIB) initiated during electrophysiologic study of a patient with anterograde conduction over the accessory pathway. Simultaneous tracings are from electrocardiographic leads I, II, III, V_1, V_2, and V_6 as well as from intracardiac leads in the high right atrium (HRA), His bundle area (HBE), and right ventricle (RV). Atrial fibrillation is evidenced by the rapid, irregular rhythm recorded on the HRA lead. At the left, the wide, grossly irregular QRS complexes are caused by conduction over the accessory pathway. At the right, ventricular fibrillation (VFIB) has occurred. (From Prystowsky and coworkers [24]; with permission.)

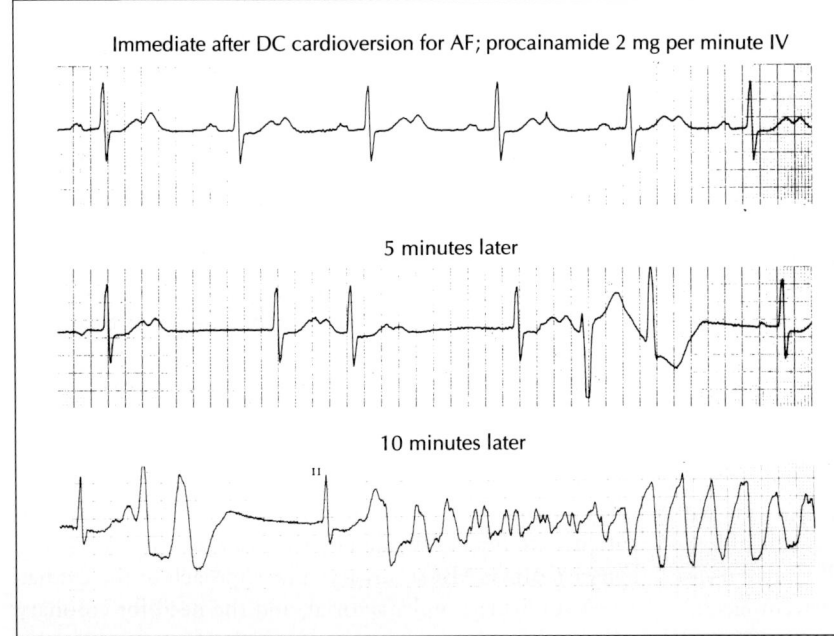

FIGURE 4 Development of torsade de pointes ventricular proarrhythmia in a patient treated with procainamide for atrial fibrillation (AF). IV—intravenous. (From Prystowsky and Klein [18]; with permission.)

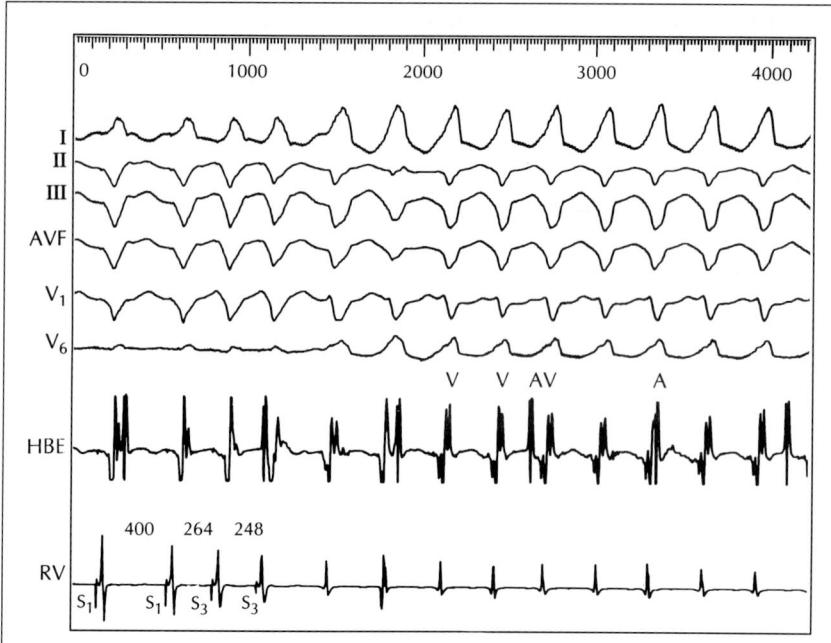

Figure 5 Initiation of sustained rapid ventricular tachycardia during programmed ventricular stimulation. Simultaneous tracings are electrocardiogram leads I, II, III, aVF, V_1, V_6, and intracardiac electrograms from the His bundle (HBE) and right ventricle (RV). The RV is paced at cycle length 400 msec (150/min) for eight beats, and two premature stimuli (S_2, S_3) are introduced with coupling of intervals of 264 and 248 msec, respectively. After the second premature stimulus, sustained ventricular tachycardia occurs and ventriculoatrial dissociation is noted on the HBE lead, with more ventricular (V) than atrial (A) electrograms.

(S_3) or atrial gallop (S_4), suggesting the possibility of systolic or diastolic dysfunction. Significant cardiac murmurs may be heard, and evidence for systemic diseases (*eg*, thyromegaly) that affect the heart also may be present.

Extensive laboratory investigation is required. Serial cardiac enzymes and electrocardiograms are necessary to diagnose an acute myocardial infarction. The electrocardiogram also may uncover the long-QT syndrome, a previous MI, nonspecific findings that suggest cardiomyopathy, or the presence of ventricular preexcitation. Serum electrolyte testing may diagnose severe hypokalemia. Other blood tests are usually unrevealing but are occasionally helpful; for example, a substantially elevated erythrocyte sedimentation rate may reveal acute myocarditis.

Echocardiography is a requisite part of the work-up. Myocardial size and function as well as valvular abnormalities are easily evaluated with this technique. Cardiac catheterization should be performed in all patients unless the cause of cardiac arrest is obvious, for example, an acute MI [18••]. Treadmill exercise testing may be useful in patients with suspected coronary artery disease to evaluate functional status or in those who had cardiac arrest during exertion. In my experience, VT-S rarely emerges during the exercise test in patients who are referred for cardiac arrest [19].

A complete electrophysiologic evaluation should be done for patients in whom an unequivocal precipitating cause of cardiac arrest has not been identified. Atrial pacing tests sinus node function and atrioventricular (AV) conduction, as well as evaluates the inducibility of supraventricular tachycardia. Most importantly, pacing the ventricle with introduction of premature beats may initiate VT-S or ventricular fibrillation [20•] (Fig. 5). Sustained monomorphic ventricular tachycardia is induced more commonly in patients with coronary artery disease compared with other forms of heart disease or idiopathic ventricular fibrillation [20•]. In a review of 1233 survivors of cardiac arrest who underwent electrophysiologic evaluation, 42% had sustained monomorphic ventricular tachycardia initiated, whereas 16% had sustained polymorphic ventricular tachycardia or ventricular fibrillation induced [20•].

Treatment

An approach to therapy is summarized in Figure 6. Patients with a clearly reversible etiology for cardiac arrest are given specific therapy for that condition. An example is routine post-MI care for patients with ventricular fibrillation that occurred within the first 48 hours after MI. Most patients do not have an obvious cause for the cardiac arrest, and treatment depends on the type of heart disease present. The overwhelming majority of patients have either coronary artery disease or cardiomyopathy. Data are sparse on patients with idiopathic ventricular fibrillation, however, but early defibrillator implantation should be considered in these cases [17]. The accessory pathway should be ablated in cardiac arrest survivors with Wolff-Parkinson-White syndrome and rapid preexcited ventricular rates during atrial fibrillation induced at electrophysiologic study [18••]. This is usually accomplished with endocardial catheter ablation techniques. Patients with cardiomyopathy should undergo electrophysiologic evaluation; results may affect the choice of antiarrhythmic therapy. Little information is available regarding the accuracy of serial electrophysiologic–pharmacologic drug testing to determine the efficacy of treatment in patients with cardiomyopathy; thus, I recommend an implantable cardioverter defibrillator (ICD) as part of their therapy [18••].

Patients with coronary artery disease are dichotomized into those with and those without sustained ventricular tachyarrhythmias initiated at electrophysiologic study. These patients are further divided by the need for coronary artery bypass graft (CABG) surgery. The approach to the cardiac arrest survivor is multifactorial, and the need for coronary revascularization should be considered. However, it is uncommon for revascularization alone to prevent recurrent cardiac arrest.

For patients in whom VT-S or ventricular fibrillation is not induced, an ICD is recommended as initial therapy for all patients except those with no evidence of myocardial dysfunction [20•]. This is a small subgroup who tend to have severe three-vessel coronary artery disease and well-preserved left ventricular function. The assumption is that this patient had an ischemic cardiac arrest without MI, although proof is almost always lacking in these instances. Few patients fall into this category, but I have had success with revascularization only in these individuals.

Patients who have VT-S or VF initiated and require CABG surgery are recommended for ICD therapy at the time of surgery. However, with the more recent use and high success of nonthoracotomy lead systems, one may want to delay ICD implantation in some patients until after CABG. If CABG or other cardiac surgery is not required, these patients are subgrouped according to the left ventricular ejection fraction. Wilbur and coworkers [21] demonstrated that recurrence of cardiac arrest was unacceptably high in patients with lower ejection fractions, and who had suppression of their ventricular arrhythmias during serial electrophysiologic–pharmacologic drug testing. For this reason, I recommend early consideration for an ICD in these individuals; however, I do routinely begin with antiarrhythmic drug therapy in patients with ejection fractions of 40% or more. Efficacy is evaluated with electrophysiologic testing. In these individuals, programmed ventricular stimulation is repeated in the presence of antiarrhythmic drugs. The patient is discharged and receives the drug if only a few repetitive ventricular beats can be initiated with an aggressive pacing protocol. Overall, most cardiac arrest survivors are treated with an ICD.

PREVENTION OF CARDIAC ARREST

Patients often have symptoms that are possibly related to an arrhythmia. These include palpitations, presyncope, dizziness, and syncope. The aggressiveness of the work-up depends not only on the symptom but also on the underlying cardiac condition; an approach to these patients is demonstrated in Figure 7. Patients without any structural heart disease and no electrocardiographic abnormalities should undergo ambulatory electrocardiographic monitoring, usually with a handheld or loop event recorder, to evaluate palpitations. Syncope or presyncope in patients without heart disease is often caused by neurally mediated syncope, which is

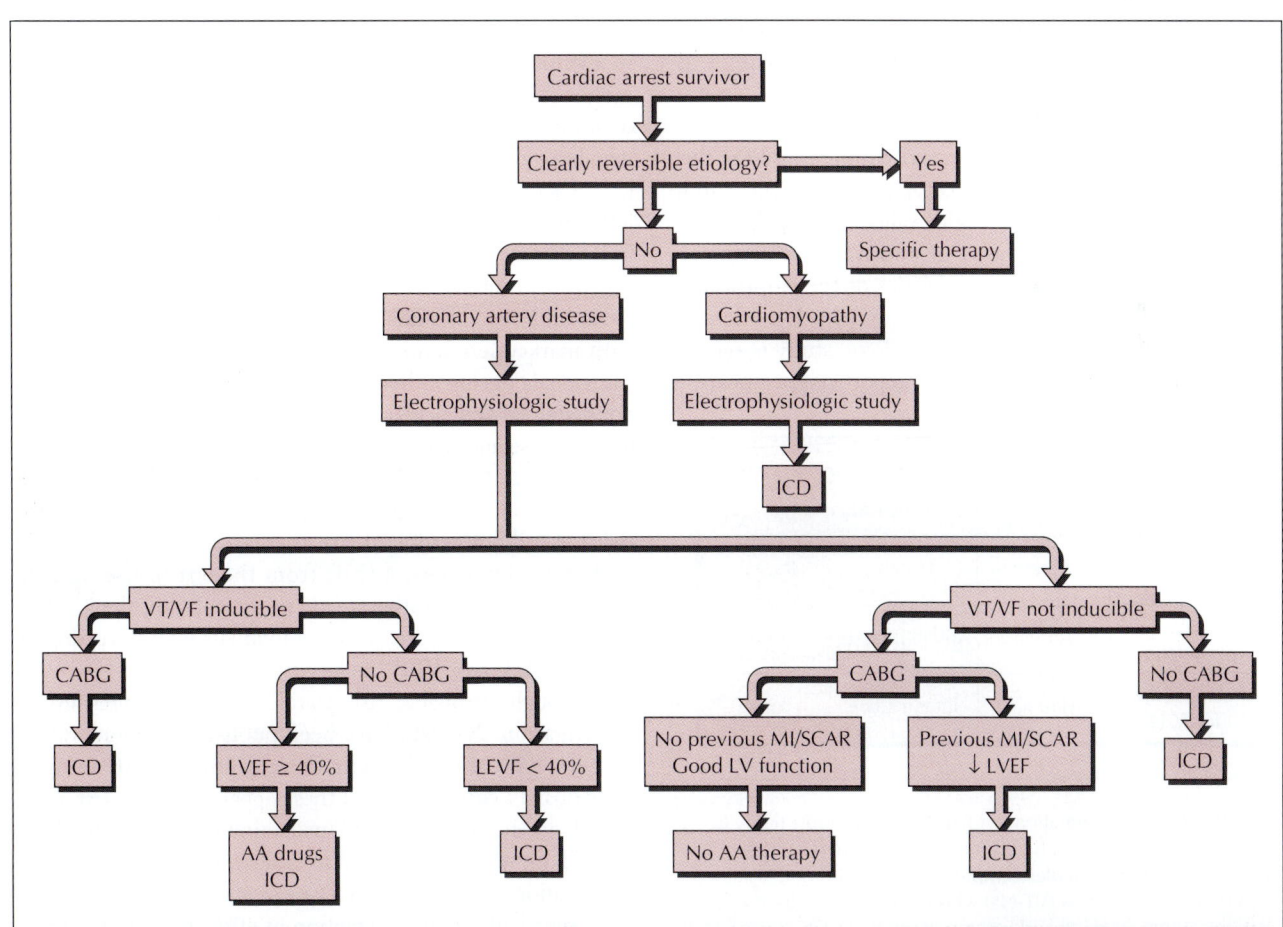

FIGURE 6 Approach to therapy for cardiac arrest survivors. AA—antiarrhythmic; CABG—coronary artery bypass graft surgery; ICD—implantable cardioverter defibrillator; LVEF—left ventricular ejection fraction; MI—myocardial infarction; SCAR—myocardial scar; VF—ventricular fibrillation; VT—sustained ventricular tachycardia.

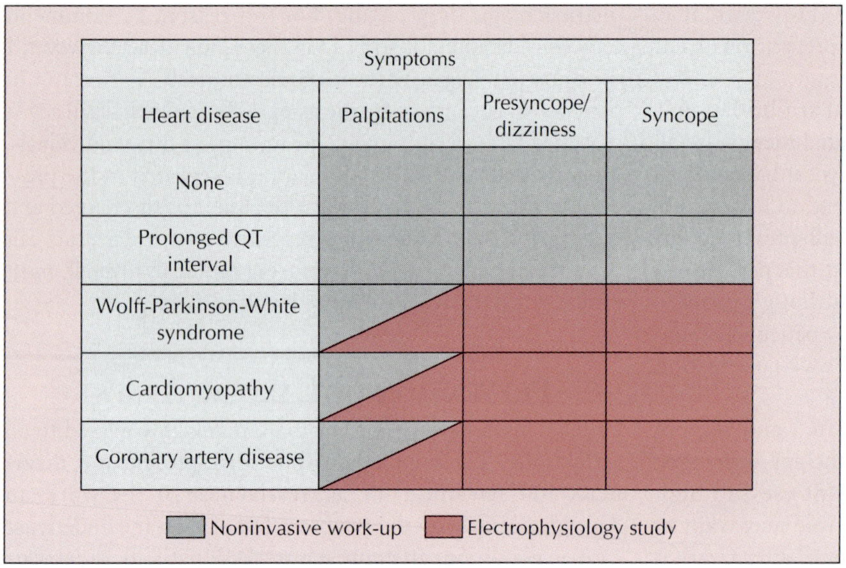

FIGURE 7 Initial work-up of patients with possible arrhythmic symptoms.

Symptoms			
Heart disease	Palpitations	Presyncope/dizziness	Syncope
None			
Prolonged QT interval			
Wolff-Parkinson-White syndrome			
Cardiomyopathy			
Coronary artery disease			

Noninvasive work-up ▨ Electrophysiology study

best uncovered during tilt-table evaluation. Patients with a prolonged QT interval and potential arrhythmic symptoms should undergo electrocardiographic monitoring to correlate symptoms with an electrocardiographic tracing. Electrophysiologic study is usually not helpful in these individuals; causes other than arrhythmias for dizziness or syncope should be sought. Therapy should be initiated if any suspicion exists that the symptoms relate to a ventricular arrhythmia. β-blockers are the initial treatment of choice.

Patients with WPW syndrome, cardiomyopathy, or coronary artery disease likely have an arrhythmic cause for their symptoms. Presyncope, dizziness, or syncope in these individuals requires electrophysiologic evaluation. If palpitations are present, either a noninvasive or invasive work-up may be done, depending on the characteristics of the palpitations. For example, if the patient relates a rapid, long-lasting episode of palpitations, electrophysiologic study is recommended. Alternatively, a patient may report skipped beats, in which case ambulatory electrocardiographic recordings are the initial recommendation. Therapy is directed by the findings of the work-up.

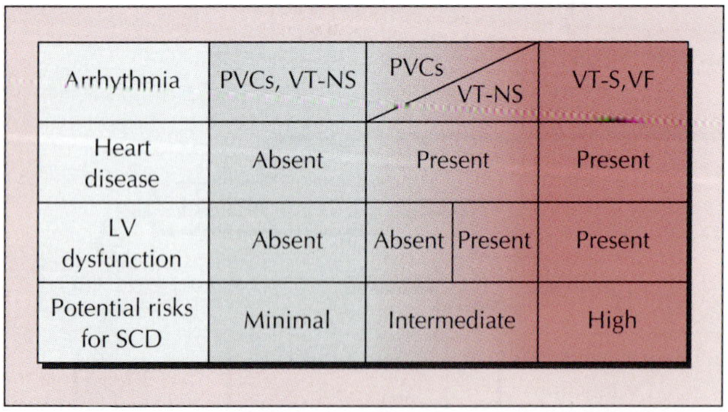

Few patients with out-of-hospital cardiac arrest are resuscitated early enough to allow survival and discharge from the hospital with minimal brain damage. Thus, risk stratification is a reasonable attempt to prevent the first cardiac arrest event in asymptomatic individuals; an approach to risk stratification is shown in Figure 8. The concept of risk stratification is to determine which individuals most closely resemble patients who have already had a cardiac arrest because of VT-S or VF [22]. Factors considered are the arrhythmia, heart disease, and left ventricular dysfunction. Asymptomatic patients without heart disease are at minimal risk for sudden cardiac death. Survivors of cardiac arrest and patients with a history of VT-S are at high risk for sudden cardiac death. Heart disease, often with marked left ventricular dysfunction, is usually present. Individuals having either premature ventricular complexes or nonsustained ventricular tachycardia with variable degrees of heart disease and left ventricular dysfunction are at intermediate risk for sudden cardiac death. This is the group for which risk stratification is suggested. In this intermediate group, the risk for sudden cardiac death increases as left ventricular dysfunction worsens, a shift from the left to the right in Figure 8. On the righthand side of the column, the patients have similar characteristics to individuals who have already suffered a VT-S or VF.

Although reasonable, risk stratification still requires further investigation. No data have been published demonstrating that any type of prophylactic therapy prolongs life in these individuals. I currently enroll these apparently high-risk individuals in the Multicenter Unsustained Tachycardia Trial (MUSTT), which is intended to evaluate one approach to risk stratification in patients who have coronary artery disease with a left ventricular ejection fraction of 40% or less in the presence of minimally symptomatic, nonsustained ventricular tachycardia. Data from MUSTT may determine whether electrophysiologic testing is useful in stratifying risk in this patient group.

Arrhythmia	PVCs, VT-NS	PVCs / VT-NS	VT-S, VF
Heart disease	Absent	Present	Present
LV dysfunction	Absent	Absent / Present	Present
Potential risks for SCD	Minimal	Intermediate	High

FIGURE 8 Risk stratification to identify patients most likely to have cardiac arrest. The first column (light) includes patients with premature ventricular complexes (PVCs) and nonsustained ventricular tachycardia (VT-NS) who have no heart disease. Patients in the far righthand column (dark) have a history of sustained ventricular tachycardia (VT-S) or ventricular fibrillation (VF). Risk stratification involves the patients in the middle column (shaded). LV—left ventricular; SCD—sudden cardiac death. (From Prystowsky [22••]; with permission.)

When to Refer

If not treated properly, survivors of cardiac arrest are usually at high risk for a recurrent episode. These individuals should be referred to a clinical electrophysiologist. Patients with long-QT syndrome may be evaluated initially by a cardiologist, but they also may require input from a clinical electrophysiologist, especially if defibrillator therapy is contemplated. Patients with syncope or presyncope who have heart disease or WPW syndrome should be referred to an electrophysiologist. Palpitations thought to be primarily extrasystoles can be evaluated by the primary-care physician or cardiologist. If the clinician is concerned about a more serious arrhythmia, the patient should be referred to an electrophysiologist.

References and Recommended Reading

Recently published papers of particular interest have been highlighted as:
- Of interest
- Of outstanding interest

1.• Cupples LA, Gagnon DR, Kannel WB: Long- and short-term risk of sudden coronary death. *Circulation* 1992, 85:11–18.
2. Gillum FR: Sudden coronary death in the United States, 1980–1985. *Circulation* 1989, 79:756–765.
3. Prystowsky EN, Heger JJ, Zipes DP: The recognition and treatment of patients at risk for sudden death. In *Cardiac Emergencies*. Edited by Eliot RS, Saenz A, Forker AD. Kisco, NY: Futura Publishing; 1982:353–384.
4. Cobb LA, Werner JA, Trobaugh GB: Sudden cardiac death. I. A decade's experience with out-of-hospital resuscitation. *Mod Concepts Cardiovasc Dis* 1980, 49:31–36.
5. Liberthson RR, Nagel EL, Hirschman JC, Nussenfeld SR: Pre-hospital ventricular defibrillation. Prognosis and follow-up course. *N Engl J Med* 1974, 291:317–321.
6. Myerburg RJ, Conde CA, Sung RJ, *et al.*: Clinical, electrophysiologic and hemodynamic profile of patients resuscitated from pre-hospital cardiac arrest. *Am J Med* 1980, 68:568–576.
7. Luu M, Stevenson WG, Stevenson LW, *et al.*: Diverse mechanisms of unexpected cardiac arrest in advanced heart failure. *Circulation* 1989, 80:1675–1680.
8.•• Cobb LA, Weaver WD, Fahrenbruch CE, *et al.*: Community-based interventions for sudden cardiac death. Impact, limitations, and changes. *Circulation* 1992, 85(I):98–102.
9. Kellermann AL, Hackman BB, Somes G, Kreth TK: Impact of first-responder defibrillation in an urban emergency medical services system. *JAMA* 1993, 270:1708–1713.
10. Liberthson RR, Nagel EL, Hirschman JC, *et al.*: Pathophysiologic observations in pre-hospital ventricular fibrillation and sudden cardiac death. *Circulation* 1974, 49:790–798.
11. Reichenbach DD, Moss NS, Meyer E: Pathology of the heart in sudden cardiac death. *Am J Cardiol* 1977, 39:865–872.
12. Cobb LA, Werner JA, Trobaugh GB: Sudden cardiac death. II. Outcome of resuscitation; management, and future directions. *Mod Concepts Cardiovasc Dis* 1980, 49:37–42.
13.• Myerburg RJ, Kessler KM, Mallon SM, *et al.*: Life-threatening ventricular arrhythmias in patients with silent myocardial ischemia due to coronary artery spasm. *N Engl J Med* 1992, 326:1451–1455.
14. Maron BJ, Roberts WC, Epstein SE: Sudden death in hypertrophic cardiomyopathy: a profile of 78 patients. *Circulation* 1982, 65:1388–1394.
15. Klein GJ, Prystowsky EN, Yee R, *et al.*: Asymptomatic Wolff-Parkinson-White. Should we intervene? *Circulation* 1989, 80:1902–1905.
16.• Moss AJ, Robinson J: Clinical features of the idiopathic long QT syndrome. *Circulation* 1992, 85(I):140–144.
17. Wever EFD, Hauer RNW, Oomen A, *et al.*: Unfavorable outcome in patients with primary electrical disease who survived an episode of ventricular fibrillation. *Circulation* 1993, 88:1021–1029.
18.•• Prystowsky EN, Klein GJ: *Cardiac arrhythmias: an integrated approach for the clinician.* New York: McGraw-Hill; 1994.
19. Evans JJ, Skale BT, Windle JR, *et al.*: Comparison of ventricular tachycardia induction between exercise and electrophysiologic testing in patients with ventricular tachycardia [abstract]. *Circulation* 1984, 70:423.
20.• Knilans TK, Prystowsky EN: Antiarrhythmic drug therapy in the management of cardiac arrest survivors. *Circulation* 1992, 85:118–124.
21. Wilbur DJ, Garan H, Finkelstein D, *et al.*: Out-of-hospital cardiac arrest: use of electro-physiologic testing in the prediction of long-term outcome. *N Engl J Med* 1988, 318:19–24.
22. Prystowsky EN: Antiarrhythmic therapy for asymptomatic ventricular arrhythmias. *Am J Cardiol* 1988, 61:102A–107A.
23. Prystowsky EN: Tachyarrhythmias: the role of antiarrhythmic drugs in the therapeutic hierarchy. In *Tachycardias: Mechanisms and Management*. Edited by Josephson ME, Wellens HJJ. 1993, 375–389.
24. Prystowsky EN, Knilans TK, Evans JJ: Diagnostic evaluation and treatment strategies for patients at risk for serious cardiac arrhythmias. Part 2: Ventricular tachyarrhythmias and Wolff-Parkinson-White syndrome. *Mod Concepts Cardiovasc Dis* 1991, 60:55–59.

Select Bibliography

Cummins RO, Ornato JP, Thies WH, Pepe PA: Improving survival from sudden cardiac arrest: the "chain of survival" concept. *Circulation* 1991; 83:1832–1847.

Mirowski M, Reid PR, Mower MM, *et al.*: Termination of malignant ventricular arrhythmias with an implanted automatic defibrillator in human beings *N Engl J Med* 1980; 303:322–324.

Prystowsky EN: Electrophysiologic-electropharmacologic testing in patients with ventricular arrhythmias. *PACE* 1988; 11:225–251.

Risk Factors for and Prevention of Atherosclerotic Cardiovascular Disease

Pantel S. Vokonas
William B. Kannel

Key Points

- Atherosclerotic cardiovascular disease (CVD), in all its clinical manifestations, represents the leading cause of disability and mortality throughout much of the industrialized world.
- Epidemiologic studies have identified several important risk factors for CVD including hypertension, hyperlipidemia, cigarette smoking, diabetes, obesity, and physical inactivity.
- Cardiovascular risk is assessed in the outpatient setting using standard clinical procedures and simple laboratory tests followed by appropriate measures to modify relevant factors.
- Information available from intervention studies has already validated the efficacy and safety of preventive management of several risk factors in reducing the toll of CVD in the population.

Atherosclerotic cardiovascular disease (CVD) encompasses a broad spectrum of disease conditions of the heart and circulation that include coronary heart disease (CHD), cerebrovascular disease, and peripheral vascular disease (PVD). Because congestive heart failure often shares antecedents of atherosclerotic and hypertensive heart disease, it is also included under the heading of CVD.

The incidence of almost all cardiovascular events increases dramatically with advancing age (Fig. 1), serving to emphasize the heavy toll of disability and death attributable to CVD throughout life as well as the need for preventive attention for persons of all ages.

Because these conditions represent leading causes of morbidity and mortality in the United States and throughout much of the industrialized world, a working knowledge of risk factors for CVD and potential benefits of their modification on the part of primary care physicians and other health care professionals would make an important contribution to the future clinical and preventive management of this constellation of diseases.

RISK FACTORS FOR CARDIOVASCULAR DISEASE

Evidence from epidemiologic investigations indicates that a number of identifiable factors are associated with enhancement or acceleration of the underlying atherosclerotic process [1•] and thus, contribute to the development of clinical manifestations of CVD. This represents the central concept of the so-called risk-factor hypothesis, which constitutes the mainstay of modern cardiovascular prevention.

In this context, advanced age and male gender are two of the most important such risk factors; however, both factors are considered irremediable. Attention, therefore, focuses on attributes that can be potentially modified. These factors can be broadly classified in two categories: 1) atherogenic personal traits such as hypertension, hyperlipidemia, and glucose intolerance; or 2) lifestyle influences

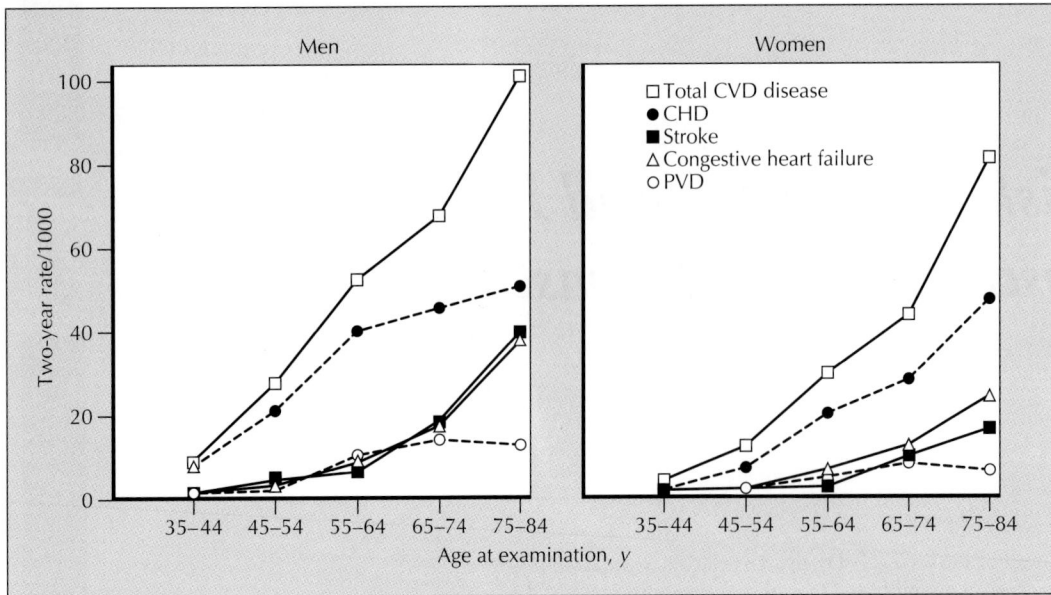

FIGURE 1 Age trends in incidence of total cardiovascular disease (CVD) and component CVD outcomes including coronary heart disease (CHD), stroke, congestive heart failure, and peripheral vascular disease (PVD) for men and women. Framingham Study, 26-year follow-up.

such as smoking, physical inactivity, and dietary patterns. Several well-established risk factors for CVD are considered in detail below.

Blood Pressure and Hypertension

Although conventional clinical wisdom emphasizes hypertensive risk related to elevations of diastolic blood pressure (diastolic hypertension), evidence from Framingham and other studies indicates an equal if not more potent risk for CVD associated with elevations of systolic blood pressure [2]. This is particularly relevant in older persons in whom progressive vascular stiffening results in significant elevations of systolic blood pressure and high prevalence of isolated systolic hypertension.

Relations between CVD occurrence and systolic and diastolic components of blood pressure are illustrated in Figures 2 and 3, respectively. Absolute risk, based on CVD incidence rates, is usually two to three times higher in older persons at corresponding levels of blood pressure, and tends to be higher in men than in women.

Risk gradients for CVD are generally similar in direction and magnitude when individuals are classified according to hypertensive status instead of absolute levels of blood pressure (Table 1). Overall risk of CVD tends to be two to three times higher in subjects with definite hypertension than in normotensive subjects, whereas risk is intermediate for those patients with mild hypertension. Similar patterns of risk attributable to hypertension have been documented specifically for CHD, stroke, congestive heart failure, and PVD (Table 2). When considered alone, isolated systolic hypertension also confers substantial risk of CVD events.

Previous data from randomized clinical trials have established a strong case for the efficacy of treating combined elevations of systolic and diastolic blood pressure in hypertensive patients at all ages, although considerable uncertainty remained regarding the treatment of isolated systolic hypertension. The findings of the Systolic Hypertension in the Elderly Program (SHEP) [3••], however, have served to dispel much of this uncertainty. This study documented impressive reductions in total numbers of fatal and nonfatal strokes in the

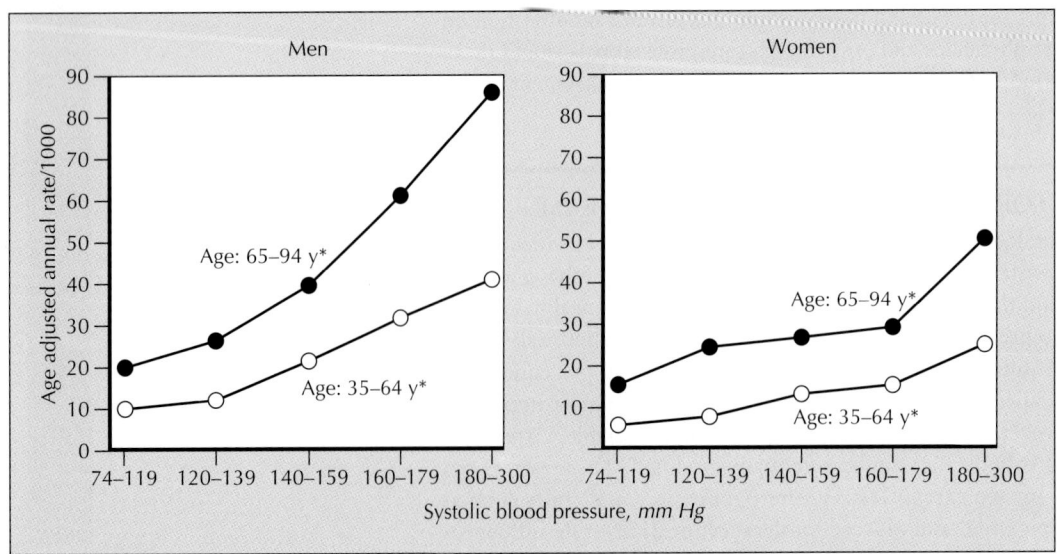

FIGURE 2 Risk of cardiovascular disease by age, sex, and level of systolic blood pressure. Framingham Study, 30-year follow-up. *$P < 0.001$ (age-adjusted Wald statistic for logistic regression analysis). (From Vokonas et al. [2]; with permission.)

active treatment group compared with the placebo group. Statistically significant reductions in nonfatal myocardial infarctions plus coronary death, as well as combined CHD and total CVD outcomes, were also noted in the treatment group. There appears to be little or no evidence from this study that lowering of systolic or diastolic blood pressure results in an increased risk of CHD events or mortality, particularly at the lower end of the distribution for blood pressure, the so-called J-shaped curve [4].

Two other recent clinical trials of drug therapy for hypertension in the elderly that included patients with isolated systolic hypertension also demonstrated beneficial effects [5,6].

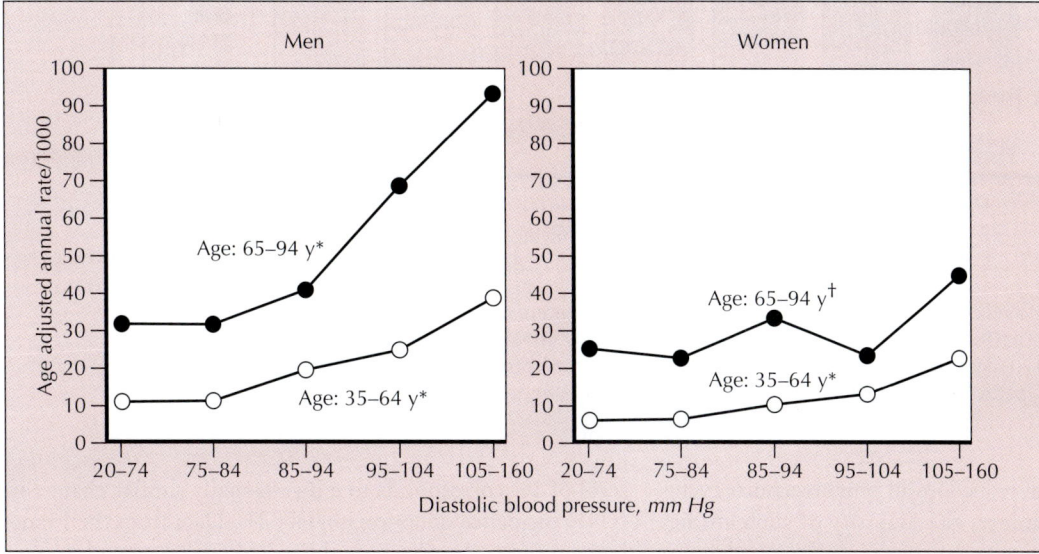

FIGURE 3 Risk of cardiovascular disease by age, sex, and level of diastolic blood pressure. Framingham Study, 30-year follow-up. *$P< 0.001$, †$P< 0.05$ (age-adjusted Wald statistic for logistic regression and analysis. *From* Vokonas *et al.* [2]; with permission.)

TABLE 1 RISK OF CARDIOVASCULAR DISEASE BY HYPERTENSIVE STATUS ACCORDING TO AGE AND SEX: FRAMINGHAM STUDY, 30-YEAR FOLLOW-UP

	Average annual age-adjusted rate per 1000, CVD			
	35–64 y*		65–94 y*	
Hypertensive status	**Men**	**Women**	**Men**	**Women**
Normal (<140/90 mm Hg)	11	5	22	19
Mild (140–160/90–95 mm Hg)	20	10	40	26
Definite (>160/95 mm Hg)	31	17	73	35

*All trends significant at $P<0.001$.
From Vokonas *et al.* [2]; with permission.

TABLE 2 RISK OF CARDIOVASCULAR EVENTS BY HYPERTENSIVE STATUS: FRAMINGHAM STUDY, 30-YEAR FOLLOW-UP

	Age-adjusted risk ratio*			
	35–64 y		65–94 y	
Cardiovascular event	**Men**	**Women**	**Men**	**Women**
Coronary heart disease	2.6§	3.3§	2.9§	2.0§
Stroke	6.0§	3.0§	3.1§	3.0§
Peripheral vascular disease	2.5§	3.0§	1.5	1.7‡
Congestive heart failure	3.0§	3.0§	3.8§	2.0§
CVD†	2.8§	3.4§	3.3§	1.8§

*Ratio of definite hypertension: normotension; hypertension defined as blood pressure greater than 160/95 mm Hg.
†In persons free of any CVD at the initial visit: ‡$P<0.05$, §$P<0.001$, hypertensives versus normotensives.
From Kannel *et al.* [15]; with permission.

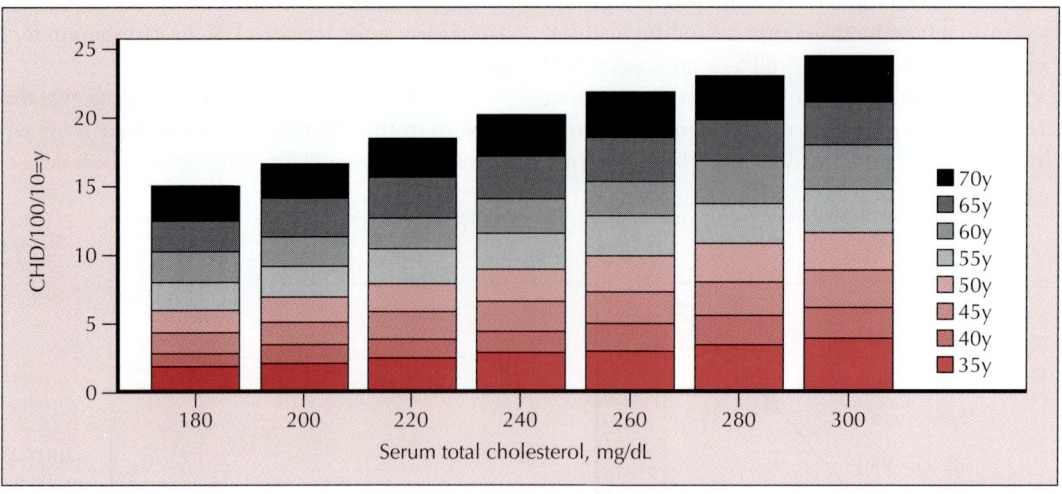

FIGURE 4 Relation of serum cholesterol to coronary heart disease (CHD) in men who have systolic blood pressures of 120 mm Hg or less, no diabetes, no left ventricular hypertrophy as determined by electrocardiogram, no cigarette smoking, and average high-density lipoprotein cholesterol levels at 45 mg/dL. (*Adapted from* Castelli *et al.* [10]; with permission.) *Data from* Anderson *et al.* [29].)

In addition to substantial reductions in cerebrovascular events and congestive heart failure, the majority of such studies performed in older persons to date have consistently demonstrated beneficial trends or significant reductions in CHD events and mortality. Such results appear to be considerably less apparent in clinical therapeutic trials in predominantly middle-aged hypertensive patients [7•].

Blood Lipids

Abnormalities of blood lipids represent well-established risk factors for at least two components of CVD, namely CHD and PVD. Regarding CHD, evidence from population studies indicate that overall incidence rates for CHD correlate well with serum total cholesterol levels [8,9••,10••]. The character of this relation further suggests that a change in serum cholesterol of 1% corresponds to a directionally similar change in CHD incidence of approximately 2%. Data from the Framingham Study that illustrate this relation for men and women at varying ages are shown in Figures 4 and 5.

Although useful in screening large populations for dyslipidemias, serum cholesterol cannot be considered the sole measure of risk for CHD attributable to serum lipids. This is based on our current understanding of lipoprotein cholesterol subfractions and the availability of standardized laboratory methods to measure them in clinical practice [11]. Serum total cholesterol tends to index low-density-lipoprotein (LDL) cholesterol, which varies directly with CHD risk (Fig. 6) and is considered atherogenic. High-density-lipoprotein (HDL) cholesterol varies inversely with CHD incidence (Fig. 7) and is considered anti-atherogenic or

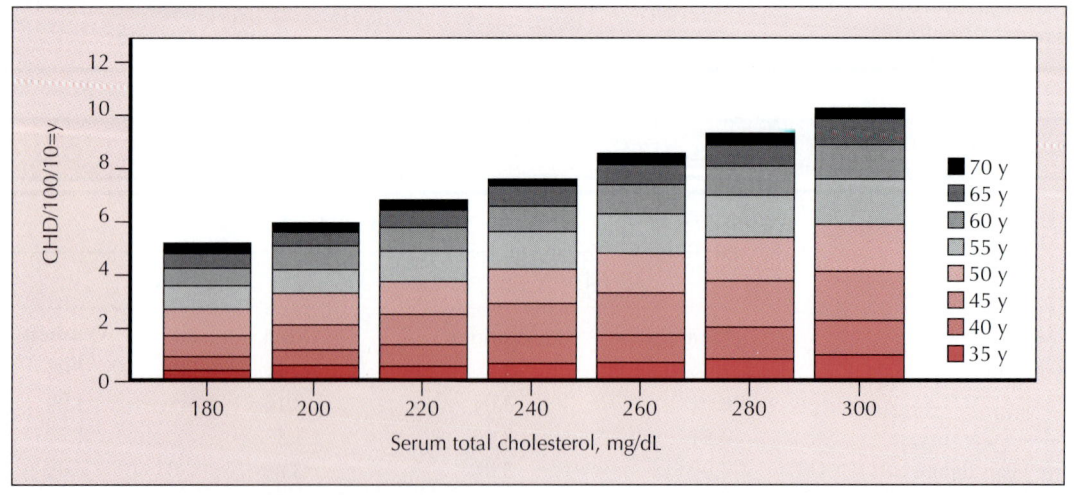

FIGURE 5 Relation of serum cholesterol to coronary heart disease (CHD) in women with systolic blood pressures of 120 mm Hg or less, no diabetes, no left ventricular hypertrophy as determined by electrocardiogram, no cigarette smoking, and average high-density lipoprotein cholesterol levels at 55 mg/dL. (*Adapted from* Castelli *et al.* [10]; with permission. *Data from* Anderson *et al.* [29].)

protective. This lipid moiety adds substantial precision in assessing coronary risk at limited additional cost. Construction of a serum cholesterol–to-HDL ratio provides a highly accurate characterization of CHD risk in subjects of the Framingham Study, as illustrated in Figure 8. Indeed, additional data from Framingham and other studies confirm the overall reliability of the cholesterol/HDL ratio in assessing CHD risk in younger and older persons, and also in men and women. The rationale for this approach is that the ratio reliably captures the effect of a dynamic equilibrium of lipid

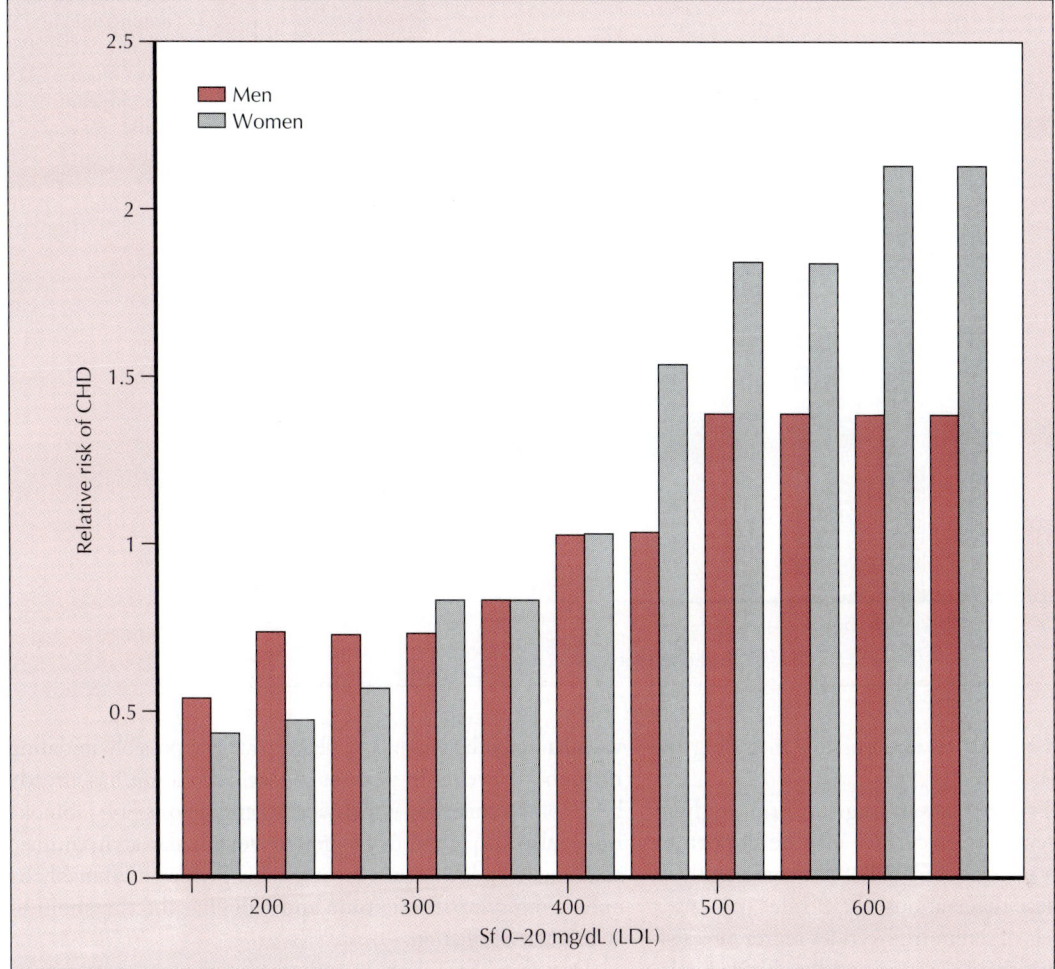

FIGURE 6
Relation of low-density-lipoprotein (LDL) cholesterol to relative risk of coronary heart disease (CHD) occurrence. Framingham Study, 30-year follow-up. (*From* Castelli *et al.* [8]; with permission.) Sf—Svedberg flotation units.

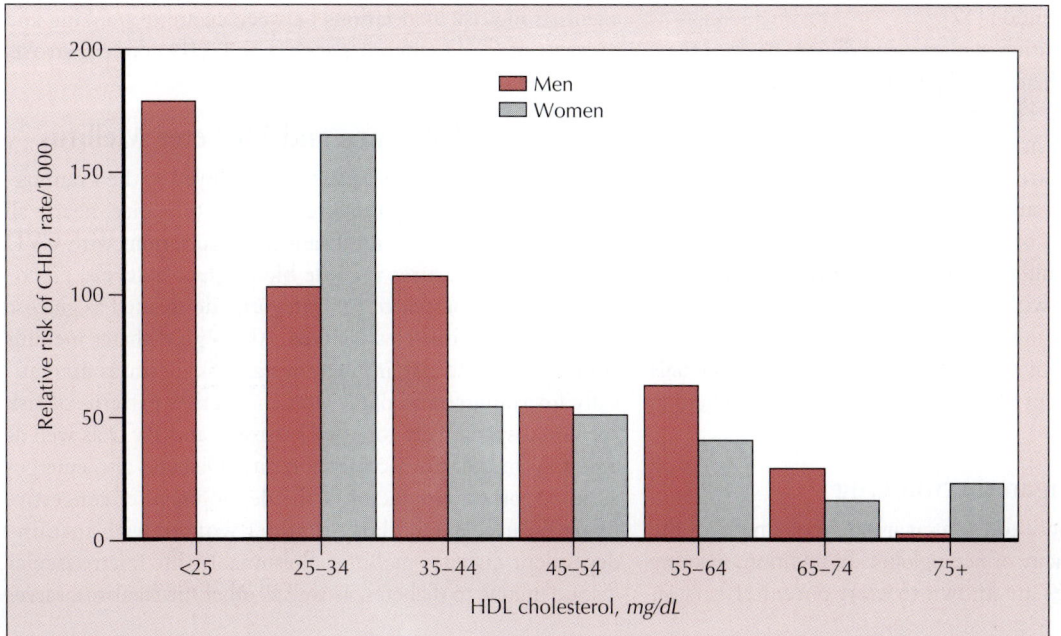

FIGURE 7
Relation of high-density-lipoprotein (HDL) cholesterol to coronary heart disease (CHD) incidence in 4 years. Framingham Study. *From* Castelli *et al.* [8]; with permission.)

Risk Factors for and Prevention of Atherosclerotic Cardiovascular Disease

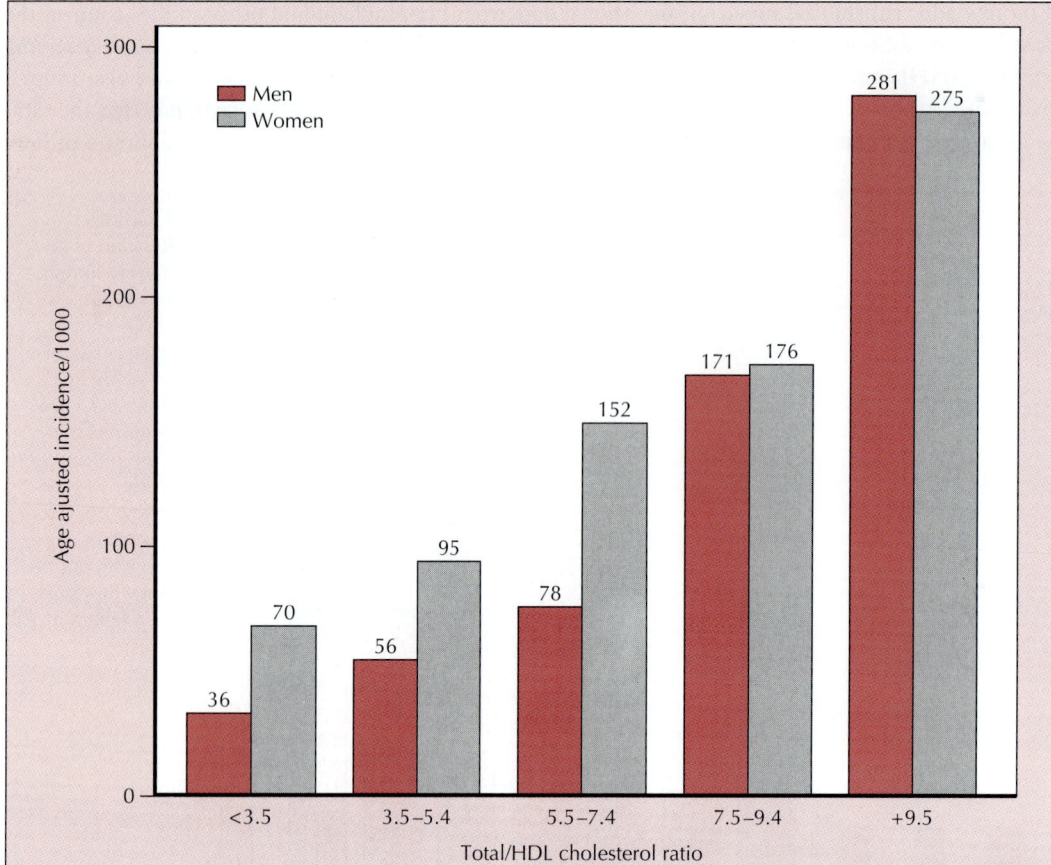

FIGURE 8 Risk of coronary heart disease (CHD) by total to high-density lipoprotein (HDL) cholesterol ratios among men and women 50 to 90 years of age. Framingham Study, 26-year follow-up.

transport into and out of body tissues, possibly including the intima of blood vessels.

Data from several studies, including the Framingham Study, suggest that serum triglycerides may be important predictors for CHD in men or women, but not consistently in both sexes. Despite these observations, the current consensus holds that elevated levels of serum triglycerides represent a risk marker for obesity, glucose intolerance, and low HDL levels, all of which confer risk for CHD and, to the extent possible, deserve preventive attention [12].

Data from intervention studies using dietary or drug therapy demonstrate the benefit of lipid alteration in reducing risk of CHD events [13•]. However, nearly all such investigations have been conducted in middle-aged men, leaving considerable uncertainty regarding the efficacy and safety of such measures in women and in older persons of both sexes. Current management of hyperlipidemia in a person considered to be at risk should consist of a highly individualized approach beginning with appropriate dietary measures and weight control before initiating a trial of specific drug therapy to achieve a carefully monitored lipid-lowering effect. Details regarding the treatment of dyslipidemias appear elsewhere in this volume.

Cigarette Smoking

Carbon monoxide derived from cigarette smoke reduces the oxygen-carrying capacity of hemoglobin. In addition, nicotine and other substances are known to exert potent effects on vascular smooth muscle and blood platelets, possibly initiating thrombotic events in persons whose circulation has already been compromised by underlying atherosclerosis [14•]. Smoking is also suspected of triggering ventricular arrhythmias, resulting in sudden death in vulnerable persons presumably by enhancing sympathetic tone and reducing the threshold to ventricular fibrillation.

Data from Framingham and other studies are quite consistent with the effects of such mechanisms and actually document strong risk associations between cigarette smoking and an array of CVD outcomes including CHD (Fig. 9), stroke, PVD, and death [15].

Glucose Tolerance and Diabetes Mellitus

A number of clinical measures are employed in the Framingham Study to identify impaired glucose tolerance, nearly all of which demonstrate significant risk associations with CVD [16]. These measures include blood glucose levels, glycosuria, and the composite risk categories designated as glucose intolerance and diabetes mellitus. Although diabetes mellitus confers enhanced risk in men, overall risk increases dramatically for younger and older women. Similar patterns of risk are noted specifically for CHD, stroke, and PVD as well as coronary and cardiovascular mortality. Diabetes also emerges as an important risk factor in the development of congestive heart failure, particularly in older women with insulin-dependent diabetes mellitus. Presumably, the microvascular disease unique to diabetes, as well as other mechanisms, serves to produce progressive damage to heart muscle, ultimately resulting in compromised ventricular function and heart failure.

There is limited evidence that control of hyperglycemia by oral hypoglycemic agents or insulin effectively forestalls the development or complications of CVD, although encouraging trends in this regard were identified in the recently completed Diabetes Control and Complications Trial [17•]. Available information would, therefore, continue to support the concept that there is more to be gained in reducing risk by correcting associated cardiovascular risk factors in persons with diabetes than by attention confined to early detection and control of hyperglycemia.

Left Ventricular Hypertrophy

Left ventricular hypertrophy as determined by the electrocardiogram emerges as a strong risk factor for CHD in both sexes. Modest increases in CHD incidence are noted for voltage criteria for LVH alone with marked additional risk conferred by definite LVH which, in addition to voltage criteria, includes repolarization (ST and T wave) abnormalities consistent with LVH. These ECG findings presumably reflect derangements of myocardial structure and function related to early compromise of the underlying coronary circulation that appear before the development of clinical manifestations of CHD [18].

In this context, LVH (LV mass) as determined by cardiac echocardiography has emerged as an extremely potent independent predictor of CHD as well as other CVD events, especially in older persons [19•].

Body Weight

Progressive increases in body weight resulting in obesity represent important risk factors for CVD in men and women at all ages. Increases in body weight translate into directionally similar changes in several risk factors considered to be more directly related to the pathogenesis of atherosclerosis than obesity [20]. These include increases in blood pressure, serum cholesterol and triglycerides, and blood glucose. The exception is HDL cholesterol, which varies inversely with body weight. Recent data from Framingham and other studies, however, document the independent contribution of obesity in the development of CVD and its component outcomes [16,21•]. Such observations serve to emphasize the need to incorporate measures ultimately designed to control or, if necessary, to gradually reduce body weight as part of comprehensive risk management. When coupled with appropriate dietary measures, weight control is particularly useful in the initial management of patients with hypertension, dyslipidemia, and diabetes or combinations of these conditions.

Recent studies also indicate that character of fat distribution is as important as total adiposity in conferring risk for developing CVD. Thus, the pattern of increased abdominal or truncal obesity, which appears to be closely related to the phenomenon of insulin resistance, is also associated with hypertension, hyperlipidemia, and glucose intolerance, all factors that enhance CVD risk [22•].

Physical Activity

Accumulating evidence now suggests that lifetime vigorous physical activity may forestall CHD in men, although similar evidence is not yet available for women [23,24•]. Previously reported data from the Framingham Study indicating that overall mortality (including coronary mortality) was inversely related to level of physical activity in middle-aged men support these findings. Although a program of regular physical activity coupled with appropriate dietary and weight-control measures should be strongly encouraged for persons of all ages, it would be unwise to place undue emphasis on this approach alone in attempting to reduce the risk for CVD.

Other Risk Factors

Several hematologic or hemostatic factors are described as risk variables in the Framingham Study. Hematocrit appeared to contribute to CVD in middle-aged men and women, but not in older persons [16]. White blood cell count—which is strongly correlated with the number of cigarettes smoked per day, hematocrit, and vital capacity—is also associated with enhanced risk for CVD in men (both smokers and nonsmokers), but only in women smokers [25]. These data are consistent with reports from other studies. Plasma fibrinogen showed strong risk associations for CVD in men similar to findings from other studies [26]. Significant risk associations, however, are not apparent in women.

An extensive array of psychosocial, occupational, dietary, and other factors are described as putative risk parameters for CVD in the Framingham Study; however, limited

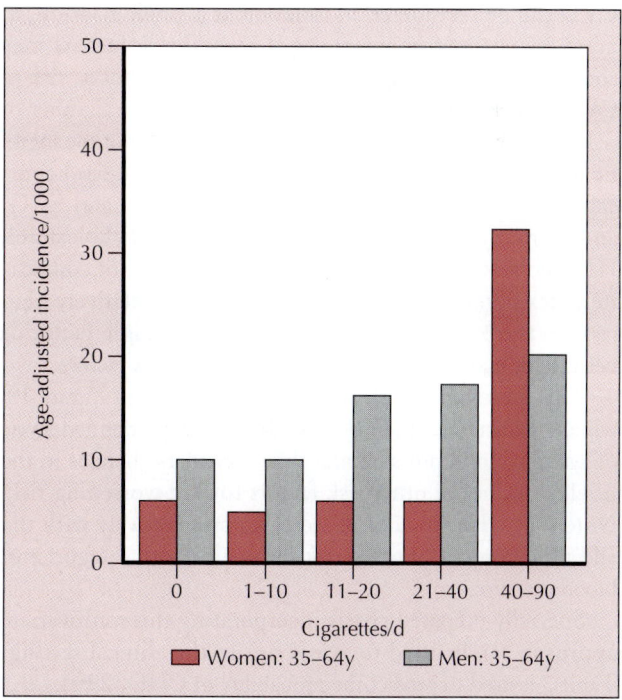

FIGURE 9 Risk of coronary heart disease based on cigarette consumption, age-adjusted incidence rates. Framingham Study, 30-year follow-up. *Data from* Cupples and D'Agostino [16].)

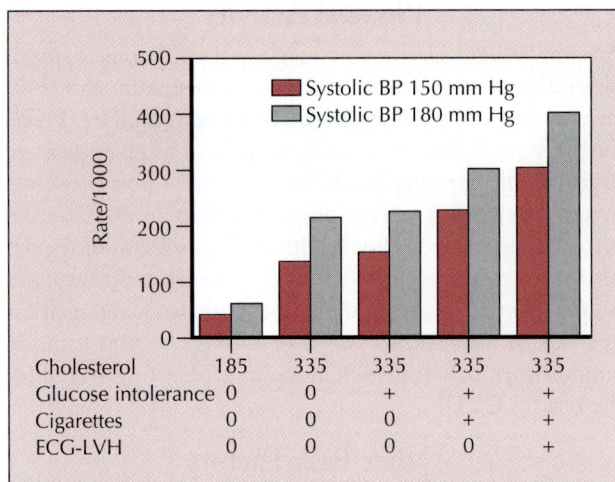

FIGURE 10 Risk of coronary heart disease in 8 years at systolic blood pressures (BPs) of 150 and 180 mm Hg according to the intensity of other factors, men 45 years of age. Framingham Study, 26-year follow-up. ECG-LVH—left ventricular hypertrophy as determined by electrocardiogram.

information is available regarding specific associations of these factors with CVD in young or older persons. A recent report characterized the independent contribution of parental history as a risk factor for CHD in the Framingham Study [27].

Cardiovascular Risk Profiles

Although associations between a specific risk factor and CVD can be considered in isolation as a single relation, in many instances combinations of several risk factors may constitute the observed risk profile. In such instances, risk of CVD can be reliably estimated by synthesizing a number of risk factors into a composite score, based on a multiple logistic function [28]. Risk factors are assessed by standard clinical procedures (smoking history, blood pressure, and ECG) and by routine laboratory studies (serum total cholesterol, HDL cholesterol, and blood glucose). This type of composite index permits detection of individuals at relatively high risk on the basis of marked elevation of a single factor or because of marginal abnormalities of several risk factors.

This multivariate risk scenario is illustrated in Figure 10, which characterizes the risk of CHD at two predefined levels of systolic blood pressure and then considers changes in the levels or values of other risk factors toward worsening risk. Note that CHD incidence increases progressively with the additional impact of other risk factors for both categories of blood pressure.

Specially prepared charts incorporating this multivariate approach can be used to assess risk in the clinical setting; Table 3 is used to predict the probability of CHD [29••].

Perspectives for Primary Prevention of Cardiovascular Disease

Effective prevention of a specific disease or cluster of diseases such as CVD often requires two basic approaches, and primary care physicians can play important roles in implementing both. The first approach focuses on individuals identified to be at risk for CVD. These persons usually require additional assessment of risk factors, extensive counselling, and the initiation of appropriate measures to reduce the probability of CVD outcomes. Continued medical surveillance is necessary to maintain long-term control of operative risk factors. The objective is to delay or prevent the development of disease in that individual.

The second approach addresses a defined population. In this approach, community-based screening programs focusing on risk factors such as hypertension or hyperlipidemia are used to identify susceptible persons for individualized medical attention. Public education efforts and other techniques are employed to curb cigarette smoking and to encourage less atherogenic diets, regular exercise, and other beneficial measures. The objective with this approach is to shift the overall distribution of risk factors to one favoring a lower rate of occurrence of CVD in the population.

Such considerations are more relevant today than ever before. Recently, a marked and progressive decline in mortality due to CHD and CVD has occurred in the United States and several other industrialized nations. Age-specific trends indicate decreasing mortality due to CVD, including CHD and stroke, across the entire age span. Similar trends in cardiovascular mortality have been identified in the Framingham population [30•]. At the same time, the prevalence of several CVD risk factors such as untreated hypertension, elevated serum cholesterol levels, and cigarette smoking has diminished in the general population, while impressive improvements have occurred in the diagnosis and treatment of CVD. Although the available information supports the contention that both of these potentially beneficial effects have contributed to the observed decline in mortality from CVD, the current consensus gives greater weight to the success of widespread primary preventive strategies, resulting in lowered levels of major risk factors that contribute to disease, rather than to improved diagnosis and treatment of established disease [31•].

Acknowledgment

The authors thank Ms. Claire Chisholm for her invaluable assistance in preparing this manuscript. This work was supported by the Health Services Research and Development Service of the Department of Veterans Affairs, the Visiting Scientist Program of the Framingham Heart Study and grant nos. N01-HV-92922, N01-HV52971, and 5T32-HL-07374-13 of the National Institutes of Health.

TABLE 3 CORONARY HEART DISEASE RISK FACTOR PREDICTION TABLE

1. Find points for each risk factor

Age (if female)		Age (if male)		HDL-cholesterol		Total-cholesterol		Pressure		Other	
Age (y)	n	Age (y)	n	HDL-C	n	Total-C	n	SBP	n		n
30	-12	30	-2	25–26	7	139–151	-3	98–104	-2	Cigarettes	4
31	-11	31	-1	27–29	6	152–166	-2	105–112	-1	Diabetic–male	3
32	-9	32–33	0	30–32	5	167–182	-1	113–120	0	Diabetic–female	6
33	-8	34	1	33–35	4	183–199	0	121–129	1	ECG-LVH	9
34	-6	35–36	2	36–38	3	200–219	1	130–139	2		
35	-5	37–38	3	39–42	2	220–239	2	140–149	3	0 points for each NO	
36	-4	39	4	43–46	1	240–262	3	150–160	4		
37	-3	40–41	5	47–50	0	263–288	4	161–172	5		
38	-2	42–43	6	51–55	-1	289–315	5	173–185	6		
39	-1	44–45	7	56–60	-2	316–330	6				
40	0	46–47	8	61–66	-3						
41	1	48–49	9	67–73	-4						
42–43	2	50–51	10	74–80	-5						
44	3	52–54	11	81–87	-6						
45–46	4	55–56	12	88–96	-7						
47–48	5	57–59	13								
49–50	6	60–61	14								
51–52	7	62–64	15								
53–55	8	65–67	16								
56–60	9	68–70	17								
61–67	10	71–73	18								
68–74	11	74	19								

2. Sum points for all risk factors

___ Age + ___ HDL-C + ___ Total-C + ___ SBP + ___ Smoker + ___ Diabetes + ___ ECG-LVH = ___ Point Total*

3. Look up risk corresponding to point total

	Probability			Probability	
n	5-y (%)	10-y (%)	n	5-y (%)	10-y (%)
≤1	<1	<2	17	6	13
2	1	2	18	7	14
3	1	2	19	8	16
4	1	2	20	8	18
5	1	3	21	9	19
6	1	3	22	11	21
7	1	4	23	12	23
8	2	4	24	13	25
9	2	5	25	14	27
10	2	6	26	16	29
11	3	6	27	17	31
12	3	7	28	19	33
13	3	8	29	20	36
14	4	9	30	22	38
15	5	10	31	24	40
16	5	12	32	25	42

4. Compare to average 10-y risk

	Probability	
Age (y)	Women (%)	Men (%)
30-34	<1	3
35-39	<1	5
40-44	2	6
45-49	5	10
50-54	8	14
55-59	12	16
60-64	13	21
65-69	9	30
70-74	12	24

These tables were prepared with the help of William B. Kannel, MD, Ralph D'Agostino, PhD, Keaven Anderson, PhD, Daniel McGee, PhD. Framingham Heart Study.
*Minus points subtract from total.
ECG-LVH—left ventricular hypertrophy as determined by electrocardiogram; HDL—high-density lipoprotein; SBP—systolic blood pressure.
From Anderson *et al.* [29]; with permission.

References and Recommended Reading

Recently published papers of particular interest have been highlighted as:
- Of interest
- •• Of outstanding interest

1. • Ross R: The pathogenesis of atherosclerosis: a perspective for the 1990s. *Nature* 1993, 362:801–809.
2. Vokonas PS, Kannel WB, Cupples LA: Epidemiology and risk of hypertension in the elderly: the Framingham Study. *J Hypertens* 1988, 8(suppl I):53–59.
3. •• SHEP Cooperative Research Group: Prevention of stroke by antihypertensive drug treatment in older persons with isolated systolic hypertension: final results of the Systolic Hypertension in the Elderly Program (SHEP). *JAMA* 1991, 265:3255–3264.
4. Wilhelmsen L: J-shaped curves. *J Hum Hypertens* 1990, 4(suppl 2):21–25.
5. Dahlof B, Lindholm LH, Hausson L, *et al.*: Morbidity and mortality in the Swedish Trial in Old Patients with Hypertension (STOP-Hypertension). *Lancet* 1991, 338:1281–1285.
6. MRC Working Party: Medical Research Council trial of treatment of hypertension in older adults: principal results. *Br Med J* 1992, 304:405–412.
7. • Kaplan NM: Antihypertensive therapy to maximally reduce coronary risk. *Am Heart J* 1993, 125:1487–1493.
8. Castelli WP, Wilson PW, Levy D, Anderson K: Cardiovascular risk factors in the elderly. *Am J Cardiol* 1989, 63:12H–19H.
9. •• Pikkanen J, Linn S, Heiss G, *et al.*: Ten-year mortality from cardiovascular disease in relation to cholesterol level among men with and without preexisting cardiovascular disease. *N Engl J Med* 1990, 322:1700–1707.
10. •• Castelli WP, Anderson K, Wilson PWF, *et al.*: Lipids and risk of coronary heart disease. The Framingham Study. *Ann Epidemiol* 1992, 2:23–28.
11. Steinberg D, Witztum JL: Lipoproteins and atherogenesis: current concepts. *JAMA* 1990, 264:3047.
12. Gotto AM Jr: Hypertriglyceridemia: risks and perspectives. *Am J Cardiol* 1992, 70:19H–25H.
13. • Montague T, Tsuyuki R, Burton J, *et al.*: Prevention and regression of coronary atherosclerosis. Is it safe and efficacious therapy? *Chest* 1994, 105:718–726.
14. • Muller JE, Abela GS, Nesto RW, *et al.*: Triggers, acute risk factors and vulnerable plaques: the lexicon of a new frontier. *J Am Coll Cardiol* 1994, 23:809–813.
15. Kannel WB, Higgins M: Smoking and hypertension as predictors of cardiovascular risk in population studies. *J Hypertens* 1990, 8(suppl 5):S3–S8.
16. Cupples LA, D'Agostino RB: Some risk factors related to the annual incidence of cardiovascular disease and death using pooled repeated biennial measurements: Framingham Heart Study, a 30-year follow-up. In *The Framingham Study: An Epidemiological Investigation of Cardiovascular Disease*. Edited by Kannel WB, Wolf PA, Garrison RJ: National Heart, Lung and Blood Institute; 1987: NIH Publication No. 87–2703.
17. • Diabetes Control and Complications Trial Research Group: The effect of intensive treatment of diabetes in the development and progression of long-term complications in insulin-dependent diabetes mellitus. *N Engl J Med* 1993, 329:997–986.
18. Kannel WB Dannenberg AL, Levy D: Population implications of electrocardiographic left ventricular hypertrophy. *Am J Cardiol* 1987, 60:851–931.
19. • Levy D, Garrison RJ, Savage DD, *et al.*: Prognostic implications of echocardiographically determined left ventricular mass in the Framingham Heart Study. *N Engl J Med* 1990, 322:1561–1566.
20. Borkan GA, Sparrow D, Wisnieski C, *et al.*: Body weight and coronary risk: patterns of risk factor change associated with long-term weight change. The Normative Aging Study. *Am J Epidemiol* 1986, 124:410–419.
21. • Manson JE, Colditz GA, Stampfer MJ, *et al.*: A prospective study of obesity and risk of coronary heart disease in women. *N Engl J Med* 1990, 322:882–889.
22. • Reaven GM: Role of insulin resistance in human disease (Syndrome X): an expanded definition. *Ann Rev Med* 1993, 44:121–131.
23. Berlin JA, Colditz GA: A meta-analysis of physical activity in the prevention of coronary heart disease. *Am J Epidemiol* 1990, 132:612–628.
24. • Paffenbarger RS Jr, Hyde RT, Wing AL, *et al.*: The association of changes in physical activity level and other lifestyle characteristics with mortality among men. *N Engl J Med* 1993, 328:533–537.
25. Kannel WB, Anderson K, Wilson PWF: White blood cell count and cardiovascular disease. *JAMA* 1992, 267:1253–1256.
26. Ernst E: Fibrinogen: its emerging role as a cardiovascular risk factor. *Angiology* 1994, 45:87–93.
27. Myers RH, Kiely DK, Cupples LA, *et al.*: Parental history is an independent risk factor for coronary artery disease: The Framingham Study. *Am Heart J* 1990, 120:963–969.
28. Chambless LE, Dobson AJ, Patterson CC, *et al.*: On the use of a logistic risk score in predicting risk of coronary heart disease. *Stat Med* 1990, 9:385–396.
29. •• Anderson KM, Wilson PWF, Odell PM, *et al.*: An updated coronary risk profile. A statement for health professionals. *Circulation* 1991, 83:357–363.
30. • Sytkowski PA, Kannel WB, D'Agostino RB: Changes in risk factors and the decline in mortality from cardiovascular disease. The Framingham Heart Study. *N Engl J Med* 1990, 322:1635–1641.
31. • Goldman L: Cost-effectiveness perspectives in coronary heart disease. *Am Heart J* 1990, 119:733–739.

Select Bibliography

Hunninghake DB: Diagnosis and treatment of lipid disorders. *Med Clin North Am* 1994, 78:247–257.

Pinkney JH, Yudkin JS: Antihypertensive drugs: issues beyond blood pressure control. *Prog Cardiovasc Dis* 1994, 36:397–415.

Schaefer EJ: New recommendations for the diagnosis and treatment of plasma lipid abnormalities. *Nutr Rev* 1993, 51:246–253.

Summary of the Second Report of the National Cholesterol Education Program (NCEP) Expert Panel on Detection, Evaluation, and Treatment of High Blood Cholesterol in Adults (Adult Treatment Panel II). *JAMA* 1993, 269:3015–3023.

The Fifth Report of the Joint National Committee on Detection, Evaluation, and Treatment of High Blood Pressure. National High Blood Pressure Education Program, National Heart, Lung, and Blood Institute; 1993: NIH Publication No. 93–1088.

Approach to the Patient with Hyperlipidemia

Neil J. Stone

> **Key Points**
> - Damage to the endothelium initiates a cascade of events leading to cholesterol-rich, atherosclerotic plaque.
> - Both total and high-density lipoprotein (HDL) cholesterol should be measured in all adults over 19 years of age at least once every 5 years; the intensity of the evaluation and treatment depends on coronary risk status and other health conditions.
> - Intervention focuses on low-density lipoprotein (LDL) cholesterol calculated by measurement of fasting cholesterol, triglycerides, and HDL.
> - Risk factors include age, menopausal status, hypertension, diabetes mellitus, cigarette smoking, and family history of premature cardiovascular disease (before 65 years of age in female and 55 in male relatives); sedentary lifestyle and obesity are targets for intervention that should improve one or more risk factors.
> - Secondary causes of hyperlipidemia should always be ruled out before treatment begins; diet, drugs, and diseases affecting lipid levels should be reviewed.
> - Diet is the initial treatment, emphasizing low fat (< 30% of calories), low saturated fat, and low dietary cholesterol; calories should be restricted and regular aerobic exercise encouraged for overweight patients.
> - In patients with coronary disease, significantly lowering LDL cholesterol can slow progression or cause regression of existing atherosclerotic plaques as seen by angiography.
> - Major drugs to lower elevated LDL cholesterol in high-risk patients include bile-acid sequestering resins, niacin, and hydroxymethylglutaryl–coenzyme A reductase inhibitors (or statins); others include gemfibrozil and probucol.

The atherosclerotic process begins with a cholesterol-rich fatty streak that can be seen in coronary arteries as early as the second decade of life. In patients with risk factors for atherosclerosis, this streak can progress to a fibrous plaque whose main components are intra- and extracellular cholesterol, smooth muscle cells, and cellular elements from the vessel wall contained by a thin fibrous cap. This fibrous plaque can evolve into a complicated plaque with hemorrhage, necrosis, calcification, and overlying thrombosis.

The initiating event of atherosclerosis is endothelial injury caused by turbulence of blood flow (explaining the predilection for atherosclerotic worsening at the branch points) or merely hypercholesterolemia resulting in excess low-density lipoprotein (LDL). The damaged surface attracts platelets that release growth factors leading to the involvement of smooth muscle cells. The hallmark of accelerated atherosclerotic syndromes is damaged intimal and medial layers, as seen in venous coronary bypass grafts, angioplasty, and heart transplantation.

Low-density lipoprotein oxidation is critical in this process, which allows the LDL to be taken up easily by monocytes and macrophages that become foam cells. Even in minimally modified form, the usual LDL-receptor mechanism does not function to limit excess cholesterol uptake by the cell. Steinberg and coworkers [1] showed the interrelationships between theories about lipids and response to injury.

The Multiple Risk Factor Intervention Trial studied 360,000 men and showed convincingly that risk of coronary death correlates with serum cholesterol over a wide range of values [2]. The lowest risk was seen in those with cholesterol values under 200 mg/dL, and there was increasing risk with values above 240 mg/dL. Other risk factors also may be implicated in the atherosclerotic process (Table 1). Every patient evaluated for hyperlipidemia should have a checklist of risk factors on his or her chart. Not only are risk factors associated with dyslipidemia (*eg*, lipid abnormalities are more likely in patients with diabetes, hypertension, and obesity), but the presence of associated risk factors increases cardiac risk.

Nonmodifiable risk factors include age and gender (*ie*, men and postmenopausal women are at increased risk). Modifiable risk factors include excess LDL, low levels of high-density lipoprotein (HDL), hypertension (including systolic hypertension in elderly patients), diabetes mellitus, cigarette smoking, sedentary lifestyle, and abdominal or male-pattern obesity. Femoral-gluteal obesity is primarily a cosmetic problem, whereas abdominal obesity is associated with hyperinsulinemia and attendant hypertension, hyperglycemia, low HDL cholesterol (HDL-c), and hypertriglyceridemia [3]. Figure 1 shows the value of assessing cholesterol in light of associated risk factors [2]. For example, a nonsmoker with cholesterol in the 221 to 244 range has a lower risk than a smoker with hypertension and cholesterol in the 182 to 202 range. Hence, a high-risk individual would be one with two or more risk factors or the presence of coronary or vascular disease elsewhere.

Secondary causes of elevated blood lipids should always be determined. A useful mnemonic is to think of the three D's: *diet*, *drugs*, and *diseases* (Table 2). If secondary causes are not seen, consider primary hyperlipidemia and screen the patient's family.

MEASUREMENT OF LIPIDS AND LIPOPROTEINS

Serum cholesterol can be obtained in the nonfasting state and has been recommended as a screening test. Many patients with desirable cholesterol values but low HDL-c will be

TABLE 1 HOW RISK FACTORS AFFECT ATHEROSCLEROSIS

Biology	Hyperlipidemia	Hypertension	Smoking	Genetics	Other
Endothelial injury	Excess LDL	+	+	Homocystinuria	Immune complexes
Lipoproteins, monocytes	++	–	–	++	
Platelets	+	–	++	–	
Smooth cell proliferation	+	+	–	++	
Plaque disruption	++	+	–	++	
Thrombosis	+	–	++	+	
Associated with oxidized LDL	Low HDL		Depletes vitamin C	Small, dense LDL	

Adapted from Badimon and coworkers [35]; with permission.
HDL—high-density lipoprotein; LDL—low-density lipoprotein; –—mild reductions; ——moderate reductions; +—mild increments; ++—moderate increments.

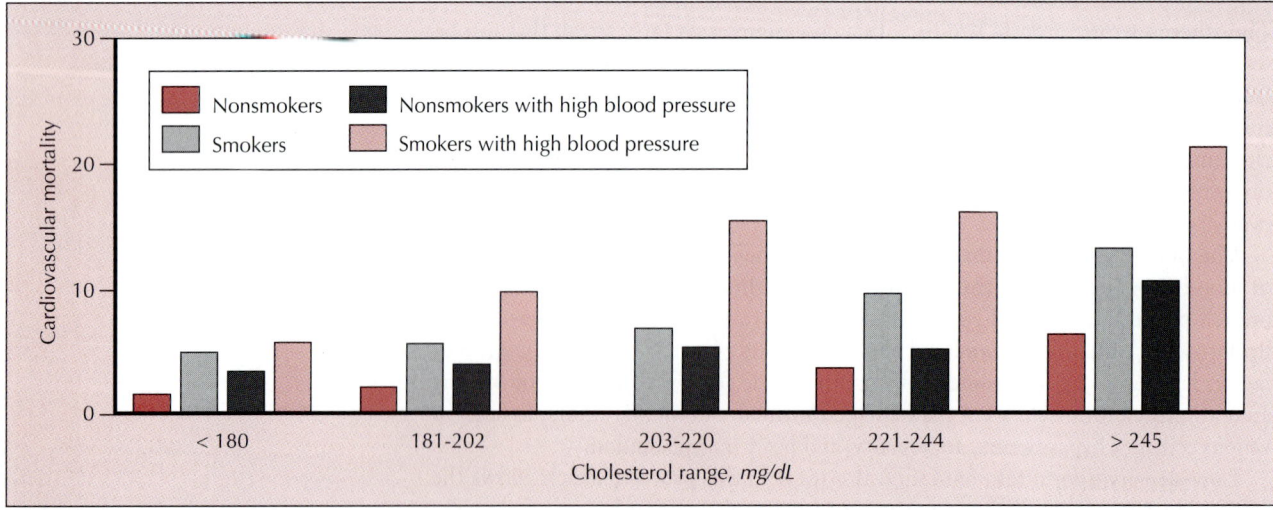

FIGURE 1 Effect of risk factors on modifying risk of cardiovascular mortality in the Multiple Risk Factor Intervention Trial (MRFIT) Study.

Table 2. Secondary causes of hypercholesterolemia and high triglycerides

Cause	Procedure or test
Hypercholesterolemia	
Diet	Dietary history (focus on saturated fats, dietary cholesterol)
Drugs	Diuretics, steroids, anabolic steroids
Hypothyroidism	TSH test
Nephrotic syndrome	Urine analysis, serum albumin
Obstructive liver disease	Abnormal alkaline phosphatase and enzymes
Diabetes mellitus	FBS, glycated hemoglobin
Transplantation	Multiple causes including drugs like steroids
High triglycerides	
Diet	Dietary history (focus on calorie excess, alcohol)
Drugs	Diuretics, steroids, estrogens, retinoic acid, beta-blockers
Hypothyroidism	TSH test
Nephrotic syndrome (severe)	Urine analysis, serum albumin
Chronic renal disease	BUN, creatinine
Diabetes mellitus	FBS, glycated hemoglobin

BUN—blood urea nitrogen; FBS—fasting blood sugar; TSH—thyroid-stimulating hormone.

---

missed using the original Adult Treatment Panel's criteria: 240 mg/dL or greater is high, 200 to 239 mg/dL is borderline, and under 200 mg/dL is desirable [4••]. This is important, because low serum cholesterol levels (< 200 mg/dL) and low HDL-c (< 35 mg/dL) are frequently seen in those who either have or are suspected of having coronary artery disease (CAD). This combination is often noted in men with a family history of premature CAD [5]. Thus, screening may be best accomplished with nonfasting cholesterol and HDL-c. If abnormal values are found, repeat the tests. This should be done in the fasting state 12 to 14 hours after the meal. This allows measurement of triglycerides, which are so highly variable that the patient should be fasting and at a steady weight. A nonfasting value is only useful in the patient with abdominal pain and suspected pancreatitis; here, values over 1000 mg/dL suggest chylomicronemia as a cause of the pancreatitis. Measurement of total cholesterol and HDL-c is also performed. Laboratories can then calculate LDL cholesterol (LDL-c) by the following formula:

$$\text{LDL-c} = \text{Total cholesterol} - \text{HDL-c} - (\text{Triglycerides}/5)$$

This formula is valid if triglycerides are less than 400 mg/dL and the rare type III abnormality is not present. LDL-c values are used to determine risk and if further evaluation and therapy are needed (Table 3). As with lipids, these values need to be repeated at least once to establish a true baseline.

Secondary causes of hyperlipidemia also need to be considered. Dietary causes include a diet too rich in saturated fat, cholesterol, and excess calories. Drugs implicated in hyperlipidemia include steroids, androgens, diuretics, beta-blockers, and retinoic-acid derivatives. Diseases commonly found to cause hyperlipidemia include hypothyroidism (measure thyroid-stimulating hormone to find subclinical hypothyroidism that can elevate cholesterol levels), obstructive liver disease, chronic renal disease, nephrosis, and diabetes mellitus.

Family screening is mandatory if lipid levels are diet-resistant, because several familial syndromes such as familial hypercholesterolemia and familial combined hyperlipidemia may be present. The former often has cholesterol deposits in tendons, most notably the Achilles tendons, called *xanthomas*. The latter is associated more with abnormalities of triglyceride metabolism.

Low HDL-c (< 35 mg/dL) increases coronary risk and is also a target for therapy. Excess body weight, cigarette smoking, hypertriglyceridemia, and sedentary lifestyle (which are often interrelated) should be corrected so that elevated HDL-c may result. Exercise must be regular and sustained over many months before elevated HDL-c is seen. Alcohol raises HDL-c, but it cannot be recommended for this purpose because of the negative aspects associated with excess usage (especially in women and younger persons). High HDL-c (> 70 mg/dL) is linked to longevity syndromes, and in a low-risk person, it suggests a more conservative approach to drug therapy.

Hypertriglyceridemia drops out as an independent risk factor in multivariate analysis, yet triglycerides are a valuable indicator that associated metabolic abnormalities may be present. Dense, triglyceride-rich LDL particles characterize those patients with greater coronary artery disease by angiography [6]. Those with small, dense LDL usually have triglyceride levels over 150 mg/dL (Table 4). The clinician should have a clue that triglycerides will be elevated, because the serum is often turbid (*eg*, you cannot read newsprint clearly through it) (Fig. 2). If triglycerides exceed 1000 mg/dL, the serum is often creamy, representing chylomicronemia. The cream means that the patient is either nonfasting (triglycerides mildly elevated) or has a major disorder of triglyceride removal with increased risk of pancreatitis (triglycerides > 1000 mg/dL).

How accurate are these measurements? Most laboratories now show a precision and accuracy level of 95% or more for

Table 3. Low-density lipoprotein cholesterol decision cutoffs

LDL-c, *mg/dL*	Impression	Comments
≥ 160	High-risk	Evaluate for therapy
130–159	Borderline	Evaluate if risk factors
< 130	Desirable	Goal if no evidence of CAD
100	Optimal	Goal for those with CAD

CAD—coronary artery disease.

Table 4 Triglyceride decision cutoffs	
Triglyceride, *mg/dL*	Significance
< 200	Desirable; some think coronary risk is less if under 150
200–399	Borderline; if associated with low HDL-c, high LDL-c, diabetes or personal/family history of CAD, it is significant
≥ 400	High; avoid estrogens, steroids, and excess alcohol as they can trigger marked triglyceride rise and pancreatitis

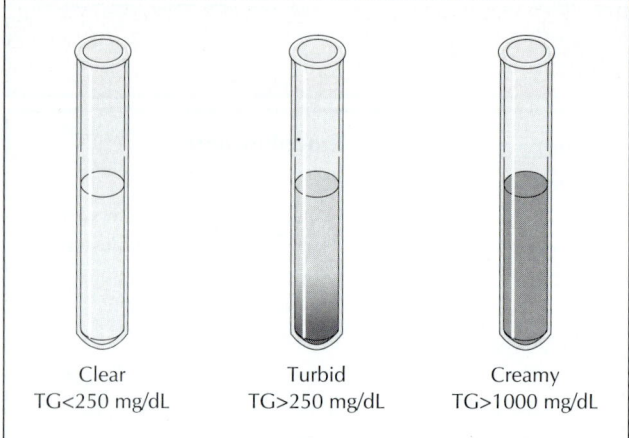

Figure 2 Visual inspection of triglyceride-rich lipoproteins. Turbidity shows if large, triglyceride-rich lipoproteins are present. TG—triglycerides.

cholesterol. Table 5 shows factors that must be considered when the clinician evaluates lipid measurements. Screening values can be nonfasting because one is only trying to see if a potential lipid/lipoprotein problem exists. For detailed evaluation or determining response to therapy, it is useful to require the individual to fast for 12 to 14 hours and not consume alcohol within the preceding 24 hours. Also, the individual should be at a stable weight and without intercurrent illness or stress. Lipids should be determined in outpatients using the sitting position without an overly tight tourniquet. Nonetheless, there can be significant sources of error; Table 5 gives a brief listing [7••]. A common source of confusion occurs when an individual starts total fat and saturated fat restriction but HDL-c decreases along with LDL-c. The LDL:HDL ratio, however, is improved, and it may improve more if regular aerobic exercise is added.

It has been known for two decades that cholesterol levels decrease and triglyceride levels increase over a several-week period after a myocardial infarction (MI). Cholesterol measured within the first 24 hours does reflect pre-event lipid values [8], yet cholesterol values decrease markedly in the week after MI [9]. How soon after MI should plasma lipid values be assessed? In one study, cholesterol fell 31% and LDL-c 48% in the week after MI [10]. Physicians and patients often are first aware of lipids in the post-MI state. Every patient with MI requires a fasting lipoprotein profile before discharge, but the patient should be cautioned that it may take 2 to 3 months before lipid values return to their pre-event stage. Because these patients generally undergo dietary and activity counseling before leaving the hospital (with the goal of achieving LDL-c values of approximately 100 mg/dL and HDL-c values of over 45 mg/dL), in many cases the patient and physician will never learn how bad the lipids were if no previous values are available.

Patients with CAD who are admitted electively have lipid and lipoprotein values that must be interpreted critically as well. HDL (and also apolipoprotein A-I) values are lower at cardiac catheterization [11]. This is significant, because HDL-c values are important predictors of the presence and extent of CAD [12].

Dietary Therapy

Nonpharmacologic Modification Trials

The Oslo Dietary and Smoking Intervention Trial studied men without overt CAD and showed that those randomized to a modified fat diet and counseling to reduce smoking had a 47% lower incidence of sudden death and heart attack than

Table 5 Sources of laboratory variation in lipid measurements			
Behavioral		**Sampling sources**	
Diet	Fats raise TC, HDL; saturated fats raise LDL	Fasting	Essential for triglycerides
Obesity	Increases TG; lowers HDL	Nonfasting	After eating, see increased VLDL and lower LDL; total cholesterol changes to small degree
Smoking	Decreases HDL (*eg*, 11% in one study)		
Exercise	Lowers TG; increases HDL	Posture	Approximately 9% higher for TC and LDL and 10% for HDL-c when lying down compared with standing
Alcohol	Increases TG; increases HDL		
		Fingerstick	Can see unreliable values if technician not well trained or machine not calibrated regularly

HDL—high-density lipoprotein; LDL—low-density lipoprotein; TC—total cholesterol; TG—triglyceride; VLDL—very-low-density lipoprotein.

those in the control group [13]. Further analysis showed that the net difference of 10% in serum cholesterol between the intervention and control groups was the main cause for the 47% reduction in first events of CAD. At 5 years, the difference between both groups in total mortality became significant, with a 33% lower mortality in the intervention group.

The Multiple Risk Factor Intervention Trial (MRFIT) studied 12,866 high-risk men from 35 to 57 years of age who were hypercholesterolemic, hypertensive, or smokers [14]. There was an insignificant difference of 7.1% in mortality between special-intervention and usual-care groups after 8 years. Although quit rates for cigarette smokers clearly improved in the trial and dietary change was evident, the mean net differences between special intervention and usual care for diastolic blood pressure was only 4%, and for serum cholesterol was only 2%. A possibly unfavorable response to high-dose, diuretic, antihypertensive medication in the treated group (especially those with electrocardiographic abnormalities at baseline) may explain some of the differences as well. At 10 years, the small differences achieved in risk factors finally resulted in significant differences between clinical end points.

The Los Angeles Veterans Administration Study randomized patients to a treatment group with an intake of 50% less cholesterol and significantly lower saturated fat than the control group [15]. At the end of the study, the treatment group had 12.7% lower cholesterol and significantly lower coronary and cerebrovascular events ($P < 0.01$) than the control group.

Ornish and coworkers [16] looked at a selected (randomization here was really a failed effort) group of individuals who on a strict, very low-fat diet demonstrated regression on quantitative coronary angiography performed at 1 year. LDL levels decreased from 152 to 95 mg/dL in the treatment group. Other interventions in this trial included exercise, meditation, stress management, and smoking cessation.

The St. Thomas Atherosclerosis Regression Trial showed the benefits of diet on coronary dimensions in patients with CAD [17•]. After 39 months, the proportion showing an increased luminal diameter was 4% for the usual-care group, 38% for the diet group, and 33% for the diet-and-cholestyramine-resin group. The mean absolute width of the coronary segments correlated independently and significantly with LDL-c change during the trial.

Practical Aspects of Diet

A diet with a low percentage of calories derived from total fat and saturated fat and low in dietary cholesterol has been recommended for the American public. Current dietary figures are from the US Surgeon General's report in 1988 [18] (Table 6).

The diet recommended for the general population is the Step 1 Diet. The MRFIT trial showed that certain high-fat eating behaviors are easier for patients to alter than others. Those changes made with relative ease include increasing consumption of fish and poultry, having less red meat, using skim or low-fat milk products, using margarine instead of butter, and reducing egg yolks. Those that were much harder were decreasing the quantity of meat consumption to 6 or 7 ounces daily and avoiding high-fat cheese, snacks, crackers, chips, processed sausage, and luncheon meats [19]. Patients also should be advised that before they add psyllium, modified fat foods, or even garlic, they must subtract dietary fat from their diet. These items can help to lower cholesterol as adjuncts, not substitiutes, to a low-saturated-fat diet [20].

The lipid-lowering therapeutic diet is the Step 2 Diet, and it is particularly recommended for patients at high risk of CAD. Here, a dietitian is required to help the patient not only achieve a very low saturated fat intake but also to choose and prepare balanced, nutritious, and nonrepetitious meals.

Dietary assessment is required to determine progress and can be used to involve the patient in behavioral change. Ask if the patient has the specific skills needed to be on a good cholesterol-lowering diet, such as knowing how to read labels, order when dining out, prepare low-fat foods, and alter familiar recipes to comply with the diet. If the patient cannot do these things, referral to a dietitian is crucial. You may wish to have the patient bring a written, 24- to 72-hour dietary diary to the next visit; with this, it is easy to tell at a glance if the patient understands the diet. Another option is having the patient fill out a food-frequency questionnaire designed to review dietary adherence. A useful one is the MEDICS questionnaire; the letters of this mnemonic stand for the sources of dietary fat (Table 7).

Soluble fiber is a useful adjunct to a cholesterol-lowering therapy and can be obtained in oatmeal, oatbran, or in fruits and vegetables. In addition, fruits and vegetables are a good source of antioxidants. Finally, a good diet can make it easier for a given dosage of medication to facilitate the attainment of LDL-c goals [21•]. Drugs should be added to the diet and never prescribed in place of it.

DRUG TREATMENT

Clinical Intervention Trials

Primary-prevention clinical trials have shown that lipid-lowering drugs can affect the incidence of CAD. The first was the Lipid Research Clinics Primary Prevention Trial, which showed that using cholestyramine resin for every 1% that the

TABLE 6 CURRENT AND RECOMMENDED US DIETS			
	Current diet	Step 1	Step 2
Total fat, %		< 30	< 30
Men	36		
Women	37		
Saturated fat, %		< 10	< 7
Men	13		
Women	13		
Dietary cholesterol, *mg*		< 300	< 200
Men	435		
Women	304		

cholesterol was lowered resulted in a 2% lowering of coronary risk [22]. The Helsinki Heart Trial used a different medication, gemfibrozil, which raised HDL-c as much as it lowered LDL-c [23]; this trial also showed a significant reduction in fatal and nonfatal MI. Most of the benefit in this trial occurred in men with a lipid profile characterized by high cholesterol, high triglycerides, and low HDL-c. Both trials have been criticized as not affecting the total mortality rate, but they were not designed (each having too few subjects) to do so. One disturbing feature has been an increase in accidental deaths and violence in each of the drug treatment arms; however, this has not been seen in the smaller but more aggressive lipid-lowering, secondary-prevention trials. Also, many of those dying violently in these trials were not receiving cholesterol-lowering treatment when they died.

The largest clinical trial aimed at men after MI was the Coronary Drug Project [24]. This used niacin, clofibrate, estrogens, and D-thyroxine; the last two drugs were found to be harmful during the trial and discontinued. Data showed that niacin and clofibrate both lowered nonfatal MI rates, but did not lower total mortality. Many clinicians were unconvinced of the value of lipid-lowering after MI, because short-term prognosis seemed to relate strongly to the amount of jeopardized and damaged myocardium. A later look at survivors of the niacin trial at 15 years, however, showed an 11% increased survival in the niacin group compared with the control group.

The case for lowering cholesterol after MI has become more compelling [25]. Blood cholesterol levels appear to add to the already high absolute risk of another MI in the postinfarction period, even after adjustment for the myocardial impairment dominating the short-term prognosis. Other important risk factors in long-term prognosis include HDL-c, hypertension, and cigarette smoking. Also, lowered cholesterol after MI is associated with an approximately 25% reduction in recurrent infarction. This is approximately the same benefit obtained from β-blockers given after MI. Moreover, concern regarding noncoronary deaths is less, because cardiovascular deaths predominate (82%). Therefore, aggressive lipid management with the goal of lowering LDL-c to 100 mg/dL and raising HDL-c to over 35 mg/dL (as a minimum) seems to be as reasonable a management strategy as aspirin, β-blockers, and angiotensin-converting enzyme inhibitors [26].

Drug studies using angiography as an end point have shown that aggressive, lipid-lowering therapy can reduce progression or even cause regression. The Cholesterol-Lowering Atherosclerosis Study (CLAS) evaluated 162 post–coronary bypass patients randomly assigned to placebo or treatment with colestipol and niacin [27]. Combined coronary, femoral, and carotid angiograms were obtained initially and after 2 years. Drug treatment resulted in a 26% decrease in cholesterol, 43% decrease in LDL-c, and 37% increase in HDL-c. Of the treatment group, 61% showed favorable outcomes (either nonprogression of coronary lesions or reversal) versus 39% of the placebo group. Atherosclerosis regression was observed in 16.2% of the drug group versus 2.4% of the placebo group ($P < 0.002$). Results were even more impressive at 4-year follow-up.

The Familial Atherosclerosis Treatment Study (FATS) [28•] used quantitative coronary angiography in 146 patients with hypercholesterolemia treated in a double-blind, randomized trial with lovastatin and colestipol, niacin and colestipol, or placebo and colestipol over a 2-year period (Fig. 3). The two treatment groups had less progression and more regression, and clinical cardiac events were markedly reduced.

In the University of California–San Francisco Familial Hypercholesterolemia trial, Kane and coworkers [29] showed that aggressive LDL-lowering therapy involving two and even three drugs resulted in decreased progression and even regression on serial angiography in asymptomatic men and women

TABLE 7 THE MEDICS QUESTIONNAIRE*	
Meats	How often and how much red meat, sausage, and organ meats? Fried foods? Know how to order when dining out?
	Advise more fish, skinless poultry. Have meats broiled with sauces on the side. Avoid high-fat meats, hot dogs, sausage, and organ meats. Try to keep total meat quantity to under 6 oz daily.
Eggs	How many egg yolks per week?
	Use egg yokes sparingly; egg whites are preferred.
Dairy	How many high-fat cheese, milk, and cream products per week? Do you add cheese to burgers or nachos?
	Low-fat cheese and milk products are advised.
Invisible fats	How many baked goods per week?
	Stick with whole-grain products and avoid high-fat doughnuts, coffee cakes, croissants, and muffins.
Cooking dairy fats	What cooking or table fat do you use and how much?
	Avoid butter; use soft margarine, avoiding hardened forms. Avoid fried foods. Use canola, safflower, corn oil, and olive oil. Avoid coconut, palm, and palm kernel oils, which are highly saturated. Know how to modify recipes.
Snacks	What snacks and how often?
	Advise fruits, vegetables, pretzels; avoid high-fat dips, candy bars.
	Physician may add questions about distilled spirits (hard liquor, wine, or beer) and salt, if applicable.

*Can be given to patients at each visit to fill out and circle those lipid-lowering habits (in italics) that they need to work on.

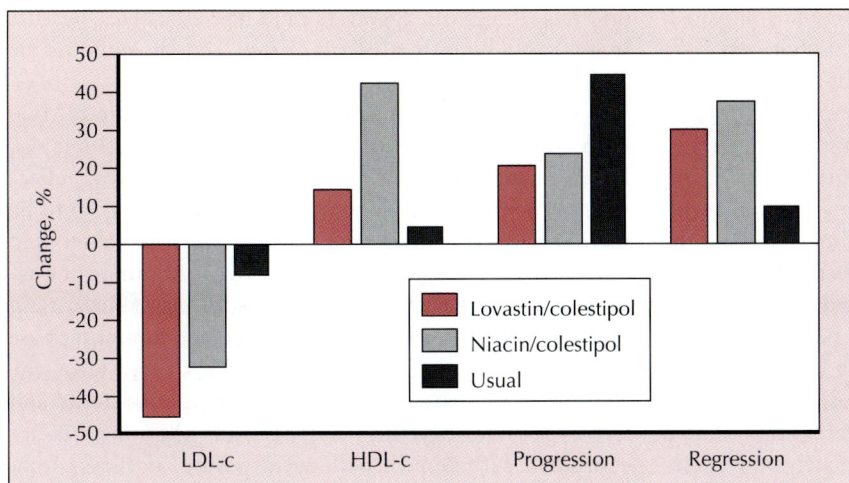

FIGURE 3 Effect of lipid lowering on coronary artery disease. HDL-c—high-density lipoprotein cholesterol; LDL-c—low-density lipoprotein cholesterol. (*Data from* Brown and coworkers [28].)

with familial hypercholesterolemia. This study was the first to show a significant effect from lipid lowering on atherosclerosis in women. These patients were heterozygous for familial hypercholesterolemia. This is a diet-resistant genetic syndrome in which untreated cholesterol values average approximately 360 mg/dL. Because a recent review [30] noted that over two thirds of relatives of patients with known familial hypercholesterolemia are not properly diagnosed (and thus are denied treatment shown to alter their coronary risk), this represents an important clinical challenge.

The Program on the Surgical Control of the Hyperlipidemias (POSCH) investigated the effect of partial ileal bypass on blood cholesterol reduction, coronary morbidity, and mortality in 838 survivors of MI and followed for a mean of 9.7 years [31]. These patients were not chosen on the basis of their lipids. Cholesterol reduction was greater in the treatment group, and at repeat coronary arteriography, progression of coronary disease was significantly reduced in the surgery group ($P < 0.001$). This was almost a pure trial of LDL-c lowering, because HDL-c values were not greatly affected.

In summary, these coronary angiographic trials show that regression and stabilization are 1.5 to 2.0 times more common in patients with intervention than in control patients, and progression is likewise reduced by approximately 50% in those with intensive lipid lowering. Lesions with a narrowing of 50% luminal diameter or greater at baseline seem to be more responsive, but reduction in subsequent coronary events is related to the stabilization of lesions to less than 50% luminal narrowing [32]. The Scandinavian Simvastatin Survival Study was a landmark clinical trial of 4444 men and women with coronary disease. The treatment group was given diet and simvastatin which lowered the average LDL-c from approximately 190 mg/dL to 130 mg/dL. The results were striking: there was a 30% decline in total mortality, as well as significant declines in cardiovascular risk. This was seen for women as well as men [33].

Choice of Drugs

Before starting drug therapy, determine if the patient has made a concerted effort regarding diet and exercise. Referral to a dietitian may provide the information necessary to obtain a good dietary response. Consumption of food and especially alcohol may be underreported, and physical activity may be overestimated. Also, check if menopausal women have been prescribed estrogens, which can reverse the menopausal changes of raised LDL-c and lowered HDL-c. Estrogen treatment may lower LDL-c by 10% or more, but this will not occur if progestins are used as well. Available evidence suggests that protection of postmenopausal estrogens against CAD, however, is not dependent on the lipid effects.

Finally, review the benefits, disadvantages, and risks of drug therapy with the patient. Drug therapy will most likely benefit those at highest risk of coronary disease, such as patients with known vascular disease or a risk factor status putting them at risk in the short-term for coronary events. Men under 45 years of age and women under 55 years are thought to have a lower immediate risk of a coronary event. Therefore, gender is a risk factor when a man is 45 years or older and a woman is 55 years or older. (An exception is when the woman has an early menopause and then is at higher risk.) A young patient with elevated total cholesterol and LDL-c but a normal HDL-c and no other risk factors may be managed better with diet. Those at highest risk (*eg*, positive family history, two or more risk factors, familial hypercholesterolemia with LDL over 225 mg/dL despite diet, or known vascular disease) should be considered for drug therapy if the LDL-c is over 190 mg/dL and the HDL-c less than 35 mg/dL. An overview of drug therapy is given in Table 8.

Bile-acid sequestrants (*eg*, cholestyramine, colestipol) are used primarily for patients with hypercholesterolemia and normal triglyceride levels. Bile-acid sequestrants must be started slowly (one scoop daily), and the patient must have a clear understanding of the anticipated gastrointestinal side effects such as constipation. Those on a high-fiber diet seem to do best. Low-dose resin therapy is a useful choice, because it is well tolerated and results in LDL-c lowering in the 15% to 20% range.

Fibric-acid derivatives such as gemfibrozil (600 mg twice daily) can be employed in patients with hypertriglyceridemia and low HDL-c but elevated total cholesterol, or in the patient with marked triglyceride excess (> 500 mg/dL). Do not prescribe gemfibrozil if renal or hepatic function is impaired. While not as lithogenic as the first-generation fibric acid clofibrate, it does present a small, increased risk for gallstones.

Nicotinic acid preparations offer excellent lipid-lowering alternatives, because they raise HDL-c and lower LDL-c and triglycerides. These drugs must be given slowly and incrementally. Very low-dose initial therapy (100 mg) with increasing of the initial dose two or three times daily may be required every 2 to 4 weeks for up to 6 months, until the therapeutic dose has been achieved. At low doses, HDL-c is favorably affected, but higher doses are needed to lower LDL-c [34]. Concomitant aspirin ingestion helps to prevent flushing, which is a prostaglandin-mediated reaction. Patients should be warned about this flushing; they should take niacin with food, one aspirin approximately 30 minutes before, and slowly increase the dose. This may allow many to avoid the more expensive (and possibly with more gastrointestinal side effects) sustained-release preparations. A recent report noted that using sustained-release niacin to lower LDL-c resulted in a high incidence of hepatotoxicity. Immediate-release niacin was preferred and recommended for patients who agree to be monitored by health professionals [35]. Niacinamide is another form of the vitamin, but it is not a lipid-lowering drug and should not be substituted for niacin. Niacin may cause gout in patients with hyperuricemia. It also can aggravate mild type 2 diabetes, because it increases hepatic glucose output and thus should be avoided in most diabetics.

The most powerful drugs to lower LDL-c are HMG-CoA reductase inhibitors. For the patient with multiple risk factors or coronary disease, they may be the most cost-effective, because a low dose may allow the LDL-c goal to be met. With increasing dosage, there is less incremental lipid lowering. As a rough guide, 20 mg of lovastatin or pravastatin offers similar LDL-c lowering as 10 mg of simvastatin or 40 mg of fluvastatin. When considering a further increase in dosage above the equivalent of 40 mg of lovastatin, the addition of low-dose resin therapy is often more useful and less expensive. Myositis is seen when these agents are combined with gemfibrozil, cyclosporine, and less often, niacin. This can lead to rhabdomyolysis if not caught early, so this combination should not be used routinely. The dosage of reductase inhibitors must be kept low if used with cyclosporine (*ie*, under 20 mg of lovastatin).

Probucol is a drug that lowers LDL-c mildly and also lowers HDL-c. It is a strong antioxidant. Because no clinical trials have been reported, it is not possible to recommend this drug.

Combination therapy is most valuable in several specific situations. First, when LDL-c is so high that very large

TABLE 8 OVERVIEW OF LIPID-LOWERING THERAPY

Drug	Lipid effects	Negative aspects	Comments
Bile-acid sequestrants Cholestyramine Colestipol	TC, LDL–; TG+; HDL+	At higher dosages, gastrointestinal side effects (*eg*, constipation, rectal bleeding)	Avoid if TG > 250 mg/dL; use psyllium if constipation a problem; low-dose resin (two scoops per day) most useful
Fibric-acid derivative Gemfibrozil	TC, LDL–; TG—; HDL++	May predispose to gallstones	Drug of choice for those with marked hypertriglyceridemia; for primary prevention of CAD, use only in those with high TC, TG, and low HDL-c
Niacin Nicotinic acid or vitamin B_3 Niacinamide is *not* a substitute for niacin (minimal lipid lowering)	TC, LDL–; TG—; HDL++	Flushing in all initially; must monitor liver function tests; can exacerbate ulcer disease, elevates glucose, and cause gout; acanthosis nigricans can be seen—abates if niacin stopped	Unmodified form is inexpensive; an aspirin can be used to mitigate flushing; avoid in diabetics, if possible; if niacin well tolerated, don't change brands!
HMG-CoA reductase inhibitors Lovastatin, pravastatin Simvastatin, fluvastatin	TC, LDL—; TG-; HDL+	Few side effects at low doses; liver function tests should be monitored; myositis risk in certain situation (*eg*, with cyclosporine or gemfibrozil)	Expensive, but may be most cost-effective; lovastatin should be taken with food (not so with the others)
Combination therapy Niacin and resin Statin and resin	TC, LDL—; TG–; HDL++	Must still watch individual drug's effects	May be better for those with combined hyperlipidemia or severe hyperlipidemia

HDL—high-density lipoprotein; HMG-COA—hydroxymethylglutaryl–coenzyme A; LDL—low-density lipoprotein; TC—total cholesterol; TG—triglycerides; +—mild increments; ++—moderate increments; +++—largest increments; - —mild reductions; – —moderate reductions; ——largest reductions.

dosages of a single drug would be needed, possibly increasing toxicity, a resin and niacin or a resin and hydroxymethylglutaryl–coenzyme A (HMG-CoA) reductase inhibitor are useful combinations for the marked excess LDL-c (*eg*, in familial hypercholesterolemia). Second, when lower doses of two drugs would minimize cost or side effects, or multiple lipid abnormalities prevent a single lipid-lowering drug from sufficing, combination therapy is indicated. This is often seen in familial combined hyperlipidemia. Combinations such as niacin and resin, niacin and an HMG-CoA reductase inhibitor, and niacin and gemfibrozil have been used. There is increased risk of liver toxicity with niacin and HMG-CoA reductase inhibitors (as well as increased myositis), so these patients must be watched carefully. If diet and exercise regimens to control triglycerides and HDL-c are strictly adhered to, combination therapy is sometimes not needed.

Treatment of isolated, low HDL-c is a controversial subject. Although these individuals may be at risk, not all with low HDL-c are at increased risk. Vegetarians are a good example; they have both low HDL-c and LDL-c. If low HDL-c is not accompanied by hypertriglyceridemia, the benefit from drug therapy is uncertain. A possible approach is to keep LDL-c low with a low-saturated-fat diet rich in fruits and vegetables (a good source of antioxidants) and to reserve niacin therapy (for those with coronary disease) or gemfibrozil or niacin (if triglycerides are also elevated).

References and Recommended Reading

Recently published papers of particular interest have been highlighted as:
- Of interest
- •• Of outstanding interest

1. Steinberg D, Parthasarathy S, Carew TE, *et al*.: Beyond cholesterol: modifications of low density lipoprotein that increase its atherogenicity. *N Engl J Med* 1989, 320:915–924.

2. Stamler J, Wentworth D, Neaton JD, *et al*.: Is the relationship between serum cholesterol and risk of premature death from coronary heart disease continuous and graded? *JAMA* 1986, 256:2823–2826.

3. Kaplan NM: The deadly quartet: upper-body obesity, glucose intolerance, hypertriglyceridemia, and hypertension. *Arch Intern Med* 1989, 149:1514–1520.

4.•• Expert Panel on Detection, Evaluation, and Treatment of High Blood Cholesterol in Adults: Summary of the Second Report of the National Cholesterol Education (NCEP) Expert Panel on Detection, Evaluation, and Treatment of High Blood Cholesterol in Adults (Adult Treatment Panel II). *JAMA* 1993, 269:3015–3023.

5. Ginsburg GS, Safran C, Pasternak RC: Frequency of low serum high density lipoprotein cholesterol levels in hospitalized patients with "desirable" total cholesterol levels. *Am J Cardiol* 1991, 68:187–192.

6. Tornvall P, Bavenholm P, Landou C, *et al*.: Relation of plasma levels and composition of apolipoprotein B–containing lipoproteins to angiographically defined coronary artery disease in young patients with myocardial infarction. *Circulation* 1993, 88(part 1):2180–2189.

7.•• Cooper GR, Myers GL, Smith J, Schlant RC: Blood lipid measurements: variations and practical utility. *JAMA* 1992, 267:1652–1660.

8. Gore JM, Goldberg RJ, Matsumoto AS, *et al*.: Validity of serum total cholesterol level obtained within 24 hours of acute myocardial infarction. *Am J Cardiol* 1984, 54:722–725.

9. Ryder REJ, Hayes TM, Mulligan IP, *et al*.: How soon after myocardial infarction should plasma lipid values be assessed? *BMJ* 1984, 289:165–173.

10. Avogaro P, Bon GB, Cazzolato G, *et al*.: Variations in apolipoproteins B and A1 during the course of myocardial infarction. *Eur J Clin Invest* 1978, 8:121–129.

11. Genest JJ, Corbett HM, McNamara JR, *et al*.: Effect of hospitalization on high-density lipoprotein cholesterol in patients undergoing elective coronary angiography. *Am J Cardiol* 1988, 61:998–1000.

12. Hearn JA, DeMaio SJ, Roubin GS, *et al*.: Predictive value of lipoprotein (a) and other serum lipoproteins in the angiographic diagnosis of coronary artery disease. *Am J Cardiol* 1990, 66:1176–1180.

13. Hjermann I, Holme I, Velve Byre K, Leren P: Effect of diet and smoking intervention on the incidence of coronary heart disease. *Laucet* 1981, ii:1303–1310.

14. The Multiple Risk Factor Intervention Trial Research Group: Mortality rates after 10.5 years for participants in the multiple risk factor intervention trial: findings related to a priori hypotheses of the trial. *JAMA* 1990, 263:1795–1801.

15. Dayton S, Pearce ML, Hashimoto S, *et al*.: A controlled clinical trial of a diet high in unsaturated fat in preventing complications of atherosclerosis. *Circulation* 1969, 40(suppl II):II-1–II-63.

16. Ornish D, Brown SE, Scherwitz LW, *et al*.: Can lifestyle changes reverse coronary heart disease? The Lifestyle Heart Trial. *Lancet* 1990, 336:129–133.

17.• Watts GF, Lewis B, Brunt JNH, *et al*.: Effects on coronary artery disease of lipid-lowering diet, or diet plus cholestyramine, in the St. Thomas Atherosclerosis Regression (STARS) Study. *Lancet* 1992, 339:563–569.

18. *The Surgeon General's Report on Nutrition and Health* U.S. Department of Health and Human Services. Public Health Service. USDHHS (PHS) Publication No. 88-50210, 1988.

19. Gorder DD, Dolecek TA, Coleman GG, *et al*.: Dietary intake in the Multiple Risk Factor Intervention Trial (MRFIT): nutrient and food group changes over 6 years. *J Am Diet Assoc* 1986, 86:744–751.

20. Pearson TA: The quest for a cholesterol-decreasing diet: should we subtract, substitute, or supplement? *Ann Intern Med* 1993, 119:627–628.

21.• Cobb MM, Teitelbaum HS, Breslow JL: Lovastatin efficacy in reducing low-density lipoprotein cholesterol levels on high- vs. low-fat diets. *JAMA* 1991, 265:997–1001.

22. Lipid Research Clinics Program: The Lipid Research Clinics Coronary Primary Prevention Trial Result. I. Reduction in incidence of coronary heart disease. *JAMA* 1984, 251:351–364.

23. Frick MH, Eto O, Haapa K, *et al*.: Helsinki Heart Study: primary prevention trial with gemfibrozil in middle-aged men with dyslipidemia. *N Engl J Med* 1987, 317:1237–1245.

24. The Coronary Drug Project Research Group: Clofibrate and niacin in coronary heart disease. *JAMA* 1975, 231:360–381.

25. Rossouw JE, Lewis B, Rifkind BM: The value of lowering cholesterol after myocardial infarction. *N Engl J Med* 1990, 323:1112–1119.

26. LaRosa J, Cleeman JI: Cholesterol lowering as a treatment for established coronary heart disease. *Circulation* 1992, 85:1229–1235.

27. Cashin-Hemphill L, Mack WJ, Pogoda JM, *et al.*: Beneficial effects of colestipol-niacin on coronary atherosclerosis. A 4-year follow-up. *JAMA* 1990, 264:3013–3017.

28.• Brown G, Albers JJ, Fisher LD, *et al.*: Regression of coronary artery disease as a result of interim lipid-lowering therapy in men with high levels of apolipoprotein B. *N Engl J Med* 1990, 323:1289–1298.

29. Kane JP, Malloy MJ, Ports TA, *et al.*: Regression of coronary atherosclerosis during treatment of familial hypercholesterolemia with combined drug regimens. *JAMA* 1990, 264:3007–3012.

30. Bild DE, Williams RR, Brewer HB, *et al.*: Identification and management of heterozygous familial hypercholesterolemia: summary and recommendations from an NHLBI workshop. *Am J Cardiol* 1993, 72:1D–5D.

31. Buchwald H, Varco RL, Matts JP, *et al.*: Effect of partial ileal bypass surgery on mortality and morbidity from coronary heart disease in patients with hypercholesterolemia. *N Engl J Med* 1990, 323:946–955.

32. Blankenhorn DH, Hodis HN: Arterial imaging and atherosclerosis reversal. *Arterioscler Thromb* 1994, 14:177–192.

33. Scandinavian Simvastatin Study Group: Randomised trial of cholesterol lowering in 4444 patients with coronary artery disease: the Scandinavian Simvastatin Survival Study (4S). *Lancet* 1994, 344:1383–1389.

34. Squires RW, Allison TG, Gau GT, *et al.*: Low-dose, time-release nicotinic acid: effects in selected patients with low concentrations of high-density lipoprotein cholesterol. *Mayo Clin Proc* 1992, 67:855–860.

35. McKenney JM, Proctor JD, Harris S, Chinchili VM: A comparison of the efficacy and toxic effects of sustained vs. immediate-release niacin in hypercholesterolemic patients. *JAMA* 1994, 271:672–677.

Select Bibliography

Badimon JJ, Fuster V, Chesebro JH, Badimon L: Coronary atherosclerosis. A multifactorial disease. *Circulation* 1993, 87(suppl II):II-3–II-16.

Genest J, McNamara JR, Ordoras JM, *et al.*: Lipoprotein cholesterol, apolipoprotein A-I and B and lipoprotein (a) abnormalities in men with premature coronary disease. *J Am Coll Cardiol* 1992, 19:792–802.

MAAS Investigators: Effect of simvastatin on coronary atheroma: the Multicentre Anti-Atheroma Sudy (MAAS). *Lancet* 1994, 344:633–638.

Rath M, Niendorf A, Reblin T, *et al.*: Detection and quantification of lipoprotein (a) in the arterial wall of 107 coronary bypass patients. *Arteriosclerosis* 1989, 9:579–592.

Waters D, Higginson L, Gladstone P, *et al.* Effects of monotherapy with an HMGCoa reductase inhibitor on the progression of coronary atherosclerosis as assessed by serial quantitative arteriography: the Canadian Coronary Atherosclerosis Intervention Trial. *Circulation* 1994, 89:959–968.

Chronic Ischemic Heart Disease

Susan Simandl
Peter F. Cohn

Key Points
- The pathophysiology of myocardial ischemia is related to a mismatch between coronary blood flow and myocardial oxygen requirements.
- In most patients with coronary artery disease, the angina threshold is not fixed but varies throughout the day.
- The exercise test is probably still the most important noninvasive diagnostic test.
- Patients with chronic ischemia may or may not demonstrate painful symptoms during ischemic episodes.
- Prognosis in patients with chronic ischemia relates to the severity of coronary artery disease and the degree of left ventricular dysfunction plus objective documentation of ischemia.
- Major therapeutic agents for patients with chronic ischemia are antianginal drugs (nitrates, β-blockers, calcium blockers), antiplatelet drugs (aspirin), and revascularization procedures (coronary angioplasty, coronary artery surgery).

Myocardial ischemia occurs when the coronary blood supply cannot meet the myocardial demands. This discrepancy is termed a supply–demand mismatch. Coronary blood supply is determined by the oxygen-carrying capacity and the coronary blood flow, which is regulated by numerous interacting factors. Myocardial demands are affected by changes in heart rate, contractility, and systolic wall tension; increasing heart rate is believed to be the single most important determinant of increased myocardial oxygen consumption.

In the normal heart, the coronary blood supply increases to match increasing myocardial demands. In the patient with significant coronary atherosclerotic disease, however, myocardial oxygen consumption may exceed the coronary blood supply, resulting in myocardial ischemia. Because it is at the end of the arterial blood supply, the subendocardium is the most vulnerable to ischemia.

CLINICAL PRESENTATION

The clinical presentation of myocardial ischemia resulting from coronary artery disease ranges from asymptomatic silent ischemia to atypical angina to classic angina pectoris. Classic angina has been defined as transient precordial discomfort provoked by exertion and relieved by rest or nitroglycerin. The discomfort can be heaviness, pressure, or tightness in the chest. It also can radiate to the arm, neck, jaw, or back and may be provoked by exercise; cold, hot, or humid weather; heavy meals; or emotional stress. The discomfort begins gradually and reaches maximal intensity over several minutes before resolving. Classic angina eases after rest or 2 to 3 minutes after nitroglycerin is taken. Most importantly, angina is *not* described as a brief, sharp, pleuritic, stabbing, localized, or migratory discomfort.

Atypical angina is a syndrome that has some similar symptoms, but lacks one or more of the criteria for classic angina [1••]. Angina equivalents are symptoms of

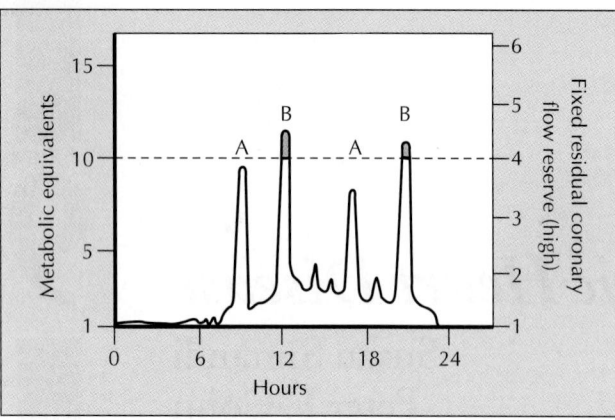

FIGURE 1 Fixed coronary artery obstructions not adequately compensated by collateral flow may reduce coronary flow reserve. In this diagram, it is reduced to only four times the resting values. The patient can exercise up to approximately 10 metabolic equivalents without having ischemia (A); however, if the patient exercises above approximately 10 metabolic equivalents, he or she will consistently develop ischemia (B). (From Maseri and coworkers [18]; with permission.)

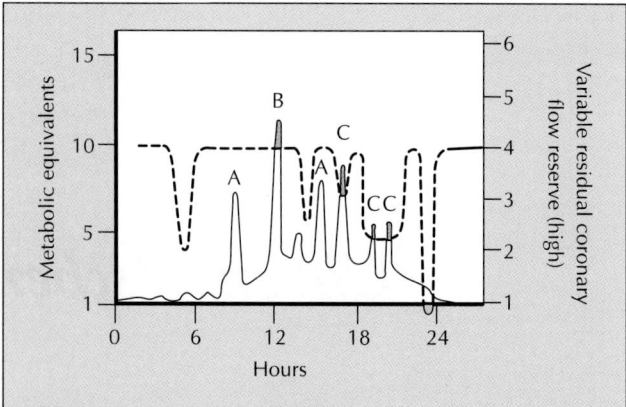

FIGURE 2 Residual coronary flow reserve may have an upper limit that is indeed fixed, but it can decrease because of mechanisms that transiently interfere with coronary blood flow. Thus, residual coronary flow reserve can vary throughout the day. Under these conditions, if the patient exercises beyond the maximal residual coronary flow reserve, the patient will always develop ischemia (B). However, the patient may also develop ischemia on other occasions after smaller degrees of exercise when residual coronary flow reserve is decreased by these functional factors (C). Occasionally, coronary flow reserve can decrease so that resting flow is impaired and ischemia occurs at rest. At other times of the day, this patient can exercise below the level of maximal residual coronary flow reserve without experiencing ischemia (A). In this case, the coronary flow reserve is fixed at approximately four times resting levels, so that the patient can exercise to approximately 10 metabolic equivalents in the absence of transient impairment of coronary flow. This level of work is compatible with most activities of daily life; hence, if the episodes of transient impairment of coronary flow reserve could be prevented, the patient would develop angina only after efforts of unusual intensity. (From Maseri and coworkers [18]; with permission.)

myocardial ischemia other than angina. Exertional dyspnea is often referred to as an anginal equivalent. Others use the term to describe pain in a referred location, such as isolated exertional arm or neck discomfort not accompanied by discomfort in the chest [1••]. Variant angina is chest discomfort occurring at rest secondary to coronary vasospasm and associated with ST-segment elevation (rather than depression) on electrocardiography (ECG).

The angina threshold is the level of metabolic activity (physical or emotional) at which myocardial ischemia ensues. If this threshold is fixed, the same amount of exertion, often expressed in metabolic equivalents or as a rate–pressure product (heart rate multiplied by systolic blood pressure), provokes the patient's angina (Fig. 1). In other patients, the threshold varies throughout the day. These patients sometimes have angina at rest or with minimal exertion; at other times, they are able to exercise more vigorously (Fig. 2). Many patients have both fixed- and variable-threshold angina, which is described as mixed angina pectoris.

The clinical history may give clues to the mechanism of a patient's angina (increasing myocardial demands as seen in exertional angina and decreasing coronary blood supply in patients with angina without precipitant). This information may help to guide the physician in choosing a medication (Fig. 3).

DIAGNOSIS

The diagnosis of coronary artery disease cannot be made on physical examination; however, some findings may increase clinical suspicion of coronary artery disease. One such example is systemic hypertension. Skin xanthomas are found in patients with familial hypercholesterolemia who have an increased incidence of premature coronary artery disease. Arcus cornealis (an opaque, grayish ring at the periphery of the cornea found in young white patients) is a predictor of subsequent coronary events. The presence of carotid or femoral bruits, which is suggestive of peripheral vascular disease, increases the likelihood that the patient also has atherosclerotic heart disease. Cardiac examination may give clues to underlying organic heart disease (eg, if pathologic murmurs or gallops are noted) but it is by no means sensitive or specific for the diagnosis of coronary artery disease.

Noninvasive tests include exercise ECG, ambulatory ECG monitoring, nuclear imaging, and echocardiography. The exercise stress test is best used in patients who have normal findings on resting ECG. The patient exercises, commonly with either a treadmill or a stationary bicycle, and the patient's exercise duration, symptoms, blood pressure, heart rate, heart rhythm, physical examination findings, and ECG findings are analyzed. In the context of the clinical history, these parameters are evaluated to formulate a diagnostic impression.

The pretest risk (the probability of disease in the patient having the test) can be ascertained on clinical examination. Pryor and coworkers [2] concluded that the type of chest pain (typical, atypical, or nonanginal) was the most important predictor of significant coronary artery disease, followed by evidence of a prior myocardial infarction, gender, age, tobacco use, hyperlipidemia, ST-T segment changes on ECG, and a history of diabetes. Figures 4 and 5 are nomograms for estimating the likelihood of significant coronary artery disease. The posttest risk (the probability of disease in a patient with a positive test result) is assessed in light of the pretest risk and the test results (Table 1).

Exercise radionuclide ventriculography, thallium-201 stress testing, and stress echocardiography have increased the sensitivity for detecting coronary artery disease [3,4]. These specialized tests are commonly used in patients with abnormal baseline ECG results that make the exercise ECG findings difficult to interpret. Radionuclide and echocardiographic studies are also commonly used in patients with poor exercise capacity and those who are unable to exercise. In these circumstances, pharmacologic stress agents such as dipyridamole, dobutamine, or adenosine have been employed. The sensitivity and specificity of dipyridamole-thallium stress testing are nearly comparable to those of exercise thallium stress testing [5]. Because of their increased cost and time of performance as well as the marginal benefit for improved detection in some patients, however, nuclear and echocardiographic stress tests are not routinely recommended as screening procedures.

In patients with chronic stable angina, the stress test has been said to provide little diagnostic information after clinical parameters are taken into account. However, the stress test can be used to monitor disease progression and the patient's response to medication. It also can assess the functional significance of a lesion detected angiographically, assess the benefits of revascularization via surgery or angioplasty, and perhaps most importantly, provide a prognostic assessment (aid in risk stratification).

PROGNOSIS

The prognosis in patients with chronic stable angina can be determined by the patient history, physical examination, noninvasive data, and coronary angiographic results. Some investigators believe that severe angina is consistent with a poorer outlook. Thus, the angina score, which takes into account the severity and frequency of the angina as well as the results of resting ECG, has been shown to be an independent predictor of prognosis [6]. Clinical findings suggestive of poor left ventricular function are also associated with a worse prospect.

With information obtained from the clinical examination, the clinician decides if the patient is in a low- or high-risk group. In high-risk patients (those with frequent episodes of angina and evidence of left ventricular dysfunction on clinical examination), coronary angiography with an eye toward revascularization should be performed. In low-risk patients or those in a poorly defined risk category on clinical examination, stress data have helped to delineate high- and low-risk groups. The specific criteria vary from report to report, but the conclusion remains the same: patients with poor exercise capacity and those with severe ischemia by ST response at a low workload compose a high-risk cohort (Table 2).

Radionuclide stress tests (either with ventriculography demonstrating poor resting left ventricular function or failure of the left ventricular ejection fraction to increase with exercise [7,8] or with perfusion imaging showing severe ischemia as evidenced by multiple reversible thallium defects), thallium uptake in the lungs, and transient postexercise left ventricular dilatation identify patients at higher risk for cardiac events [9–11]. Although left ventricular function

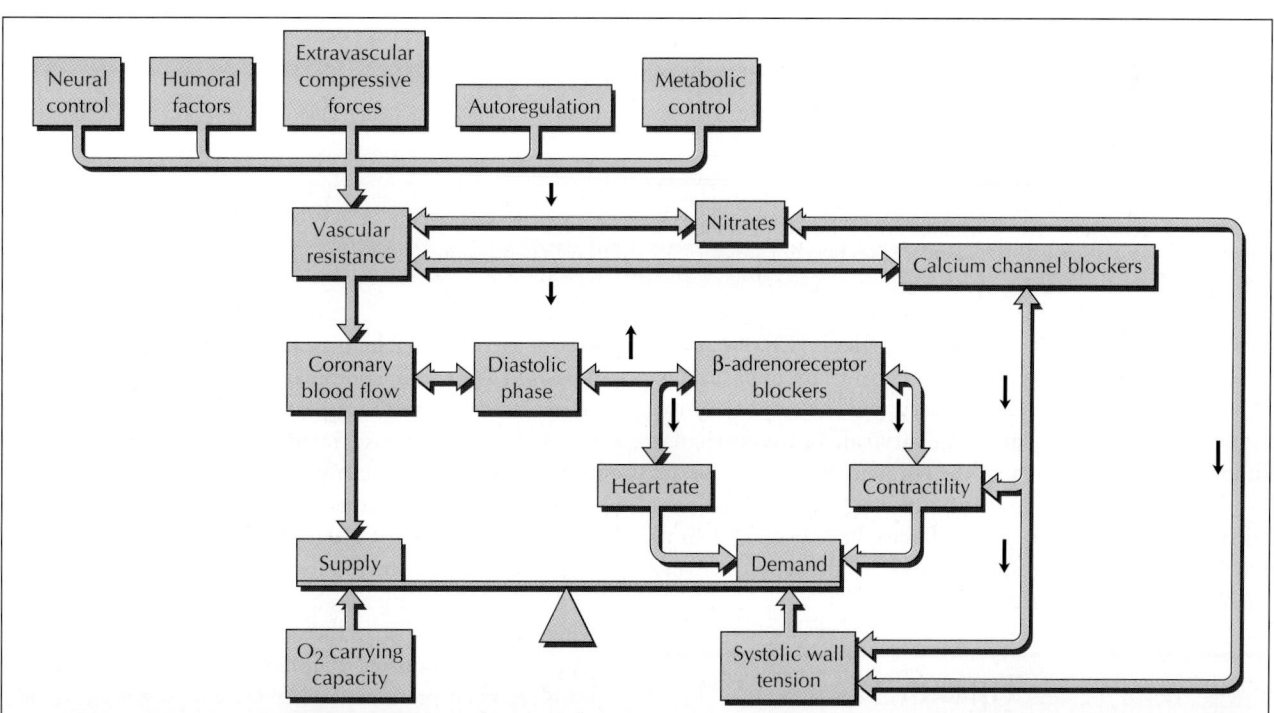

FIGURE 3 Effect of nitrates, beta-adrenoreceptor blockers, and calcium channel blockers on myocardial oxygen supply and demand. Reflex effects are not shown. (From Ardehali and Ports [19]; with permission.)

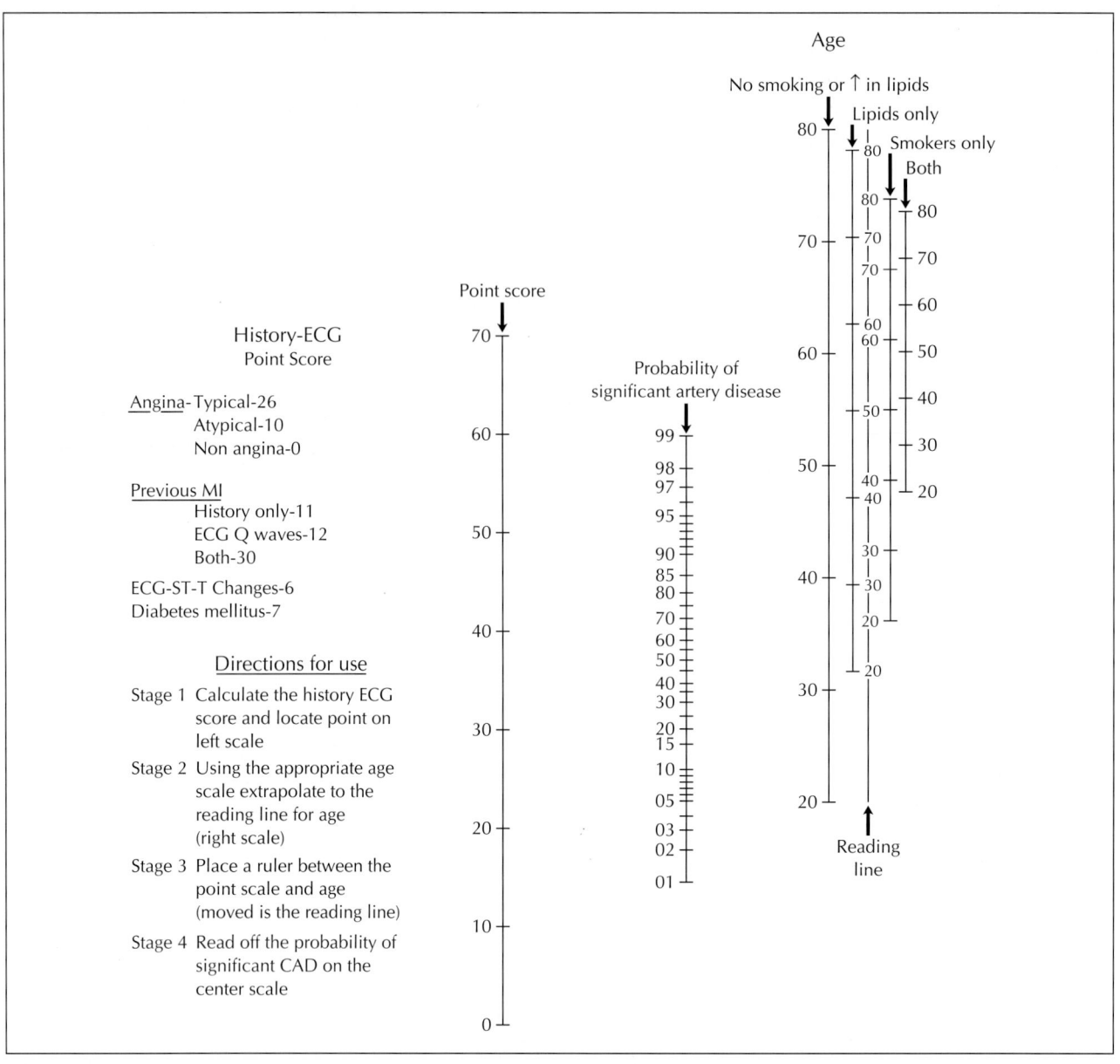

FIGURE 4 Nomogram for estimating the likelihood of significant coronary artery disease (CAD) in men. ECG—electrocardiographic; MI—myocardial infarction. (From Pryor and coworkers [2]; with permission.)

is probably the strongest predictor of prognosis [12], the severity of the coronary artery disease has significant implications. Both the number of diseased vessels and the severity of the stenosis [12,13] correlate with survival. Left ventricular function and the severity of the coronary artery disease act synergistically in determining survival [12], and patients with left main coronary artery disease have been shown to have the worst prognosis, followed by those with severe three-vessel coronary artery disease [14].

THERAPY

The goals of therapy in managing chronic stable angina are to prolong survival, reduce the incidence of disease progression, alleviate symptoms, and improve exercise capacity. Nitrates, β-blockers, and calcium antagonists are the three classes of agents available to treat chronic stable angina. They can be used alone or in combination.

Nitrates dilate coronary arteries and decrease cardiac preload. Their use is associated with reflex tachycardia, an effect that may increase myocardial demands and can be blunted by concomitant use of a β-blocker. Short-acting nitrates, which are most often administered in sublingual or buccal mucosa spray form, are often used to treat an acute episode of angina. Patients should be told to sit down when they take this type of agent, because the vasodilatation may be associated with transient hypotension and dizziness. This effect is especially prominent when there is preexistent vasodilatation, as in very hot, humid weather or after a hot shower. Most patients with chronic stable angina have a short-acting nitrate preparation prescribed for them to take on an "as-needed" basis. They also may be on a daily regimen of a

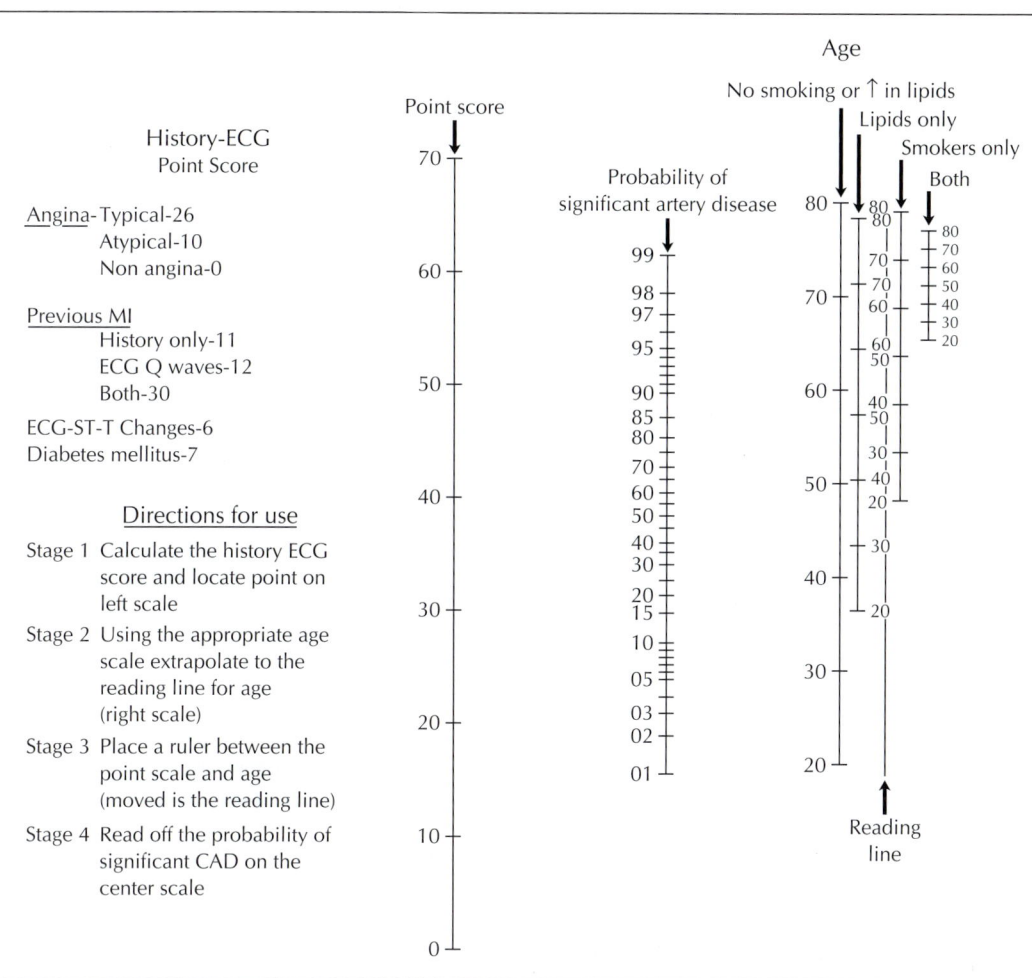

FIGURE 5
Nomogram for estimating the likelihood of significant coronary artery disease (CAD) in women. ECG—electrocardiographic; MI—myocardial infarction. (From Pryor and coworkers [2]; with permission.)

longer-acting nitrate. At present, a multitude of preparations are available in different forms and with different half-lives. The most important aspect of long-term nitrate therapy is to ensure an adequate nitrate-free interval, which will prevent nitrate tolerance.

β-Blockers decrease heart rate and contractility. They must be used with caution in patients who have significant bradyarrhythmias, asthma, congestive heart failure, or hypotension. They also must be used prudently in patients with diabetes mellitus and peripheral vascular disease. Because they blunt the tachycardia associated with exercise, these agents are well suited for patients with exertional or effort-induced angina. In addition, they are effective therapy for patients with angina who also have coexisting hypertension.

Calcium channel antagonists are a diverse group of agents, all of which act as vasodilators. Like β-blockers, many can be used as antianginal and antihypertensive agents. Diltiazem and verapamil can be used in patients with coexistent supraventricular arrhythmias, but unlike nifedipine, they must be used cautiously in patients with bradyarrhythmias. Verapamil is a potent negative inotrope and is not recommended in patients with poor left ventricular systolic function.

TABLE 1 POSTTEST RISK OF OBSTRUCTIVE CORONARY DISEASE AFTER A SYMPTOM-LIMITED EXERCISE TEST*

Clinical presentation	Men, %		Women, %	
	ECG abnormal[†]	ECG normal[‡]	ECG abnormal	ECG normal
Typical angina	95	50	80	30
Probable angina	85	25	55	15
Nonspecific chest pain	40	10	10	5
Asymptomatic	30	5	5	< 1

From Chaitman [20]; with permission.
*Patients without myocardial infarction.
[†]Horizontal or downsloping ST-segment depression of 1 mm or more.
[‡]Heart rate that is 85% or more of the age-predicted maximum.
ECG—electrocardiogram.

Table 2. Risk stratification by exercise testing

Study	Patients, n	Low	Intermediate	High
McNeer et al. [22]	1472	< 1 mm ST ↓ FS ≥ IV Peak HR ≥ 160 bpm		≥ 1 mm ST ↓ FS I or II
Bruce et al. [23] (Seattle Heart Watch)	2001	< 1 mm ST ↓ No LV dysfunction	≥ 1 mm ST ↓ No LV dysfunction	FS ≤ I Peak SBP < 130 mm Hg Cardiomegaly
Dagenais et al. [24]	107	≤ 2 mm ST ↓ FS ≥ IV	≤ 2 mm ST ↓ FS ≥ III	≥ 2 mm ST ↓ FS ≤ I
Schneider et al. [25]	80			> 1 mm ST ↓ FS I or II
Weiner et al. [26]	292	≤ 2 mm ST ↓ No LV dysfunction		LV dysfunction or ≥ 2 mm ST ↓ beginning in stage I
Weiner et al. [27] Coronary Artery Surgery Study	4083	< 1 mm ST ↓ FS ≥ III	≥ 1 mm ST ↓ FS ≥ III	≥ 1 mm ST ↓ FS ≤ I

From Deering and Weiner [21]; with permission.
FS—final exercise stage (Bruce protocol); HR—heart rate; LV—left ventricular; SBP—systolic blood pressure; ST ↓—ST-segment depression.

All three classes of antianginal drugs decrease the incidence of ischemia and improve exercise performance. These agents can be used as the sole therapy for patients stratified by noninvasive methods to a low-risk group for cardiac events or who are good candidates for revascularization. They are also often used as adjuncts to revascularization. In addition, because of its proven benefit in post–myocardial infarction, unstable angina, and post–coronary bypass patients, daily aspirin use is often recommended. Finally, risk modification with diet counseling, antilipemic therapy, smoking cessation, and exercise programs is strongly advised. All of these measures can be initiated by the generalist; when revascularization is indicated by refractory symptoms or markedly abnormal stress test results, referral to a specialist is appropriate.

Coronary artery bypass graft surgery is performed to improve quality of life and prolong survival. Coronary artery bypass grafting has been shown to relieve angina more effectively than medical therapy [15] and is effective when angina is refractory to medical therapy. The poorer the prognosis (ie, severe ischemia combined with poor left ventricular function), the greater the benefits of revascularization (albeit possibly at a higher operative risk).

The role of coronary angioplasty in the treatment of chronic stable angina is evolving. A randomized trial comparing angioplasty with medical therapy in patients with single-vessel coronary artery disease reported a statistically significant improvement in exercise tolerance and anginal symptoms among the angioplasty group [16]. The angioplasty patients had a greater number of hospital days, however, as well as a higher incidence of repeated angioplasty (with its associated risks) and a higher cost than the medically treated patients. Another randomized study, which compared angioplasty with coronary artery bypass surgery, showed no difference in the rate of death or nonfatal myocardial infarction between the two groups 2.5 years after enrollment. However, the angioplasty group had a statistically significant increase in subsequent revascularization procedures (repeated angioplasty, bypass surgery, or both) and the need for repeated coronary arteriography [17••]. Surgical patients had less angina and required less antianginal therapy in this study.

References and Recommended Reading

Recently published papers of particular interest have been highlighted as:
• Of interest
•• Of outstanding interest

1.•• Shub C: Stable angina pectoris: I. Clinical patterns. *Mayo Clin Proc* 1990, 64:233–242.
2. Pryor DB, Harrell FE Jr, Lee KL, *et al.*: Estimating the likelihood of significant coronary artery disease. *Am J Med* 1983, 75:771–780.
3. Epstein SE: Implication of probability analysis on the strategy used for noninvasive detection of coronary artery disease. *Am J Cardiol* 1985, 46:441–449.
4. Armstrong WF, O'Donnell J, Dillon JC, *et al.*: Complementary value of two-dimensional exercise echocardiography to routine treadmill exercise testing. *Ann Intern Med* 1986, 105:829–835.
5. Francisco DA, Collins SM, Go RT, *et al.*: Tomographic thallium-201 myocardial perfusion scintigrams after maximal coronary artery vasodilation with intravenous dipyridamole: comparison of qualitative and quantitative approaches. *Circulation* 1982, 66:370–379.
6. Califf RM, Mark DB, Harrell FE Jr, *et al.*: Importance of clinical measures of ischemia in the prognosis of patients with documented coronary artery disease. *J Am Coll Cardiol* 1988, 11:20–26.

7. Taliercio CP, Clements IP, Zinsmeister AR, Gibbons RJ: Prognostic value and limitations of exercise radionuclide angiography in medically treated coronary artery disease. *Mayo Clin Proc* 1988, 63:573–582.

8. Bonow RO, Kent KM, Rosing DR, *et al.*: Exercise-induced ischemia in mildly symptomatic patients with coronary artery disease and preserved left ventricular function. *N Engl J Med* 1984, 311:1339–1345.

9. Ladenheim ML, Pollock BH, Rozanski A, *et al.*: Extent and severity of myocardial reperfusion as predictors of prognosis in patients with suspected coronary artery disease. *J Am Coll Cardiol* 1986, 7:464–471.

10. Gill JB, Ruddy TD, Newell JB, *et al.*: Prognostic importance of thallium uptake by the lung during exercise in coronary artery disease. *N Engl J Med* 1987, 317:1486–1489.

11. Weiss AT, Berman DS, Lew AS, *et al.*: Transient ischemic dilatation of the left ventricle on stress thallium-201 scintigraphy: a marker of severe and extensive coronary artery disease. *J Am Coll Cardiol* 1987, 9:752–759.

12. Mock MB, Ringqvist I, Fisher LD, *et al.*: Survival of medically treated patients in the Coronary Artery Surgery Study (CASS) Registry. *Circulation* 1982, 66:562–568.

13. Harris PJ, Behar VS, Conley MJ, *et al.*: The prognostic significance of 50 percent stenosis in medically treated patients with coronary artery disease. *Circulation* 1980, 62:240–248.

14. Proudfit WJ, Bruschke AV, MacMillan JP, *et al.*: Fifteen year survival study of patients with obstructive coronary artery disease. *Circulation* 1983, 68:986–997.

15. CASS Principal Investigators and Their Associates: Coronary Artery Surgery Study (CASS): A randomized trial of coronary artery bypass surgery. Quality of life in patients randomly assigned to treatment groups. *Circulation* 1983, 68:951–960.

16. Parisi AF, Folland ED, Hartigan P: A comparison of angioplasty with medical therapy in the treatment of single-vessel coronary artery disease. *N Engl J Med* 1992, 326:10–16.

17.•• Coronary angioplasty versus coronary artery bypass surgery: the Randomized Interaction Treatment of Anginal (RITA) Trial. *Lancet* 1993, 341:573–580.

18. Maseri A, Chierchia S, Kaski JC: Mixed angina pectoris. *Am J Cardiol* 1985, 56:30E–33E.

19. Ardehali A, Ports TA: Myocardial oxygen supply and demand. *Chest* 1990, 90:699–705.

20. Chaitman BR: The changing role of the exercise electrocardiogram as a diagnostic and prognostic test for chronic ischemic heart disease. *J Am Coll Cardiol* 1986, 1195–1210.

21. Deering TF, Weiner DA: Prognosis of patients with CAD. *J Cardiopulmonary Rehabil* 1985, 5:352–331.

22. McNeer JF, Margolis JR, Lee KL, *et al.*: The role of the exercise test in the evaluation of patients for ischemic heart disease. *Circulation* 1979; 57:64–70.

23. Bruce RA, DeRouen TA, Hammermeister KE: Noninvasive screening criteria for enhanced 4-year survival after aortocoronary bypass surgery. *Circulation* 1979; 60:638–646.

24. Dagenais GR, Rouleau JR, Christen A, Fabia J: Survival of patients with a strongly positive exercise electrogram. *Circualation* 1982; 65:452–456.

25. Schneider RM, Seaworth JF, Dohnman ML, *et al.*: Anatomic and prognostic implications of an early positive treadmill exercise test. *Am J Cardiol* 1982; 50:682–688.

26. Weiner DA, McCabe CH, Ryan TJ: Prognostic assessment of patients with coronary artery disease by exercise testing. *Am Heart J* 1983; 105:749–755.

27. Weiner DA, Ryan TJ, McCabe CH, *et al.*: The prognostic importance of a clinical profile and exercise test in medically treated patients with coronary heart disease. *J Am Coll Cardiol* 1984; 3:772–779.

SELECT BIBLIOGRAPHY

Braunwald E, ed: *Heart Disease: A Textbook of Cardiovascular Medicine*, edn 4. Philadelphia: WB Saunders; 1992.

Detrano R, *et al*. The diagnostic accuracy of exercise electrocardiogram: a meta-analysis of 22 years of research. *Prog Cardiovasc Dis* 1989, 31:173–206.

Unstable Angina and Non–Q Wave Myocardial Infarction

John Speer Schroeder

> ### Key Points
> - Unstable angina and non-Q wave myocardial infarction are important diagnoses to establish because of a high infarction/death rate that occurs over the next few months.
> - These acute coronary syndromes are caused by atherosclerosis plaque rupture with varying degrees of occlusion because of platelet thrombus at the rupture site.
> - Diagnosis is established by a history of prolonged angina chest pain, electrocardiographic changes, and serial creatine kinase and creatine kinase MB enzyme testing.
> - Therapy is directed at the platelet thrombus (aspirin and heparin), prevention of coronary spasm (intravenous or topical nitroglycerin, rate-lowering calcium blockers), and treatment of contributing factors such as hypertension and tachycardia.

The syndromes of unstable angina pectoris (UAP) and non–Q wave myocardial infarction (NQMI) are referred to as intermediate coronary syndromes, because they sit between predictable exertional angina on the one hand and an acute transmural myocardial infarction on the other. The diagnosis is important [1,2]. These syndromes frequently precede a more serious cardiovascular event that can now be prevented with aggressive medical therapy and, in many instances, coronary interventional procedures or coronary bypass surgery.

Unstable angina has had many clinical terms through the years, including impending myocardial infarction, rest angina, angina decubitus, crescendo angina, preinfarction angina, and acute coronary syndrome. It is important for the physician to recognize the diagnosis, rapidly initiate aggressive treatment, and in most instances, obtain a cardiology consultation to assist with the patient's care.

PATHOPHYSIOLOGY

This change from an asymptomatic to an unstable state is thought to result from a rupture of an atherosclerotic plaque in the coronary artery [3••,4••]. As shown in Figure 1, once the plaque ruptures, exposure of the plaque contents to the blood stream results in platelet thrombosis as part of a "repair process." Platelet aggregation releases vasoactive substances that can cause local vasoconstriction, which can further reduce the coronary lumen diameter. This complex combination of platelet thrombosis, threatening to close off the coronary artery, coronary vasospasm, and counteractive natural lytic mechanisms, attempting to lyse the platelet thrombus combine to cause dynamic, changing degrees of coronary occlusion that lead to the unstable angina syndrome. If this process is not reversed, complete occlusion may occur, leading to a transmural Q-wave myocardial infarction.

DIAGNOSIS

Unstable angina pectoris should be suspected or included in the differential diagnosis when a patient relates a changing or crescendo pattern of chest pain consistent with myocardial ischemia. The character of the chest pain is typical for angina pectoris, (*ie*, squeezing or pressure), usually in the substernal area that may radiate into the neck, jaw, or inner aspect of either arm. Relief of the pain within 5 minutes by sublingual nitroglycerin assists in the diagnosis. NQMI should be suspected when the patient has a more prolonged episode of ischemic chest pain (> 15–30 minutes) that resolves spontaneously or with subsequent therapy.

Examples include the following:
1. A patient with known, stable, five-block exertional angina being treated with β-blockers and isosorbide dinitrate reports that pain suddenly began with simply walking across the room.
2. A patient calls and reports that her angina has been occurring at 3 AM the past two nights instead of just during marked exertion.
3. A patient reports that his exertional angina attacks are much more severe and may take three or four nitroglycerin tablets to relieve.
4. A woman with coronary artery disease risk factors calls at 5 AM and reports a 30-minute episode of severe substernal chest pain radiating into her left elbow.
5. A 59-year-old man who has smoked for the past 40 years comes to your office at 9 AM to get treatment for "heartburn." He relates recurring neck pain that has occurred off and on for the past 3 hours.
6. A 65-year-old man who had coronary artery bypass surgery 10 years ago reports sudden onset of "that old chest pain."
7. A patient with known hypertension reports trouble breathing and "maybe a little chest pressure" whenever she climbed three or four steps for the past week.
8. A 72-year-old woman reports two episodes of heaviness in her chest, each lasting approximately 1 hour and associated with mild diaphoresis.

These simple examples reflect the fact that UAP or NQMI can occur in the setting of known coronary artery disease or *de novo* disease, but the characteristics are frequently similar.

Initial Assessment

The initial assessment of a patient presenting with symptoms that may represent UAP or NQMI should include a thorough history, physical examination, laboratory studies, and electrocardiography.

History

The physician should obtain a thorough patient history. Is the chest pain from myocardial ischemia? Is it typical versus atypical pain? Are there known coronary artery disease risk factors? Is there known coronary artery disease? Does nitroglycerin (TNG) relieve or reduce the chest pain?

Physical examination and laboratory studies

Physical examination and laboratory studies should concentrate on whether other factors contributed to the myocardial ischemia. Is there decreased oxygen delivery (*eg*, anemia)? Is there increased oxygen demand, such as tachycardia secondary to new arrhythmia (*eg*, atrial fibrillation with rapid ventricular rate), increased heart rate, increased blood pressure, or hyperthyroidism?

Electrocardiography

Electrocardiography should establish whether ST segment elevation is present. This would be an indication for consideration of immediate thrombolytic therapy.

Diagnostic Testing

If the patient is having acute chest pain during your interview, a trial of sublingual nitroglycerin can be helpful.

Electrocardiography

The electrocardiogram is an essential tool in evaluating not only the cause of the patient's chest pain but also its severity. The finding of the ST-segment elevation or T-wave peaking suggests acute transmural ischemia, and the patient generally would be considered for thrombolytic therapy. If the ST

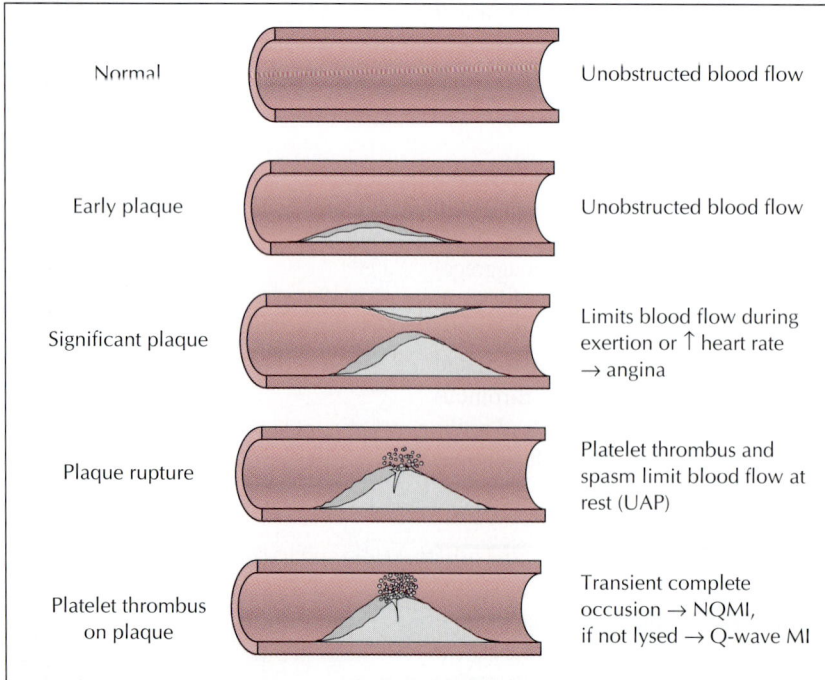

FIGURE 1 Atherosclerotic plaque in a coronary artery as it relates to clinical syndromes. NQMI—non–Q wave myocardial infarction; MI—myocardial infarction.

elevation resolves with sublingual nitroglycerin, this suggests that coronary spasm was playing a significant role, but that the setting likely is still a ruptured, unstable atherosclerotic plaque. ST depression and abnormal T waves are consistent with myocardial ischemia, particularly if it is a change from previous electrocardiograms or disappears with relief of chest pain after nitroglycerin. T-wave inversion suggests a recent subendocardial ischemic event that would be consistent with UAP or NQMI (Fig. 2). Serial electrocardiograms are valuable in making the diagnosis of UAP or NQMI, because a

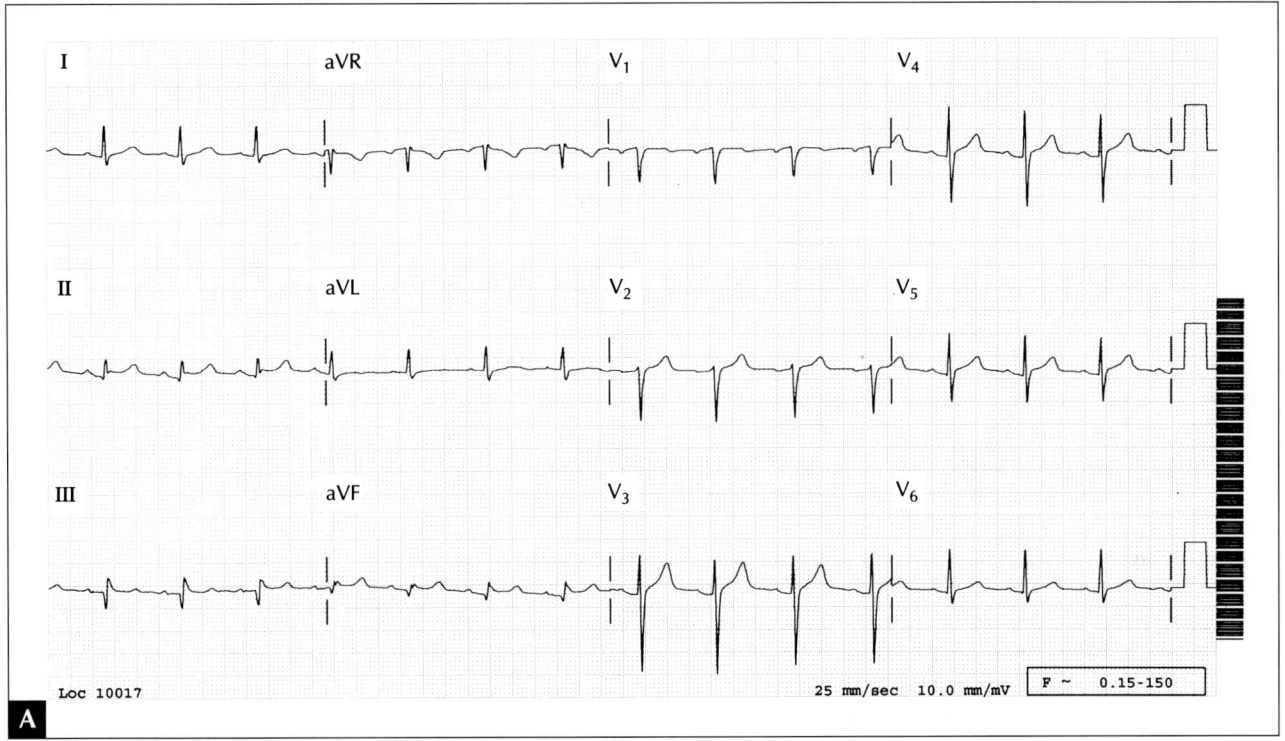

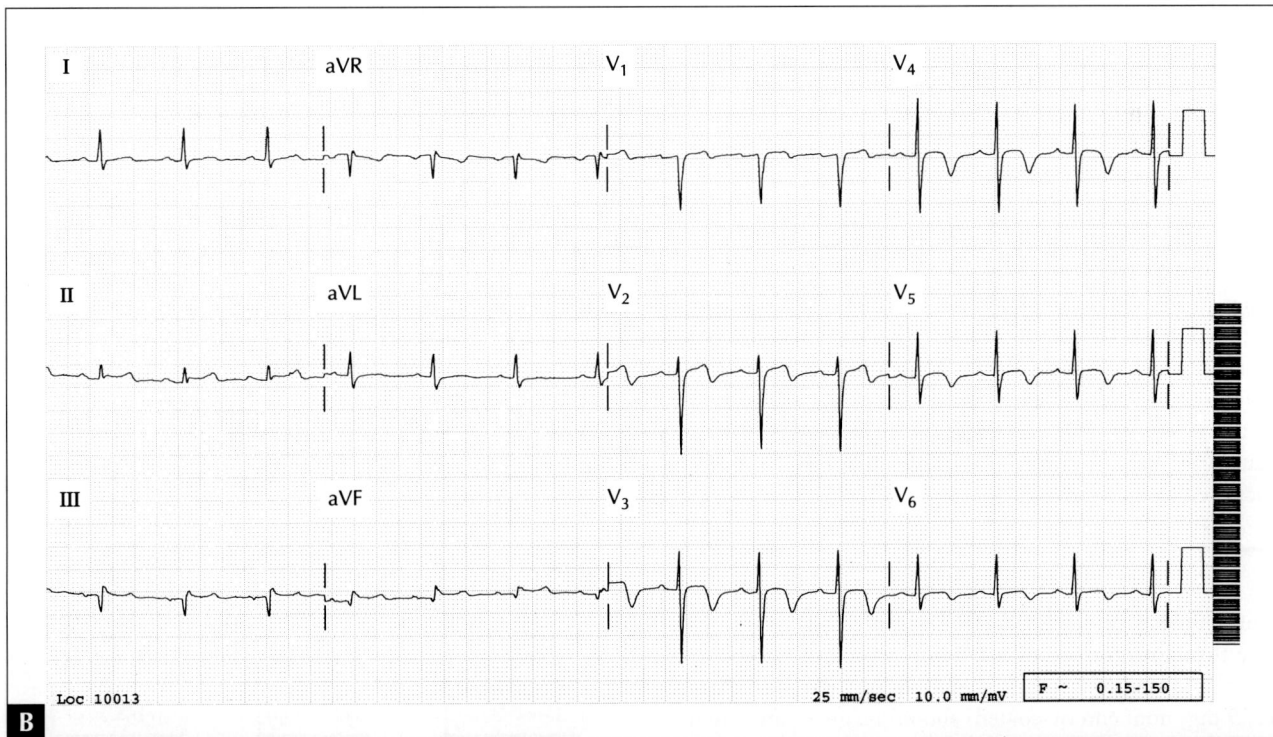

FIGURE 2 **A,** Twelve-lead electrocardiogram (ECG) in a patient complaining of crescendo angina chest pain. Leads qIII and AVG as well as ST-segment elevation in leads II, III, and AVF suggest an acute or recent inferior myocardial infarction. **B,** Twelve-lead ECG of the same patient taken 24 hours later. There is no change in the inferior leads. However, there is new T-wave inversion in anterior leads V_2 through V_6 consistent with severe anterior ischemia and/or a non–Q wave myocardial infarction if serial creatine kinase or creatine kinase–MB enzyme levels become elevated.

TABLE 1 SERUM ENZYME CHANGES IN UNSTABLE ANGINA AND NON–Q WAVE MYOCARDIAL INFARCTION.

Time, h	Unstable angina		NQMI CK rise		NQMI MB rise only	
	CK	MB, %	CK	MB, %	CK	MB, %
Normal value	< 160	< 5	< 160	< 5	< 160	< 5
0	100	3	100	3	100	3
8	120	4	260	8	160	9
24	110	3	150	7	150	7

CK—creatine kinase; MB—myocardial band; NQMI—non–Q wave myocardial infarction.

rapidly changing pattern of ST-T waves suggests a dynamic ongoing process.

A normal electrocardiogram can be useful to rule out myocardial ischemia, but it also can be misleading. A normal electrocardiogram can be consistent with a noncardiac cause for the chest pain in approximately 10% of the patients presenting with a history consistent for unstable angina. However, a normal electrocardiogram also may reflect true posterior ischemia or be associated with a dissecting thoracic aneurysm. Exercise testing may be useful if the diagnosis at this point is still not clear. It is best to review the findings with a cardiologist before initiating exercise testing, however, because stress testing in the setting of UAP or NQMI may be hazardous to the patient.

Creatine kinase enzymes

Serial creatine kinase enzyme levels are most useful in differentiating UAP from NQMI (Table 1). Generally, total and MB creatine kinase are drawn at the time of patient encounter and 8 and 24 hours after the initial patient encounter if the patient had a prolonged (> 15 minute) episode of chest pain that may have resulted in myocardial necrosis. Some patients may not have an elevated total creatine kinase, but still show evidence of NQMI based an abnormal increase in the MB fraction that reflects death of myocardial tissue.

If the episode of prolonged pain occurred more than 24 hours previously, a creatine kinase elevation may have already returned to normal. In this instance, the MB fraction may still be elevated, or LDH isoenzyme levels can help to establish a diagnosis of NQMI. Other laboratory testing should be used to rule out extracardiac causes of excess oxygen use that have caused the heart to increase its oxygen demand and need for increased coronary blood flow.

TREATMENT

Initial therapy should be directed toward preventing progressive thrombus formation that could completely occlude the vessel and lead to transmural myocardial infarction. Aspirin (325 mg, non–enteric coated) should be given immediately whether the initial contact is by telephone, in the office, or in the emergency room. The basis for this therapy is a 12-week study of 1266 veterans given Alka-Seltzer (Miles Inc, West Haven, CT) containing aspirin (325 mg) or placebo for 12 weeks following diagnosis of UAP [5]. The 12-week death rate was 3.3% in the placebo group and 1.6% in the aspirin group—a 51% reduction. Similar decreases occurred in fatal and nonfatal myocardial infarctions.

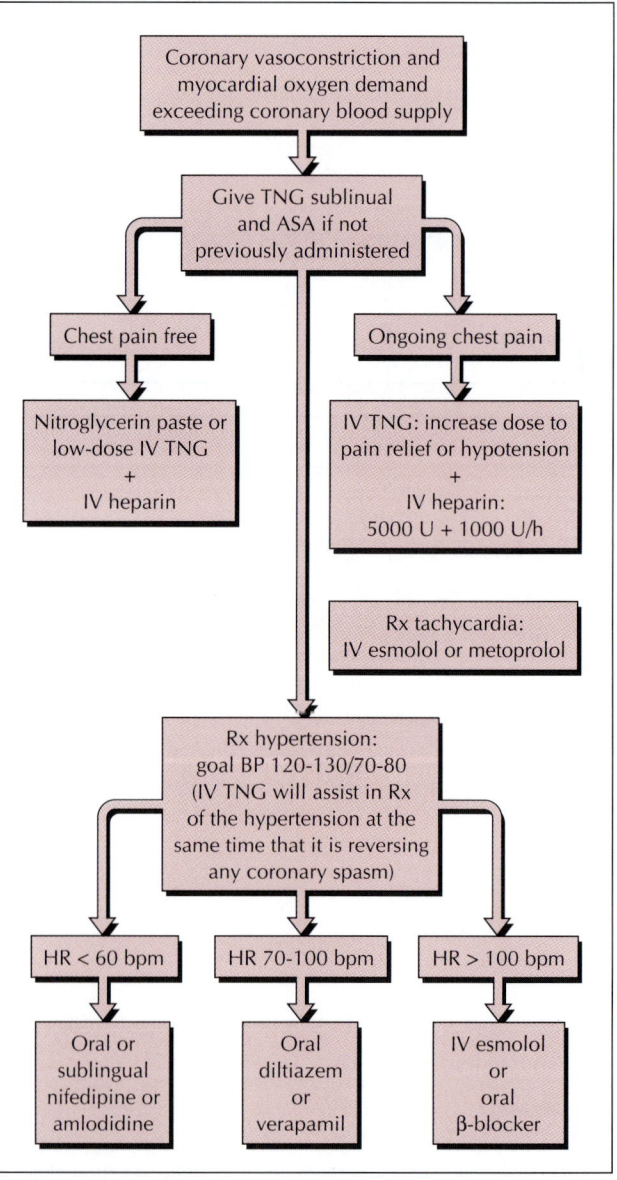

FIGURE 3 Approach to patients presenting with unstable angina or non–Q wave myocardial infarction. ASA—aspirin; BP—blood pressure; HR—heart rate; IV—intravenous; TNG—nitroglycerin.

Nitroglycerin (usually one tablet sublingually every 5 minutes three times or until dizziness or severe headache occurs) should be used if the patient has it available and has not used it at the time of initial contact. If not available at home, this therapy should be used early during assessment of the patient in the office or the emergency department. The basis for nitroglycerin therapy includes reversal of any local coronary vasoconstriction related to the platelet thrombus as well as causing preload and afterload reduction, resulting in lessened myocardial oxygen demand by the heart.

In the Emergency Department

Once the initial assessment has established a probable diagnosis of UAP or NQMI, therapy should be directed toward treating the three ongoing processes: platelet thrombus formation, coronary vasoconstriction, and myocardial oxygen demand exceeding coronary blood supply (Fig. 3). Give TNG sublingually and aspirin if not previously administered. Thrombolytic therapy has not been shown to be therapeutic for the UAP and NQMI syndromes despite the fact that early platelet thrombus formation plays a pathogenic role [6,7].

After initial emergency room therapy, the patient should be reassessed if there is continued diffuse ST-segment depression on electrocardiography, consider emergency coronary angiography. If there is continued ischemic chest pain, increase intravenous TNG to blood pressure tolerance and consider emergency coronary angiography. If there is a progression to ST-segment elevation, consider thrombolytic therapy.

Hospitalization

Generally, all patients with UAP or NQMI should be hospitalized for initiation of medical therapy and to monitor their course over the next 24 hours. An electrocardiographically monitored bed is useful for assessing heart rate response to therapy and to watch for ischemia-related arrhythmias.

On the first day of hospitalization, continue daily aspirin (plain or enteric-coated). Also, initiate diltiazem therapy if not already started for NQMI. Continue intravenous heparin until the patient is pain-free for 24 to 48 hours or the decision to proceed with angiography has been made.

Cardiology Consultation

Depending on whether it is immediately available, cardiology consultation will always be necessary to assist in the initial care of the patient, particularly if myocardial ischemic chest pain is persistent. Decision points are usually based on:
- Serial electrocardiograms and enzyme tests;
- Ongoing pain—reassessment after maximizing intravenous TNG and/or β-blocker;
- Severe pain or progressive electrocardiogram change—urgent assessment by coronary angiography.

Initiate additional antiischemic therapy if the patient has not been on antianginal therapy. Consider oral diltiazem if the heart rate is over 70 bpm; the PR interval is less than 0.20, blood pressure is over 110/70 mm Hg, and there is no congestive heart failure. Oral diltiazem has been shown to reduce the frequency of recurrent myocardial infarction and ischemia events in NQMI patients [8,9•,10,11].

Subsequent Therapy

The great majority of patients with UAP or NQMI "cool down" on hospitalization and initial medical therapy. Further therapeutic decisions are based on response to initial therapy and laboratory assessment. Generally, a decision will be made on whether the patient is a candidate for coronary intervention based on functional status, personal desires, and availability of results.

Long-term medical therapy is directed toward maintaining good blood pressure control in addition to antiplatelet and antiischemic therapy. Typical regimens include the following:

1. Enteric-coated aspirin, 80 mg qd;
2. Long-acting diltiazem, 120–360 mg qd;
3. Angiotensin-converting enzyme inhibitor if additional antihypertensive prescription is required; and
4. Hygienic measures such as low saturated fat diet, walking program, and antioxidants.

Coronary Arteriography and Intervention

Because the patient with UAP or NQMI is at increased risk for a major cardiovascular event over the next 12 months, assessment of the coronary anatomy is usually performed. Decisions regarding subsequent therapy are based on coronary anatomy, suitability for interventional techniques, left ventricular function, and suitability of patient for functional restoration. Figure 4 shows a tight stenosis detected by coronary angiography and treated with coronary angioplasty.

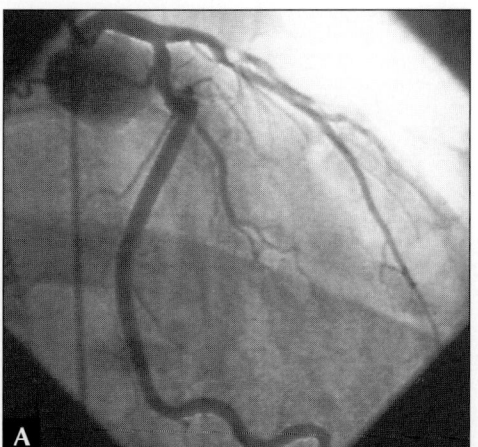
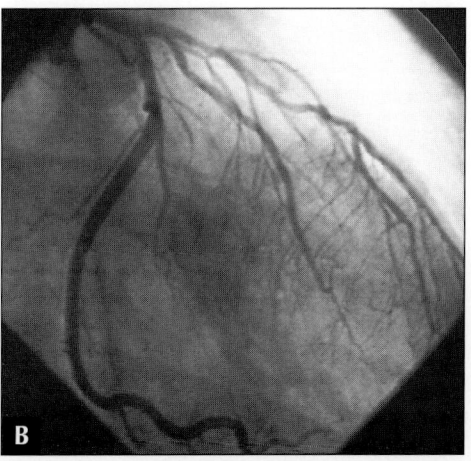

Figure 4 Coronary angiogram in the RAO position showing a tight proximal stenosis of the left anterior descending coronary artery before (**A**) and after (**B**) angioplasty.

References and Recommended Reading

Recently published papers of particular interest have been highlighted as:
- Of interest
- •• Of outstanding interest

1. Braunwald E: Unstable angina. *Circulation* 1989, 80:410–414.
2. Theroux P: A pathophysiologic basis for the clinical classification and management of unstable angina. *Circulation* 1987, 75(suppl V):V103–V109.
3. •• Fuster V, Badimon L, Badimon JJ, *et al.*: Mechanisms of disease: the pathogenesis of coronary artery disease and the acute coronary syndromes (first of two parts). *N Engl J Med* 1992, 326:242–250.
4. •• Fuster V, Badimon L, Badimon JJ, *et al.*: Mechanisms of disease: the pathogenesis of coronary artery disease and the acute coronary syndromes (second of two parts). *N Engl J Med* 1992, 326:310–318.
5. Lewis HD Jr, Davis JW, Archibald JD, *et al.*: Protective effects of aspirin against acute myocardial infarction and death in men with unstable angina: results of a veterans cooperative study. *N Engl J Med* 1983, 309:396–403.
6. Freeman MB, Langer A, Wilson RF, *et al.*: Thrombolysis in unstable angina: randomized double-blind trial of t-PA and placebo. *Circulation* 1992, 85:150–157.
7. Ambrose JA, Hjemdahl-Monsen C, Borrico S, *et al.*: Quantitative and qualitative effects of intracoronary streptokinase in unstable angina and non–Q-wave infarction. *J Am Coll Cardiol* 1987, 9:1156–1165.
8. Gibson RS: Non-Q wave myocardial infarction: diagnosis, prognosis and management. *Curr Probl Cardiol* 1988, 13:1–72.
9. • Boden WE, Roberts R: Prognosis and management of patients with non–Q-wave myocardial infarction. *Prog Cardiol* 1991:143–160.
10. The Multicenter Diltiazem Postinfarction Trial Research Group: The effect of diltiazem on mortality and reinfarction after myocardial infarction. *N Engl J Med* 1988, 318:385–392.
11. Gibson RS, Young PM, Boden WE, *et al.*: Prognostic significance and beneficial effect of diltiazem: results from the Multicenter Diltiazem Reinfarction Study. *Am J Cardiol* 1987, 60:203–209.

Select Bibliography

Clinical Practice Guidelines, Unstable Angina: Diagnosis and Management AH CPR Publication #94-0602. Available from Unstable Angina Guidelines AHCPR Clearinghouse, PO Box 8547, Silver Spring, MD 20907.

Quick Reference Guide for Clinicians. AH CPR, Publication #94-0603. Available from Unstable Angina Guidelines AHCPR Clearinghouse, PO Box 8547, Silver Spring, MD 20907.

Q-Wave Myocardial Infarction

Haim Hammerman
Robert A. Kloner

> **Key Points**
> - Q-wave myocardial infarction is defined as presence of Q wave on the electrocardiogram.
> - The key symptom is severe substernal chest pain.
> - Thrombolytic therapy plus aspirin is the treatment of choice.
> - Early thrombolytic therapy yields the best results.
> - Adjunctive therapy includes heparin and, in some patients, β-blockers and angiotensin-converting-enzyme inhibitors.
> - Ongoing research is assessing the effects of newer antithrombin and adjunctive therapy.

Acute myocardial infarction (MI) is classified for prognostic purposes into two groups: 1) Q-wave MI, in which a Q wave develops on the electrocardiogram (ECG), and 2) acute MI without a Q wave. Presence of a Q wave does not reliably correlate with pathologic findings of transmural MI; however, non–Q-wave MI is often pathologically nontransmural or subendocardial. Q-wave MI tends to be larger in size than non–Q-wave MI and has a higher in-hospital mortality [1•,2•].

DIAGNOSIS

Clinical Criteria

Typically, a patient with acute MI suffers from severe substernal, pressing chest pain, not relieved by rest. The pain may radiate to the left arm, neck, jaw, epigastrium, or back. The pain usually lasts for over 30 minutes. Chest pain may be accompanied by diaphoresis, weakness, anxiety, restlessness, or altered mentation. Symptoms of nausea, vomiting, and abdominal pain may occur, particularly in acute inferior MI. When heart failure exists, shortness of breath and cough with frothy sputum are prominent.

Syncope and sudden death may be the initial presentation of acute MI [1•,2•]. Several studies have revealed circadian variation for the onset time of acute MI, with a peak incidence in the morning at approximately 9 AM [3].

Physical Examination

The patient appears restless, pale, anxious, and diaphoretic. The skin may be cold. Pulse rate and blood pressure may be reduced because of vasovagal reaction. In approximately 20% of cases, hypertension and tachycardia exist in the first hours because of excessive sympathetic discharge. If pump failure is present, tachypnea, hypotension, tachycardia, and pulmonary rales may be present. The pulse is irregular when there are arrhythmias. Low-grade fever is common. Jugular venous distension may be observed as part of biventricular failure or may suggest right ventricular MI. A dyskinetic cardiac impulse may be palpated, a fourth heart sound (S_4) is usually present, and a third heart sound (S_3) is heard with heart failure and mitral regurgitation. There may be a holosystolic murmur with either papillary muscle ischemia or rupture because of mitral regurgitation or ventricular septal rupture. If pericarditis is present, a transient pericardial rub may be auscultated.

Laboratory Findings

After myocardial injury, the cells release cardiac enzymes into the bloodstream that can be detected and measured.

Creatine kinase

Onset of increased creatine kinase (CK) activity in the circulation starts 4 to 8 hours after infarction, with a peak as early as 8 hours after the onset of pain, if there is successful and early reperfusion. Creatine kinase levels may be elevated for up to 50 hours, with a mean peak at 24 hours in nonreperfused infarcts; they decline to normal within 72 hours. This is a highly sensitive enzyme for myocardial infarction, but it is not specific. Creatine kinase levels may be elevated in severe muscle trauma and rhabdomyolysis, strenuous exercise, surgery, intramuscular injection, seizures, myxedema, hypothermia, cerebrovascular accident, and diabetic ketoacidosis. In addition, CK levels may be elevated in several cardiac conditions that are not MI, including postelectric cardioversion or defibrillation, myocarditis, cardiac surgery, and cardiac contusion.

Creatine kinase isoenzyme MB is more specific to myocardium; thus, it can help to rule out noncardiac causes of elevated CK levels. Time of onset, peak, and decline are the same as for CK.

Some CK isoforms (of MB and MM) are released early and permit early detection of necrosis and reperfusion. For example, if the MB2 level is elevated or MB2:MB1 ratio is over 3.8 within 75 minutes of symptoms, there is reperfusion. MM3 levels increase as soon as 1 hour after symptoms. In reperfusion, the MM3 level and MM3:MM1 ratio are elevated.

Aspartate aminotransferase

Aspartate aminotransferase (AST) activity has an onset of 8 to 12 hours, peaks at 18 to 36 hours, and declines to normal within 4 to 5 days. This enzyme has a high sensitivity and poor specificity; it is elevated in many conditions (*eg*, liver disease).

Lactate dehydrogenase

Lactate dehydrogenase (LDH) activity has a late onset of 24 to 48 hours, peaks at 4 to 5 days, and declines to normal within 8 to 10 days. It has high sensitivity but poor specificity. LDH levels may be elevated in hemolysis, leukemia, hepatic disorders, and pulmonary disease. LDH1 isoenzyme is more specific and may be elevated in cardiac necrosis and hemolysis.

In acute MI, the LDH1:LDH2 ratio is over 1. LDH and its isoenzymes are of diagnostic value in patients who present late after the onset of symptoms.

Other enzymes

Other enzymes used infrequently for the diagnosis of infarction include myoglobin, troponin, and myosin light chains. Nonspecific laboratory findings include leukocytosis, elevated erythrocyte sedimentation rate, and hyperglycemia [4,5].

Electrocardiographic Findings

In the early stage of acute MI (often called the *hyperacute phase*), there are giant, positive peaked T waves with initially taller R waves than normal (Fig. 1). These are followed by ST segment elevation with a decrease in amplitude of the R waves and development of deep negative (pathologic) Q waves that last 0.04 seconds and have over 25% of R-wave amplitude.

The R waves may be lost and replaced by QS waves. Over time, the ST-segment may return to normal with T-wave inversion; with time, the T waves may return to be positive. Occasionally, in cases of left ventricular dyskinesis or aneurysm, the ST-segment remains elevated (Fig. 1). Determination of MI location according to ECG leads is listed in Table 1.

Imaging Techniques

Echocardiography

Echocardiography is of value in localizing and quantifying regional wall-motion abnormalities associated with infarcts [6•]. Echocardiography can detect thinning or lack of wall thickening, but cannot necessarily differentiate severe ischemia from necrosis. In patients with complications, echocardiography is of value in identifying factors such as

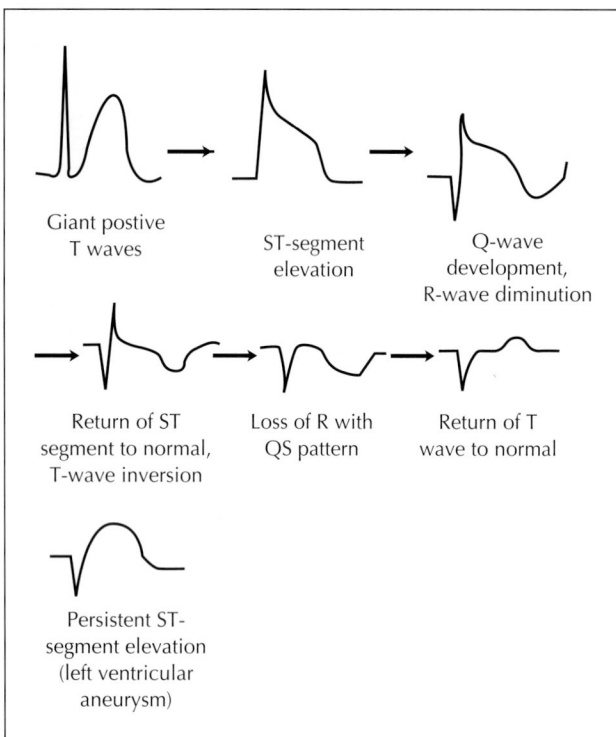

FIGURE 1 Electrocardiographic findings in myocardial infarction. Giant positive T waves are shown in hyperacute phase, followed by ST-segment elevation, then Q-wave development and R-wave diminution. Over time, the ST segment returns to normal, with loss of R wave, T-wave inversion, and sometimes T-wave pseudonormalization. There is persistent ST elevation in left ventricular aneurysm.

Table 1. Location of myocardial infarction according to electrocardiogram leads

Location	ECG leads
Anteroseptal	V_1 through V_4
Lateral	I, aVL, V_6
High lateral	I, aVL
Anterolateral	I, aVL, V_3 through V_6
Extensive anterior	I, aVL, V_1 through V_6
Inferior	II, III, aVF
Posterior	V_1 through V_2 (mirror image)
Right ventricular	V_1, V_{3R}, V_{4R}

ECG—electrocardiogram.

early infarct expansion, mitral insufficiency, papillary muscle rupture, ventricular septal defect, and free wall rupture with tamponade as responsible for pump failure, hemodynamic instability, and tachycardia. Echocardiography is also useful for identifying left ventricular thrombi, aneurysms, pseudoaneurysms, and pericardial effusion.

Radionuclide ventriculography

Radionuclide ventriculography is useful for assessing global and regional function. Use of this technique is limited because of the risks of radiation exposure and, in some facilities, the need to transport the patient out of the coronary care unit. Radionuclide ventriculography is superior to echocardiography in the quantification of global ventricular function [4].

Radionuclide scintigraphy

Infarct-avid agents such as technetium-99m pyrophosphate can sensitively detect infarction and define its location. Reliable detection is possible only after 24 hours from MI onset. Perfusion scintigraphy using an agent such as thallium-201 can detect hypoperfused or necrotic myocardium, but it sometimes fails to differentiate between severe ischemia and necrosis. Technetium-99m isonitril (99m sestamibi) is used for myocardial perfusion imaging and may become useful for assessing myocardium at risk and the success of reperfusion [4,7].

Arrhythmic Complications

The incidence of arrhythmias is high in patients suffering acute MI and may be as high as 100% in those who are monitored in the early phase. The most commonly encountered arrhythmias are premature ventricular beats. The most serious arrhythmia is ventricular fibrillation, which may be primary if it occurs early. Ventricular fibrillation is caused by acute ischemia and usually does not have a negative long-term prognosis if treated quickly.

Secondary ventricular tachycardia or fibrillation occurs late in the course of MI (over 48 hours after onset), is associated with severe left ventricular dysfunction, and has a poor long-term prognosis. In general, arrhythmias occurring during MI should be treated if they cause hemodynamic deterioration, increase oxygen consumption, or deteriorate to life-threatening arrhythmias. Ventricular fibrillation is treated by electrical defibrillation and cardiopulmonary resuscitation. Ventricular tachycardia with hemodynamic compromise is treated by electrical cardioversion. Lidocaine is indicated mainly for patients with symptomatic or sustained ventricular arrhythmias. If this drug fails, other antiarrhythmic drugs should be considered (*eg*, procainamide, bretylium tosylate, amiodarone). Prophylactic use of lidocaine in patients with acute MI is no longer common practice. Although late ventricular arrhythmias are associated with poor prognosis, long-term treatment with agents such as flecainide and encainide after infarction were associated with a worse outcome in the Cardiac Arrhythmias Suppression Trial [8].

Sinus bradycardia is common in inferior MI, secondary to sinoatrial node ischemia or vagal stimulation. It often is asymptomatic and does not need treatment, unless it is accompanied by hemodynamic impairment. Sinus tachycardia is common and may be caused by pain, anxiety, catecholamine release, reduced left ventricular function and heart failure, and pericarditis. It is important to recognize the cause to avoid tachycardia, which increases oxygen demand.

Premature atrial beats are common and may be associated with heart failure. Atrial fibrillation occurs in approximately 20% of infarctions. It is often transient, is more commonly observed in anterior MI, and may be associated with heart failure, atrial ischemia, or pericarditis. These arrhythmias should be treated as in other conditions. Atrial tachycardia and flutter are uncommon [1•,2•,9••].

Conduction Disturbances

The type of conduction disturbance depends on the location of MI. In anterior-wall MI, blocks are usually secondary to injury in intraventricular bundle branches. In inferior MI, blocks are usually above the His bundle in the atrioventricular (AV) node.

Temporary Pacing

Temporary pacing should be instituted with the following conditions:

Asystole
Complete heart block
Right bundle-branch block with left anterior or left posterior hemiblock
New left bundle-branch block
Mobitz type 2 second-degree AV block
Symptomatic bradycardia resistant to atropine
Atrial or ventricular overdrive pacing for incessant ventricular tachycardia [1•,2•,9••]

Hemodynamic Complications

Table 2 summarizes the major mechanical complications of MI. Table 3 summarizes the hemodynamic complications of acute MI and approach to therapy.

MANAGEMENT

The patient is admitted to the coronary care unit for ECG and vital-sign monitoring. A thrombolytic agent is administered intravenously (Table 4), and the patient chews one aspirin as soon as possible after admission according to indications and contraindications. Heparin is also administered following thrombolysis in most centers. If admission to the coronary care unit is delayed, this therapy should be considered in the emergency ward. In some centers primary angioplasty rather than thrombolysis is the therapy of choice. The patient should have bed rest for 24 hours or until becoming stable. All patients with acute ischemic pain should have supplemental oxygen. Food should be restricted in the first hours to avoid vomiting and aspiration; the patient should receive a light, low-sodium diet for the first days.

An analgesia-morphine sulfate is given intravenously in repeated doses of 2 to 5 mg every 5 to 30 minutes as needed but before signs of toxicity (depressed respiration and hypotension) appear. Large cumulative doses of 2 to 3 mg/kg are rarely required. Efforts to control pain should include reperfusion therapy and administration of oxygen, nitrates, β-blockers, and in refractory circumstances, intraaortic balloon counterpulsation. For sedation, diazepam (2 to 10 mg) may be given two to three times daily. β-blocking agents may be used to limit myocardial damage, reinfarction, and mortality. There is a reported reduction of 14% in 7-day mortality rates if β-blockers (without thrombolysis) are begun within 12 hours of symptoms [10]. Early administration of β-blockers with thrombolysis may reduce the incidence of nonfatal reinfarction and recurrent ischemia. One large study used metoprolol (15 mg) intravenously in three divided doses (at 2-minute intervals), then 50 mg orally four times daily followed by 100 mg twice daily [9••,10]. Late therapy (from the third day) is with captopril in patients with ejection fractions of 40% or less; target dosage is 50 mg

TABLE 2 MECHANICAL COMPLICATIONS OF ACUTE MYOCARDIAL INFARCTION

Complications	Management
Left-sided heart failure	Hemodynamic monitoring If wedge pressure is high and BP stable, give diuretics, vasodilators; if wedge pressure is high and BP low, give dobutamine, dopamine, intraaortic balloon pump Consider long-term captopril
Right-sided heart failure	Hemodynamic monitoring Consider RV infarction May require volume to maintain forward output; if forward output is adequate, apply cautious use of diuretics
Cardiogenic shock	Hemodynamic monitoring If wedge pressure is low, volume load; if wedge pressure is high, use inotropic support (dopamine, dobutamine), intraaortic balloon counterpulsation Early angioplasty may improve survival
Papillary muscle rupture/ventricular septal defect	Hemodynamic monitoring Use afterload reduction (nitroprusside) if BP is stable, intraaortic balloon pump, emergency surgery
Cardiac rupture	Emergency pericardiocentesis, then emergency surgery
Papillary muscle dysfunction (mitral regurgitation)	Afterload reduction, diuretics If mitral regurgitation is severe, consider surgery
Pericarditis	Aspirin, analgesia (avoid steroids and potent nonsteroidal antiinflammatory agents, which may impede healing)
LV thrombus	Anticoagulate acutely; oral anticoagulation is recommended for 3–6 mo
Postinfarction angina	Nitrates, β-blockers, heparin, aspirin Consider angiography and revascularization
Infarct extension (increase of necrosis)	Analgesia, β-blockers, nitrates Consider thrombolysis, angiography, and revascularization
Infarct expansion (thinning and dilation of infarct). Early phase of LV aneurysm.	Treat heart failure, avoid steroids and nonsteroidal agents, avoid increase in afterload Treat with ACE inhibitors, anticoagulation
LV remodeling (late ventricular dilation)	Treat heart failure There is reduction of mortality, recurrent MI, and heart failure with captopril therapy [24]

ACE—angiotensin-converting enzyme; BP—blood pressure; LV—left ventricular; MI—myocardial infarction; RV—right ventricular.

TABLE 3 HEMODYNAMIC SUBSETS IN ACUTE MYOCARDIAL INFARCTION AND SPECIFIC THERAPY			
	CI, $L/min/m^2$	PCW, $mm\,Hg$	Therapy*
No pulmonary congestion or hypoperfusion	> 2.2	< 18	—
Hyperdynamic state	> 2.2	< 18	β-blockade
Pulmonary congestion	> 2.2	> 18	Diuretic, vasodilators (nitroglycerin or arteriolar dilators); consider ventilation and circulatory assist in severe cases†
Peripheral hypoperfusion	< 2.2	< 18	Replacement of volume
Pulmonary congestion and peripheral hypoperfusion	< 2.2	> 18	Sympathomimetic agents (dopamine, dobutamine), ventilation, intraaortic balloon, assist device†, consider PTCA for shock

*In every patient with acute myocardial infarction, consider thrombolytic, heparin, aspirin, and β-blockade.
†Consider surgical correction for mitral regurgitation, ventricular septal defect, and correction of ischemia by emergency revascularization.
CI–cardiac index; PCW—pulmonary capillary wedge pressure.

three times daily, at least. Late therapy with captopril reduces the 4-year mortality rate, heart failure, and recurrent MI. Tables 5 and 6 list drugs used in MI therapy.

Thrombolytic Therapy

Acute coronary thrombotic occlusion is found in most patients with Q-wave MI. Thrombolytic therapy can dissolve the clot, restore coronary flow, reduce infarct size, and improve survival, especially if administered within the first 6 hours of the onset of pain [11••]. The large GISSI trial [12] compared therapy with intravenous streptokinase (1.5 million IU) to placebo in patients presenting within 12 hours of infarct onset. This study showed an 18% reduction of 21-day mortality in the streptokinase group; the earlier treatment was started, the more effective it was. If therapy was given within 1 hour of symptoms, mortality reduction was as high as 47%. Similar results were observed in the ISIS-2 study [13], which showed benefit in survival of patients treated between 12 and 24 hours after onset. In comparing anistreplase, duteplase (double-chain tissue-plasminogen activator [tPa]), and strep-

tokinase, the ISIS-3 investigators [14••] showed that the rate of death plus nonfatal stroke was similar in the three groups at approximately 11% at 5 weeks. Two large randomized studies, GISSI-2 [15••] and the International Study Group [16••], demonstrated similar results. The incidence of early reocclusion after successful thrombolysis ranges from 4% to 33% in various trials [11••,17•].

There is debate regarding which thrombolytic agent is superior in acute MI. The GUSTO study of 41,000 patients with acute MI [18] revealed that front-loading of tPA plus administration of heparin intravenously resulted in a slight (1%) but statistically significant reduction in deaths (6.3%) over administration of streptokinase plus heparin (7.4%) at 30 days after MI. There was a slightly greater stroke rate in the tPA plus heparin group (1.55%) compared with the streptokinase plus heparin group (1.40%). The slight benefits of tPA over streptokinase must be weighed against the significantly higher cost of tPA. Despite the debate over which thrombolytic agent is superior, thrombolytics have reduced mortality from MI by approximately 50%. In the United States, only

TABLE 4 COMMONLY USED THROMBOLYTIC AGENTS							
Agents	Half-life, min	Anti-genicity	Mode of action	Dose (bolus)	Infusion	Total dose	Comment
Streptokinase	14–20	Yes	Activator complex	—	1.5 million IU given IV for 60 min	1.5 million IU given IV	Produced by β-hemolytic streptococci
Tissue-plasminogen activator	4	No	Direct	15 mg	50 mg for 30 min and 35 mg for 60 min, IV	100 mg or according to body weight	Produced by recombinant methods; single-chain alteplase; double-chain duteplase
Anistreplase APSAC	70–120	Yes	Direct	30 mg	—	30 mg	A complex of streptokinase and plasminogen
Urokinase	14–20	No	Direct	—	6000 IU (4 mL/min) for up to 2 h given IC	—	Found in urine; double-chain form; prourokinase is a single-chain form that has to be activated

APSAC—anisoylated plasminogen streptokinase activator complex; IC—intracoronary; IV—intravenously.

Table 5 Commonly used drugs in acute myocardial infarction			
Drug	**Indication and mode of action**	**Dose**	**Comments**
Atropine	For severe bradycardia and low output Parasympathetic agent	IV 0.5–1 mg every 5 min up to 2 mg	Careful observation after administration because of tachycardia. If no response to atropine, consider pacemaker insertion
Lidocaine	Drug of choice for ventricular arrhythmias in acute MI (multiple VPBs, VT, VF)	Initial IV bolus, 1 mg/kg, then 0.5 mg/kg every 10 min to a total of 4 mg/kg. Maintenance, 20–50 µg/kg/min	High doses may cause CNS toxicity. Prophylactic use of lidocaine in acute MI is no longer recommended
Dopamine	For severe pump failure. Dopaminergic, α- and β-adrenergic agent. In low doses, increases coronary flow, contractility, renal blood flow and rate. High doses—systemic vasoconstriction	IV 2–5 µg/kg/min for optimal effect. > 5–10 µg/kg/min—vasoconstriction	Consider in cases with hemodynamic deterioration. Increases myocardial oxygen consumption
Dobutamine	For severe pump failure. Synthetic sympathomimetic agent. $\beta_1 > \beta_2$; $\alpha_1 > \alpha_2$	IV 2–10 µg/kg/min increases contractility. Less arrythmogenic and less chronotropic than dopamine	As with dopamine
Nitroglycerin	Rapid onset nitrate for acute myocardial ischemia and venous dilation (preload reduction)	IV 5–15 µg/min and may be increased according to pain relief, blood pressure drop, tachycardia, or headache	Headache, flushing, hypotension, and reflex tachycardia are main side effects
Nitroprusside	Arteriolar and venous dilator. Heart failure and hypertension	IV 10–25 µg/min; maximal dose up to 300 µg/min	Thiocyanate toxicity and methemoglobinemia are main side effects

CNS—central nervous system; IV—intravenous; MI—myocardial infarction; VF—ventricular fibrillation; VPB—ventricular premature beats; VT—ventricular tachycardia.

approximately 30% to 50% of patients with MI ever receive thrombolytic therapy.

In some studies, tissue-plasminogen activator and anistreplase have been associated with a higher risk of cerebral hemorrhage (0.66% and 0.55%, respectively) compared with streptokinase (0.24%) [14••]. There was a significant excess of strokes with tPA (1.39%) versus streptokinase (1.04%) in the ISIS study [14••]. The large randomized trials reported a 0.8% to 1.0% bleeding rate requiring transfusion. The reinfarction rate differs in various trials: 3.5% in patients treated with streptokinase, and 2.9% in those treated with tPA. tPA is associated with significantly fewer reports of allergy (which causes persistent symptoms) and hypotension (requiring drug treatment) [11••,14••,15,16,17•].

Early Adjunctive Therapy With Thrombolysis

Antiplatelet therapy with aspirin plays a major role in the treatment of acute MI, as shown in the ISIS-2 study [13]. Aspirin demonstrated a beneficial effect on survival similar to that of streptokinase, and concurrent use of aspirin and streptokinase showed better effect on survival than each agent alone [13]. The recommended dose of aspirin is 80 to 325 mg daily, starting as soon as possible after admission and preferably given as a chewable preparation at admission.

Results from some studies suggest that it is clinically important to start full-dose heparin infusion during or after thrombolysis; although this is common practice among many cardiologists, many unanswered questions exist regarding heparin therapy [11••,17•]. Ongoing studies are investigating newer antithrombin agents such as hirudin and hirulog as adjunctive therapy.

Recommendation for Thrombolytic Therapy

Patients who present with chest pain suggestive of MI within 6 hours from onset and have at least 1 mm of ST-segment elevation in at least two contiguous ECG leads should receive thrombolytic therapy if no contraindications exist. Thrombolysis should be considered in patients with more than 6 hours of symptom onset with a "stuttering" pattern of pain. Although thrombolytic therapy generally is not used with non-Q-wave infarcts, it is an area of investigation.

Absolute contraindications to thrombolysis include:
Active internal bleeding
Suspected aortic dissection
Prolonged or traumatic cardiorespiratory resuscitation
Recent head trauma or intracranial neoplasm
Diabetic hemorrhagic retinopathy
Pregnancy

Previous allergic reaction to streptokinase or anistreplase
Recorded blood pressure of over 200/120
History of hemorrhagic cerebrovascular accident
Relative contraindications to thrombolysis include:
Recent trauma or surgery of more than 2 weeks
History of chronic severe hypertension
Active peptic ulcer
History of cerebrovascular accident
Known bleeding diathesis or current use of anticoagulants
Significant liver dysfunction
Prior exposure to steptokinase or anistreplase (does not apply to re-use of tPA or urokinase) [1•,2•,9••,12,19••]

Angioplasty

Several studies have shown that routine angioplasty performed immediately within 1 to 2 days (or within 3 to 14 days after thrombolysis) does not preserve more myocardium or reduce the incidence of reinfarction or death compared with a more conservative approach, in which angioplasty is performed only in patients with evidence of ischemia [19••,20••]. Early revascularization was beneficial and improved survival in cardiogenic shock complicating acute MI [21]. Studies comparing immediate angioplasty to thrombolysis in acute MI show a lower incidence of reocclusion, reinfarction, recurrent ischemia, and death in patients treated with angioplasty [22•].

Postinfarction Evaluation

Prognosis after acute MI is related to three main factors:
1. Extent of left ventricular dysfunction, including degree of left ventricular dilatation;
2. Presence of residual myocardial ischemia; and
3. Degree of electrical instability of myocardium.

Various techniques can be used to evaluate these factors, and the clinician must choose the most effective and suitable test according to the patient's condition and the clinician's judgment. Patients with clinical indicators of high risk for ischemic events should be directed to cardiac catheterization before discharge from the hospital. Other patients can be managed according to one of three strategies recommended by the American College of Cardiology/American Heart Association Task Force as shown in Figure 2.

Long-Term Adjunctive Therapy

Early treatment with enalapril in patients within the first 24 hours of an acute MI did not demonstrate any survival benefit [23]. Patients with low ejection fractions benefit from late therapy with captopril. Long-term therapy reduces the 4-year mortality rate, heart failure, and recurrent infarction rates [24••]. Long-term β-blocker therapy in patients who can tolerate these drugs improves long-term survival, possibly because there is less ischemic arrhythmia [10]. Aspirin therapy also may reduce post-MI recurrent infarction.

Table 6. Chronic therapy for secondary prevention

Drug	Mode of action	Dose*	Comments
Aspirin	Antiplatelet agent	80–325 mg/d as soon as patient is admitted, then long-term 160–350 mg/d	Caution in peptic ulcer disease or other bleeding diasthesis
Heparin and warfarin	Anticoagulant together or immediately after thrombolysis Patient with large anterior MI should be given full-dose heparin and then considered for oral anticoagulant (warfarin) for 3 months, especially if LV thrombus is present	IV heparin with APTT 1.5–2.0 times control for 48 hours	Side effects of bleeding
β-blockade (various studies)	Reduces risk of reinfarction or mortality after completed MI	Propranolol 180–240 mg/d Metaprolol 200 mg/d Timolol 20 mg/d or other drug that shows evidence of secondary prevention	Contraindications: bradycardia, hypotension, moderate to severe LV failure, AV conduction disturbance, obstructive pulmonary disease
Captopril [24]	Angiotensin-converting enzyme reduces mortality rate by 19% in patients with systolic dysfunction ≤ 40% EF [23] There is no evidence of improvement with early treatment of enalapril in acute MI [23]	Target dose of 50 mg at least 3 times a day	Treatment begins 3–16 d after MI

*May be given in divided doses in some cases. APTT—activated partial thromboplastin time; AV—atrioventricular; EF—ejection fraction; IV—intravenous; LV—left ventricular; MI—myocardial infarction.

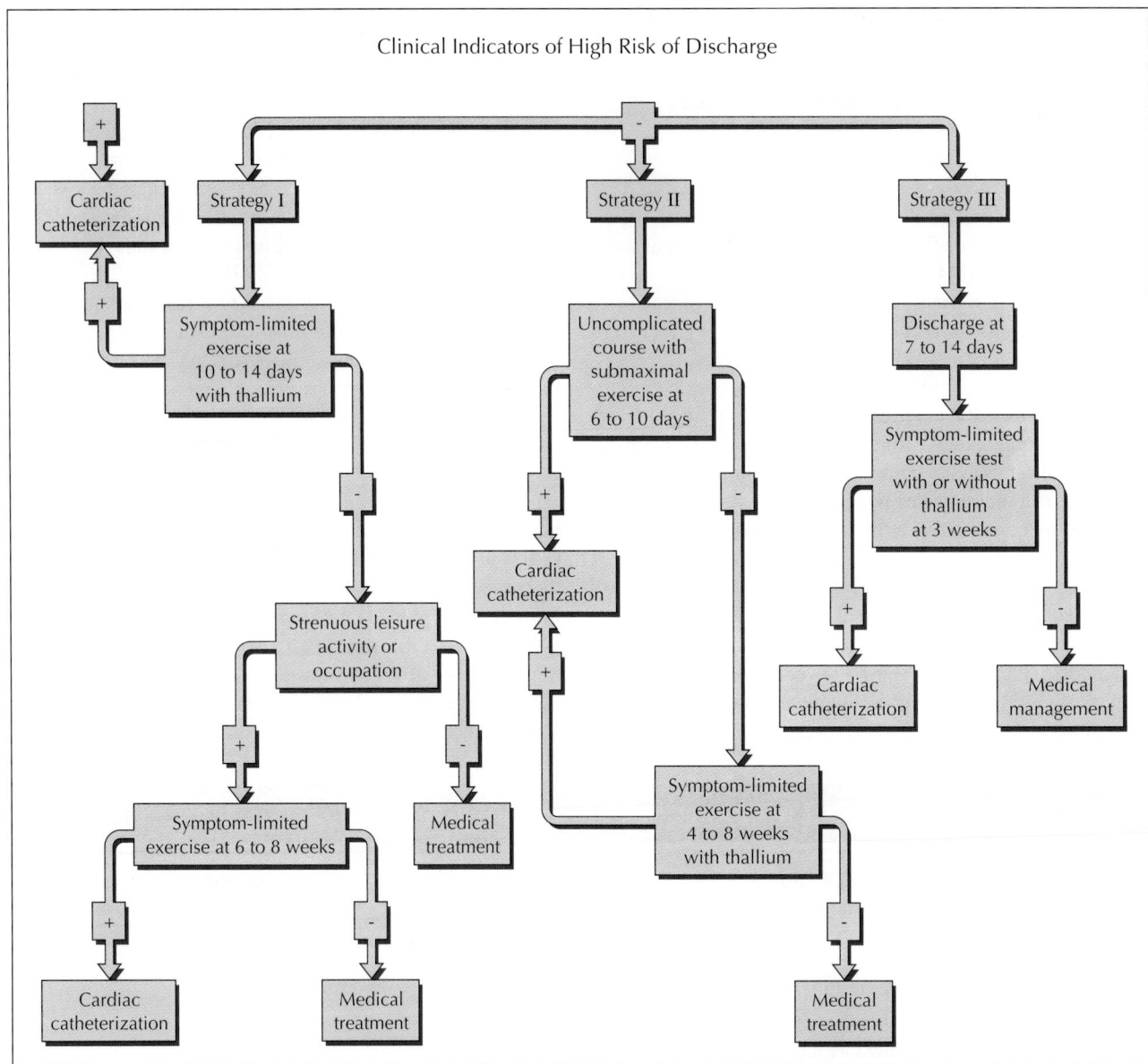

FIGURE 2 Strategies for exercise test and evaluation according to existence of clinical indicators. + indicates evidence of ischemia; - indicates lack of ischemia. (*From* American College of Cardiology/American Heart Association [9••], with permission.)

REFERENCES AND RECOMMENDED READING

Recently published papers of particular interest have been highlighted as:
- Of interest
- •• Of outstanding interest

1.• Pasternak RC, Braunwald E, Sobel BE: Acute myocardial infarction. In *Heart Disease: A Textbook of Cardiovascular Medicine*, edn 4. Edited by Braunwald E. Philadelphia: WB Saunders; 1992:1200–1291.

2.• Hagar JM, Kloner RA: Acute myocardial infarction. In *The Guide to Cardiology*, edn 2. Edited by Kloner RA. New York: LeJacq Communications; 1990:207–239.

3. Ridker PM, Manson JAE, Buring JE, *et al.*: Circadian variation of acute myocardial infarction and the effect of low-dose aspirin in a randomized trial of physicians. *Circulation* 1990, 82:897–902.

4. Blackwell GG, Pohost GM: Diagnosis and quantitation of myocardial infarction. *Curr Opin Cardiol* 1991, 6:559–566.

5. Puleo PR, Perryman B: Noninvasive detection of reperfusion in acute myocardial infarction based on plasma activity of creatine kinase MB subforms. *J Am Coll Cardiol* 1991, 17:1047–1052.

6.• Peels CH, Visser CA, Kupper AJF, *et al.*: Usefulness of two-dimensional echocardiography for immediate detection of myocardial ischemia in the emergency room. *Am J Cardiol* 1990, 65:687–691.

7. Christian TF, Clements IP, Gibbons RJ: Noninvasive identification of myocardium at risk in patients with acute myocardial infarction and nondiagnostic electrocardiogram with technetium-99m-sestamibi. *Circulation* 1991, 83:1615–1620.

8. The Cardiac Arrhythmias Suppression Trial II Investigators (CAST II): effect of the antiarrhythmic agent moricizine on survival after myocardial infarction. *N Engl J Med* 1992, 327:227–233.

9.•• American College of Cardiology/American Heart Association: task force guidelines for the early management of patients with acute myocardial infarction. *Circulation* 1990, 82:664–707.

10. Yusuf S, Peto R, Lewis J, *et al.*: β blockade during and after myocardial infarction: an overview of the randomized trials. *Prog Cardiovasc Dis* 1985, 27:335–371.

11.•• Granger CB, Califf RM, Topol EJ: Thrombolytic therapy for acute myocardial infarction. A review. *Drugs* 1992, 44:293–325.

12. Gruppo Italiano per lo Studio della Streptochinasi nell'Infarto Miocardico (GISSI): effectiveness of intravenous thrombolytic treatment in acute myocardial infarction. *Lancet* 1986, i:397–401.

13. ISIS-2 (Second International Study of Infarct Survival) Collaborative Group: randomised trial of intravenous streptokinase, oral aspirin, both, or neither among 17,187 cases of suspected acute myocardial infarction. *Lancet* 1988, ii:349–360.

14.•• ISIS-3 (Third International Study of Infarct Survival) Collaborative Group: ISIS-3: a randomized comparison of streptokinase vs. tissue plasminogen activator vs. anistreplase and of aspirin plus heparin vs. aspirin alone among 41,299 cases of suspected acute myocardial infarction. *Lancet* 1992, 339:753–766.

15.•• Gruppo Italiano per lo Studio della Sopravivenza nell'Infarto Miocardico: GISSI-2: a factorial randomised trial of alteplase versus streptokinase and heparin versus no heparin among 12,490 patients with acute myocardial infarction. *Lancet* 1990, 336:65–71.

16.•• The International Study Group: In-hospital mortality and clinical course of 20,891 patients with suspected acute myocardial infarction randomised between alteplase and streptokinase with or without heparin. *Lancet* 1990, 336:71–75.

17.• Kirshenbaum JM: Therapy for acute myocardial infarction: an update. *Heart Dis Stroke* 1992, 1:211–217.

18. GUSTO Investigators: An international randomized trial comparing four thrombolytic strategies for acute myocardial infarction. *N Engl J Med* 1993, 329:673–682.

19.•• Rogers WJ, Baim DS, Wackers FJT, *et al.*: Comparison of immediate invasive, delayed invasive, and conservative strategies after tissue type plasminogen activator. *Circulation* 1990, 81:1457–1476.

20.•• Baim DS, Braunwald E, Feit F, *et al.*: The Thrombolysis in Myocardial Infarction (TIMI) Trial phase II: additional information and perspectives. *J Am Coll Cardiol* 1990, 15:1188–1192.

21. Moosvi AR, Khaja F, Villanueva L, *et al.*: Early revascularization improves survival in cardiogenic shock complicating acute myocardial infarction. *J Am Coll Cardiol* 1992, 19:907–914.

22.• Lange RA, Hillis LD: Immediate angioplasty for acute myocardial infarction. *N Engl J Med* 1993, 328:726–728.

23. Swedberg K, Held P, Kjekshus J, *et al.*: Effects of the early administration of enalapril on mortality in patients with acute myocardial infarction—results of the Cooperative New Scandinavian Enalapril Survival Study II (Consensus II). *N Engl J Med* 1992, 327:678–684.

24.•• Pfeffer MA, Braunwald E, Moye LA, *et al.*: Effect of captopril on mortality and morbidity in patients with left ventricular dysfunction after myocardial infarction—results of the survival and ventricular enlargement trial. *N Engl J Med* 1992, 327:669–677.

SELECT BIBLIOGRAPHY

Antman EM, Berlin JA: Declining incidence of ventricular fibrillation in myocardial infarction: implications for the prophylactic use of lidocaine. *Circulation* 1992, 86:764–773.

Fuster V, Stein B, Ambrose JA, *et al.*: Atherosclerotic plaque rupture and thrombosis: evolving concepts. *Circulation* 1990, 82(suppl II):47–59.

LATE Study Group: Late Assessment of Thrombolytic Efficacy (LATE) Study with alteplase 6–24 hours after onset of acute myocardial infarction. *Lancet* 1993, 342:759–766.

Mitral Stenosis and Regurgitation

Sidney C. Smith, Jr.
Park W. Willis, IV

> ### Key Points
> - Advanced diagnostic techniques such as color flow Doppler echocardiography, and new therapeutic approaches, such as balloon mitral valvuloplasty, left ventricular unloading therapy, and direct mitral valve repair offer improved care for patients with mitral valve disease.
> - Rheumatic heart disease remains the major cause of mitral stenosis, and outbreaks of rheumatic fever have been recently reported in the United States.
> - An echocardiographic scoring system identifies patients most likely to benefit from balloon mitral valvuloplasty.
> - Physicians should make patients with mitral valve disease familiar with the new American Heart Association guidelines for and prevention of infective endocarditis.
> - Resting ejection fraction remains preserved late in the course of mitral regurgitation, and exercise radionuclide ejection fractions may assist in selecting patients who are candidates for mitral valve surgery.

Over the past 20 years our understanding of the pathophysiology of mitral valve disease has increased substantially. Advanced echocardiographic methods have expanded our diagnostic capability. New therapeutic approaches such as balloon mitral valvuloplasty, left ventricular unloading therapy, and direct mitral valve repair have improved the treatment and prognosis for patients with mitral valve disease. This chapter details current trends in the diagnosis and therapy of mitral stenosis and regurgitation from the standpoint of the clinician.

MITRAL STENOSIS

Etiology and Pathophysiology

Most cases of mitral stenosis are caused by rheumatic heart disease (Table 1) [1•]. Less frequently, severe mitral annular calcification, malignant carcinoid, or rheumatoid arthritis may be the underlying cause. The clinical presentation and physical findings of left atrial myxoma can mimic rheumatic mitral stenosis. Congenital forms of mitral stenosis are rare and usually present in childhood, associated with other congenital lesions. Two thirds of patients with rheumatic mitral stenosis are female.

Because of the strong association of rheumatic heart disease with mitral stenosis, the practicing physician should be familiar with current diagnostic criteria for acute rheumatic fever. The American Heart Association has recently published updated Jones criteria for the diagnosis of acute rheumatic fever (Table 2) [2••]. These changes emphasize the importance of establishing the initial attack of rheumatic fever and expand on the available tools to diagnose streptococcal pharyngitis with clarification of available antibody tests. Echocardiographic abnormalities without accompanying auscultatory findings are considered insufficient to be the sole criteria for valvulitis in acute rheumatic fever.

Patients with mitral valve stenosis often have no definite history of rheumatic fever in childhood or as a young adult and are usually asymptomatic until the third or fourth decade. Multiple episodes of rheumatic fever during childhood may result in an accelerated disease course causing the patient to present with mitral stenosis at an earlier age. This is especially common in patients living in underdeveloped areas and temperate zones where the disease often presents during adolescence. In general, approximately 10 years will elapse between an episode of acute rheumatic fever and the first appearance of the murmur of mitral stenosis.

The rheumatic process, presumably through an autoimmune mechanism, results in fibrosis and scarring, especially at the margins of the mitral valve leaflets. This results in fusion of the valve leaflets and shortening and thickening of the chordae tendineae. The result is progressive narrowing of the mitral valve orifice with increasing left atrial and pulmonary venous pressures. Left atrial enlargement and progressive calcification of the mitral valve follow as this process progresses. The normal valve area of 4 to 6 cm^2 is reduced to less than 2 cm^2. Severe hemodynamic changes occur at valve areas less than 1 cm^2.

Clinical Presentation

The most common presenting symptom of mitral stenosis is exertional dyspnea secondary to pulmonary venous hypertension. The majority of patients with mitral stenosis are women, symptoms often appear initially during the second trimester of pregnancy, when blood volume and cardiac output peak. Patients also may experience orthopnea, paroxysmal nocturnal dyspnea, and progressive fatigue and weakness. Pulmonary hypertension may be associated with chest pain and hemoptysis. Approximately 50% of patients with mitral stenosis are older than 30 years of age and may have significant coronary artery disease. Therefore, it is important to consider multiple causes for chest pain. Hoarseness (Ortner's syndrome) may occur because of compression of the left recurrent laryngeal nerve between the enlarged pulmonary artery, aorta, and ligamentum arteriosum. Unfortunately, systemic embolism may be the first symptom of mitral stenosis, especially in association with the development of atrial fibrillation. Although infective endocarditis is uncommon, it can complicate the clinical course of mitral stenosis [3].

The classic physical findings of mitral stenosis are a loud first heart sound (S_1) associated with a low-pitched diastolic rumble best heard at the apex, with the bell of the stethoscope, in the left lateral decubitus position. Positional variation in the intensity of the diastolic rumble may indicate that left atrial myxoma is present. A high-pitched opening snap (OS) may be heard just after the second heart sound (S_2). The S_2-OS interval narrows as the severity of mitral stenosis increases. When pulmonary hypertension develops, the amplitude of the pulmonic component of S_2 increases and a right ventricular heave may be detected. Pulmonary rales, jugular venous distention, hepatic enlargement, and peripheral edema may be present, representing generalized findings for congestive heart failure. With severe pulmonary hypertension, pulmonary regurgitation may be present (Graham Steell murmur), which should be distinguished from aortic regurgitation. Atrial fibrillation is often present as mitral stenosis progresses in severity, and characteristic ruddy cheeks (mitral facies) may be noted.

Laboratory Findings

Echocardiography is the most valuable clinical test in the management of mitral stenosis. It is useful in gauging the severity of mitral stenosis, distinguishing left atrial myxomas, and identifying coexisting atrial septal defects, thrombi, and valvular vegetations (Fig. 1). In addition, associated valvular lesions such as mitral regurgitation, aortic stenosis or regurgitation, and pulmonary and tricuspid valvular disease, which are also associated with rheumatic heart disease, may be identified. Color flow Doppler echocardiography is useful in assessing the extent of associated mitral regurgitation. Transesophageal echocardiography may help to detect left atrial thrombi (Fig. 2).

Recently, a scoring system based on the results of echocardiography has been devised to assist in identifying patients who may best benefit from balloon mitral valvuloplasty. The scoring system grades from 0 to 4+ the following four echocardiographic factors: valvular rigidity, valvular calcification, valvular thickening, and the amount of subvalvular disease; a score of 4+ represents a severely abnormal finding. Thus, a valve with severe rigidity, extensive calcification, severe thickening, and substantial subvalvular thickening would receive a score of 4 for each category, for a total score

Table 1 Mitral stenosis

Etiology
Rheumatic heart disease (most common)
Congenital
Mitral annular calcification
Malignant carcinoid
Rheumatoid arthritis
Exclude
Left atrial tumor (usually myxoma)
Cor triatriatum
Associated atrial septal defect

Table 2 Guidelines for diagnosis of rheumatic fever (Jones Criteria, Updated 1992)

Major manifestations
Carditis
Polyarthritis
Chorea
Erythema marginatum
Subcutaneous nodules

Minor manifestations
Arthralgia
Fever
Elevated erythrocyte sedimentation rate
Elevated C-reactive protein
Prolonged PR interval
Evidence of antecedent group A streptococcal infection
Positive throat culture or rapid streptococcal antigen test
Elevated or increasing streptococcal antibody titer

From Dajani and coworkers [2••]; with permission.
Note: When supported by evidence of antecedent group A streptococcal infection, two major or one major and two minor manifestations indicate a high probability of rheumatic fever.

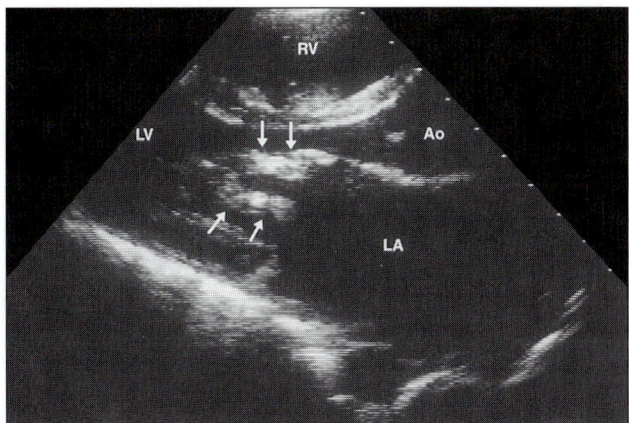

FIGURE 1 Mitral stenosis. Mid-diastolic frame from a transthoracic two-dimensional echocardiogram, in the parasternal long-axis plane, showing a thickened mitral valve with limited leaflet excursion and left atrial enlargement. Note that leaflet calcification and marked subvalvular thickening (*arrows*) would predict a suboptimal outcome after balloon dilatation. Ao—aorta; LA—left atrium; LV—left ventricle; RV—right ventricle.

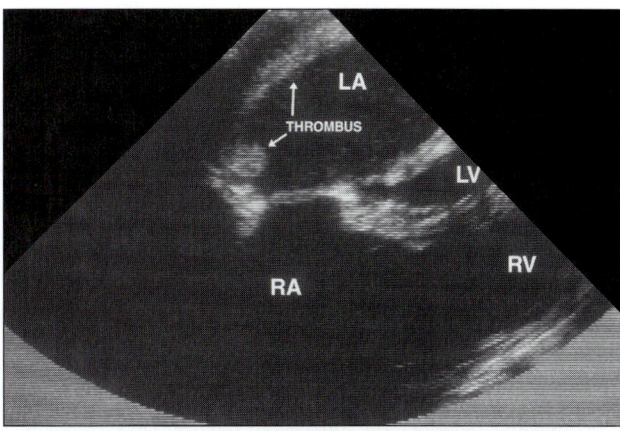

FIGURE 2 Mitral stenosis. Late diastolic frame from an intraoperative transesophageal echocardiogram, in the short-axis plane, showing left atrial mural thrombus. The finding of left atrial thrombus in a patient with mitral stenosis is a contraindication to balloon valvuloplasty. LA—left atrium; LV—left ventricle; RA—right atrium; RV—right ventricle.

of 16. Patients with mitral valve scores of 8 or less generally have the best results from balloon mitral valvuloplasty.

The electrocardiogram is useful in identifying left atrial enlargement with terminal negative P waves in V_1 and the presence of right ventricular hypertrophy pattern with increased R wave in V_1 and a rightward axis. Both of these findings reflect increasing severity of mitral stenosis. It is important to identify the presence of atrial fibrillation, because these patients will require anticoagulation therapy.

Chest x-ray may be useful in identifying left atrial enlargement with elevation of the left mainstem bronchus, pulmonary venous hypertension, and the presence of mitral calcification. In general, and especially during pregnancy, the echocardiogram provides more precise and clinically valuable information for the management of patients with mitral stenosis than other noninvasive tests.

Other adjuncts to the echocardiogram in the diagnosis and management of patients with mitral stenosis include exercise testing and cardiac catheterization. Exercise testing either in association with cardiac catheterization or separately is sometimes valuable in developing management strategies for those patients with mitral stenosis of borderline severity. Cardiac catheterization before surgical intervention for mitral stenosis is generally required to identify coronary artery disease in older patients and to assess the severity of mitral stenosis using hemodynamic parameters [4]. Many patients will be identified as candidates for balloon mitral valvuloplasty and undergo cardiac catheterization for this reason.

Management

Medical therapy for mitral stenosis includes 1) antibiotic prophylaxis for infective endocarditis and recurrent rheumatic fever; 2) management of pulmonary venous hypertension and right heart failure; 3) control of atrial fibrillation; and 4) anticoagulation for prevention of thromboembolism.

The recently published American Heart Association guidelines for antibiotic prophylaxis for infective endocarditis at the time of dental and surgical procedures should be carefully reviewed with the patient (Table 3) [5••]. Wallet-sized summary cards are available from the American Heart Association to assist the patient in this regard. The guidelines for duration of long-term antibiotic therapy using 1.2 million units benzathine penicillin G monthly as prophylaxis against recurrent rheumatic fever are not well established. Generally, continuation to age 40 or later is advisable if the patient is in an occupation such as teaching, where frequent exposure to younger children with streptococcal infection may occur.

Diuretic therapy is useful in managing the symptoms of pulmonary venous congestion and right heart failure; however,

TABLE 3 ANTIBIOTIC PROPHYLAXIS FOR PREVENTION OF ENDOCARDITIS

Regimens for dental, oral, or upper respiratory tract procedures

Amoxicillin 3 g PO 1 h before procedure, then 1.5 g PO 6 h after initial dose

*Erythromycin ethylsuccinate 800 mg or erythromycin stearate 1 g PO 2 h before procedure, then one half the dose 6 h after initial dose

*Clindamycin 300 mg PO 1 h before procedure and 150 mg 6 h after initial dose

Regimens for genitourinary and gastrointestinal procedures

Ampicillin 2 g IV (or IM) plus gentamicin 1.5 mg/kg IV (or IM) (not to exceed 80 mg) 30 minutes before procedure, followed by amoxicillin 1.5 g PO 6 h after the initial dose. Alternatively repeat parenteral regimen may be repeated once 8 hours after initial dose

*Vancomycin 1 g IV over 1 h plus gentamicin 1.5 mg/kg IV (or IM) (not to exceed 80 mg) 1 h before procedure. May be repeated once 8 hours after initial dose

†Amoxicillin 3 g PO 1 h before procedure; then 1.5 g PO 6 hours after initial dose

From Dajani and coworkers [5••]; with permission.
*For patients allergic to amoxicillin, ampicillin, and/or penicillin.
†Alternate oral regimen for low-risk patients.

vigorous diuresis in the presence of significant mitral stenosis may markedly decrease cardiac output.

It is important to control the heart rate when atrial fibrillation occurs, because rapid ventricular response may increase pulmonary congestion due to shortened diastolic filling time. Thus, prompt therapy should be instituted with digoxin to control ventricular response when atrial fibrillation develops. Digoxin is not helpful in treating patients with mitral stenosis who remain in normal sinus rhythm without atrial fibrillation. β-blockers or calcium channel antagonists may be added to digoxin therapy when the ventricular rate remains poorly controlled. In patients who require prompt control of ventricular rate because of hemodynamic deterioration, intravenous diltiazem or esmolol will provide a more rapid reduction in the ventricular response than digoxin. Anticoagulation therapy should be initiated promptly when atrial fibrillation or a documented thromboembolic event has occurred. Once the ventricular rate is controlled and the patient has completed 3 weeks of anticoagulation therapy, elective pharmacologic or electrical cardioversion may be attempted.

When to Refer

Because the natural history of mitral stenosis is related to symptomatic status, the patient should be evaluated for mechanical intervention such as balloon valvuloplasty, open commissurotomy, or valve replacement as the symptoms progress beyond New York Heart Association (NYHA) Class II. In patients with NYHA Class II symptoms, valve area is usually less than 1.0 cm_2/m_2 body surface area. Balloon valvuloplasty provides an acceptable alternative to open commissurotomy, with the best results occurring in patients with pliable leaflets, minimal calcification, mild leaflet thickening, and mild subvalvular fibrosis as demonstrated on echocardiography [6,7]. In patients in whom such findings are absent, mitral valve replacement or open commissurotomy should be considered [8]. Because anticoagulation with coumadin is required after valve replacement, valvuloplasty or commissurotomy are the procedures of choice for women of child-bearing age. Findings of significant mitral regurgitation or a heavily calcified valve argue for mitral valve replacement. Bioprostheses in the mitral position carry a significant risk for embolic events in the absence of anticoagulation.

Because the volume of procedures performed and the operating physician's experience have a significant impact on the outcome for both surgical and cardiac interventional procedures, physicians and patients should base the final decision regarding the choice of mechanical procedure on the results at their local institution. Published mortality rates for mitral valve replacement or open commissurotomy are generally 1% to 4%, whereas the reported mortality for balloon mitral valvuloplasty has ranged from 0% to 4%. Approximately 35% of patients undergoing balloon mitral valvuloplasty will be left with a small residual atrial septal defect which, in the majority of cases, will decrease in size or close. Ten percent of patients undergoing balloon mitral valvuloplasty will develop restenosis after 1 to 2 years. At present, balloon mitral valvuloplasty appears to be the treatment of choice for carefully selected patients with mitral stenosis [9].

MITRAL REGURGITATION
Etiology and Pathophysiology

Mitral regurgitation may result from a disorder of any of the components of the mitral valve, which include the annulus, anterior and posterior leaflets, chordae tendineae, and papillary muscles (Table 4). Mitral regurgitation may also be caused by mitral valve prolapse. Mitral regurgitation due to involvement of the leaflets is common secondary to rheumatic heart disease and occurs more often in men than in women. With acute rheumatic fever, severe mitral regurgitation is more likely to involve the anterior leaflet, whereas chordal rupture, either primary or myxomatous in etiology, and papillary muscle ischemia generally involve the posterior leaflet. Endocarditis and Marfan's syndrome are important causes of mitral regurgitation. Degenerative annular calcification, more common in women, may also result in mitral regurgitation. Annular dilatation secondary to cardiomyopathy is an increasingly frequent cause of mitral regurgitation and varying degrees of mitral regurgitation are found in up to 30% of patients undergoing coronary artery bypass surgery [10]. Finally, prosthetic mitral valve dysfunction is becoming a more frequent cause of clinically encountered mitral regurgitation.

Mitral regurgitation results in significant backflow during systole from the left ventricle into the left atrium. The result is chronic progressive enlargement of both chambers to accommodate the regurgitant volume, which may be four to five times the forward flow when severe. Because regurgitant flow occurs at relatively low impedance into the left atrium, the left ventricular ejection fraction may be preserved late into the course of mitral regurgitation. The ejection fraction in mitral regurgitation may not serve as an accurate index of left ventricular function, and thus, may lead to an erroneously favorable estimate of myocardial performance.

The sudden increase in left atrial volume and pressure associated with acute mitral regurgitation may result in severe pulmonary congestion, often in the presence of preserved left ventricular ejection fraction. Atrial fibrillation may cause significant hemodynamic compromise when it occurs in the course of either acute or chronic mitral regurgitation.

TABLE 4 MITRAL REGURGITATION: ETIOLOGY

Acute
Ruptured chordae tendineae
Papillary muscle rupture
Endocarditis
Trauma
Prosthetic valve dysfunction

Chronic
Rheumatic heart disease
Papillary muscle dysfunction
Severe left ventricular dilatation
Endocarditis
Mitral valve prolapse
Associated with hypertrophic obstructive cardiomyopathy
Congenital abnormalities
Marfan's syndrome
Prosthetic valve dysfunction

Clinical Presentation

Patients with chronic mitral regurgitation may enjoy a relatively asymptomatic course for 20 to 30 years, but finally present with symptoms of progressive weakness and fatigue. Orthopnea and systemic embolism are uncommon presenting symptoms in mitral regurgitation [1]. In contrast with mitral stenosis, the S_1 in mitral regurgitation is usually diminished. The S_2 may be widely split and an apical third heart sound (S_3) may be present. With left ventricular enlargement, the apical impulse becomes diffuse and is displaced laterally. The most prominent finding in mitral regurgitation is a holosystolic murmur beginning with S_1 and extending into the aortic component of S_2. The murmur radiates from the apex to the axilla, but may be heard at the left external edge and at the aortic area when there is marked posterior leaflet prolapse. With marked anterior leaflet prolapse, the murmur may be directed to the posterior wall of the left atrium and may be more prominent over the spine. There is little correlation between the intensity of the murmur and the severity of mitral regurgitation. The murmur may be increased in intensity by isometric exercise, which serves to distinguish it from that of aortic stenosis and hypertrophic obstructive cardiomyopathy. The location of the murmur distinguishes it from the murmur of a ventricular septal defect, which is loudest along the left sternal border and is often associated with parasternal thrill. With pulmonary hypertension, the pulmonic component of S_2 is increased and the systolic murmur of tricuspid regurgitation may be present along the left sternal border.

Laboratory Findings

As with mitral stenosis, color flow Doppler echocardiography has contributed greatly to the management of patients with mitral regurgitation (Fig. 3). It usually aids in establishing the diagnosis and helps to quantify the severity of mitral regurgitation, thereby assisting with patient management. With acute mitral regurgitation, left ventricular and left atrial chamber size may be normal. The left ventricular ejection fraction is usually preserved unless the regurgitation occurs in the setting of acute myocardial infarction, in which case regional wall motion abnormalities and impaired ejection fraction may occur. Echocardiography may be particularly valuable in confirming the presence of flail mitral leaflet or endocarditis. In chronic mitral regurgitation, both left ventricular and left atrial chamber sizes are increased. Assessment of left ventricular wall stress and systolic volume may be more valuable in predicting the patient's suitability for valve replacement than the ejection fraction. Left ventricular dimensions can be followed serially in association with the regurgitant mitral jet volume to assess the results of unloading therapy. Transesophageal echocardiography is especially valuable in assessing patients undergoing mitral valve surgery as possible candidates for direct reconstructive repair rather than mitral replacement.

No electrocardiographic abnormalities are diagnostic for mitral regurgitation. Progressive left ventricular hypertrophy and left atrial enlargement are observed as the mitral regurgitation worsens. Atrial fibrillation generally occurs late in the course of mitral regurgitation. In patients with suspected acute mitral regurgitation, the electrocardiogram results may be normal, except for sinus tachycardia and evidence of acute infarction or ischemia, if that is the underlying etiology.

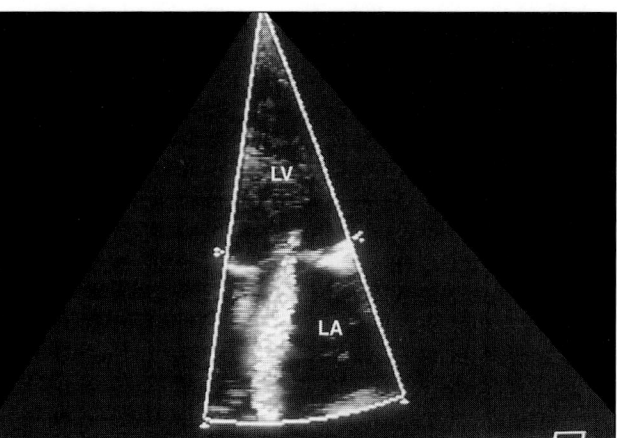

FIGURE 3 Mitral regurgitation. Late systolic frame from a transthoracic color flow Doppler study, in the apical four-chamber plane, showing turbulent flow in the left atrium caused by a high velocity jet of mitral regurgitation. LA—left atrium; LV—left ventricle. (*See* Color Plate.)

The chest radiograph generally demonstrates left ventricular and left atrial enlargement as chronic mitral regurgitation increases in severity. Pulmonary venous congestion may be seen as the clinical course worsens. In patients with acute mitral regurgitation, pulmonary venous hypertension may be the only finding, while left atrial and left ventricular size are normal.

Cardiac catheterization is useful in evaluating older patients with mitral regurgitation to rule out coronary artery disease, before proceeding with mitral valve surgery. In much younger patients with isolated mitral regurgitation, sufficient data may be obtained from echocardiography such that cardiac catheterization is usually unnecessary. In those with acute mitral regurgitation, marked elevation of pulmonary capillary wedge pressure may be noted with prominent regurgitant V waves. As previously mentioned, it is not unusual to find normal or above-normal ejection fractions in patients with acute regurgitation unless myocardial infarction with papillary muscle rupture is the cause, in which case regional wall-motion abnormalities usually are present. Angiographic assessment of mitral regurgitation is the most reliable system for grading mild and severe degrees of mitral regurgitation. However, angiography may not be accurate in assessing moderate regurgitation due to variation in techniques of angiographic injection or left-ventricular-loading conditions. This makes decisions regarding surgery more difficult when moderate regurgitation is noted and other factors previously mentioned should be carefully considered. The V wave amplitude may also be misleading as a guide to severity of mitral regurgitation and should not be used as a reference for surgical decisions.

In patients with moderate mitral regurgitation in whom resting left ventricular ejection fraction appears preserved, exercise radionuclide ejection fractions may help to assess possible candidacy for mitral valve surgery. The inability to elevate ejection fraction with exercise may signal left ventricular dysfunction and a need for surgical intervention.

Management

Patients with acute severe mitral regurgitation should be stabilized with diuretics and afterload reduction. Nitroprusside, which acts as an arteriolar and venous dilator, should be instituted promptly and titrated to optimize systemic vascular resistance, forward cardiac output, and pulmonary capillary wedge pressures. Digoxin and inotropic agents generally are not useful, because ventricular function is usually preserved with acute mitral regurgitation.

Patients with chronic mitral regurgitation who are asymptomatic should be given antibiotic prophylaxis for infective endocarditis as outlined in the discussion for patients with mitral stenosis [5]. The incidence of embolic events is lower than that for mitral stenosis, but anticoagulation should be initiated for those patients in atrial fibrillation and patients with previous embolic events. Patients with minimal or no symptoms should receive follow-up echocardiography on a yearly basis to assess left ventricular size and function unless the mitral regurgitation is mild and ventricular dimensions are normal, in which case follow-up at longer intervals is indicated. Patients who develop symptoms should be considered for therapy with vasodilators, especially the angiotensin-converting-enzyme (ACE) inhibitors and diuretics. Digoxin should be instituted for atrial fibrillation to control ventricular rate and in patients with progressive left ventricular dysfunction who are not candidates for mitral valve replacement. Symptomatic patients with left ventricular dysfunction and mitral regurgitation who are not candidates for mitral valve surgery should be considered for combined diuretic, ACE inhibitor, and digoxin therapy.

Intraaortic balloon counterpulsation is indicated when severe hemodynamic instability is present. Surgical therapy with mitral valve replacement or repair is pursued promptly when patients cannot be stabilized hemodynamically. In cases of endocarditis, if patients can be stabilized, antibiotic therapy is started before proceeding with mitral valve replacement for acute mitral regurgitation.

When to Refer

Surgery for mitral regurgitation has evolved over the past 10 years such that reconstructive repair is performed as frequently as mitral valve replacement. The advantages of repair include lower operative mortality; preservation of the annular-chordal-papillary muscle continuity, which maintains left ventricular function; elimination of thromboembolic risk, thus obviating the need for anticoagulation; and a lower risk of late failure than might be encountered with the bioprostheses. Transesophageal echocardiography is necessary preoperatively to assess candidates for reconstructive surgery, and intraoperative Doppler color flow mapping is extremely useful in assessing the adequacy of reconstruction.

Both bioprosthetic and mechanical valves have an embolic risk and require anticoagulation in the mitral position, although the risk of emboli with a bioprosthetic valve is lower when normal sinus rhythm is present. Bioprosthetic valves generally calcify and become dysfunctional after 7 to 10 years; thus, mechanical valve replacement is preferred if reconstructive surgery is not feasible. The operative mortality in active centers for isolated mitral valve replacement ranges from 2% to 7% in patients with NYHA Class II or III symptoms undergoing elective valve replacement and 1% to 4% for similar patients undergoing reconstructive surgery. Mortality is higher for patients with NYHA Class IV symptoms as well as patients undergoing surgery for acute mitral regurgitation or those with concomitant coronary bypass surgery. Because of the improved outcome with earlier surgery, surgery is recommended for most patients with isolated severe mitral regurgitation who remain symptomatic NYHA Class II in association with medical therapy and have elevated end-systolic volumes of greater than 30 mL/m^2. End-systolic volume should be monitored carefully in those asymptomatic patients with ejection fractions between 55 and 70. Surgical intervention should be performed in these patients as left ventricular function deteriorates. Specifically, elective mitral valve surgery should be considered in this group of patients before ejection fraction is less than 0.50 and the end-systolic volume index greater than 50 mL/m^2.

REFERENCES AND RECOMMENDED READING

Recently published paper of particular interest have been highlighted as:
- Of interest
- •• Of outstanding interest

1. • Braunwald E: Valvular heart disease. In *Heart Disease*, edn 4. Philadelphia: WB Saunders; 1992:1007–1035.
2. •• Dajani AS, Ayoub E, Bierman FZ, *et al.*: Guidelines for the diagnosis of rheumatic fever: Jones Criteria, updated 1992. *Circulation* 1993, 87:302–307.
3. McHenry MM: Systemic arterial embolism in patients with mitral stenosis and minimal dyspnea. *Am J Cardiol* 1966, 18:169–174.
4. Reis R, Roberts W: Amounts of coronary arterial narrowing by atherosclerotic plaques in clinically isolated mitral valve stenosis: analysis of 76 necropsy patients older than 30 years. *Am J Cardiol* 1986, 57:1119.
5. •• Dajani AS, Bisno AL, Chung KJ, *et al.*: Prevention of bacterial endocarditis. *Circulation* 1991, 83:1174–1178.
6. Wilkins GY, Weyman AE, Abascal VM, *et al.*: Percutaneous balloon dilatation of the mitral valve: an analysis of echocardiographic variables related to outcome and the mechanism of dilatation. *Br Heart J* 1988, 60:299–308.
7. Abascal VM, Wilkins GT, O'Shea JP, *et al.*: Prediction of successful outcome in 130 patients undergoing percutaneous balloon mitral valvotomy. *Circulation* 1990, 82:448–456.
8. Cosgrove DM, Stewart WJ: Mitral valvuloplasty. *Curr Prob Cardiol* 1989, 14:359–415.
9. Kirklin JW: Percutaneous balloon versus surgical closed commissurotomy for mitral stenosis. *Circulation* 1991, 83:1450–1451.
10. Olson LJ, Subramanian R, Ackerman DM: Surgical pathology of the mitral valve: a study of 712 cases spanning 21 years. *Mayo Clin Proc* 1987, 62:22.

SELECT BIBLIOGRAPHY

Bisno A, Shulman S, Dajani A: The rise and fall of rheumatic fever. *JAMA* 1988, 249:728.

Cohen DJ, Kuntz RE, Gordon SPF, *et al.*: Predictors of long-term outcome after percutaneous balloon mitral valvuloplasty. *N Engl J Med* 1992, 327:1329–1335.

Crawford MD, Souchek J, Oprian CA, *et al.*: Determinants of survival and left ventricular performance after mitral valve replacement. *Circulation* 1990, 81:1173–1181.

Fenster MS, Feldman MD: Mitral regurgitation: an overview. *Curr Probl in Cardiol* 1995, 20:195–280.

Reyes VP, Rasju BS, Wynne J, *et al.*: Percutaneous balloon valvuloplasty compared with open surgical commissurotomy for mitral stenosis. *N Engl J Med* 1994, 331:961–967.

Mitral Valve Prolapse

Richard B. Devereux

> **Key Points**
> - Mitral valve prolapse is usually a primary, dominantly inherited condition with more consistent gene expression in women than in men or children.
> - Diagnosis is by midsystolic click/late systolic murmur; echocardiography confirms and documents severity.
> - True mitral valve prolapse syndrome is characterized by low body weight and blood pressure, minor skeletal abnormalities, orthostatic hypotension, palpitations, and mitral regurgitation of variable degree.
> - Complications are progressive mitral regurgitation, infective endocarditis, and possible risk of arrhythmic sudden death and orthostatic syncope.
> - Risk factors for complications include older age, male gender, mitral regurgitant murmur, and possibly greater weight and higher blood pressure.
> - Presence and severity of mitral regurgitation govern frequency and intensiveness of follow-up.

Mitral valve prolapse (MVP) is the most common abnormality of the heart in industrialized nations, affecting 3% to 4% of adults. By definition, MVP reflects abnormal systolic displacement of the mitral valve leaflets superiorly and posteriorly from the left ventricle into the left atrium. That may occur because the mitral leaflets, anulus, and chordae tendineae are enlarged in relation to left ventricular size (Fig. 1) or because they are abnormally distensible [1].

Although MVP has been reported to have many causes, most cases occur as a primary condition. Extensive studies [2,3] have shown that the primary condition is passed from affected mothers and fathers to children of both genders in a pattern indicative of autosomal dominant inheritance. Family studies show that the age of onset is between 10 and 16 years, is more consistently expressed in women than men, and may become undetectable after middle age in mildly affected women [3]. As a result of the gender difference in the expression of primary MVP, nearly two thirds of adults with this condition are women. A small percentage of cases occur secondarily to other inheritable connective tissue diseases such as Marfan syndrome or Ehlers-Danlos syndrome. Mitral valve prolapse also may be produced by conditions, including anorexia nervosa or atrial septal defect, that make the left ventricle abnormally small.

DIAGNOSIS

In clinical practice, MVP is most commonly first recognized by auscultation. Typical auscultatory features are a midsystolic click and late systolic murmur, which is separated from the first heart sound by a silent interval but continues until the second heart sound. These sounds are best heard by listening over the left ventricular impulse and medial to it, with the patient in the supine, left decubitus, and sitting positions. Because systolic clicks may have other causes and mitral annular calcification may produce a late systolic murmur in older persons, it is important to perform physical maneuvers during auscultation that take advantage of the key role of valvular-ventricular disproportion in producing the manifestations of MVP [3].

As Figure 2 shows, maneuvers that reduce left ventricular chamber size will cause the click and onset of the murmur to move closer to the first heart sound, whereas the loudness of the click and murmur are affected by changes in blood pressure independent of changes in timing. Figure 3 shows how

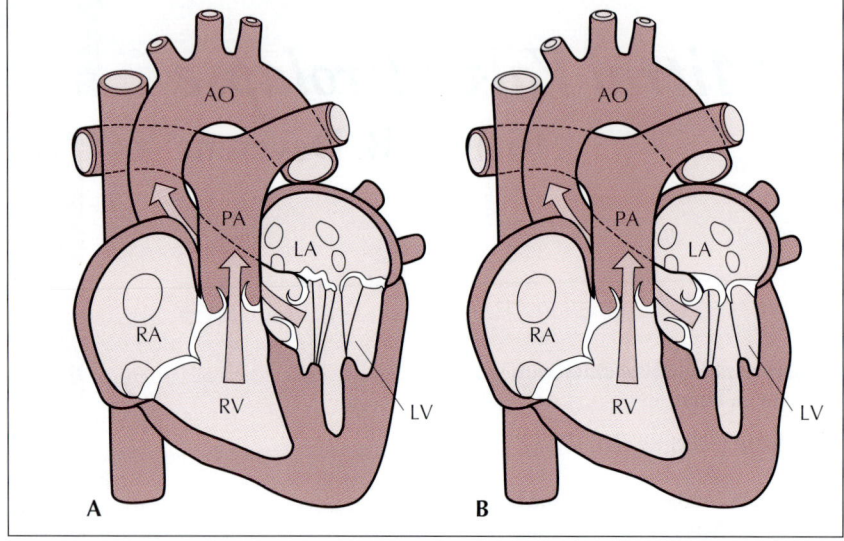

FIGURE 1 Diagram showing enlargement of mitral leaflets, annulus, and chordae **A**, in patients with mitral valve prolapse compared with **B**, findings in healthy persons. AO—aorta; LA—left atrium; LV—left ventricle; PA—pulmonary artery; RA—right atrium; RV—right ventricle.

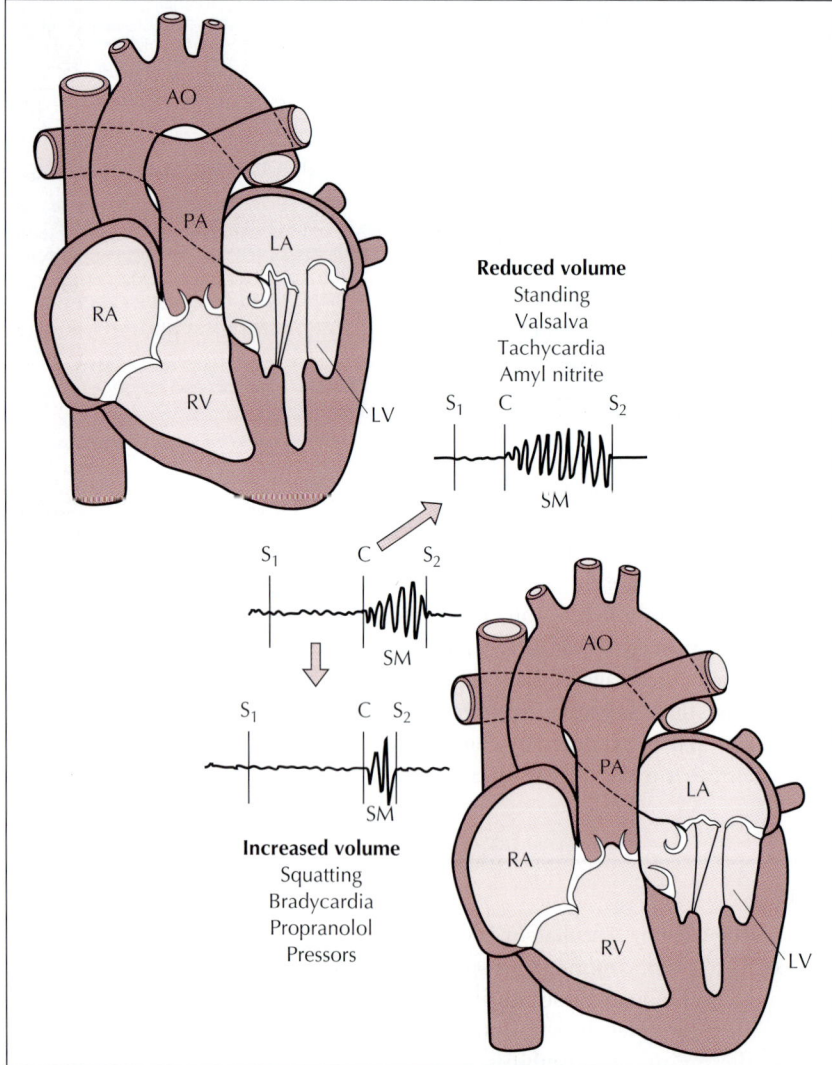

FIGURE 2 Effect of maneuvers that change left ventricular (LV) volume on the timing of the click (C) and murmur (SM) of mitral valve prolapse. The onset of the murmur and occurrence of the click move closer to the first heart sound (S_1) when LV volume is reduced and farther from it when LV volume is increased. AO—aorta; LA—left atrium; PA—pulmonary artery; RA—right atrium; RV—right ventricle; S_2—second heart sound. (*From* Devereux and coworkers [24]; with permission.)

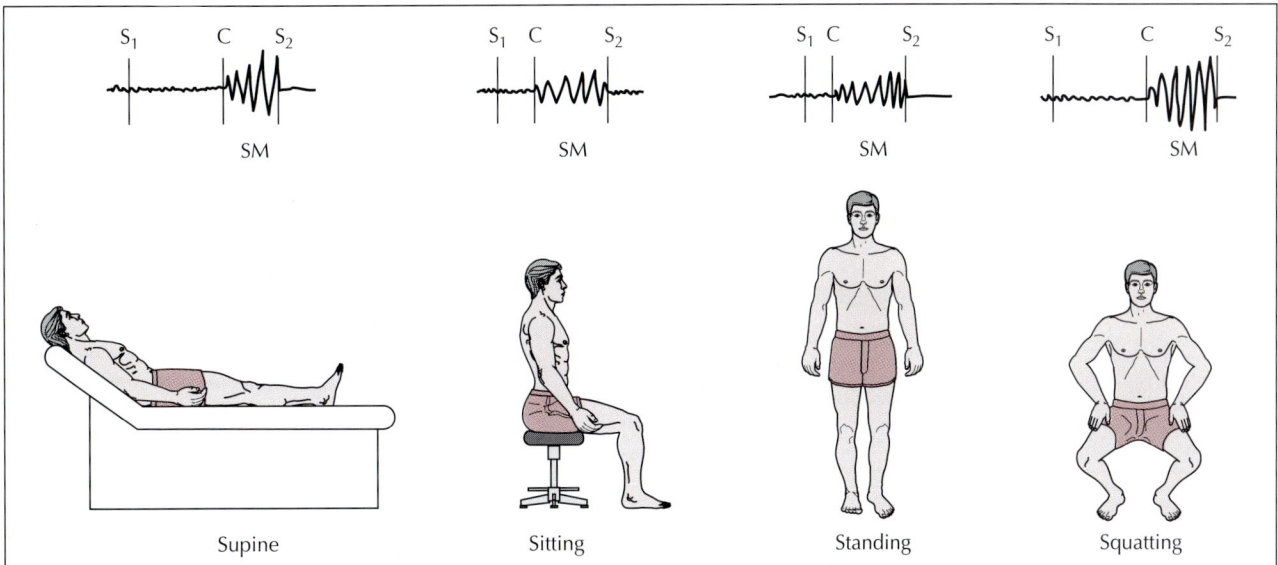

FIGURE 3 Effect of maneuvers during physical examination that change left ventricular chamber volume on the timing of the click (C) and murmur (SM) of mitral valve prolapse. (*From* Devereux and coworkers [24]; with permission.)

standard maneuvers during physical examination affect the click and murmur. It is especially important to time the onset after the first sound and continuation until the second sound of the late systolic murmur, as miscategorization of midsystolic murmurs caused by normal blood flow in thin-chested persons or aortic sclerosis in older patients is a common cause of false-positive diagnoses of MVP (Fig. 4) [4•]. When both a midsystolic click and late systolic murmur are present and respond appropriately to these maneuvers, the diagnosis of MVP can be made confidently by physical examination.

Late-systolic buckling of mitral leaflets on M-mode echocardiographic tracings occurs simultaneously with the midsystolic click and onset of the late systolic murmur (Fig. 5).

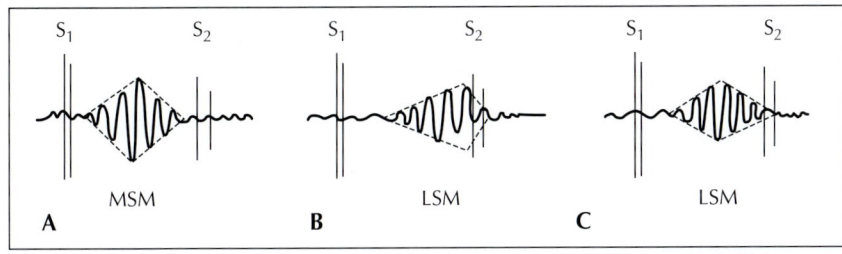

FIGURE 4 Timing of a midsystolic murmur (MSM, **A**) which begins after the first heart sound (S_1) and ends before the second heart sound (S_2) and of late systolic murmurs (LSM, **B** and **C**) which begin after S_1 but continue to or through S_2. Note that both types of murmur may have a crescendo-decrescendo configuration.

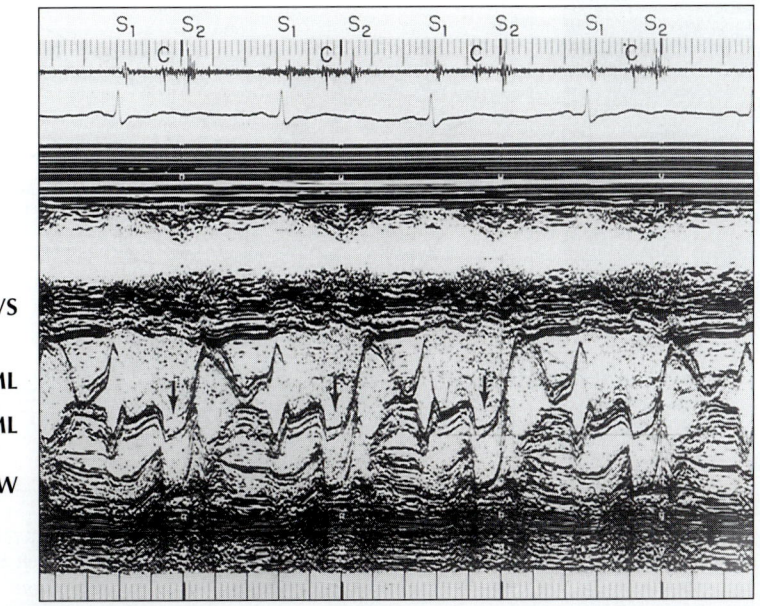

FIGURE 5 M-mode echocardiographic recording of the mitral valve demonstrating late systolic prolapse (*arrows*) and simultaneous phonocardiogram showing a midsystolic click (C) and late systolic murmur. AML—anterior mitral leaflet; IVS—interventricular septum; PML—posterior mitral leaflet; PW—posterior wall; S_1—first heart sound; S_2—second heart sound.

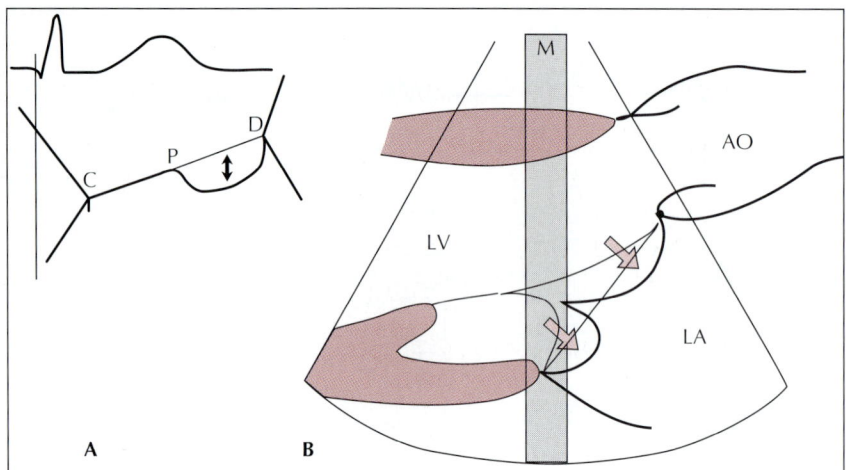

FIGURE 6 **A**, M-mode and **B**, two-dimensional echocardiographic diagnostic criteria of mitral valve prolapse. The condition is diagnosed when there is at least 2 mm of posterior displacement of continuous mitral leaflet interfaces behind the valve's C-D line in late systole on high-quality M-mode recordings (Figure 5) or protrusion of one or both mitral leaflets across the line connecting the hinging points of the mitral leaflets in two-dimensional long-axis views (Figure 7). AO—aorta; LA—left atrium; LV—left ventricle; M—course of M-mode beam. (*From* Devereux and coworkers [5]; with permission.)

An accurate diagnosis can be made on M-mode recordings when continuous mitral leaflet interfaces "turn around" and move at least 2-mm posterior to the valve's C-D line in late systole (Fig. 6) [3,5]. Holosystolic posterior motion of mitral leaflets on M-mode recordings is no longer used to diagnose MVP because it may be produced artifactually by errors in ultrasound beam angulation.

Two-dimensional echocardiography has greatly enhanced recognition and assessment of the severity of MVP. The condition can be accurately diagnosed by two-dimensional echocardiography when one or both mitral leaflets are seen to protrude or "billow" into the left atrium in systole in the parasternal or apical long-axis view (Figs. 6 and 7) [3,6]. Careful assessment of mitral leaflet motion on two-dimensional echocardiograms has revealed that the posterior motion of MVP seen on M-mode recordings may be produced both by billowing of leaflets into the left atrium and by posterior motion of the mitral leaflets because of exaggerated systolic distensibility of the mitral anulus in some persons (Fig. 8) [1]. It is important *not* to diagnose MVP based on apparent protrusion of the mitral leaflets into the left atrium that is seen only in the apical, four-chamber, two-dimensional view; this is a common normal consequence of the "saddle" shape of the mitral anulus (Fig. 9) [6].

Two-dimensional echocardiography is especially useful for identifying several mitral valve abnormalities associated with more severe forms of MVP. These include enlargement of the mitral leaflets and anulus [7] and prominent leaflet thickening [8], both of which are associated with severe mitral regurgitation. Billowing of one mitral leaflet segment that is so prominent it loses apposition with the appropriate segment of the other mitral leaflet is an anatomic cause of severe mitral regurgitation that can be readily visualized on two-dimensional echocardiography (Fig. 10) [9•]. Although conventional and color-flow Doppler echocardiography are not useful for diagnosing MVP, as there are many etiologies for mitral regurgitation, they are of great value for grading the severity of regurgitation, which in turn is the most important factor in determining the risk of major complications.

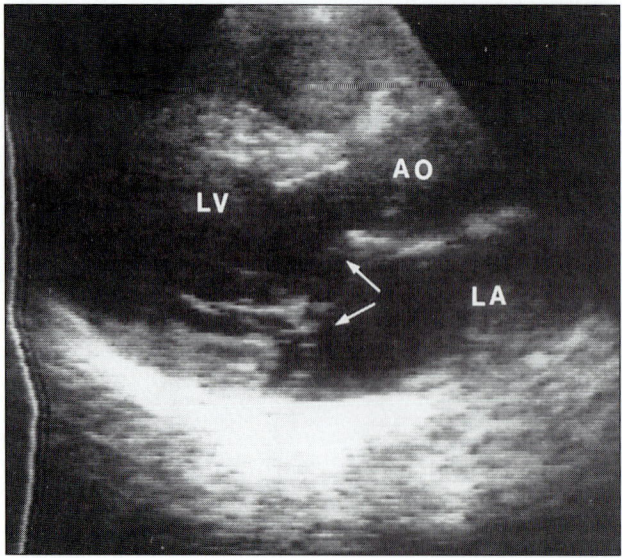

FIGURE 7 Two-dimensional echocardiogram in parasternal long-axis view showing late-systolic billowing of both mitral leaflets (*arrows*) into the left atrium (LA). AO—aorta; LV—left ventricle.

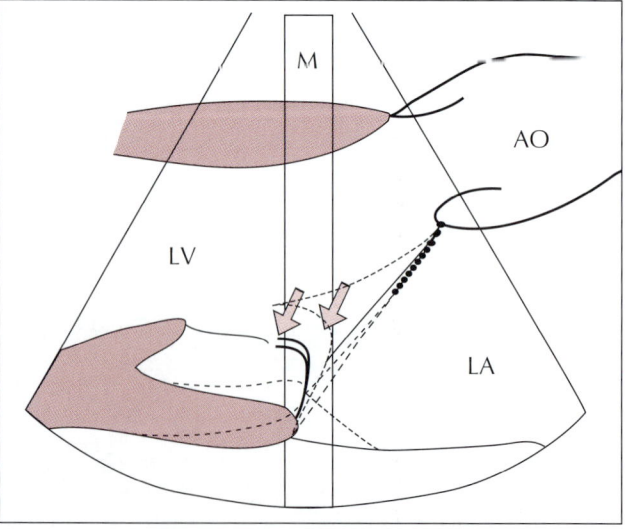

FIGURE 8 Production of M-mode prolapse by exaggerated annular distention during systole. AO—aorta; LA—left atrium; LV—left ventricle; M—course of M-mode beam. (*From* Pini and coworkers [1]; with permission.)

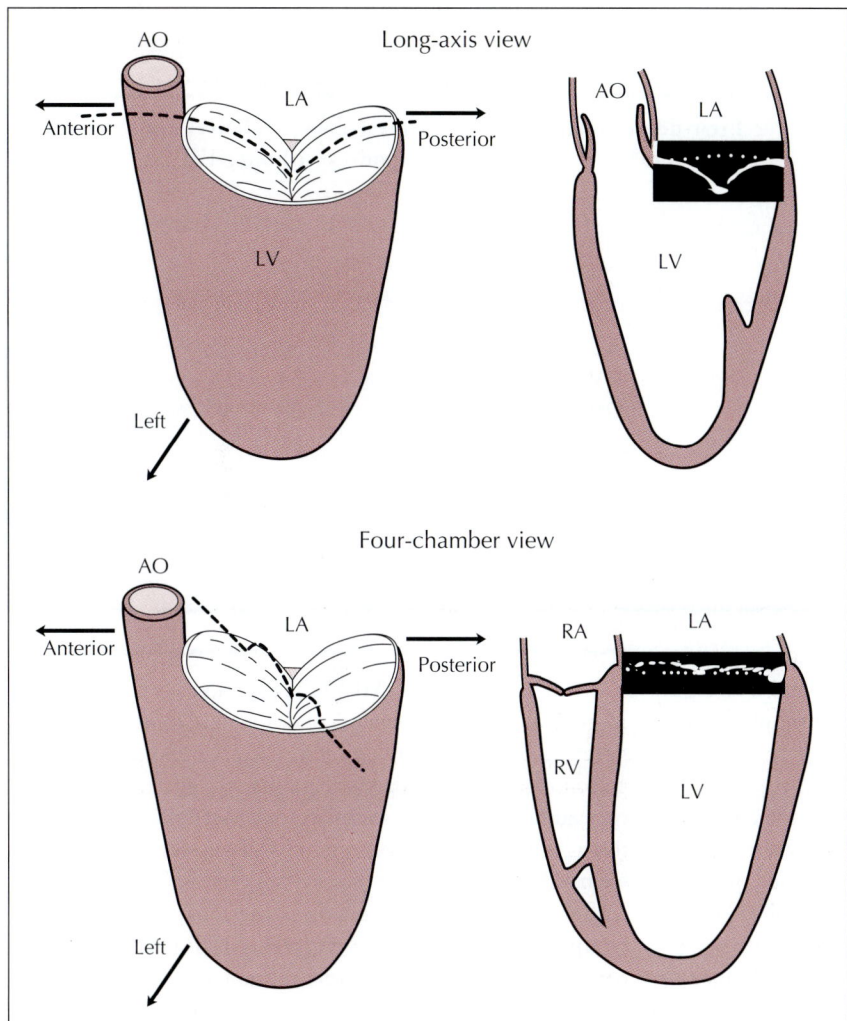

FIGURE 9 Artifactual mitral valve prolapse in the apical four-chamber view resulting from the saddle shape of the mitral anulus. AO—aorta; LA—left atrium; LV—left ventricle; RA—right atrium; RV—right ventricle. (*From* Levine and coworkers [6]; with permission.)

CLINICAL FEATURES

The typical auscultatory features of MVP are useful in making a diagnosis, but these features may vary considerably from one careful examination to another. Consequently, up to one fifth of patients with clinically recognized MVP confirmed by echocardiography and one third of unselected persons with this condition may have "silent" MVP on a single examination (Table 1) [10]. As a result, it is important to examine a patient several times to determine whether a murmur is intermittently present.

Extracardiac features of primary MVP have been shown in both family studies (Table 1) and clinical series. These include a tendency to have low body weight and low blood pressure [11], which may constitute the "selective advantage" that accounts for the high population prevalence of

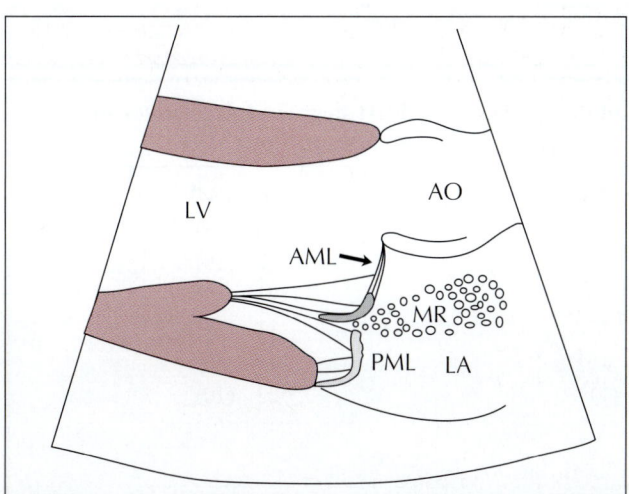

FIGURE 10 Severe posterior mitral leaflet (PML) prolapse into the left atrium (LA) producing loss of coaptation with the anterior mitral leaflet (AML) and allowing severe mitral regurgitation (MR). AO—aorta; LV—left ventricle.

TABLE 1 PREVALENCE OF AUSCULTATORY FEATURES AND EXTRACARDIAC MANIFESTATIONS OF MITRAL VALVE PROLAPSE IN INDEX CASES AND AFFECTED FAMILY MEMBERS

	First-degree relatives with MVP		First-degree relatives and spouses without MVP	
	n	(%)*	n	(%)§
Midsystolic click only	27	(33)†	7	(3)
Late systolic murmur only	14	(17)‡	8	(4)
Click and late systolic murmur	13	(16)†	1	(< 1)
Holosystolic murmur only	1	(1)†	0	(0)
Thoracic bony abnormalities	33	(41)†	34	(15)†
Body weight < 90% of ideal	26	(32)†	29	(13)†
Systolic blood pressure < 120 mm Hg	43	(53)†	65	(28)†

*n=81.
†$P < 0.01$;
‡$P < 0.001$.
§n=232.
MVP—mitral valve prolapse.

this inherited condition. Also, thoracic bony abnormalities (including pectus excavatum, mild scoliosis, and a straight thoracic spine) occur several times more commonly among adults with MVP than among members of the general population.

A variety of symptoms were associated with the condition often enough in initial clinical reports to suggest a distinct MVP syndrome that included chest pain, dyspnea, palpitations, anxiety, and panic attacks. Carefully controlled studies have found little or no evidence, however, that these symptoms—with the exception of palpitations—are truly linked to MVP (Table 2). The erroneous conclusion of previous studies appears to have resulted from selection bias, which causes more symptomatic patients to seek experts who perform clinical studies, and from a true tendency of women to report more of these symptoms than men regardless of whether they have MVP (Table 3).

Another set of symptoms that appears to be truly associated with MVP in controlled studies is syncope or presyncope caused by orthostatic hypotension [12]. The mechanism of this phenomenon is uncertain, but it may relate to the low resting blood pressure found in some patients with MVP.

COMPLICATIONS

In general, MVP is a benign condition, and most patients will never have an important complication. A minority of affected persons develop severe mitral regurgitation, infective endocarditis, neurologic ischemic episodes, or sudden death. Because of the high population prevalence of MVP, however, an appreciable number of adults have these complications (Table 4) [4•].

Severe mitral regurgitation is the most common major complication of MVP; conversely, MVP is now the most common valvular cause of severe mitral regurgitation in industrialized nations. Severe mitral regurgitation in a patient with MVP can be suspected on physical examination by a holosystolic or nearly holosystolic mitral regurgitant murmur associated with an audible third heart sound and leftward displacement of an enlarged, dynamic, left ventricular impulse (Fig. 11). Objective confirmation of this complication can be obtained by demonstrating a large mitral regurgitant jet by pulsed or color-flow Doppler echocardiography (Fig. 12). Imaging echocardiography usually reveals left ventricular and left atrial enlargement, and it also demonstrates a spectrum of morphologic valvular abnormalities, including leaflet and annular enlargement,

TABLE 2 PREVALENCE OF SYMPTOMS IN ADULT FAMILY MEMBERS WITH AND WITHOUT MITRAL VALVE PROLAPSE

	First-degree adult relatives with MVP		First-degree adult relatives and spouses without MVP	
	n	(%)*	n	(%)†
Palpitations	32	(40)	53	(23)
Atypical chest pain	14	(17)	37	(16)
Dyspnea	5	(6)	21	(9)
Panic attacks	6	(7)	11	(5)
Trait anxiety score > 50	5	(6)	14	(6)
Inferior lead electrocardiogram repolarization abnormalities	9	(11)	23	(10)

*n=81.
†n=232.

TABLE 3 RELATIONSHIP OF GENDER TO CLINICAL FEATURES OF MITRAL VALVE PROLAPSE

	Women	Men	
	n (%)*	n (%)	P
Nonanginal chest pain	63 (29)	24 (13)	< 0.001
Dyspnea	50 (23)	15 (8)	< 0.001
Panic attacks	29 (13)	4 (2)	< 0.001
High trait anxiety	23 (11)	6 (3)	< 0.01
Inferior lead ST-T abnormalities	44 (20)	12 (6)	< 0.001

*$n=216$.
‡$=185$.

TABLE 4 ANNUAL OCCURRENCE IN THE UNITED STATES OF COMPLICATIONS ASSOCIATED WITH MITRAL VALVE PROLAPSE

Complication	Patients per year, n	Patients with mitral valve prolapse, n	Annual events attributable to mitral valve prolapse, n
Mitral valve surgery	16,000	25	4000
Infective endocarditis	9000	13	1150
Sudden death*	400,000	1	4000

*Figures for sudden death are less stable than for other complications, because they are based on a single study.

distortion and thickening of leaflet segments, and redundancy or rupture of chordae tendineae [7,8,9•,13••].

The likelihood of developing severe mitral regurgitation increases with age and is greater for men than for women [14,15]. By the age of 75 years, approximately 1.5% to 2.0% of women with MVP and 5.5% of affected men will develop regurgitation of sufficient severity to require surgical valve repair or replacement. Initially mild regurgitation may become severe during prolonged follow-up of these patients [16]. In addition to the irreversible risk factors of age and gender, some evidence exists that high blood pressure or increased body weight may promote the progression of regurgitation.

Infective endocarditis occurs in approximately 25% as many patients with MVP as develop severe regurgitation (Table 4), implying a cumulative risk of less than 1% by age 75. The risk of endocarditis is increased about threefold in men compared with women, in persons older than 45 years of age compared with younger persons, and in patients with a mitral regurgitant murmur (Table 5) [17]. Whether mitral leaflet thickening or other specific morphologic abnormalities

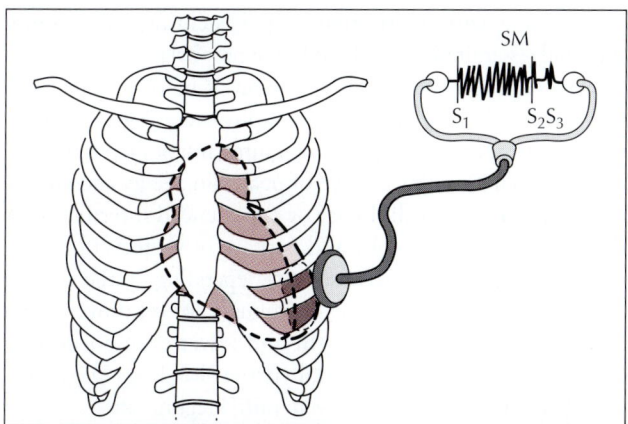

FIGURE 11 Schematic diagram of a nearly holosystolic mitral regurgitant murmur with a third heart sound and leftward displacement of an enlarged left ventricular impulse, which is felt to the left of the midclavicular line in the fifth and sixth intercostal spaces, instead of being smaller than a quarter in diameter and being limited to one interspace in normal persons. S_1—first heart sound; S_2—second heart sound; SM—systolic murmur.

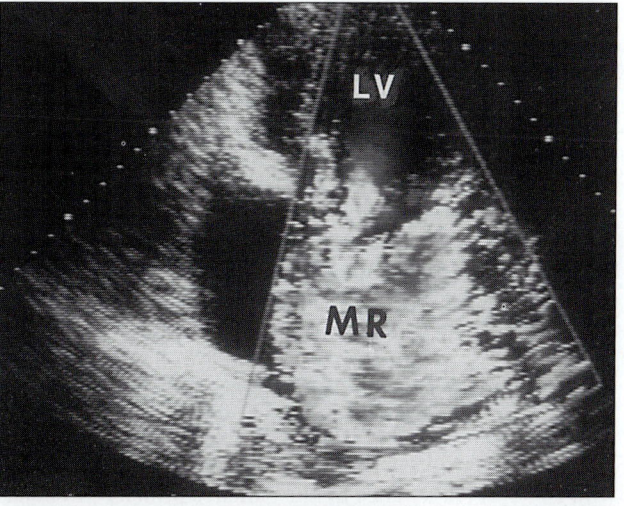

FIGURE 12 Severe mitral regurgitation (MR) demonstrated by color flow Doppler echocardiography. The multicolored MR jet fills almost the entire left atrium, which is nearly 10 cm in diameter. (*See* Color Plate.)

Table 5. Relative risk of infective endocarditis in persons with mitral valve prolapse by gender, age, and history of murmur

	Total, n	Male	> 45 y, n	History of murmur, n
Cases	21	13	13	15*
Controls	102	36	31	41

	Male vs. female	≥ 45 y vs. < 45 y	Present vs. absent
Odds ratio	2.98	3.72	3.72
P	0.023	0.006	0.009
95% CI	1.35, 7.86	1.40, 9.88	1.33, 10.38

Adapted from MacMahon and coworkers [17]; with permission.
*History of a murmur before development of endocarditis.
CI—confidence interval.

Table 6. Matching risk and management in mitral valve prolapse

Low risk
Subjects without mitral regurgitant murmurs or Doppler regurgitation, especially women younger than 45 years.
Management: reassurance; no clear need for antibiotics; reevaluation and echocardiography at moderate intervals (5 years).

Moderate risk
Subjects with intermittent or persistent mitral murmurs and mild Doppler regurgitation.
Management: antibiotic prophylaxis with amoxicillin or erythromycin; treat even mild established hypertension; reevaluation and echocardiography more frequently (2 to 3 years).

High risk
Subjects with moderate or severe mitral regurgitation.
Management: antibiotic prophylaxis with amoxicillin (unless allergic); optimize afterload (arterial pressure); reevaluate with Doppler echocardiography and other tests if needed annually.
Consider valve repair or replacement for exertional dyspnea or decline of left ventricular function into low-normal range.

---

increase the risk of endocarditis independent of their role in causing mitral regurgitation has not yet been established. About one third of endocarditis cases are of dental origin, which is similar to the experience with other predisposing valvular lesions. During long-term follow-up, a majority of patients with MVP who develop endocarditis require valve surgery or suffer cardiac death [18••].

Neurologic ischemic events appear to occur more commonly among persons with MVP than among members of the general population, but the association is sufficiently weak that it can be clearly identified only in groups at low risk of stroke, such as young women [19]. Thrombotic lesions on denuded segments of endothelium at the junction between the mitral leaflets and left atrial wall have been identified pathologically in patients with MVP who suffered strokes, but clinical clues to which patients are at risk for neurologic events are not yet known.

Sudden death is the most feared, least understood, and perhaps the rarest major complication of MVP. An increased risk of sudden death is well established in patients with severe mitral regurgitation, but this appears to relate to the degree of regurgitation rather than MVP [20]. Instances of sudden death in patients without known severe mitral regurgitation are often associated with severe valvular deformity but also increased heart weight, suggesting that unrecognized regurgitation or some other hemodynamic overload may have been present [21,22]. To date, neither specific arrhythmias nor other electrocardiographic features such as repolarization abnormalities have been documented to identify the patient with MVP who is at increased risk of sudden death.

MANAGEMENT

The proper starting point of management for most patients with MVP is reassurance by the patient's primary physician that they have a condition that is generally benign and may even be marginally beneficial if they have inherited the common tendency to low body weight and low blood pressure. For a person with only a midsystolic click and no mitral regurgitant murmur on several examinations, and no evidence of mitral regurgitation by Doppler echocardiography if it is performed, no clear evidence exists that peridental endocarditis prophylaxis or other specific medication is needed. It is reasonable to reevaluate such patients at 5-year intervals.

The presence and severity of mitral regurgitation are the best indicators of the need for active treatment and more frequent follow-up (Table 6) [4•]. This may be assessed directly by Doppler echocardiography or indirectly by auscultation. Persons with intermittent or persistent mitral murmurs and mild regurgitation need antibiotic prophylaxis with amoxicillin or erythromycin [23•], treatment of mild hypertension, and reevaluation and echocardiography every 2 to 3 years. A person with severe regurgitation requires antibiotic prophylaxis with amoxicillin in the absence of penicillin allergy and annual reevaluation by a cardiologist or experienced internist with Doppler echocardiography and perhaps other tests (24-hour electrocardiography or exercise test) depending on the clinical circumstances. It is also logical, although not yet proven to be beneficial, to avoid overweight and lower even borderline elevated arterial pressure by antihypertensive drugs in patients with MVP and moderate or severe mitral regurgitation.

Patients with other manifestations of MVP may need other forms of specific management. When distressing palpitation is from frequent, single premature ventricular contractions or self-terminating paroxysms of supraventricular tachycardia at rates that do not cause hemodynamic embarrassment, treatment with a long-acting β-adrenoreceptor blocker or digoxin may give symptomatic relief. Sustained, re-entrant, supraventricular tachycardias now often can be caused by radiofrequency ablation of accessory pathways in the electrophysiology laboratory. Rate-control with β-blockers, digoxin, or both, and anticoagulation with sodium warfarin to prevent stroke is needed if sustained atrial fibrillation develops, usually with hemodynamically important mitral regurgitation or after mitral valve surgery. Patients with MVP and orthostatic hypotension may benefit from stopping low-salt diets, adding sodium chloride in tablet form, or if the above are not successful, taking fluorine 0.05 to 0.10 mg/d to induce expansion of the blood volume.

Acknowledgment

The author thanks Virginia Burns for her assistance in preparing this manuscript.

References and Recommended Reading

Recently published papers of particular interest have been highlighted as:
- Of interest
- •• Of outstanding interest

1. Pini R, Greppi B, Kramer-Fox R, *et al.*: Mitral valve dimensions and motion and familial transmission of mitral valve prolapse with and without mitral leaflet billowing. *J Am Coll Cardiol* 1988, 12:1423–1431.
2. Devereux RB, Brown WT, Kramer-Fox R, *et al.*: Inheritance of mitral valve prolapse: effect of age and sex on gene expression. *Ann Intern Med* 1982, 97:826–832.
3. Devereux RB, Kramer-Fox R, Shear MK, *et al.*: Diagnosis and classification of severity of mitral valve prolapse: methodologic, biologic and prognostic considerations. *Am Heart J* 1987, 113:1265–1280.
4. • Devereux RB, Kramer-Fox R, Shear MK, Kligfield P: Relation of panic attacks and midsystolic murmurs to over-diagnosis of mitral valve prolapse. *Cardiovasc Rev Reports* 1994, 15:11–15.
5. Devereux RB, Kramer-Fox R, Kligfield P: Mitral valve prolapse: etiology, clinical manifestations and management. *Ann Intern Med* 1989, 111:305–317.
6. Levine RA, Triulzi MO, Harrigan P, *et al.*: The relationship of mitral annular shape to the diagnosis of mitral valve prolapse. *Circulation* 1987, 75:756–767.
7. Pini R, Devereux RB, Greppi B, *et al.*: Comparison of mitral valve dimension and motion in mitral valve prolapse with severe mitral regurgitation to uncomplicated mitral valve prolapse and to mitral regurgitation without mitral valve prolapse. *Am J Cardiol* 1988, 62:257–263.
8. Levine RA, Stathogiannis E, Newell JB, *et al.*: Reconsideration of echocardiographic standards for mitral valve prolapse: lack of association between leaflet displacement isolated to the apical four chamber view and independent echocardiographic evidence of abnormality. *J Am Coll Cardiol* 1988, 11:1010–1019.
9. • Grayburn PA, Berk MR, Spain MG, *et al.*: Relation of echocardiographic morphology of the mitral apparatus to mitral regurgitation in mitral valve prolapse: assessment by Doppler color flow imaging. *Am Heart J* 1990, 119:1095–1102.
10. Devereux RB, Kramer-Fox R, Brown WT, *et al.*: Relation between clinical features of the "mitral prolapse syndrome" and echocardiographically documented mitral valve prolapse. *J Am Coll Cardiol* 1986, 8:763–772.
11. Devereux RB, Brown WT, Lutas EM, *et al.*: Association of mitral valve prolapse with low body-weight and low blood pressure. *Lancet* 1982, ii:792–795.
12. Weissman NJ, Shear MK, Kramer-Fox R, Devereux RB: Contrasting patterns of autonomic dysfunction in patients with mitral valve prolapse and panic attacks. *Am J Med* 1987, 82:880–888.
13. •• Weissman NJ, Pini R, Roman MJ, *et al.*: In vivo mitral valve morphology and function in mitral valve prolapse. *Am J Cardiol* 1994, 73:1080–1088.
14. Devereux RB, Hawkins I, Kramer-Fox R, *et al.*: Complications of mitral valve prolapse: disproportionate occurrence in men and older patients. *Am J Med* 1986, 81:751–758.
15. Wilcken DE, Hickey AJ: Lifetime risk for patients with mitral prolapse of developing severe valve regurgitation requiring surgery. *Circulation* 1988, 78:10–14.
16. Kolibash AJ Jr, Kilman JW, Bush CA, *et al.*: Evidence for progression from mild to severe mitral regurgitation in mitral valve prolapse. *Am J Cardiol* 1986, 58:762–767.
17. MacMahon SW, Roberts JK, Kramer-Fox R, *et al.*: Mitral valve prolapse and infective endocarditis. *Am Heart J* 1987, 113:1291–1298.
18. •• Frary CJ, Devereux RB, Kramer-Fox R, *et al.*: Clinical and health-care cost consequences of infective endocarditis in mitral valve prolapse. *Am J Cardiol* 1994, 73:263–267.
19. Barnett HJ, Boughner DR, Taylor DW, *et al.*: Further evidence relating mitral valve prolapse to cerebral ischemic events. *N Engl J Med* 1980, 302:139–144.
20. Kligfield P, Hochreiter C, Niles N, *et al.*: Relation of sudden death in pure mitral regurgitation with and without mitral valve prolapse, to repetitive ventricular arrhythmias and right and left ventricular ejection fraction. *Am J Cardiol* 1987, 60:397–399.
21. Farb A, Tang AL, Atkinson JB, *et al.*: Comparison of cardiac findings in patients with mitral valve prolapse who die suddenly to those who have congestive heart failure from mitral regurgitation and to those with fatal noncardiac conditions. *Am J Cardiol* 1992, 70:234–239.
22. Morales AR, Remanelli R, Boncek RJ, *et al.*: Myxoid heart disease: an assessment of extraordinary cardiac pathology in severe mitral valve prolapse. *Hum Pathol* 1992, 23:129–137.
23. • Dajani AS, Bisno AL, Chung DJ, *et al.*: Prevention of bacterial endocarditis: recommendations by the American Heart Association. *JAMA* 1990, 264:2919–2922.
24. Devereux RB, Perloff JK, Reichek N, *et al.*: Mitral valve prolapse. *Circulation* 1976, 54:3–14.

Selected Bibliography

Barlow JE, Pocock WA, Marchand P, *et al.*: The significance of late systolic murmurs. *Am Heart J* 1963, 66:443–452.

Leatham A, Brigden W: Mild mitral regurgitation and the mitral prolapse fiasco. *Am Heart J* 1980, 99:659–664.

Nishimura RA, McGoon MD, Shub C, *et al.*: Echocardiographically documented mitral-valve prolapse: long-term follow-up of 237 patients. *N Engl J Med* 1985, 313:1305–1309.

Wooley CF, Boudoulas H, eds.: *Mitral Valve Prolapse and the Mitral Valve Prolapse Syndrome*. Mt. Kisco, NY: Futura; 1988.

Aortic Stenosis and Regurgitation

14

Michael A. Fifer

> **Key Points**
> - Aortic stenosis and, less often, aortic regurgitation may cause angina in the absence of coronary artery disease.
> - Sudden death is rare among truly asymptomatic patients with aortic stenosis or regurgitation.
> - The "classic" physical examination findings of aortic regurgitation may be absent when regurgitation develops acutely.
> - Doppler echo examination for aortic regurgitation is so sensitive that many false-positive findings occur.
> - Aortic valve replacement for aortic stenosis is generally reserved for symptomatic patients, whereas surgery for aortic regurgitation may be indicated for low or decreasing left ventricular ejection fraction, even for patients without symptoms.

The clinical manifestations of aortic valve disease are heart failure, angina, syncope, and death. Aortic stenosis is particularly prevalent in the elderly population [1]. It has been increasingly appreciated that aortic regurgitation may result from diseases of the aorta rather than of the aortic valve per se [2]. Clinical recognition of aortic valve disease is critical because properly timed valve replacement may dramatically improve symptoms and prolong life.

AORTIC STENOSIS

Etiology and Pathophysiology

There are three causes of valvular aortic stenosis in adults [3]; these causes are illustrated, along with a normal valve, in Figure 1. The prevalence of congenitally bicuspid aortic valves is approximately 1%, with a male preponderance. Stenosis resulting from fibrosis, calcification, and stiffening of a bicuspid valve is the usual cause of isolated aortic stenosis in patients younger than 60 years of age. Less commonly, bicuspid aortic valves cause aortic regurgitation. A substantial fraction of bicuspid valves cause no hemodynamic abnormality throughout life [4]. Rheumatic aortic stenosis is characterized by thickening of the valve cusps, fusion of the commissures, and calcification. Usually, the central orifice is relatively fixed, so that some degree of regurgitation is present as well. The majority of patients with rheumatic aortic valve disease also have clinically evident mitral valve disease. Senile calcific aortic stenosis is the most common type occurring in patients older than 70 years of age, and results from progressive scarring, calcification, and stiffening of the valve without fusion of the commissures. The consequences of aortic stenosis for systole are a gradient across the aortic valve, high intraventricular pressure, a compensatory increase in ventricular wall thickness and, for a minority of patients, a decrease in ejection fraction (systolic dysfunction). The consequences of aortic stenosis for diastole are diminished distensibility of the ventricle (diastolic dysfunction) caused by the increase in wall thickness,

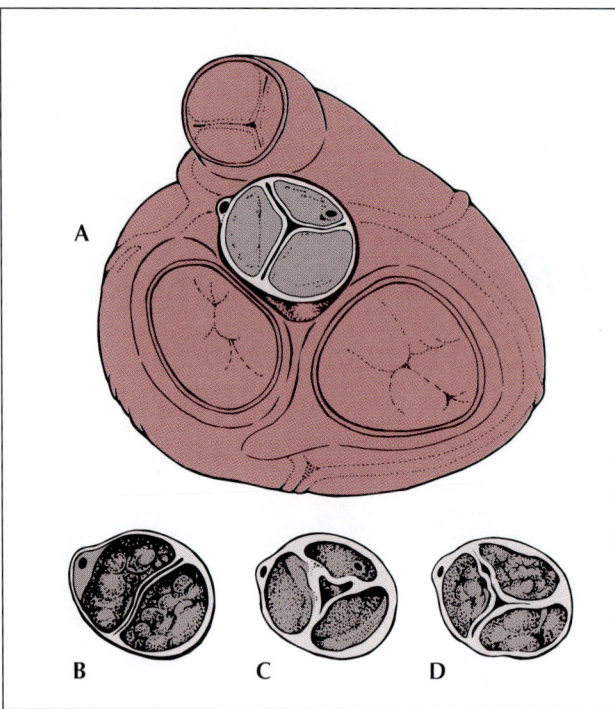

FIGURE 1 Schematic drawings showing **A**, a normal aortic valve; **B**, a calcified bicuspid valve with calcific deposits on the cusps; **C**, a rheumatic valve with commissural fusion; and **D**, a calcific tricuspid "senile" valve with calcific deposits on the cusps without commissural fusion. (*Adapted from* Sutton and Fox [26]; with permission.)

enhanced importance of the atrial kick for ventricular filling, and the potential for sudden decompensation if the atrial kick is lost, as with atrial fibrillation.

Evaluation

Symptoms of left-side heart failure resulting from aortic stenosis may be caused by systolic or diastolic dysfunction, or both. Whereas resting myocardial blood flow is increased, the capacity to augment flow at times of stress is correspondingly diminished, which may lead to angina, subendocardial infarction (even with no coronary artery disease), and fibrosis. Angina is induced by exertion or emotion, and may be relieved by nitroglycerin whether or not coronary artery disease is present; rest angina generally indicates concomitant coronary artery disease. Lightheadedness and syncope typically occur during or immediately after exertion and may result from an exercise-induced decrease in systemic vascular resistance without a proportionate increase in cardiac output or from bradyarrhythmias caused by extension of aortic valve calcification into the conduction system. Clinically apparent embolization from the aortic valve and endocarditis are both rare [5]. There is an association between aortic stenosis and gastrointestinal bleeding originating from angiodysplasia, usually of the ascending colon [6].

Hypertension may coexist with severe aortic stenosis. The pulse pressure is usually normal but may be wide, especially in older patients [7,8]. The carotid upstroke is usually weak and delayed but may be normal or nearly so in patients with hypertension and in elderly patients with atherosclerotic, noncompliant arteries. In low-output states, the carotid volume is diminished, so that it is difficult to judge the rate of increase of the upstroke. A thrill is often felt over the carotid arteries, in the suprasternal notch, or in the second right intercostal space.

The left ventricular impulse is forceful and sustained; it is displaced leftward and downward when the ejection fraction is low. The second heart sound (S_2) is single or narrowly or paradoxically split; normal splitting suggests that severe aortic stenosis is not present. A fourth heart sound (S_4) is common and reflects left ventricular diastolic dysfunction. A third heart sound (S_3) is less common and indicates systolic dysfunction [9]. An ejection click is caused by checking of the upward movement of a domed aortic valve and is best heard after the first heard sound (S_1) at the lower left sternal border or apex in the young patient with a mobile valve. It is rare in adults older than 30 years of age, who have calcified, immobile valves. The crescendo-decrescendo (diamond-shaped) systolic murmur of

TABLE 1 DIFFERENTIAL DIAGNOSIS OF AORTIC STENOSIS

	Aortic stenosis	Hypertrophic cardiomyopathy	Mitral regurgitation
Carotid upstroke	Delayed	Brisk or bisferiens, or both	Brisk
S_2	Single	Split	Split
Ejection click	Sometimes present	Absent	Absent
Murmur location	Right upper sternal border, left sternal border, apex, carotids	Left lower sternal border, apex	Apex, axilla, left sternal border
Murmur during Valsalva maneuver	Softer	Louder	Louder
Murmur of aortic regurgitation	Common	Rare	Unusual
Aortic valve calcification on chest roentgenography	Usual	Absent	Absent
Dilation of ascending aorta on chest roentgenography	Usual	Absent	Absent

aortic stenosis is typically described as harsh, rough, or grunting. It is usually best heard in the second right intercostal space and may radiate widely to the neck, left sternal border, and apex. In elderly patients, it is often heard best at the apex, so that mitral regurgitation is erroneously suspected. The intensity of the murmur does not correlate with the severity of stenosis; it may be soft with severe stenosis and low cardiac output. A prolonged crescendo phase with a late peak suggests significant stenosis. The murmur of aortic stenosis must be distinguished from that of other cardiac lesions (Table 1). A diastolic murmur of aortic insufficiency is useful in establishing valvular aortic stenosis as opposed to hypertrophic cardiomyopathy as the cause of a systolic murmur.

The cardinal finding on the electrocardiogram (Fig. 2) is left ventricular hypertrophy, often with a "strain" pattern: ST-segment depression and T-wave inversion, usually in leads I, aV_L, and V_{4-6}. The absence of hypertrophy by electrocardiographic criteria, however, does not exclude hemodynamically significant stenosis. Other, more variable findings are left atrial abnormality, left axis deviation, and left bundle branch block. The chest roentgenogram may show calcification in the region of the aortic valve, although the technique is insensitive; on the other hand, no calcification of the valve seen by fluoroscopy in a patient older than 40 years of age virtually excludes severe aortic stenosis [7]. Poststenotic dilation of the ascending aorta is often seen. A "left ventricular configuration" (*ie*, rounding of the left ventricular border and apex), indicates left ventricular hypertrophy, whereas left ventricular enlargement suggests systolic dysfunction.

There is considerable variation among physicians in the use of exercise testing to evaluate aortic stenosis. Because of the possibility of inducing angina, severe dyspnea, hypotension, or syncope, some have considered severe aortic stenosis to be a contraindication to exercise testing. Others have suggested that exercise testing is useful to establish safe levels of physical activity in asymptomatic patients with aortic stenosis. Exercise may produce ST-segment and T-wave abnormalities and even thallium defects in the absence of coronary artery disease.

Echocardiography (Fig. 3) is the mainstay of the noninvasive evaluation of aortic stenosis. The valve is seen to be thickened and calcified, and leaflet excursion is reduced. In younger patients, the valve leaflets may be mobile, but tethering of their tips results in "doming" of the valve. In some patients, the valve is bicuspid, although this finding is often obscured by thickening and calcification. The echocardiogram is more sensitive than the electrocardiogram for detecting left ventricular hypertrophy. Left ventricular ejection fraction may be calculated from a technically adequate echocardiogram. The echocardiogram is also useful for distinguishing between valvular aortic stenosis and other causes of outflow gradients, such as hypertrophic cardiomyopathy.

The noninvasive assessment of the severity of aortic stenosis has been revolutionized by Doppler echocardiography. The peak and mean aortic valve gradients are calculated from the simplified Bernoulli equation as $4v^2$, for which v is the velocity of blood flow across the valve in m/sec. The gradient may be underestimated if the Doppler beam is not aligned correctly to measure the maximum blood flow velocity. It should be

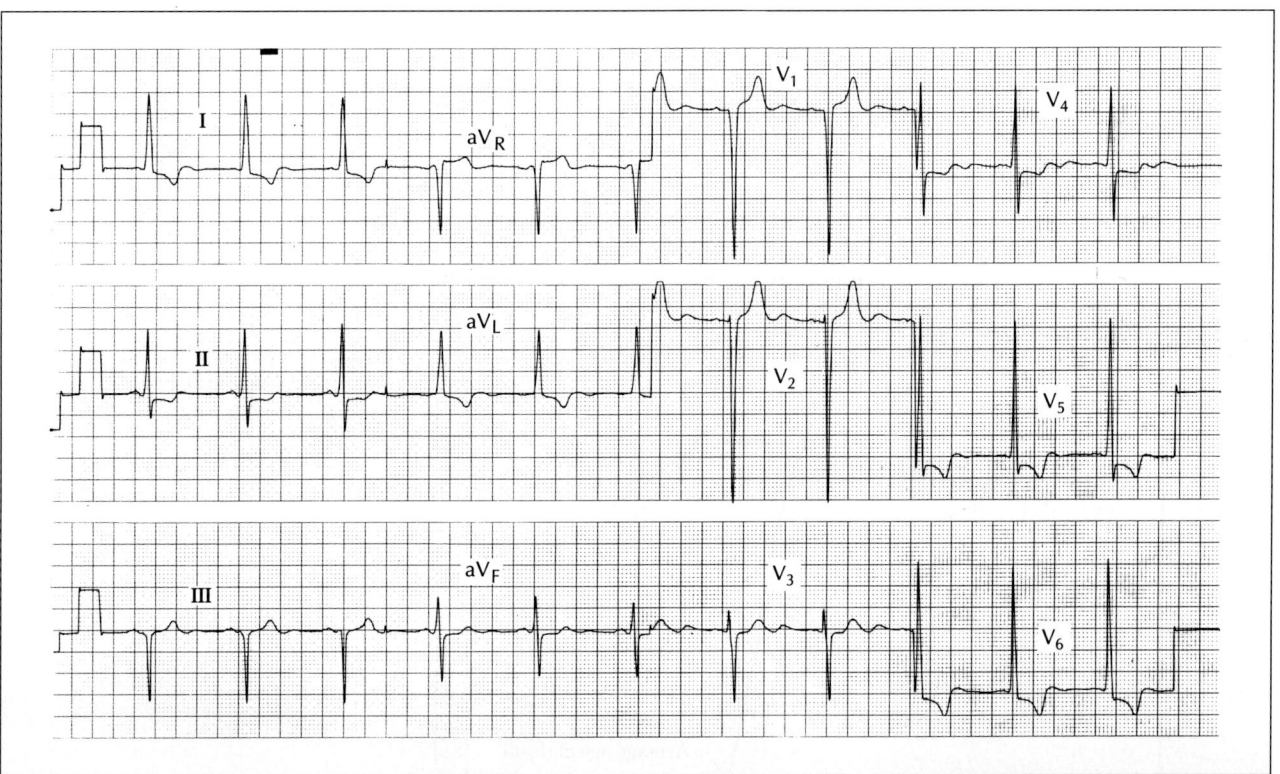

FIGURE 2 Electrocardiogram of a 77-year-old woman with senile calcific aortic stenosis reveals left ventricular hypertrophy, with a "strain" pattern (ST-segment depression and T-wave inversion) in leads I, aV_L, and V_{4-6}.

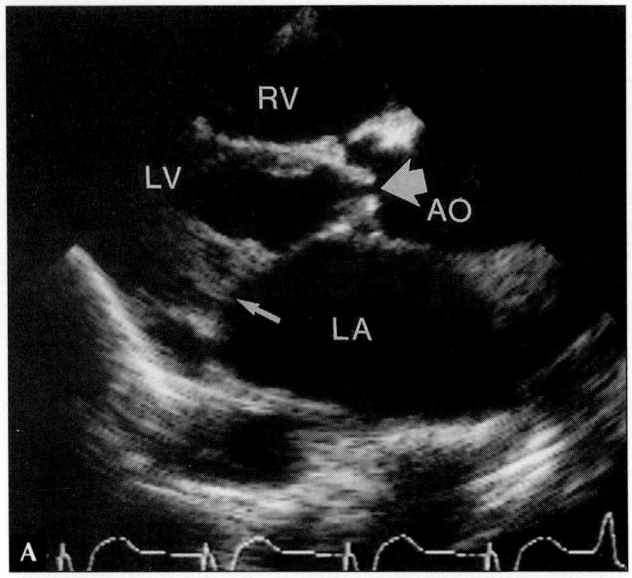 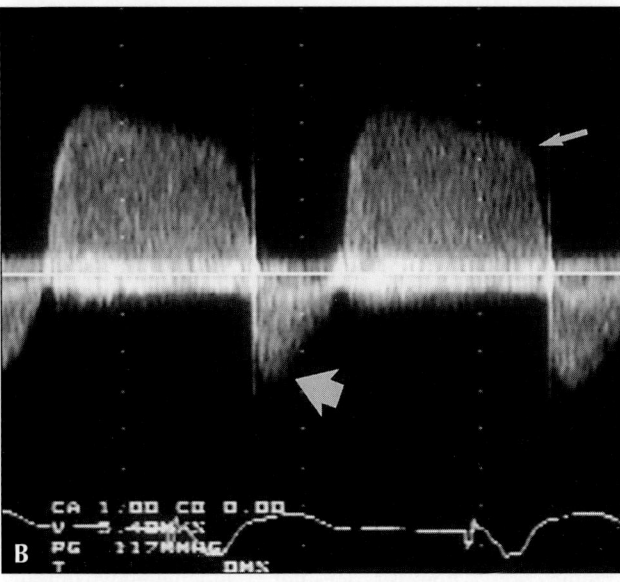

FIGURE 3 **A**, Two-dimensional echocardiogram and **B**, Doppler velocity tracing in a 70-year-old woman with rheumatic heart disease. The two-dimensional long-axis view in **A** shows the right ventricle (RV), left atrium (LA), left ventricle (LV), and aorta (AO). Two of the aortic valve leaflets (*thick arrow*) are thickened and have restricted openings. The mitral valve (*thin arrow*) is thickened and stenotic. The Doppler tracing in **B**, recorded from the left ventricular outflow tract, shows a peak velocity of 2.9 m/s and mean velocity of 2.1 m/s (*thick arrow*), corresponding to peak and mean gradients of 33 and 18 mm Hg, respectively. The Doppler signal in the opposite direction (*thin arrow*) demonstrates aortic regurgitation. (Courtesy of Michael H. Picard, MD.)

recognized that the peak gradient measured by Doppler differs from (and is greater than) the peak-to-peak gradient measured during cardiac catheterization; the mean gradient may be measured by either technique and is the most useful. Doppler echocardiography may also be used to estimate aortic valve area. A technically optimal echocardiogram in a young patient who does not have risk factors for coronary artery disease may preclude the need for cardiac catheterization before aortic valve replacement.

Management

Although patients with aortic stenosis may be asymptomatic for many years, the prognosis for symptomatic patients with significant stenosis is poor, with death usually occurring within 5 years of symptom onset [10,11•,12]. Symptoms of heart failure are the most ominous, followed by syncope and then angina (Fig. 4). Although sudden death may occur, it is almost always preceded by other symptoms in adults with aortic stenosis; the risk of sudden death in truly asymptomatic patients is low [10,13•].

Patients with aortic stenosis should be questioned closely at 3- to 6-month intervals for the occurrence of angina, light-headedness, syncope, or symptoms of heart failure and instructed to contact the physician if symptoms appear between visits. Although careful physical examination usually distinguishes aortic stenosis from other conditions and indicates its severity, the work-up usually includes echocardiography for confirmation. Once significant aortic stenosis is estab-

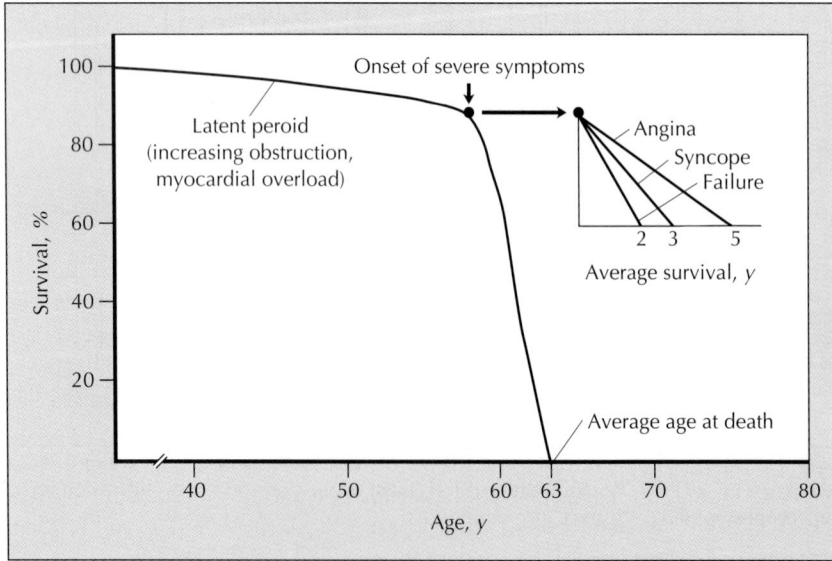

FIGURE 4 The natural history of aortic stenosis. (*From* Ross and Braunwald [27]; with permission.)

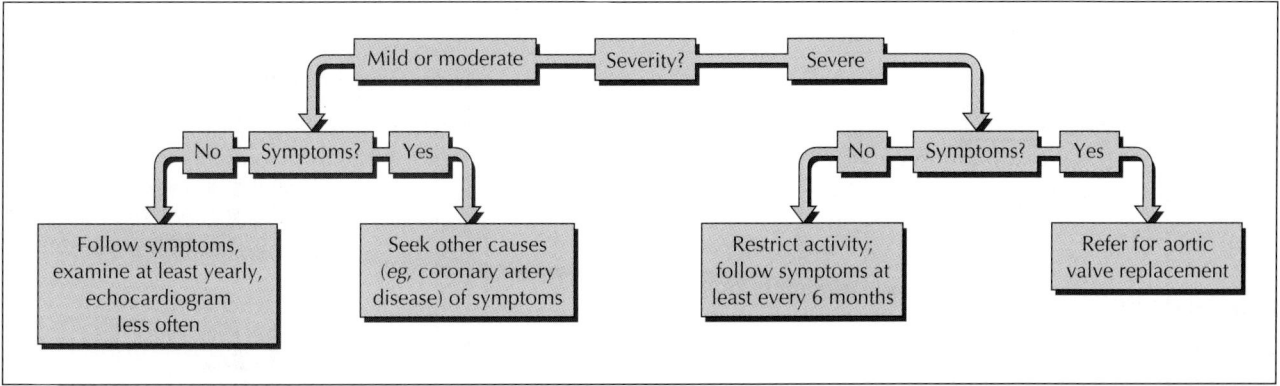

FIGURE 5 Management of aortic stenosis.

lished, repeat echocardiography is generally not necessary because the indication for surgery is usually the appearance of symptoms (see the following paragraphs). The management of aortic stenosis is diagrammed in Figure 5.

Endocarditis prophylaxis should be administered according to the guidelines of the American Heart Association; this recommendation also applies to patients with bicuspid aortic valves without significant stenosis or regurgitation. Asymptomatic patients with hemodynamically significant stenosis should be prohibited from occupations and sports that require heavy exertion. Most patients with asymptomatic aortic stenosis tolerate noncardiac surgery without complications [14]. Digoxin should be used for rapid supraventricular tachyarrhythmias. If nitrates are needed for concomitant coronary artery disease, they must be used cautiously for fear of inducing hypotension. Drugs with negative inotropic effects, such as β-blockers and calcium channel blockers, should be avoided. Treatment with digoxin and the careful use of diuretics may be indicated to stabilize a patient with heart failure before valve replacement. Vasodilators are relatively contraindicated. Cardiogenic shock caused by aortic stenosis should be managed with dobutamine for inotropic support, intraaortic balloon counterpulsation if necessary, and urgent mechanical relief of aortic stenosis.

When to Refer

The patient should be referred to a cardiologist for consideration of cardiac catheterization if cardiac symptoms are present and there is clinical or echocardiographic evidence of at least moderately severe aortic stenosis. In patients with cardiac symptoms and only mild aortic stenosis, cardiology consultation may be helpful for diagnosing concomitant cardiac conditions, such as coronary artery disease or excessive left ventricular hypertrophy. Cardiology referral should also be considered, even in the absence of symptoms, if aortic stenosis is severe, so that the cardiologist may participate in the decision regarding the timing of surgery.

At cardiac catheterization, the peak-to-peak and mean aortic valve gradients are usually estimated from a catheter advanced in retrograde fashion across the stenotic valve and another in a peripheral (*eg*, femoral) artery. Valve area is calculated from the mean gradient and cardiac output by means of the Gorlin equation. The normal aortic valve area is 3 to 4 cm^2; symptoms do not occur until the valve area decreases to less than 1.0 cm^2. Surgery for aortic stenosis is generally indicated for symptomatic patients with a mean gradient of 40 mm Hg or greater and an aortic valve area of 0.8 cm^2 or less. Patients with low cardiac output, low gradient, and low calculated valve area present a thorny management problem that is beyond the scope of this chapter [15]. Right-side heart catheterization and—if indicated and considered safe—left ventriculography are also performed. If it is necessary to assess the severity of coexisting aortic regurgitation, supravalvular aortography is performed. Because much information may be obtained from a technically optimal echocardiogram, the principal indication for cardiac catheterization in adults is to assess the severity of coexisting coronary artery disease by coronary arteriography; this approach is generally deemed necessary in patients older than the age of 40 years and in younger patients with risk factors for atherosclerosis.

Aortic valve replacement is indicated for patients with even mildly symptomatic severe aortic stenosis if they have no major concomitant noncardiac conditions. Coronary bypass grafting is a generally accepted, if unproven, adjunct to valve replacement in patients with coronary artery disease. Advanced age is not in itself a contraindication to surgery because otherwise healthy octogenarians undergo valve replacement with acceptable mortality and morbidity (Fig. 6) [16]. Similarly, even severe left ventricular systolic dysfunction is not a contraindication to valve replacement if the depression of ejection fraction is caused by severe aortic stenosis and not by another condition, such as coronary artery disease, because clinical outcome is almost invariably good and the ejection fraction improves postoperatively in such cases (Fig. 7) [17]. Surgery is sometimes advocated for asymptomatic patients with aortic stenosis if 1) they are young and have very vigorous lifestyles; 2) they have a markedly abnormal response to exercise during formal testing; 3) they have progressive cardiac enlargement or depression of left ventricular ejection fraction; or 4) they have left heart filling pressures that are markedly elevated at rest or with exercise. These indications for valve replacement are not established [18•].

Whereas mechanical valves require life-long anticoagulation therapy with warfarin, bioprosthetic valves degenerate more quickly than mechanical valves, especially in younger patients. For these reasons, young and middle-aged patients usually receive mechanical valves, whereas elderly patients and

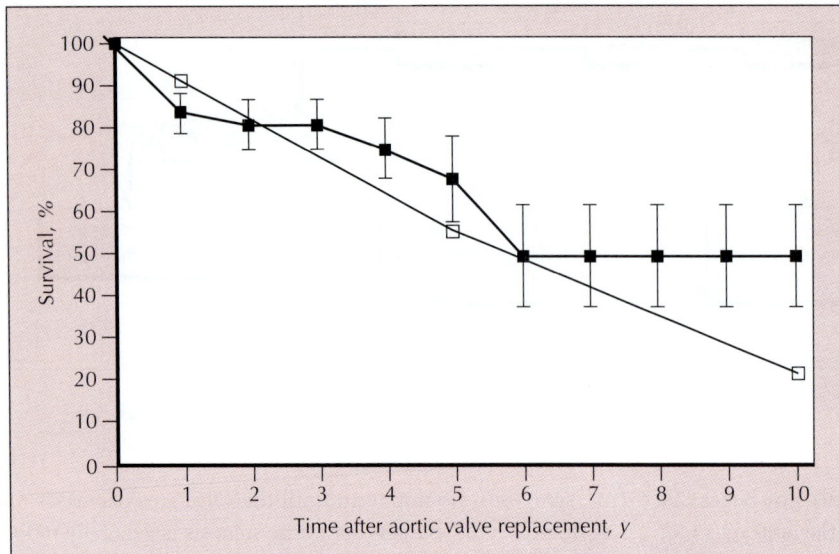

FIGURE 6 Actuarial survival curve for octogenarians undergoing aortic valve replacement for aortic stenosis (*closed squares*). For comparison, actuarial survival curve for unselected 80-year-old persons (*open squares*) from US census data is also shown. (From Levinson and coworkers [16]; with permission).

patients with contraindications to anticoagulation usually receive bioprosthetic valves.

In patients with absolute contraindications to aortic valve replacement (*eg*, metastatic cancer or severe emphysema), percutaneous balloon aortic valvuloplasty may be offered as palliative therapy. Although this technique may provide lasting benefit for young patients with congenital aortic stenosis, it provides only temporary relief for adults with calcific aortic stenosis; restenosis of the valve within 1 year is the rule. Percutaneous aortic valvuloplasty may also have a role as a "bridge" to valve replacement in moribund patients with severe aortic stenosis.

AORTIC REGURGITATION

Etiology and Pathogenesis

Aortic regurgitation may result from diseases causing deformity of the valve leaflets or, alternatively, from diseases causing dilation or distortion of the aortic root, with resultant failure of the leaflets to coapt. This distinction is vital because the causes of aortic regurgitation associated with the two mechanisms differ substantially (Table 2) [2,19]. Like rheumatic aortic stenosis, rheumatic aortic regurgitation is usually accompanied by clinically important rheumatic mitral stenosis or regurgitation, or both. The manifestations of chronic and acute aortic regurgitation are disparate (Table 3) [20•]. With chronic aortic regurgitation, there is a gradual and marked increase in left ventricular end-diastolic volume. Left ventricular distensibility is increased, such that there is only a modest increase in end-diastolic pressure. Total left ventricular stroke volume increases, forward stroke volume (total stroke volume minus the volume regurgitated across the aortic valve back into the ventricle) is maintained, ejection fraction is initially normal, and heart rate does not increase markedly. Aortic systolic pressure is high, diastolic pressure is low, and pulse pressure is wide. With long-standing volume overload of the ventricle, there is an eventual loss of myocardial contractility, with consequent increase in end-systolic volume and decrease in ejection fraction. The loss of myocardial contractility may be irreversible. In acute aortic regurgitation (as caused by endocarditis or aortic dissection), regurgitation into an unprepared left ventricle results in a marked increase in end-diastolic pressure, which is transmitted backward to the left

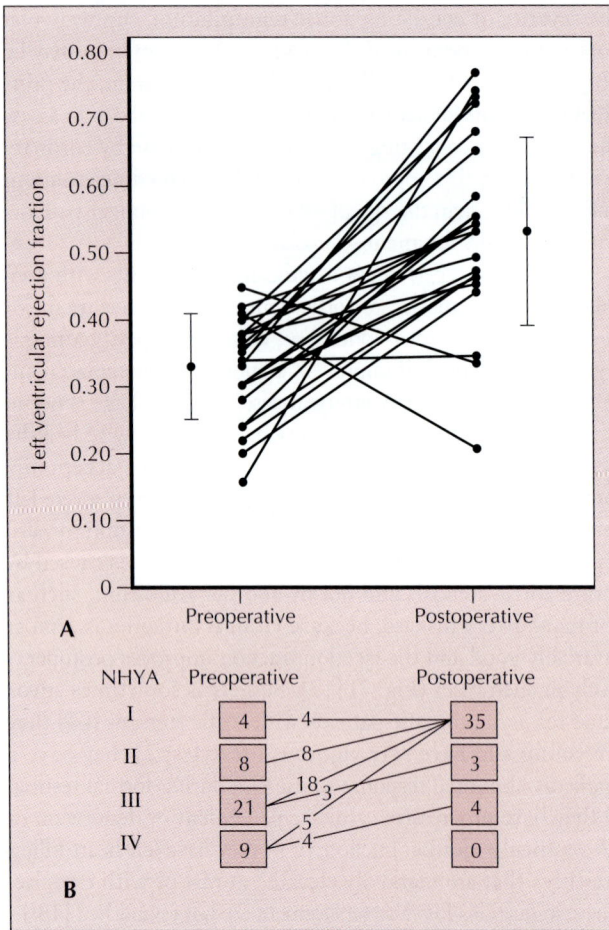

FIGURE 7 Change in **A**, New York Heart Association (NYHA) class and **B**, left ventricular ejection fraction after aortic valve replacement for aortic stenosis in patients with low preoperative ejection fraction and no significant associated cardiac abnormalities. (*From* Rediker and coworkers [17]; with permission.)

Table 2 Causes of aortic regurgitation

Diseases causing deformity of aortic valve leaflets	Diseases causing dilation or dissection of aortic root
Congenitally bicuspid valve	Idiopathic (annuloaortic ectasia)
Rheumatic fever	Aortic dissection
Endocarditis	Chronic, severe hypertension
Trauma	Inflammatory diseases (*eg*, ankylosing spondylitis)
Myxomatous ("floppy") valve with prolapse	Connective tissue diseases (*eg*, Marfan syndrome)
Inflammatory diseases (*eg*, systemic lupus erythematosus)	Syphilitic aortitis
	Nonspecific aortitis

atrium and pulmonary circulation, resulting in pulmonary congestion. Total left ventricular stroke volume increases minimally, forward stroke volume falls, and there is compensatory tachycardia in an attempt to maintain cardiac output. Prominent widening of the pulse pressure (and the corresponding physical signs of chronic aortic regurgitation; see the following paragraphs) is absent. The manifestations of aortic regurgitation described in the following paragraphs are of the chronic form unless otherwise noted.

Evaluation

Patients with chronic aortic regurgitation may have no symptoms until left ventricular contractile dysfunction and marked cardiomegaly are apparent. The most common symptoms are those of left-side heart failure: dyspnea on exertion, orthopnea, paroxysmal nocturnal dyspnea, and fatigue. Angina is much less common than that in aortic stenosis but may be caused by increased myocardial oxygen demand associated with hypertrophy in the face of a decreased supply associated with low perfusion (aortic diastolic) pressure. Syncope is rare. Prominent neck pulsations may be noted by the patient, and the high stroke volume may be experienced as uncomfortable palpitations, especially when the patient lies down. Patients with acute aortic regurgitation may have severe dyspnea, weakness, hypotension, and cardiovascular collapse.

In cases of severe chronic aortic regurgitation, the aortic diastolic pressure is usually 60 mm Hg or less. The pulse pressure (which should be measured by the physician) is wide, with muffled sounds continuing to a pressure as low as 0 mm Hg; in such cases, the aortic diastolic pressure correlates best with the onset of muffled (phase IV) Korotkoff sounds. The wide pulse pressure manifests as various peripheral signs, such as Corrigan's pulse (rapid rise and collapse), Quincke's pulse (flushing and blanching of the capillary bed in the fingertips, seen by transmitting a light through the fingers), Duroziez's sign (systolic and diastolic murmurs over a femoral artery lightly compressed by the stethoscope), and "pistol shot" systolic sounds over the femoral artery. The peripheral arterial pulsation may be bisferiens.

The left ventricular impulse is displaced downward and leftward. An S_3 may indicate left ventricular systolic dysfunction [21] or merely left ventricular dilation [9]. A systolic murmur is usually present and reflects the increased total stroke volume traversing the left ventricular outflow tract. A relatively soft, high-pitched, blowing decrescendo diastolic murmur is best heard with the diaphragm of the stethoscope in held expiration with the patient sitting up and leaning forward. It is typically heard at the mid or lower left sternal border in primary valve disease; auscultation predominantly at the right upper sternal border suggests root disease. The

Table 3 Chronic versus acute aortic regurgitation

	Chronic	Acute
Symptoms	Often none; exertional dyspnea, orthopnea, paroxysmal nocturnal dyspnea	Dyspnea, often severe and at rest; weakness
Appearance	Often normal	Dyspneic, pale, diaphoretic
Heart rate	Normal	Fast
Pulse pressure	Wide	Normal or slightly widened
Peripheral signs of aortic regurgitation	Present	Absent
Left ventricular impulse	Heaving, displaced laterally and inferiorly	Normal
Murmur	Long	Short
Left ventricular hypertrophy on electrocardiogram	Present	Absent
Cardiomegaly on chest roentgenography	Present	Absent
Pulmonary congestion on chest roentgenography	Absent	Present
Pulmonary capillary wedge pressure	Normal or mildly elevated	Markedly elevated

Aortic Stenosis and Regurgitation

length of the murmur correlates with the severity of regurgitation, except in acute aortic regurgitation. Aortic regurgitation may cause a mid and late diastolic rumble at the apex (Austin-Flint murmur), which is distinguished from the murmur of mitral stenosis by the absence of an opening snap and of a loud S_1. In acute aortic regurgitation, there is tachycardia, peripheral vasoconstriction, normal pulse pressure without the peripheral signs of chronic aortic regurgitation, a normal left ventricular impulse, and a short, relatively soft diastolic murmur.

The electrocardiogram shows left ventricular hypertrophy in most patients with chronic aortic regurgitation but not in patients with acute aortic regurgitation. ST-segment and T-wave abnormalities, left atrial abnormality, left axis deviation, or left bundle branch block may be present. Chest roentgenogram shows left ventricular enlargement. The ascending aorta is dilated, markedly so if root disease is the cause of regurgitation. Acute aortic regurgitation produces a roentgenogram characterized by pulmonary edema with normal heart size.

The echocardiogram (Figs. 3 and 8) images both the valve leaflets and the aortic root and is the most useful test, invasive or noninvasive, for determining the cause of regurgitation. Valve abnormalities that may be detected include thickening of cusps, prolapsed or flail leaflets, and vegetations. Transthoracic and, in particular, transesophageal echocardiography are useful for detecting proximal aortic dissection. The echocardiogram may be used for serially assessing left ventricular size and systolic function, which are critical for determining the timing of aortic valve replacement in asymptomatic or minimally symptomatic patients. Doppler echocardiography is so sensitive for detecting valvular regurgitation that it generates "false positives"; a useful rule is that if aortic regurgitation is not discernible by careful cardiac auscultation (see the preceding paragraphs), then it is not responsible for symptoms. Doppler echocardiography is moderately useful for grading the severity of regurgitation. Radionuclide ventriculography provides the ratio of stroke volume ejected by the left ventricle to that ejected by the right ventricle, a useful estimate of the severity of aortic regurgitation in the absence of shunts or other regurgitant lesions. Failure of the ejection fraction to increase during exercise has been proposed as a test of left ventricular reserve in patients with aortic regurgitation, but the validity of this criterion for determining the timing of aortic valve surgery has not been established.

Management

Like patients with aortic stenosis, patients with aortic regurgitation may be asymptomatic for many years. Sudden death may occur, but it is rare in asymptomatic patients [10,22•]. Although low left ventricular ejection fraction in aortic stenosis is usually reversed with relief of afterload excess by valve replacement, low ejection fraction in aortic regurgitation often reflects irreversible loss of myocardial contractility.

The work-up of aortic regurgitation includes carefully questioning the patient for symptoms of heart failure, inquiring into the cause of regurgitation, and meticulously assessing left ventricular systolic function. When indicated on clinical grounds or by echocardiography, the erythrocyte sedimentation rate for inflammatory disease, serology for syphilis, and blood cultures for endocarditis should be obtained. The patient should be evaluated clinically every 3 to 6 months, and left ventricular systolic function should be assessed by echocardiography or radionuclide ventriculography (one or the other should be performed consistently, rather than switching from one to the other) every 6 to 12 months. The management of chronic aortic regurgitation is shown schematically in Figure 9.

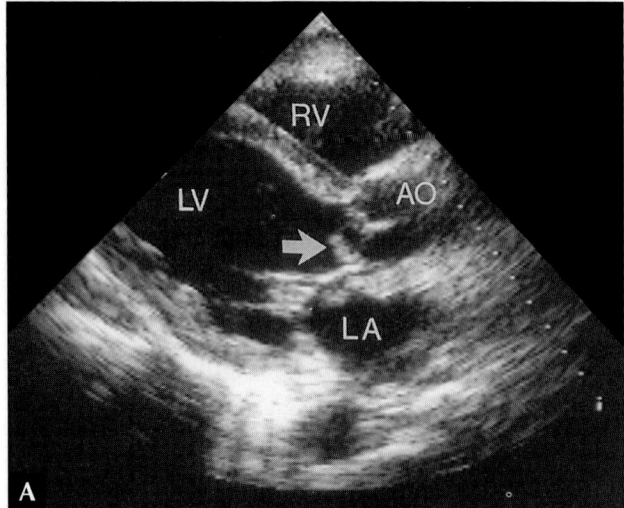 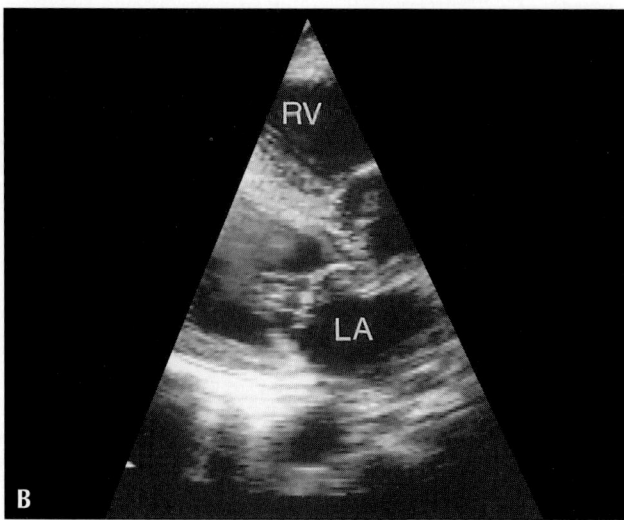

FIGURE 8 Two-dimensional echocardiogram **A**, without and **B**, with a superimposed color Doppler signal from a 49-year-old man with severe aortic regurgitation and an aortic root abscess. The right ventricle (RV), left atrium (LA), left ventricle (LV), and aorta (AO) are shown. The left ventricle is dilated. One aortic valve leaflet visualized in end-diastolic frame is in the normal position in the aorta, but the other (*arrow*) has prolapsed into the left ventricular outflow tract. The thickened area between the aorta and the left atrium is the abscess. The light blue color Doppler signal depicts the jet of regurgitation through the aortic valve into the left ventricle (*see* Color Plate). (Courtesy of Michael H. Picard, MD.)

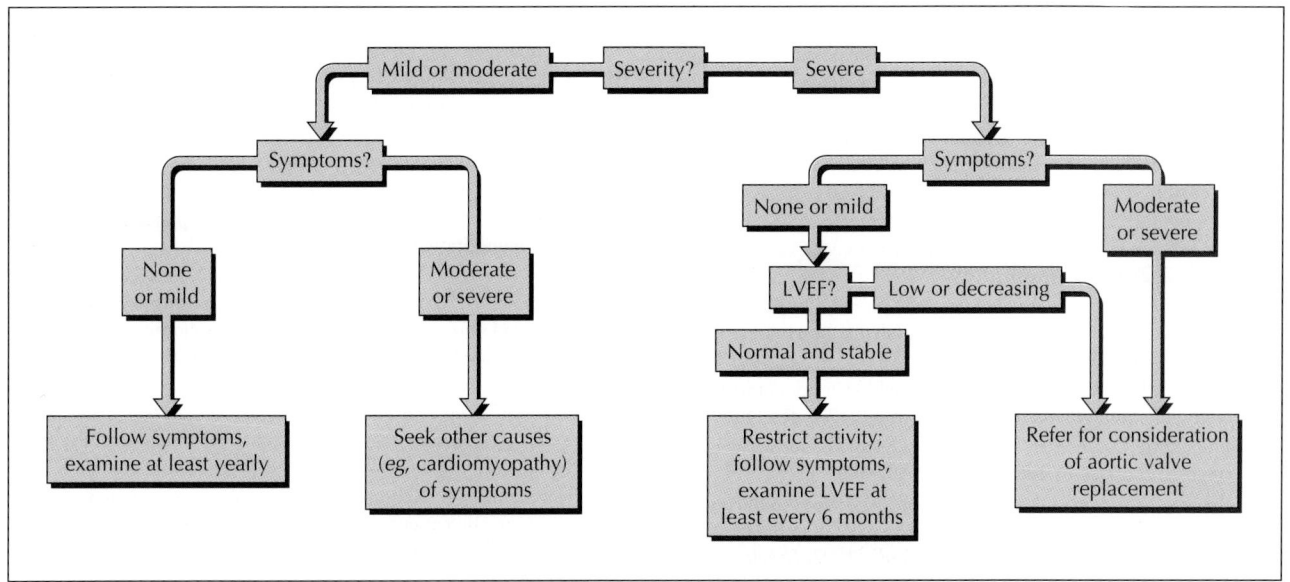

FIGURE 9 Management of aortic regurgitation. Serial left ventricular ejection fraction (LVEF) determinations for an individual patient should be obtained consistently from either echocardiography or radionuclide ventriculography.

Patients with asymptomatic but severe aortic regurgitation should avoid heavy exertion, including competitive sports. Systolic hypertension should be treated, usually with an angiotensin-converting enzyme inhibitor. Long-term therapy with vasodilators (hydralazine, 3 mg/kg/d [23], or enalpril, 20 mg bid [24]) reduces left ventricular volume. It has recently been reported that treatment with nifedipine, 20 mg bid, delays the need for aortic valve replacement [25]. Endocarditis prophylaxis is necessary. Digoxin, diuretics, and vasodilators are indicated for symptomatic patients with contraindications to cardiac surgery or in preparation for surgery. Drug therapy for acute aortic regurgitation includes diuretics, oral and intravenous vasodilators (in particular, afterload reduction with drugs such as nitroprusside), and, as indicated, inotropic support (usually with dobutamine). Urgent or emergency aortic valve surgery, even with active endocarditis, may be lifesaving. Intra-aortic balloon counterpulsation is not useful because inflation of the balloon in diastole worsens regurgitation across the aortic valve.

When to Refer

Patients should be referred to a cardiologist if they have symptoms or signs of heart failure and aortic regurgitation is evident on physical examination. Asymptomatic patients with aortic regurgitation should be promptly referred if left ventricular ejection fraction is low or in the low-normal range or if serial noninvasive studies indicate that it is decreasing over time.

The definitive test for grading aortic regurgitation is supravalvular aortography performed as part of cardiac catheterization. The regurgitant fraction, derived from a comparison of total (angiographic) and forward (*eg*, thermodilution) left ventricular stroke volume, is fraught with error and is a less useful index of the severity of regurgitation. Right-side heart catheterization, left ventriculography, and—for patients older than 40 years of age or for younger patients with atherosclerosis risk factors—coronary arteriography are also performed.

If there is no noncardiac contraindication, surgery is performed if aortic regurgitation is severe and symptoms are more than minimal. Surgery should be strongly considered for asymptomatic or minimally symptomatic patients if left ventricular ejection fraction is mildly or moderately impaired, if there is a decline in left ventricular ejection fraction within the normal range, or if there is very marked left ventricular dilation [22•]. Patients with severe depression of ejection fraction may not benefit from valve surgery.

The usual operation for valve disease is aortic valve replacement, although a minority of patients are successfully treated with valve repair. The considerations regarding type of valve prosthesis are similar to those for surgery for aortic stenosis. Patients with root disease require aortic repair, usually accompanied by valve replacement, often with a composite graft.

References and Recommended Reading

Recently published papers of particular interest have been highlighted as:
- Of interest
- •• Of outstanding interest

1. Lindroos M, Kupari M, Heikkila J: Prevalence of aortic valve abnormalities in the elderly: an echocardiographic study of a random population sample. *J Am Coll Cardiol* 1993, 21:1220–1225.
2. Olson LT, Subramanian R, Edwards WD: Surgical pathology of pure aortic insuffficiency: a study of 225 cases. *Mayo Clin Proc* 1984, 59:835–841.
3. Subramanian R, Olson LJ, Edwards WD: Surgical pathology of pure aortic stenosis: a study of 374 cases. *Mayo Clin Proc* 1984, 59:683–690.
4. Fenoglio JJ, McAllister HA, DeCastro CM, *et al.*: Congenital bicuspid aortic valve after age 20. *Am J Cardiol* 1977, 39:164–169.

5. Selzer A: Changing aspects of the natural history of valvular aortic stenosis. *N Engl J Med* 1987, 317:91–98.

6. King RM, Pluth JR, Giuliani ER: The association of unexplained gastrointestinal bleeding with calcific aortic stenosis. *Ann Thorac Surg* 1987, 44:514–516.

7. Levinson GE: Aortic stenosis. In *Valvular Heart Disease*, edn 2. Edited by Dalen JE, Alpert JS. Boston: Little, Brown and Company; 1987:197–282.

8. Lombard JT, Selzer A: Valvular aortic stenosis: a clinical and hemodynamic profile of patients. *Ann Intern Med* 1987, 106:292–298.

9. Folland ED, Kriegel BJ, Henderson WG, *et al*.: Implications of third heart sounds in patients with valvular heart disease. *N Engl J Med* 1992, 327:458–462.

10. Turina J, Hess O, Sepulci F, Krayenbuehl HP: Spontaneous course of aortic valve disease. *Eur Heart J* 1987, 8:471–483.

11.• Horstkotte D, Loogen F: The natural history of aortic valve stenosis. *Eur Heart J* 1988, 9(suppl E):57–64.

12. Aronow WS, Ahn C, Kronzon I, Nanna M: Prognosis of congestive heart failure in patients aged ≥ 62 years with unoperated severe valvular aortic stenosis. *Am J Cardiol* 1993, 72:846–848.

13.• Pellikka PA, Nishimura RA, Bailey KR, Tajik AJ: The natural history of adults with asymptomatic, hemodynamically significant aortic stenosis. *J Am Coll Cardiol* 1990, 15:1012–1017.

14. O'Keefe JH, Shub C, Rettke SR: Risk of noncardiac surgical procedures in patients with aortic stenosis. *Mayo Clin Proc* 1989, 64:400–405.

15. Carabello BA: Advances in the hemodynamic assessment of stenotic cardiac valves. *J Am Coll Cardiol* 1987, 10:912–919.

16. Levinson JR, Akins CW, Buckley MJ, *et al*.: Octogenarians with aortic stenosis: outcome following aortic valve replacement. *Circulation* 1989, 80(suppl I):I-49–I-56.

17. Rediker DE, Boucher CA, Block PC, *et al*.: Degree of reversibility of left ventricular systolic dysfunction after aortic valve replacement for isolated aortic stenosis. *Am J Cardiol* 1987, 60:112–118.

18.• Braunwald E: On the natural history of severe aortic stenosis. *J Am Coll Cardiol* 1990, 15:1018–1020.

19. Guiney TE, Davies MJ, Leech GJ, Leatham A: The aetiology and course of isolated severe aortic regurgitation: a clinical, pathological, and echocardiographic study. *Br Heart J* 1987, 58:358–368.

20.• Morganroth JM, Perloff JK, Zeldis SM, Dunkman WB: Acute severe aortic regurgitation: pathophysiology, clinical recognition, and management. *Ann Intern Med* 1977, 87:223–232.

21. Abdulla AM, Frank MJ, Erdin RAJ, Canedo MI: Clinical significance and hemodynamic correlates of the third heart sound gallop in aortic regurgitation: a guide to optimal timing of cardiac catheterization. *Circulation* 1981, 64:464–471.

22.• Bonow RO, Lakatos E, Maron BJ, *et al*.: Serial long-term assessment of the natural history of asymptomatic patients with chronic aortic regurgitation and normal left ventricular systolic function. *Circulation* 1991, 84:1625–1635.

23. Greenberg B, Massie B, Bristow JD, *et al*.: Long-term vasodilator therapy of chronic aortic insufficiency: a randomized double-blinded, placebo-controlled clinical trial. *Circulation* 1988, 78:92–103.

24. Lin M, Chiang H, Lin S, *et al*.: Vasodilator therapy in chronic asymptomatic aortic regurgitation: enalapril versus hydralazine therapy. *J Am Coll Cardiol* 1994, 24:1046–1053.

25. Scognamiglio R, Rahimtoola SH, Fasoli G, *et al*.: Nifedipine in asymptomatic patients with severe aortic regurgitation and normal left ventricular function. *N Engl J Med* 1994, 331:689–694.

26. Sutton GC, Fox KM: *A Color Atlas of Heart Disease: Pathological, Clinical and Investigatory Aspects*. London: Current Medical Literature; 1990:136–137.

27. Ross J Jr, Braunwald E: Aortic stenosis. *Circulation* 1968, 37(suppl V):V-61–V-67.

SELECT BIBLIOGRAPHY

Braunwald E: Valvular heart disease. In *Heart Disease*, edn 4. Edited by Braunwald E. Philadelphia: WB Saunders Company; 1992:1035–1053.

Rahimtoola SH: Perspective on valvular heart disease: an update. *J Am Coll Cardiol* 1989, 14:1–23.

Waller BF, Howard J, Fess S: Pathology of aortic valve stenosis and pure aortic regurgitation: a clinical morphologic assessment—Parts I and II. *Clin Cardiol* 1994, 17:85–92, 150–156.

Tricuspid and Pulmonic Valve Disease

D. Brent Glamann
Mark J. Pirwitz
L. David Hillis

> ### Key Points
> - Congenital anomalies of the tricuspid and pulmonic valves constitute 10% to 15% of all congenital heart disease.
> - Pulmonic stenosis is the most common congenital right-sided valvular abnormality and is effectively treated by balloon valvuloplasty.
> - Pulmonic regurgitation usually results from pulmonary arterial hypertension, and its prognosis is largely determined by the underlying disease process.
> - Tricuspid stenosis is nearly always caused by rheumatic disease and is never seen without concomitant mitral or aortic involvement.
> - Tricuspid regurgitation (TR) usually results from right ventricular dilatation; patients with TR present with right-sided heart failure.

The tricuspid and pulmonic valves are often overlooked during evaluation of suspected cardiac disease. This is particularly true in the United States, where the incidence of rheumatic valvular disease has declined and other disease processes involving the right-sided valves (*eg*, infective endocarditis in intravenous drug abusers) have increased in frequency.

TRICUSPID VALVE DISEASE

Congenital

Congenital anomalies of the tricuspid valve are uncommon, accounting for only 1% to 3% of congenital heart disease. Only tricuspid atresia and Ebstein's anomaly are of clinical importance, and almost all patients with tricuspid atresia are diagnosed and surgically corrected in infancy or early childhood.

In Ebstein's anomaly, the septal and inferior tricuspid valve leaflets are displaced away from the tricuspid annulus into the right ventricle. The anterior leaflet retains its normal attachment to the atrioventricular groove and is typically large and redundant. The displacement of the valve apparatus divides the right ventricle into 1) an inlet portion, which is functionally part of the right atrium (the so-called *atrialized* portion) and 2) a distal, functionally small right ventricular chamber. Associated anomalies include an interatrial communication (atrial septal defect or patent foramen ovale) in 50% to 75% of cases, ventricular septal defect, pulmonary stenosis, and mitral valve prolapse [1]. In addition, as many as 25% of patients with Ebstein's anomaly have ventricular preexcitation, most commonly via a right-sided accessory atrioventricular pathway [2].

Most patients with Ebstein's anomaly survive to adulthood, and an occasional patient lives into the seventh or eighth decade. The patient is often asymptomatic until the third or fourth decade, when dyspnea, fatigue, or cyanosis appear insidiously. In 15% to 20% of cases, sudden cardiac death caused by tachydysrhythmias

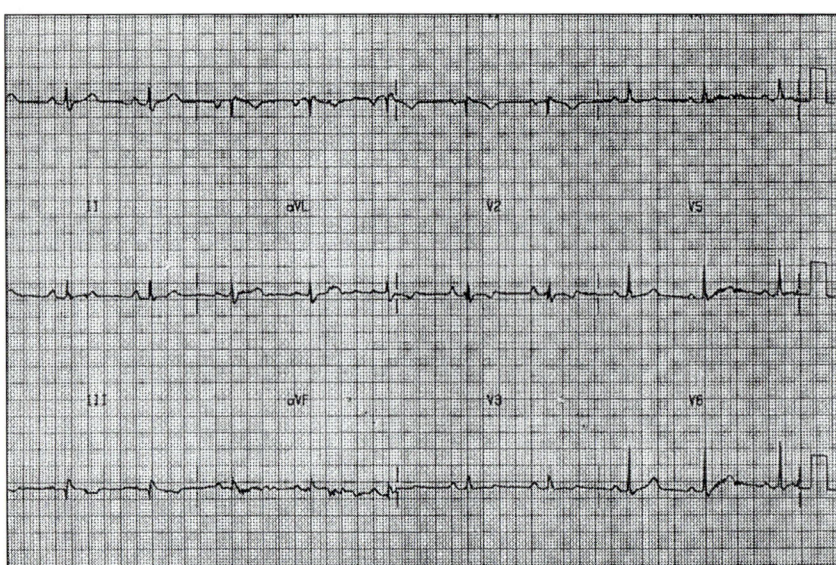

FIGURE 1 Electrocardiogram from a patient with Ebstein's anomaly demonstrating a prolonged PR interval, peaked P waves, and an incomplete right bundle-branch block.

may be the presenting manifestation. The onset of right heart failure portends a poor prognosis and is the most common cause of death.

On physical examination, the arterial and jugular venous pulses are usually normal, although regurgitant V waves are not uncommon. The right ventricular impulse is typically absent. The first heart sound (S_1) is usually loud and widely split, as is the second heart sound (S_2), and multiple systolic clicks as well as right-sided gallops may be heard. A murmur of tricuspid regurgitation is invariably present at the left lower sternal border and characteristically increases with inspiration. A scratchy, diastolic murmur that may be confused with a pericardial friction rub is commonly present as well.

The electrocardiogram (ECG) usually reveals normal sinus rhythm, although supraventricular arrhythmias are not uncommon. Tall and peaked P waves, a prolonged PR interval, and a complete or incomplete right bundle-branch block are common (Fig. 1). Chest radiography usually demonstrates globular cardiomegaly caused by the enlarged right atrium. Echocardiography is extremely valuable in identifying the anatomic relationship between the tricuspid valve apparatus and right heart chambers as well as in assessing right ventricular function, tricuspid regurgitation, and intracardiac shunting [3]. Finally, the diagnosis of Ebstein's anomaly may be made at catheterization by recording a simultaneous intracardiac pressure and electrogram with a single catheter. When this catheter is withdrawn from the right ventricle to the right atrium, a right ventricular electrical potential continues to be recorded after the pressure contour has changed to a right atrial waveform. In addition, right ventricular angiography is usually diagnostic.

Management of the patient with Ebstein's anomaly is based on the severity of disease. An acyanotic patient with minimal symptoms is managed conservatively, whereas the patient with class III or IV heart failure, a cardiothoracic ratio of 0.65 or higher, severe cyanosis, or paradoxic embolization may benefit from surgical repair [4,5]. Refractory tachydysrhythmias may be treated at the time of surgery.

Acquired

Tricuspid stenosis

Tricuspid stenosis (TS) is uncommon and results almost exclusively from rheumatic scarring; other causes of functional and anatomic TS are listed in Table 1. Hemodynamically insignificant TS occurs in up to 15% of patients with rheumatic heart disease, but is clinically important in only 3% to 5% [6]. Isolated rheumatic TS in the absence of concomitant mitral involvement, aortic involvement, or both is extremely rare. As with rheumatic mitral stenosis, rheumatic TS is more common in young or middle-aged women.

TABLE 1 CAUSES OF FUNCTIONAL OR ANATOMIC TRICUSPID STENOSIS
Tricuspid valve vegetations
Tumor (myxoma, leiomyoma, metastatic melanoma)
Thrombus (ball valve)
Carcinoid syndrome
Löffler's endocarditis
Postsurgical (following tricuspid annuloplasty)
Constrictive pericarditis
Methysergide

TABLE 2 SYMPTOMS OF TRICUSPID STENOSIS
Easy fatigability (because of reduced cardiac output)
Right upper quadrant abdominal discomfort (because of hepatic congestion)
Anorexia, nausea, vomiting, and eructation (because of passive congestion of the gastrointestinal tract)
Syncope/near syncope
Periodic cyanosis (because of right-to-left intracardiac shunting through a patent foramen ovale)
Vague retrosternal chest discomfort

TABLE 3 COMPARISON OF AUSCULTATORY FEATURES IN MITRAL AND TRICUSPID STENOSIS		
	Mitral stenosis	Tricuspid stenosis
Location	Apex	Left lower sternal border
Quality	Rumbling	Rumbling
Intensity	Louder	Softer
Pitch	Lower	Higher
Timing	Mid-diastole	Mid-diastole
Duration	Longer	Shorter
Opening snap	Earlier	Later and increases with inspiration

Patients with TS usually have symptoms related to their predominant left-sided valvular abnormality. Indeed, the absence of pulmonary congestion in a patient with severe mitral stenosis should raise the suspicion of concomitant TS. Symptoms that are primarily related to TS result from peripheral venous congestion or a reduced cardiac output (Table 2).

On physical examination, the patient with TS has jugular venous distention with prominent A waves and hepatojugular reflux. Hepatomegaly with presystolic pulsation, ascites, peripheral edema, and pleural effusions are common, and in some subjects, mild scleral icterus or cyanosis may be present. The auscultatory findings are usually dominated by concomitant left-sided disease. S_1 is increased in intensity, as is the pulmonic component of S_2 (because of pulmonary hypertension induced by left-sided valvular disease). The murmur of TS may be confused with that of mitral stenosis, but careful auscultation can usually distinguish them (Table 3).

Electrocardiographically, the patient with TS usually has right atrial enlargement, with tall, peaked P waves in standard lead II. The PR interval is often slightly prolonged, and ECG evidence of mitral stenosis is often present. Atrial fibrillation is common, although some patients remain in sinus rhythm even with severe mitral stenosis. On chest radiography, the patient has right atrial enlargement with rightward displacement of the right lower cardiac contour. Coexisting left atrial enlargement (because of mitral stenosis) may produce concentric contours on the right side of the cardiac silhouette. Tricuspid valve calcification, which may be identified on the lateral chest film, is difficult to distinguish from mitral valve calcification. Echocardiography and Doppler ultrasound provide a qualitative assessment of the severity of TS, but the echocardiographic assessment of tricuspid leaflet dynamics has limitations [7]. Assessment of the severity of TS is best done by catheterization, where right atrial and ventricular pressures are recorded simultaneously (Fig. 2). A mean diastolic gradient across the tricuspid valve of 2 to 3 mm Hg is suggestive of TS, but gradients as high as 5 mm Hg have been reported in patients with predominant tricuspid regurgitation. Provocative maneuvers during catheterization (*eg*, deep inspiration, exercise, volume infusion) may magnify a small resting gradient.

The patient with isolated TS may be asymptomatic for years. Once symptoms develop, sodium restriction and diuretics are effective in relieving peripheral venous congestion. Once medically refractory symptoms develop, tricuspid balloon valvuloplasty with a mobile valve having an orifice area of 3.0 cm^2 or less may be considered. If the valve is unsuitable for valvuloplasty or the orifice area is 1.5 cm^2 or less, surgical commissurotomy or valve replacement should be recommended. If valve replacement is required, a bioprosthesis is preferable because of 1) its proven durability in the tricuspid position and 2) the increased risk of a thromboembolic complication with a mechanical prosthesis in this position [8,9]. If a mechanical prosthesis is necessary, a St. Jude valve should be used [10].

Tricuspid regurgitation

Tricuspid regurgitation (TR) may be functional or organic. Functional TR is more common than organic TR and results from right ventricular dilatation, which in turn may result from pulmonary hypertension of any cause, right ventricular outflow obstruction (valvar, supravalvar, or infundibular), right ventricular infarction, or dilated cardiomyopathy. Organic TR

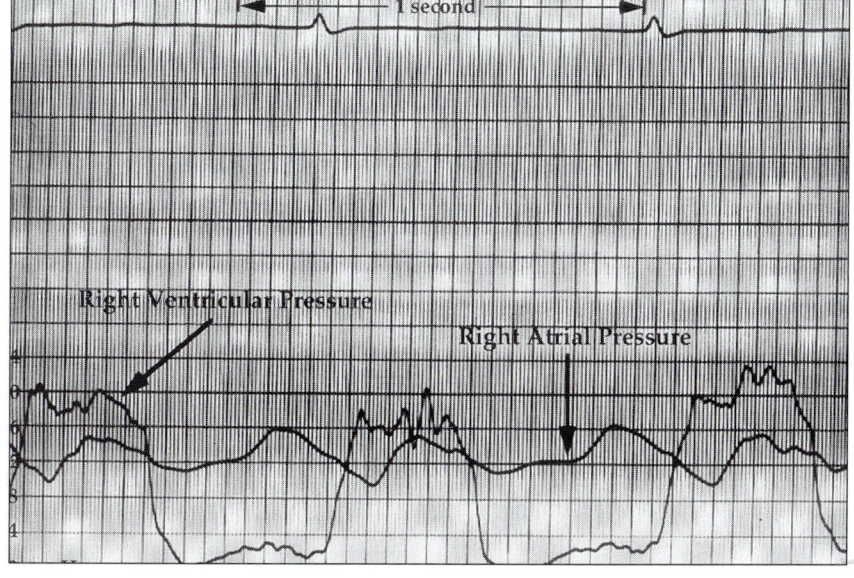

FIGURE 2 Simultaneous right atrial and ventricular pressure tracings in a patient with tricuspid stenosis. There is a gradient of 11 mm Hg across the tricuspid valve during diastole.

TABLE 4 CAUSES OF ORGANIC TRICUSPID REGURGITATION
Rheumatic
Infective endocarditis
Ebstein's anomaly
Right ventricular papillary muscle dysfunction
Myxomatous degeneration
Carcinoid syndrome
Trauma
Tricuspid valve prolapse
Connective tissue disorders (rheumatoid arthritis, systemic lupus erythematosus, Marfan syndrome)
Right atrial myxoma
Methysergide
Endomyocardial fibrosis
Thyrotoxicosis

may result from a variety of disease processes (Table 4). Recently, TR caused by infective endocarditis has appeared with increasing frequency, most commonly in intravenous drug abusers. The causative organism is usually *Staphylococcus aureus*. Fortunately, most of these patients respond to medical therapy and have a better prognosis than those with left-sided endocarditis. Vegetation size may be an important predictor of outcome, in that a patient with a vegetation greater than 2.0 cm in diameter has an increased mortality [11•]. Organic TR is generally well tolerated in the absence of elevated right ventricular systolic pressure; indeed, the surgical procedure of choice in the patient with right-sided endocarditis refractory to medical therapy is tricuspid or pulmonic valve excision *without* replacement [12].

Symptoms of TR are similar to those of tricuspid stenosis. On physical examination, the patient usually has distended neck veins with prominent V waves, hepatomegaly that may be pulsatile, ascites, and peripheral edema. Cardiac examination may reveal a seesaw motion of the anterior chest wall and rightward displacement of the right heart border. On auscultation, S_1 is typically diminished, and the pulmonic component of S_2 may be prominent in the presence of pulmonary hypertension. A holosystolic murmur is present at the left lower sternal border and characteristically increases in intensity with inspiration (Carvallo sign). In addition, a right ventricular gallop (S_3) and a diastolic rumble ("relative" tricuspid stenosis) may be audible.

Common ECG features include right-axis deviation, right-atrial enlargement, and right ventricular hypertrophy. Chest radiography reveals right atrial and right ventricular enlargement. Two-dimensional echocardiography with Doppler color-flow mapping is useful for detecting TR and estimating right ventricular peak-systolic pressure, but it is limited in its ability to quantitate the magnitude of regurgitation [13]. Some degree of TR is detected in up to 83% of normal subjects using Doppler color-flow mapping [14,15]. At cardiac catheterization, right atrial and right ventricular diastolic pressures are elevated. A right ventricular systolic pressure greater than 60 mm Hg suggests a functional etiology of TR, whereas a systolic pressure less than 40 mm Hg implies organic disease. Although right ventricular angiography will demonstrate regurgitation of contrast material into the right atrium, quantitation of TR by this method is imprecise.

Treatment of functional TR is directed at the underlying disease process. In the absence of pulmonary hypertension, TR usually does not require surgical treatment; when surgical therapy is necessary, tricuspid annuloplasty with (Carpentier) or without (De Vega) a prosthetic ring may be performed [16]. When valve replacement is indicated, a bioprosthesis (preferably a large, porcine heterograft) should be inserted for reasons outlined previously. If surgery is not feasible, medical therapy with sodium restriction, digoxin, and diuretics should be employed.

PULMONIC VALVE DISEASE

Congenital

Valvular pulmonic stenosis (PS) is a congenital abnormality in almost all patients and constitutes 10% to 12% of congenital heart disease. Acquired PS is exceedingly rare but may result from rheumatic scarring, infective endocarditis, trauma, malignant carcinoid syndrome, cardiac tumors, or an aneurysm of a sinus of Valsalva.

The patient with PS is frequently asymptomatic. He or she eventually may note exertional dyspnea, fatigue, syncope, or anterior chest pain, and peripheral edema and other evidence of peripheral venous congestion may develop if right ventricular decompensation occurs. If the foramen ovale is patent, intermittent or continuous right-to-left intracardiac shunting with resultant clubbing or cyanosis may occur.

On physical examination, the patient may have evidence of right ventricular failure (peripheral edema, hepatomegaly, jugular venous distention), right ventricular lift at the left sternal border, and a systolic thrill over the pulmonic area (second left intercostal space). On auscultation, S_1 is normal, and S_2 is widely split but moves with respiration. The pulmonic component is soft and markedly delayed. A harsh, crescendo–decrescendo systolic murmur is audible along the left sternal border and loudest over the pulmonic area. An ejection click that softens or even disappears with inspiration may be heard at the pulmonic area. As the severity of stenosis increases, the murmur peaks later in systole, and the ejection click moves closer to or even blends with S_1.

The ECG may reveal right-axis deviation, right ventricular hypertrophy, right atrial enlargement, and complete or incomplete right bundle-branch block (Fig. 3). Chest radiography demonstrates diminished pulmonary vascular markings and a markedly dilated main pulmonary artery. Mild to massive cardiomegaly may be present. Two-dimensional echocardiography with Doppler ultrasound is useful to visualize the pulmonic valve, to assess the severity of stenosis, and to identify coexisting anomalies [17]. Cardiac catheterization demonstrates a pressure gradient during systole

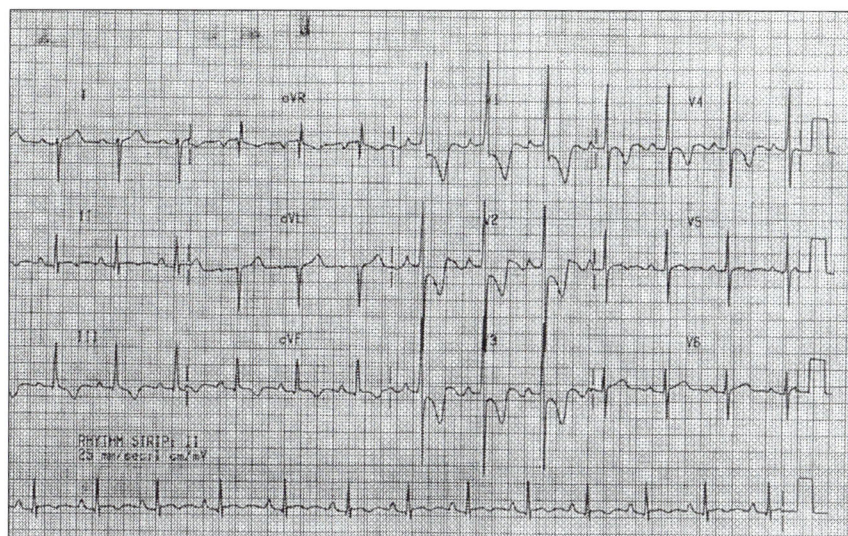

FIGURE 3 Electrocardiogram from a patient with congenital pulmonic stenosis showing right-axis deviation, right atrial enlargement, and right ventricular

between the right ventricle and pulmonary artery. The severity of PS is quantitated according to the right ventricular peak-systolic pressure (Table 5).

Many adults with mild or moderate PS are asymptomatic and require no treatment. Surgical valvotomy, balloon valvuloplasty, or (rarely) valve replacement is warranted for the indications outlined in Table 6. Balloon valvuloplasty is currently the procedure of choice for relief of valvular PS; its results are excellent and comparable to surgical valvotomy [18,19•].

Acquired

Similar to TR, acquired pulmonic regurgitation (PR) may be functional or organic. Functional PR usually results from pulmonary arterial hypertension, regardless of etiology. Rarely, it occurs with idiopathic dilatation of the pulmonary artery [20]. Organic PR is relatively rare; it may occur with infective endocarditis, rheumatic scarring, chest trauma, carcinoid syndrome, syphilis, or following balloon valvuloplasty or surgical valvotomy.

The patient with functional PR presents with symptoms induced by the underlying disease. Organic PR in the absence of pulmonary hypertension may be well tolerated for many years. When severe and long-standing, it may cause symptoms and signs of right ventricular failure.

Cardiac examination may reveal a palpable pulsation over the pulmonic area. On auscultation, S_2 is widely split, with an accentuated pulmonic component. A blowing, decrescendo diastolic murmur is audible in the second and third left intercostal spaces and increases in intensity with inspiration. A systolic ejection murmur caused by increased flow across the pulmonic valve is frequently heard. If right ventricular dilatation and decompensation have occurred, a right-sided S_3 and holosystolic murmur of TR may be present.

The ECG demonstrates right-axis deviation, right ventricular hypertrophy, and possibly right bundle-branch block. Chest radiography shows right ventricular enlargement and dilatation of the pulmonary artery. Echocardiography may reveal right ventricular dilatation, paradoxic motion of the interventricular septum during systole, and occasionally, diastolic fluttering of the tricuspid valve. As with TR, a small amount of PR is seen in most normal subjects (93%) with Doppler color-flow mapping [14]. At cardiac catheterization, right ventricular systolic and diastolic pressures are similar to pulmonary arterial pressures provided that PS is not present. With pulmonary angiography, there is reflux of contrast material into the right ventricle.

The prognosis of a patient with functional PR is largely determined by the underlying disease process, and therapeutic measures should be tailored accordingly. Organic PR is usually benign. In the occasional patient in whom severe PR causes right ventricular failure despite medical therapy, surgical intervention is warranted.

TABLE 5 GRADING OF VALVULAR PULMONIC STENOSIS	
Right ventricular peak-systolic pressure, *mm Hg**	Grade
30–49	Mild
50–99	Moderate
≥100	Severe

*As determined at cardiac catheterization.

TABLE 6 INDICATIONS FOR BALLOON PULMONIC VALVULOPLASTY OR SURGICAL TREATMENT
Symptoms attributable to the stenosis
Intermittent or continuous cyanosis
Right ventricular peak-systolic pressure >100 mm Hg, even without symptoms

References and Recommended Reading

Recently published papers of particular interest have been highlighted as:
• Of interest

1. Giuliani ER, Fuster V, Brandenberg RO, Mair DD: Ebstein's anomaly: the clinical features and natural history of Ebstein's anomaly of the tricuspid valve. *Mayo Clin Proc* 1979, 54:163–173.
2. Smith WM, Gallagher JJ, Kerr CR, *et al.*: The electrophysiologic basis and management of symptomatic and recurrent tachycardia in patients with Ebstein's anomaly of the tricuspid valve. *Am J Cardiol* 1982, 49:1223–1234.
3. Shiina A, Seward JB, Tajik AJ, *et al.*: Two-dimensional echocardiographic-surgical correlation in Ebstein's anomaly: preoperative determination of patients requiring tricuspid valve plication vs. replacement. *Circulation* 1983, 68:534–544.
4. Driscoll DJ, Mottram CD, Danielson GK: Spectrum of exercise intolerance in 45 patients with Ebstein's anomaly and observations on exercise tolerance in 11 patients after surgical repair. *J Am Coll Cardiol* 1988, 11:831–836.
5. Mair DD, Seward JB, Driscoll DJ, Danielson GK: Surgical repair of Ebstein's anomaly: selection of patients and early and late operative results. *Circulation* 1985, 72(suppl 2):70–76.
6. Yousof AM, Shafei MZ, Endrys G, *et al.*: Tricuspid stenosis and regurgitation in rheumatic heart disease: a prospective cardiac catheterization study in 525 patients. *Am Heart J* 1985, 110:60–64.
7. Pearlman AS: Role of echocardiography in the diagnosis and evaluation of severity of mitral and tricuspid stenosis. *Circulation* 1991, 84(suppl 1):193–197.
8. Guerra F, Bortolotti U, Thiene G, *et al.*: Long-term performance of the Hancock bioprosthesis in the tricuspid position. A review of 45 patients with 14-year follow-up. *J Thorac Cardiovasc Surg* 1990, 99:838–845.
9. Cobanoglu A, Ott GY: Tricuspid valve surgery: indications, methods, and results. In *Cardiovascular Clinics. Valvular Heart Disease: Comprehensive Evaluation and Treatment*, edn 2. Edited by Frankl WS, Brest AN. Philadelphia: FA Davis; 1993:265–271.
10. Singh AK, Feng WC, Sanofsky SJ: Long-term results of St. Jude medical valve in the tricuspid position. *Ann Thorac Surg* 1992, 54:538–540.
11. • Hecht SR, Berger M: Right-sided endocarditis in intravenous drug users. Prognostic features in 102 episodes. *Ann Intern Med* 1992, 117:560–566.
12. Arbulu A, Holmes RJ, Asfaw I: Tricuspid valvulectomy without replacement. Twenty years' experience. *J Thorac Cardiovasc Surg* 1991, 102:917–922.
13. Simpson IA, Sahn DJ: Quantification of valvular regurgitation by Doppler echocardiography. *Circulation* 1991, 84(suppl 1):188–192.
14. Maciel BC, Simpson IA, Valdes-Cruz LM, *et al.*: Color-flow Doppler mapping studies of "physiologic" pulmonary and tricuspid regurgitation: evidence for true regurgitation as opposed to a valve closing volume. *J Am Soc Echocardiogr* 1991, 4:589–597.
15. Yoshida K, Yoshikawa J, Shakudo M, *et al.*: Color Doppler evaluation of valvular regurgitation in normal subjects. *Circulation* 1988, 78:840–847.
16. McGrath LB, Gonzalez-Lavin L, Bailey BM, *et al.*: Tricuspid valve operations in 530 patients. Twenty-five year assessment of early and late phase events. *J Thorac Cardiovasc Surg* 1990, 99:124–133.
17. Richards KL: Assessment of aortic and pulmonic stenosis by echocardiography. *Circulation* 1991, 84(suppl 1):182–187.
18. McCrindle BW, Kan JS: Long-term results after balloon pulmonary valvuloplasty. *Circulation* 1991, 83:1915–1922.
19. • Rao PS: Transcatheter treatment of pulmonary outflow tract obstruction: a review. *Prog Cardiovasc Dis* 1992, 35:119–158.
20. Ansari A: Isolated pulmonary valvular regurgitation: current perspectives. *Prog Cardiovasc Dis* 1991, 33:329–344.

Select Bibliography

Braunwald E: Valvular heart disease. In *Heart Disease. A Textbook of Cardiovascular Medicine*, edn 4. Edited by Braunwald E. Philadelphia: WB Saunders; 1992:1053–1060.

Hypertrophic Cardiomyopathy

Gregg M. Yamada
Joseph S. Alpert

> ### Key Points
> - Familial hypertrophic cardiomyopathy (HCM) is a rare autosomal dominant disorder linked to mutations of the cardiac myosin heavy chain genes.
> - In obstructive HCM, systolic anterior motion of the mitral valve leaflet creates a subaortic pressure gradient.
> - Echocardiography is the most useful study in the diagnosis of HCM, providing both anatomic and physiologic information.
> - Sudden death is the most devastating consequence of HCM, associated with a 2% to 3% annual mortality rate in patients younger than 30 years of age.
> - Medical therapy, including β-blockers, calcium channel blockers, and antiarrhythmic agents, is the initial treatment for most patients with HCM.
> - Surgical therapy is considered for patients refractory to medical therapy.

The most characteristic morphologic feature of hypertrophic cardiomyopathy (HCM) is idiopathic left ventricular hypertrophy. Hypertrophy of the nondilated left ventricle results in abnormal diastolic function and produces a dynamic subaortic pressure gradient. The pattern of left ventricular hypertrophy is typically asymmetrical, primarily involving the anterior and basal septum; however, other segments may be selectively involved.

ETIOLOGY

Hypertrophic cardiomyopathy occurs in less than 0.2% of the population, and approximately 45% of these cases are sporadic [1]. Familial HCM is transmitted in an autosomal dominant pattern, although the anatomic distribution and severity of ventricular hypertrophy may vary within a single family.

The etiology of HCM is unknown; however, familial patterns have been linked genetically to the cardiac myosin heavy chain genes on chromosome 14 band q1. Different mutations within this gene can be identified in approximately 50% of families with HCM [2,3].

PATHOPHYSIOLOGY

Hypertrophic cardiomyopathy may be either obstructive or nonobstructive depending on the presence or absence of a dynamic subaortic pressure gradient (Fig. 1). In obstructive HCM, it is uncertain if forceful ventricular contraction produces this gradient or if a true mechanical obstruction to flow exists. Systolic anterior motion of the mitral valve leaflet is the proposed mechanism of mechanical outflow obstruction. In this hypothesis, hypertrophy of the ventricular septum results in narrowing of the left ventricular outflow tract. Consequently, during ventricular systole, blood is expelled at a higher velocity, creating a Venturi effect near the anterior mitral leaflet. The mitral leaflet is drawn into contact with the ventricular septum, creating

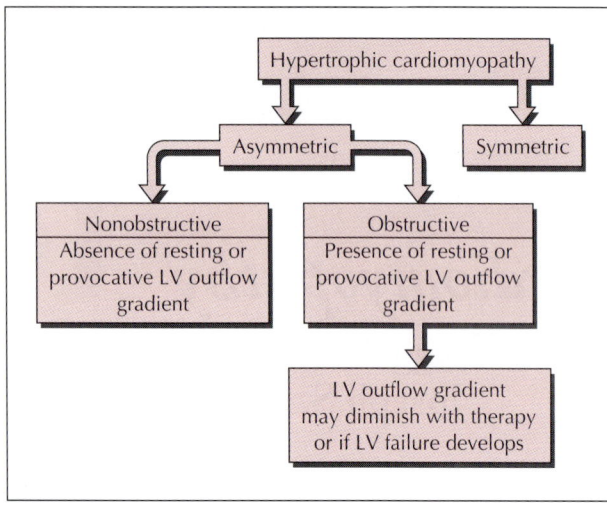

FIGURE 1 Classification of hypertrophic cardiomyopathy (HCM). LV—left ventricular.

a subaortic gradient and resulting in ventricular outflow obstruction (Fig. 2). The severity of the pressure gradient may vary at rest, during exercise, or after pharmacologic therapy.

Nonobstructive HCM is characterized by left ventricular hypertrophy in the absence of a resting pressure gradient. Diastolic dysfunction, due to decreased compliance and incomplete relaxation of the hypertrophied ventricle, leads to impaired early diastolic filling and increased left ventricular end-diastolic pressure (LVEDP). Myocardial ischemia may result from increased myocardial oxygen demand in the absence of coronary artery disease (Fig. 3).

CLINICAL MANIFESTATIONS

The clinical presentation of HCM is variable. Many patients are asymptomatic. The most common symptoms include dyspnea (diastolic dysfunction), exertional angina (myocardial ischemia), fatigue, near syncope, and syncope (decreased cardiac output or arrhythmias). The morphologic and functional severity of the cardiomyopathy are not necessarily correlated with the severity of the clinical symptoms. Patients with minimal hypertrophy may have severe complaints, whereas those with marked hypertrophy may be relatively asymptomatic.

The cardiac examination is abnormal in patients with significant subaortic pressure gradients. The characteristic systolic murmur of HCM is harsh, in character with a crescendo–decrescendo pattern. The murmur is heard best between the left sternal border and the cardiac apex and often radiates to the axilla. In patients with prominent gradients, the murmur tends to be holosystolic at the cardiac apex because of accompanying mitral regurgitation. Abrupt standing and Valsalva's maneuver accentuate the murmur of HCM, whereas squatting and isometric handgrip diminish it. The apical impulse is displaced laterally, and a systolic thrill is often palpable. Additionally, forceful atrial contraction combined with interrupted systolic flow due to left ventricular outflow obstruction may generate a triple apical impulse (Fig. 4).

DIAGNOSIS

Echocardiography is the most useful study in the diagnosis of HCM, providing morphologic and functional information (Fig. 5). The most characteristic finding is asymmetrical septal hypertrophy, which contributes to the narrowing of the left ventricular outflow tract. As previously mentioned, it is unclear if systolic anterior motion of the mitral valve leaflet is solely responsible for the subaortic pressure gradient; however, when present, a high incidence of outflow obstruction is seen. Variable degrees of mitral regurgitation are present in patients with outflow gradients. Diastolic dysfunction occurs in most patients with HCM, even in the absence of a ventricular

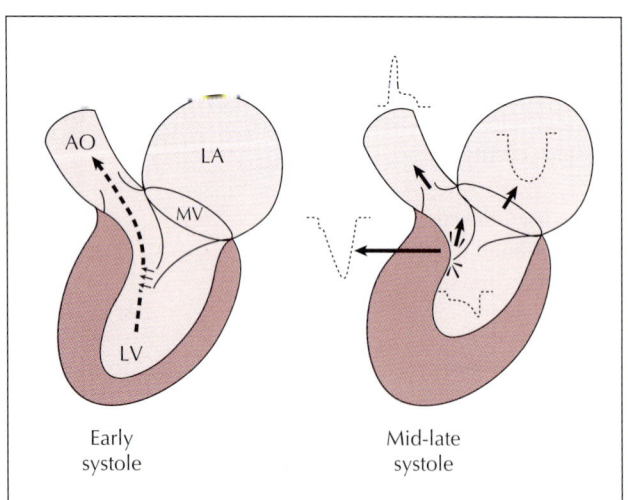

FIGURE 2 Mechanism of systolic anterior motion of the mitral leaflet in obstructive hypertrophic cardiomyopathy. AO—aorta; LA—left atrium; LV—left ventricle; MV—mitral valve. (*From* Wigle [24]; with permission.)

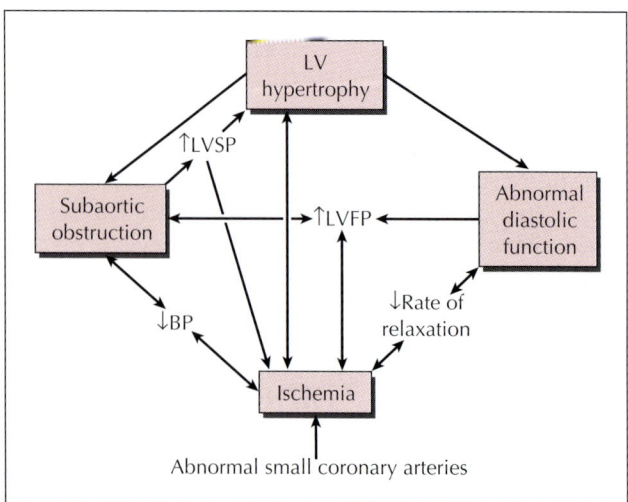

FIGURE 3 Pathophysiologic interrelationships of left ventricular (LV) hypertrophy, subaortic obstruction, diastolic dysfunction, and myocardial ischemia in hypertrophic cardiomyopathy. BP—blood pressure; LVFP—left ventricular filling pressure; LVSP—left ventricular systolic pressure. (*From* Maron *et al.* [25]; with permission.)

	HCM	MR, AS
Decreased LV cavity size Valsalva, standing, excercise, tachycardia, hypovolemia, inhalation of amyl nitrite	↑	↓
Increased LV cavity size Squatting, passive elevation of patient's legs, isometric handgrip, administration of phenylephrine	↓	No change or slight ↑

FIGURE 4 Response of murmurs of hypertrophic cardiomyopathy (HCM), aortic stenosis (AS), and mitral regurgitation (MR) to various maneuvers.

outflow gradient, but the presence of diastolic dysfunction does not always correlate with clinical symptoms [4].

The most characteristic electrocardiographic features include nonspecific ST segment and T wave changes, left ventricular hypertrophy, abnormal Q waves in the anterolateral and inferior leads (pseudoinfarction pattern), and left atrial enlargement. Large amplitude (> 10 mm), inverted T waves in the left precordial leads may identify patients with apical HCM, but the clinical significance of these T-wave inversions is uncertain [5].

The chest radiograph often is unrevealing. The left ventricle may be prominent, but the cardiac silhouette usually is not enlarged. The left atrium and atrial appendage may be prominent secondary to increased pressure and associated mitral regurgitation.

Cardiac catheterization is performed if surgery is contemplated or if the diagnosis remains uncertain despite noninvasive assessment. Typically, a left ventricular outflow gradient is detected, and LVEDP is increased. Variable degrees of atherosclerosis may be present.

Electrophysiologic study is indicated in high-risk patients, including those with a history of previous syncope, cardiac arrest, and symptomatic ventricular tachycardia. Induction of sustained ventricular tachycardia (predominantly polymor-

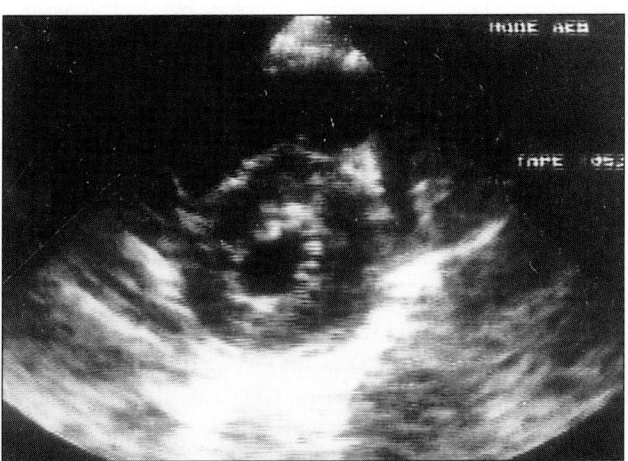

FIGURE 5 Echocardiogram of hypertrophic cardiomyopathy as seen in the short-axis view (*Courtesy of* Linda A. Pape, MD).

phic) is associated with cardiac arrest in 77% of patients and syncope in 49% [6]. The role of electrophysiologic testing in other subsets of patients with HCM is unclear. Signal-averaged electrocardiography helps to identify high-risk patients with HCM, but its utility remains uncertain [7].

COURSE AND PROGNOSIS

The clinical course is variable. It is not known why some patients remain clinically stable for years and only mildly symptomatic, whereas others deteriorate more rapidly [8]. Sudden death is the most devastating sequelae of HCM, with an annual mortality rate of 2% to 3% in patients younger than 30 years of age [9]. Much of the published literature, however, has originated from tertiary care centers and may overestimate the actual mortality rate in the general population because of selection bias [10]. Risk factors for sudden death include nonsustained ventricular tachycardia on Holter monitor, age less than 30 years, syncope, and a family history of sudden death.

The predictive value of a large resting outflow gradient is uncertain; however, decreased left ventricular end-diastolic volume is associated with future syncopal events and sudden death [11,12••]. Nonsustained ventricular tachycardia on Holter monitor is associated with an 8% annual mortality rate [13]. However, ventricular tachycardia is poorly predictive of sudden death in the absence of presyncope, syncope, or inducible sustained ventricular tachycardia on electrophysiologic study [14••]. Although ventricular arrhythmias are the most common cause of sudden death, acute hemodynamic derangements (both physiologic and pharmacologic) that augment the outflow gradient and diminish diastolic filling also may play a role.

Patients with mild hypertrophy without resting outflow gradients, or nonobstructive HCM, have a more favorable prognosis [15]. The prognosis in patients older than 60 years of age is similar to that in younger patients and appears related to cardiac function [16]. Patients with HCM who are symptomatic or who have a family history of sudden death should be referred to a cardiologist. Patients with asymptomatic HCM also should be restricted from competitive athletics; however, noncompetitive athletics are not contraindicated (*eg*, walking, bicycling).

TREATMENT

The clinical spectrum of disease in HCM is variable. Because of the lack of prospective, randomized, controlled trials, therapeutic comparisons are difficult, and treatment must be individualized. Medical therapy is the initial treatment of choice for most patients. Those who remain refractory to therapy or who are unable to tolerate medications are then evaluated for possible surgical correction.

Medical Therapy

The most commonly used drugs, all with proven efficacy in alleviating symptoms, are β-blockers, calcium channel blockers, and antiarrhythmic agents.

β-blockers are effective in alleviating angina, dyspnea, and other symptoms of HCM. Overall clinical improvement, however, may be seen in only one third to one half of all patients treated. Mechanisms of action include a decrease in myocardial oxygen consumption (negative inotropy), increased diastolic filling time (decreased heart rate), and inhibition of sympathetic stimulation during exercise. The effect of β-blockers on the incidence of sudden death has not been determined conclusively.

Verapamil is the most frequently used calcium channel blocker for the treatment of HCM. It alleviates symptoms and improves exercise function in approximately two thirds of patients who have failed β-blocker therapy [17]. A more recent report has corroborated symptomatic improvement observed in patients with HCM taking verapamil, but found no increase in exercise capacity [18]. Mechanisms of action include a decrease in the systolic left ventricular outflow gradient through negative inotropic effects and an improvement in diastolic function. Verapamil should be used with great caution in patients with severe left ventricular outflow gradients and elevated left ventricular end-diastolic pressures [19]. The effect of verapamil on sudden death remains undetermined. Only limited information is available on the use of other calcium channel blockers in the treatment of HCM.

Disopyramide is a type IA antiarrhythmic agent with negative inotropic properties that effectively relieves symptoms of HCM and improves exercise capacity [20]. Although disopyramide is potentially effective in treating supraventricular and ventricular arrhythmias in patients with HCM, a clear survival benefit remains to be proved [21••].

In addition to its antiarrhythmic effects, amiodarone may relieve symptoms and improve exercise capacity in patients refractory to β-blockers and calcium channel blockers through an undefined mechanism. Although amiodarone effectively suppresses supraventricular and ventricular tachycardia, its role in preventing sudden death remains unknown.

Surgical Therapy

Patients refractory to medical therapy are considered for ventricular septal myotomy–myectomy or mitral valve replacement following cardiac catheterization. The operative mortality rate is approximately 5%, and a majority of patients report long-term symptomatic improvement [22]. Dual-chamber pacing also can abolish left ventricular outflow obstruction in selected patients.

References and Recommended Reading

Recently published papers of particular interest have been highlighted as:
- Of interest
- • Of outstanding interest

1. Maron BJ, Bonow RO, Cannon RO, *et al.*: Hypertrophic cardiomyopathy: interrelations of clinical manifestations, pathophysiology, and therapy. *N Engl J Med* 1987, 316:780–789.
2. Watkins H, Rosenzweig A, Hwang DS, *et al.*: Characteristics and prognostic implications of myosin missense mutations in familial hypertrophic cardiomyopathy. *N Engl J Med* 1992, 326:1108–1114.
3. Garcia JA, McKenna W, Pare P, *et al.*: Mapping a gene for familial hypertrophic cardiomyopathy to chromosome 14q1. *N Engl J Med* 1989, 321:1372–1378.
4. Nihoyannopoulos P, Karatasakis G, Frenneaux M, *et al.*: Diastolic function in hypertrophic cardiomyopathy: relation to exercise capacity. *J Am Coll Cardiol* 1992, 19:536–540.
5. Alfonso F, Nihoyannopoulos P, Stewart J, *et al.*: Clinical significance of giant negative T waves in hypertrophic cardiomyopathy. *J Am Coll Cardiol* 1990, 15:965–971.
6. Fananapazir L, Tracy CM, Leon MB, *et al.*: Electrophysiologic abnormalities in patients with hypertrophic cardiomyopathy: a consecutive analysis in 155 patients. *Circulation* 1989, 80:1259–1268.
7. Cripps TR, Counihan PJ, Frenneaux MP, *et al.*: Signal-averaged electrocardiography in hypertrophic cardiomyopathy. *J Am Coll Cardiol* 1990, 15:956–961.
8. McKenna WJ: The natural history of hypertrophic cardiomyopathy. *Cardiovasc Clin* 1988, 19:135–142.
9. McKenna WJ, England D, Doi YL, *et al.*: Arrhythmia in hypertrophic cardiomyopathy. I: Influence on prognosis. *Br Heart J* 1981, 46:168–172.
10. Spirito P, Chiarella F, Carratino L, *et al.*: Clinical course and prognosis of hypertrophic cardiomyopathy in an outpatient population. *N Engl J Med* 1989, 320:749–755.
11. Maron BJ, Bonow RO, Cannon RO, *et al.*: Hypertrophic cardiomyopathy: Interrelations of clinical manifestations, pathophysiology and therapy. *N Engl J Med* 1987, 316:780–789.
12.•• Nienaber CA, Hiller S, Spielmann RP, *et al.*: Syncope in hypertrophic cardiomyopathy: multivariate analysis of prognostic determinants. *J Am Coll Cardiol* 1990, 15:948–955.
13. Maron BJ, Savage DD, Wolfson JK, Epstein SE: Prognostic significance of 24 hour ambulatory electrocardiographic monitoring in patients with hypertrophic cardiomyopathy: a prospective study. *Am J Cardiol* 1981, 48:252–257.
14.•• Fananapazir L, Chang AC, Epstein SE, McAreavey D: Prognostic determinants in hypertrophic cardiomyopathy: prospective evaluation of a therapeutic strategy based on clinical, Holter, hemodynamic and electrophysiological findings. *Circulation* 1992, 86:730–740.
15. Aron LA, Hertzeanu L, Enrique FZ, *et al.*: Prognosis of nonobstructive hypertrophic cardiomyopathy. *Am J Cardiol* 1991, 67:215–216.
16. Pelliccia F, Cianfrocca C, Romeo F, Reale A: Natural history of hypertrophic cardiomyopathy in the elderly. *Cardiology* 1991, 78:329–333.
17. Rosing DR, Idanpaan-Heikkila U, Maron BJ, *et al.*: Use of calcium-channel blocking drugs in hypertrophic cardiomyopathy. *Am J Cardiol* 1985, 55(Suppl):185B–195B.
18. Gilligan DM, Chan WL, Joshi J, *et al.*: A double-blind, placebo-controlled crossover trial of nadolol and verapamil in mild and moderately symptomatic hypertrophic cardiomyopathy. *J Am CollCardiol* 1993, 21:1627–1629.
19. Epstein S, Rosing D: Verapamil: Its potential for serious complications in patients with hypertrophic cardiomyopathy. *Circulation* 1981, 64:437–439.
20. Hartmann A, Kuhn J, Hopf R, *et al.*: Effect of propranolol and disopyramide on left ventricular function at rest and during exercise in hypertrophic cardiomyopathy. *Cardiology* 1992, 80:81–88.
21.•• Blanchard DG, Ross J: Hypertrophic cardiomyopathy: prognosis with medical or surgical therapy. *Clin Cardiol* 1991, 14:11–19.
22. McIntosh CL, Maron BL: Current operative treatment of obstructive hypertrophic cardiomyopathy. *Circulation* 1988, 78:487–494.
23. Maron BJ, Wolfson JK, Ciro E, Spirito P: Relation of electrocardiographic abnormalities and patterns of left ventricular hypertrophy identified by 2-dimensional echocardiography in patients with hypertrophic cardiomyopathy. *Am J Cardiol* 1983, 51:189–194.

24. Wigle ED: Hypertrophic cardiomyopathy: a 1987 viewpoint (editorial). *Circulation* 1987, 73:311–322.
25. Maron BJ, Bonow RO, Cannon RO, *et al.*: Hypertrophic cardiomyopathy: Interrelations of clinical manifestations pathophysiology, and therapy. *N Engl J Med* 1987, 316:844–852.
26. Chou TC: *Electrocardiography in Clinical Practice*. Philadelphia: WB Saunders; 1991:250–251.

Select Bibliography

Blanchard DG, Ross J: Hypertrophic cardiomyopathy: Prognosis with medical or surgical therapy. *Clin Cardiol* 1991, 14:11–19.

Fananapazir L, Chang AC, Epstein SE, McAreavey D: Prognostic determinants in hypertrophic cardiomyopathy: Prospective evaluation of a therapeutic strategy based on clinical, Holter, hemodynamic and electrophysiological findings. *Circulation* 1992, 86:730–740.

Maron BJ, Bonow RO, Cannon RO, *et al.*: Hypertrophic cardiomyopathy: Interrelations of clinical manifestations, pathophysiology, and therapy. *N Engl J Med* 1987, 316:780–789.

McKenna WJ: The natural history of hypertrophic cardiomyopathy. *Cardiovasc Clin* 1988, 19:135–142.

Nienaber CA, Hiller S, Spielmann RP, *et al.*: Syncope in hypertrophic cardiomyopathy: Multivariate analysis of prognostic determinants. *J Am Coll Cardiol* 1990, 15:948–955.

Congestive Cardiomyopathy

Sanjiv Sobti
Timothy J. Regan

> ### Key Points
> - Alcohol consumption is one of the most common, identifiable causes of congestive cardiomyopathy.
> - Diastolic dysfunction accounts for up to 40% of heart failure cases.
> - Endomyocardial biopsy provides no diagnostic information and is not recommended in most patients with congestive cardiomyopathy.
> - The single most powerful predictor of mortality is low ejection fraction.
> - A selective subset of patients with congestive cardiomyopathy may respond to the use of β-blockers.
> - A pure lusitropic drug to treat isolated diastolic heart failure is not currently available.
> - Use of vasodilators to treat congestive cardiomyopathy has decreased the mortality rate associated with this disease.

Congestive cardiomyopathy is usually associated with impaired systolic function of the left ventricle (Fig. 1). In some patients, diastolic function may be the predominant abnormality and require a different therapeutic approach. More often, however, this alteration is combined with systolic dysfunction. Consideration of the etiologic factors that may precipitate or play a role in the development of the diffuse myocardial disease is crucial to preventing or ameliorating the process (Table 1). More frequent etiologies include hypertension, alcohol consumption, age, viral infection, and drug toxicity.

Hypertension is a leading cause of heart failure resulting from both systolic and diastolic dysfunction, even without significant coronary atherosclerosis. Early symptoms are often caused by diastolic dysfunction of the left ventricle [1••]. Many patients with hypertension have evidence of abnormal left ventricular relaxation and filling, even without left ventricular hypertrophy [2].

Alcoholism is one of the most common, identifiable causes of cardiomyopathy. Over time, excessive alcohol consumption can lead to heart muscle disease without evident malnutrition. Although no specific cardiovascular markers exist, plasma tests used in the diagnosis of liver injury and urinary ethanol levels may be helpful. Progression of heart disease may be delayed or even reversed in patients who abstain from alcohol.

The normal aging process may be associated with a decline of ventricular diastolic function, whereas ventricular systolic function is unaltered at rest. Elderly persons are more prone to develop diastolic heart failure if they also have hypertension. The prevalence of systolic hypertension attributable to increased arterial stiffness is high among the elderly.

Presentation of patients with heart muscle disease caused by a viral infection is quite varied [3••,4•]. Patients may have a distinct viral syndrome with severe cardiovascular compromise that may be fatal or may spontaneously resolve. Acute fulmi-

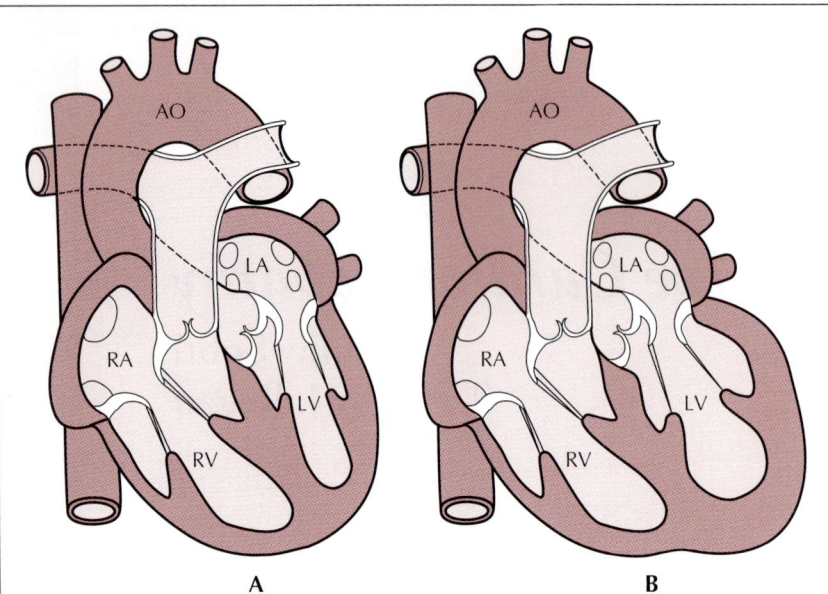

FIGURE 1 Schematic presentation of normal (**A**) and dilated (**B**) left heart. AO—aorta; LA—left atrium; LV—left ventricle RA—right atrium; RV—right ventricle.

nating myocarditis is usually associated with left ventricular dysfunction, which may progress to dilated cardiomyopathy. Chronic active myocarditis tends to have clinical relapses. Despite persistent infiltrates with chronic persistent myocarditis, normal ventricular function may be maintained even though it is associated with chest pain or arrhythmias [4•].

Doxorubicin and other anthracycline antitumor agents are causes of dose-related and irreversible toxic cardiomyopathy. Evidence also supports the concept that a specific diabetic cardiomyopathy without accelerated coronary atherosclerosis or hypertension increases the incidence of heart failure, more so in females than males [5]. Finally, morbid obesity may cause circulatory congestion associated with increased blood volume and arterial pressure as well as eccentric hypertrophy [6].

FUNCTIONAL ABNORMALITIES

During the early stages of the disease, stroke volume is maintained despite decreased ejection fraction by increased end-diastolic volume. Increased ventricular wall stress stimulates myocyte hypertrophy, which may normalize wall stress. With further reductions of the ejection fraction, ventricular volume and stress increase and stroke volume decreases (Table 2). Increased heart rate may sustain normal cardiac output. Fluid retention, which is initially adaptive, may further increase ventricular volume, leading to pulmonary and systemic venous congestion. Multiple neurohumoral mechanisms, including the release of circulating norepinephrine and stimulation of the renin-angiotensin system (Fig. 2), are activated. Atrial natriuretic factor partly counteracts the undesirable fluid retention promoted by vasopressin. During the advanced stage, these neurohumoral mechanisms override serum osmolarity homeostasis, causing a decrease in serum sodium levels and resistance to medical therapy.

Up to 40% of symptomatic patients have diastolic heart failure. The mechanisms responsible for diastolic dysfunction despite normal systolic function are decreased compliance (increased stiffness) and impaired ventricular relaxation (Fig. 3). Hence, the left ventricle is unable to fill adequately at normal diastolic pressures. Reduced left ventricular filling volume leads to decreased stroke volume and symptoms of low cardiac output, whereas increased filling pressure leads to pulmonary congestion.

CLINICAL PRESENTATION

Symptoms usually develop gradually after an asymptomatic period with cardiac dysfunction. There are three cardinal symptoms, any of which may be predominant: fatigue (caused by low cardiac output), dyspnea, and weight gain (often with venous and hepatic congestion). Some patients have noncongestive symptoms including palpitations, chest pains, fainting spells, and lightheadedness. Orthopnea, paroxysmal nocturnal dyspnea, chronic cough, abdominal distention, right upper quadrant pain, or nausea also may be present. Occasionally, the first symptom to occur is secondary to an embolic event.

Physical Examination

Physical signs vary according to when a patient is seen during the natural history of congestive cardiomyopathy. Commonly, the patient has tachypnea, tachycardia, and usually sinus but occasionally atrial fibrillation. Systolic blood pressure may be normal, high, or low. Pulse pressure is narrow, reflecting a diminished stroke volume; there may be pulsus alternans. Jugular veins are frequently distended with a prominent V wave, a sign of tricuspid regurgitation. The liver may be enlarged and pulsatile, and ascites and peripheral edema may be present. The apical impulse is usually displaced laterally and inferiorly. The most prominent and useful finding on auscultation is a loud third heart sound, best heard with the bell of the stethoscope placed lightly over the cardiac apex with the patient in the left lateral position. During diastolic heart failure, however, a fourth heart sound is most common.

TABLE 1 ETIOLOGIES OF CONGESTIVE CARDIOMYOPATHY

Frequent incidence
Hypertension
Ethyl alcohol abuse
Viral infection
Age
Idiopathic

Less frequent incidence
Metabolic
  Nutritional–obesity, thiamine
  Endocrinologic–diabetes mellitus, myxedema
  Uremia
  Amyloid
  Electrolyte imbalance
Infectious
  Bacterial
  Mycobacterial
  Parasitic
  Spirochetal
  Rickettsial
  Fungal
Immune
  Transplantation rejection
  Autoimmune disease (collagen diseases)
  Peripartum
Toxic
  Chemotherapeutic agents
  Catecholamines
  Cocaine
  Cobalt
Familial
  Myotonia dystrophica
  Progressive muscular dystrophy
  Neuromyopathic
Hypersensitivity
  Methyldopa
  Penicillin
  Sulfonamides
  Tetracycline
  Phenylbutazone

TABLE 2 FUNCTIONAL ABNORMALITIES IN CONGESTIVE CARDIOMYOPATHY

Parameter	Congestive cardiomyopathy
Systolic function	
Ejection fraction (only with systolic dysfunction)	Decreased
Wall stress	Increased
Diastolic function	
Muscle stiffness	Increased or normal
End-diastolic pressure/volume	Increased or normal
Left ventricular volume	
End-systolic volume	Increased
End-diastolic volume	Increased
Left ventricular mass	Increased
Volume:mass ratio	Increased

Systolic murmurs of functional mitral and tricuspid regurgitation may be present. Patients may have physical signs of congested lungs and pleural effusion if seen before treatment.

Laboratory Evaluation

Chest radiography reveals varying degrees of cardiomegaly and pulmonary venous congestion, ranging from pulmonary venous redistribution to frank pulmonary edema in the acutely ill patient (Fig. 4). Kerley's B lines and peribronchial cuffing as signs of interstitial edema are common during the acute phase.

Electrocardiography (ECG) commonly reveals sinus tachycardia with nonspecific ST-T wave changes. Other ECG abnormalities are shown in Figures 5 and 6. Holter monitoring shows a high incidence of ventricular extrasystoles, which are frequently complex. More than 70% of patients have multiformed ventricular extrasystole or ventricular couplets, and 30% to 70% have episodic nonsustained

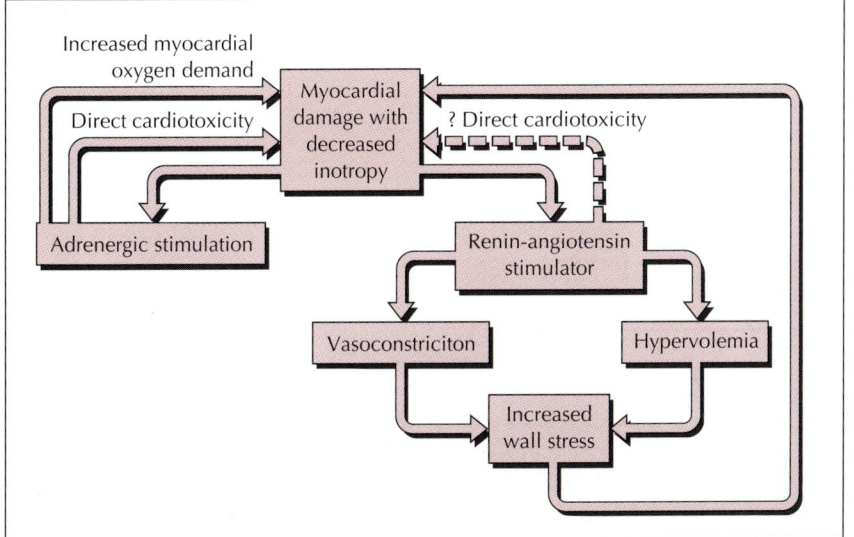

FIGURE 2 Activated neurohumoral mechanisms in heart failure.

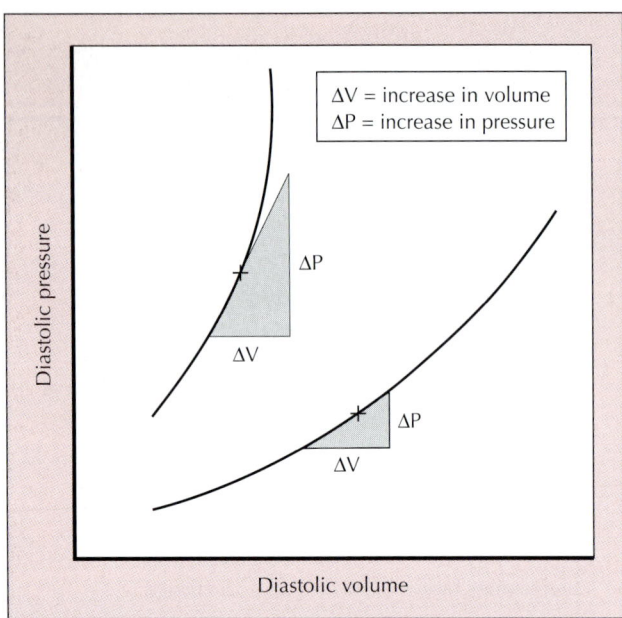

FIGURE 3 Left ventricular diastolic volume pressure relationship in healthy persons and patients with diastolic dysfunction. For the same volume, the increase in filling pressures is greater for patients with diastolic dysfunction (the curve is shifted to the left and the slope is steeper).

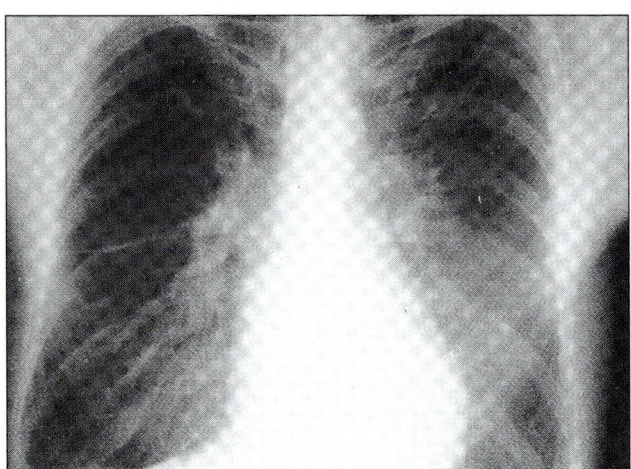

FIGURE 4 Chest radiograph of a patient with diastolic heart failure but a normal ejection fraction, borderline cardiomegaly with bilateral pulmonary edema, and fluid in the minor fissure.

(≥ 3 beats in series and < 30 seconds) or sustained (> 30 seconds) ventricular tachycardia [7]. Less common, but by no means infrequent, are atrial extrasystole and supraventricular tachycardia. There is no consensus that complex or frequent ventricular arrhythmias predict sudden (presumably arrhythmic) death, but they do appear to predict total mortality. At least one annual baseline 24-hour Holter recording with repeat monitoring is recommended. Unfortunately, an unremarkable Holter recording (≤ 1000 ventricular extrasystole per 24 hours) does not exclude the possibility of future sudden death.

Electrophysiologic studies may be helpful for patients with repeated runs of sustained monomorphic tachycardia or arrhythmia-induced syncope or near-syncope who have reliably induced ventricular tachycardia. In these patients, electrophysiologic study can be used to select the optimal antiarrhythmic drugs [8•]. If these antiarrhythmic drugs fail to suppress the arrhythmia, the patient should have an automatic cardioverter/defibrillator device implanted.

The echocardiographic features of congestive cardiomyopathy are characteristic (Figs. 7 through 9; Table 3). Echocardiography is very useful for excluding heart failure

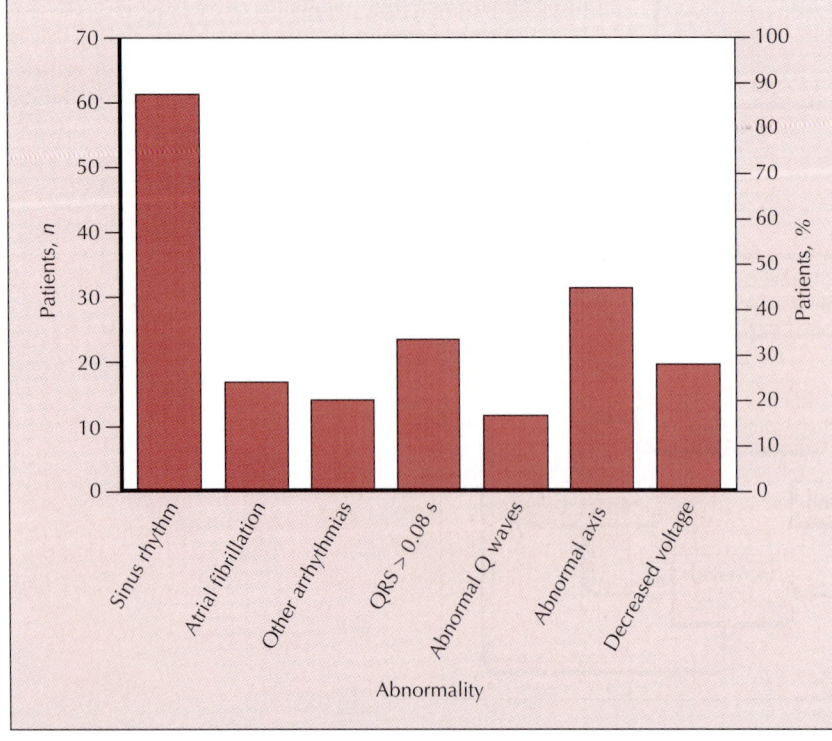

FIGURE 5 Electrocardiographic findings in a series of 74 patients with congestive cardiomyopathy. (*Adapted from* Kristinsson [18]; with permission.)

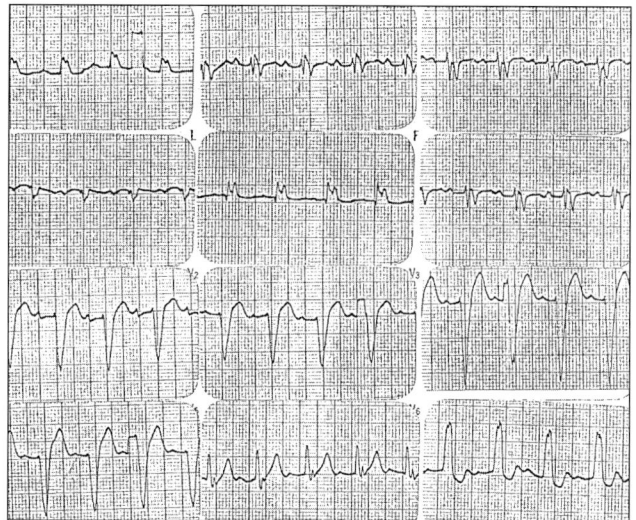

FIGURE 6 Electrocardiogram from a patient with congestive cardiomyopathy showing left bundle-branch block.

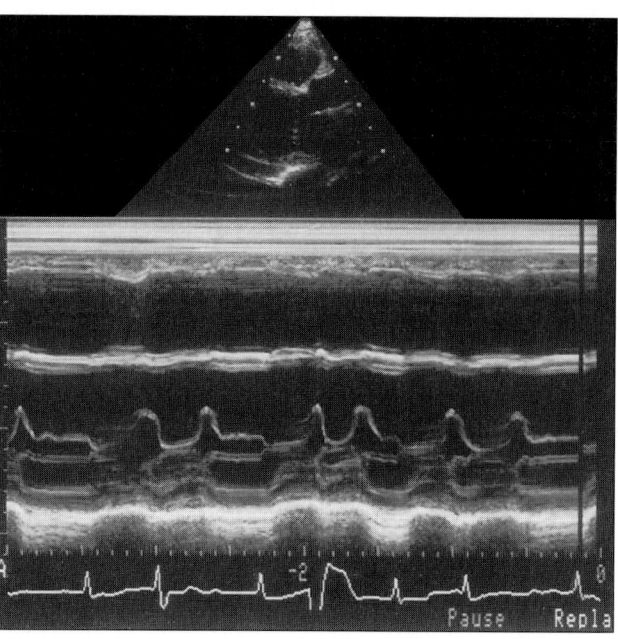

FIGURE 7 M-mode echocardiogram of a patient with congestive cardiomyopathy. The left ventricular (LV) and right ventricular (RV) cavities are dilated, and systolic motion of the interventricular septum and the LV posterior wall is decreased. Note the increased E–to–septal point separation. LV cavity in diastole = 60 mm; RV cavity in diastole = 35 mm.

secondary to a primary valvular disease. It is sometimes difficult to distinguish between this cardiomyopathy and ischemic left ventricular failure, because segmental wall-motion abnormalities characteristic of ischemic disease are also observed in cardiomyopathy. Radionuclide ventriculography is usually not needed unless the echocardiographic study is inadequate.

Cardiac catheterization is not routinely done unless a question exists of ischemic heart disease. Parameters obtained from right- and left-side heart catheterization are listed in Table 4. Endomyocardial biopsy is not useful except when a diagnosis of myocarditis is considered.

Assessment of Functional Status

Severity of heart failure is estimated by clinical and radiographic examination, measures of ventricular performance (ejection fraction and serial hemodynamic parameters measured with right heart catheterization), and exercise capacity. All these methods have limitations when used independently. In practice, the most frequently used methods are clinical, radiographic, and echocardiographic.

Patients are often classified according to the New York Heart Association scheme (Table 5). This classification is relatively subjective, however, and only assesses functional capacity and the degree of disability. It is not a measure of the

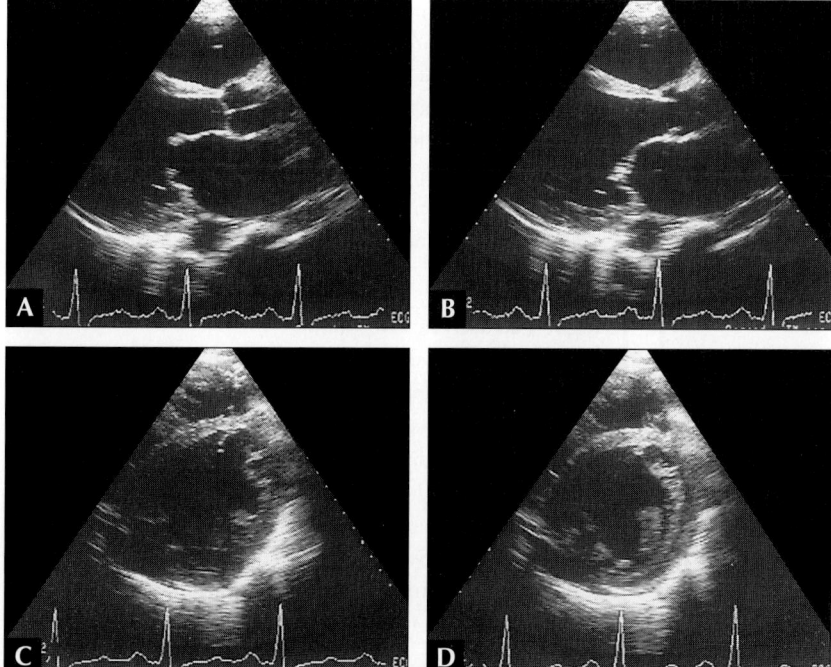

FIGURE 8 Two-dimensional echocardiogram of a patient with congestive cardiomyopathy in the parasternal long axis view in diastole (**A**), and systole (**B**). The left ventricular cavity, right ventricular outflow tract, and left atrium are enlarged. During systole, there is minimal contraction of the interventricular septum and the left ventricular posterior wall. Note the short-axis view of the left ventricle at the level of midcavity (**C**) and the lack of significant contraction during systole (**D**).

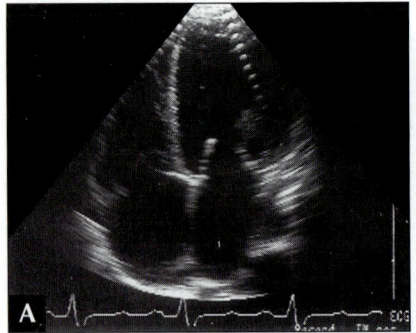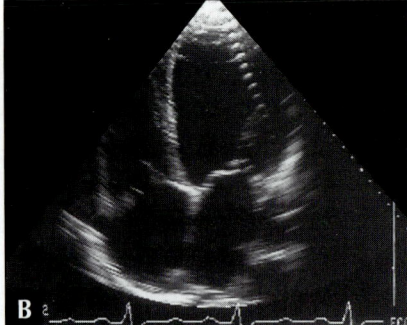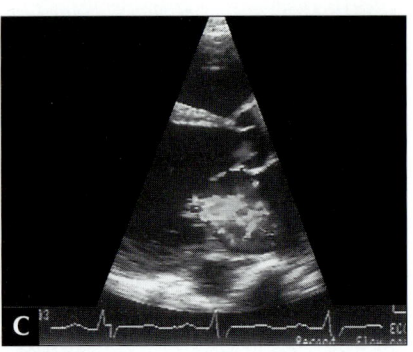

FIGURE 9 Four-chamber view in diastole (**A**), and systole (**B**) of the same patient shown in Figure 8. Note the dilation of all four chambers of the heart. Color Doppler study (**C**) in the parasternal long-axis view shows functional mitral regurgitation (*See* Color Plate.)

severity of left ventricular dysfunction. Estimation of the severity of heart failure using exercise testing with or without measurement of oxygen consumption also has its limitations. Some patients with severe left ventricular dysfunction can achieve normal levels of exercise, so normal exercise capacity does not indicate that the heart failure is mild. However, serial measurements of ejection fraction and ventricular dimensions by echocardiography are helpful.

Differential Diagnosis

The differential diagnosis includes all causes of congestive heart failure. Organic valvular or congenital heart disease usually can be readily differentiated; principal differential causes include coronary artery disease with ischemic left ventricular failure, restrictive cardiomyopathy, hypertrophic cardiomyopathy, pulmonary disease, rheumatic heart disease, and effusoconstrictive pericardial disease (Table 6). Heart muscle disease secondary to specific etiologies must be recognized early to enhance the potential for reversibility.

In coronary heart disease, there often is a history of angina or myocardial infarction. Electrocardiograms can show evidence of previous myocardial infarction but may be misleading, because Q waves are present in some patients with congestive cardiomyopathy and normal coronary arteries on coronary angiography.

Clinical Course and Prognosis

The clinical course of congestive cardiomyopathy is usually steadily downhill over a period of 3 to 6 years (an average) during which time progressive deterioration in exercise tolerance occurs and the heart size increases. Patients become increasingly refractory to diuretics, leading to escalating dose requirements and, in turn, progressive electrolyte imbalance and a further increase in plasma catecholamine levels. A sudden, symptomatic deterioration should alert the clinician

TABLE 3 ECHOCARDIOGRAPHIC FINDINGS IN DILATED CARDIOMYOPATHY

M-mode
Increased diastolic dimensions of left ventricular and possibly right ventricular cavity
Decreased left ventricular fractional shortening
Decreased mitral valve opening in diastole
Increased E-to-septal point separation
Increased left atrial size
Pericardial effusion

Two-dimensional
Four-chamber dilation
Decreased ejection fraction
Possible mural thrombus (any chamber)
Pericardial effusion

Doppler studies (including color Doppler)
Demonstrate tricuspid and mitral regurgitation
Estimate pulmonary hypertension

TABLE 4 HEMODYNAMIC PARAMETERS IN CONGESTIVE CARDIOMYOPATHY

Systolic failure
Right-side heart catheterization
  Increased systemic and pulmonary vascular resistance
  Increased right ventricular end-diastolic pressure
  Increased mean pulmonary artery pressure
  Increased pulmonary capillary wedge pressure (reflects left ventricular filling pressure)
  Decreased cardiac index
Left-side heart catheterization
  Increased left ventricular end-diastolic pressure
  Increased left ventricular systolic and diastolic volume
  Decreased ejection fraction

Diastolic failure
Right-side heart catheterization
  Increased right ventricular end-diastolic pressure
  Increased mean pulmonary artery pressure
  Increased pulmonary capillary wedge pressure
  Decreased cardiac index
Left-side heart catheterization
  Increased left ventricular end-diastolic pressure
  Normal left ventricular systolic volume
  Normal left ventricular diastolic volume
  Normal ejection fraction

Table 5. New York Heart Association Functional Classification

Class I
No limitation during ordinary physical activity. Does not cause undue fatigue, dyspneas, or palpitation.

Class II
Slight limitation of physical activity. Ordinary physical activity results in fatigue, palpitation, dyspnea, or angina.

Class III
Marked limitation of physical activity. Although patients are comfortable at rest, less than ordinary activity will lead to symptoms.

Class IV
Inability to carry on any physical activity without discomfort. Symptoms of congestive failure are present even at rest; with any physical activity, discomfort is increased.

The single most powerful prognostic factor is ejection fraction, and in patients with ejection fractions under 20%, the 1-year mortality rate is more than 50% (Table 7). Half of all deaths from severe congestive cardiomyopathy occur suddenly, associated with a tachy- or bradyarrhythmia. Less common (but important) in patients who are subjectively well with less severe ventricular dysfunction is sudden death from a major thromboembolic event.

Treatment

Systolic Failure

Clinicians treating patients with congestive cardiomyopathy primarily caused by systolic failure are confronted with four major therapeutic concerns:

1. The hemodynamic state of the heart;
2. The risk of life-threatening ventricular arrhythmias and systemic emboli;
3. Persistent myocardial inflammation; and
4. Ultimately, the proper selection of patients for cardiac transplantation (Table 8) [9].

For some patients, specific therapy can be tailored to the specific etiology. Blood pressure control for patients with hypertension and ethanol abstinence for persons with addiction can significantly improve cardiac function and reduce mortality. The majority of patients with demonstrable myocardial inflammation have passed the acute tissue-invasive stage. As many as 50% of biopsy-proven cases of myocarditis show spontaneous improvement, and immunosuppressive treatment in general has not yet proven to be effective.

General measures that should be encouraged for all patients with heart failure include appropriate moderation of

to look for exacerbating factors, including physical, emotional, and environmental stress; systemic infection; sinus tachycardia and arrhythmias (atrial and ventricular); noncompliance with low-sodium diet or medications; pulmonary embolism; development of a second form of heart disease (*eg*, coronary artery disease); or conditions causing high-output states (*eg*, anemia). The most useful means of following the clinical course of the disease is a careful history and physical examination, including body-weight measurements. Serial chest radiographs, echocardiographs, or both to evaluate increasing heart size are helpful.

Table 6. Differential characteristics of the cardiomyopathies

Morphologic feature	Dilated	Hypertrophic	Restrictive
Dilated ventricular cavities	+	–	–
Dilated atrial cavities	+	+	±
Hypertrophied left ventricular walls	±	+	±
Asymmetric septal hypertrophy	–	±	–
Increased heart weight	+	+	+
Abnormally thickened intramural arteries	–	+	±
Intracardiac thrombus	+	–	±
Thickened anterior mitral valve leaflet	–	+	±
Myocardial fiber disarray	–	+	–
Functional			
Systolic function	D	I	N
Diastolic function	N or abnormal	Abnormal	Abnormal
Dynamic left ventricular outflow gradient	–	±	–
Systolic anterior motion of the mitral valve	–	±	–
"Square root sign" in ventricular pressure tracings	–	–	+

D—decreased; I—increased; N—normal.

TABLE 7 FACTORS ASSOCIATED WITH A POOR PROGNOSIS IN CONGESTIVE CARDIOMYOPATHY
Ejection fraction < 20%
Cardiac index less than 2.5 L/min/m²
Cardiothoracic ratio > 0.55%
Conduction delay on electrocardiogram
Diminished left ventricular wall thickening
Marked elevation of right and left ventricular filling pressures (LVEDP > 20 mm Hg)*
Ventricular arrhythmias
Marked elevation of plasma catecholamines (> 800 pg/mL)
Decreased serum sodium levels
Age > 55 y
LVEDP–left ventricular end-diastolic pressure

TABLE 8 CONTRAINDICATIONS TO HEART TRANSPLANTATION
Age > 65 y
Severe pulmonary hypertension
Severe hepatic or renal dysfunction
Active systemic infection
Any systemic disease considered likely to limit or preclude survival and rehabilitation after transplantation
Severe peripheral or cerebrovascular disease
Insulin-requiring diabetes with severe retinal or renal small vessel disease
A history of behavior pattern or psychiatric illness likely to interfere significantly with compliance following a disciplined medical regimen
No adequate external psychosocial support

physical activity and diet. Bed rest is recommended for acutely ill patients, but during the chronic, compensated stage, gradual progression of frequency and duration of walking is recommended. Regarding diet, modest restriction of sodium intake, with fluid retention controlled by the diuretic regimen, is a standard approach.

Digitalis and diuretics have been the linchpins of traditional therapy for congestive heart failure. For the acutely failing heart, digitalis provides demonstrable inotropic benefit. For the chronically failing heart, the efficacy of digitalis has been attributed less to its inotropic property than to control of the ventricular response to atrial fibrillation or a slowed sinus rate. Some patients in sinus rhythm improve clinically with chronic digitalis therapy, but patients with mild heart failure tolerate the cessation of digitalis therapy. A high incidence of toxicity mandates that digitalis be used cautiously in a patient population subject to multiple drug interactions, fluctuating potassium levels, and predisposition to life-threatening arrhythmias. Use of loop diuretics such as furosemide and ethacrynic acid has enabled many patients with severe heart failure to remain free of edema. In refractory cases of heart failure, diuresis can be maintained by the intermittent use of a proximal tubular diuretic such as metalozone combined with a loop diuretic.

In large, randomized, clinical trials, vasodilator therapy has proven to be effective in reducing mortality. For most patients with symptomatic heart failure, the initial regimen includes a combination of a diuretic, digitalis, and a vasodilator (preferably one with both arteriolar and venodilator properties). Hemodynamic and clinical improvement with afterload reduction in severe heart failure has been achieved with a number of vasodilators. The most widely used are the angiotensin-converting enzyme (ACE) inhibitors and direct-acting arteriolar dilators, such as hydralazine, combined with nitrates (which act predominately as venodilating agents). A word of caution, however: potassium-sparing diuretics and ACE inhibitors used together can cause fatal hyperkalemia.

In patients with asymptomatic left ventricular dysfunction (ejection fraction, < 35%), ACE inhibitors significantly

TABLE 9 SHORT-TERM HEMODYNAMIC EFFECTS OF SYMPATHOMIMETIC AGENTS AND PHOSPHODIESTERASE INHIBITORS

	Receptors Stimulation				Inotropy		Chronotropy	Systemic vascular resistance	Renal blood flow
	B_1	B_2	DA	α	Short term	Long term			
Sympathomimetics									
Dobutamine	++	+	–	±	+	–	+	D	–
Dopamine									
> 2 μg/kg/min	–	–	+	–	–	–	–	D	++
2–5 μg/kg/min	+	+	+	–	+	–	+	D,N	+
> 5 μg/kg/min	+	+	+	+	++	–	++	I	±
Phosphodiesterase inhibitors									
Amrinone	–	–	–	–	++	?	–	D	

D—decreased; I—increased; N—normal.

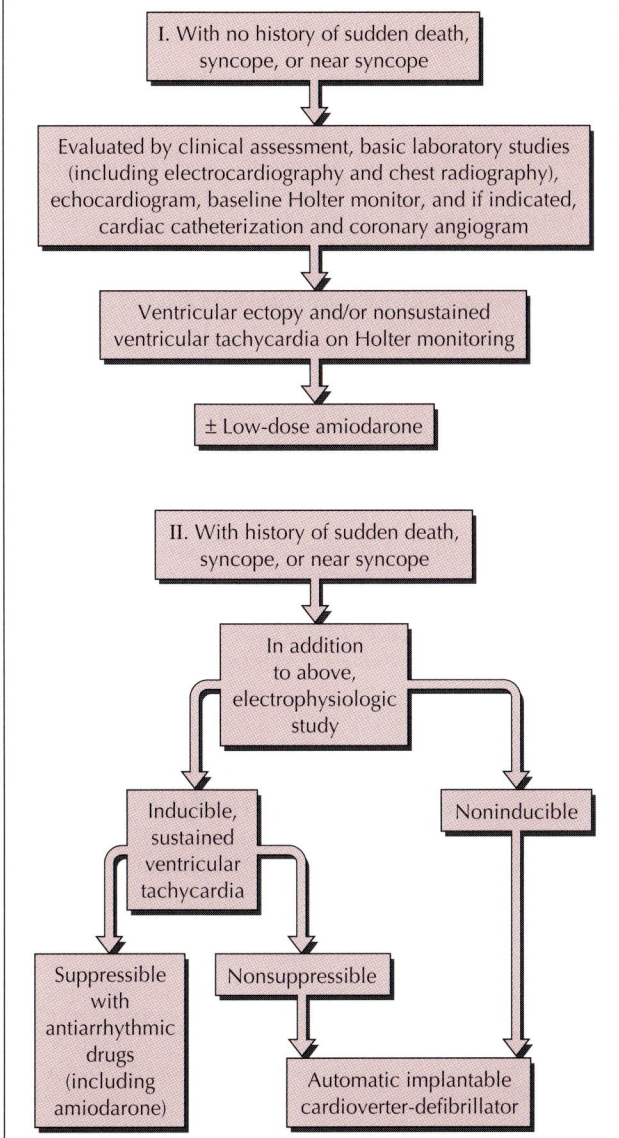

FIGURE 10 Management plan for patients with congestive cardiomyopathy at high risk for sudden death.

decrease the incidence of heart failure compared with placebo [10•]. Currently available non digitalis inotropes are listed with their mechanism of action in Table 9. These inotropic agents are only useful in acute situations, and none has been shown to reduce mortality. Milrinone, the only orally available phosphodiesterase inhibitor, has been associated with an increased mortality [11].

β-adrenergic blockade for treating certain subsets of patients has gained advocacy [12•,13,14]. Because of evidence that activation of the sympathetic nervous system may have deleterious cardiac effects, β-blockade (usually with metoprolol, a β_1-selective agent) has been suggested to improve symptoms and prolong survival. When administered long term (> 2 months), β-blockers improve, rather than depress, systolic function. Other likely mechanisms for the beneficial effects of β-adrenergic blockers are its negative inotropic effect, its inducement of improved diastolic relaxation and increased myocardial β-receptor density, and its reduction in myocardial damage caused by catecholamine release. The initial starting dose is small (metoprolol, 5 mg orally twice a day) and is gradually increased over 6 months to the conventional dose (metoprolol, 50 mg twice a day) provided the patient can tolerate it. This has been demonstrated for metoprolol [13] and bucindolol [14]; bucindolol (a β-blocker with vasodilator properties) has also been shown to improve diastolic function [14]. An assessment of the true clinical efficacy of β-blockade and its impact on survival in congestive cardiomyopathy must await the results of ongoing multicenter trials.

Systemic emboli arising from intracardiac thrombi occur in as many as 30% of patients with congestive cardiomyopathy and may be more common with atrial fibrillation. The strongest predictive factor for systemic embolization appears to be a previous embolus. Chronic oral sodium warfarin therapy is essential for patients with congestive cardiomyopathy with intracardiac thrombi (especially pedunculated), a previous embolic event, or atrial fibrillation.

Perhaps the most controversial issue in the treatment of congestive cardiomyopathy is management of ventricular arrhythmias. Antiarrhythmic drugs have not yet been shown to decrease mortality, and certain agents actually decrease systolic function and can be proarrhythmic [15]. A reasonable policy (Fig. 10) is to limit antiarrhythmic therapy to patients with inducible ventricular tachycardia or symptomatic arrhythmias, especially those with a history of sudden death. Implantable defibrillators decrease the recurrence rate in patients with symptomatic ventricular tachycardia or fibrillation. The decision to recommend an implantable device should be made carefully, however, because most of the currently used devices require thoracotomy, which is by no means a benign procedure [16•,17•].

Patients who remain symptomatic despite maximal medical therapy with a combination of vasodilators, diuretics, and digitalis should be referred to a cardiologist for evaluation and further management (including use of β-blockers for a selected group of patients).

Diastolic Failure

An ideal agent with purely "lusitropic" properties that selectively enhance myocardial relaxation without associated effects on left ventricular contractility or the peripheral vasculature is not available. Diuretics should be used judiciously because of the volume sensitivity of patients with increased left ventricular stiffness. Excessive diuresis carries the risk of reduced stroke volume and cardiac output; however, β-blockers and calcium channel blockers can counteract the inappropriate reduction of ventricular volume by enhancing relaxation and prolonged diastolic filling period resulting from slowing of the heart rate. Although digitalis and vasodilators are generally not useful for treating heart failure with normal systolic function, their exact role for treating diastolic heart failure is currently under investigation.

References and Recommended Reading

Recently published papers of particular interest have been highlighted as:
- Of interest
- •• Of outstanding interest

1. •• Bonow KO, Udelson JE: Left ventricular diastolic dysfunction as a cause of congestive heart failure. *Ann Intern Med* 1992, 117:502.

2. Cuocola A, Sax FL, Brush JE, *et al*.: Left ventricular hypertrophy and impaired diastolic filling in essential hypertension: diastolic mechanisms for systolic dysfunction during exercise. *Circulation* 1990, 81:978.

3. •• Peters NS, Poole-Wilson PA: Myocarditis: continuing clinical and pathologic confusion. *Am Heart J* 1991, 121:942.

4. • Leiberman EB, Hutchins GM, Herskowitz A, *et al*.: Clinicopathologic description of myocarditis. *J Am Coll Cardiol* 1991, 18:1617.

5. Lapa AS, Regan TJ: Direct effects of diabetes on heart muscle. *Coronary Artery Dis* 1992, 3:42.

6. Alexander JK: The cardiomyopathy of obesity. *Prog Cardiovasc Dis* 1985, 27:325.

7. Gradman A, Deedwanai P, Cody R, *et al*.: Predictors of total mortality and sudden death in mild to moderate heart failure. *J Am Coll Cardiol* 1989, 14:564.

8. • Kulick DL, Bhandari AK, Hong R, *et al*.: Effect of acute hemodynamic decompensation on electrical inducibility of ventricular arrhythmias in patients with dilated cardiomyopathy and complex nonsustained ventricular arrhythmia. *Am Heart J* 1990, 119:878.

9. Kriett JM, Kaye MR: The registry of the International Society for Heart Transplantation: 7th Official Report, 1990. *J Heart Transplant* 1990, 9:323.

10. • The SOLVD Investigators: Effect of enalapril on mortality and the development of heart failure in asymptomatic patients with reduced left ventricular ejection fraction. *N Engl J Med* 1992, 327:685.

11. Packer M, Carver JR, Rodheffer RJ, *et al*. and the PROMISE Study Investigators and Coordinators: Effects of milrinone on mortality in severe chronic heart failure. The Prospective Randomized Milrinone Survival Evaluation (PROMISE). *N Engl J Med* 1991, 325:1468.

12. • Waagstein F, Bristow MR, Swedberg K, *et al*.: Beneficial effects of metoprolol in idiopathic dilated cardiomyopathy. *Lancet.* 1993; 342:1441–1446.

13. Sachdev V, Moore CK, Das SK, Starling MR: Effects of β-blocking therapy on left ventricular systolic function in heart failure. *Circulation* 1992, 86:I-119.

14. Eichhorn EJ, Bedotto JB, Malloy CR, *et al*.: Effect of β-adrenergic blockade on myocardial function and energetics in congestive heart failure. *Circulation* 1990, 82:473.

15. Stevenson WG, Weiss JN, Stevenson LW, *et al*.: Risk of conversion from non-inducible to inducible ventricular tachycardia by procainamide in patients with dilated heart failure. *J Am Coll Cardiol* 1987, 9A:246.

16. • Dreifus LS, Fisch C, Griffin J, *et al*.: Guidelines for implantation of cardiac pacemakers and antiarrhythmia devices, July 1991. A report of the American College of Cardiology/American Heart Association Task Force on Assessment of Diagnostic and Therapeutic Cardiovascular Procedures (Committee on Pacemaker Implantation). *J Am Coll Cardiol* 1991, 18:1; *Circulation* 1991, 84:455.

17. • Fogoros RN, Elson JJ, Bonnet CA, *et al*.: Long-term outcome of survivors of cardiac arrest whose therapy is guided by electrophysiological testing. *J Am Coll Cardiol* 1992, 19:782.

18. Kristinsson A: *Diagnosis, Natural History, and Treatment of Congestive Cardiomyopathy*. PhD Thesis: University of London, 1969.

Select Bibliography

Cohn JN: Nitrates versus angiotensin-converting enzyme inhibitors for congestive heart failure. *Am J Cardiol* 1993, 72:216.

Garg R, Packer M, Pitt B, *et al*.: Mechanisms and management of heart failures: Implications of clinical trials for clinical practice. *J Am Coll Cardiol* 1993, 22 (suppl A):3A–205A.

Lessmeier TJ, Lehmann MH, Steinman RT, *et al*.: Outcome with implantable cardioverter-defibrillator therapy for survivors of ventricular fibrillation secondary to idiopathic dilated cardiomyopathy or coronary artery disease without myocardial infarction. *Am J Cardiol* 1993, 72:991.

Restrictive Cardiomyopathy

Martin E. Goldman
Edward A. Fisher

> **Key Points**
> - The hallmark of restrictive cardiomyopathy is abnormal diastolic filling of the ventricles, which are stiff because of fibrosis, hypertrophy, or secondary infiltration.
> - The classic Doppler echocardiographic finding is rapid diastolic ventricular inflow and early cessation of diastolic flow.
> - Differential diagnosis includes congenital, valvular, hypertensive, and pericardial disease (especially constrictive pericarditis).
> - Endomyocardial biopsy can differentiate restriction from constriction and other causes of heart failure.
> - Conventional treatment can temporize by relieving symptoms caused by restricted diastolic ventricular filling and subsequent passive right- and left-sided congestion.

Cardiomyopathies (diseases affecting the myocardium) are categorized as restrictive, hypertrophic, or dilated. Of these, restrictive cardiomyopathies are more common in Africa, the tropics, and subtropics than in North America and Europe. The etiology of restrictive cardiomyopathy may be primary, including idiopathic, or secondary, resulting from a known cause or associated with a disease affecting other organ systems.

The hallmark of restrictive cardiomyopathies is abnormal diastolic filling of the ventricles, which are stiff because of fibrosis, hypertrophy, or secondary infiltration. Right and left ventricular chamber size is usually normal, and systolic function may be preserved until late in the disease course. Importantly, the diagnosis of restrictive cardiomyopathy is made in the absence of congenital, valvular, hypertensive, or pericardial disease, and it is essential to differentiate it from constrictive pericarditis as the latter may be surgically treated. Clinical presentation and hemodynamic data of the two may be very similar, but echocardiography, cardiac catheterization, endomyocardial biopsy, computed tomography (CT), and magnetic resonance imaging (MRI) may assist in differentiating the two diseases.

Idiopathic causes of restrictive cardiomyopathy include "primary restriction," endomyocardial fibrosis, and eosinophilic myocardial disease. Common secondary causes of restrictive physiology include amyloidosis, sarcoidosis, glycogen storage disease (including Fabry's disease), carcinoid, hemachromatosis, and less frequently, fibroelastosis, tumors, pseudoxanthoma elasticum, and collagen-vascular diseases.

CLINICAL MANIFESTATIONS

Patients may be asymptomatic or, rarely, present with extreme dyspnea and heart failure. Because of the diastolic filling abnormality and limited ability to increase cardiac output, decreased exercise tolerance is common. Elevated jugular venous pressure, which paradoxically may increase with inspiration (Kussmaul's sign), and prominent third and fourth heart sounds may be present because of restricted left ventricle filling. Apical impulse is often palpable in patients with restrictive cardiomyopathy but not in those with constrictive pericarditis. Chronically elevated venous pressure often produces peripheral edema, ascites, and hepatosplenomegaly late in the disease course. Cardiac transplant rejection is clinically difficult to differentiate.

Diagnosis

The most common and characteristic electrocardiographic (ECG) findings are low voltage, left-axis deviation, and pseudomyocardial infarction (Q waves mimicking infarction). Chest radiography may show an enlarged cardiac silhouette (often from atrial enlargement) and peripheral vascular redistribution characteristic of congestive heart failure; there is no pericardial calcification.

M-mode and two-dimensional echocardiography generally confirm normal left and right ventricular size and are important in excluding hypertrophic cardiomyopathy and valvular heart disease. The classic Doppler finding is rapid ventricular inflow and early cessation of flow in diastole. This produces a tall E wave. Atrial inflow (A wave) is blunted, because ventricular filling is limited during atrial systole. Therefore, the E:A ratio is high. Doppler findings may vary, however. For example, in early amyloidosis, there may be abnormal ventricular relaxation and a resultant smaller E wave and taller A wave (compliance abnormality). Unfortunately, echocardiographic diagnosis of pericardial thickening is technique-dependent (gain, and so on) and does not correlate well with pericardial thickness of pathologic specimens [1,2].

With constriction, the abnormal pericardium impedes normal ventricular filling and elevates end-diastolic pressures, whereas with restriction, the abnormal myocardium elevates diastolic pressures. During inspiration, the right ventricle fills as its free wall bulges out; however, with constriction, this occurs at the expense of left ventricular filling. The rigid pericardial restraint inhibits diastolic expansion of the right ventricular free wall, and the pliant interventricular septum bulges into the left ventricle, limiting its filling. With expiration, the opposite occurs: the left ventricle fills as the septum bulges into the right ventricle. These respiratory variations in ventricular filling can be detected by two-dimensional and Doppler echocardiography. There are greater respiratory-dependent changes in inflow velocity filling patterns across the mitral and tricuspid valves in patients with constriction than with restrictions [3,4], and patients with constriction have earlier and more complete diastolic ventricular filling. Patients with restriction, however, are more likely to have diastolic mitral or tricuspid regurgitation, a classic finding in restrictive physiology indicating marked elevation of ventricular diastolic pressure.

Ultrasonic tissue characterization uses quantitative backscatter imaging to detect abnormal cardiac tissues and can identify the soft-tissue acoustic characteristics of the restrictive cardiomyopathies. Sound waves are attenuated and reflected differently by the denser fibrosed and infiltrated myocardium. Backscatter imaging estimates the amount of ultrasound energy reflected from the myocardium back to the transducer [5]. Application in patients with amyloid, sarcoid, and primary restriction may be useful in detecting cardiac involvement before ventricular function has been affected and when treatment of the cardiomyopathy may be possible.

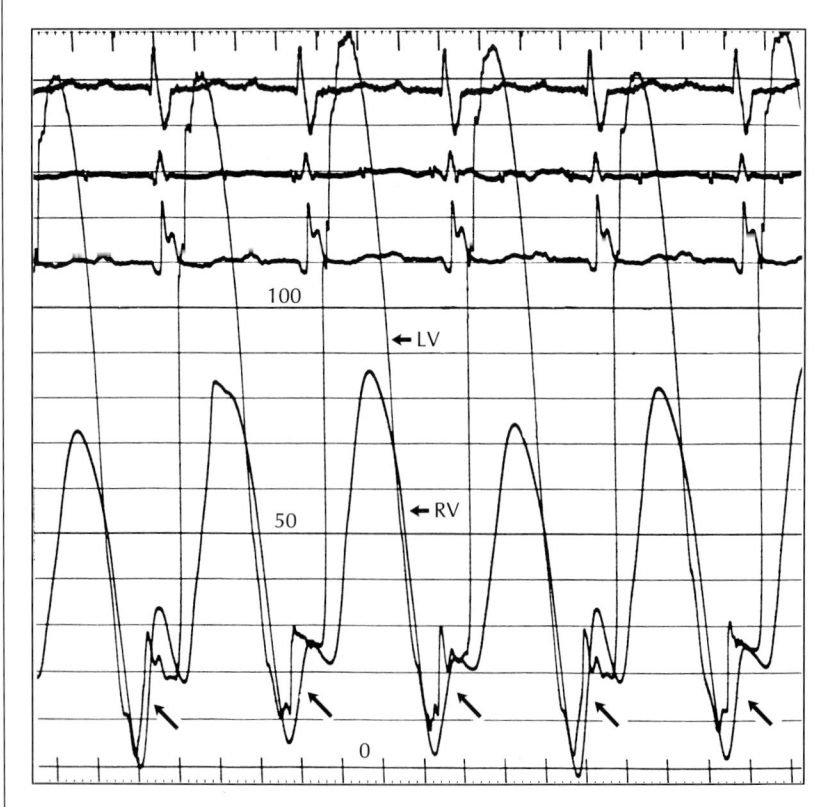

FIGURE 1 Restrictive cardiomyopathy. Hemodynamic tracings demonstrating a sharp pressure increase (*arrows*) in mid-diastole in both the left (LV) and right ventricles (RV). Note that diastolic pressures in the two ventricles are similar.

Magnetic resonance imaging also has been used to diagnose restrictive cardiomyopathy. Although MRI demonstrates a thickened pericardium in constriction, suggestive findings of restriction include enlarged atrial chambers, thick ventricular walls, impaired ventricular filling (demonstrated by a prominent signal within the atria at all phases of the cardiac cycle consistent with stasis of blood secondary to elevated ventricular diastolic pressure), and normal pericardial thickness [6]. Computed tomography can detect the pericardial abnormalities of constriction.

Hemodynamic and angiographic evaluation during cardiac catheterization shows that both constriction and restriction manifest preserved systolic function, prominent and rapid decline in ventricular pressures at the onset of diastole, and a rapid increase in pressure forming a dip and plateau suggestive of a square-root sign (Fig. 1) [7•,8]. In restriction, left atrial pressure may exceed that of the right by 9 mm Hg, and left ventricular filling pressure usually exceeds that of the right by more than 5 mm Hg [8]. Also in restriction, the left ventricle is usually more involved than the right; with constriction, the abnormal pericardium constrains both ventricles equally. Pulmonary artery systolic pressure is usually elevated (> 45 mm Hg) with restriction and lower with constriction [9].

Endomyocardial biopsy is the definitive method to differentiate restriction from constriction and other causes of heart failure; a specific etiology of restriction was identified in 15 of 30 patients studied with class III or IV heart failure, with 11 patients with amyloidosis [10]. Myocyte diameter, nuclear area, and severity of fibrosis can be measured on the biopsy specimen. Myocyte hypertrophy and interstitial fibrosis are frequently found in restriction as well as hypertrophic cardiomyopathy, but without the latter's myocardial disarray [11•].

Treatment and Prognosis

Conventional treatment of restrictive cardiomyopathy is directed toward relief of symptoms caused by restricted diastolic ventricular filling and subsequent passive right- and left-sided congestion. Diuretics are used to reduce peripheral edema and ascites. Angiotensin-converting enzyme (ACE) inhibitors should be used with caution, because they may reduce ventricular filling to an excessive degree, reducing cardiac output [12]. Calcium blocking agents have been useful in treating diastolic abnormalities in patients with hypertensive or hypertrophic cardiomyopathy, but these agents also must be used with caution in patients with restriction because of their vasodilating effects. Glucocorticoid steroids and cytotoxic agents may play a role in specific causes of restrictive cardiomyopathy.

Patients with primary restrictive cardiomyopathy have a reasonably good 5-year survival rate, which may result from early diagnosis and recognition by noninvasive techniques. Of 26 Japanese patients, only 2 with idiopathic restriction died within 1 year, 2 died within 5 years, and 6 others died after 10 years [13]. Once the onset of heart failure occurs, however, mean survival decreases significantly. Mean survival has been reported to be 9 years after the onset of initial symptoms, but only 5 years following the onset of heart failure [14]. Of eight children studied (age range, 1 to 10 years), those having evidence of heart failure with systemic venous congestion and whose biopsies were consistent with idiopathic restrictive cardiomyopathy had a median survival of only 1.4 years [15].

Primary Causes

Endomyocardial Fibrosis

Besides idiopathic causes, there are two primary causes of restrictive cardiomyopathy. Endomyocardial fibrosis is a progressive disease most commonly occurring in children and young adults living in Africa, particularly Uganda and Nigeria, as well as in India, Brazil, and other tropical regions, where it may cause up to 25% of deaths from heart disease [16]. Clinically, patients present with pulmonary and venous congestion. Pathologically, ventricular involvement predominates, with extensive fibrous endocardial lesions of the inflow portion of the right and left ventricles and involvement of the mitral and tricuspid valves. Mural thrombi occur in up to 41% of patients [17].

ST-segment and T-wave abnormalities, decreased voltage, and right atrial enlargement are found on ECG. Atrial arrhythmias are frequent. Echocardiography may demonstrate dilated atria, thickened right ventricle with obliteration of the apex, and increased echo density of the myocardium. Thrombi may be also seen in both ventricles. Varying degrees of tricuspid and mitral regurgitation are also seen. Unlike Chagas' disease, in which apical aneurysms form, the apex is involved with the fibrous process, and systolic ventricular function may be preserved.

Endomyocardial biopsy can confirm the diagnosis. Two-year mortality rate is approximately 50% [18], and medical therapy is not very successful. Surgical excision and stripping of the fibrous endothelial layer of endocardium and valve replacement have been successful, but this carries a high operative mortality (15% to 25%) [19].

Hypereosinophilic Syndrome

Hypereosinophilia (> 1500 eosinophils/mL) is seen as a response to parasitic infections, allergies and hypersensitivity, connective tissue diseases, neoplasias, autoimmune disorders, and cutaneous diseases. When no underlying cause is found, it is called idiopathic. The clinical diagnosis of idiopathic hypereosinophilic syndrome connotes end-organ (heart, central nervous system, kidney, lung, gastrointestinal, and skin) dysfunction. Cardiac involvement, occurring in approximately 50% of cases, is the most serious clinical presentation [20]. The disease may be due to local deposition of toxic eosinophillic proteins, including cationic protein and major basic protein, which ultimately cause fibrosis (Fig. 2).

In 1936, Löffler and coworkers [21] described "fibroplastic parietal endocarditis with blood eosinophilia in two patients with blood eosinophilia (70%), severe chronic congestive heart failure, and mitral regurgitation." At autopsy, there was extensive fibrous thickening of the endocardium of both ventricles with overlying thrombus in the left ventricle. In 1948, Davies and coworkers [22] described patients with endomyocardial

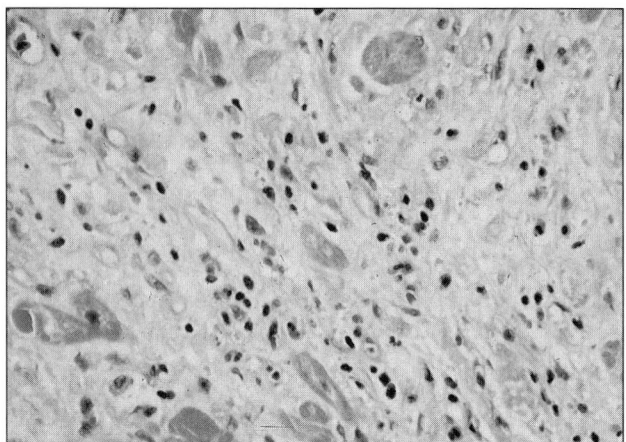

FIGURE 2 Hypereosinophilic syndrome. Endomyocardial biopsy demonstrating areas of scarring with mixed inflammatory infiltrate containing scattered eosinophils.

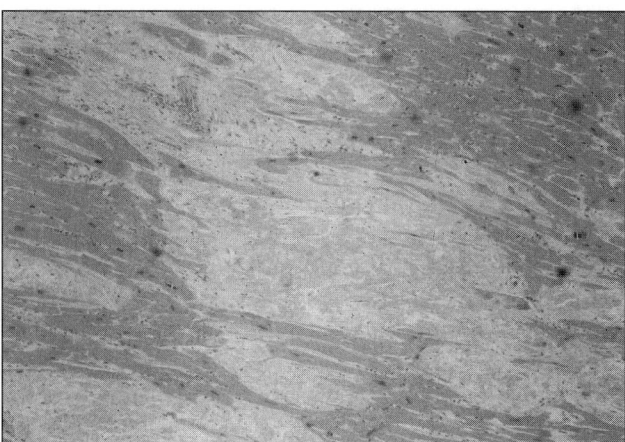

FIGURE 3 Cardiac amyloidosis. Nodular interstitial deposits of amyloid separating myocytes. This pattern is seen with AL amyloid.

fibrosis in West Africa. In 1956, Gerbaux and coworkers [23] suggested that endomyocardial fibrosis and Löffler's endocarditis were essentially the same disease, and indeed, autopsied hearts from patients with these disorders were found to be indistinguishable by Fauci and coworkers [20]. It is possible these disorders are the same disease seen at different stages of development.

The characteristic cardiac lesion of the hypereosinophilic syndrome is endocardial fibrosis and thrombus formation. Most evidence suggests that the endothelial damage initiates thrombosis. Large mural thrombi may occur in either ventricle, impairing filling and serving as a potential thromboembolic source, despite preserved systolic function. Atrioventricular valves often become regurgitant. Heart failure and restrictive symptoms progress rapidly, and both medical treatment (digitalis, diuretics, afterload-reducing agents, and anticoagulation therapy) and surgical treatment may be beneficial. Glucocorticoid steroids and cytotoxic agents (hydroxyurea) have improved the prognosis of hypereosinophilic syndromes, which has traditionally been poor [20].

SECONDARY CAUSES

Amyloidosis

Amyloidosis is a systemic disease caused by extracellular deposition of insoluble amyloid protein fibrils that accumulate in tissues and cause pressure atrophy and dysfunction of the infiltrated organs. Cardiac involvement is the most common cause of death in primary amyloidosis [24], which is composed of an NH_2-terminal portion of an immunoglobulin light chain (designated AL amyloid) originating from a monoclonal population of plasma cells (Fig. 3). AA amyloid (G nonimmunoglobulin protein produced in secondary amyloidosis) is found with various chronic inflammatory diseases. Of 153 patients with primary amyloidosis studied by Cohen and coworkers [24], 41% had cardiac involvement and 27% evidence of heart failure. These patients had the worst prognosis: median survival was 7.7 months and 5-year survival 2.4%. In contrast, the 48% of patients who presented with renal symptoms and primary nephrotic syndrome had a 5-year survival rate of 20%. Cardiac involvement is less common in secondary or familial amyloidosis (AF) [25]. Cardiac deposition is common in senile amyloidosis (Fig. 4) and may contribute to diastolic dysfunction, which is commonly seen, or to significant systolic dysfunction, which is rarely seen [26].

Amyloid deposition between myocardial fibers may involve all cardiac chambers as well as the media of the intramural coronary arteries (Fig. 5) [27]. Patients may present with evidence of restriction with venous congestion and heart failure, arrhythmias, and orthostatic hypotension (probably on the basis of neuropathy [25]). In contrast to the thick walls observed on echocardiography, ECG may show diffusely diminished voltage because of the replacement of normal myocardium by amyloid [27]. Left-axis deviation, atrial fibrillation, and ventricular arrhythmias are seen, particularly with more severe infiltration.

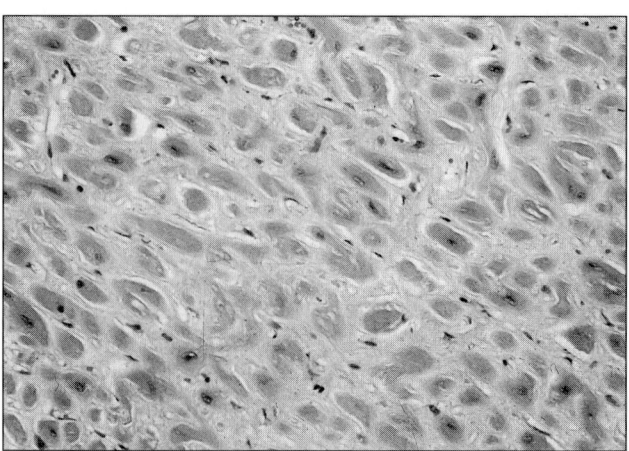

FIGURE 4 Cardiac amyloidosis. Interstitial pattern of amyloid deposition surrounding individual myocytes. This pattern is seen with senile amyloidosis.

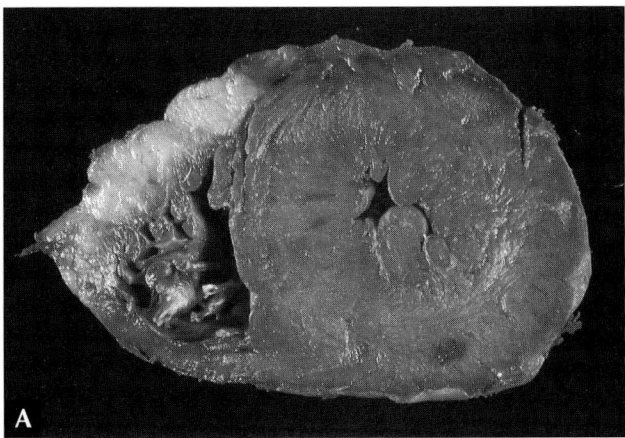
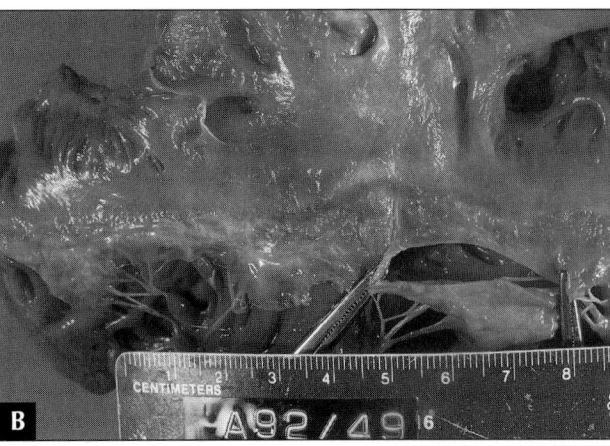

FIGURE 5 Cardiac amyloidosis. **A**, Cross-section through right and left ventricles (LV) demonstrating thickening of LV wall. The myocardium has a somewhat pale and waxy appearance. **B**, Endocardial amyloid deposits of right atrium and tricuspid valve. Note the waxy appearance.

Two-dimensional echocardiography is extremely sensitive for detecting cardiac amyloid and documenting increased myocardial-wall thickness, increased atrial septal thickness, increased right ventricular thickness, and the distinctive, patchy, ground-glass appearance of the myocardium (Fig. 6). Interatrial septal thickening is often noted. Importantly, clinical heart failure correlates strongly with greater wall thickness, ground-glass appearance, and left atrial enlargement. Patients with the greatest mean ventricular wall thickness have the poorest survival rates [28].

The ground-glass appearance of the myocardium, which has a greater impedance mismatch than normal interstitial material, may result from the amorphous amyloid deposition that replaces collagen bundles in the myocardium [29,30]. Newer techniques of tissue characterization and quantitative ultrasonic imaging may identify the acoustic abnormalities of cardiac amyloidosis.

Although distinctive echocardiographic features are adequate evidence for the diagnosis of amyloidosis, definitive diagnosis is made by tissue biopsy (rectal mucosa, gingiva, fat pad, liver, and kidney). Transvenous endomyocardial biopsy confirms cardiac amyloidosis.

Clinical management of amyloidosis is based on treatment of symptoms. Diuretics reduce venous congestion. Calcium blockers are relatively contraindicated because of their negative inotropic effect [30]. Additionally, ACE inhibitors should be used with caution, because they may significantly reduce ventricular filling and cardiac output. Patients may be sensitive to digitalis, which may predispose to significant arrhythmias because of the selective binding of digoxin to amyloid fibers in the heart [27]. Although several regimens have been used to treat amyloidosis, including melphalan, prednisone, and colchicine, none has been effective [31,32]. Of two published cases of heart trans-

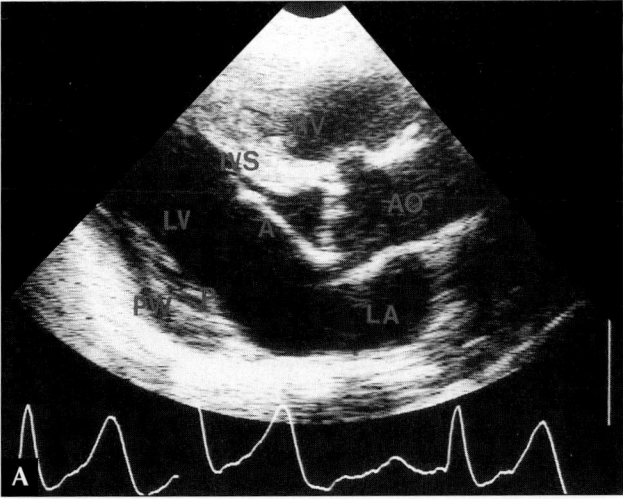
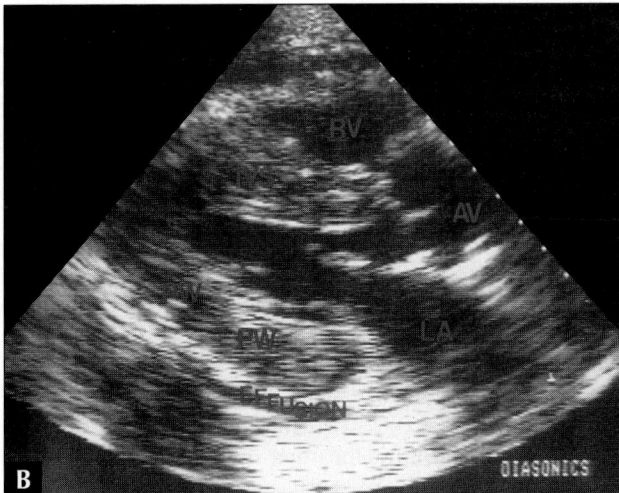

FIGURE 6 Two-dimensional echocardiogram, long-axis view, diastole. **A**, Normal diastolic expansion of the left ventricular cavity (note open mitral valve and closed aortic valve confirming diastole). **B**, Amyloidosis. The ventricular wall is markedly thickened with increased echo density (ground-glass appearance). Note the restricted diastolic expansion of the LV cavity because of myocardial infiltration. A—anterior leaflet of the mitral valve; Ao—aortic valve; IVS—interventricular septum; LA—left atrium; LV—left ventricle; P—pericardium; PW—posterior LV wall; RV—right ventricle.

plantation for amyloidosis, one patient died postoperatively and one had recurrence of amyloidosis in the allograft [33,34].

Sarcoidosis

Sarcoidosis is a multisystem granulomatous disorder of unknown etiology. The disease occurs most commonly in adults and is more common in blacks than in whites. Involvement is manifested by bilateral hilar adenopathy, pulmonary infiltrates, and typical cutaneous and ocular lesions.

Although cardiac involvement is clinically recognizable in only 5% of patients with proven sarcoidosis, pathologic evidence of myocardial noncaseating granulomas (predominantly in the left ventricular free wall and basal interventricular septum) is found in approximately 25% of cases. Antemortem diagnosis is made with endomyocardial biopsy, but a negative biopsy does not rule out the disease because of its patchy involvement. The granuloma is eventually fibrose, and ventricular aneurysms may occur [35]. The clinical spectrum ranges from asymptomatic to arrhythmias (especially ventricular), conduction abnormalities, heart failure (right and/or left sided), or sudden death.

The prognosis is much worse if myocardial involvement exists. The most common cause of death is sudden cardiac arrest, presumably on the basis of ventricular tachycardia, which may occur in 23% of patients [36], and complete heart block. Patients also develop pulmonary fibrosis with respiratory failure and cor pulmonale [37]. Syncope may be common, either because of cardiac arrhythmias or pulmonary dysfunction.

Repolarization abnormalities, ST-segment and T-wave abnormalities, arrhythmias, varying degrees of atrioventricular block, and Q waves mimicking myocardial infarction may be found on ECG [36]. Echocardiography can detect left ventricular systolic dysfunction [38] and localized thinning and dilatation, usually at the base. Thallium-201 scanning has been used to detect myocardial perfusion defects [39], and gallium scanning may detect regions of myocardial involvement.

Patients are treated with appropriate conventional therapy, including heart-failure medications, pacemaker implantation, and antiarrhythmic agents. Because the 1-year mortality rate of cardiac sarcoidosis may be 60%, with many patients dying suddenly, aggressive investigation and management of the ventricular arrhythmias may improve the overall mortality [37]. Additionally, steroids may be beneficial in improving pulmonary and cardiac manifestations. Transplantation is probably not a viable alternative because of the risk of recurrence.

Fabry's Disease

Fabry's disease is an X-linked disorder of glycosphingolipid metabolism from an enzyme deficiency (ceramide trihexosidase) leading to lipid deposition in vasculature of various organs, precipitating myocardial, cerebral, and renal dysfunction. Accumulation of glycosphingolipid in the lysosomes of cardiac tissue can cause increased ventricular wall thickness, simulating hypertrophic cardiomyopathy, mitral valve prolapse, ascending aortic dilatation [40], heart failure, hypertension, or mitral regurgitation. Patients usually have noncardiac presentation, including paresthesias and typical skin lesions (angiokeratomas).

A patient with Fabry's disease and evidence of endothelial infiltration of the coronary arteries presented with angina and myocardial ischemia, and he was treated with successful coronary artery bypass graft surgery [41]. Diagnosis of Fabry's disease is confirmed by a very low level of α-galactosidase activity and endomyocardial biopsy. Enzyme replacement therapy, which is currently available for Gaucher's disease (an inherited deficiency of glycosides that rarely causes ventricular dysfunction), may soon be available for Fabry's disease.

Carcinoid Heart Disease

Carcinoid heart disease occurs in 50% to 70% of patients with classic carcinoid syndrome and metastatic tumors [42]. Carcinoid tumor, most commonly originating in the appendix, secretes serotonin, which causes cutaneous flushing and bronchoconstriction. Usually, serotonin is inactivated by the liver, but hepatic metastasis facilitates development of carcinoid heart disease. The right side of the heart is affected more than the left because of pulmonary inactivation of the humeral substances. Grossly visible, focal, fibrous lesions can be seen on the mural endocardium of the right atrium, right ventricle, or left ventricle, and diffuse or focal thickening of the tricuspid and pulmonic valves can be seen with rare involvement of left-sided valves. Histologic examination reveals fibrous tissue devoid of elastic fibrils [43].

Two-dimensional echocardiography may reveal dilated right-sided chambers with a thickened, echodense, tricuspid valve that is severely incompetent because of immobile leaflets. The pulmonic valve is also thickened and may be stenotic [44]. Patients are managed with α-adrenergic receptor and serotonin blockers. Diuretics may be useful in reducing symptoms of severe tricuspid regurgitation. Replacement of the tricuspid and/or pulmonic valve with heterografts has been successful [42]. Interferon treatment has been attempted with some success.

Hemochromatosis

Hemochromatosis results from excessive iron deposition because of increased iron absorption (primary hemochromatosis) or excessive transfusions or oral intake. Clinical manifestations result from deposition in the liver, pancreas, heart, and pituitary, causing fibrosis and organ failure. Hemochromatosis is one of the most common genetic diseases inherited as an autosomal recessive trait, and clinical manifestations include skin hyperpigmentation, diabetes mellitus, cardiac impairment, arthropathy, and hypogonadism.

Cardiac involvement is the presenting manifestation in approximately 15% of patients. Iron deposition is greater in the ventricles than the atria [45,46]. Congestive heart failure is common and is the principal cause of death in untreated patients. The heart may be enlarged and misdiagnosed as idiopathic cardiomyopathy. ECG may show ST-segment and T-wave abnormalities and arrhythmias, particularly supraventricular. Endomyocardial biopsy can document cardiac involvement. Patients with hemochromatosis have been successfully treated with venesection [47]; chelation therapy has also been used successfully in the treatment of congestive cardiomyopathy resulting from iron overload [48].

Conclusions

Restrictive cardiomyopathy is the least common of the major primary cardiomyopathies; however, restriction should be suspected in patients with unexplained diastolic dysfunction. Two-dimensional and Doppler evaluation are frequently diagnostic, but endomyocardial biopsy is definitive. Unfortunately, therapeutic modalities are limited for management of most patients with restrictive heart disease. Because of the similar presentation of constrictive heart disease, however, which is surgically treatable, a full investigation of the underlying disease of a patient presenting with elevated end-diastolic pressure and suspected restrictive disease is warranted.

References and Recommended Reading

Recently published papers of particular interest have been highlighted as:
• Of interest

1. Voelkel AG, Pietro DA, Follard ED, *et al.*: Echocardiographic features of constrictive pericarditis. *Circulation* 1978, 58:871–875.
2. Plehn JF, Friedman BJ: Diastolic dysfunction in amyloid heart disease: restrictive cardiomyopathy or not? *J Am Coll Cardiol* 1989, 13:54–56.
3. Janos GG, Kalavathy A, Meyer RA, *et al.*: Differentiation of constrictive pericarditis and restrictive cardiomyopathy using digitized echocardiography. *J Am Coll Cardiol* 1983, 1:541–549.
4. Hatle LK, Appleton CP, Popp RL, *et al.*: Differentiation of constrictive pericarditis and restrictive cardiomyopathy by Doppler echocardiography. *Circulation* 1989, 79:357–370.
5. Skorton DJ, Miller JG, Wickline SA, *et al.*: Ultrasonic characterization of cardiovascular tissue. In *Cardiac Imaging*. Edited by Marcus ML, Schelbert HR, Skorton DJ, Wolf GL. Philadelphia: WB Saunders; 1991:886–895.
6. Sechtem U, Higgins CB, Sommerhoff BA, *et al.*: Magnetic resonance imaging of restrictive cardiomyopathy. *Am J Cardiol* 1987, 59:480–482.
7.• Vaitkus PT, Kussmaul WG: Constrictive pericarditis versus restrictive cardiomyopathy: a reappraisal and update of diagnostic criteria. *Am Heart J* 1991, 122:1431–1441.
8. Meaney E, Shabetai R, Bhargava V, *et al.*: Cardiac amyloidosis, constrictive pericarditis and restrictive cardiomyopathy. *Am J Cardiol* 1976, 38:547–556.
9. Child JS, Perloff JK, *et al.*: The restrictive cardiomyopathies. *Cardiol Clin* 1988, 6:289–316.
10. Schoenfeld MH, Supple EW, Dec GW Jr, *et al.*: Restrictive cardiomyopathy versus constrictive pericarditis: role of endomyocardial biopsy in avoiding unnecessary thoracotomy. *Circulation* 1987, 75:1012–1017.
11.• Katritsis D, Wilmshurst PT, Wendon JA, *et al.*: Primary restrictive cardiomyopathy: clinical and pathologic characteristics. *J Am Coll Cardiol* 1991, 18:1230–1235.
12. Bengur AR, Beekman RH, Rocchini AP, *et al.*: Acute hemodynamic effects of captopril in children with a congestive or restrictive cardiomyopathy. *Circulation* 1991, 83:523–527.
13. Hirota Y, Shimizu G, Kita Y, *et al.*: Spectrum of restrictive cardiomyopathy: report of the national survey in Japan. *Am Heart J* 1990, 120:188–194.
14. Siegel RJ, Shan PK, Fishbein MC, *et al.*: Idiopathic restrictive cardiomyopathy. *Circulation* 1984, 70:165–169.
15. Lewis AB: Clinical profile and outcome of restrictive cardiomyopathy in children. *Am Heart J* 1992, 123:6.
16. Gupta PN, Valiathan MS, Balakrishnan KG, *et al.*: Clinical course of endomyocardial fibrosis. *Br Heart J* 1989, 62:450–454.
17. Martinez EE, Venturi M, Buffolo E, *et al.*: Operative results in endomyocardial fibrosis. *Am J Cardiol* 1989, 63:627–629.
18. Barretto AC, da Luz PL, de Oliveira SA, *et al.*: Determinants of survival in endomyocardial fibrosis. *Circulation* 1989, 80(suppl 1):177–182.
19. Mady C, Pereira Barretto AC, de Oliveira SA, *et al.*: Effectiveness of operative and non-operative therapy in endomyocardial fibrosis. *Am J Cardiol* 1989, 15:1281.
20. Fauci AS, Harley JB, Roberts WC, *et al.*: The idiopathic hypereosinophilic syndrome: clinical, pathologic, and therapeutic considerations. *Ann Intern Med* 1982, 97:78–92.
21. Löffler W, *et al.*: Endocarditis Parietalis Fibroplastica mit Bluteosinophile. Ein Eigenartiges Krankheitsbild. *Schweiz Med Wochenschr* 1936, 66:817–820.
22. Davies JNP, *et al.*: Endocardial fibrosis in Africans. *East Afr Med J* 1948, 25:10–14.
23. Gerbaux A, de Brux J, Bennaceur M, *et al.*: L'endocardite parietale fibroplastique avec eosinophile sanguine endocardite de Löffler. *Bull Men Soc Med Hop Paris* 1956, 72:456–465.
24. Cohen AS: Amyloidosis. *N Engl J Med* 1967, 277:522–530.
25. Gertz MA, Kyle RA: Primary systemic amyloidosis: a diagnostic primer. *Mayo Clin Proc* 1989, 64:1505–1519.
26. Pomerance A: Senile cardiac amyloidosis. *Br Heart J* 1965, 27:711–718.
27. Falk RH: Cardiac amyloidosis. In *Progress in Cardiology*. Edited by Zipes DP and Rowlands DJ. Philadelphia: Lea & Febiger; 1989:143.
28. Cueto-Garcia L, Reeder GS, Kyle RA, *et al.*: Echocardiographic findings in systemic amyloidosis: spectrum of cardiac involvement and relation to survival. *J Am Coll Cardiol* 1985, 6:737–743.
29. Pinamonti B, Picano E, Ferdeghnin EM, *et al.*: Quantitative texture analysis in two-dimensional echocardiography: application to the diagnosis of myocardial amyloidosis. *J Am Coll Cardiol* 1989, 14:666–671.
30. Gertz MA, Falk RH, Skinner M, *et al.*: Worsening of congestive heart failure in amyloid heart disease treated by calcium channel-blocking agents. *Am J Cardiol* 1985, 55:1645.
31. Kyle RA, Greipp PR: Primary systemic amyloidosis: comparison of melphalan and prednisone versus placebo. *Blood* 1978, 52:818–827.
32. Cohen AS, Rubinow A, Anderson JJ, *et al.*: Survival of patients with primary (AL) amyloidosis colchicine-treated cases from 1976 to 1983 compared with cases seen in previous years (1961–1973). *Am J Med* 1987, 82:1182–1190.
33. Conner R, Hosenpud JD, Norman DJ, *et al.*: Heart transplantation for cardiac amyloidosis: successful one-year outcome despite recurrence of the disease. *J Heart Transplant* 1988, 7:165–167.
34. Moulin G, Cognat T, Delaye J, *et al.*: Amylose disseminee primitive familiale (nouvelle forme clinique?). *Ann Dermatol Venerol* 1988, 115:565–570.
35. Temple-Camp CR: Sarcoid myocarditis: a report of three cases. *N Z Med J* 1989, 102:501–502.
36. Roberts WC, McAllister HA Jr, Ferrans VJ, *et al.*: Sarcoidosis of the heart. *Am J Med* 1977, 63:86–108.
37. Roberts WC, McAllister HA, Ferrans VJ, *et al.*: Sarcoidosis of the heart. A clinicopathologic study of 35 patients (group I) and review of 78 previously described necropsy patients (group II). *Am J Med* 1977, 63:86.
38. Burstow DJ, Tajik AJ, Bailey KR, *et al.*: Two-dimensional echocardiographic findings in systemic sarcoidosis. *Am J Cardiol* 1989, 63:478–482.

39. Kinney EL, Jackson GL, Reeves WC, *et al.*: Thallium-scan myocardial defects and echocardiographic abnormalities in patients with sarcoidosis without clinical cardial dysfunction. An analysis of 44 patients. *Am J Med* 1980, 68:497–503.

40. Goldman ME, Cantor R, Schwartz MF, *et al.*: Echocardiographic abnormalities and disease severity in Fabry's disease. *J Am Coll Cardiol* 1986, 7:1157–1161.

41. Fisher EA, Desnick RJ, Gordon RE, *et al.*: Fabry disease: an unusual cause of severe coronary artery disease in a young man. *Ann Intern Med* 1992, 117:221–223.

42. Lundin L, Hansson HE, Landelius J, *et al.*: Surgical treatment of carcinoid heart disease. *J Thorac Cardiovasc Surg* 1990, 100:552–561.

43. Ross EM, Roberts WC: The carcinoid syndrome: comparison of 21 necropsy subjects with carcinoid heart disease to 15 necropsy subjects without carcinoid heart disease. *Am J Med* 1985, 79:339–354.

44. Lundin L, Landelius J, Andren B, *et al.*: Transesophageal echocardiography improves the value of cardiac ultrasound in patients with carcinoid heart disease. *Br Heart J* 1990, 64:190–194.

45. Short EM, Winkle RA, Billingham ME, *et al.*: Myocardial involvement idiopathic hemochromatosis. Morphologic and clinical improvement following venesection. *Am J Med* 1981, 70:1275–1279.

46. Vigorita VJ, Hutchins GM: Cardiac conduction system in hemochromatosis: clinical and pathologic features of six patients. *Am J Cardiol* 1979, 44:418–423.

47. Easley RM, Schreiner BF, Yu PN, *et al.*: Reversible cardiomyopathy associated with hemochromatosis. *N Engl J Med* 1972, 287:866–867.

48. Rahko PS, Salerni R, Uretsky BF: Successful reversal by chelation therapy of congestive cardiomyopathy due to iron overload. *J Am Coll Cardiol* 1986, 8:436–440.

Infectious Myocarditis

Martin E. Goldman

> **Key Points**
> - Infectious myocarditis has an acute phase with a clinical spectrum ranging from no symptoms to severe heart failure.
> - The chronic phase of illness may result from autoimmune mechanisms triggered by the initial infection without residual evidence of the inciting agent.
> - Endomyocardial biopsies have limited value in most patients and should be reserved for specific subgroups.
> - The value of immunosuppressive therapy has not been established.
> - Therapy should be directed to the inciting infectious agent if specific therapy is available and to alleviating symptoms of heart failure and treating arrhythmias if life-threatening.

Myocarditis is an inflammation of the heart muscle, primarily associated with an infectious agent, although other substances also may precipitate an inflammatory response by the myocardium. Most episodes of infectious myocarditis are clinically silent and resolve spontaneously, but noninvasive technologies such as cardiac ultrasound facilitate recognition and diagnosis of even mild, asymptomatic cases. The other end of the spectrum is an acute presentation with severe heart failure. Additionally, some patients may develop dilated cardiomyopathy years after their silent episode of myocarditis. A review of 673 consecutive patients with dilated cardiomyopathy found the disease etiology to be idiopathic in 47%, idiopathic myocarditis in 12%, and coronary disease in 11% of patients [1]. Because of its varied presentation, the actual incidence of infectious myocarditis is difficult to assess. The estimated incidence of cardiac involvement in all viral infections is 5% [2] and the autopsy incidence of myocarditis of suspected viral origin 2.5% to 5.0% [2,3].

DISEASE MECHANISM

In animal models, viral myocarditis is a two-component disease. The initial phase of direct cytopathogenic myocardial damage, viral replication, minimal myocyte necrosis, or cellular infiltrate is an infectious phase and may last 7 to 14 days, usually followed by complete recovery. The second phase, which develops as the virus is cleared, involves a T-lymphocytic response against a myocardial/viral antigen, resulting in myocyte destruction and, ultimately, congestive failure (Fig. 1). Sole and Liu [4••] propose a multifactoral mechanism of myocarditis, including microvascular constriction and spasm, which causes dissolution of the myocardial matrix and diffuse loss of cardiac muscle mass ultimately leading to myocardial failure.

Indirect evidence of infectious etiology in humans is suggested by an elevated coxsackievirus B–antibody titer in 30% of patients with dilated cardiomyopathy compared with only 2% of controls [5]. Investigators have also described defects suppressor lymphocyte function in patients with myocarditis and dilated myopathy.

An autoimmune mechanism of acute and chronic myocarditis that may be primary or triggered by a viral infection was demonstrated by Lauer and coworkers [6]. They used enzyme-linked immunosorbent assay (ELISA) and Western blot tests and found that 17 of 40 (42%) of serum samples of patients with myocarditis showed antibody binding against myosin compared with only 1 of 39 (2.5%) in healthy controls [6]. Unfortunately, endomyocardial biopsies have not fully elucidated the etiology of most myocarditis or the complex relationship between histopathologic findings and clinical manifestations.

VIRAL INFECTIOUS MYOCARDITIS

Infectious myocarditis can be caused by bacterial, fungal, parasitic, rickettsial, or spirochetal organisms, although viral agents are the most common infectious etiology (Table 1). The spectrum of clinical manifestations ranges from a totally asymptomatic response to severe congestive heart failure. Symptoms may consist of a viral prodrome, myalgia, rhinorrhea, mild fatigue, shortness of breath, palpitations, chest pain, and fever. Importantly, symptoms may mimic an acute myocardial infarction (MI). Dec and coworkers [7•] reported that 11 of 34 patients with clinical signs and symptoms consistent with acute MI but normal coronary arteries had histologic evidence of myocarditis. Three of these 11 patients developed cardiogenic shock, and two patients had pathologic Q waves.

More recently, Narula and coworkers [8] reported eight patients with normal coronary arteries who experienced severe precordial chest pain, with electrocardiographic (ECG) changes in the anterior leads in four patients and inferior leads in one consistent with MI. Creatine kinase muscle and brain (CK-MB) isoenzyme fractions ranged from 4% to 22% (normal, < 5%). Antimyosin myocardial scintigraphy revealed diffuse, heterogeneous, global left ventricular uptake in seven of the eight patients, whereas 45 other patients with acute MI and angiographic evidence of coronary occlusion had intense, discrete, localized uptake. Thus, myocarditis should be included in the differential diagnosis of acute MI if coronary arteries are normal.

Physical examination may be normal or include sinus tachycardia and ventricular gallops and evidence of pulmonary congestion. Chest radiograph may demonstrate normal or enlarged cardiac silhouette with evidence of pulmonary congestion.

Electrocardiography may demonstrate sinus tachycardia, ST-T wave abnormalities, Q waves, atrial abnormalities, or conduction defects. Morgera and coworkers [9] reviewed ECGs from 45 consecutive patients with histologic diagnosis of active myocarditis; the ECG pattern was abnormal in 43 patients. Normal P waves, atrioventricular (AV) block, and repolarization abnormalities were common among patients with cardiac symptoms of short duration (< 1 month). Patients with a longer clinical history, however, had atrial abnormalities (left atrial enlargement and atrial fibrillation), left ventricular hypertrophy, and left bundle-branch block (LBBB). Supraventricular arrhythmias were noted in 20% of patients. Complete and advanced AV block was observed in 15% and was not a reliable marker of myocardial damage. Analysis of the QRS pattern was an excellent measure of the degree of left ventricular damage. Patients with abnormal QRS complexes had more severe left ventricular impairment and higher frequency of hypertrophy and fibrosis. The ECG abnormality that correlated best with the most severe left ventricular dysfunction was LBBB. Patients with right bundle-branch block had a shorter clinical history and higher right ventricular filling pressures. ST-segment abnormalities alone did not appear to have a negative prognostic value; however, abnormal Q waves and ST-segment elevation seen in three patients were associated with a fulminant progressive fatal course in two of the three. In the group of 13 patients who died, sudden death occurred in 4 of the 9 patients with abnormal QRS complexes. Thus, presence of an abnormal QRS or LBBB

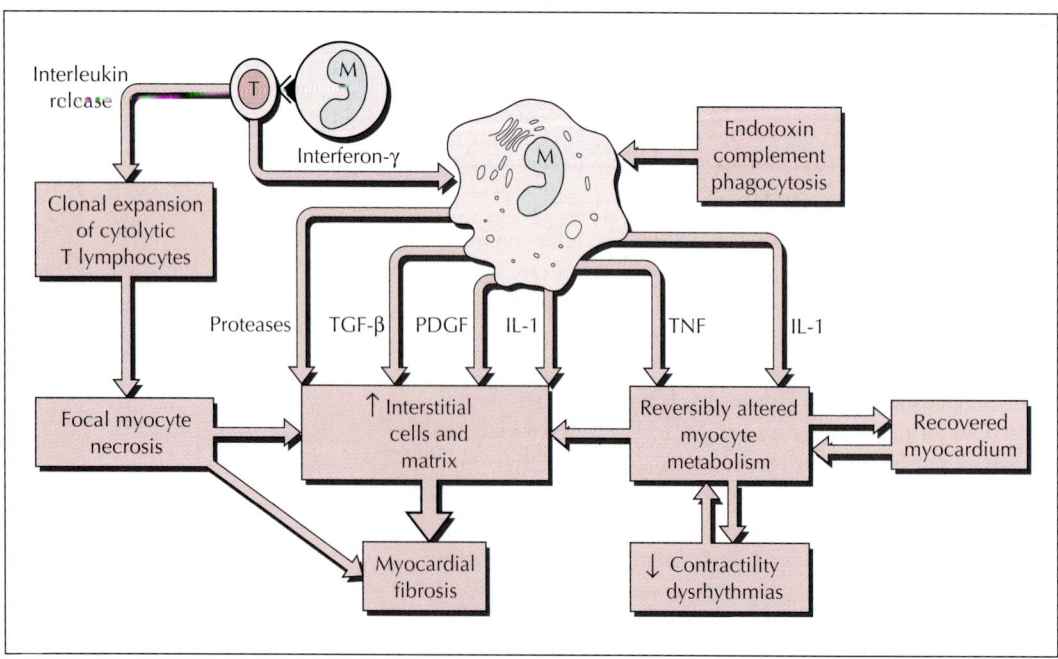

FIGURE 1
Cellular pathways mediating reversible and irreversible immune injury to the heart. IL—interleukin; M—macrophage; PDGF—platelet-derived growth factor; TGF-β—transforming growth factor–β; TNF—tumor necrosis factor. (*From* Lange and Schreiner [42]; with permission.)

TABLE 1 INFECTIOUS ETIOLOGIES OF MYOCARDITIS

Viral	Bacterial	Metazoal
Coxsackievirus	Brucellosis	Cysticercosis
Cytomegalovirus	Diphtheria	Echinococcus
Echo virus	Clostridia	Schistosomiasis
Epstein-Barr virus	Endocarditis-associated myocarditis	Trichinosis
Hepatitis	Gonococcus	**Fungal**
Human immunodeficiency virus	Meningococcus	Actinomycosis
Influenza	*Salmonella typhi*	Aspergillosis
Mumps	Staphylococcus	Blastomycosis
Mycoplasma *pneumoniae*	Streptococcus	Candidiasis
Poliomyelitis	Tuberculosis	Histoplasmosis
Rabies	**Spirochetal**	**Rickettsial**
Retrovirus	Leptospirosis	Q fever
Rubella	Lyme disease	Rocky Mountain spotted fever
Rubeola	Syphilis	Typhus
Varicella	**Protozoal**	
	Amebiasis	
	Chagas' disease (*Trypanosoma cruzi*)	
	Toxoplasmosis	

on the ECG of a patient with myocarditis implies more severe myocardial damage and a poorer prognosis. AV block may be transient, but if unrecognized, it may cause sudden death. Significant ventricular arrhythmias are another serious complication of myocarditis and may be the initial presentation.

Echocardiography facilitates initial diagnosis and frequent noninvasive monitoring of the patient's clinical course. The echocardiogram may be normal or demonstrate varying degrees of left ventricular dysfunction, which may be focal or global (Fig. 2). Doppler findings may include mild valvular regurgitation or diastolic dysfunction, which may precede systolic abnormalities. Importantly, diffuse myocardial damage may be documented by involvement of the right and left ventricles and dilation of all four chambers, but some patients may have only minimal or focal left ventricular dysfunction. Radionuclide imaging may confirm biventricular involvement. An abnormal left ventricle response to exercise, by either radionuclear-gated blood pool scanning (multiple-

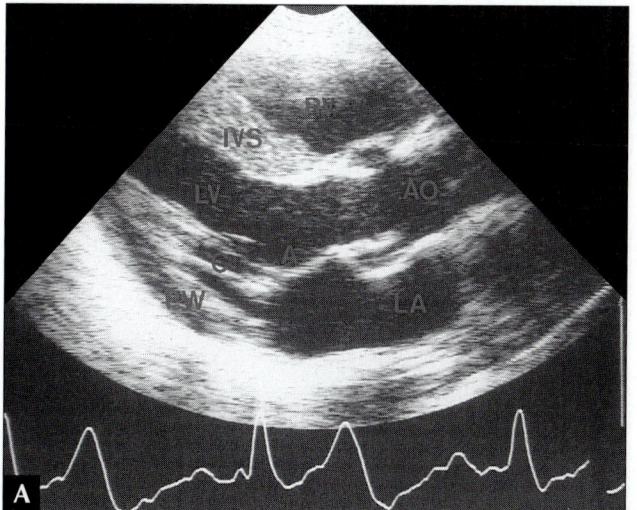
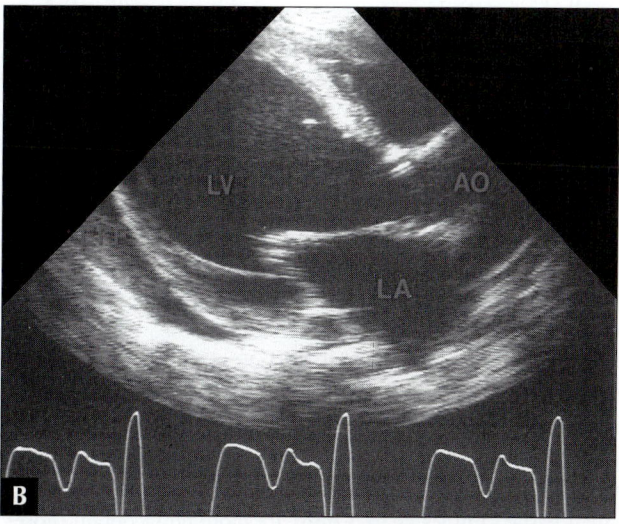

FIGURE 2 Two-dimensional echocardiogram. **A,** Long-axis view, systolic frame: normal wall thickening and cavity size. **B,** Dilated and severely hypocontractile left ventricle. A—anterior leaflet of the mitral valve; Ao—aorta; C—chordae tendonae; EFF—pericardial effusion; IVS—interventricular septum; LA—left atrium; LV—left ventricle; PW—posterior LV wall; RV—right ventricle.

gated acquisition [MUGA]) or exercise echocardiography, may demonstrate abnormal ventricular reserve even with normal resting function.

Monoclonal antimyosin antibody radiolabeled with indium-111 may reveal diffuse uptake, because cellular myosin is released into the extracellular fluid due to myocardial necrosis and cellular disruption. In a study of patients with suspected myocarditis, antimyosin antibody imaging had a sensitivity of 100% and specificity of 58% [10]. Gallium-67 also may demonstrate diffuse uptake but has high sensitivity and low specificity. The potential value of nuclear magnetic resonance imaging and positron-emission tomography in the diagnosis of myocarditis has not yet been defined.

Serologic studies including CK-MB fractions may be abnormal, indicating of myocardial damage. Identification of viral particles in throat swabbing, stool, or blood and increased viral antibody titers may be useful but are not specific for the diagnosis of viral myocarditis.

With recent analysis of the genome of cardiotropic viruses, radiolabeled genetic probes can identify a viral signal in biopsy specimens even if no evidence of an inflammatory response exists. Bowles and coworkers [11] using a coxsackie B viral probe, found virus-specific RNA sequences in up to 50% of patients with myocarditis or dilated cardiomyopathy. The polymerase chain reaction (PCR) is a sensitive method to detect residual viral genome and persistence in endomyocardial biopsy specimens. Using PCR, Keeling and coworkers [11] detected enteroviral genome in 6 of 50 (12%) patients with dilated cardiomyopathy compared with 13 of 75 (17%) of controls. Although this study suggests that persistent enteroviral infection itself causes dilated myopathy, an autoimmune reaction to an initial infection is possible. Thus, genetic probe techniques may elucidate the complex relationship between viral infections and myocarditis.

Endomyocardial Biopsy

Sutton and coworkers [13] first described the transthoracic needle biopsy technique in human subjects in 1956. Subsequently, Sakakibara and Konno [14] reported the currently used technique of performing endomyocardial biopsy via a fluoroscopically guided transvenous bioptome to sample the apex, free wall, and septum of the right ventricle. Usually, the right internal jugular vein is the preferred entry site, with the subclavian veins as alternatives.

In more than 4000 biopsies performed at Stanford University in the 1970s, the morbidity rate was less than 1%, and there were no deaths [15]. Rare complications of transvenous endomyocardial biopsy include pneumothorax, ventricular or atrial arrhythmias, bradycardia, hypotension, and perforation of the right ventricular free wall and tricuspid regurgitation because of damaged chordae tendineae. Echocardiographic guidance can substantially reduce the incidence of complications as well as radiation exposure. Usually, more than five small tissue samples (1 to 3 mm) are required to obtain representative samples of the myocardium. Importantly, myocardial tissue more than 5 mm below the endocardial surface is not sampled by the bioptome. Because myocarditis may be a focal disease involving only 5% of the myocardium, sampling error accounts for most false-negative diagnoses and may occur in up to 40% of patients [16]. A larger number of biopsy specimens has a greater diagnostic yield. Histologically defined myocarditis has been diagnosed in only 5% to 30% of patients clinically suspected of having myocarditis, up to 41% of patients with acutely dilated cardiomyopathy, and up to 63% of patients with chronic dilated myopathy [16]. The incidence of biopsy-confirmed myocarditis in unexplained congestive heart failure has ranged from 0% to 67%. In a study of 100 consecutive right ventricular endomyocardial biopsies, a positive biopsy was found in only 11% of patients clinically thought to have myocarditis [18].

Because of differing patient populations, sampling error, and conflicting criteria for defining myocarditis, the Dallas criteria were established to standardize histologic criteria [19] (Table 2). This classification, based on findings of the first biopsy, was defined by the type, distribution, and extent of cellular infiltrate and fibrosis (Fig. 3). Specific lymphocyte counts, formerly considered critical, were no longer recommended; however, this morphologic criterion lacks clinical correlation and is prone to sampling error and interobserver variability. Thus, Lieberman and coworkers [20••] introduced a clinicopathologic description of myocarditis combining clinical and histologic findings. Their four categories were fulminant myocarditis, acute, chronic active, and chronic persistent patients.

The fulminant group had acute onset of symptoms with significant left ventricular dysfunction. Their endomyocardial biopsy demonstrated foci of active myocarditis, and patients went on to complete recovery or death. Immunosuppressive therapy was of no benefit. Patients with acute myocarditis had

TABLE 2 DALLAS CRITERIA

Initial biopsy
Myocarditis, with or without fibrosis
Borderline
No myocarditis

Inflammation
Type: eosinophilic, giant cell, granulomatous, lymphocytic, neutrophilic, mixed
Distribution: interstitial, endocardial
Extent: mild, moderate, severe

Fibrosis
Type: pericellular, perivascular, replacement
Distribution: interstitial, endocardial
Extent: mild, moderate, severe

Subsequent biopsies
Ongoing (persistent)
Resolving (healing)
Resolved (healed)

Adapted from Aretz [18]; with permission.

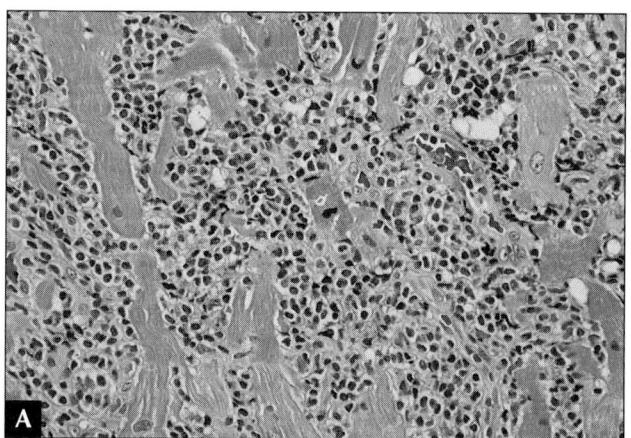
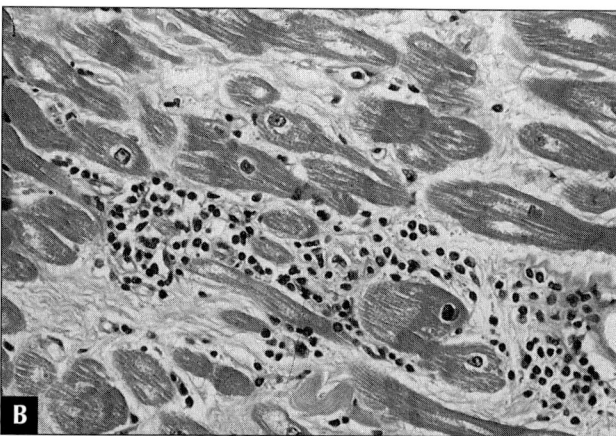

FIGURE 3 Viral myocarditis. **A,** First biopsy showing severe lymphocytic myocarditis with myocyte necrosis. **B,** Follow-up biopsy 6 months later showing resolving myocarditis with fibrosis and residual lymphocytic infiltrate.

distinct onset of cardiac symptoms with varying degrees of congestive heart failure. Their biopsies demonstrated active or borderline myocarditis according to the Dallas criteria, and they usually had resolution of their myocarditis. Immunosuppressive therapy was sometimes beneficial. The chronic active patients had varying degrees of left ventricular dysfunction, with biopsies demonstrating active or borderline myocarditis. They developed dilated cardiomyopathy, and immunosuppressant therapy was of no benefit. Patient with chronic persistent myocarditis had varying degrees of left ventricular dysfunction and no significant symptoms of congestive heart failure. Their biopsies also demonstrated active or borderline myocarditis. The classification of Lieberman and coworkers is similar to that used for viral hepatitis and attempts to integrate clinical and pathologic findings.

NATURAL HISTORY AND TREATMENT OF VIRAL MYOCARDITIS

The natural history of myocarditis varies with etiology. The vast majority of patients with viral myocarditis have few or no symptoms and a totally benign course. Treatment should be geared to manage specific clinical symptoms with the standard regimen for heart failure and arrhythmias. In the early phases of myocarditis, bed rest may be beneficial in limiting myocardial oxygen consumption and ventricular wall stress. Congestive heart failure is treated with diuretics, vasodilators, angiotensin-converting enzyme inhibitors, and digitalis. Patients with myocarditis may be sensitive to digitalis during the acute stages of myocarditis. By blocking replication of certain viruses, inhibition of interleukin-2 (IL-2) messenger RNA, and preventing the microvascular spasm, the calcium channel–blocking agent verapamil improved the clinical and pathological course of experimental murine myocarditis [21•]. Captopril, which besides being an afterload 3-reducing agent can also neutralize oxygen free radicals, had a similar beneficial effect in another animal model [22]. Human studies have not yet confirmed these findings. If the patient presents with symptomatic bradyarrhythmias, a temporary pacemaker should be inserted. If prolonged and symptomatic, ventricular arrhythmias may require electrophysiological study for selection of appropriate management. Consideration of prolonged observation in a monitored setting to determine if the inflammatory process is transient may obviate treatment with potential proarrhythmic agents or even antifibrillary devices.

Immunosuppressive therapy has been used for many years but has not been documented to be of substantial benefit. Corticosteroids, azathioprine, antithymocyte globulin, and cyclosporine have been used with varying success in patients with biopsy-proven myocarditis. O'Connell and Mason [23•] accumulated 13 different studies with a total of 118 patients and improvement in 52% of those undergoing immunosuppressive therapy. Because some patients may improve spontaneously, however, definitive conclusions regarding the benefits of immunosuppressive therapy were not possible. OKT3 (a murine monoclonal antibody directed to the T-cell CD3 antigen) also has been used with some success.

Because of the varying criteria used and the small number of patients reported from individual centers, the National Institutes of Health (NIH)–sponsored myocarditis treatment trial was established [24]. Enrollment was initiated in 1986 and completed in 1990. Approximately 10% of the 2200 patients screened with suspected myocarditis had a positive biopsy. Patients with unexplained congestive heart failure and endomyocardial biopsy demonstrating myocarditis were randomized to conventional therapy for congestive heart failure or a combination of conventional therapy and prednisone and cyclosporine, the rationale being that myocarditis is initiated by an immune response against a myocardial/viral antigen (or even an autoimmune reaction). Patients were followed-up until 1 year after the initial randomization. After 1 year, no difference existed in mortality rates between the conventionally treated group or the immunosuppressive arm [25••]. There was also no significant difference in left ventricular ejection fraction at baseline or 1 year after randomization between the two treatment groups. Subset analysis is still pending. High-dose intravenous gammaglobulin may be beneficial in children presenting with presumed myocarditis. Twenty-one children treated with intravenous immunoglobulin, 2 g/kg over 24 hours, had better ventricular function at 1 year and had a tendency towards better survival than a historical control group [26].

Because of the variation in diagnostic yield from biopsies and the controversy regarding appropriate therapeutic response, indications for endomyocardial biopsy for suspected myocarditis should be limited to patients with unexplained heart failure and normal coronary arteries who are experiencing progressive deterioration in their clinical course or present with significant ventricular ectopy. A positive biopsy in those patients with extremely poor prognosis may warrant a 2-month trial of immunosuppressive therapy. Unfortunately, based on current data, one cannot predict which patients with myocarditis will respond to such treatment.

In a limited trial, intravenous rabaviran (an antiviral agent) was useful in reducing viral shedding; however, all three patients died within 8 months of treatment [27]. Antiviral therapy with interferon has also shown some promise as a potential therapy of acute myocarditis.

CARDIAC TRANSPLANTATION

Currently, cardiac transplantation is offered to patients with end-stage cardiomyopathy. Early cardiac transplantation may be an alternative for patients with acute myocarditis and a fulminant course who do not respond to conventional therapy or a trial of immunosuppressive agents. However, two studies comprising 38 patients demonstrated a higher rejection rate and lower survivor rates in patients with acute myocarditis treated with transplantation compared with controls [28,29].

SPECIFIC AGENTS OF VIRAL MYOCARDITIS

Coxsackievirus A and B, echovirus, and influenza are the most common viruses causing myocarditis, with coxsackievirus the most frequent [30]. Clinical manifestations such as pleurodynia, generalized myalgias, and arthralgic and upper respiratory symptoms should raise suspicion of a viral etiology. Patients may have pleuritic or pericarditic chest pain and diffuse ST-T wave abnormalities on ECG. Elevated antibody titers to cardiotrophic viruses are reported in over 50% of asymptomatic adults (probably from silent viral infection) and are of little value in establishing the diagnosis of myocarditis [31]. Atrioventricular block may require temporary pacemaker implantation. Treatment is geared to specific symptoms.

Immunosuppressive therapy in the acute phase may be deleterious, and its benefit in the second phase of illness is unclear. In most patients, viral myocarditis is a benign illness, and there is complete recovery without sequelae. Approximately 50% of patients with left ventricular dysfunction may stabilize or even demonstrate spontaneous improvement [32].

Human Immunodeficiency Virus

In 1989, Levy and coworkers [33] reported that 32 of 62 patients (52%) infected with human immunodeficiency virus (HIV) had evidence of cardiac abnormalities either by echocardiogram, ECG, or Holter monitoring. Echocardiography can detect asymptomatic pericardial effusions or biventricular dysfunction. Clinical congestive heart failure may occur in 10% to 25% of patients with AIDS.

The mechanism of myocardial involvement in AIDS may be related to primary viral infection with HIV or secondary to cytomegalovirus or other cardiotropic viruses, other infectious agents (tuberculosis or toxoplasmosis), ischemic cardiomyopathy, malnutrition, cytokines such as tumor necrosis factor, and in intravenous drug abusers, cocaine-related damage (Table 3). Baroldi and coworkers [34] found evidence of cardiac lymphocytic infiltrate in 20 of 26 patients (77%) with AIDS; although nine of the 26 met the Dallas criteria for myocarditis, none had cardiac symptoms. In a study by Anderson and Virmani [35] of 71 patients with AIDS, necropsy demonstrated the incidence of fungal, mycobacterial, and protozoal opportunistic pathogens to be 58%, 42%, and 80%, respectively, with no evidence of direct HIV involvement. Kaposi's sarcoma was found in 49% of heart specimens, and 52% of patients had histologic evidence of myocarditis.

Mortality secondary to progressive heart failure, lethal ventricular arrhythmias, or pericardial tamponade may be as high as 18%. Symptoms and manifestations of heart failure are treated with digoxin, diuretics, afterload reduction, and vasodilators. Treatment alternatives are limited in patients with AIDS because of their underlying immunodeficiency. However, when the cardiac manifestations are disproportionate to other clinical signs of disease and treatable fungal or mycobacterial involvement is suspected, myocardial biopsy may be worthwhile to direct specific treatment. Pentamidine, which is used to treat *Pneumocystis carinii* pneumonia, may precipitate ventricular arrhythmias and should be used with caution because of the frequency of clinical and subclinical cardiac involvement in AIDS.

Giant Cell Myocarditis

Giant cell myocarditis, identified by the presence of giant cells in the myocardium, aorta, and other major arteries, is part of the spectrum of systemic giant cell arthritis (temporal arthritis). It is occasionally associated with autoimmune diseases such as myasthenia gravis, lupus, and thyrotoxicosis, and has an acute course manifested by chest pain and dyspnea. bradyarrhythmias and tachyrhythmias are common. The disease may respond to corticosteroid therapy adjusted to the erythrocyte sedimentation rate.

TABLE 3 CARDIAC INVOLVEMENT IN ACQUIRED IMMUNODEFICIENCY SYNDROME

Myocarditis	Malignant
Viral	Kaposi's sarcoma
Opportunistic infections	Lymphoma
Autoimmune	
	Toxicity
Pericarditis	Cocaine
Autoimmune	Pentamidine
Infectious	Other drugs

Bacterial Myocarditis

Diphtherial myocarditis may occur in up to 20% of cases of diphtheria infection. Dilated cardiomyopathy with congestive heart failure may develop rapidly and is the most common cause of death in diphtheria. Antitoxin therapy, erythromycin, or penicillin G and diuretics are the mainstays of treatment. Streptococcal myocarditis is a major manifestation of acute rheumatic fever pancarditis following a β-hemolytic streptococcal infection and may be the etiology of left ventricular dysfunction seen many years after the initial infection. Although ECG abnormalities (primarily ST-T and Q-Tc) may be frequent in typhoid fever (*Salmonella typhi*), clinical myocarditis is rare. Bradycardia may be a harbinger of myocarditis. Treatment of typhoid fever includes trimethoprim-sulfamethoxazole or ceftriaxone.

Lyme Carditis

Lyme disease is a nonfatal multiorgan disorder caused by *Borrelia burgodorferi* and may involve the heart, nervous system, skin, and muscles. The spirochete is transmitted by a tick *Ixodes dammini*; *Ixodes pacificus* is found in the western United States. The white-tailed deer is the dominant host for the adult tick. The initial manifestation of Lyme disease is a characteristic skin rash, erythema nicum migraines, which occurs in 60% to 80% of cases and may clear without therapy. Additional symptoms include fever, myalgias, arthralgias, headache, lymphadenopathy, and fatigue [36]. Late persistent infection is manifested by arthritis in 40% to 50% of patients and clinical nerve palsies and meningoencephalitis in 7% to 19%. Cardiac involvement may be seen 2 to 6 weeks after the tick bite in 1.6% to 10% of patients [36].

The ECG may demonstrate no abnormality or mild ST-T abnormalities. The most common cardiac manifestation is varying degrees of AV block at the level of the AV node; McAllister and coworkers [37] found an incidence of AV block in 87% of 52 cases of Lyme carditis that they reviewed. The AV block usually resolves without requiring a permanent pacemaker. Gallium-67 or indium-111 antimyosin antibody scanning may be positive. Lyme carditis is usually treated with penicillin G 20 mμ or ceftriaxone 2 gm/d intravenously for 10 to 20 days, or oral tetracycline 250 mg four times a day [36].

Trypanosomiasis (Chagas' Disease)

Chagas' disease is caused by the hemoflagellate *Trypanosoma cruzi* and is the leading cause of cardiac disease in South and Central America, especially Brazil, Chile, and Argentina [38]. The clinical course is triphasic and includes an acute, latent, and chronic stage. Acute disease follows a parasitic infection transmitted to humans through the bite of a blood-sucking insect (the reduviid bug), which harbors the parasite in its gastrointestinal tract. At night, while the bug feeds on humans by piercing the skin, the bug may defecate, releasing trypanosomes that may enter the skin after the affected person scratches the bite. Localized swelling of the infected area is called a *chagoma*. The bug may bite around the human eye, leading to a conjunctival infection, unilateral periorbital edema, and swelling of the eyelid called *Romaña's sign* [38]. The acute phase results from trypanosomal transformation to a flagellate form in which they enter the bloodstream and infect the myocardial and muscle cells and the glia of the nervous system. Acute disease manifestations include fever, myalgias, vomiting, diarrhea, meningeal irritation, lymphadenopathy, hepatosplenomegaly, and myocarditis. During this phase, parasites are seen in the cardiac fibers with a marked lymphocytic infiltrate and contraction band necrosis (Fig. 4).

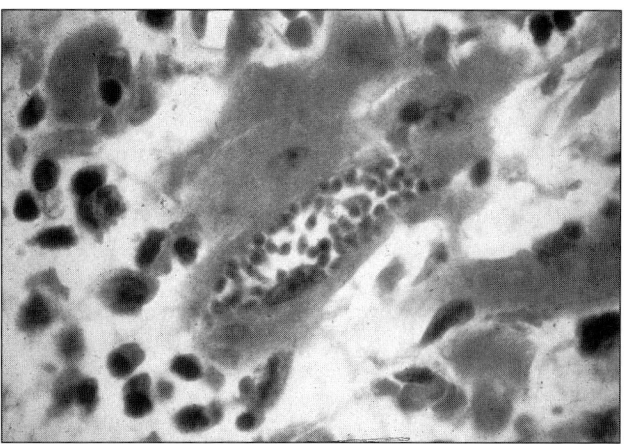

FIGURE 4 Myocarditis in acute Chagas' disease. Parasites forming a pseudocyst are seen within a cardiac myocyte. Note the surrounding inflammatory infiltrate.

Acute myocarditis may develop with prolongation of the PR interval, low QRS voltage, and heart failure. Symptoms of the acute phase resolve spontaneously within 3 to 4 months in over 85% of cases. Following a latent period of clinical quiescence that may last for 10 to 50 years after the initial infection (average, 20 years), approximately 30% will develop chronic Chagas' disease. Cardiac manifestations of the chronic phase include congestive heart failure (the most common), arrhythmias, conduction defects, thromboemboli, and sudden death [39]. Megaesophagus or megacolon may develop as well.

Diagnosis is confirmed by parasites in the myocardium (Fig. 3), the complement fixation test (Machado-Guerreiro test), and enzyme-linked immunosorbent assay. Xenodiagnosis, in which the patient suspected of having Chagas' disease is bitten by a reduviid bug sucking parasites into its intestine, may be positive in 30% to 40% of patients with chronic Chagas' disease. Echocardiography may demonstrate dilated cardiomyopathy with the distinctive appearance of preserved ventricular septum function, posterior-wall hypocontractility, and apical aneurysm with possible thrombus.

Chronic Chagas' cardiomyopathy may result from several factors. These include an intense allergic response to the parasite, autoimmune response, microvascular pathology from an infection of endothelial cells and myocytes altering synthetic function, inflammatory response, parasitic-associated fibroblast stimulation, and other factors [38].

The most common ECG changes in patients with chronic Chagas' disease are right bundle-branch block (30% to 60% of cases) and left anterior hemiblock. Ajmaline, a conduction-depressing antiarrhythmic agent, may evoke fascicular block in an infected patient before the disease is clinically manifest [39]. Atrial fibrillation and ventricular arrhythmias are common, the latter being a major cause of sudden death among patients with chronic Chagas' disease. The overall 10-year mortality is reported to be 36% and the incidence of sudden death 17.6% [40].

Treatment includes management of the clinical symptoms of congestive heart failure with anticoagulation and antiarrhythmic therapy when indicated. Analogues of primaquine may clear parasites from the blood in the early stage of infection but may have no impact on the inexorable development of the chronic phase. Currently recommended antibiotic treatment is nifurtimox, 8 to 10 mg/kg by mouth in four divided doses for 120 days. A recent study reported the beneficial effects of benznidazole (5 mg/kg/d for 30 days [6]. The 131 treated patients were compared with 70 untreated patients and demonstrated less ECG changes (4.2% vs, 30%) and lower frequency of clinical deterioration (2.1% vs. 17%) in an 8-year follow-up. Amiodarone, mexiletine, electrophysiologic studies appear to be useful in treating the ventricular arrhythmias of Chagas' disease.

Toxoplasmosis

Toxoplasmosis is a parasitic infection caused by *Toxoplasma gondii*. Three patterns of infection are seen: diffuse, miliary type; glandular, involving only the lymph nodes; and organ infiltration. Myocyte infection may be of little consequence until a cyst ruptures, causing myocytic necrosis, lymphocytic infiltration, and interstitial fibrosis. Symptoms may include chest pain, arrhythmias, and heart failure. The diagnosis is confirmed by a toxoplasma-antibody titer greater than 1256. Currently recommended treatment is pyrimethamine 25 mg once a day and sulfadiazine 4 g/d in four divided doses for 3 to 4 weeks [41].

Helminthic Myocarditis

Trichinosis, caused by *Trichinella spiralis*, is fatal in 5% of cases, primarily because of myocardial involvement. Chest pain and heart failure may develop because of lymphocytic and eosinophillic infiltration. Treatment includes mebendazole 200 to 400 mg orally three times a day for 3 days, then 400 to 500 mg three times a day for 10 days, with corticosteroids [40]

Echinococcosis occurs primarily in sheep-raising areas of the world and is caused by *Echinococcus granulosus*. Dogs are the primary host, sheep the intermediate host, and human infection results from accidental ingestion of infected feces. Infestation in the liver, lung, or heart may result in a hydatid cyst. Cysts developing in the left or right ventricle may obstruct flow, rupture and embolize, or cause an anaphylactic reaction. A calcified cyst may be seen on chest radiography or two-dimensional echocardiography. Careful surgical resection is recommended if feasible. Medical therapy is with albendazole 400 mg orally twice a day for 28 days [41].

Conclusions

Myocarditis remains a challenging dilemma both in its diagnosis and management. Endomyocardial biopsy may prove beneficial in patients with fulminant heart failure unresponsive to conventional therapy or in whom an opportunistic or unusual treatable infection is suspected. Management is supportive to relieve symptoms, and when available, specific treatment is directed to the infectious agent.

References and Recommended Reading

Recently published papers of particular interest have been highlighted as:
- Of interest
- Of outstanding interest

1. Kasper EK, Hutchins GM, Deckers JW, *et al*. Causes of dilated cardiomyopathy: A clinicopathologic review of 673 consecutive patients. *J Am Coll Cardiol* 1994, 23:586–590.
2. Woodruff JF: Viral myocarditis: a review. *Am J Pathol* 1980, 101:427–484.
3. Gore I, Saphir O: Myocarditis: a classification of 1402 cases. *Am Heart J* 1947, 34:827–830.
4.•• Sole MJ, Liu P: Viral myocarditis: A paradigm for understanding the pathogenesis and treatment of dilated cardiomyopathy. *J Am Coll Cardiol* 1993, 22 [suppl A]:99A–105A.
5. Cambridge E, MacArthur CG, Waterson AP, *et al*.: Antibodies to coxsackie B virus in congestive cardiomyopathy. *Br Heart J* 1979, 41:692–696.
6. Lauer B, Padberg K, Schultheiss H, Strauer B: Autoantibodies against human ventricular myosin insera of patients with acute and chronic myocarditis. *J Am Coll Cardiol* 1994, 23:146–153.
7.• Dec GW Jr, Waldman H, Southern J, *et al*.: Viral myocarditis mimicking acute myocardial infarction. *J Am Coll Cardiol* 1992, 20:85–89.
8. Narula J, Khaw BA, Dec GW, *et al*.: Brief report: recognition of acute myocarditis masquerading as acute myocardial infarction. *N Engl J Med*, 1993, 328:100–104.
9. Morgera T, Dilenarda A, Dreas L, *et al*.: Electrocardiography of myocarditis revisited. *Am Heart J*, 1992, 124:456–467.
10. Yasuda T, Palacios IF, Dec W, *et al*.: Indium^{111} monoclonal antimyosin antibody imaging in the diagnosis of acute myocarditis. *Circulation* 1987, 76:306–310.
11. Bowles N, Richardson P, Olsen E, Archard L: Detection of coxsackie B virus specific RNA sequences in myocardial biopsy samples from patients with myocarditis and dilated cardiomyopathy. *Lancet* 1986, i:1120–1123.
12. Keeling PJ, Jeffery S, Laforio ALP, *et al*.: Similar prevalence of enteroviral genome within the myocardium from patients with idiopathic dilated cardiomyopathy and controls by the polymerase chain reaction *Br Heart J* 1992, 68:554–559.
13. Sutton DC, Sutton GC, Kent G: Needle biopsy of the human ventricular myocardium. *Q Bull Northwest Univ Med Sch* 1956, 30:213–219.
14. Sakakibara S, Konno S: Endomyocardial biopsy. *Jpn Heart J* 1962, 3:537–543.
15. Mason JW: Techniques for right and left ventricular endomyocardial biopsy. *Am J Cardiol* 1978, 41:887–892.
16. Chow LH, Radio SJ, Sears TD, McManus BM: Insensitivity of right ventricular endomyocardial biopsy in the diagnoses of myocarditis. *J Am Coll Cardiol* 1989, 14:1915.
17. Dec GW Jr, Palacios IF, Fallon JT, *et al*.: Active myocarditis in the spectrum of acute dilated cardiomyopathies: clinical features, histologic correlates, and clinical outcome. *N Engl J Med* 1985, 312:885–890.
18. Nippoldt TB, Edwards WD, Holmes DR Jr, *et al*.: Right ventricular endomyocardial biopsy: clinicopathologic correlates in 100 consecutive patients. *Mayo Clin Proc* 1982, 57:407–418.

19. Aretz HT: The Dallas criteria. *Hum Pathol* 1987, 18:619–624.
20.•• Lieberman EB, Hutchins GM, Herskowitz A, *et al.*: Clinicopathologic description of myocarditis. *J Am Coll Cardiol* 1991, 18:1617–1626.
21.• Dong R, Liu P, Wee I, *et al.*: Verapamil ameliorates the clinical and pathological course of murine myocarditis. *J Clin Invest* 1992, 90:2022–2030.
22. Rezkalla S, Kloner RA, Khatib G, Khatib R: Beneficial effects of captopril in acute coxsackie B_3 murine myocarditis. *Circulation* 1990, 81:1039–1046.
23.• O'Connell JJ, Mason JW: Inflammatory myocarditis. In *Congestive Heart Failure*. Edited by Hosenpud J, Greenberg B. New York: Springer-Verlag; 1994:223–233
24. O'Connell JB, Mason JW. The applicability of results of streamlined trials in clinical practice: the Myocarditis Treatment trial *Stat Med* 1990:9:193–197.
25.•• Mason JW, O'Connell JB, Herskowitz A, *et al.*: A clinical trial of immunosuppressive therapy for myocarditis. *N Engl J Med* 1995, 333:269–275.
26. Drucker NA, Colan SD, Lewis AB, *et al.*: Gamma-globulin treatment of acute myocarditis in the pediatric population. *Circulation* 1994, 89:252–257
27. Ray CG, Licenogle TB, Minnicha LL: The use of intravenous rabaviran to treat influenza virus associated myocarditis. *J Infect Dis* 1989, 1589:829.
28. O'Connell JB, Dec GW, Goldenberg JF, *et al.*: Results of heart transplantation for active lymphocytic myocarditis. *J Heart Transplant* 1990, 9:351–356.
29. Pham JM, Kormos RL, Armitage JM, *et al.*: Cardiac transplantation in patients with active myocarditis. *J Heart Lung Transplant* 1993, 12:A146.
30. Reyes MP, Lerner AM: Coxsackievirus myocarditis—with special reference to acute and chronic effects. *Prog Cardiovasc Dis* 1985, 27:373.
31. Eggers HJ, Mertens T: Viruses and myocardium: notes of a virologist. *Eur Heart J* 1987, 8(suppl J):129–133.
32. Weiss MB, Marboe CC, Escala EL, *et al.*: Natural history of untreated chronic myocarditis (active myocarditis with fibrosis). *Eur Heart J* 1987, 8(suppl J):247.
33. Levy WS, Simon GL, Rios JC, Ross AM: Prevalence of cardiac abnormalities in human immunodeficiency virus infection. *Am J Cardiol* 1989, 63:86.
34. Baroldi G, Corallo S, Moroni M, *et al.*: Focal lymphocytic myocarditis in acquired immunodeficiency syndrome (AIDS): a correlative morphologic and clinical study in 26 consecutive fatal cases. *J Am Coll Cardiol* 1988, 12:463.
35. Anderson DW, Virmani R: Emerging patterns of heart disease in human immunodeficiency virus infection. *Hum Pathol* 1990, 21:253.
36. Steere AC: Lyme disease. *N Engl J Med* 1989, 321:586–596.
37. McAlister HF, Klementowicz PT, Andrews C, *et al.*: Lyme carditis: an important cause of reversible heart block. *Ann Intern Med* 1989, 110:339–345.
38. Morris SA, Tannowitz HB, Wittner M, Bilezikian JP: Pathological and physiological insights into the cardiomyopathy of Chagas' disease. *Circulation* 1990, 82:1900–1909.
39. Chiale PA, Przybylski J, Laino RA, *et al.*: Electrocardiographic changes evoked by ajmaline in chronic Chagas' disease without clinical manifestations. *Am J Cardiol* 1982, 49:14–20.
40. McGuire JH, Hoff R, Sherlock I, *et al.*: Cardiac morbidity and mortality due to Chagas' disease: prospective electrocardiographic study of a Brazilian community. *Circulation* 1987, 75:1140–1145.
41. Viotti R, Vigliano C, Armenti H, Segura E: Treatment of chronic Chagas' disease with benznidazole: clinical and serologic evolution of patients with long follow-up. *Am Heart J* 1994, 127:151–162.
42. Lange LG, Schreiner GF: Immune mechanisms of cardiac disease. *N Engl J Med* 1994, 330:1129–1135.

Infectious Endocarditis

Gordon A. Ewy

Key Points
- The diagnostic criteria for infectious endocarditis now include echocardiographic features.
- The classic triad of findings in patients with infectious endocarditis is fever, organic heart murmur, and positive blood culture.
- Cardiac auscultation is important in the prevention, diagnosis, and assessment of severity in patients with infectious endocarditis.
- Echocardiography is used to identify vegetations or perivalvular abscesses and to determine chamber size and function and condition of the valves.
- Infectious endocarditis is a potentially lethal disease; patients should be referred when this diagnosis is seriously considered.

DIAGNOSTIC CRITERIA

The annual incidence of infectious endocarditis varies from 2 to 4 per 100,000 people. Proposed diagnostic criteria [1••] are outlined in Table 1.

Typical organisms include *Streptococcus viridans*, *Streptococcus bovis*, enterococcus, staphylococcus, or the HACEK group (*Haemophilus*, *Actinobacillus*, *Cardiobacterium*, *Eikenella*, and *Kingella* species). A single positive culture positive for any of these organisms fulfills the criterion of positive culture with a typical organism, except that the frequency of short-lived bacteremia in patients without endocarditis requires two positive cultures for *Streptococcus viridans*. If there is another focus of infection (eg, skin abscess, pneumonia), a positive blood culture becomes a minor criterion.

Persistently positive blood cultures are two positive cultures at least 12 hours apart. Persistently positive cultures are necessary if the organism is not one typically associated with infectious endocarditis.

The echocardiographic criteria are straightforward but cannot be preexistent if they are to be used as a major criterion. Nonoscillating masses are a minor echocardiographic criterion.

Predisposing conditions include the presence of an organic regurgitant cardiac murmur, prosthetic heart valves, immunologic compromise, intravenous drug use, and previous endocarditis. Vascular phenomena include embolus, Osler's nodes, Janeway lesions, and conjunctival petechiae; splinter hemorrhage or petechiae elsewhere are not specific enough. Immunologic phenomena include glomerulonephritis, positive rheumatoid factor, and C-reactive protein.

CLINICAL PRESENTATION

The classic triad of infectious endocarditis is fever, organic heart murmur, and positive blood culture; however, one, two, or (rarely) all three may be absent. Fever, the most frequent finding, may be absent in debilitated patients, but the most frequent

TABLE 1 PROPOSED CLINICAL CRITERIA FOR DIAGNOSIS OF INFECTIOUS ENDOCARDITIS*
Major
Positive blood culture (typical organism or persistently positive)
Echocardiographic (oscillating mass, abscess, or dehiscence of a prosthetic valve)
Minor
Predisposition
Fever greater than 38.0°C
Vascular phenomena
Immunologic phenomena
Echocardiographic (when not used as major criterion)
Microbiologic (one positive culture with typical organism)

*Both major criteria, one major criterion and three minor criteria, or five minor criteria are required for a definitive diagnosis.

cause of absent fever is previous antibiotic use. A heart murmur may be absent very early in the disease, especially when a normal valve is infected by a virulent organism. Murmurs of tricuspid or pulmonary valve involvement are often soft, low frequency, or atypical, and they can be easily overlooked. Patients who have undergone cardiac transplantation can have an infection at the atrial suture line. Other immunocompromised patients can have endocarditis without organic murmurs, as may occur with infection on a lead of a permanently implanted cardiac pacemaker. These are rarer causes of infectious endocarditis without a heart murmur. As discussed later, blood culture is negative in approximately 5% of patients with infectious endocarditis.

Constitutional symptoms of fatigue, malaise, anorexia, and weight loss are variable and relate to the state of the patient, the infecting organism, and (most importantly) to the duration of the infection. Peripheral manifestations, such as petechiae, splinter hemorrhages, Osler's nodes (vasculitis vs. bacteremia), Janeway lesions, and Roth spots in the fundi, are directly related to the duration of the infection.

Other findings, such as splenomegaly, anemia, and embolic phenomena, are likewise related in part to the duration of the infection. Thromboembolic phenomena may be pulmonary (from right-sided endocarditis) or systemic (central nervous

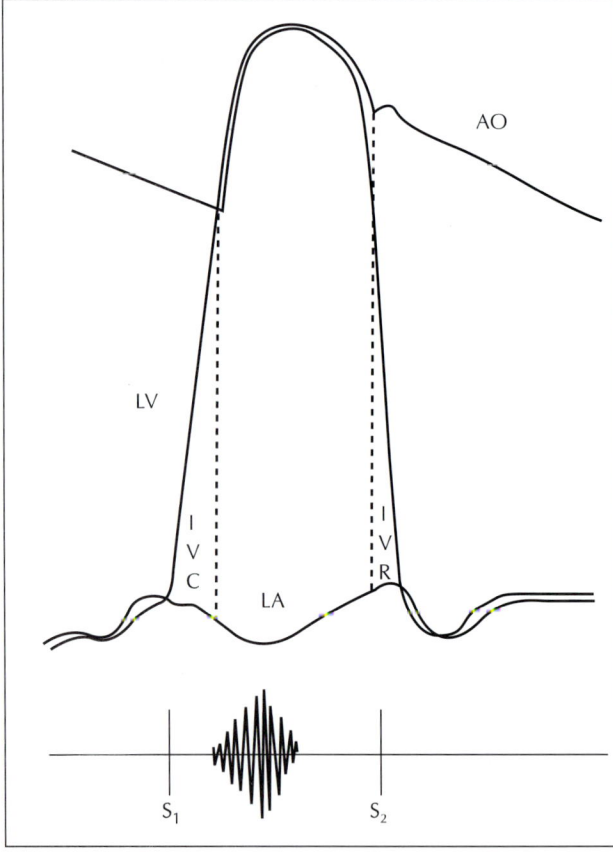

FIGURE 1 Flow murmurs have a distinct period of silence between the heart sounds and the murmur. During the isovolumetric contraction (IVC) period (the time between the closure of the atrioventricular [AV] valve and the opening of the semilunar valve), all valves are closed. Any murmur during this period must result from an abnormality. All valves are also closed during the isovolumetric relaxation (IVR) period (the time between the closure of the semilunar valves and the opening of the AV valves). This produces the silent periods right after the first heart sound (S_1) and right before the second heart sound (S_2). AO—aortic pressure; LA—left atrial pressure; LV—left ventricular pressure.

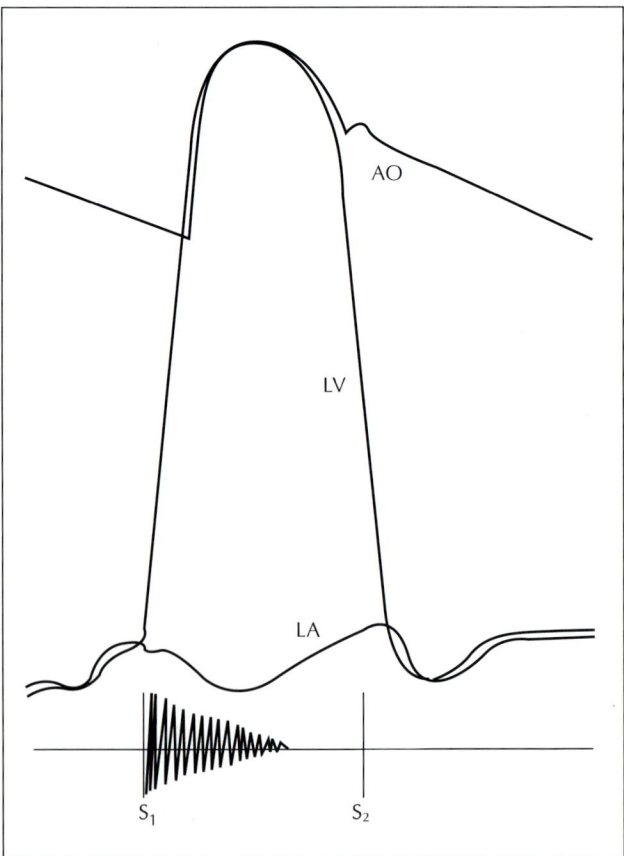

FIGURE 2 Murmurs that begin with the first heart sound (S_1) and therefore involve the isovolumetric contraction period (when all heart valves are closed) are regurgitant and therefore require endocarditis prophylaxis. AO—aortic pressure; LA—left atrial pressure; LV—left ventricular pressure; S_2—second heart sound.

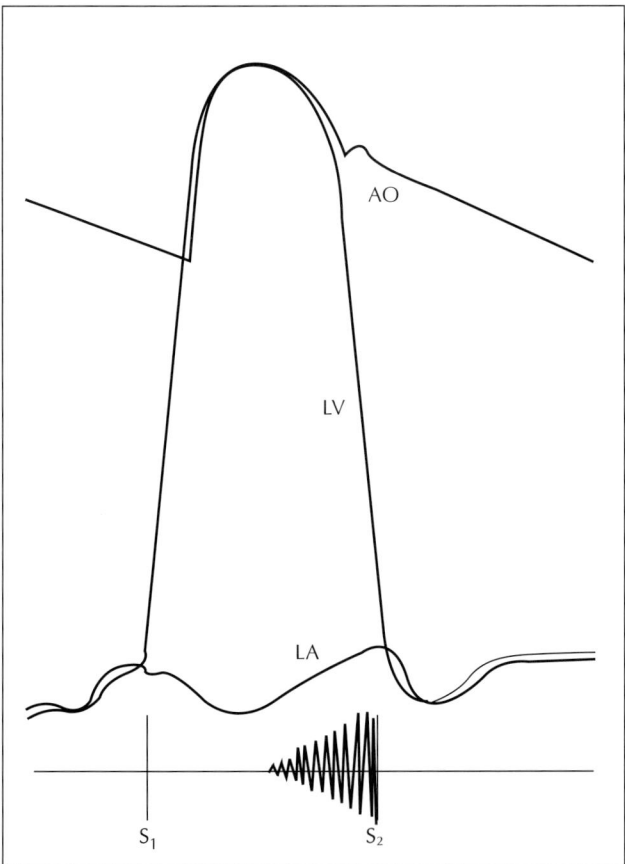

FIGURE 3 Systolic murmurs that are coincident with the second heart sound (S_2), and thus involve the isovolumetric relaxation period (a period when all heart valves are closed) and are regurgitant, require endocarditis prophylaxis. AO—aortic pressure; LA—left atrial pressure; LV—left ventricular pressure; S_1—first heart sound; S_2—second heart sound.

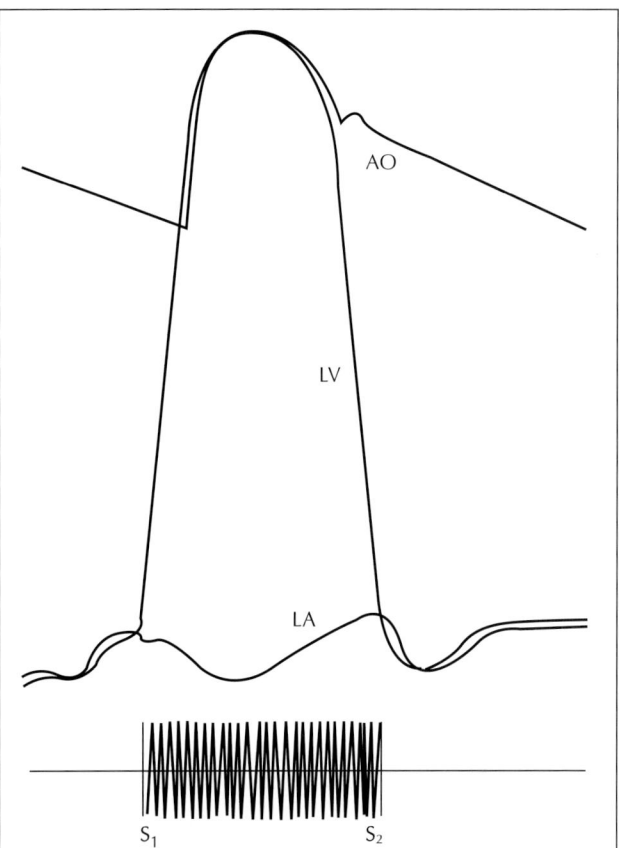

FIGURE 4 Pansystolic or holosystolic murmurs are always regurgitant, because they involve both isovolumetric periods (times when all of the heart valves are closed). AO—aortic pressure; LA—left atrial pressure; LV—left ventricular pressure; S_1—first heart sound; S_2—second heart sound.

system, renal, or other peripheral sites) from left-sided endocarditis. Mycotic aneurysms result from peripheral infection of an arterial wall and may rupture.

Auscultation

Cardiac auscultation plays an important role in infectious endocarditis. It not only allows for the identification of patients at increased risk for infectious endocarditis (those with regurgitant valvular lesions) but also identifies organic lesions and changing lesions in patients with endocarditis, helping to identify the state of cardiac function during the course of the illness.

Prevention

Patients with flow or ejection murmurs are not at risk for infectious endocarditis, but patients with regurgitant murmurs should have endocarditis prophylaxis. Therefore, it is important to identify by auscultation the presence of clinically significant regurgitant murmurs. The emphasis is on auscultation, because Doppler echocardiography frequently identifies valvular regurgitation that is not clinically significant, especially in elderly patients. Likewise, "echo-only" mitral valve prolapse without a thickened mitral valve is a benign condition. Overdiagnosis of mitral valve prolapse by echocardiography is less frequent since Weyman and associates [2] pointed out the saddle shape of the normal mitral ring and the fact that, in normal patients, apparent mitral valve prolapse is frequently present in the apical four-chamber view but not in the two-chamber view.

A flow murmur across the aortic or pulmonary valve is confined to the early and midsystolic period. There is a distinct period of silence between the first heart sound and the onset of the murmur, and another between the end of the murmur and the second heart sound (Fig. 1). Flow murmurs during ventricular ejection are early systolic. In patients with normal ventricular function, two thirds of the left ventricular volume is ejected in the first one third of systole. Mild obstruction results in little change. Moderate to severe aortic or pulmonary valve obstruction prolongs the duration of maximal flow, and the duration of the murmur increases.

In contrast, regurgitant murmurs involve either the isovolumetric contraction period or the isovolumetric relaxation period, producing a murmur that begins coincident with the first heart sound (Fig. 2), the second heart sound (Fig. 3), or both. In the latter, the murmur is pan- or holosystolic (Fig. 4),

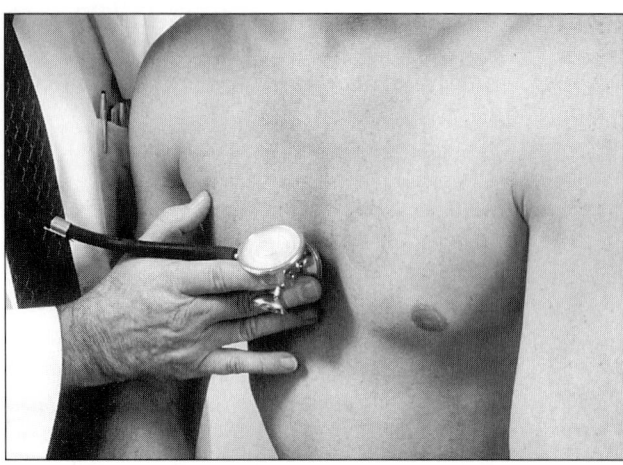

FIGURE 5 The pressure on the stethoscope should be such that an imprint from the stethoscope diaphragm remains on the skin when removed. One listens for a soft diastolic murmur; at times, this murmur is so soft that it simulates the sound of a gentle wind in the trees.

because during the isovolumetric contraction period (the time between the closure of the atrioventricular [AV] valve and the opening of the semilunar valves) all valves are closed. Any murmur during this period must result from an abnormality. The same holds for the isovolumetric relaxation period, thus the silent periods right after the first heart sound and before the second heart sound.

As in systole, not all diastolic murmurs result from an organic abnormality of the heart. Diastolic murmurs include regurgitation of the semilunar (aortic or pulmonic) valves, and obstruction of the AV (mitral or tricuspid) valves. Functional diastolic murmurs result from enhanced flow across the AV valves from another defect.

The technique of cardiac auscultation must be done carefully so as not to overlook murmurs that make the individual susceptible to infectious endocarditis. The room should be quiet, the stethoscope of top quality, and the patient examined in several positions. When listening for the murmur of aortic regurgitation, one must place the diaphragm of the stethoscope firmly against the chest wall in the third left intercostal space (Fig. 5). The patient should be auscultated in the supine, sitting, standing, and squatting (Fig. 6) positions during normal respiration and leaning forward during forced full expiration.

Likewise, when auscultating for mitral regurgitant murmurs, the patient must be examined with the stethoscope placed at the apex with the patient in the supine, left lateral, sitting, standing, squatting, and restanding positions. It is often only on restanding after squatting (Fig. 7) that the murmur of mitral valve prolapse or hypertrophic obstructive cardiomyopathy becomes apparent.

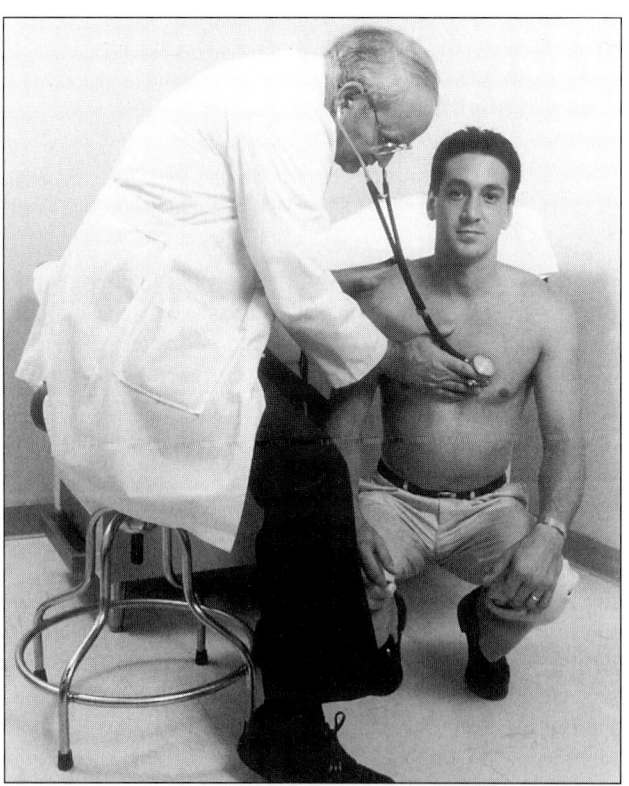

FIGURE 6 Auscultation with patient in the squatting position (note physician sitting on a stool) is an important maneuver, as squatting increases venous return (preload) and blood pressure (afterload), accentuates the murmur of aortic regurgitation, and decreases the murmur of hypertrophic obstructive cardiomyopathy.

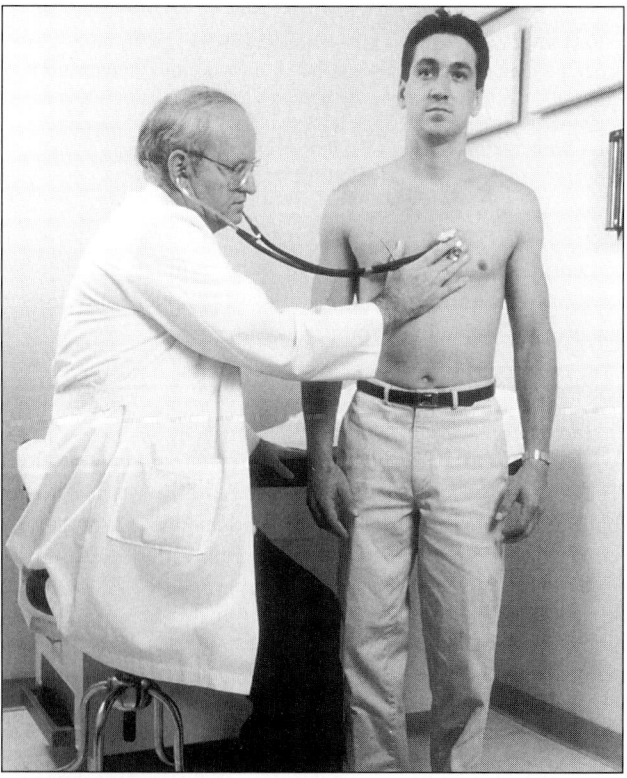

FIGURE 7 Auscultation of the patient standing after squatting is an important provocative maneuver, because this maneuver decreases venous return and thereby results in less filling of the left ventricle (decreased preload). This maneuver also decreases the blood pressure (decreased afterload). The resultant decrease in left ventricular volume increases or unmasks the murmur of mitral valve prolapse and hypertrophic obstructive cardiomyopathy.

Is the presence of a single systolic click an indication for antibiotic prophylaxis? The opinion of cardiologists is divided. My practice guidelines, and the current American Heart Association (AHA) guidelines [3•] are not to recommend antibiotic prophylaxis for clicks only. The caveat is that the patient must be examined carefully and thoroughly in appropriate positions without eliciting a murmur. Although endocarditis has been described in patients with clicks only, these descriptions were from an era when patients were not routinely examined in the standing, squatting, and restanding positions.

In addition, there are a number of sounds that can be mistaken for clicks that do not originate from the mitral valve (Table 2). The characteristic of a systolic click of mitral valve prolapse is its variable position in systole depending on the left ventricular volume. The smaller the left ventricular volume (as with abrupt standing), the earlier the click; the larger the ventricular volume (as with squatting), the later the click. Endocarditis prophylaxis is also recommended for patients at very high risk without regurgitant murmur, such as those with prosthetic heart valves or severely immunocompromised patients.

Diagnosis

Cardiac auscultation is also an important aspect of the diagnosis of infectious endocarditis. Exact interpretation of auscultatory findings is not as critical for diagnosis as it is in prevention, because echocardiography is an essential diagnostic tool in the diagnosis of infectious endocarditis.

Rarely, a murmur will be absent in the early days of endocarditis, especially when endocarditis occurs on a normal valve, such as endocarditis from staphylococci. These virulent organisms soon destroy enough of the valve that a murmur appears.

In the appropriate clinical setting, the sudden appearance of a new regurgitant murmur is nearly diagnostic of infectious endocarditis. Regurgitant apical systolic murmurs in infectious endocarditis may result from AV valve perforation, rupture of chordae tendineae, destruction of the valve, or functional AV incompetence. Regurgitant diastolic murmurs are caused by aortic or pulmonary valve perforation or destruction secondary to aortic-ventricular or aortic-atrial connections resulting from abscess-induced connections.

The auscultatory findings of tricuspid valve incompetence are more subtle. The murmur may not be typically regurgitant. The murmur may increase with inspiration (the Caravallo sign) [4], but these diagnostic features are frequently absent. The jugular venous pulse should be carefully observed for the presence of regurgitant CV waves.

Low-frequency diastolic murmurs can result from inflow obstruction caused by large vegetations or flow from increased AV valve incompetence or nonpulmonary hypertensive pulmonary valve incompetence. Inflow obstructions are rare in infectious endocarditis and most commonly result from fungal vegetation or clot formation on vegetations. The development of an apical diastolic flow murmur in a patient with preexisting mitral regurgitation usually indicates an increased degree of mitral regurgitation. The diastolic murmur of pulmonary artery insufficiency in a patient with normal pulmonary artery pressures is also low frequency but is best heard along the left sternal border.

High-frequency diastolic murmurs from the pulmonary valve occur in patients with preexisting pulmonary hypertension, such as in patients with Eisenmenger syndrome. The usual cause of a high-frequency diastolic murmur in infectious endocarditis is destruction or perforation of the aortic valve. These murmurs likewise are best heard along the left sternal border, but on occasion, perforation may lead to an eccentrically directed jet producing a high-frequency murmur best heard in the third or fourth right intercostal space compared with the third or fourth left intercostal space. Right-sided murmurs of aortic regurgitation suggest unusual causes of aortic regurgitation such as infectious endocarditis.

Determining Severity

Low-frequency third and fourth heart sounds indicate deterioration of ventricular function, usually from increasing severity of the lesions. Third heart sounds are heard with the development of heart failure. They occur at the peak of the rapid filling wave of the left ventricular pressure curve and the peak of the Doppler transmitral velocity wave (E point).

Development of a fourth heart sound suggests acute valvular incompetence, myocarditis, or a hyperkinetic state. This sound occurs at the height of the A wave in the left ventricular pressures trace and the *A* point on the Doppler transmitral velocity tracing. These low-frequency sounds are best heard with the bell of the stethoscope placed lightly on the skin, just making an air seal. Firm pressure stretches the skin, making it a diaphragm and filtering out low-frequency sounds.

The auscultatory findings of acute severe aortic and mitral regurgitation are quite different from those of chronic aortic and mitral regurgitation. These are described in Tables 3 and 4, respectively.

TABLE 2 CLICK-LIKE SOUNDS NOT CAUSED BY MITRAL OR TRICUSPID VALVE PROLAPSE

Early systolic	**Early diastolic**
Pulmonic ejection sound	Opening snap
Aortic ejection sound	**Late diastolic**
Split first heart sound	Pacemaker chest wall sound
Late systolic	**Variable systolic and diastolic**
Wide split second heart sound	Extracardiac (pneumothorax)
Variable systolic	
Atrial septal aneurysm	

TABLE 3 MANIFESTATIONS OF SEVERE AORTIC REGURGITATION

	Acute	Chronic
First heart sound	Absent	Present
Diastolic murmur	Short	Long
Pulse pressure	Normal	Increased
Ejection sound	Absent	Present
Heart rate	Fast	Normal

TABLE 4 MANIFESTATION OF SEVERE MITRAL REGURGITATION

	Acute	Chronic
Rhythm	Sinus	Atrial fibrillation
Left atrial size	Normal	Enlarged
Fourth heart sound	Present	Absent
Third heart sound	Present or absent	Present
Pulmonary component S$_2$	Increased	Normal
Murmur	Late systolic attenuation	Pansystolic
Pulmonary congestion	Early	Late

TABLE 5 ECHOCARDIOGRAPHY IN INFECTIOUS ENDOCARDITIS

Visualization of vegetations: evaluate valvular anatomy and function
Detect abscess, fistula, or perforation
Evaluate hemodynamic consequences
Negative transesophageal echocardiography, very high probability of not having infectious endocarditis
Bacteremia without endocarditis in patients with valvular heart disease are treated much differently
Transesophageal echocardiography should be repeated in patients; a negative study if the clinical course dictates

ECHOCARDIOGRAPHY

The sensitivity of echocardiography for identifying vegetations in patients with infectious endocarditis is approximately 55% for M-mode techniques, 70% to 80% for two-dimensional, and over 90% for transesophageal echocardiography [5]. The role of echocardiography is outlined in Table 5. Echocardiography can identify a vegetation or a perivalvular abscess, and it can document chamber size and function as well as the condition of the valves. Identification of a mobile or oscillating mass, an abscess, or dehiscence of a prosthetic valve are components of definite clinical criteria for the diagnosis of infectious endocarditis.

The echocardiographic size of the vegetation in some series has important prognostic significance. In right-sided endocarditis, lesions over 20 mm were associated with a 33% 6-month mortality rate, whereas 6-month mortality was only 1% if the mass was smaller [6].

The prognostic implications of vegetation size remain controversial. Some studies of left-sided endocarditis found a worse prognosis with large-sized vegetation. In some studies, emboli are more likely with a vegetation size of 10 mm or more, especially when they are mobile (*ie*, have a stalk) [5–7]. It appears that the mobility of the vegetation or those with a stalk have a higher risk on systemic emboli.

Emboli may depend on factors other than size and mobility. Some studies have implicated the organism (more common with streptococcus), the antibiotic used, and the response of vegetation size to therapy.

BLOOD CULTURES

Blood cultures are critically important to the diagnosis and management of infectious endocarditis. It is recommended that three blood cultures be taken 1 hour apart with at least 10 mL of blood for each. The reason for drawing the cultures 1 hour apart is that transient bacteremia from *Streptococcus viridans* endocarditis is not uncommon. Bacteremia from endocarditis is relatively constant, so most of the cultures are usually positive. Contamination is less likely if three separate cultures are taken.

Culture-Negative Endocarditis

Blood cultures are negative in 5% to 10% of patients with the infectious endocarditis. Common causes of culture-negative endocarditis are listed in Table 6. The major cause of negative blood cultures in patients with infectious endocarditis is prior antibiotic therapy. The longer the therapy with effective antibiotics before they are discontinued, the longer it takes for bacteremia to reappear.

TABLE 6 CATEGORIES OF CULTURE-NEGATIVE ENDOCARDITIS

Prior antimicrobial therapy before culture
Infection by fastidious microorganisms
   HACEK group
   Nutritionally deficient streptococci
   Brucella spp.
   Neisseria spp.
   Anaerobes
   Corynebacterium spp.
   Legionella spp.
   Fungi
Q fever (*Coxiella burnetti*)
Chlamydia sp.
Subacute right-sided endocarditis

HACEK—*Haemophilus*, *Actinobacillus*, *Cardiobacterium*, *Eikenella*, and *Kingella* species.

TABLE 7 NONINFECTIOUS ENDOCARDITIS OR MASSES

Myxoma
Papilloma
Acute rheumatic carditis
Lupus nonbacterial verrucous endocarditis
Marantic endocarditis
Endocardial fibroelastosis
Fibroblastic endocarditis (Löffler's endocarditis)
Carcinoid

TABLE 8 PROCEDURES AND CONDITIONS FOR WHICH ENDOCARDITIS PROPHYLAXIS IS RECOMMENDED

Dental procedures likely to cause gingival bleeding
Surgical operations that involve intestinal or respiratory mucosa
Esophageal dilation
Gallbladder surgery
Cystoscopy
Urethral dilation
Prosthetic surgery
Incision and drainage abscess
Vaginal hysterectomy
Vaginal delivery during an infection
Prosthetic cardiac valves
Previous endocarditis
Rheumatic valve dysfunction
Mitral valve prolapse with mitral regurgitation
Hypertrophic cardiomyopathy

TABLE 9 PROCEDURES AND CONDITIONS FOR WHICH INFECTIOUS ENDOCARDITIS PROPHYLAXIS IS NOT RECOMMENDED

Dental procedures not likely to produce gingival bleeding
Bronchoscopy with flexible scope
Endoscopy without biopsy
Cesarean section
Cardiac catheterization
Isolated secundum atrial septal defect
Atrial septal defect, ventricular septal defect, and patent ductus arteriosus repair after 6 months
Coronary artery bypass surgery
Mitral valve prolapse without mitral regurgitation
Functional heart murmurs
Implanted pacemakers

Bacteremia Versus Endocarditis

A major diagnostic dilemma may occur in a patient with organic heart disease who presents with fever. The problem is compounded if there are positive blood cultures or the patient has an endocardial mass or endocarditis of noninfectious origin (Table 7).

Antibiotic Prophylaxis

The AHA recommendations for who should and should not receive prophylactic therapy are outlined in Tables 8 and 9, respectively. Recommendations for antibiotic therapy for endocarditis prophylaxis are outlined in Table 10.

When to Refer

Infectious endocarditis is a potentially lethal disease. Accordingly, patients should be referred whenever this diagnosis is seriously considered. All patients should be followed up by a team consisting of the patient's primary-care physician, cardiologist, infectious disease specialist, and cardiovascular surgeon.

Complications and Prognosis

Complications are not uncommon in infectious endocarditis. Table 11 lists the more common complications in order of frequency [8•]. Although cardiac complications are the most common, fatality rates may be higher from neurologic or septic complications.

TABLE 10 BACTERIAL ENDOCARDITIS PROPHYLAXIS IN ADULTS

Dental/oral/upper respiratory tract procedures for patients at high risk
Amoxicillin 3.0 g orally 1 h before procedure, then 1.5 g six hours after initial dose

For amoxicillin/penicillin allergic patients
Erythromycin ethylsuccinate 800 mg or erythromycin stearate 1.0 g orally 2 hours before procedure, then one half this dose 6 hours after initial dose

Genitourinary/gastrointestinal procedures
Ampicillin 2.0 q IV plus gentamycin 1.5 mg/kg IV (not to exceed 80 mg) 30 minutes before procedure, followed by amoxicillin 1.5 g orally 6 hours after the initial dose

Adapted from Dajani and coworkers [3•]; with permission.

TABLE 11 COMPLICATIONS OF INFECTIOUS ENDOCARDITIS

Cardiac
Neurologic
Septic
Associated with medical treatment
Renal
Extracranial systemic emboli
Septic pulmonary emboli
Complications related to surgery
Acute prosthetic heart valve insufficiency

References and Recommended Reading

Recently published papers of particular interest have been highlighted as:
• Of interest
•• Of outstanding interest

1. •• Durack DT, Luke AS, Bright DK, and the Duke Endocarditis Service: New criteria for diagnosis of infective endocarditis: Utilization of specific echocardiographic criteria. *Am J Med* 1994, 96:200–209.

2. Levine RA, Triulzi MO, Harrigan P, *et al.*: The relationship of mitral annular shape to the diagnosis of mitral valve prolapse. *Circulation* 1987, 75:756–767.

3. • Dajani AS, Bisno AL, Chung KJ, *et al.*: Prevention of bacterial endocarditis. Recommendations by the American Heart Association. *JAMA* 1990, 264:2919–2922.

4. Gooch AS, Maranchao V, Scampardonis G, *et al.*: Prolapse of both mitral and tricuspid leaflets in systolic murmur-click syndrome. *N Engl J Med* 1972, 287:1218–1222.

5. Heinle SK, Durack DT, Longabaugh JP, *et al.*: Can echocardiography predict risk of embolic events in infectious endocarditis? *Choices Cardiol* 1992, 7:79–81.

6. Hecht SR, Berger M: Right-sided endocarditis in intravenous drug users. Prognostic features in 102 episodes. *Ann Intern Med* 1992, 117:560–566.

7. Khandheria BK: Suspected bacterial endocarditis: to TEE or not TEE. *J Am Coll Cardiol* 1993, 21:222–224.

8. • Mansur AJ, Grinberg M, da Luz PL, *et al.*: The complications of infectious endocarditis: a reappraisal in the 1980s. *Arch Intern Med* 1992, 152:2428–2432.

Selected Bibliography

Kay D. *Infectious Endocarditis*, edn 2. New York: Raven Press; 1992.

Reid CL, Chandraratna PAN, Rahimtoola SH: Infectious endocarditis: improved diagnosis and treatment. *Curr Probl Cardiol* 1985, 10:1–51.

Pericardial Disease

Paul T. Vaitkus
Martin M. LeWinter

> **Key Points**
> - Pericarditis is a disease of diverse origins; treatment consists of administering a combination of antiinflammatory drugs and therapy directed at the specific underlying disease.
> - Purulent pericarditis remains an underdiagnosed medical emergency; tuberculous pericarditis may increase in frequency with the reemergence of multiple drug–resistant strains.
> - Cardiac tamponade constitutes an emergency that requires prompt recognition and treatment.
> - Constrictive pericarditis is a curable disease that should be considered in patients with unexplained heart failure; evaluation with a combination of noninvasive testing and cardiac catheterization can accurately establish the diagnosis in most patients.

The pericardium is not essential for sustaining life or health, as evidenced by a lack of cardiac dysfunction when it is congenitally absent or surgically opened. Normal functions of the pericardium include maintenance of an optimal cardiac shape, promotion of cardiac chamber interaction, restraint of overfilling of the heart, reduction of friction between the beating heart and adjacent structures, provision of a physical barrier to infection, and limitation of cardiac displacement during the cardiac cycle. The pericardium also modulates neural control of cardiac electrophysiologic mechanisms. Most often, however, the clinical importance of the pericardium manifests through its involvement in a number of significant disease states.

ACUTE PERICARDITIS

Pathophysiology

Acute pericarditis is an inflammatory condition of the pericardium that may be caused by a variety of agents and disease states (Table 1). The most common etiologic agents are viral and likely account for most cases of "idiopathic" pericarditis. With the recent epidemic of multiple drug–resistant tuberculosis in urban populations, tuberculous pericarditis may very well become an increasing problem after decades of declining incidence [1•,2]. Tuberculous pericarditis most commonly occurs in the absence of demonstrable pulmonary or extrapulmonary tuberculosis. Patients with AIDS can develop pericarditis as a result of infection with a large number of opportunistic organisms [3,4]. Pericarditis can be clinically identified in 7% to 23% of patients with myocardial infarction [5,6], and the risk for pericarditis is proportional to the size of the infarction [5,6]. Bacterial pericarditis often develops in the context of significant extracardiac infections, particularly intrathoracic infections [7•].

TABLE 1 CAUSES OF PERICARDITIS

Idiopathic
Viral
Purulent (Most common organisms in recent series are
   Pneumococcus, *Streptococcus*, *Staphylococcus*, gram-negative
   bacilli, and fungi)
Tuberculosis
Uremia
Myocardial infarction
   Acute pericarditis
   Dressler's syndrome (postmyocardial infarction syndrome)
Neoplastic disease
Radiation therapy
Autoimmune diseases
Trauma (cardiac catheterization, chest trauma, pacemaker
   insertion, thoracic surgery)
Drugs (daunorubicin, diphenylhydantoin, hydralazine,
   isoniazid, methysergide, penicillin, phenylbutazone,
   procainamide)

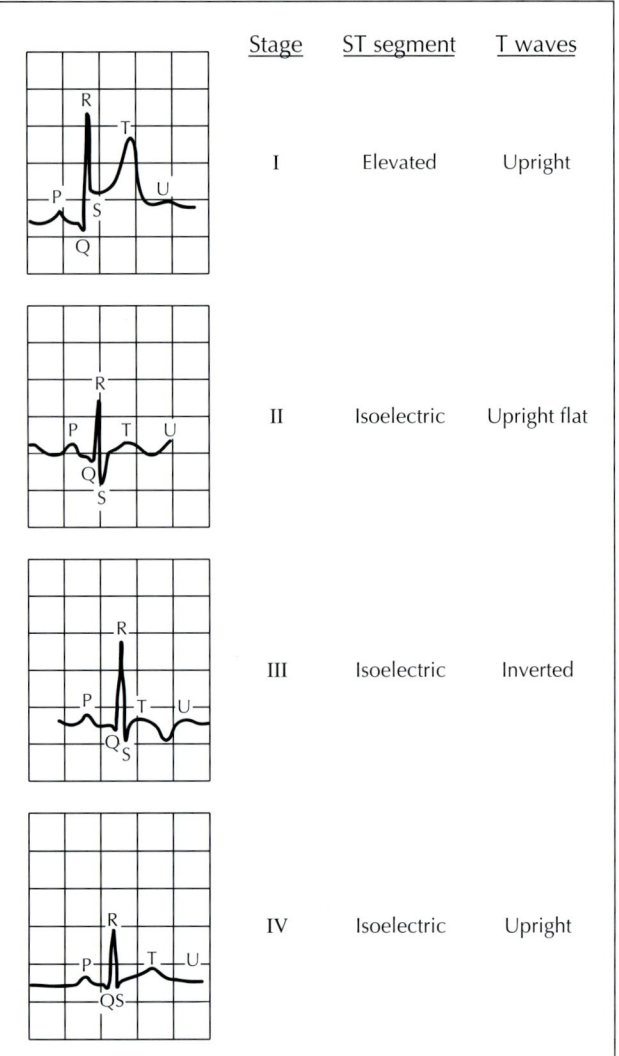

FIGURE 1 The four stages of electrocardiographic changes in acute pericarditis.

Clinical Manifestations

The cardinal clinical features of acute pericarditis are chest pain, friction rub, and electrocardiographic (ECG) changes. Many patients relate prodromal symptoms suggestive of a viral infection. The chest pain of pericarditis varies in location, intensity, and character; it may be described as sharp or dull. Most often, it is precordial or retrosternal and may be referred to the trapezius ridge. It may be aggravated by inspiration, coughing, or recumbency, and it is lessened by sitting upright and leaning forward. Although typically taking 1 or 2 hours to develop fully, at times the pain can appear with remarkable abruptness. Patients with pericarditis may be febrile and tachycardic. The pericardial friction rub is the pathognomonic auscultatory finding. It is typically scratchy and characteristically has three components, although it is not unusual for only one or two components to be audible. The systolic component is most consistently present. The friction rub may be evanescent or influenced by the patient's position; thus, repeated auscultation, and auscultation with the patient in several positions, is essential.

Bacterial pericarditis should be suspected in the presence of high fevers, chills, or night sweats. Patients with bacterial pericarditis frequently lack pleuritic chest pain or pericardial friction rubs.

Laboratory Findings

Evaluation of a patient with suspected pericarditis should routinely include ECG, chest radiography, a complete blood count, and echocardiography. Serial ECGs are valuable in establishing or confirming the diagnosis of pericarditis; four stages of ECG evolution have been described (Fig. 1). Although ECG abnormalities occur in 90% of cases, all four stages can be serially identified only in approximately 50% of patients. Early ECG changes of pericarditis must be distinguished from the normal variant of early repolarization and from myocardial ischemia or infarction. In early repolarization, the distribution of the ST-segment elevation may be very similar to that in pericarditis, but the elevation remains unchanged and does not evolve through the serial changes seen in acute pericarditis. The ST:T ratio in lead V_6 can help in differentiating early repolarization from pericarditis. If the ratio of ST-segment elevation to T-wave amplitude is less than 1:4, early repolarization is more likely; if this ratio is greater than 1:4, pericarditis is more likely (Fig. 2). The ST-segment elevation of pericarditis differs from that of myocardial ischemia in that it is typically concave upward and present in all leads except aVR and V_1, where the ST segment frequently will be depressed. Furthermore, ST segments typically return to normal before the T waves become inverted in patients with pericarditis, whereas in those with myocardial infarction, T-wave inversion evolves while the ST segments are still elevated. Finally, the ECG in patients with pericarditis often demonstrates depression of the PR segment in those leads with ST elevation.

Mild leukocytosis and mild elevation of the erythrocyte sedimentation rate are common in viral or idiopathic pericarditis. These findings are less common in the pericarditis of uremia or connective tissue disorders. A significant leukocytosis with a shift to the left raises the possibility of bacterial pericarditis. Cardiac enzyme levels may be slightly elevated in cases where the inflammatory process involves subepicardial myocardium. Chest radiography usually reveals no abnormalities in uncomplicated pericarditis, but it may show an enlarged cardiac silhouette if a significant pericardial effusion is present. Echocardiography may reveal a pericardial effusion, but absence of an effusion by no means excludes the diagnosis.

When the suspicion of bacterial or tuberculous pericarditis is high, a diagnostic pericardiocentesis is indicated. The pericardial fluid should be examined with Gram and acid-fast bacillus stains and cultured for bacteria, mycobacteria, and fungi. Tubercle bacillus is demonstrated by stain or culture in only one third to one half of patients with tuberculous pericarditis. The diagnosis is often based on a history of contact or conversion of a purified protein derivative (PPD) skin test. The presence of reduced levels of adenosine deaminase in pericardial fluid has been proposed as a specific test for tuberculous pericarditis [8].

Management

Idiopathic and viral pericarditis

In most cases of idiopathic acute pericarditis, antiinflammatory treatment with nonsteroidal antiinflammatory agents usually suppresses the clinical manifestations within 24 hours. For patients in whom nonsteroidal agents fail to ameliorate symptoms, steroid therapy can be initiated. In most patients, a single course of antiinflammatory therapy controls the illness, and the pericarditis resolves without sequelae. In some patients, the pericarditis may recur over weeks or months after the initial episode [9]. These episodes can be treated with repeated courses of nonsteroidal or steroidal antiinflammatory agents. Colchicine is promising as prophylaxis for cases of recurrent pericarditis [10], and immunosuppressive drugs (*eg*, azathioprine) have been used occasionally [9]. In rare cases, frequent and severe recurrences despite aggressive drug therapy have prompted the need for pericardiectomy [9]. Unfortunately, this procedure is often ineffective, either because of residual pericardial tissue or a shift of the inflammatory process to the pleura [9].

Bacterial and tuberculous pericarditis

Bacterial pericarditis is a medical emergency that must be treated with drainage and antibiotic agents. Mortality rates range from 56% to 77% [7•]. The presence of gram-negative organisms in particular indicates a poor prognosis. Untreated tuberculous pericarditis is associated with 80% mortality rates. Management involves administration of three antituberculous drugs for at least 9 months. The role of corticosteroid therapy and early surgical pericardiectomy in patients with tuberculous pericarditis has been a source of controversy [1•]. In the only prospective controlled trial addressing this question, prednisolone therapy was associated with a reduction in mortality and the need for emergent repeat pericardiocentesis; the rates of subsequent constrictive pericarditis did not differ between patients receiving prednisolone and placebo [11]. Complete open drainage reduced the need for subsequent urgent pericardiocentesis but did not influence development of subsequent constriction or mortality [11].

Uremia

Pericarditis developing in patients with uremia before the initiation of chronic dialysis almost always responds to the initiation of dialysis. Pericarditis in patients already receiving chronic dialysis is a more complex challenge. The pericarditis may have an identifiable cause with a specific remedy in a significant proportion of these patients. In the majority of cases, however, no specific cause will be identified, and the pericarditis typically responds to intensification of the dialysis regimen [12]. Pericardial effusions, however, will not consistently resolve with intensive dialysis [13]. Lack of response to intensive dialysis may be predicted by several clinical variables (Table 2) [12]. Nonsteroidal antiinflammatory agents can be used in these patients. Also, indomethacin has been successful in alleviating fevers but did not influence the duration of chest pain, pericardial rub, or the subsequent development of tamponade [14].

Myocardial infarction and thrombolytic therapy

Pericarditis can be mistaken for acute myocardial infarction, leading to inappropriate administration of thrombolytic agents with potentially catastrophic results [15]. Indeed, pericarditis is a relative contraindication to both thrombolytic therapy and anticoagulation treatment. Most cases of pericarditis complicating myocardial infarction, however, develop later in the

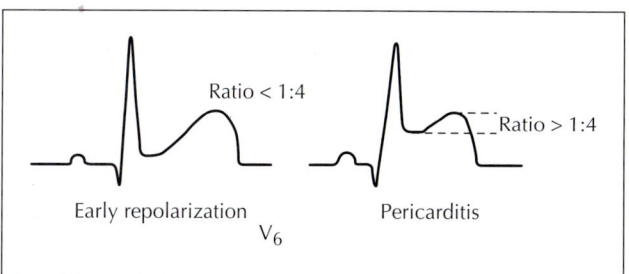

FIGURE 2 The ratio of the ST-segment elevation to the T-wave amplitude in lead V_6 is useful in differentiating early repolarization (*left*) from pericarditis (*right*).

TABLE 2 FACTORS PREDICTING FAILURE OF INTENSIVE DIALYSIS IN TREATMENT OF UREMIC PERICARDITIS
Temperature > 102°F
Rales
Jugular venous distension
Peritoneal dialysis as sole modality
WBC > 15,000 mm^3
WBC shift to the left
Large pericardial effusion by echocardiography
WBC—white-blood-cell count

Table 3 Physical findings in cardiac tamponade	
Physical finding	Frequency, %
Jugular venous distention	100
Tachypnea	80–97
Tachycardia	77–100
Pulsus paradoxus	77–89
Arterial pulse pressure < 40 mm Hg	46
Systolic blood pressure < 100 mm Hg	36–42
Diminished heart sounds	34–88
Pericardial friction rub	22–29

Table 4 Chest radiographic findings in pericardial effusion		
	Size of effusion	
Radiographic sign	Moderate and large	Small
Enlarged cardiac silhouette	78%	68%
Pericardial fat stripe	22%	8%
Left-sided pleural effusion	43%	12%
Increase in cardiac diameter since last chest radiograph	27%	54%

illness and are not a confounding factor in the early hours, when decisions concerning thrombolytic therapy are being made [5,6]. Thrombolytic therapy has been consistently shown to be associated with a reduced incidence of pericarditis, probably because it reduces the size of the infarction [5]. When pericarditis occurs after infarction, it usually resolves promptly and does not require therapy beyond the use of analgesic drugs. The incidence of Dressler's syndrome (postmyocardial infarction syndrome consisting of fever, malaise, and pleural and pericardial effusions associated with pleuropericardial pain) appears to have decreased, a trend some authorities attribute to decreased use of anticoagulation agents in patients who have had myocardial infarction [16]. If this latter observation is true, the incidence may well increase again with the resurgent use of such agents in patients with myocardial infarction.

Pericardial Effusion and Cardiac Tamponade

Pericardial effusion may develop as a result of pericarditis or as a response to injury of any cause to the parietal pericardium. Once the relatively small reserve volume of the pericardium is filled, intrapericardial pressure rises precipitously with the addition of more fluid. Pericardial effusions may be encountered in the absence of pericarditis in many clinical settings, including uremia, cardiac trauma or chamber rupture, malignancy, AIDS, and hypothyroidism. Clinical manifestations relate to the pressure in the pericardium, which in turn depends on the rapidity of accumulation and the absolute volume of the effusion. Rapid accumulation of even modest volumes can be associated with increased intrapericardial pressures and life-threatening hemodynamic compromise. With a slowly accumulating effusion, the pericardium can accommodate 1 to 2 L of fluid without a clinically significant elevation in intrapericardial pressure. Cardiac tamponade ensues when the accumulation of fluid compromises the filling of the heart and, consequently, impairs cardiac output.

Clinical Manifestations

The widespread availability of echocardiography has led to the identification of small effusions in asymptomatic patients in a wide variety of clinical settings. Small, incidentally discovered effusions rarely cause symptoms or complications. Large effusions may become clinically manifest by compressing adjacent structures, and they may cause dysphagia, cough, dyspnea, hiccups, hoarseness, nausea, or a sense of abdominal fullness. Signs of pericardial effusion are absent in patients with small effusions without increased pressure. Large effusions may muffle the heart sounds or cause rales or dullness on auscultation of the chest as a result of compression of the lung parenchyma. The typical signs of cardiac tamponade include high venous pressure, low systemic arterial pressure, diminished pulse pressure, tachycardia, tachypnea, and pulsus paradoxus. The frequency of these physical findings is somewhat variable (Table 3). A paradoxic pulse may be absent in certain clinical situations (*eg*, tamponade coexisting with atrial septal defect or aortic insufficiency). This absence can be an important confounding variable in cases of proximal aortic dissection, which can cause both acute severe aortic insufficiency and cardiac tamponade. The jugular venous pressure usually is markedly elevated, with obliteration of the normal Y-descent.

Laboratory Findings

Chest radiography can demonstrate a number of findings in patients with pericardial effusion (Table 4, Fig. 3) [17]. Because these radiographic signs are inconsistently present, however, chest radiography cannot reliably confirm or exclude the diagnosis [17]. Chest radiography also may offer clues to important coexisting conditions such as aortic dissection or malignancy. The ECG may be entirely normal or include changes typical of pericarditis; large effusions can cause a reduction in QRS voltage and electrical alternans.

Echocardiography is the most rapid and accurate means to diagnose a pericardial effusion. The effusion appears as an echofree space between the moving epicardium and stationary pericardium. Small effusions tend to be imaged only posteriorly; however, a posterior echo-free space in some cases may reflect subepicardial fat rather than pericardial effusion. Larger effusions are distributed anteriorly as well as posteriorly. Large effusions can be associated with an excessive swinging motion of the heart within the fluid-filled pericardium—the mechanism of electrical alternans. Diastolic collapse of the right atrium and right ventricle is a useful echocardiographic sign indicating increased intrapericardial pressure. In a recent analysis, however, the size of the pericardial effusion was the most important predictor of subsequent tamponade or emergent drainage, but no echocardiographic sign was uniformly successful in predicting the presence or absence of tamponade [18•]. Cardiac catheterization in the setting of tamponade will reveal elevated and equal (or near-equal) filling pressures in all four chambers as well as a depressed cardiac output. Examination of the atrial pressure wave forms reveals the loss of the normal Y-descent. The initial presentation and hemodynamic profile of tamponade may be altered by a concomitant state of intravascular volume depletion, a scenario termed *low-pressure cardiac tamponade*. In most cases of cardiac tamponade, however, cardiac catheterization is not necessary to establish the diagnosis.

Fluid obtained by pericardiocentesis should be sent for culture and cytologic examination except in the case of clear-cut traumatic tamponade. The gross appearance of the fluid is not helpful in establishing the cause, and cell counts and chemistries are of limited value. Fluid cytologic smears will be abnormal in approximately 80% of malignant effusions; the remainder are usually identified via surgical biopsy of the pericardium.

Management

Management of pericardial effusions is largely dictated by the presence or absence of hemodynamic compromise from increased pericardial pressure and the nature of the underlying disorder. In most cases, a small or incidentally discovered effusion warrants no specific intervention. Once an effusion of a certain magnitude is present, however, accumulation of even small additional amounts of fluid may result in a marked increase of intrapericardial pressure and rapid clinical deterioration. Thus, patients with any evidence of increased intrapericardial pressure or rapidly accumulating effusions must be monitored closely.

Drainage of pericardial fluid is the cornerstone of therapy for cardiac tamponade. Administration of fluids and vasopressor agents may be useful temporizing measures, but they are not a substitute for drainage and should never delay prompt removal of the pericardial fluid. Most commonly, drainage is achieved by percutaneous pericardiocentesis performed via the subxiphoid route. The procedure is effective and safe but may be complicated by laceration or puncture of the heart. Echocardiography, by confirming the presence of a sufficiently large volume of fluid in an anterior location, can decrease the risk of cardiac puncture. At least 1 cm of an echofree space anterior to the heart should be present before percutaneous pericardiocentesis is undertaken. Pericardiocentesis is ideally carried out in the cardiac catheterization laboratory with fluoroscopic guidance and concomitant right-heart catheterization. On occasion, emergency pericardiocentesis may need to be performed at the bedside. Rarely are circumstances sufficiently emergent to preclude confirmation of the diagnosis with echocardiography. Evacuation of the pericardial fluid also can be achieved via a subxiphoid surgical pericardiotomy; this procedure permits pericardial biopsy in cases of suspected malignant effusion.

In some cases, a single pericardiocentesis is effective in fully alleviating the effusion, but in most cases, consideration should be given to temporarily leaving a catheter in the pericardium for continued drainage. Subsequent management of the patient is largely dictated by the specific cause of the effusion. For malignant effusions, potential treatment modalities include chemotherapy, radiation therapy, intrapericardial sclerosis with tetracycline, indwelling pericardial drainage catheters, surgery, or percutaneous balloon pericardiotomy [19]. No clinical trials have directly compared these various options, but success rates have been similar in individual reports [19]. The specific tumor type and the severity of hemodynamic compromise caused by the effusion must be taken into account when deciding among the various treatment options [19].

Constrictive Pericarditis

The major physiologic perturbation of constrictive pericarditis is thickening of the pericardium, causing it to encase the heart in a solid, noncompliant envelope and impairing diastolic filling. The rigid pericardium markedly increases intracardiac fill-

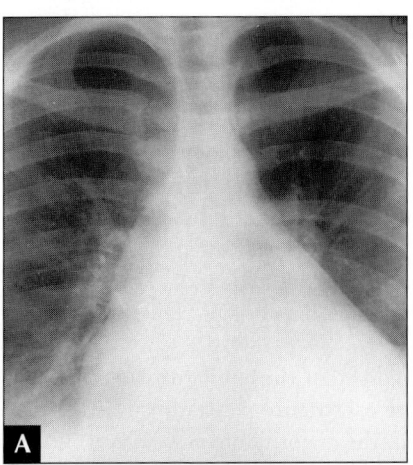
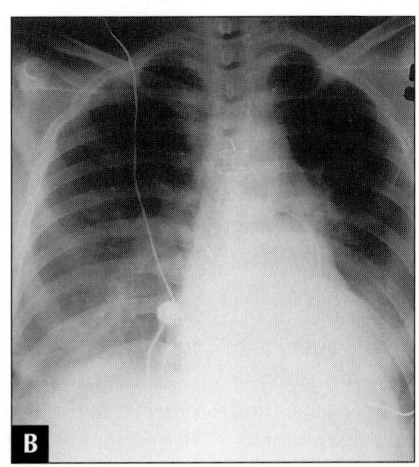
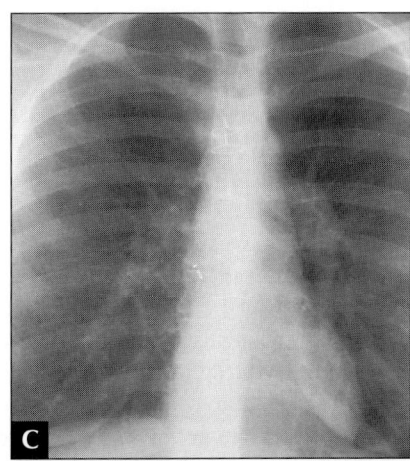

Figure 3 Chest radiographs illustrating the characteristic enlarged cardiac silhouette in a large pericardial effusion (**A**), after therapeutic pericardiocentesis (**B**), and several months later, after complete resolution of the pericardial effusion (**C**). The shape of the heart in the patient with a large effusion (**A**) has been likened to a water bottle.

TABLE 5 CAUSES OF CONSTRICTIVE PERICARDITIS	
Cause	**Frequency %**
Idiopathic	42
Radiation therapy	28
Previous open heart surgery	20
Infectious (nontuberculous)	4
Neoplasia	3
Dialysis	2
Tuberculosis	1

ing pressures. Effusive-constrictive pericarditis is a syndrome with features of both effusion and constriction. The patient initially presents with clinical symptoms most consistent with a pericardial effusion, but after the effusion is relieved, clinical and hemodynamic features of coexistent constriction appear. This syndrome may represent an intermediate step in the development of constrictive pericarditis.

Pathophysiology

Constrictive pericarditis may result from virtually any cause of pericardial injury or inflammation; the most common causes are outlined in Table 5. Tuberculous constriction may again become more common as the incidence of tuberculosis increases [2]. Intervals of many years between the inciting event and clinical manifestations of constriction are common.

Clinical Manifestations

Many symptoms of constrictive pericarditis are nonspecific and relate to chronically elevated cardiac filling pressures and chronically depressed cardiac output. Patients usually develop ascites, peripheral edema, dyspepsia, anorexia, and postprandial fullness. Cardiac cirrhosis may develop. Symptoms of left-sided congestion such as exertional dyspnea, orthopnea, and cough may occur, but these are much less prominent. The chronically low cardiac output results in fatigue and wasting.

Physical examination may reveal the patient to have a massively swollen abdomen and edematous lower extremities combined with a cachectic, wasted upper torso. The liver is frequently enlarged and pulsatile. The presence of predominant right-side failure or ascites out of proportion to peripheral edema may be clues to the presence of constriction rather than other causes of heart failure.

Patients with constrictive pericarditis have marked jugular venous distention with prominent X- and Y-descents, typically resulting in an M or W shape of the venous waves. Kussmaul's sign, which consists of the loss of normal inspiratory decrease in the jugular venous pressure with inspiration, may be present. Arterial pulse pressure may be diminished or normal, and a pulsus paradoxus is present in perhaps one third of cases. Auscultation of the heart can reveal a characteristic, early diastolic sound: the pericardial knock. The knock occurs slightly earlier in diastole than the third heart sound and is of a higher acoustic frequency.

Laboratory Findings

The ECG abnormalities seen in patients with constrictive pericarditis include low voltage, T-wave inversions, P mitrale, atrial fibrillation, atrioventricular and intraventricular conduction delays, and the development of Q waves. The cardiac silhouette on a chest radiograph may be small, normal, or enlarged. The presence of pericardial calcification is helpful in confirming the diagnosis and suggests tuberculosis as the cause. Only 50% of patients with constriction will have pericardial calcification, however, and conversely, a calcified pericardium does not automatically connote constriction.

Echocardiography can demonstrate pericardial thickening in most cases of constriction, although the presence or absence of echocardiographic pericardial thickening does not establish or exclude the diagnosis with certainty. The suspicion of constrictive pericarditis in a patient with heart failure is sometimes first raised when the echo demonstrates preserved left ventricular systolic function and normal cardiac chamber sizes. Left ventricular systolic function may be impaired in some cases of constriction. Preserved systolic function therefore is not a prerequisite for diagnosis.

Differentiation of constrictive pericarditis from restrictive cardiomyopathy is a major diagnostic challenge of paramount importance. Constrictive pericarditis is an eminently treatable disease, whereas restriction usually carries a poor prognosis despite therapy. Restriction is most commonly caused by infiltrative diseases of the myocardium such as amyloidosis, sarcoidosis, and hemochromatosis. Both constrictive pericarditis and restrictive cardiomyopathy are characterized by impaired diastolic filling of the ventricles. A variety of criteria has been employed to distinguish between constrictive pericarditis and restrictive cardiomyopathy [20••]; these indices are based on detecting differences in ventricular diastolic filling patterns in the two conditions. Because they have been evaluated only in small groups of patients, these indices have not been widely adopted [20••]. Computed tomography and magnetic resonance imaging are more accurate for detecting pericardial thickening than echocardiography and are therefore important diagnostic modalities in differentiating restriction from constriction [20••].

Cardiac catheterization demonstrates elevated and virtually equal diastolic pressures in both ventricles. The individual hemodynamic criteria that have been used to differentiate constriction from restriction have varying degrees of accuracy and are capable of providing the correct diagnosis in approximately 75% of patients [20••]. Catheterization also provides the opportunity to perform endomyocardial biopsy to search for evidence of infiltrative cardiomyopathy. The finding of amyloids, sarcoids, or hemochromatosis precludes the need for further investigation [20••].

With the combined use of these diagnostic tests, it is possible to differentiate constrictive pericarditis from restrictive cardiomyopathy in the majority of cases (Fig. 4) [20••]. When the diagnosis remains ambiguous, it is often necessary to perform a thoracotomy to permit direct inspection of the pericardium.

Management

Despite an initially effective relief of symptoms, long-term prognosis with drug therapy alone is limited. The natural history in most cases is one of advancing severity. Pericardiectomy is the definitive treatment for constrictive pericarditis. In most cases, patients will exhibit dramatic and sustained improvement, although several months may elapse before complete improvement is noted. The outcome is not uniformly favorable, because hepatic or cardiac failure may be irreversible or the myocardium atrophied because of long-standing compression, leading to a persistent low-cardiac-output state after pericardiectomy. Constrictive physiologic features and symptoms also may recur because of involvement of the epicardial layers by the inflammatory and fibrotic process.

WHEN TO REFER

Because these various pericardial disorders can occur in a wide variety of clinical contexts, patients typically will first undergo evaluation by generalists or noncardiology subspecialists. The history, physical examination, and ECG and radiographic features of these illnesses should be familiar to all family practitioners, internists, and internal medicine subspecialists. Indeed, the primary-care physician will most often be the one who identifies the possibility of a pericardial emergency (tamponade and bacterial pericarditis).

When percutaneous pericardial drainage procedures are contemplated, either for diagnostic or therapeutic reasons, echocardiographic evaluation should in most cases precede pericardiocentesis. Echocardiography and subsequent pericardiocentesis should ideally be performed by physicians experienced in these procedures. In hospitals with cardiac catheterization laboratories, pericardiocentesis is best performed in this arena so as to permit the opportunity to obtain confirmatory hemodynamic measurements and any other adjuvant diagnostic information. It is also the setting best equipped to respond to complications or unexpected developments.

The patient with suspected constriction should be referred to a cardiologist for evaluation. Although the diagnosis may be firmly established in some cases with radiographic imaging, the patient often will require cardiac catheterization to confirm the diagnosis and to evaluate the possibility of associated conditions before referral to a cardiothoracic surgeon for thoracotomy.

Management of the patient whose pericardial disease relates to a systemic illness (including uremia, connective tissue disorders, malignancy, or AIDS) will usually necessitate participation of the appropriate subspecialist. In most of these circumstances, treatment of the pericardial disease is but one component of managing a complicated illness, and management will frequently entail use of specialized procedures such as dialysis or antitumor therapy.

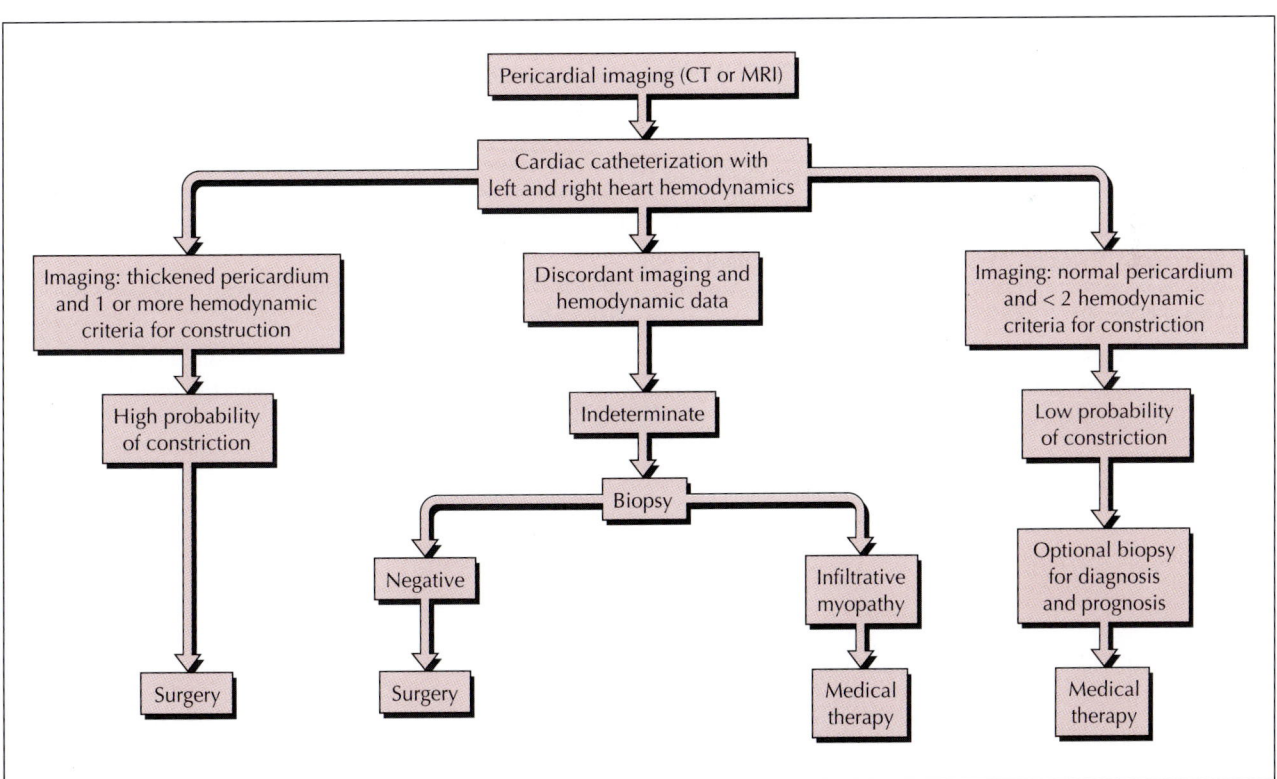

FIGURE 4 An algorithm for distinguishing restriction from constriction. If pericardial calcification is evident on chest radiography, more sophisticated imaging modalities are unnecessary. (*From* Vaitkus and Kussmaul [20••]; with permission.)

References and Recommended Reading

Recently published papers of particular interest have been highlighted as:
- Of interest
- •• Of outstanding interest

1. • Fowler NO: Tuberculous pericarditis. *JAMA* 1991, 266:99–103.
2. Bloom BR, Murray CJ: Tuberculosis: commentary on a reemergent killer. *Science* 1992, 257:1055–1064.
3. Acierno LJ: Cardiac complications in acquired immunodeficiency syndrome (AIDS): a review. *J Am Coll Cardiol* 1989, 13:1144–1154.
4. Dacso SS: Pericarditis in AIDS. *Cardiol Clin* 1990, 8:697–699.
5. Correlae E, Maggioni AP, Romano S, *et al.*: Comparison of frequency, diagnostic and prognostic significance of pericardial involvement in acute myocardial infarction treated with and without thrombolytics. *Am J Cardiol* 1993, 71:1377–1381.
6. Tofler GH, Muller JE, Stone PH, *et al.*: Pericarditis in acute myocardial infarction: characterization and clinical significance. *Am Heart J* 1989, 117:86–90.
7. • Sagrista-Sauleda J, Barrabes JA, Permanyer-Miralda G, Soler-Soler J: Purulent pericarditis: review of a 20-year experience in a general hospital. *J Am Coll Cardiol* 1993, 22:1661–1665.
8. Sagrista-Sauleda J, Permanyer-Miralda G, Soler-Soler J: Tuberculous pericarditis: ten-year experience with a prospective protocol for diagnosis and treatment. *J Am Coll Cardiol* 1988, 11:724–728.
9. Fowler NO, Harbin AD: Recurrent acute pericarditis: follow-up study of 31 patients. *J Am Coll Cardiol* 1986, 7:300–305.
10. Guindo J, de la Serna AR, Ramio J, *et al.*: Recurrent pericarditis: relief with colchicine. *Circulation* 1990, 82:1117–1120.
11. Strang JI, Gibson DG, Mitchison DA, *et al.*: Controlled clinical trial of complete open surgical drainage and of prednisolone in treatment of tuberculous pericardial effusion in Transkei. *Lancet* 1988, ii:759–764.
12. De Pace NL, Nestico PF, Schwartz AB, *et al.*: Predicting success of intensive dialysis in the treatment of uremic pericarditis. *Am J Med* 1984, 76:38–46.
13. Frommer JP, Young JB, Ayus JC: Asymptomatic pericardial effusion in uremic patients: effect of long-term dialysis. *Nephron* 1985, 39:296–301.
14. Spector D, Alfred H, Siedlecki M, Briefel G: A controlled study of the effect of indomethacin in uremic pericarditis. *Kidney Int* 1983, 24:663–669.
15. Renkin KJ, DeBruyne B, Benit E, *et al.*: Cardiac tamponade early after thrombolysis for acute myocardial infarction: a rare but not reported hemorrhagic complication. *J Am Coll Cardiol* 1991, 17:280–285.
16. Lichstein E, Arsura E, Hollander G, *et al.*: Current incidence of postmyocardial infarction (Dressler's) syndrome. *Am J Cardiol* 1982, 50:1269–1271.
17. Eisenberg MJ, Dunn MM, Kanth N, *et al.*: Diagnostic value of chest radiography for pericardial effusion. *J Am Coll Cardiol* 1993, 22:588–593.
18. • Eisenberg MJ, Oken K, Guerrero S, *et al.*: Prognostic value of echocardiography in hospitalized patients with pericardial effusion. *Am J Cardiol* 1992, 70:934–939.
19. Vaitkus PT, Herrmann HC, LeWinter MM: Treatment of malignant pericardial effusion. *JAMA* 1994, 272:59–64.
20. •• Vaitkus PT, Kussmaul WG: Constrictive pericarditis versus restrictive cardiomyopathy: a reappraisal and update of diagnostic criteria. *Am Heart J* 1991, 122:1431–1441.

Select Bibliography

Cimino JJ, Kogan AD: Constrictive pericarditis after cardiac surgery: report of three cases and review of the literature. *Am Heart J* 1989, 118:1292–1301.

Feigenbaum H: Pericardial disease. In *Echocardiography*, edn 4. Edited by Feigenbaum H. Philadelphia: Lea & Febiger; 1986:548–578.

Fowler NO: *The Pericardium in Health and Disease*. New York: Futura Publishing; 1985.

Gregoratos G: Pericardial involvement in acute myocardial infarction. *Cardiol Clin* 1990, 8:601–608.

Lorell BH, Grossman W: Profiles in constrictive pericarditis, restrictive cardiomyopathy, and cardiac tamponade. In *Cardiac Catheterization, Angiography, and Intervention*, edn 4. Edited by Grossman W. Philadelphia: Lea & Febiger; 1991:633–653.

Rostand SG, Rutsky EA: Pericarditis in end-stage renal disease. *Cardiol Clin* 1990, 8:701–707.

Spodick DH: Pericarditis in systemic diseases. *Cardiol Clin* 1990, 8:709–716.

Congenital Heart Disease, Including Unrepaired Lesions in the Adult

22

Melvin D. Cheitlin

Key Points
- More patients with congenital heart disease will be seen by the internist than ever in the past; patients with congenital heart disease are living to have children with congenital heart disease.
- In adult patients, congenital heart disease is frequently not recognized and is misdiagnosed.
- Atrial septal defect is the most common significant congenital heart defect seen in the adult and is unrecognized because the physical findings are subtle.
- The pregnant patient with Eisenmenger's syndrome has a high maternal and fetal mortality rate.
- The most common cause of a continuous murmur is a patent ductus arteriosus; clinicians should remember that patent ductus arteriosus is not the *only* cause of continuous murmur.
- With the exception of the patient with a septal defect or patent ductus arteriosus with pulmonary vascular disease, cyanotic congenital heart disease is very unusual and is unexpected in the adult. However, it can occur and can frequently be corrected if recognized.
- Doppler echocardiography is the single most important diagnostic tool in congenital heart disease and frequently makes cardiac catheterization unnecessary.

Congenital heart disease is usually the province of the pediatrician and the pediatric cardiologist. Most significant lesions are found in children and are identified or surgically "corrected" by the time the internist sees the patient. However, the conditions of some patients are not discovered in childhood, and the internist sees congenital heart disease most often in the five ways listed in Table 1 [1]. This chapter deals with the first two categories of congenital cardiac lesions.

MINOR LESIONS

A good example of a minor lesion is the bicuspid aortic valve. Most bicuspid aortic valves of normal histology are competent or have only minor regurgitation; however, occasionally these valves can be severely incompetent. Of the two complications seen with these valves, the most important is infective endocarditis. Antibiotic prophylaxis for dental procedures or surgery through contaminated areas is required to decrease the possibility of endocarditis developing. The second complication is the development of calcification and severe aortic stenosis at 40 to 50 years of age. A large proportion of people with bicuspid aortic valves never have any complications and can live a normal life span without problems.

Clues that the valve is bicuspid come from physical examination. Because the valve does not open properly, these patients can have an ejection click and a short systolic ejection murmur. The murmur is similar to an innocent ejection murmur, but if it is associated with an ejection click, a diagnosis of abnormal aortic valve is

TABLE 1 MOST COMMON PRESENTATIONS OF CONGENITAL HEART DISEASE IN ADULTS
Minor lesions without hemodynamic consequence Major lesions that were not diagnosed previously Major lesions that were previously diagnosed but at present are unamenable to surgery, including irreversible pulmonary vascular disease and cyanotic patients with extremely small pulmonary arteries that would not support a shunt Lesions recognized, operated on, and anatomically and/or physiologically "corrected" Lesions operated on and "cured," an extremely small category consisting of some secundum atrial septal defects and patent ductus arteriosus that are closed

probable. Because there is difficulty with coaptation at the aortic leaflets, minimal aortic regurgitation may be present, the murmur of which can be increased in loudness by a handgrip or by squatting. The diagnosis can be made with Doppler echocardiography. When this lesion is recognized, the major appropriate treatment is prophylaxis at the time of dental procedure and at other times of bacteremia to prevent endocarditis.

Other lesions that can be problems in differential diagnosis are 1) dextrocardia and situs inversus and 2) a pulmonary varix (or pulmonary varicose vein), which may appear as a solitary nodule on the chest roentgenogram. The varix presents as a rounded density in the lung, usually near the cardiac silhouette on the left or the right side and frequently in association with a disease that increases left atrial pressure, such as mitral stenosis. Under fluoroscopy, the Valsalva maneuver collapses the lesion and it disappears.

Many other minor lesions are important to recognize, such as the right-sided aortic arch that can be mistaken for a paratracheal mass. The major challenge with most is recognizing the lesion, and thus, avoiding the mistake of diagnosing a more serious problem.

RECOGNITION OF COMMON CONGENITAL HEART DISEASE PROBLEMS

The unoperated, hemodynamically important congenital heart disease problems likely to be seen in the adult are relatively few. Adult patients with pulmonary atresia and tetralogy of Fallot can be seen previously undiagnosed. McNamara and Latson [2], looking at the number of children born with congenital heart disease, showed that atrial septal defect, interventricular septal defect, patent ductus arteriosus (PDA), tetralogy of Fallot, and coarctation of the aorta constituted approximately 60% of the cases of congenital heart disease in adults. If Ebstein's disease, aortic stenosis, pulmonic valve stenosis, and bicuspid aortic valve are added, the vast majority of the important congenital heart disease lesions seen in adulthood are accounted for.

Predominant Left-to-Right Shunts with Normal or Moderately Increased Pulmonary Vascular Resistance

Predominant left-to-right shunts with normal or moderately increased pulmonary vascular resistance can occur at the atrial level, the ventricular level, or the pulmonary artery level. All of these shunts result in the return of pulmonary venous blood to the right side of the heart. This increase in pulmonary blood flow increases pulmonary vascular markings on chest roentgenography (Fig. 1). If the shunt is large, ventricular enlargement along with pulmonary hypertension results, leading to right ventricular hypertrophy and finally right-sided heart failure.

Interatrial septal defect

Anatomy

Three types of atrial septal defects are 1) ostium secundum (the most common type), 2) ostium primum (results in a low-lying atrial septal defect where the atrial septum joins the confluence of the mitral and tricuspid rings), and 3) sinus venosus defects (the least common type, it is most often either superior near the entrance of the superior vena cava or inferior near the inferior vena cava and the ostium of the coronary sinus).

Pathophysiology

Because the right ventricle is more compliant than the left ventricle, it fills more readily. In diastole, blood just returning from the lung to the left atrium goes through the defect into the right side of the heart, resulting in a right ventricular end-diastolic volume and subsequent stroke volume that are larger than those on the left. The blood flow through the lung is markedly increased. The pathophysiology is similar in the three types of atrial septal defects.

Physical, electrocardiographic, and roentgenographic findings

The physical, electrocardiographic, and chest roentgenographic findings in atrial septal defect are listed in Table 2.

Doppler echocardiography

There is an increased right ventricular volume and a flattening of the interventricular septum at end-diastole, with systolic paradoxical motion of the septum. Doppler echocardiography shows a continuous flow across the atrial septum (Fig. 2). With the intravenous injection of agitated saline (intravenous contrast injection), microbubbles are seen filling the right atrium and right ventricle, and a negative-contrast jet may be seen flowing across the atrial septum from right to left.

Complications

Pulmonary hypertension. The most important complication of atrial septal defect is the development of severe pulmonary vascular disease, which occurs only with large atrial septal defects with large left-to-right shunts and produces a form of Eisenmenger's syndrome. It occurs in fewer than 10% of

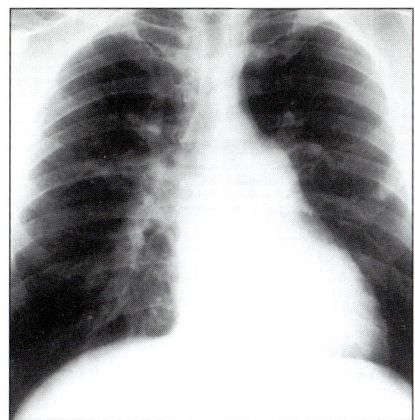

FIGURE 1 Chest x-ray, posterior-anterior projection of 40-year-old man with a secundum atrial septal defect with a pulmonary blood flow/systemic blood flow ratio of 2:1.

TABLE 2 PHYSICAL, ELECTROCARDIOGRAPHIC, AND CHEST ROENTGENOGRAPHIC FINDINGS IN ATRIAL SEPTAL DEFECT

Finding	Comment
Systolic ejection murmur in the second left intercostal space	Produced by the increased right ventricular stroke volume
Increase in the pulmonary vascular markings on chest roentgenography	Caused by the increased pulmonary blood flow
Diastolic flow rumble at the left sternal border	Produced by an increase in flow across the tricuspid valve
Wide, fixed splitting of the second heart sound	Caused by the increased right ventricular filling in diastole, which is unaffected by respiration
rSR' in V_1 on the electrocardiogram	Caused by the increased right ventricular diastolic filling, which increases the size of the right atrium and the right ventricle

patients with large atrial septal defects. It almost always occurs after puberty, and if the patient reaches 30 to 40 years of age without developing pulmonary hypertension, the later development of pulmonary vascular disease is rare. There is an increase in right ventricular and pulmonary artery systolic pressure, with the subsequent development of right ventricular hypertrophy. Eventually, the shunt becomes a right-to-left one, and cyanosis occurs.

The pulmonary artery branches maintaining high even systemic pressures dilate, and they may become atherosclerotic and calcified. The patient now has the complications of systemic arterial desaturation, with polycythemia and the subsequent clotting and bleeding problems. In addition, the patient may develop syncopal episodes, probably from arrhythmias, dyspnea, hemoptysis, and anginal chest pain. Pregnancy is poorly tolerated, with fetal wastage high and the maternal mortality rate increased.

Congestive heart failure. With the increased volume load on the right ventricle, right ventricular dilatation and hypertrophy occur. Eventually, right ventricular systolic dysfunction supervenes, and the right ventricle dilates further, interfering with left ventricular filling in diastole. With failure, both the right and the left ventricle filling pressures rise together, as do the right and the left atrial pressures, which must remain equal because of the large connection between them.

Atrial arrhythmias. Atrial arrhythmias (*ie*, atrial fibrillation and atrial tachycardias) are not uncommon, especially in patients older than 40 years of age. Once they occur, surgical correction does not eliminate the possibility that they will recur.

Treatment

Young patients with an atrial septal defect of any type who have a pulmonary-to-systemic blood flow ratio of greater than or equal to 1.8:1 should have repair of their defect. If the right ventricle is dilated, even lesser-volume shunts should be repaired. The surgery is very low risk, and many of the complications mentioned will probably be avoided. In sinus venosus defects, the anomalous pulmonary veins can be redirected to drain into the left atrium.

Age is not a contraindication to repair. Most patients older than 60 years of age have become symptomatic, and there is good evidence that repair, even at this age, improves the patient's functional capacity and decreases symptoms [3].

Because there is no jet formation to disrupt the endocardium and create a site for the development of infective endocarditis and if no associated lesions such as mitral valve prolapse or clefting of the mitral valve with mitral regurgitation are present, antibiotic prophylaxis to prevent endocarditis is not needed in patients with atrial septal defect.

Alternatives to surgical closure of the secundum atrial septal defect are being developed. These approaches consist of patches, or "clam shells," which can be affixed by means of catheters. So far, this treatment is available at relatively few institutions and must still be considered to be under development.

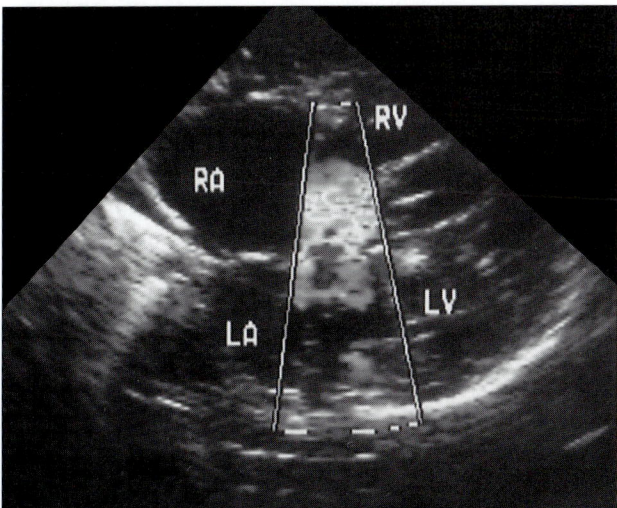

FIGURE 2 Echo-Doppler, subcostal view of a 40-year-old man with an ostium primum atrial septal defect. Doppler signal shows abnormal continuous jet from left atrium to right atrium across the low-lying atrial septal defect. RA—right atrium; RV—right ventricle; LA—left atrium; LV—left ventricle. (*See* Color Plate.)

Interventricular septal defect

Interventricular septal defect is the most commonly recognized congenital heart lesion in infants. A large percentage of these defects close in early infancy; therefore, only approximately 10% of adult patients with congenital heart disease have a large ventricular septal defect (VSD) [4].

Pathophysiology
The effect of the VSD depends on its size, its position, and the relative ratio of pulmonary vascular resistance to systemic vascular resistance. Ventricular septal defects can be 1) perimembranous, 2) supracristal, 3) a posterior or atrioventricular canal defect, or 4) muscular.

Small ventricular septal defect. With small VSDs, there is a connection between the high-pressure left ventricle and the low-pressure right ventricle. In systole, a high-velocity, small-volume jet of blood is directed from the left to the right ventricle. This left-to-right shunt adds little to the pulmonary blood flow. Therefore, the effect is to create a loud pansystolic murmur without any change in cardiac size or ventricular function. This type of defect, called *Roger's disease*, is commonly seen in the adult.

Moderate-sized ventricular septal defect. With the moderate-sized VSD, the left-to-right shunt is larger, but the defect is not large enough to create a common chamber with equal pressure between the right and the left ventricles. The right-to-left shunt is determined by the size of the VSD and the magnitude of the pulmonary vascular resistance relative to that of the systemic vascular resistance. The right ventricular pressure can be raised owing to the increased pulmonary blood flow, but it is not equal to the left ventricular pressure because the size of the defect is too small.

Large ventricular septal defect. With the large VSD, the area of the VSD is more than half of the area of the aortic ring, making the right ventricle and the left ventricle a common chamber. With the large VSD, the increased pulmonary blood flow and high pulmonary artery pressure result in irreversible pulmonary vascular disease and Eisenmenger's syndrome, usually by the end of the first or the second decade of life.

Physical findings
Small ventricular septal defect. Because the left-to-right shunt is small, there is no volume overload of the ventricles, no cardiac enlargement, and no increase in pulmonary vascular markings. The major finding is the presence of a loud pansystolic murmur along the left sternal border, usually in the third and fourth interspace and usually of grade IV to VI intensity.

The supracristal VSD murmur can simulate a pulmonic stenosis murmur, except that it is pansystolic and not ejection in type. If aortic regurgitation develops, a diastolic murmur comes directly off of the second heart sound (S_2) and can be confused with the murmur of PDA and other lesions causing continuous murmurs.

Moderate-sized ventricular septal defect. In addition to the pansystolic murmur along the left sternal border, enlargement of the left atrium and dilatation and hypertrophy of the left ventricle may be noted on chest roentgenography and electrocardiography (ECG). The S_2 may be increased in intensity, and in adolescents and thin adults, a diastolic flow rumble of increased blood flow across the mitral valve may be heard at the apex. A ventricular gallop (S_3) resulting from an increased rate of left ventricular filling is not unusual.

Large ventricular septal defect. By the time patients reach adolescence or adulthood, they most often have severe pulmonary hypertension. If they still have an appreciable left-to-right shunt, a pansystolic murmur is still present. The pulmonic heart sound (P_2) is always increased and now may be coincident with the aortic second sound (A_2), so that there is a single loud S_2. The left ventricle is laterally displaced and hypertrophied, as is the right ventricle.

As the pulmonary vascular resistance increases relative to the systemic vascular resistance, the left-to-right shunt decreases. The size of the left ventricle decreases; the systolic murmur decreases in intensity and is no longer present throughout systole, finally disappearing altogether. At this point, predominant right ventricular hypertrophy may be present. With pulmonary hypertension, pulmonic valvular regurgitation causes a high-frequency blowing diastolic murmur that is heard along the left sternal border, similar to the murmur of aortic regurgitation. With right ventricular failure and dilatation, the tricuspid ring dilates and tricuspid regurgitation occurs, causing a systolic murmur along the left sternal border that may increase with inspiration.

Diagnosis
With the left-to-right shunt, pansystolic murmur is the best clue to the diagnosis. The enlarged left ventricle and left atrium and increased pulmonary vascular markings are seen on chest roentgenography. Echocardiography identifies the chamber enlargement and the increased left ventricular stroke volume, and Doppler echocardiography demonstrates the position of the jet across the interventricular septum (Fig. 3). From the velocity of the jet, the gradient in systole can be estimated. With low pressure in the right ventricle, the jet is high velocity. As the systolic gradient between the right and the left ventricles decreases as the VSD becomes larger, the velocity of the jet also decreases.

Complications
The development of irreversible pulmonary vascular disease is the most common complication of the large VSD (Table 3). High pulmonary blood flow and pressure, and high shear forces damage the intima of the small pulmonary arteries, resulting in intimal hyperplasia, medial hypertrophy of the small pulmonary arteries, and fewer small pulmonary vessels. All of these changes, which are irreversible, result in pulmonary vascular disease and pulmonary hypertension with left-to-right shunting and cyanosis with its complications. Eventually, dilatation of the right ventricle occurs, as does severe left- and right-sided heart failure.

With large left-to-right shunts, left ventricular failure can occur. In my experience, the high-flow, low-pressure VSD, sufficient to cause heart failure, is extremely unusual in adults. With large VSDs, the most common presentation in the adult is that of Eisenmenger's syndrome.

In some patients, hypertrophy of the crista supraventricularis causes infundibular stenosis, converting the clinical picture to that of a "pink" tetralogy of Fallot. The severity of the obstruction caused by the infundibular stenosis is such that a right-to-left shunt may occur through the VSD, and the clinical picture becomes that of a tetralogy of Fallot.

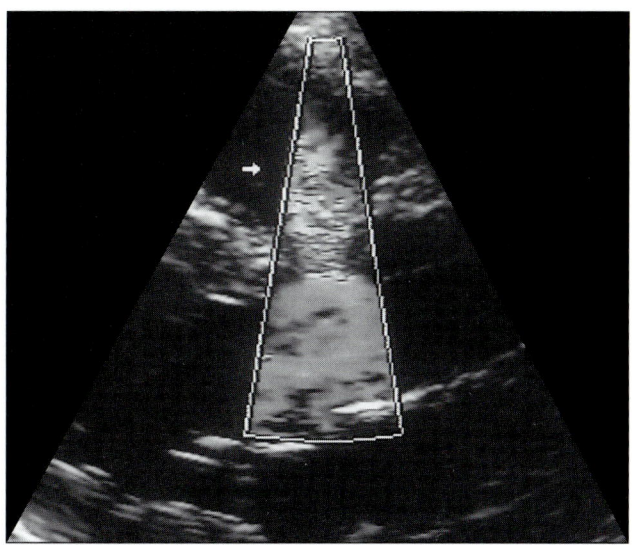

FIGURE 3 Echo-Doppler, parasternal long-axis view of a 32-year-old man with a moderate sized ventricular septal defect. Systolic jet is seen through the ventricular septal defect from left ventricular outflow tract to right ventricle. (*See* Color Plate.)

TABLE 3 COMPLICATIONS OF VENTRICULAR SEPTAL DEFECT

Ventricular septal defect	Complication
Small VSD	Infective endocarditis
Supracristal VSD	Progressive aortic regurgitation
Moderate and large VSD	Congestive heart failure
	Infective endocarditis
	Pulmonary vascular disease

VSD—ventricular septal defect.

Infective endocarditis. The high-velocity jet injures the endocardium. Vegetations occur on the right ventricular side of the VSD or on the tricuspid or pulmonic valve. Emboli therefore occur most often to the lungs.

Prolapse of the right coronary cusp of the aortic valve and aortic regurgitation with supracristal VSD.

Treatment

Small VSDs without hemodynamic significance need only antibiotic prophylaxis to prevent endocarditis. If infective endocarditis recurs in a patient with a small VSD despite adequate antibiotic prophylaxis, then consideration should be given to closing the VSD.

In patients with large VSDs with a large left-to-right shunt and with a pulmonary blood flow–to–systemic blood flow ratio of 2:1 or greater, surgical closure is indicated. This type of VSD is unusual in the adult. With pulmonary hypertension, if a left-to-right shunt is still present in the range of 1.8:1, the pulmonary vascular resistance is not greater than 7.5 Wood units, and the arterial saturation is greater than 90%, then closure can be considered.

With the Eisenmenger's syndrome and cyanosis, operative closure is contraindicated because it would require all the systemic venous return to go through the lungs and would precipitate severe right-sided heart failure. Phlebotomy is indicated only for a very high hematocrit level (> 65) or if the "polycythemic syndrome" of headache, lethargy, and excessive fatigue occurs. The only hope that these patients have is lung transplantation with or without heart transplantation. This approach is still available in only a few centers.

Patent ductus arteriosus

Anatomy

Patent ductus arteriosus completes the "big three" of left-to-right shunts. It is by far the most common cause of a continuous murmur and results from persistent patency of the fetal ductus arteriosus, which connects the proximal descending aorta just beyond the takeoff of the left subclavian artery with the pulmonary artery just to the left of the bifurcation [5].

Pathophysiology

With a small PDA, the high-pressure aorta is connected with the pulmonary artery, which results in a high-velocity jet of low volume into the pulmonary artery. The larger the ductus, the more the shunt is determined by the ratio of pulmonary vascular resistance to systemic vascular resistance. If the patent ductus is large enough, there is equalization of pressure in the pulmonary artery and the aorta; then, the size of the shunt depends completely on the ratio of pulmonary vascular resistance to systemic vascular resistance. As with the VSD, the high pressure and high flow result in irreversible changes in the pulmonary vasculature, an irreversible increase in pulmonary vascular resistance, and Eisenmenger's syndrome.

Physical findings

Small patent ductus arteriosus. The continuous jet from the aorta to the pulmonary artery results in a high-pitched, continuous murmur, with peaking of the murmur at the time of the S_2. The murmur is best heard in the second interspace to the left of the sternum and under the left clavicle. If the shunt is small, there is no increase in heart size and no increase in pulmonary vascular markings.

Moderate-sized patent ductus arteriosus. The volume of the left-to-right shunt is increased; the murmur becomes louder and coarser, still peaking at the S_2; and the pulmonary artery pressure may be increased, causing an increased P_2. Because of the increased flow across the mitral valve, there may be a mitral diastolic flow rumble and an S_3 at the apex. Left ventricular hyperactivity and possibly a right ventricular lift are present because of the high right ventricular pressure.

Patent ductus arteriosus with pulmonary hypertension. As the pulmonary artery and aortic pressures equalize, the left-to-right shunt is totally dependent on the ratio of pulmonary vascular resistance to systemic vascular resistance. As the pulmonary vascular resistance approaches the systemic vascular resistance, the murmur may be heard only in late systole. Finally, with a further increase in pulmonary vascular resistance, there is little left-to-right shunt and no murmur is heard. The P_2 is then loud and coincident with the A_2, creating a loud single S_2. The findings are those of pulmonary hypertension, frequently with a diastolic decrescendo murmur of pulmonic regurgitation. With right ventricular dilatation, right-sided heart failure and tricuspid regurgitation may result.

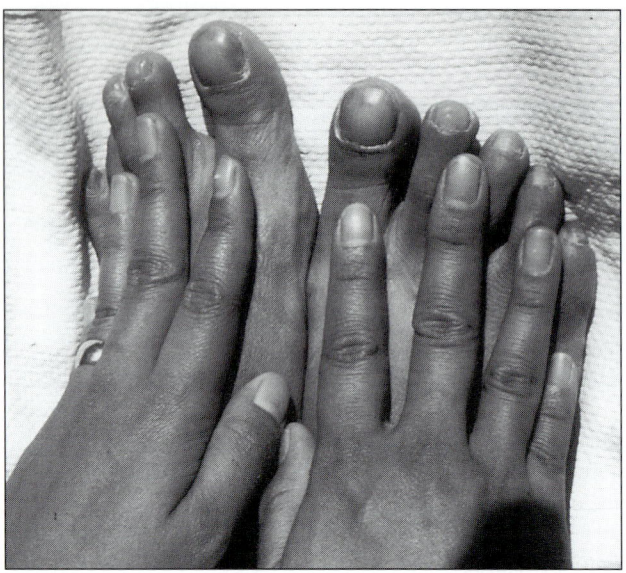

FIGURE 4 Hands and feet of a 20-year-old woman with patent ductus arteriosus and pulmonary vascular disease. Note cyanosis and clubbing of the toes, and pink nonclubbed fingers. (*See* Color Plate.)

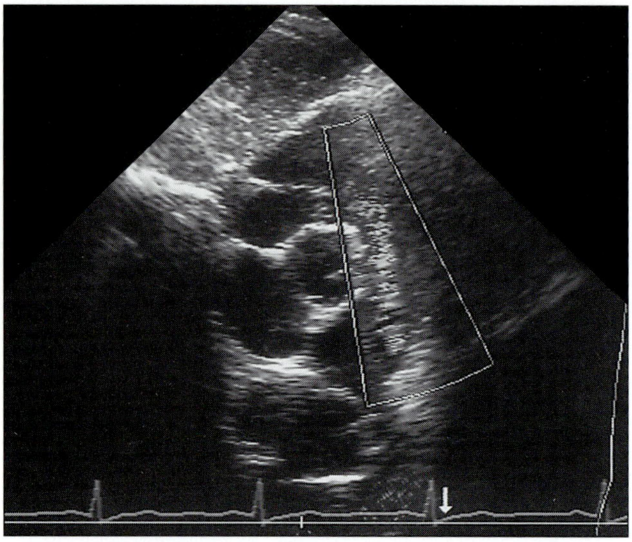

FIGURE 5 Echo-Doppler, short-axis view at level of aortic valve. The color of Doppler shows an abnormal jet in the main pulmonary artery which, on motion, showed that jet through the patent ductus entered at the bifurcation of the pulmonary artery and went down the main pulmonary artery. (*See* Color Plate.)

With pulmonary vascular disease, a right-to-left shunt occurs, with arterial desaturation occurring downstream from where the patent ductus enters. This event results in the finding of "differential cyanosis," pink fingers and cyanosis and clubbing of the toes (Fig. 4).

Diagnosis
The best clue to the presence of a PDA is the continuous murmur. With the larger shunts, the ascending aorta, the left atrium, and the left ventricle should be dilated and hypertrophied, which can be seen on both chest roentgenography and ECG. Echocardiography reveals the chamber enlargement, and Doppler echocardiography demonstrates the abnormal high-velocity jet entering the main pulmonary artery, swirling down one side of the pulmonary artery and up the other, that is characteristic of a PDA (Fig. 5).

As pulmonary vascular resistance increases, the jet may be less obvious or even absent, and the findings are those of pulmonary hypertension and right ventricular failure, with an increased S_2, pulmonic regurgitation, tricuspid regurgitation, right-sided S_3 and artrial gallop (S_4) sounds, and an elevated jugular venous pressure. Here, the presence of differential cyanosis can make the diagnosis.

The differential diagnosis of a continuous murmur is important and consists of problems that create a continuous murmur at the base of the heart to the left of the sternum (Table 4). Four conditions must be considered when a continuous murmur is heard: 1) aorta–pulmonary artery window, in which a connection exists between the ascending aorta and the main pulmonary artery; 2) ruptured sinus of Valsalva aneurysm into the outflow tract of the right ventricle; 3) supracristal VSD with aortic regurgitation; and 4) coronary artery–pulmonary artery fistula. Of all of these conditions, PDA is by far the most common.

Another lesion that is important to exclude is a venous hum loud enough to be heard in the second interspace on the left. The murmur can be obliterated by pressing firmly over the internal jugular vein and occluding it. In addition, a mammary souffle in the pregnant or postpartum woman with lactating breasts can be confusing. Blood flow to the breasts is markedly increased, creating continuous bruits; here, finding the position of the loudest bruit and pressing firmly with the stethoscope can obliterate the bruit. Other causes of continuous murmur, such as coronary arteriovenous fistulas, coronary-cameral fistulas, pulmonary arteriovenous fistulas, and systemic arteriovenous fistulas, are usually loudest in different areas of the chest and are usually not confused.

TABLE 4 DIFFERENTIAL DIAGNOSIS OF A CONTINUOUS MURMUR

Confusion with PDA
Aortic-pulmonary window
Sinus of Valsalva aneurysm rupturing into the right atrium or right ventricle
Supracristal VSD with aortic regurgitation
Coronary artery to pulmonary artery fistula
Venous hum

Other causes of continuous murmurs
Mammary souffle in pregnant women with lactating breasts
Coronary arteriovenous fistula
Coronary cameral fistula
Pulmonary arteriovenous fistula
Systemic arteriovenous fistula

PDA—patent ductus arteriosus; VSD—ventricular septal defect.

Complications

The complications of PDA are similar to those of VSD, although a large left-to-right shunt and a lower-pressure pulmonary artery are more often seen in adults with PDA than in those with VSD. The danger of a small PDA is the development of infective endarteritis, and its presence requires antibiotic prophylaxis at the time of dental or other procedures causing bacteremias.

Treatment

A small PDA should be closed in children and young adults because the perioperative mortality rate is low and the operation is curative. As the patient gets older, the ductus becomes atherosclerotic and is therefore more easily torn at surgery, increasing the danger of a surgical mishap. In patients older than 60 years of age, the danger of the surgery is similar to or greater than the danger of developing infective endarteritis, and I do not recommend surgery. With a large PDA and a large shunt, especially in a symptomatic patient, I recommend surgery at any age.

In a patient with pulmonary vascular disease and little or no left-to-right shunt, surgical closure is contraindicated, and lung transplantation is the patient's only hope.

Pure Valvular Lesions
Aortic stenosis

Anatomy

Congenital aortic stenosis can occur at any level of the left ventricular outflow tract and ascending aorta. The most common type is caused by valvular abnormalities. If its histology is normal, the bicuspid aortic valve does not create severe aortic stenosis, but it may be incompetent, resulting in aortic regurgitation. Severe aortic stenosis may occur with the bicuspid valve early in infancy if the valve is dysplastic. If the histology of the valve is normal, a minority of patients with bicuspid aortic valve will develop fibrosis and calcification and severe aortic stenosis between 40 and 50 years of age [6].

The aortic valves that are congenitally stenotic in childhood are those with only one commissure; the bicuspid valve with a fused commissure or a unicuspid valve; and those without any normally formed commissures, the so-called acommissural valves. Much less often, left ventricular outflow tract obstruction above (supravalvular) or below (subvalvular) the aortic valve occurs. Supravalvular aortic stenosis can be caused by a discrete membrane, an hourglass constriction, or a hypoplastic ascending aorta. These obstructions are usually above the takeoff of the coronary arteries. The subvalvular obstructions can be discrete and membranous, caused by abnormal hypertrophy (so-called hypertrophic cardiomyopathy), or caused by a fibromuscular tunnel involving both the interventricular septum and the anterior leaflet of the mitral valve. These problems are more difficult to treat surgically.

Pathophysiology

The obstruction to the left ventricular outflow tract results in a systolic afterload burden to the left ventricle, which causes left ventricular hypertrophy, and the pathophysiologic consequences are similar in all ways to those seen in the adult with acquired aortic stenosis.

The increase in left ventricular mass, the high left ventricular systolic pressure, the relatively low aortic diastolic pressure, and the high extramural pressure on the intramural coronary arteries all result in an increase in myocardial oxygen demand and a decrease in coronary blood supply. The pathophysiologic factors result in myocardial ischemia, which can lead to angina pectoris and myocardial infarction.

Ventricular arrhythmia and sudden death can result from myocardial ischemia. Exertional syncope can be caused by an inability to increase stroke volume with exercise and therefore a decrease in systolic blood pressure, but it may be caused by sudden self-limited ventricular arrhythmias or inappropriate reflexes that cause vasodilation and bradycardia at a time when the aortic systolic pressure is falling.

Physical findings

The systolic ejection murmur at the base, which radiates into the carotid arteries, is the most valuable diagnostic sign of aortic stenosis. With valvular aortic stenosis, because the valve is flexible in the young adult, there is frequently a systolic ejection click. In half of the patients, minimal aortic regurgitation is audible. If the chest wall has a normal configuration and the cardiac output is normal, the murmur is usually loud enough to create a systolic thrill. Therefore, in a young person, the absence of a thrill is powerful evidence against severe aortic stenosis. However, in an older person, who may have decreased cardiac output and an increased anteroposterior diameter of the chest, the absence of a systolic thrill is less valuable in predicting the absence of severe aortic stenosis.

Left ventricular hypertrophy is the natural compensation for severe aortic stenosis, so a sustained point of maximal impulse and an S_4 are also good evidence of the increased severity of aortic stenosis. With left ventricular failure, there is dilatation of the left ventricle and an S_3, but they are present very late in the natural history of the disease. The absence of a systolic ejection click should lead the clinician to suspect calcification of the aortic valve or an unusual type of aortic stenosis, either supravalvular or subvalvular.

Diagnosis

The systolic ejection murmur is the best clue to the diagnosis of aortic stenosis. Chest roentgenography usually shows poststenotic dilatation of the ascending aorta, but the cardiac silhouette is usually normal. The ECG in severe aortic stenosis usually demonstrates left ventricular hypertrophy (Fig. 6), although approximately 15% to 20% may show only ST-T wave changes or be within normal limits. In these situations, echocardiography shows left ventricular hypertrophy if the aortic stenosis is severe, usually without dilatation of the left ventricle. In young adults, left ventricular contractility is usually preserved. Supravalvular aortic stenosis, subvalvular aortic stenosis, and hypertrophic cardiomyopathy can be diagnosed with echocardiography, which is the best way to visualize the discrete membranous type of subaortic stenosis. Doppler echocardiography can reliably identify minimal-velocity and high-velocity jets, and therefore minimal and large systolic gradients, and is a good way of detecting an increase in the severity of the lesion over the years.

Complications and treatment
The complications of congestive heart failure, angina pectoris including non–Q wave myocardial infarction, exertional syncope, arrhythmias, sudden death, and infective endocarditis are all similar to those seen with acquired aortic stenosis. In adolescents and young adults, the presence of severe aortic stenosis with a systolic gradient of 50 mm Hg, or an aortic valve area of less then 0.8 cm², is an indication for surgical correction. With commissurial fusion and an uncalcified valve, correction can be achieved by repair rather than by replacement. In children and some young adults, balloon valvotomy can be just as effective as surgical valve repair. If the valve is calcified, as it is in almost all patients older than 40 years of age, valvular replacement is necessary.

When valve repair is possible, it is highly likely that a second surgical procedure, and even replacement of the valve, will be necessary after 15 to 20 years.

Valvular pulmonary stenosis

Anatomy
Valvular pulmonary stenosis is a relatively uncommon problem in adults. Although stenosis of the right ventricular outflow tract can be at, below, or above the pulmonic valve, valvular pulmonary stenosis is by far the most common as an isolated lesion. Infundibular stenosis without a VSD and supravalvular pulmonary stenosis are extremely rare.

Pathophysiology
The abnormally formed pulmonic valve is the pathology causing valvular pulmonary stenosis. The obstruction to right ventricular outflow causes an afterload burden on the right ventricle, resulting in right ventricular hypertrophy. There is a large gradient across the pulmonic valve, and the jet causes poststenotic dilatation of the main pulmonary artery and frequently of the left pulmonary artery but not of the right.

Physical findings
The obstruction across the pulmonic valve results in a high-velocity jet created by the entire stroke volume. This jet results in a loud ejection murmur, best heard in the second intercostal space to the left of the sternum. It radiates into the lung fields and less well into the neck. The flexible stenotic valve and poststenotic dilatation result in an ejection click.

Right ventricular hypertrophy results in a systolic precordial lift. A prominent "A" wave may also be present in the jugular venous pulse. If there is a right-to-left shunt through a patent foramen ovale, cyanosis may be present.

Diagnosis
The systolic ejection murmur in the second interspace to the left of the sternum is the first clue to the diagnosis. The ejection click, especially with changes in respiration, is an excellent clue to the valvular abnormality. With severe pulmonic valve stenosis, right ventricular hypertrophy is seen on the ECG. Doppler echocardiography demonstrates right ventricular hypertrophy and the high-velocity jet across the pulmonic valve, allowing for an estimation of the systolic gradient.

Complications
Valvular pulmonary stenosis is a rare disease in adults. If it occurs in adults severely enough to cause right ventricular hypertrophy, then repair of the pulmonic valve is indicated. If the patient has signs of right ventricular failure, the lesion should be repaired at any age. If pulmonic valvular stenosis is present, even if it is mild, antibiotic prophylaxis to prevent endocarditis is indicated.

Coarctation of the aorta

Anatomy
In adults, coarctation of the aorta constitutes approximately 5% of cases of congenital cardiovascular disease. The most common form consists of a relatively short constriction of the descending aorta just beyond the takeoff of the left subclavian artery at the level of the ligamentus arteriosus. Occasionally, the aorta proximal to this point can be markedly hypoplastic, resulting in a longer length of constriction.

A bicuspid aortic valve is the most commonly associated abnormality and may be present in up to 80% of patients. In addition, associated congenital aneurysms may be present in the aorta either proximal or distal to the coarctation or in

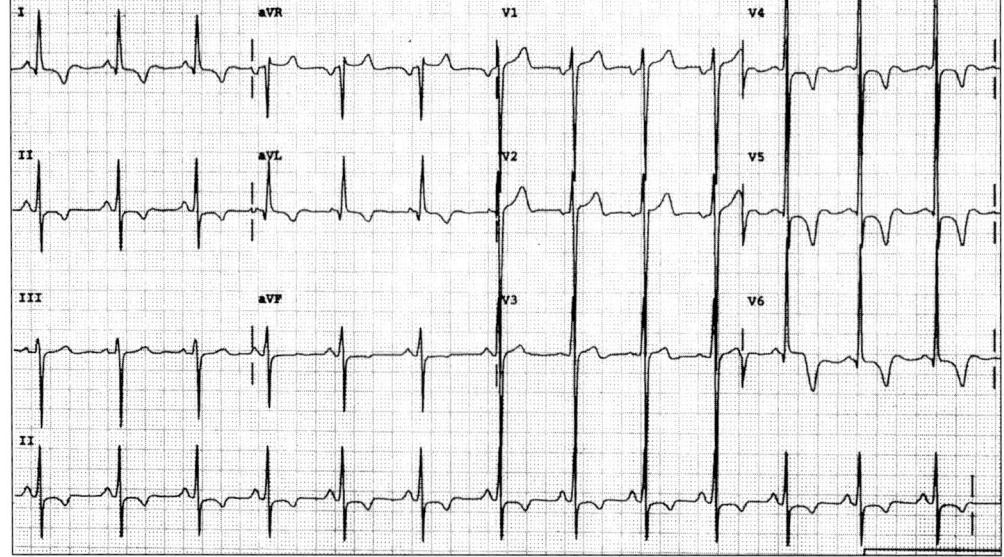

FIGURE 6 Electrocardiogram showing left ventricular hypertrophy and left atrial abnormality in a 45-year-old man with a calcified bicuspid aortic valve and a mean systolic gradient across the aortic valve of 80 mm Hg.

arteries of the circle of Willis (so-called berry aneurysms). Associated abnormalities such as PDA, aortic valve and subvalvular stenosis, and mitral valve abnormalities are not uncommon.

Pathophysiology

Coarctation of the aorta results in higher blood pressure in the aorta and arteries proximal to the obstruction and lower blood pressure distally. With severe coarctation of the aorta, collateral circulation develops that bypasses the obstruction. This collateral circulation involves the branches of the subclavian and cervical arterial system, the intercostal arteries, and the internal mammary and periscapular arteries, all of which have connections to arteries arising distal to the coarctation. These vessels dilate and elongate, becoming enlarged and tortuous.

The variables that determine the clinical picture depend on the severity of the obstruction. Minor obstructions cause almost no collateral formation and produce only a dampening of the distal aortic pressure, whereas severe to total occlusion of the aorta causes marked damping of the pulse beyond the coarctation and decreases in distal arterial blood pressure. The size and number of collaterals are also important. The collaterals can be so large and extensive that distal aortic flow is not impaired, and even distal pulse pressure and mean blood pressure might be only mildly decreased. The proximal aortic hypertension results in left ventricular hypertrophy and can eventually cause congestive heart failure.

Physical findings

The diagnosis of coarctation of the aorta is easily made by noting a decreased or an absent femoral arterial pulse compared with the brachial pulse. In some patients, the femoral pulses may be difficult to feel; in this case, the diagnosis can be made by comparing the systolic blood pressure in the right arm with the blood pressure in the leg, with both being taken with appropriately sized cuffs. It is important to take the blood pressure in both arms to pick up the unusual coarctation that begins proximal to the takeoff of the left subclavian artery. Normally, the indirect systolic blood pressure by cuff should be 10 mm Hg or higher in the leg than in the arm. If the systolic blood pressure is lower in the leg than in the arm, a diagnosis of aortic obstruction is made; in the proper setting, the etiology is coarctation of the aorta.

The murmur generated by flow past the obstruction is a late systolic bruit heard at the base of the heart anteriorly and as well or better in the interscapular area to the left of the spine. If the patient has a bicuspid aortic valve, an ejection click, a blowing diastolic murmur of aortic regurgitation, or both may also be heard. With the patient leaning forward with the arms crossed over the chest, intercostal and periscapular arterial pulsations can be felt with palpation over the posterior chest wall, and systolic bruits may be heard over the enlarged, tortuous collateral vessels.

Diagnosis

The ECG findings can be within normal limits or show left ventricular hypertrophy. On chest roentgenography, the ascending aorta is frequently dilated; there is a large aortic "knob" because of the lateral displacement of the left subclavian artery. At times, notching of the descending aorta can be seen at the point of the constriction, and poststenotic dilatation can be noted below the coarctation. Rib notching, especially of the third rib and lower, is seen because of the enlarged tortuous intercostal arteries. On barium swallow, a proximal and distal impingement on the barium-filled esophagus of the aorta above and below the coarctation can be seen. On two-dimensional echocardiography, only hypertrophy of the left ventricle and abnormalities of the aortic valve may be seen. With transesophageal echocardiography, the area of the coarctation can be visualized. Doppler or transesophageal echocardiography can reveal the high-velocity jet of blood across the coarctation.

Complications and treatment

Eventually, left-sided heart failure can occur, as can infective endarteritis distal to the coarctation and infective endocarditis on the bicuspid aortic valve. Berry aneurysm rupture can cause a cerebrovascular bleed, and dissection of the aorta proximal to the coarctation has been reported.

In coarctation of the aorta that is severe enough to cause an increase in proximal aortic blood pressure and the development of collateral circulation, resection of the coarctation should be done, especially in young people. If the coarctation is mild, without collateral formation and with minimal difference in blood pressure proximal and distal to the coarctation, there is little evidence that resection of the coarctation is better than treatment with antihypertensive agents.

Even after coarctation repair, antibiotic prophylaxis to prevent infective endocarditis is recommended.

Cyanotic Lesions (Lesions with Right-to-Left Shunts)

Cyanotic lesions are characterized by a right-to-left shunt large enough to cause arterial desaturation. For a patient to be cyanotic, the reduced hemoglobin concentration must be at least 5 g/dL. Lesser concentrations, for instance in patients with anemia, will not result in cyanosis. The right-to-left shunting can occur at any cardiac level. Table 5 lists examples of lesions in this group and the cardiac level at which shunting occurs.

Although several congenital heart lesions are included in this group, relatively few are seen in the adult without previous surgery.

Eisenmenger's syndrome

Eisenmenger's syndrome lesions have already been discussed under the section dealing with atrial septal defects, VSDs, and PDA. When pulmonary hypertension occurs, it is clinically difficult to make a distinction between these lesions. All are characterized by the findings of pulmonary hypertension (*ie*, a loud P_2, right ventricular hypertrophy, possibly pulmonic valve regurgitation, right-sided heart failure, dilatation of the right ventricle with tricuspid regurgitation, and right-sided S_3 and S_4 sounds). The murmurs are no longer characteristic, the pulmonary arteries are large, and the peripheral lung fields are clear

TABLE 5 RIGHT-TO-LEFT SHUNTS CLASSIFIED BY CARDIAC LEVEL	
Level at which shunting occurs	Examples of lesions
Venous	Total anomalous pulmonary venous drainage; anomalous drainage of the superior vena cava into the left atrium
Atrial	Atrial septal defect with pulmonary hypertension; tricuspid atresia; Ebstein's disease; valvular pulmonary stenosis with blown-open foramen ovale
Ventricular	Ventricular septal defect with pulmonary hypertension; tetralogy of Fallot; pulmonary atresia; patent ductus with pulmonary hypertension
Arterial	Transposition of the great vessels; truncus arteriosus; double-outlet right ventricle; pulmonary arteriovenous fistula

common is valvular pulmonic stenosis alone. The other two lesions inferred from the "tetralogy" are right ventricular hypertrophy and an aortic root that overrides the VSD.

Pathophysiology

The clinical picture depends on the severity of the right ventricular outflow tract obstruction, the size of the VSD, and the systemic vascular resistance. As mentioned in the section on VSD, in patients with large VSDs and pulmonary hypertension, right ventricular hypertrophy is at times accompanied by hypertrophy of the crista supraventricularis, which can form an acquired infundibular obstruction. In many of these patients, the obstruction is mild enough so that left-to-right shunting still occurs, and although a systolic gradient is present across the infundibular obstruction, there is still a predominant left-to-right shunt.

With the congenital malformation of the right ventricular outflow tract that defines the true tetralogy of Fallot, the right ventricular outflow tract is severely stenotic, and the shunt through the VSD is from right to left. The murmur is therefore that of infundibular pulmonary stenosis and not that of VSD.

Physical findings and diagnosis

In infundibular pulmonary stenosis with hypertrophy of the crista supraventricularis and VSD, the murmur may still be pansystolic, loudest at the left sternal border. With obstruction, the predominant systolic murmur is that of infundibular pulmonary stenosis: in other words, a loud ejection murmur without an ejection click. The pulmonary arteries may still be large on roentgenography and echocardiography. In this disease, the magnitude of a right-to-left shunt is usually small at rest.

With tetralogy of Fallot, the right ventricular outflow tract is severely obstructed, the pulmonary blood flow is never large, and the main pulmonary artery and its branches

because of extreme narrowing of the pulmonary vessels, or so-called pruning (Figs. 7 and 8). The definitive differential diagnosis can be made with two-dimensional Doppler echocardiography.

Tetralogy of Fallot

Anatomy

Beyond infancy, tetralogy of Fallot is the most common lesion causing cyanosis. It is characterized by obstruction in the right ventricular outflow tract and a VSD, usually proximal to the outflow obstruction. The right ventricular obstruction is usually infundibular, with or without valvular pulmonic stenosis. Least

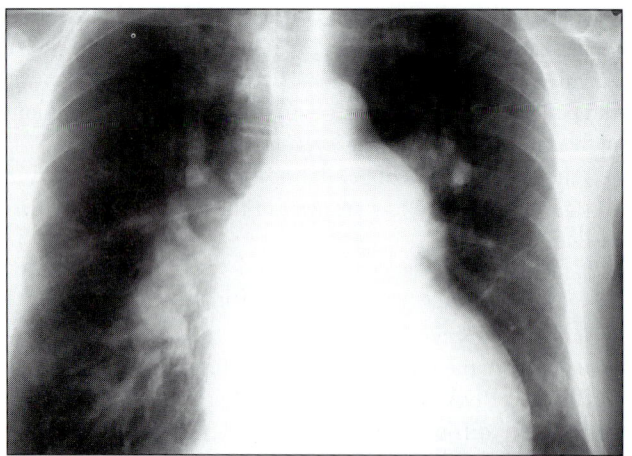

FIGURE 7 Chest x-ray, posteroanterior projection of a 50-year-old man with a large ventricular septal defect, pulmonary hypertension, and pulmonary vascular disease. Note huge main pulmonary artery, large right and left proximal pulmonary arteries, and absence of pulmonary vascular markings in the lateral one third of lung fields ("pruning"). The cardiac silhouette is enlarged, with dilated left ventricle.

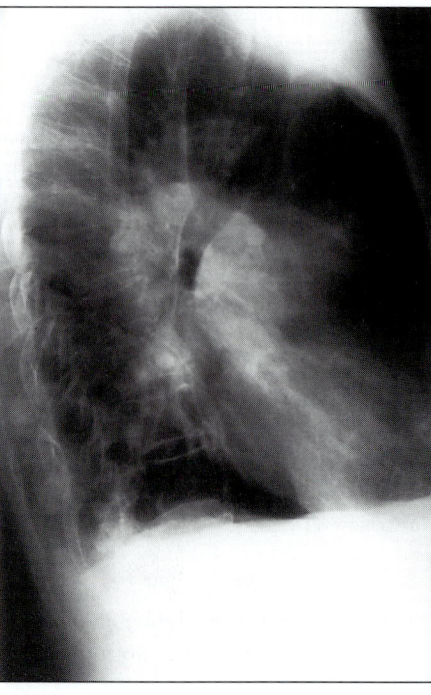

FIGURE 8 Chest x-ray, right lateral view. Same patient as in Figure 7.

are small. It is common for patients with these lesions in infancy to have cyanosis of the mucous membranes of the mouth, nail beds, and conjunctiva and to have clubbing of the fingers and toes. Right ventricular hypertrophy is invariably noted on ECG. Although a definitive diagnosis can be made with two-dimensional Doppler echocardiography, it is recommended that these patients have catheterization, mainly to look at the size of the pulmonary artery and its branches and at the origin and disposition of the coronary arteries. In 15% of cases, the left anterior descending coronary artery anomalously arises from the right coronary artery or the anterior sinus of Valsalva and crosses the right ventricular outflow tract.

Treatment
In most cases in which tetralogy of Fallot is found in the adult, complete correction is indicated. This is true even if the patient is doing well with a Blalock-Taussig or Potts shunt.

Pulmonary arteriovenous fistula

Anatomy
Pulmonary arteriovenous fistulas can be single, multiple, or even microscopic in number and size. They are often associated with hereditary hemorrhage telangiectasia (Rendu-Osler-Weber disease).

Pathophysiology
A right-to-left shunt exists because the arteriovenous fistula bypasses the pulmonary capillary bed. Because these arteriovenous fistulas are low-resistance shunts in the low-resistance pulmonary circuit, there is no afterload or preload burden on either the right or the left ventricle. The main problem is arterial desaturation and its consequences: polycythemia, clubbing, and the possibility of endarteritis. The heart itself is not abnormal from the pulmonary arteriovenous fistulas per se.

Physical findings
Telangiectasis on the mucous membranes and a personal or family history of gastrointestinal bleeding can be seen in patients with Rendu-Osler-Weber disease. The fistulas are subpleural, and if they are at the lung surface and have a large flow, they create a continuous murmur. At times, this murmur can be difficult or impossible to hear. The murmur may be mainly systolic. Because most of these fistulas are in the lower lobes, the murmur is usually in the anterior or lateral chest. Findings of cyanosis and clubbing are present.

Diagnosis
The lesions are commonly seen on plain chest films. With the roentgenographic findings and cyanosis, even without the diagnostic continuous murmur, a diagnosis can be made. Doppler echocardiography is of help in ruling out the other, more common causes of continuous murmurs and central cyanosis. With the injection of microbubbles, bubbles can be seen to fill the left side of the heart after filling the right side. It may not be possible to tell how the microbubbles get into the left side of the heart by transthoracic echocardiography.

Angiocardiography is essential in defining how many arteriovenous fistulas exist and where they are located (Fig. 9).

Complications
These fistulas create cyanosis and its complications. Hemoptysis is not uncommon. Gastrointestinal bleeding associated with Rendu-Osler-Weber syndrome can be seen. Finally, endarteritis caused by infection of arteriovenous fistulas has occurred. Systemic embolization through arteriovenous fistulas has been described.

Treatment
A single fistula or a limited number of pulmonary arteriovenous fistulas that create a large right-to-left shunt can be surgically excised by partial lobectomy. Catheter embolization of pulmonary arteriovenous fistulas can be accomplished, with elimination of or marked diminution in the shunt. This approach may be preferable to surgical excision, even with a single fistula. It is the preferential technique for multiple arteriovenous fistulas.

Ebstein's disease

Anatomy
Ebstein's disease is a congenital lesion that is characterized by displacement of a portion of the tricuspid valve attachment

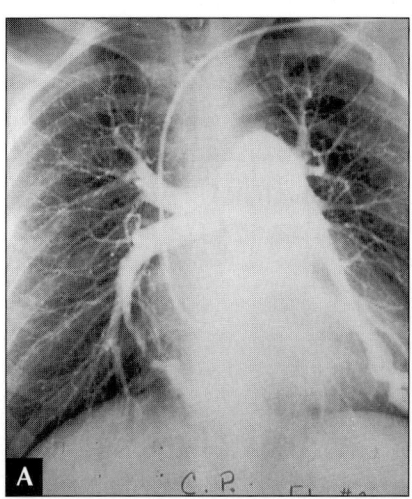
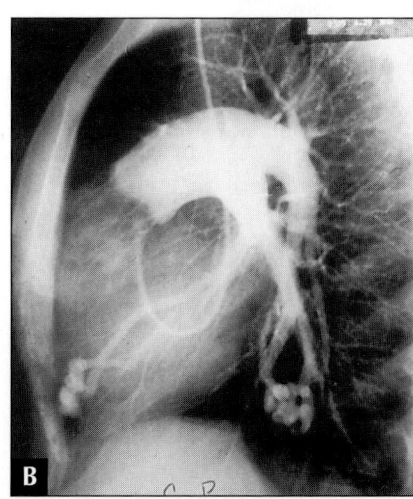

FIGURE 9 **A**, Angiocardiogram, pulmonary artery injection in the posteroanterior projection of a 30-year-old woman with pulmonary vascular disease who suddenly developed a continuous murmur lateral to the cardiac apex. Two pulmonary arteriovenous fistulae are visible, one in the right middle lobe and one on the left lower lobe. **B**, Angiocardiogram, pulmonary artery injection in the left lateral projection. Note the filling of the retrosternal space by the enlarged right ventricle as well as the two arteriovenous fistulae. Same patient as in A.

into the anatomic right ventricle. The posterior and septal leaflets are usually involved, and the displacement varies from mild to severe, resulting in enlargement of the chamber above the tricuspid valve (the "right atrium") and compromise of the chamber below (the "right ventricle"). There is frequently an atrial septal defect or an open foramen ovale.

Pathophysiology

The tricuspid valve is usually incompetent, resulting in a varying degree of tricuspid regurgitation. The "right atrium" is enlarged. If the tricuspid regurgitation is sufficient, the right atrial pressure is abnormally high, and if an atrial septal defect is present, a right-to-left shunt at the atrial level can cause arterial desaturation and even cyanosis.

There is frequently a muscle connection between the right atrium and the right ventricle, or a bundle of Kent; therefore, the anatomic substrate for Wolff-Parkinson-White syndrome exists in approximately 20% of patients.

Physical findings

The patient may have a precordial lift in the area of the outflow tract of the right ventricle. There may be signs of tricuspid regurgitation with an increased "V wave." The large anterior leaflet may move toward the atrium one or more times during ventricular systole, causing one or more nonejection clicks. The murmur of tricuspid regurgitation with its enhancement on inspiration is common. The S_1 and S_2 are frequently widely split, so that it often sounds as if there are several systolic clicks. The patient may be cyanotic with clubbing.

Approximately 20% of patients have supraventricular tachycardias.

Diagnosis

The chest roentgenogram shows a wide sweep of the right atrial border. The heart looks globular, but the pulmonary vascular markings are always normal or diminished, never plethoric. The ECG usually shows a right bundle branch block with a low-voltage rSR′ in V_1 and occasionally demonstrates first-degree atrioventricular block and Wolff-Parkinson-White syndrome, usually with a posteriorly directed delta wave. Two-dimensional Doppler echocardiography can make the diagnosis because the attachment of the posterior or septal leaflet, which is displaced toward the apex, is clearly visualized on echocardiography (Fig. 10).

Complications

Most patients with Ebstein's disease who survive to adulthood do quite well. Cyanosis in childhood is a bad prognostic sign. Symptoms are related to the degree of tricuspid regurgitation and the presence and magnitude of a right-to-left shunt. The most troublesome problem that many people experience is with paroxysmal atrial tachycardia. Evidence indicates that the bundle of Kent can be interrupted by radiofrequency catheter ablation, which should be accomplished for those with recurrent paroxysmal atrial tachycardia.

For patients who are symptomatic and have easy fatigability, cyanosis, or shortness of breath, surgical correction should be considered. Various techniques of plication of the portion of the right ventricle above the tricuspid valve have been advocated, together with closing of the atrial septal defect, and tricuspid valve replacement has also been described. In patients who are minimally symptomatic or are asymptomatic, no surgery or ablation techniques are indicated.

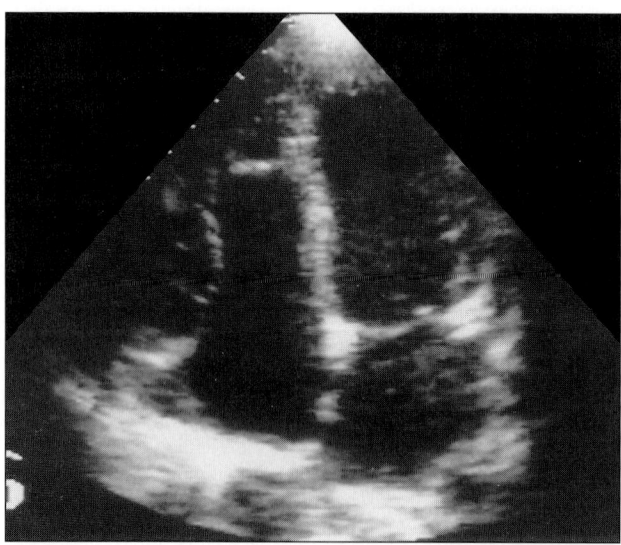

FIGURE 10 Two-dimensional echocardiogram, four-chamber view of a 50-year-old man with Ebstein's anomaly. Note displacement of the septal leaflet of the tricuspid valve down into the right ventricle almost to the apex.

REFERENCES AND RECOMMENDED READING

1. Cheitlin MD: Congenital heart disease in the adult. *Mod Concepts Cardiovasc Dis* 1986, 55:20–24.
2. McNamara DG, Latson LA: Long-term follow-up of patients with malformations for which definitive surgical repair has been available for 25 years or more. *Am J Cardiol* 1982, 50:560–568.
3. Cowen ME, Jeffrey RR, Drakeley MJ, et al.: The results of surgery for atrial septal defect in patients aged fifty years and over. *Eur Heart J* 1990, 11:29–34.
4. Ellis JH IV, Moodie DS, Sterba R, et al.: Ventricular septal defect in the adult: natural and unnatural history. *Am Heart J* 1987, 114:115–120.
5. Morgan JM, Gray HH, Miller GA, et al.: The clinical features, management and outcome of persistence of the arterial duct presenting in adult life. *Int J Cardiol* 1990, 27:193–199.
6. Fenoglio JJ Jr, McAllister HA Jr, DeCastro CM, et al.: Congenital bicuspid aortic valve after age 20. *AM J Cardiol* 1977, 39:164–169.

SELECT BIBLIOGRAPHY

Cheitlin MD, Sokolow M, McIlroy MB: Congenital heart disease (with special references to adult cardiology). In *Clinical Cardiology*, edn 6. Norwalk, CT: Appleton & Lange; 1993:358–406.

Liberthson RR: *Congenital Heart Disease: Diagnosis and Management in Children and Adults.* Boston: Little Brown; 1989.

Congenital Heart Disease in the Adult Postoperative Patient

23

John S. Child

> ### Key Points
> - Cardiac operations for congenital heart disease, now common in adults, have resulted in the survival of many previously operated infants and children to adulthood.
> - Understanding of the basic malformation, the nature of the surgical operation, and any potential residua, sequelae, and complications is mandatory for proper care of adults with operated congenital heart disease.
> - Residua and sequelae generally can be categorized as electrophysiologic or as anatomic with attendant hemodynamic consequences.
> - Superimposed, adult acquired diseases such as hypertension, aortic stenosis, or coronary artery disease may result in deterioration of ventricular function despite a good operative outcome, and they require proper diagnosis and treatment.
> - Knowledge of how to integrate sophisticated imaging and hemodynamic assessment, the mainstay being echocardiography, into the care of the patient is important.

Because of advances in cardiovascular surgical techniques during the past 25 years, there are many long-term survivors of cardiac operations during infancy and childhood, and physicians are faced with caring for an increasing number of patients with congenital heart disease [1•,2••,3]. Caring for adults with congenital heart disease requires knowledge of the original defect, the hemodynamic and anatomic problems caused by that defect, and the progressive age-related changes in anatomy and physiology. Proper patient care after catheterization or surgical palliation or repair requires intimate knowledge of the nature and effects of the intervention and of the postoperative residua, sequelae, and complications (Table 1) [1•,2••,3].

The success of these interventions is judged by the patient's quality of life, survival time, and need for reoperation. The general practitioner must be knowledgeable about currently applied techniques and materials as well as outmoded techniques previously applied during infancy and childhood. Adults who underwent surgery 20 or more years ago are alive because of their operations, but they may have had inadequate myocardial protection or have degenerating prosthetic materials.

GENERAL POSTOPERATIVE CONSIDERATIONS

Except for ligation of an uncomplicated patent ductus arteriosus and suture closure of a secundum atrial septal defect, all other surgery for cardiac anomalies leaves behind or causes some obligatory abnormality, ranging from trivial to serious (Tables 1 and 2). Postoperative residua and sequelae can be broadly categorized as electrophysiologic or anatomic (valvular, myocardial, vascular), or related to the durability of prosthetic materials and valves.

Residua (defects only partially or not corrected)	Sequelae (defects caused by the form of operative intervention)
Bicuspid aortic valve (coarctation) Cleft mitral leaflet (ostium primum atrial septal defect) Residual ventricular outflow obstruction Atrioventricular valve regurgitation (after Fontan procedure for tricuspid atresia or single ventricle) Systemic hypertension (coarctation) or pulmonary hypertension (shunts) Myocardial function—long-term ability of right ventricle (transposition) or single ventricle to function as systemic ventricle; effects of previous volume/pressure overload, prolonged cyanosis and erythrocytosis on coronary reserve and myocardial contractility Cyanosis—residual left superior vena cava to left atrium with or without coronary sinus atrial septal defect	Mechanical—ventricular function (ventriculotomy), intraventricular or venous baffle obstruction (*eg*, Mustard or Rastelli repair). Electrophysiologic—atrial arrhythmias and sinus node dysfunction (atrial septal, Mustard intraatrial baffle, Fontan) conduction defects (central right bundle-branch block or left anterior fascicular block after ventricular septal patch, *eg*, tetralogy of Fallot), ventriculotomy-induced ventricular arrhythmias or conduction defects Valvular—aortic or pulmonic regurgitation (valvotomy, tetralogy of Fallot), mitral regurgitation or stenosis after repair of cleft mitral leaflet (primum atrial septal defect) Prosthetic materials—patches (deterioration with time, ventricular septal patch leaks), conduits (kinking or progressive intraluminal obstruction), valves (bioprosthetic deterioration with stenosis/regurgitation) or disk valves with thrombosis, fracture, or stenosis; anticoagulant complications Cyanosis—pulmonary arteriovenous fistulae (Glenn shunt)

Table 1 Representative residua and sequelae after intracardiac repair for congenital heart disease

Electrophysiologic Sequelae

Electrophysiologic sequelae include atrial and ventricular arrhythmias caused by scar or aneurysm formation after atrial or ventricular incisions or patch suturing. Insertion of intracardiac patches or conduits may cause disruption of the conduction system. For example, repair of tetralogy of Fallot includes a right ventricular outflow tract incision and ventricular septal defect patch. If the right ventricular outflow tract or pulmonary artery obstruction is inadequately relieved by the operation, the resultant right ventricular pressure overload superimposed on the right ventricular outflow tract scar or aneurysm may cause ventricular arrhythmias.

Anatomic Sequelae and Residua

Important anatomic sequelae and residua must be sought. Bicuspid aortic valves are often associated with aortic coarctation and continue to pose risks of progressive stenosis, regurgitation, and endocarditis after coarctation repair. Variations on a parachute mitral valve, often found in conjunction with coarctation and other stenoses in sequence on the left-sided circulation, may have gone undetected. Repair of an ostium primum atrial septal defect includes cleft mitral valve repair; residual mitral regurgitation may exist and is occasionally progressive. Subaortic, discrete stenosis may coexist and should be recognized.

Repaired tetralogy of Fallot may have pulmonary regurgitation because of a valvulotomy or a transannular incision and patch. Isolated mild to moderate low-pressure pulmonary regurgitation is common and well-tolerated. Severe pulmonary regurgitation may cause right ventricular failure and tricuspid regurgitation, particularly if there is any residual right ventricular outflow, pulmonary valvular or arterial (*eg*, branch stenosis) obstruction. Also, muscular ventricular septal defects may have been missed preoperatively. Postoperative aortic regurgitation is common in the adult whose malformation was associated with a dilated aortic root or trunk (*eg*, tetralogy of Fallot, transposition of the great arteries, single ventricle in association with pulmonic stenosis, truncus arteriosus). Atrioventricular valve regurgitation is common preoperatively in candidates for the Fontan procedure and may progress postoperatively. These valvular lesions pose a continuing risk for endocarditis and may affect long-term ventricular performance.

Prosthetic Materials

Use of prosthetic materials such as septal patches, mechanical or bioprosthetic valves, and intracardiac and extracardiac conduits may have long-term consequences. Prosthetic valves are associated with a risk for thrombus formation and infective endocarditis. Bioprosthetic valves may undergo premature degeneration and calcification. External conduits may kink or develop internal intimal thickening ("peel formation"), and valved conduits frequently undergo valvular degeneration that may result in severe obstruction. An internal conduit holds a risk for conduit leaks, internal obstruction, and kinking, or it may partially obstruct the chamber within which it sits. Examples of procedures using external and internal conduits include the Fontan repair with an external conduit from the right atrium to the pulmonary artery (for tricuspid atresia or single ventricle with pulmonic stenosis), and the Rastelli repair with an external conduit from the right ventricle to the pulmonary artery (for D-transposition or double-outlet right ventricle) and an intraventricular conduit to route the left ventricle to the aorta via the ventricular septal defect.

Transthoracic echocardiography with Doppler and color-flow imaging is the mainstay for detailed anatomic and hemodynamic postoperative evaluation of patients with congenital heart disease. These studies are best done in laboratories having extensive experience with these abnormalities [4]. Transesophageal echocardiography (TEE) is needed

TABLE 2 POTENTIAL RESIDUA AND SEQUELAE AFTER REPAIR OF SPECIFIC COMMONLY OPERATED CONGENITAL HEART DEFECTS

Original Defect	Residua	Sequelae
Bicuspid aortic valve	Aortic regurgitation or stenosis (if valvotomy) Left ventricular enlargement or left ventricular hypertrophy	Prosthetic valve malfunction Anticoagulation
Coarctation	Bicuspid aortic valves Hypertension Residual coarctation Left ventricular hypertrophy Coronary disease Intracranial aneurysms	Recurrent coarctation
Atrial septal defect secundum	Atrial arrhythmias Mitral prolapse/mitral regurgitation Right atrial and right ventricular enlargement Right ventricular failure Tricuspid regurgitation Pulmonary hypertension	Atrial fibrillation/stroke
Atrial septal defect primum	Residual cleft mitral valve/mitral regurgitation Discrete subaortic stenosis (missed) Right ventricular, right atrial, left atrial enlargement Tricuspid regurgitation Pulmonary hypertension Atrial arrhythmias	Mitral stenosis Subaortic stenosis caused by chordal attachments to ventricular septum and suture of mitral valve cleft Patch leak Atrial arrhythmias
Tetralogy of Fallot	Right ventricular outflow tract obstruction Ventricular septal defect patch leak Branch pulmonary stenosis Right ventricular hypertrophy Aortic regurgitation (dilated aorta)	Ventricular septal defect patch right bundle-branch block (aortic regurgitation as a complication) Right ventricular outflow tract incision Pulmonary regurgitation Right bundle-branch block Ventricular arrhythmia Conduit obstruction
Transpositions	Decreased systemic right ventricular function Aortic regurgitation	Intracardiac conduit leak/obstruction Extracardiac conduit obstruction Intraatrial baffle leak or obstruction Caval or pulmonary venous obstruction Atrial and ventricular arrhythmias, sinus node dysfunction
Univentricular hearts (tricuspid atresia, single ventricle)	Atrioventricular valve regurgitation Myocardial dysfunction Aortic regurgitation	Fontan conduit obstruction/thrombus Atrial patch leak Atrial and ventricular arrhythmias Pulmonary arteriovenous fistulae (Glenn shunt)

when transthoracic echocardiography is not technically adequate and structures are not readily accessible to surface echocardiography (*eg*, aortic coarctation) [5]. Magnetic resonance imaging (MRI) is complementary for imaging abnormalities of the great vessels. If the echocardiographic and MRI data are not definitive, they conflict with the clinical picture, or reoperation is indicated, goal-directed diagnostic cardiac catheterization may be necessary. Intraoperative TEE improves results by detecting unexpected anomalies, refining known anatomic details, or allowing detection and re-repair of unsatisfactory results while the patient is still in the operating room.

SPECIFIC POSTOPERATIVE LESIONS

Congenital aortic stenosis caused by a bicuspid aortic valve is one of the most common congenital cardiac malformations, although it may go unrecognized early in life. It may be directly repaired in younger patients (< 21 years old) by valvotomy or balloon dilation using percutaneous catheter techniques if the valve is pliant and noncalcified with obstruction caused by congenital fusion of the commissures. There is often some degree of aortic regurgitation after valvotomy or balloon valvuloplasty, and the inherent abnormal valve remains a site for recurrent stenosis or infective endocarditis.

Aortic regurgitation usually progresses gradually but can suddenly increase because of infective endocarditis. Generally, recurrent aortic stenosis slowly progresses, and reoperation is often necessary. Echocardiographic quantitation of aortic valve area, aortic regurgitation, and left ventricular size and ejection fraction should be done routinely on a yearly basis. For the older patient, direct valve replacement is often preferable. Surgically important aortic regurgitation requires directly proceeding with valve replacement to remove the left ventricular volume overload and to preserve ventricular function. Despite the best attempts at selecting patients, some may exhibit late myocardial dysfunction and ventricular arrhythmias. The type of aortic prosthesis used affects its long-term durability, and the need for anticoagulation therapy and possible reoperation. Antiinfective endocarditis prophylaxis is required for life.

Valvular pulmonic stenosis (isolated) usually can be readily repaired with excellent results. Minimal residua and sequelae are expected if the valve repair is performed when the patient is young (< 21 years old), even if mild degrees of pulmonic stenosis and regurgitation remain. If severe pulmonic stenosis is operated on after 21 years of age, the outlook is excellent; however, the longstanding right ventricular pressure overload and hypertrophy can result in right ventricular failure. Balloon dilation has largely replaced surgical valvotomy, except for dysplastic valves, and short-term results have been excellent.

Ebstein's anomaly is the most common cause of surgically important congenital tricuspid valvular regurgitation. If the anterior tricuspid leaflet is shown by echocardiography to be long and mobile, a surgeon experienced with this anomaly can achieve a good repair. Residual, mild to moderate, low-pressure tricuspid regurgitation is usually well tolerated. Valvular reconstruction reduces right ventricular volume overload and improves right ventricular function. An interatrial communication (a commonly associated defect) should be closed at the same time to eliminate cyanosis and avoid future risk of paradoxic embolization. Wolff-Parkinson-White syndrome is a common association. During the same operation, right-sided atrioventricular bypass tracts are surgically interrupted to prevent the accelerated ventricular response to supraventricular arrhythmias. Postoperative supraventricular arrhythmias may still recur but usually respond to pharmacologic treatment with standard, type-I antiarrhythmic agents. If amiodarone therapy or radiofrequency ablation becomes necessary, consultation with a specialist is needed. Valve replacement, occasionally required, has a long-term mortality rate of 10% to 15%. Tissue valves are preferred because of concerns about the risk of pulmonary embolization from mechanical prostheses despite anticoagulation. Improvement after surgical intervention notwithstanding, there are obligatory residual abnormalities of ventricular size and function.

Isolated, left-sided, atrioventricular valve incompetence may occur with congenital transposition of the great arteries. The left-sided tricuspid valve may have an Ebstein-like malformation, with severe left atrioventricular valve regurgitation initially mistaken for mitral regurgitation until echocardiographic study elucidates the inverted ventricles. Replacement is usually required when regurgitation is severe. The possibility of complete heart block (approximately 2% accrued incidence per year) and right ventricular failure (the systemic subaortic ventricle) warrants annual electrocardiograms and echocardiograms.

Surgical Procedures

Intraatrial Surgery

Atrial septal defects, particularly the secundum variety, are some of the most common congenital heart defects. Early closure of these defects prevents subsequent right ventricular dysfunction or pulmonary hypertension. Surgical closure achieves excellent long-term results, particularly if performed by the age of 40 years. Nonetheless, even patients older than 60 years benefit from repair symptomatically and prognostically, but they do experience more arrhythmias and pulmonary problems than patients operated on before age 40 [6••,7,8].

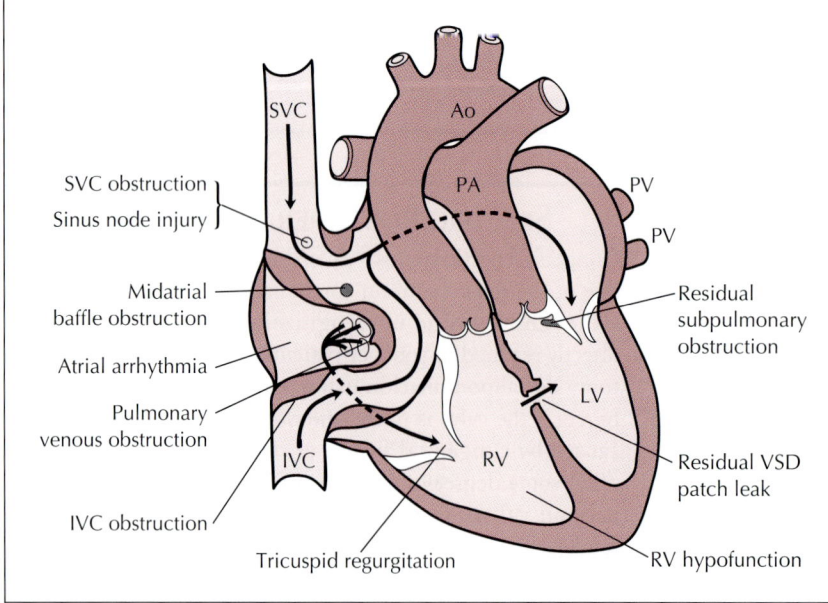

FIGURE 1. Postoperative Mustard repair procedure for D-transposition of the great arteries. The intraatrial baffle can be seen to connect the superior and inferior vena cavae (SVC, IVC) to the left ventricle (LV), which directs deoxygenated blood to the lungs via the pulmonary artery (PA). Pulmonary veins (PV) are routed to the right ventricle (RV), which directs oxygenated blood to the body via the aorta (Ao). As such, the circulation in series is reconstituted. This schematic displays the various potential sequelae or complications. VSD—ventricular septal defect.

Removal of the left-to-right shunt usually decreases the right ventricular size to normal if done during childhood, whereas adults who undergo repair usually have some residual right ventricular enlargement. Long-term right ventricular dysfunction is infrequent. Even if a patient has preoperative tricuspid regurgitation and right ventricular failure, right ventricular function usually improves postoperatively. Significantly increased pulmonary vascular resistance decreases long-term improvement and survival.

The incidence of atrial arrhythmias increases each decade in adults with an unrepaired atrial septal defect. The later the operation is performed, the less preventable these arrhythmias. With repair after age 40, as many as 50% of patients with preoperative sinus rhythm will have late postoperative atrial fibrillation.

Intraatrial "switch" surgery has primarily been performed for complete transposition of the great arteries (Fig. 1). Such procedures redirect the systemic venous flow to the left ventricle (which supplies blood to the lungs via the pulmonary artery) and the pulmonary venous flow to the right ventricle (which ejects blood to the body via the aorta). Currently, the trend is to perform an arterial switch procedure during infancy, but a large number of today's young adults have previously had a Mustard or Senning atrial switch procedure. Although approximately 80% of these patients survive to adulthood, long-term complications are the rule (Tables 1 and 2) [9,10]. Routine follow-up electrocardiograms should be obtained. Atrial arrhythmias are common; injury to the sinus node may cause bradycardias and junctional escape rhythms, which may require inserting a permanent pacemaker. Because of the unusual intracardiac pathways, the pacemaker should be inserted by a physician experienced in dealing with these patients.

Long-term concerns about the functioning of the right ventricle in the systemic subaortic position persist, with some patients developing cardiomyopathy and ventricular failure. Echocardiography should be performed at least yearly to detect this complication. Afterload reduction with angiotensin-converting enzyme (ACE) inhibitors may be needed if the right ventricular ejection fraction is decreased or systemic arterial hypertension is detected.

Intraventricular Surgery

Intraventricular surgery includes repair of ventricular septal defects and tetralogy of Fallot as well as Rastelli procedures. Intraventricular surgery may be performed via a right atriotomy or ventriculotomy. Long-term outcome is affected by the adequacy of myocardial protection, degree of residual ventricular pressure or volume overload, subsequent electrophysiologic sequelae, and durability of prosthetic conduits, valves, and patches.

The most representative malformation is tetralogy of Fallot. Patients who received palliative aortopulmonary shunts (Blalock-Taussig, Pott's, or Waterston) and subsequent intracardiac repair at approximately 2 years of age have a nearly 90% survival rate 20 years after operation. Before complete repair, these shunts may gradually obstruct and result in increased cyanosis because of decreased pulmonary

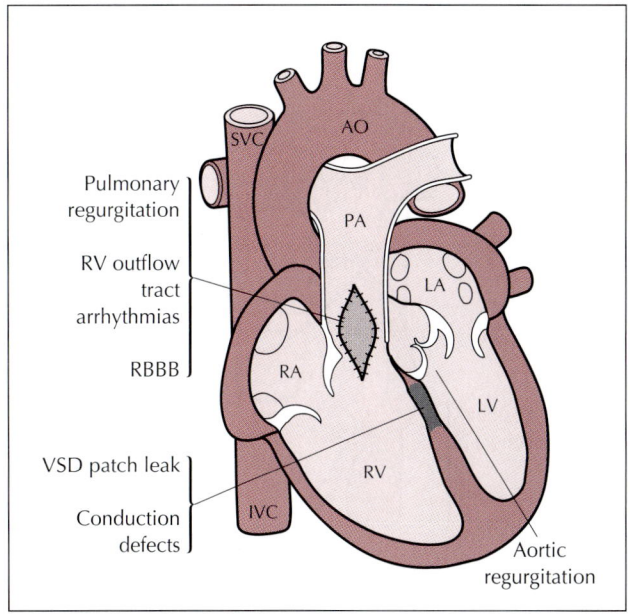

FIGURE 2 Representative corrective repair for tetralogy of Fallot. The misaligned ventricular septal defect (VSD) has been closed with a patch. Obstruction to flow from the right ventricle (RV) to the pulmonary artery (PA) may occur in the right ventricular outflow tract, pulmonary annulus or valve, or the PA. Here, a transannular patch is enlarging the right ventricular outflow tract and annulus after resection of obstructing right ventricular outflow tract muscle via the right ventricular incision. Potential sequelae or complications of the VSD patch and transannular incision and patch are shown. The aortic root, once overriding the VSD, may result in long-term aortic regurgitation. AO—aorta; LA—left atrium; LV—left ventricle; RA—right atrium; RBBB—right bundle branch block; SVC—superior vena cava.

blood flow, or they may be too large and either result in left ventricular volume overload or increased pulmonary vascular resistance and pulmonary hypertension. Adults who received palliative shunts as children benefit from complete repair. Although patients older than 40 years at the time of repair have a late mortality rate of approximately 15%, long-term survival is enhanced by intracardiac repair, and most of these patients lead essentially normal lives [11,12••].

Approximately 15% of persons with tetralogy of Fallot require reoperation for residua and sequelae of the previous intracardiac repair, including residual right ventricular outflow tract obstruction and ventricular septal defect patch leaks (Figs. 2 and 3). Severe pulmonary regurgitation may occur if the pulmonary valve is excised and can result in right ventricular failure and tricuspid regurgitation requiring reoperation to insert a bioprosthetic valve. In patients with severe hypoplasia of the pulmonary valve or pulmonary atresia, a right ventricular–to–pulmonary artery conduit may be necessary. As previously noted, this can result in late obstruction because of intimal buildup or degeneration of a tissue valve within the conduit. Such hemodynamic abnormalities cause pressure and volume overload of a right ventricle with an incisional scar and, occasionally, a right ventricular aneurysm. This is the substrate for ventricular arrhythmias and sudden death. Bundle-branch blocks or high-grade

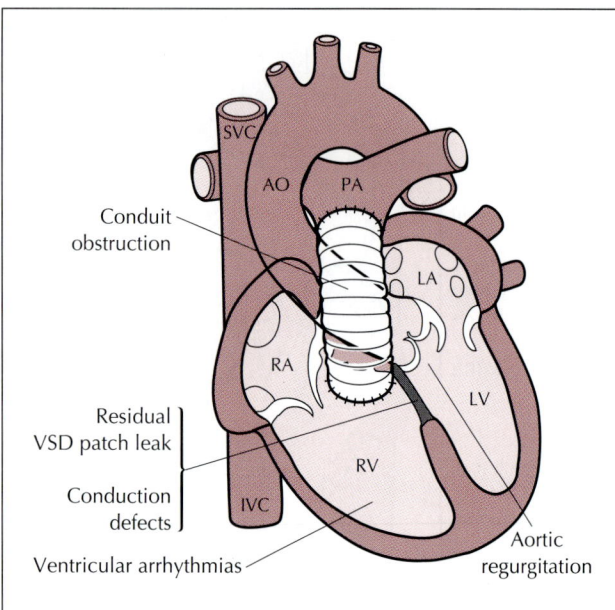

FIGURE 3 Rastelli repair of severe tetralogy of Fallot/pulmonary atresia. The ventricular septal defect (VSD) is patched, and the right ventricle (RV)–to–pulmonary artery (PA) connection is made by a conduit, usually containing a bioprosthetic valve. Potential sequelae, residua, and complications are noted.

dysfunction, even though volumes increase postoperatively. Because of concerns about long-term left ventricular function in adults with repaired tetralogy of Fallot, systemic arterial hypertension must be treated, preferably with afterload-reducing agents (ACE inhibitors). Aortic regurgitation (common in the adult with tetralogy of Fallot) may become severe and cause ventricular failure. It is also susceptible to infective endocarditis and requires lifelong prophylaxis. Two-dimensional echocardiography and Doppler evaluation are necessary to evaluate the right ventricular outflow tract and pulmonary artery anatomy for obstruction and to measure right ventricular systolic pressure and ventricular septal patch leaks.

Central Arterial Surgery

Central arterial surgery includes palliative aortopulmonary shunts and repair of patient ductus, coarction of the aorta, or sinus of Valsalva aneurysms. Surgical division of an isolated small patent ductus arteriosus in a child is an extracardiac operation and as close to a curative operation as can be performed. Currently, a potentially competing technique is transcatheter closure. If the ductus is moderate to large, surgical division in childhood usually allows regression of the left atrial and ventricular size. If a large ductus is not closed early, pulmonary hypertension and pulmonary vascular disease may occur.

heart block may result from incision and resection of the right ventricular outflow tract and insertion of the ventricular septal defect patch.

Late postoperative left ventricular function relates to the adequacy of myocardial protection at operation, age at time of repair, and degree of left-side heart volume overload from prior palliative shunt procedures. There are also concerns that the duration of cyanosis before repair may relate to progressive myocardial fibrosis and late ventricular dysfunction. Patients with severe cyanotic tetralogy of Fallot may have reduced left ventricular volume and ejection fraction. Repair after 2 years of age leaves residual left ventricular

Surgical repair of coarctation of the aorta relieves the obstructive gradient in most instances [13]. A bicuspid aortic valve often coexists and requires endocarditis prophylaxis. Even in the well-repaired aortic coarctation, yearly follow-up for late hypertension is needed. Patients should undergo treadmill stress testing with the specific goal of detecting an inordinate rise in arterial blood pressure that may occur despite normal resting blood pressure. Resting and immediate postexercise blood pressures should be taken in both the arms and legs to detect a residual coarctation gradient. Recurrent coarctation may require repeat surgery or balloon dilation if severe. Residual coarctation should be quantified by TEE or MRI of the descending thoracic aorta.

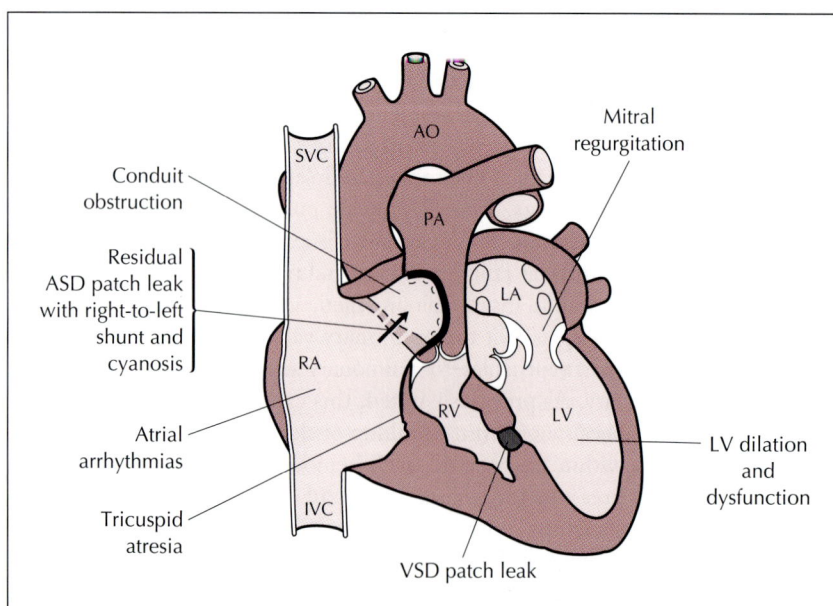

FIGURE 4 Right atrium (RA)–to–pulmonary artery (PA) connection for tricuspid atresia, functionally a univentricular heart, is a common variation on the Fontan connection seen on patients operated on within the last few years. (Now, a total cavopulmonary connection with a lateral tunnel is more commonly performed.) The obligatory atrial septal defect (ASD) is closed. Flow from the left ventricle (LV) to the PA is removed by closing a ventricular septal defect (VSD) as shown or by oversewing the pulmonary valve. Potential residua, sequelae, and complications also are

Caval to Pulmonary Arterial Connections

Fontan or Glenn shunts are performed to increase pulmonary blood flow in malformations with a basic underlying problem of a "univentricular heart" with pulmonic stenosis and intracardiac shunts (Fig. 4). Cyanosis is relieved, and symptoms are improved or alleviated [14]. Long-term problems relate mainly to arrhythmias and ventricular function; atrial fibrillation or flutter is poorly tolerated. Cardiac output and systemic venous congestion decrease. Ventricular function can deteriorate over time and may cause or be compounded by atrioventricular valve regurgitation. Routine echocardiographic evaluation of ventricular function and valvular regurgitation is necessary. The caval and right atrial connections to the right ventricle or pulmonary artery are better imaged by transesophageal echocardiography.

Infective endocarditis prophylaxis is necessary for patients with valvular regurgitation. Hypertension must be normalized with afterload reduction (by ACE inhibitors) to decrease the load on the ventricle. Ventricular dysfunction occasionally becomes sufficiently severe to require orthotopic cardiac transplantation.

References and Recommended Reading

Recently published papers of particular interest have been highlighted as:
- Of interest
- •• Of outstanding interest

1.• Perloff JK, Child JS: *Congenital Heart Disease in Adults*. Philadelphia: WB Saunders; 1991.

2.•• 22nd Bethesda Conference: Congenital heart disease after childhood: an expanding patient population. *J Am Coll Cardiol* 1991, 18:311–342.

3. Morris CD, Menashe VD: 25-Year mortality after surgical repair of congenital heart defect in childhood. *JAMA* 1991, 266:3447–3452.

4. Child JS: Echo-Doppler and color-flow imaging in congenital heart disease. *Cardiol Clin* 1990, 8:289–313.

5. Marelli AJ, Child JS, Perloff JK: Transesophageal echocardiography in congenital heart disease in the adult. *Cardiol Clin* 1993, 11:505–520.

6.•• Murphy JG, Gersh BJ, McGoon MD, *et al.*: Long term outcome of patients undergoing surgical repair of isolated atrial septal defect: follow-up at 27-32 years. *N Engl J Med* 1990, 323:1645–1650.

7. St. John Sutton MG, Tajik AJ, McGoon DC: Atrial septal defect in patients 60 years and older: operative results and long-term postoperative follow-up. *Circulation* 1981, 84:402–409.

8. Steele PM, Fuster V, Cohen M, *et al.*: Isolated atrial septal defect with pulmonary vascular obstructive disease: long term follow-up and prediction of outcome after surgical correction. *Circulation* 1987, 76:1037–1042.

9. Hayes CJ, Gersony WM: Arrhythmias after the Mustard operation for transposition of the great arteries: a long-term study. *J Am Coll Cardiol* 1986, 7:133–137.

10. Warnes CA, Somerville J: Transposition of the great arteries: late results in adolescents and adults after the Mustard operation. *Br Heart J* 1987, 58:148–155.

11. Hu DCK, Seward JB, Puga FJ, *et al.*: Total correction of tetralogy of Fallot at age 40 years or older: long-term follow-up. *J Am Coll Cardiol* 1985, 5:40–44.

12.•• Waien SA, Liu PP, Ross BL, *et al.*: Serial follow-up of adults with repaired tetralogy of Fallot. *J Am Coll Cardiol* 1992, 20:295–300.

13. Presbitero P, Demarie D, Villani M, *et al.*: Long term results (15-30) years of surgical repair or aortic coarctation. *Br Heart J* 1987, 57:462–467.

14. Driscoll DJ, Offord KP, Feldt RH, *et al.*: Five- to fifteen-year follow-up after Fontan operation. *Circulation* 1992, 85:469–496.

Pulmonary Hypertension

Stuart Rich

Key Points
- Severe pulmonary hypertension can result from many common cardiopulmonary conditions.
- The accurate diagnosis of pulmonary hypertension requires multiple tests to evaluate all possible contributing factors.
- General treatment measures appear to be helpful for patients with pulmonary hypertension of many etiologies.
- The assessment of drug effects and drug initiation should be left to experienced specialists.
- The prognosis of patients with severe primary and secondary forms of pulmonary hypertension may markedly improve with appropriately focused, aggressive treatments.

Although not common, pulmonary hypertension usually overwhelms the clinical course of a patient whether its etiology is primary or secondary. For this reason, early diagnosis of pulmonary hypertension could have important implications for patients regarding their responsiveness to treatment and clinical course. There are many causes of pulmonary hypertension that can affect the pulmonary vascular bed in similar ways. Injury to the pulmonary vascular endothelium produces a cascade of effects including pulmonary vasoconstriction and thrombosis that is self-perpetuating and can lead to extreme pulmonary hypertension and right-side heart failure. Some patients have pulmonary hypertension from more than one cause, such as chronic obstructive pulmonary disease as well as pulmonary thromboembolism. For these patients, distinguishing the relative contribution of each underlying disease to the overall clinical state can be quite difficult.

Many physicians are confused when a patient has pulmonary hypertension that appears to be out of proportion to the underlying disease. The response of the pulmonary vascular bed to all types of stimuli is markedly variable, however. Some patients may have only minimal elevations in pulmonary hypertension when exposed to hypoxia; other patients may have a pronounced effect. Appreciating the variability of the pulmonary vascular response to injury explains why many patients have pulmonary hypertension that appears to be more severe than the extent of the underlying disease process.

ROLE OF THE GENERALIST

Patients suspected of having pulmonary hypertension should be referred to a specialist in the field because of the complexity of pulmonary hypertensive disease and the morbidity associated with both diagnostic testing and therapies. Early diagnosis of pulmonary hypertension is fundamental to successfully treating the patient, however, and in this regard, heightened suspicion by the primary-care physician is

TABLE 1 CAUSES OF PULMONARY HYPERTENSION AND CONFIRMING DIAGNOSTIC TESTS	
Cause	**Test**
Lung disease (*eg*, parenchymal, hypoxic)	Chest radiography or high-resolution computed tomography Pulmonary function tests
Heart disease (*eg*, congenital, abnormal left heart filling)	Echocardiography Catheterization
Pulmonary vascular obstruction (*eg*, thromboembolism, mediastinal fibrosis)	Lung scan Pulmonary angiography
Collagen vascular diseases	Serologic tests High-resolution chest computed tomography
Primary pulmonary hypertension (diagnosis of exclusion)	Catheterization

TABLE 2 CONDITIONS ASSOCIATED WITH UNEXPLAINED PULMONARY HYPERTENSION
Exogenous substance ingestion Anorexic agents Toxic rapeseed oil L-Tryptophan Crack cocaine Human immunodeficiency virus infection (with or without AIDS) Portal hypertension

critical in making an early diagnosis. After patients with pulmonary hypertension have been evaluated and placed on long-term treatment, the generalist should be able to manage the patient, with periodic consultation from the cardiologist or pulmonologist. Because there are so few centers of excellence in this area, it is essential for the generalist to reassume day-to-day care.

DIAGNOSIS

An algorithm to diagnose the cause of pulmonary hypertension has been established through the National Institute of Health Registry on Primary Pulmonary Hypertension (Table 1) [1].

Because the underlying cause of pulmonary hypertension may not be readily apparent, a physician needs to assess all possible etiologies, even when there is no clinical history or overt signs of an underlying disease process. There also is an association between unexplained pulmonary hypertension and other conditions (Table 2).

Chest radiography is helpful in evaluating parenchymal lung disease. Pulmonary hypertension of any etiology often manifests with cardiomegaly and enlarged central pulmonary arteries (Fig. 1). Tapering of the pulmonary vasculature and oligemia are nonspecific findings and do not indicate a diagnosis. The lung fields on the chest x-ray film may appear normal in spite of interstitial lung disease; hence, if interstitial lung disease is suspected, a high-resolution chest computed tomographic (CT) scan is the test of choice. Its sensitivity for detecting interstitial abnormalities will generally preclude the need for open-lung biopsy.

Patients with pulmonary hypertension generally have limited exercise tolerance and may have exercise-induced syncope. Exercise tolerance is an important prognostic indicator, however, and assessing it may help in the early detection of patients with mild pulmonary hypertension when symp-

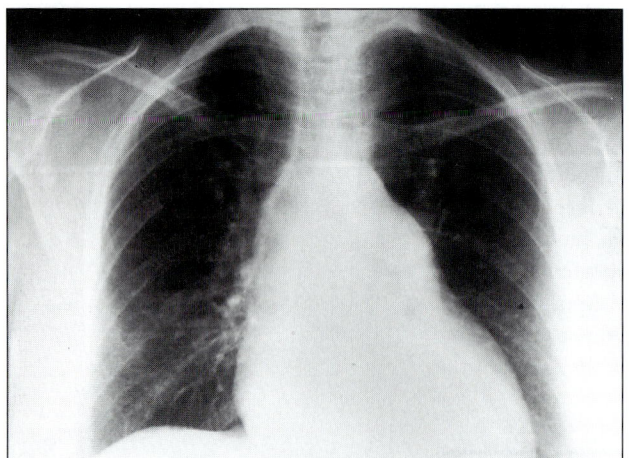

FIGURE 1 Chest radiographic (posteroanterior view) of a patient with unexplained pulmonary hypertension. Cardiomegaly with a large central pulmonary artery, prominent right descending pulmonary artery, and tapering of the vessels towards the periphery. The lung fields are clear. This could be a radiograph of a patient with pulmonary hypertension from almost any etiology.

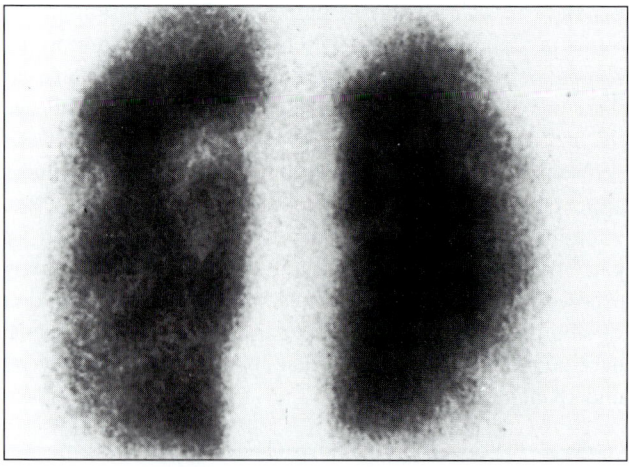

FIGURE 2 Perfusion lung scan (posterior upright view) of a patient with primary pulmonary hypertension. Patchy distribution of tagged albumin is marked but not in any anatomic segmental or subsegmental distribution suggesting pulmonary thromboembolism. This lung-scan pattern also may be seen in patients with pulmonary hypertension of other etiologies.

toms are manifest primarily with effort. The concomitant measurement of systemic oxygen saturation with pulse oximetry will confirm abnormal cardiopulmonary performance and help guide the physician toward the need for oxygen therapy. Patients whose history suggests limited effort tolerance should be studied using modified or low-level treadmill protocols.

Pulmonary Function Testing and Echocardiography

Pulmonary function tests are necessary to establish whether an obstructive airways disease or restrictive lung disease is present. Patients who develop pulmonary hypertension from obstructive airways disease should have associated clinical findings, but restrictive lung disease can be more difficult to ascertain. Increased pulmonary artery pressures produce restrictive changes in the lungs to a moderate degree. Thus, the diagnosis of restrictive lung disease requires a combination of restrictive changes on pulmonary function testing and evidence of parenchymal lung disease either by chest radiography, high-resolution CT scan, or lung biopsy. Although diffusion capacity from carbon monoxide may be reduced with pulmonary hypertension of any etiology, extremely low levels may suggest interstitial lung disease when it is not obvious from other tests.

The ventilation-perfusion lung scan will reveal patients with a high likelihood of having thromboembolism. Because thromboembolism that produces pulmonary hypertension is usually silent, this lung scan needs to be performed on every patient regardless of a history of deep-vein thrombosis or previous pulmonary embolism. Patients with primary pulmonary hypertension may have abnormal, patchy distribution of radionuclide that is not suggestive of pulmonary thromboembolism (Fig. 2). Abnormal distribution or retention of xenon in the ventilation scan may indicate underlying parenchymal lung disease.

Echocardiography is very helpful in revealing underlying congenital heart disease. Use of saline contrast and color Doppler will aid in detecting intracardiac shunts, which usually are bidirectional or reversed in patients with pulmonary hypertension. When in doubt, transesophageal echocardiography can be instrumental in differentiating an atrial septal defect from a patent foramen ovale.

Pulmonary Angiography and Cardiac Catheterization

Although pulmonary angiography carries increased risk in patients with pulmonary hypertension, it is mandatory for patients whose lung scan suggests the possibility of pulmonary thromboembolism. Hypotensive episodes after pulmonary angiography may be vagally mediated, and pretreating patients with 1 mg of atropine and using low-osmolar, nonionic agents may make the procedure safer in this regard. Making selective injections based on the abnormalities seen in the lung scan can reduce the amount of contrast needed to make the diagnosis.

Because the clinical management of the patient with pulmonary hypertension can be complex, cardiac catheterization is advised for every patient in whom the diagnosis of pulmonary hypertension is suspected. In addition to confirming the etiology, catheterization will help to establish the prognosis by directly measuring cardiac output and pulmonary artery saturation, both of which predict survival. It is also essential to accurately determine pulmonary-capillary wedge pressure to assess left ventricular end-diastolic pressure. The pulmonary-capillary wedge pressure may be difficult to obtain in these patients, but a conclusion that the patient had a "falsely elevated wedge pressure" is unacceptable. Catheterization of patients with advanced disease can be quite difficult; these patients should be referred to physicians with considerable experience.

CAUSES OF PULMONARY HYPERTENSION AND TREATMENT

Chronic thromboembolic obstruction of the proximal pulmonary arteries is an established treatable cause of pulmonary hypertension.

Primary Pulmonary Hypertension

Primary pulmonary hypertension is a diagnosis of exclusion and can be made only when all secondary causes have been eliminated. The natural history of primary pulmonary hypertension is poor, with a mean survival of 2.8 years from the time of diagnosis [1]. As many as 30% of these patients however, can return to a normal lifestyle and have improved survival if they are diagnosed early and respond to high doses of calcium channel blockers (Fig. 3) [2•]. The titration of calcium block-

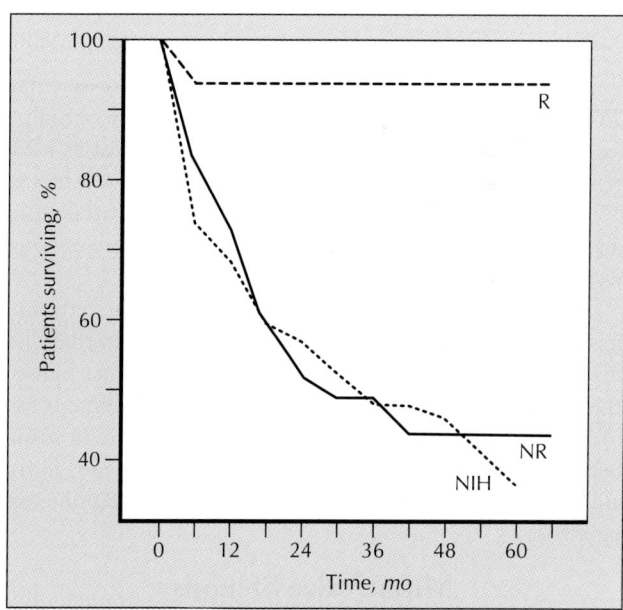

FIGURE 3 The 5-year survival rate of patients with primary pulmonary hypertension treated using high doses of calcium channel blockers (R) compared with the 5-year survival rate of patients followed-up over the same interval who were nonresponders (NR). The survival of patients who responded to high doses of calcium channel blockers was markedly improved. Survival data for historical controls (NIH) were provided by the National Institutes of Health Registry on Primary Pulmonary Hypertension. (*Adapted from* Rich and coworkers [2•]; with permission.)

ers at high doses can be extremely hazardous and should be done by physicians with established experience and expertise. Patients who fail to respond to calcium channel blockers should be given intravenous prostacyclin therapy although long-term experience is limited, it appears that most patients have improved quality of life and survival [3•]. Patients who continue to deteriorate in spite of medical management should be considered for lung transplantation [4]. The use of single- or bilateral lung transplantation is still controversial and may differ from center to center.

Obstructive Lung Disease

The development of pulmonary hypertension in patients with chronic obstructive pulmonary disease results in increased mortality. The only established, effective treatment of pulmonary hypertension in these patients has been chronic supplemental oxygen therapy [5]. Although it rarely reduces pulmonary artery pressure in the short term, oxygen retards progression of the pulmonary hypertension. Monitoring the response to oxygen therapy with arterial blood gases is important to check for carbon dioxide retention.

Vasodilators have been tested in patients with pulmonary hypertension from chronic obstructive pulmonary disease, but little documentation of their effectiveness exists. More importantly, however, vasodilators may worsen gas exchange, reduce arterial oxygen saturation, and cause pronounced systemic hypoxemia [6]. Vasodilators are not recommended, but if they are given to patients with lung disease, careful monitoring of the arterial blood gases before and after their administration is important.

Collagen Vascular Disease

Pulmonary hypertension complicating collagen vascular disease is becoming increasingly recognized and may be multifactorial. Virtually all of the collagen vascular diseases have been reported to be associated with pulmonary hypertension [7]. The mechanism may be associated interstitial lung disease, direct effects on the pulmonary vasculature causing vasoconstriction or thrombosis, or both.

Experience with using vasodilators for these patients has been unsatisfactory, which probably reflects that the disease process had been ongoing for a long time before the pulmonary hypertension was recognized. Although use of immunosuppressive therapy may be justifiable in some patients for treating their pulmonary hypertension, more studies need to be conducted before recommendations can be made.

Mitral Valve Stenosis

Pulmonary hypertension is a common complication of mitral valve stenosis because of the increased left atrial pressure transmitted backward into the pulmonary vascular bed. The severity of pulmonary hypertension in mitral stenosis varies and it results from vasoconstriction occurring in addition to the increased left atrial pressure. The definitive treatment for these patients has been mitral valve surgery. Although operative mortality increases among patients with severe pulmonary hypertension, no level of pulmonary artery pressure precludes mitral valve replacement or valvotomy, because pulmonary artery pressure usually regresses by at least 50% postoperatively [8]. More recent experience using balloon valvuloplasty for mitral stenosis has been quite similar—the level of pulmonary hypertension usually falls to a modest degree initially and continues to fall over time [9].

Congenital Heart Disease

Pulmonary hypertension secondary to congenital heart disease is well recognized in infants and children and is occasionally seen in adults. The fundamental principle in managing congenital heart disease with pulmonary hypertension is surgical correction before the pulmonary vascular disease becomes advanced. A patent intracardiac shunt associated with pulmonary hypertension usually results in right-to-left shunting with systemic hypoxemia. Patients with pulmonary hypertension and reversed shunting (Eisenmenger's syndrome) are considered inoperable.

The right-to-left shunt may protect the right ventricle against episodes of acute right ventricular failure, particularly during periods of stress, so the natural disease course of these patients is better than that of patients with primary pulmonary hypertension of similar severity [10]. The use of vasodilators with these patients can be quite hazardous, because they may lower systemic vascular resistance and worsen the right-to-left shunting. At present, heart–lung or lung transplantation is considered to be the best therapeutic option for patients with congenital heart disease and Eisenmenger's syndrome.

Left Ventricular Diastolic Dysfunction

Physicians accept pulmonary hypertension as a result of increased left atrial pressure from mitral stenosis. It is less well appreciated that similar levels of pulmonary hypertension can develop in patients with hypertensive or ischemic heart disease (or both) who have increased left ventricular end-diastolic pressure [11]. These patients are sometimes mistakenly thought to have both left ventricular disease and primary pulmonary hypertension. The correct diagnosis can be established by cardiac catheterization demonstrating high left ventricular end-diastolic filling pressures. The treatment of these patients (as for patients with other secondary forms of pulmonary hypertension) is focused on the underlying cause. Thus, patients with hypertensive heart disease should have their systemic blood pressures aggressively treated, because the pulmonary artery pressures would be expected to respond accordingly. Similarly patients with ischemic heart disease should have the left ventricular ischemia aggressively managed. Once these patients develop right ventricular failure, managing the left ventricular dysfunction becomes extraordinarily difficult.

General Treatment Measures

General treatment measures for patients with primary and secondary pulmonary hypertension are indicated in

TABLE 3 GENERAL TREATMENT MEASURES FOR PATIENTS WITH PULMONARY HYPERTENSION

Treatment	Comments
Daily activity	General activity advised, isometric and strenuous activity should be avoided
Supplemental oxygen	Continuous in hypoxic lung disease, supplemental in instances of profound hypoxemia (exercise/altitude)
Cardiac glycosides	Unproven, may be helpful in overt right ventricular failure
Diuretics	Relieve venous congestion and edema, may require large doses or multiple drugs
Anticoagulants	Improve survival in some patients, low doses effective

Table 3. Digitalis has never been evaluated prospectively for cor pulmonale, but it is beneficial for patients with left-side heart failure, and thus, may be useful if right-side heart failure is present. Diuretics will help to relieve venous congestion and reduce dyspnea. Oxygen is of unproven benefit for treating pulmonary hypertension without chronic obstructive pulmonary disease, but it may be useful for patients with severe hypoxia. Warfarin anticoagulation therapy improves survival in patients with primary pulmonary hypertension, especially those unresponsive to oral vasodilators [2•]. Low-dose anticoagulation therapy, to prolong the international normalized ratio to 2 to 3 times the control value, appears to be effective and is associated with a minimal risk of bleeding. Patients with liver dysfunction from venous congestion may be very sensitive to anticoagulants and need particularly close monitoring.

Because patients with pulmonary hypertension often have a limited cardiac output, they need to be advised regarding changes in their lifestyle. Isometric activities in particular should be avoided as they may induce syncope. On the other hand, patients with advanced pulmonary hypertension may lead productive lives as they learn to limit their stress, and these patients should be encouraged to be as active as possible.

WHEN TO REFER

Diagnosing and managing pulmonary hypertension is highly specialized and associated with increased risks. Specifically, commonly used tests such as lung scanning and echocardiography may show subtle abnormalities that are difficult to accurately interpret for patients with severe pulmonary hypertension. Other tests, such as exercise testing, pulmonary angiography, and right-side heart catheterization are associated with increased morbidity and mortality. Therefore, patients with the clinical features of pulmonary hypertension should be referred to specialists with expertise in this area for an accurate diagnosis.

Even more important, however, is the need for referring patients with a confirmed diagnosis of pulmonary hypertension to recognized experts for treatment. Although high doses of calcium channel blockers improve survival for some patients with primary pulmonary hypertension, many physicians are uncomfortable about initiating calcium blockers at high doses, and patients who may have been helped remain chronically, inappropriately treated. Similarly, surgical interventions requiring mitral valve replacement, repair of congenital heart disease, or thromboendarterectomy require particular expertise, because operative morbidity and mortality are clearly increased in patients with pulmonary hypertension. These patients must be referred to institutions with proven experience in these specialized areas.

As pulmonary hypertension is probably more common than we appreciate, the generalist retains a critical role in making the initial diagnosis, initiating the workup, and the ongoing management of patients on therapy. Many treatment measures are both new and complex, so frequent communication between the generalist and the specialist are important to maintain a high level of day-to-day care.

REFERENCES AND RECOMMENDED READING

Recently published papers of particular interest have been highlighted as:

• Of interest

1. Rich S, Dantzker DR, Ayres SM, *et al.*: Primary pulmonary hypertension: a national prospective study. *Ann Intern Med* 1987, 107:216–223.
2.• Rich S, Kaufmann E, Levy PS: The effect of high doses of calcium-channel blockers on survival in primary pulmonary hypertension. *N Engl J Med* 1992, 327:76–81.
3.• Barst RJ, Rubin LJ, McGoon MD, *et al.*: Survival in primary pulmonary hypertension with long-term continuous intravenous prostacyclin. *Ann Intern Med* 1994, 121:409–415.
4. Pasque MK, Trulock EP, Kaiser LD, Cooper JD: Single lung transplantation for pulmonary hypertension: three month hemodynamic follow-up. *Circulation* 1991, 84:2275–2279.
5. Timms RM, Khaja FU, Williams GW, *et al.*: Hemodynamic response to oxygen therapy in chronic obstructive pulmonary disease. *Ann Intern Med* 1985, 103:29–36.
6. Melot C, Hallemans R, Naeije R, *et al.*: Deleterious effect of nifedipine on pulmonary gas exchange in chronic obstructive pulmonary disease. *Am Rev Respir Dis* 1984, 130:612–616.

7. Kasukawa R, Nishimaki T, Takagi T, *et al.*: Pulmonary hypertension in connective tissue disease. Clinical analysis of sixty patients in multi-institutional study. *Clin Rheumatol* 1990, 9:56–62.

8. Zener JC, Hancock EW, Shumway NE, *et al.*: Regression of extreme pulmonary hypertension and mitral valve surgery. *Am J Cardiol* 1972, 30:820–826.

9. Ribeiro PA, Al Zaibag M, Abdullah M: Pulmonary artery pressure and pulmonary vascular resistance before and after mitral balloon valvotomy in 100 patients with severe mitral valve stenosis. *Am Heart J* 1993, 125:1110–1113.

10. Young D, Mark H: Fate of the patient with Eisenmenger's syndrome. *Am J Cardiol* 1971, 65:655–669.

11. Kessler KM, Willens HJ, Mallon SM: Diastolic left ventricular dysfunction leading to severe reversible pulmonary hypertension. *Am Heart J* 1993, 126:234–235.

SELECT BIBLIOGRAPHY

Christman BW, McPherson CD, Newman JH, *et al.*: An imbalance between the excretion of thromboxane and prostacyclin metabolites in pulmonary hypertension. *N Engl J Med* 1992, 327:70–75.

D'Alonzo GG, Barst RJ, Ayres SM, *et al.*: Survival in patients with primary pulmonary hypertension: results from a national prospective registry. *Ann Intern Med* 1991, 115:343–349.

Kaiser LR, Cooper JD: The current status of lung transplantation. *Adv Surg* 1992, 25:259–307.

Mette SA, Palevsky HI, Pietra GG, *et al.*: Primary pulmonary hypertension in association with human immunodeficiency virus infection. *Am Rev Resp Dis* 1992, 145:1196–1200.

Rubin LJ: ACCP Consensus Statement: primary pulmonary hypertension. *Chest* 1993, 104:236–250.

Pulmonary Embolism

Paul D. Stein
Russell D. Hull

Key Points

- It is critical to employ a method of prophylaxis against deep venous thrombosis that is effective for that particular condition in which deep venous thrombosis is likely to occur: low-dose heparin is effective in only some conditions.
- Anticoagulant therapy is the primary treatment for deep venous thrombosis and pulmonary embolism; for treatment, intravenous or subcutaneous heparin should be administered in doses sufficient to prolong the activated partial thromboplastin time to a range that corresponds to a level of 0.2 to 0.4 μ/mL. Heparin and warfarin therapy can be started together, and warfarin should be administered to achieve an international normalized ratio of 2.0 to 3.0 and continued for at least 3 months.
- The bedside evaluation of pulmonary embolism is meaningful and helps determine the extent to which diagnostic tests should be pursued; a sound bedside impression also contributes strongly to formulating a noninvasive diagnosis of pulmonary embolism.
- The diagnostic validity of ventilation-perfusion lung scanning is enhanced when this technique is combined with prior clinical assessment.
- Strategies of diagnosis developed based on diagnosing and treating deep venous thrombosis as an alternative to the diagnosis of pulmonary embolism spare many patients the necessity of pulmonary angiography.
- Transvenous inferior vena cava occlusion is indicated if there is a contraindication to anticoagulant use, a continuing predisposition to pulmonary embolism, or a recurrence of pulmonary embolism on full-dose anticoagulants.
- Thrombolytic therapy for pulmonary embolism is indicated if the patient is hypotensive or hypoxic on high levels of oxygen or has acutely induced right ventricular failure.

Pulmonary embolism (PE) is a complication of deep venous thrombosis (DVT). The most frequent predisposing factor for PE (and for deep venous thrombosis) is bed rest, usually following surgery (Table 1).

DEEP VENOUS THROMBOSIS

Diagnosis

Deep venous thrombosis of the thigh veins is more likely to cause PE than thrombosis of the veins of the calves. Techniques for diagnosing DVT include impedance plethysmography, B-mode ultrasonography, magnetic resonance imaging, venography, and radionuclide scanning. Radionuclide scanning is more sensitive for detecting venous thrombosis in the calves than venous thrombosis in the thighs. Therefore, in view of the greater danger of DVT of the thighs, the value of radionuclide scanning of the legs is limited. Impedance plethysmography is sensitive for the detection of DVT of the thighs [1,2], and B-mode ultrasonography using compression has a sensitivity equal to or higher than that of impedance plethysmography for the detec-

TABLE 1 PREDISPOSING FACTORS FOR ACUTE PULMONARY EMBOLISM	
Factor	Patients with positive angiographic findings, %*
Immobilization (≤3 mo)	54
Surgery (≤3 mo)	42
Coronary artery disease (ever)	20
Thrombophlebitis (ever)	19
Malignancy	18
Myocardial infarction	13
Trauma (lower extremities)	12
Congestive heart failure (right or left)	12
Chronic obstructive pulmonary disease	10
Stroke (ever)	10
Asthma	7
Pneumonia (acute)	7
History of pulmonary embolism	6
Collagen vascular disease	4
Postpartum (≤3 mo)	2
Interstitial lung disease	2
Sickle cell disease	1
Vasculitis	1
Self-administered drug use	1

Data from the National Collaborative Study of the Prospective Investigation of Pulmonary Embolism Diagnosis (PIOPED) [18].
*Patients may have more than 1 predisposing factor; n=383.

tion of DVT [3,4,5•]. Both methods are valid alternatives to contrast venography [5•]. Most centers employ B-mode ultrasonography. Venography, which is an invasive procedure, generally does not need to be performed in view of the excellent results shown with noninvasive techniques. Magnetic resonance imaging, although useful, is expensive [6•].

Prevention

Fatal PE resulting from untreated, clinically symptomatic DVT occurs more frequently (37%) than fatal PE in patients with asymptomatic, early DVT diagnosed by refined techniques (5%) [7,8]. Recommendations for the prevention of DVT, which are based on recommendations by the American College of Chest Physicians Consensus Conference on Antithrombotic Therapy, are outlined in Table 2 [9••]. Antithrombotic prevention of DVT differs from anticoagulant therapy in that the dose of heparin is lower. Intermittent pneumatic compression is beneficial in preventing DVT, but it is not adequate for therapy. Graded-pressure elastic stockings also may be beneficial, but aspirin is generally not [9••].

Treatment

Anticoagulant therapy for DVT, again based on recommendations by the American College of Chest Physicians Consensus Conference on Antithrombotic Therapy, is outlined in Table 3 [10••]. Heparin should be administered to increase the activated partial thromboplastin time to a range that corresponds to a blood heparin level of 0.2 to 0.4 μ/mL. This level should be maintained for 5 or 6 days after the initiation of therapy with warfarin. Warfarin should be administered to maintain the international normalized ratio at 2.0 to 3.0. The international normalized ratio can be calculated if the prothrombin time ratio and the sensitivity of the thromboplastin reagent used to obtain the prothrombin time ratio are known [11•]. Warfarin therapy should be continued for at least 3 months. Warfarin should be continued longer if a predisposition to DVT exists. It is helpful to obtain an impedance plethysmogram or B-mode ultrasound image of the legs at the time that anticoagulants are about to be discontinued: this is to be certain that no continuing DVT is present.

PULMONARY EMBOLISM

Clinical Diagnosis

Regarding the clinical diagnosis of PE, it is useful to consider PE in terms of the syndrome of presentation: the syndrome of pulmonary hemorrhage or infarction, of uncomplicated PE (ie, PE not complicated by pulmonary hemorrhage or infarction and not complicated by circulatory collapse), and of circulatory collapse or shock [12]. Most patients in whom PE is diagnosed have pleuritic pain or hemoptysis. Patients with PE and circulatory collapse usually die within 1 or 2 hours, and the diagnosis of PE in most is unsuspected.

Nonspecific abnormalities, as a group and in the proper setting, form a syndrome that is suggestive of PE. The symptoms and signs of acute PE in patients with no prior cardiopulmonary disease are listed in Table 4 [13•]. Among patients with no prior cardiopulmonary disease in whom a clinical diagnosis is made, the vast majority have either dyspnea, tachypnea, or pleuritic pain. Pleuritic pain is more common than hemoptysis among patients with no prior cardiopulmonary disease, and almost all have dyspnea, tachypnea, pleuritic pain, unexplained evidence of atelectasis, or a parenchymal abnormality on the chest radiograph [14]. Conversely, clinically detectable PE is rare in patients without one of these findings. Signs of pulmonary hypertension or right ventricular failure (eg, an accentuated pulmonary component of the second sound or a right ventricular lift) are uncommon. Qualitative signs of DVT, including erythema, palpable cord, tenderness, Homans' sign, or edema, occur in less than one third of patients with PE, but the addition of calf asymmetry of 1 cm or more to these signs increased the prevalence of a detectable abnormality of the lower extremities from 27% to 56% [15]. Nevertheless, DVT is the cause of PE in most patients [16••].

Sudden, unexplained shortness of breath in a patient who is a likely candidate for PE (a patient who has had recent surgery, is debilitated, or is immobilized) is a finding that leads to a diagnosis. Electrocardiographic findings are usually abnormal [13•,17••]. The typical electrocardiographic abnormalities are nonspecific ST-segment or T-wave changes (> 40% of patients) (Table 5) [13•,17••]. Right ventricular

Table 2. Recommendations for the Prevention of Deep Venous Thrombosis

Patients undergoing general surgery

General surgery patients who are undergoing minor operations, younger than 40 y of age, and have no clinical risk factors require no specific prophylaxis other than early ambulation

General surgery patients who are older than 40 y of age and undergoing major operations but who have no additional clinical risk factors for venous thromboembolism require low-dose heparin (5000 U SQ q 12 h) or intermittent pneumatic compression; combining graded-pressure elastic stockings with low-dose heparin may give better protection than either alone

General surgery patients who are older than 40 y of age, undergoing major operations, and have additional risk factors require heparin (5000 U SQ q 8 h) or low-molecular-weight heparin

General surgery patients (as profiled in the third recommendation) prone to bleeding or wound infection should be treated with intermittent pneumatic compression or dextran

General surgery patients with multiple risk factors should be treated with low-dose heparin or low-molecular-weight heparin or dextran combined with intermittent pneumatic compression

In selected high-risk general surgery patients, perioperative warfarin may be used at an INR of 2.0–3.0.

Aspirin is not recommended for prophylaxis in patients undergoing general surgery

Patients undergoing orthopedic surgery

In patients undergoing total hip replacement, warfarin (INR, 2.0–3.0), low-molecular-weight heparin, and subcutaneous heparin in doses adjusted to keep the activated partial thromboplastin time in the upper-normal range (31–36 s) 6 h after injection are the most effective prophylactic agents; in patients with a high risk for bleeding, intermittent pneumatic compression is recommended as an alternative

In patients with hip fractures, warfarin (INR, 2.0–3.0) or low-molecular-weight heparin is recommended

In patients undergoing knee surgery, either low-molecular-weight heparin or intermittent pneumatic compression is recommended

In selected high-risk orthopedic and multiple-trauma patients in whom other forms of prophylaxis would be contraindicated or ineffective, placement of a prophylactic inferior vena cava filter may be considered

In multiple-trauma patients, intermittent pneumatic compression, warfarin, and low-molecular-weight heparin are recommended when feasible

Patients who have neurologic disorders or have had neurosurgery

In patients undergoing intracranial neurosurgery, intermittent pneumatic compression with or without elastic stockings is recommended

In patients with acute spinal cord injury with paralysis, subcutaneous heparin in doses adjusted to keep the activated partial thromboplastin time in the upper-normal range (31–36 s) 6 h after injection or low-molecular-weight heparin is recommended for prophylaxis; warfarin also may be effective; low-dose heparin and intermittant pneumatic compression when used alone appear to be ineffective and are not recommended

In patients with ischemic stroke and lower extremity paralysis, low-dose heparin and low-molecular-weight heparin are effective; warfarin is probably effective. Intermittent pneumatic compression is an effective alternative in patients with hemorrhagic complications of stroke

Medical patients

In patients with clinical risk factor, low-dose heparin (5000 U q 8 h or q 12 h) or low-molecular-weight heparin are recommended

In patients with long-term indwelling central venous catheters, warfarin (1 mg/d) is recommended to prevent axillary-subclavian venous thrombosis

Adapted from Clagett and coworkers [9••]; with permission.
INR—international normalized ratio; q 8 h—every 8 hours; q 12 h—every 12 hours; SQ—subcutaneously.

Table 3. Recommendations for the Treatment of Deep Venous Thrombosis, Pulmonary Thromboembolism, or Both

Patients with deep venous thrombosis or pulmonary embolism should be treated with intravenous or subcutaneous heparin sufficient to prolong the activated partial thromboplastin time to a range that corresponds to a blood heparin level of 0.2 to 0.4 µ/mL

Heparin and warfarin therapy can be started together; heparin therapy should be discontinued on day 5 or 6 if the prothrombin time is therapeutic; for massive pulmonary embolism or ileofemoral thrombosis, a longer period of heparin therapy may be considered

Therapy should be continued for at least 3 mo using oral anticoagulants to prolong the prothrombin time to an international normalized ratio of 2.0–3.0; heparin to prolong the activated partial thromboplastin time to a range that corresponds to a blood heparin level of 0.2 to 0.4 µ/mL may be used when oral anticoagulants are either contraindicated (*eg*, pregnancy) or inconvenient

Patients with multiple episodes of recurrent venous thrombosis or a continuing risk factor should be treated indefinitely

Symptomatic isolated calf vein thrombosis should be treated with anticoagulation for 3 mo; if for any reason anticoagulation cannot be given, serial noninvasive studies of the lower extremity should be performed to assess for proximal extension of thrombus

Adapted from Hyers and coworkers [10••]; with permission.

hypertrophy, right bundle-branch block, right-axis deviation, P pulmonale, and an $S_1Q_2T_3$ pattern are uncommon [13•,17••]; in fact, new left-axis deviation occurs more often than right-axis deviation. Rhythm disturbances are uncommon [13•,17••].

Chest radiographic findings are also nonspecific. They frequently show unexplained parenchymal abnormalities, small pleural effusions, or elevation of a hemidiaphragm (Table 6) [13•]. Vascular signs on chest radiography (decreased pulmonary vascularity, a prominent central pulmonary artery, or both) are uncommon or difficult to recognize.

Ventilation-Perfusion Lung Scan

Pulmonary embolism is present in 87% of patients whose ventilation-perfusion lung scan findings show a high probabil-

TABLE 4 SYMPTOMS AND SIGNS OF ACUTE PULMONARY EMBOLISM IN PATIENTS WITH NO PREEXISTING CARDIAC OR PULMONARY DISEASE

Symptoms or signs	Patients with symptom or sign, %*
Dyspnea	73
Pleuritic pain	66
Cough	37
Leg swelling	28
Leg pain	26
Hemoptysis	13
Palpitations	10
Wheezing	9
Anginalike pain	4
Tachypnea (≥20/min)	70
Rales (crackles)	51
Tachycardia (>100/min)	30
Fourth heart sound	24
Increased pulmonary component of second sound	23
Deep venous thrombosis	11
Diaphoresis	11
Temperature >38.5°C	7
Wheezes	5
Homans' sign	4
Right ventricular lift	4
Pleural friction rub	3
Third heart sound	3
Cyanosis	1

Adapted from Stein and coworkers [13•]; with permission.
*n=117.

TABLE 5 ELECTROCARDIOGRAPHIC MANIFESTATIONS IN PATIENTS WITH PULMONARY EMBOLISM AND NO PRIOR CARDIAC OR PULMONARY DISEASE

Electrocardiographic finding	Patients with finding, %*
Normal electrocardiographic findings	30
Rhythm disturbances	
Atrial flutter	1
Atrial fibrillation	4
Atrial premature contractions	4
Ventricular premature contractions	4
P wave	
P pulmonale	2
QRS abnormalities	
Right-axis deviation	2
Left-axis deviation	13
Incomplete right bundle-branch block	4
Complete right bundle-branch block	6
Right ventricular hypertrophy	2
Pseudoinfarction	3
Low voltage (frontal plane)	3
ST segment and T wave	
Nonspecific ST-segment or T-wave abnormalities	49

Data from Stein and coworkers [13•]; with permission.
*Some patients had more than one abnormality; n=89.

TABLE 6 CHEST RADIOGRAPHIC FINDINGS IN PULMONARY EMBOLISM IN PATIENTS WITH NO PREVIOUS CARDIAC OR PULMONARY DISEASE

Chest radiographic finding	Patients with finding, %†
Atelectasis or pulmonary parenchymal abnormality	68
Pleural effusion	48
Pleural-based opacity	35
Elevated diaphragm	24
Decreased pulmonary vascularity	21
Prominent central pulmonary artery	15
Cardiomegaly	12
Westermark's sign*	7

Adapted from Stein and coworkers [13•]; with permission.
*Prominent central pulmonary artery and decreased pulmonary vascularity.
†n=117.

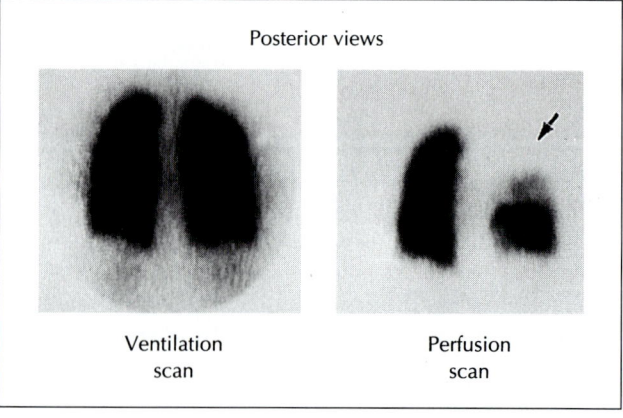

FIGURE 1 Posterior views of ventilation lung scan (*left*) and perfusion lung scan (*right*) showing normal ventilation with absent perfusion in the right upper lobe (*arrow*).

Table 7. Probability of Pulmonary Embolism Using Clinical Assessment in Combination with Ventilation-Perfusion Lung Scans

	Ratio of PE-positive patients to total patients, n/n (%)*			
Scan category	CP of 80%–100%	CP of 20%–79%	CP of 0%–19%	All probabilities
High probability	28/29 (96)	70/80 (88)	5/9 (56)	103/118 (87)
Intermediate probability	27/41 (66)	66/236 (28)	11/68 (16)	104/345 (30)
Low probability	6/15 (40)	30/191 (16)	4/90 (4)	40/296 (14)
Near-normal to normal	0/5 (0)	4/62 (6)	1/61 (2)	5/128 (4)
Total	61/90 (68)	170/569 (30)	21/228 (9)	252/887 (28)

From A Collaborative Study by the PIOPED Investigators [18••]; with permission.

*PE positive indicates an angiographic reading that shows PE or the determination of PE by the outcome classification committee on review. PE status is based on angiographic interpretation for 713 patients, on angiographic interpretation and outcome classification committee reassignment for 4 patients, and on clinical information alone (without definitive angiography) for 170 patients.
CP—clinical probability; PE—pulmonary embolism.

ity of PE [18••]. If lung scan findings are normal, PE is excluded (Fig. 1). If the probability is intermediate, there is no information, with PE being present in approximately 30% of patients. If the probability is low, PE is present in 14%. Therefore, a low-probability ventilation-perfusion lung scan does not exclude PE [18••].

Prior clinical assessment combined with interpretation of the ventilation-perfusion lung scan improves diagnostic validity (Table 7) [18••]. Similarly, if the ventilation-perfusion scan findings indicate a low probability of PE and the clinical suspicion is concordantly low, PE can be excluded in 96% of patients [18••]. The probability of PE with various ventilation-perfusion lung scan probabilities combined with various concordant and discordant clinical suspicions is shown in Table 7.

The probability of PE can be determined based on the number of mismatched perfusion defects [19•,20•]. A further refinement of probability can be made if the ventilation-perfusion lung scan is interpreted after patients are stratified according to prior cardiopulmonary disease (Fig. 2) [19•]. Fewer mismatched perfusion defects are required to diagnose PE in patients with no prior cardiopulmonary disease. Adding clinical assessment to the stratification results in a more accurate evaluation (Fig. 3 and 4) [21•].

Pulmonary Angiography

Pulmonary angiography (Fig. 5) is associated with serious complications in approximately 1% of patients [22•]. When needed, pulmonary angiography is useful, and it remains the diagnostic "gold standard" for PE. Patients in whom the risk

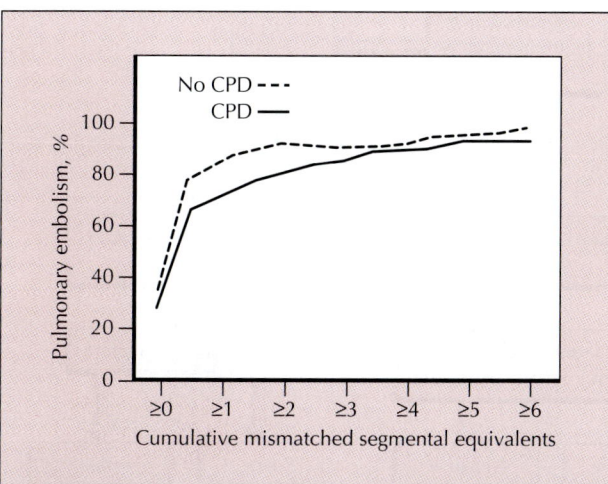

Figure 2 Predictive value of pulmonary embolism relative to the cumulative number of mismatched segmental equivalent perfusion defects among patients with no prior cardiopulmonary disease (CPD) and those with prior CPD. Significant differences occurred with 0.5 or more and 1.0 or more segmental equivalents ($P < 0.01$) and with 1.5 or more segmental equivalents ($P < 0.05$). (*From* Stein and coworkers [19•]; with permission.)

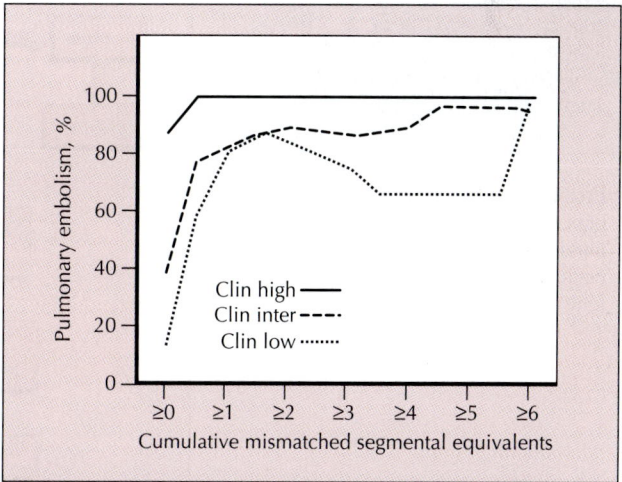

Figure 3 Predictive value of pulmonary embolism relative to the cumulative number of mismatched segmental equivalent perfusion defects among patients with no prior cardiopulmonary disease. Patients were categorized as having high-probability (Clin high), intermediate-probability (Clin inter), or low-probability clinical assessment (Clin low). The variability of the low-probability curve is because of the small numbers of patients in that group. (*From* Stein and coworkers [21•]; with permission.)

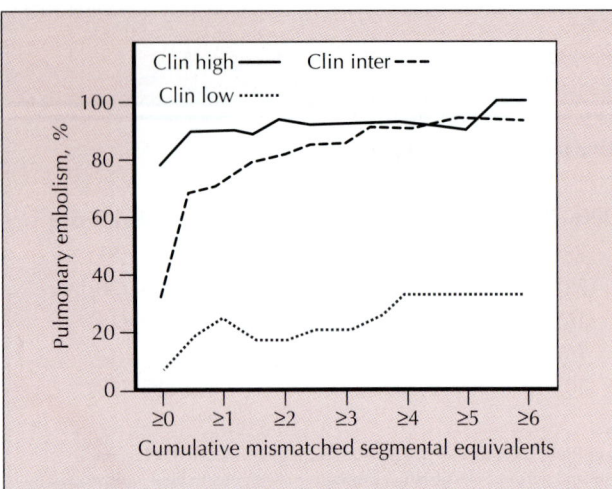

FIGURE 4 Predictive value of pulmonary embolism relative to the cumulative number of mismatched segmental equivalent perfusion defects among patients with prior cardiopulmonary disease. Patients were categorized as having high-probability (Clin high), intermediate-probability (Clin inter), or low-probability clinical assessment (Clin low). (*From* Stein and coworkers [21•]; with permission.)

of complications from PE are greatest are those referred for angiography from the medical intensive care unit. Frequently, such patients are receiving respiratory support and are in an unstable condition. The presence or absence of PE and the magnitude of pulmonary hypertension does not relate to the frequency of morbidity from angiography [22•]. Elderly patients (*ie*, 70 years of age or older) are at greater risk for renal impairment from the injection of contrast material than younger patients [23].

Residual Impairment

A residual abnormality of perfusion 1 year after acute PE is more frequent in patients with prior cardiopulmonary disease than in those with no prior cardiopulmonary disease [24]. A posttherapy baseline ventilation-perfusion lung scan is useful in the event of suspected recurrent PE. This baseline lung scan will assist in determining if abnormalities on a later ventilation-perfusion lung scan are new or residuals of prior PE.

Strategy for Diagnosis

Strategies have been developed to reduce the number of pulmonary angiograms that may be required [16••, 25•, 26••]. If

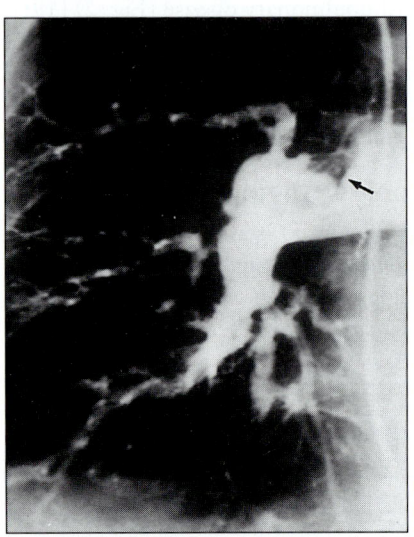

FIGURE 5 Pulmonary arteriogram of right pulmonary artery showing multiple intraluminal filling defects, one of which occludes the artery to the right upper lobe (*arrow*).

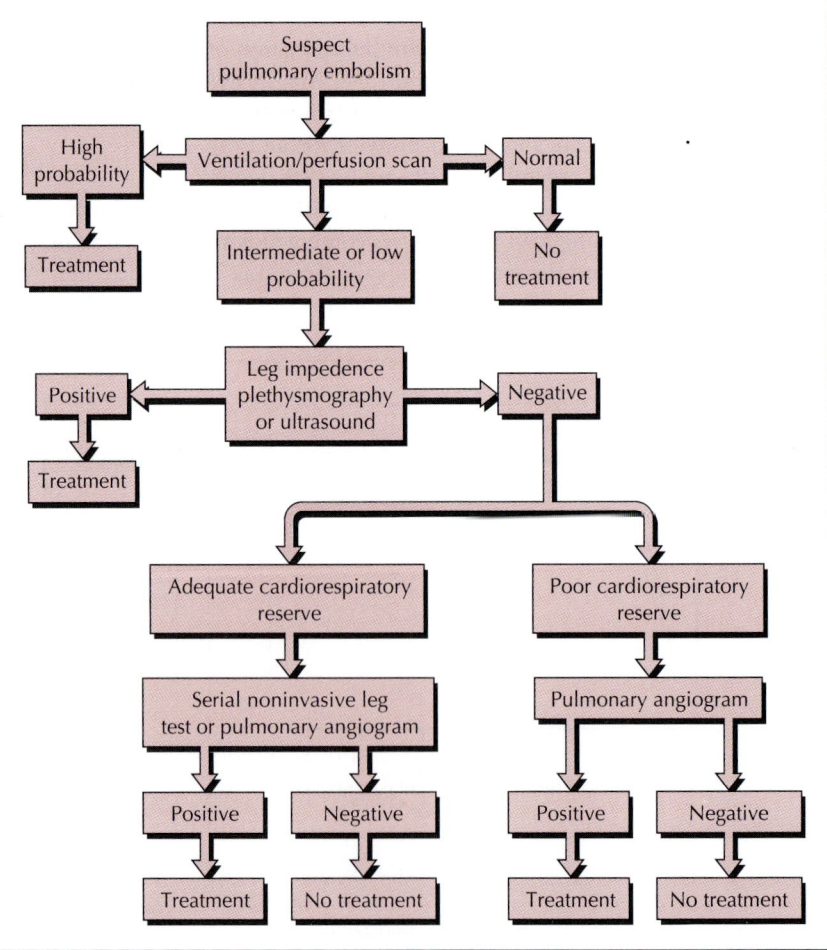

FIGURE 6 Strategy for the diagnosis and treatment of patients with suspected acute pulmonary embolism based on use of a ventilation-perfusion scan as the first diagnostic test. (*From* Stein and coworkers [26••]; with permission.)

the patient has a high-probability ventilation-perfusion scan, particularly in association with a high clinical suspicion, treatment with anticoagulants generally is indicated (Fig. 6). In patients with a high-probability ventilation-perfusion scan and an uncertain or low clinical suspicion, studies of the leg veins may assist the clinician in reaching a decision about therapy. If ventilation-perfusion lung scan findings are normal, treatment is not indicated. If lung scan findings show an intermediate or low probability of PE, a noninvasive evaluation of the proximal veins of the legs for DVT is useful. If the results of such tests for DVT are positive, then treatment is indicated; if the leg study findings are negative, the clinician should obtain either a pulmonary angiogram to clarify the diagnosis, or if cardiorespiratory reserve is adequate, follow the patient with serial studies of the legs (using impedance plethysmographic or B-mode Doppler studies) [26••]. The latter strategy is safe, and the risk of PE is low among patients in whom serial investigations of the legs show no DVT [27,•,28,29]. It may be more economical or convenient to obtain studies of the legs before ventilation-perfusion scanning. Lung scans are recommended, however, if there is a suspicion of PE, regardless of the results of leg studies.

Approximately 50% of patients with PE have negative results on noninvasive tests for DVT, even though DVT is the source of the PE [2]. This finding may reflect the possibility that the thrombi may embolize entirely, leaving no residual evidence in the deep veins. Preliminary data suggest that a D-dimer level of less than 500 µg/L would tend to exclude PE [30•]. An elevation in the D-dimers level to 500 µg/L or higher, however, provides no diagnostic information and may occur under various conditions other than PE.

Treatment

Antithrombotic therapy for PE is the same as antithrombotic therapy for DVT (Table 3). Inferior vena cava occlusion is indicated if there is a contraindication to anticoagulant use, a continuing predisposition to PE, or a recurrence of PE on full-dose anticoagulants.

Thrombolytic therapy is indicated if the patient is hypotensive or hypoxic on 100% oxygen or has echocardiographic evidence of right ventricular dysfunction [31]. Thrombolytic therapy is not indicated for the routine treatment of PE. Factors that increase the risk of thrombolytic therapy are listed in Table 8 [32]. It is generally recommended that pulmonary angiograms be obtained in patients with suspected PE who may be candidates for thrombolytic therapy. Pulmonary angiography, however, markedly increases the risk of major bleeding with thrombolytic therapy. Therefore, thrombolytic therapy perhaps may be administered to unstable patients on the basis of a strong clinical impression and a high-probability ventilation-perfusion lung scan [33].

TABLE 8 FACTORS THAT INCREASE THE RISK OF THROMBOLYTIC THERAPY FOR ACUTE PULMONARY EMBOLISM

Pregnancy at any stage and the first 10 d postpartum

Uncontrolled hypertension, *ie*, diastolic blood pressure >110 mm Hg by several measurements or hypertensive retinopathy with hemorrhages or exudates

Bleeding diathesis

History of major gastrointestinal bleeding within 6 mo or symptoms of active gastrointestinal diseases that have a propensity to bleed

Renal insufficiency (creatine level, >3.0 mg/dL)

Severe hepatic insufficiency

Evidence of a lesion associated with intracranial hemorrhage, including cerebral malignancy, aneurysm, abscess, or head trauma

History of cerebrovascular disease

Neurosurgery within 6 mo

Severe trauma within 2 mo

Any surgical or invasive procedure, including biopsies, deep tissue aspirations, depot injections, unsuccessful attempts at central line placement, and removal of successfully placed central lines (*eg*, subclavian or internal jugular) within 10 d of study entry. Previous arterial punctures of the femoral or brachial arteries are relative contraindications

Placement of a central venous line within 48 h

Ophthalmologic surgery within 6 wk

Cardiopulmonary resuscitation (≥ 1 min of external cardiac massage) within 2 wk of study entry

Adapted from A Collaborative Study by the PIOPED Investigators [32]; with permission.

REFERENCES AND RECOMMENDED READING

Recently published papers of particular interest have been highlighted as:
- Of interest
- •• Of outstanding interest

1. Moser KM, LeMoine JR: Is embolic risk conditioned by location of deep venous thrombosis? *Ann Intern Med* 1981, 94:439–444.
2. Hull RD, Hirsh J, Carter CJ, *et al.*: Pulmonary angiography, ventilation lung scanning, and venography for clinically suspected pulmonary embolism with abnormal perfusion lung scan. *Ann Intern Med* 1983, 98:891–899.
3. White RH, McGahan JP, Daschbach MM: Diagnosis of deep-vein thrombosis using duplex ultrasound. *Ann Intern Med* 1989, 111:297–304.
4. Becker DM, Philbrick JT, Abbitt PL: Real time ultrasonography for the diagnosis of lower extremity deep venous thrombosis. *Arch Intern Med* 1989, 149:1731–1734.
5.• Heijboer H, Cogo A, Buller HR, *et al.*: Detection of deep vein thrombosis with impedance plethysmography and real-time compression ultrasonography in hospitalized patients. *Arch Intern Med* 1992, 152:1901–1903.
6.• Spritzer CE, Norconk JJ, Sostman HD, Coleman RE: Detection of deep venous thrombosis by magnetic resonance imaging. *Chest* 1993, 104:54–60.
7. Byrne JJ: Phlebitis: a study of 748 cases at the Boston City Hospital. *N Engl J Med* 1955, 253:579–586.
8. Collins R, Scrimgeour A, Yusuf S, Peto R: Reduction in fatal pulmonary embolism and venous thrombosis by perioperative administration of subcutaneous heparin. *N Engl J Med* 1988, 318:1162–1173.
9.•• Clagett GP, Anderson FA Jr, Heit J, *et al.*: Prevention of venous thromboembolism. *Chest* 1995, 108(suppl):312S–334S.

10.•• Hyers TM, Hull RD, Weg JG: Antithrombotic therapy for venous thromboembolic disease. *Chest* 1995, 108(suppl):335S–351S.

11.• Hirsh J, Dalen JE, Deykin D, Poller L: Oral anticoagulants: mechanism of action, clinical effectiveness, and optimal therapeutic range. *Chest* 1992, 102(suppl):312S–326S.

12. Stein PD, Willis PW III, DeMets DL: History and physical examination in acute pulmonary embolism in patients without preexisting cardiac or pulmonary disease. *Am J Cardiol* 1981, 47:218–223.

13.• Stein PD, Terrin ML, Hales CA, *et al*.: Clinical, laboratory, roentgenographic and electrocardiographic findings in patients with acute pulmonary embolism and no pre-existing cardiac or pulmonary disease. *Chest* 1991, 100:598–603.

14. Stein PD, Saltzman HA, Weg JG: Clinical characteristics of patients with acute pulmonary embolism. *Am J Cardiol* 1991, 68:1723–1724.

15. Stein PD, Henry JW, Godalakrishman D, Relyea B: Asymmetry of the calves in the assessment of patients with suspected acute pulmonary embolism. *Chest* 1995; 107:936–939.

16.•• Stein PD, Hull RD, Saltzman HA, Pineo G: Strategy for diagnosis of patients with suspected acute pulmonary embolism. *Chest* 1993, 103:1553–1559.

17.•• Stein PD: Acute pulmonary embolism. *Dis Month* 1994; 40:465–524.

18.•• A Collaborative Study by the PIOPED Investigators: Value of the ventilation/perfusion scan in acute pulmonary embolism: results of the prospective investigation of pulmonary embolism diagnosis (PIOPED). *JAMA* 1990, 263:2753–2759.

19.• Stein PD, Gottschalk A, Henry JW, Shivkumar K: Stratification of patients according to prior cardiopulmonary disease and probability assessment based upon the number of mismatched segmented equivalent perfusion defects: approaches to strengthen the diagnostic value of ventilation/perfusion lung scans in acute pulmonary embolism. *Chest* 1993, 104:1461–1467.

20. Stein PD, Henry JW, Gottschalk A: Mismatched vascular defects: an easy alternative to mismatched segmental equivalent defects for the interpretation of ventilation/perfusion lung scans in pulmonary embolism. *Chest* 1993, 104:1468–1472.

21.• Stein PD, Henry JW, Gottschalk A: The addition of clinical assessment to stratification according to prior cardiopulmonary disease further optimizes the interpretation of ventilation/perfusion lung scans in pulmonary embolism. *Chest* 1993, 104:1472–1476.

22.• Stein PD, Athanasoulis C, Alavi A, *et al*.: Complications and validity of pulmonary angiography in acute pulmonary embolism. *Circulation* 1992, 85:462–469.

23. Stein PD, Gottschalk A, Saltzman HA, Terrin ML: Diagnosis of acute pulmonary embolism in the elderly. *J Am Coll Cardiol* 1991, 18:1452–1457.

24. Urokinase Pulmonary Embolism Trial: Chapter VIII. Perfusion lung scanning. *Circulation* 1973, 47(suppl):II-46–II–50.

25.• Dalen JE: When can treatment be withheld in patients with suspected pulmonary embolism? *Arch Intern Med* 1993, 153:1415–1418.

26.•• Stein PD, Hull RD, Pineo G: Strategy that includes serial noninvasive leg tests for diagnosis of thromboembolic disease in patients with suspected acute pulmonary embolism based on data from PIOPED. Arch Intern Med 1995 (In press).

27.• Hull RD, Raskob GE, Carter CJ: Serial impedance plethysmography in pregnant patients with clinically suspected deep-vein thrombosis. *Ann Intern Med* 1990, 112:663–667.

28. Huisman MV, Buller HR, Ten Cate JW, Vreeken J: Serial impedance plethysmography for suspected deep venous thrombosis in outpatients. *N Engl J Med* 1986, 314:823–828.

29. Hull RD, Raskob GE, Ginsberg JS, *et al*.: A noninvasive strategy for the treatment of patients with suspected pulmonary embolism. *Arch Intern Med* 1994, 154:289—297.

30.• Bounameaux H, Cirafici P, DeMoerloose P, *et al*.: Measurement of D-dimer in plasma as a diagnostic aid in suspected pulmonary embolism. *Lancet* 1991, 337:196–200.

31. Goldhaber SZ, Haire WD, Feldstein ML, *et al*.: Alteplase versus heparin in acute pulmonary embolism: randomized trial assessing right-ventricular function and pulmonary perfusion. *Lancet* 1993, 341:507–511.

32. A Collaborative Study by the PIOPED Investigators: Tissue plasminogen activator for the treatment of acute pulmonary embolism. *Chest* 1990, 97:528–533.

33. Stein PD, Hull RD, Raskob G: Risks for major bleeding from thrombolytic therapy: consideration of noninvasive management. *Ann Intern Med* 1994; 12:313–317.

Cardiac Tumors 26

Elizabeth O. Ofili
Navin C. Nanda

> ### Key Points
> - Although most primary cardiac tumors are histologically "benign," clinical manifestations can be devastating and include cerebrovascular and peripheral emboli, cardiac arrhythmias, valvular obstruction, pericardial constriction or tamponade, and death.
> - A high index of suspicion is necessary for early diagnosis. Echocardiography usually provides rapid and accurate diagnosis; chest radiography tends to be nonspecific.
> - Surgical excision is curative in most cases, although some myxomas may recur. Periodic postoperative clinical and echocardiographic surveillance is important.
> - Metastatic tumors are uniformly fatal; surgery is largely palliative.

Cardiac tumors can be primary or metastatic and can involve the heart or pericardium. Advances in diagnostic imaging now allow accurate diagnosis in most patients. Clinical manifestations and hemodynamic features of cardiac tumors can mimic virtually all other forms of heart disease. Thus, a high index of suspicion is necessary for making an accurate diagnosis.

PRIMARY CARDIAC TUMORS

Primary tumors of the heart and pericardium are rare, with an incidence of 0.002% to 0.250% in autopsy series [1,2]. Figure 1 shows the relative incidence of primary tumors of the heart. Although 75% of primary cardiac tumors are histologically benign, clinical manifestations can be quite devastating, with complications such as death caused by arrhythmia, pericardial constriction or tamponade, valvular obstruction, and cerebral arterial embolism [2].

Benign Tumors

Myxomas are the most common cardiac tumors, accounting for 30% to 50% of benign cardiac tumors in most series [3]. Over 90% of myxomas occur sporadically. Women are more commonly affected, with a typical age range of 30 to 60 years; however, patients as young as 3 years and as old as 80 years have also been reported [3]. Most myxomas are solitary tumors and are often pedunculated and attached to the limbus of the fossa ovalis of the left atrium by a short stalk. Myxomas are noted for their protean clinical manifestations. Constitutional signs and symptoms, obstructive manifestations, and embolic phenomena are the classic triad of myxoma presentation [4,5]. Presenting symptoms may include syncope, episodic dizziness, episodic dyspnea, and weight loss (Table 1). Symptoms may vary with positional change. Syncope is particularly ominous and not infrequently associated with sudden death. Multiple systemic emboli may mimic systemic vasculitis or infective endocarditis, particularly when associated with fever, weight loss, and arthralgias. The neurologic consequences of embolization include transient ischemic attacks, seizures, syncope, and cerebral infarction.

Atrial myxomas may mimic mitral or tricuspid valve disease on physical examination (Table 2). The sudden movement of tumor from atrium to the ventricle has been associated with an early diastolic sound or "tumor plop." This high-frequency diastolic sound, in addition to a diastolic murmur and (in some cases) a systolic murmur of a valvular regurgitation, has been described. Left atrial myxomas frequently mimic mitral stenosis. Right atrial myxomas may present with recurrent pulmonary emboli and right heart failure. Right atrial myxomas have been reported to mimic the carcinoid syndrome, constrictive pericarditis, tricuspid stenosis, or Ebstein's anomaly.

Familial myxomas make up 7% of all myxomas and are transmitted by an autosomal dominant trait. Compared with patients with sporadic myxomas, patients presenting with familial myxomas are usually younger (mean age in the twenties), more likely to have multiple myxomas involving chambers other than the left atrium, and more likely to have a recurrence of myxomas postoperatively [6,7]. Because cardiac myxomas may be familial, routine echocardiographic screening of first-degree relatives is appropriate, particularly in young patients who have multiple or right-sided tumors [8]. Clinical manifestations of other benign cardiac tumors are listed in Table 3.

Malignant Tumors

Malignant cardiac tumors account for 25% of all primary heart tumors. They include mesotheliomas, which typically involve the pericardium. Sarcomas involve the myocardium, and malignant vascular tumors can affect both the pericardium and the myocardium (Table 4).

METASTATIC OR SECONDARY CARDIAC TUMORS

Metastatic tumors of the heart are 25 times more common than primary cardiac tumors. All major types of tumors can metastasize to the heart, with an average frequency of 10% in autopsy series. The highest percentage of metastases to the heart occur with melanoma (64%), leukemia (43%), and malignant lymphoma (35%) [9]. Lung and breast cancers predominate as the major sites of origin for cardiac metastases because of their high prevalence and contiguous anatomic location. Pericardial metastases are most frequent, and endocardial metastases occur rarely. Discrete nodules or diffuse infiltration may occur as a result of pericardial metastases. Fibrinous pericarditis and pericardial effusion usually are present. The effusion may not be bloody. Pericardial metastases may be diffuse or present as discrete nodules.

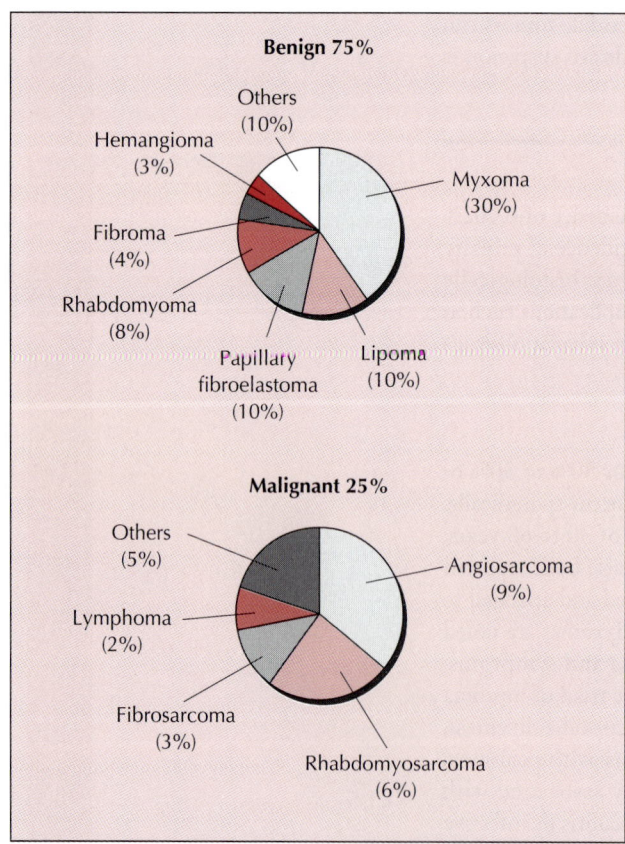

FIGURE 1 Relative incidence of primary cardiac tumors.

TABLE 1 CARDIAC MYXOMAS*

Clinical manifestations	
Symptoms	Incidence, %
Dyspnea on exertion	>75
Fever	50
Weight loss	50
Dizziness or syncope	20
Sudden death	15
Hemoptysis	15

Clinical presentation of cardiac myxoma in 130 patients	Patients, n
Signs and symptoms of mitral valve disease	57
Embolic phenomena	36
Incidental finding	16
Signs and symptoms of tricuspid valve disease	6
Sudden death	5
Pericarditis	4
Myocardial infarction	3
Signs and symptoms of pulmonary valve disease	2
Fever of unknown origin	2

Location of cardiac myxomas	
Site	Incidence, %
Left atrium	75.0
Right atrium	20.0
Left ventricle	2.5
Right ventricle	2.5
Multiple myxomas	<5.0

From McAllister and Fenoglio [20], Meller and coworkers [21], and Vidaillet and coworkers [22]; with permission.

Leukemic involvement typically causes effusion because of infiltration of the interstitium by leukemic cells. Mural thrombi and embolization secondary to metastatic cardiac tumors are quite rare. Metastatic cardiac tumors do not interfere with cardiac function until myocardial involvement is extensive. Cardiac metastases are almost always associated with widespread metastatic involvement in other organs.

The vast majority of patients with cardiac involvement because of metastatic tumor have few or no cardiac symptoms (Table 5) [1]. Despite autopsy evidence of cardiac metastases

Table 2 Conditions mimicked by atrial myxomas

Left atrium
Rheumatic mitral valve disease (stenosis, insufficiency)
Pulmonary hypertension
Cerebral emboli
Endocarditis
Myocarditis
Vasculitis

Right atrium
Rheumatic tricuspid valve disease (stenosis, insufficiency)
Pulmonary hypertension
Pulmonary emboli
Constrictive pericarditis
Ebstein's anomaly
Carcinoid heart disease

Table 3 Common manifestations of other benign cardiac tumors

Tumor	Manifestations
Rhabdomyoma	Most common childhood benign primary tumor; associated with systemic tuberous sclerosis; ventricular tachyarrhythmia
Fibroma	Second most common childhood tumor; may cause left ventricular outflow obstruction
Lipomas	Left ventricle, right atrium, and atrial septum affected in that order; rarely cause problems (valvular obstruction and conduction abnormalities)
Lipomatous hypertrophy	Adipose tissue accumulation in atrial septum; not true neoplasm; most common in the obese, elderly, and women; usually not pathologic
Papillary fibroelastoma	Affects heart valves; may embolize rarely or cause valvular dysfunction
Hemangioma and lymphangioma	Rare vascular tumors; may cause heart block and sudden death
Bronchogenic cysts, pericardial cysts, teratomas, and dermoid cysts	Most common benign pericardial tumor; usually in young children; can compress great vessels and rupture into pericardium

Table 4 Common manifestations of malignant primary cardiac tumors

Tumor	Manifestations
Sarcomas	Affect young adults; right side of heart common; rapid downhill course; death within 2 years of symptoms; local infiltration and metastases to lungs, lymph nodes, sternum and vertebral column; cardiac tamponade, right heart failure, and vena caval obstruction may occur
Angiosarcomas	Including Kaposi's sarcoma and malignant hemangioendotheliomas; 2:1 male:female ratio; usually from right atrium, attached to septum; course and clinical manifestations as for other sarcomas, including rapid downhill course
Pericardial mesothelioma	Usually affects in third to fifth decade; more in men; no association with asbestos exposure; symptomatic late in course; survival less than 1 year after diagnosis

Table 5 Clinical manifestations of cardiac metastatic tumors

Manifestation	Description
Pericardial effusion and tamponade	Most common manifestations of metastatic disease (less common but may occur with benign tumors); cytologic examination of fluid or pericardial biopsy may be diagnostic; effusive constrictive pericarditis can occur if prior irradiation
Heart failure	May be dilated or restrictive right, left, or biventricular failure; leukemic infiltration and irradiation can cause restrictive cardiomyopathy; doxorubicin cardiomyopathy is dose related (> 400–500 mg/m^2); sudden onset; resistant to conventional treatment
Myocardial ischemia and infarction	May be from large transmural tumor nodules or, rarely, tumor embolization; usually widespread metastases and poor prognosis; death within several weeks
Embolization	Most common with benign atrial myxomas but can be seen with metastatic tumors
Conduction defects and arrhythmias	Heart block is common in mesothelioma of the atrioventricular node; arrhythmias are common with metastatic myocardial disease

TABLE 6 RADIOLOGIC FINDINGS IN CARDIAC TUMORS
Cardiac enlargement (chamber enlargement; pericardial effusion)
Mediastinal widening (hilar-mediastinal adenopathy)
Calcification (rhabdomyoma, fibroma, teratoma, myxoma)

TABLE 7 DIAGNOSTIC WORK-UP OF CARDIAC TUMORS
History and physical examination (may be nonspecific)
Chest radiography
Transthoracic two-dimensional or Doppler echocardiography (left ventricular tumors, left atrial, and right atrial myxomas)
Transesophageal echocardiography (if suboptimal, inconclusive, or nondiagnostic transthoracic echocardiogram)
Computed tomography and magnetic resonance imaging (extent of myocardial invasion; pericardial or extracardiac extension)
Coronary angiography (for coronary anatomy)
Surgical exclusion or biopsy
Periodic two-dimensional echocardiogram for follow-up after surgery

in 10% to 20% of patients with widespread metastatic disease, antemortem symptoms or physical findings of cardiac involvement only occur in approximately 8% of the cases [10]. This may be because cardiac abnormalities are often overlooked by clinicians in the presence of widespread neoplastic disease.

DIAGNOSTIC TECHNIQUES

Noninvasive diagnostic cardiac evaluation is increasingly used to confirm a suspected intracardiac tumor. As a result, it is not unusual for cardiac tumors to be diagnosed and cured in patients who are totally asymptomatic or without signs of cardiovascular disease. Chest radiography tends to be nonspecific but may provide important diagnostic clues (Table 6). Careful use of noninvasive modalities such as two-dimensional echocardiography, transesophageal echocardiography, and in some instances, magnetic resonance imaging help in the preoperative localization and assessment of tumor extent; invasive procedures such as cardiac catheterization are therefore unnecessary. Table 7 summarizes a diagnostic and surveillance algorithm for evaluation of cardiac tumors. Patients presenting with clinical manifestations of cardiogenic emboli should be referred for echocardiography. A high index of suspicion is necessary for early diagnosis, particularly in patients with nonspecific symptoms such as dyspnea, atypical chest pain, or palpitations.

Echocardiography

Two-dimensional echocardiography, when carefully performed, provides adequate information regarding the presence or absence of an intracardiac tumor as well as its size, attachment, and mobility to allow for operative resection without preoperative angiography (Figs. 2 and 3). This technique is sensitive for detecting small tumors and is especially useful in the diagnosis of atrial and ventricular tumors. Furthermore, color Doppler flow studies allow for the assessment of the hemodynamic consequences of valvular obstruction or insufficiency caused by cardiac tumors [11].

Transesophageal Echocardiography

Transesophageal echocardiography provides an unimpeded view of both atria and interatrial septum. It allows a more accurate evaluation of the attachment of atrial myxomas and differentiation of atrial thrombi from cardiac tumors [12••]. Transesophageal echocardiography is complementary to the

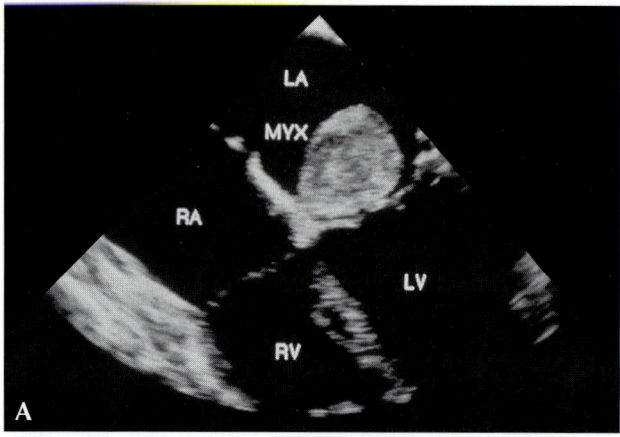
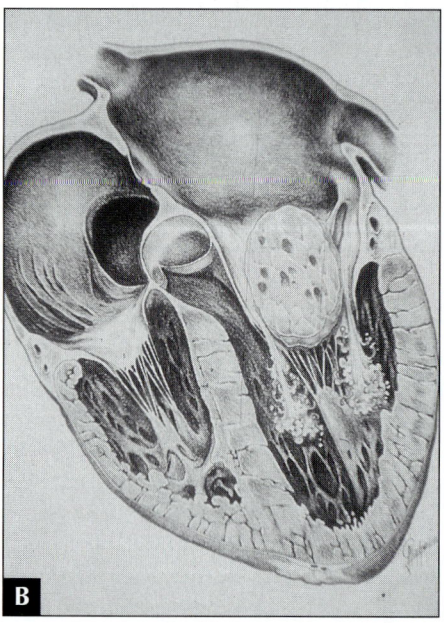

FIGURE 2 Transesophageal echocardiogram in a patient with left atrial myxoma. **A,** A large left atrial myxoma (MYX) attached to the base of interatrial septum is viewed in four-chamber view. **B,** Schematic of *panel A*. LA—left atrium; LV—left ventricle; RA—right atrium; RV—right ventricle. *From* Nanda and Mahan [23]; with permission.

transthoracic approach in providing additional visualization and superior resolution. It should be requested when the transthoracic echocardiogram is suboptimal or additional information regarding the tumor attachment and extent of involvement is needed.

Computed Tomography

Computed tomography (particularly ultrafast computed tomography) may allow tissue discrimination with definition of the degree of intramural tumor extension. It is useful for assessing the degree of myocardial invasion and involvement of pericardial and extracardiac structures [13].

Magnetic Resonance Imaging

This technique may be of considerable value in the detection and delineation of cardiac tumors, and in some cases, it may show the size, shape, and surface characteristics of the tumor more clearly than two-dimensional echocardiography [14]. The larger field-of-view with magnetic resonance imaging also may provide a better definition of tumor prolapse,

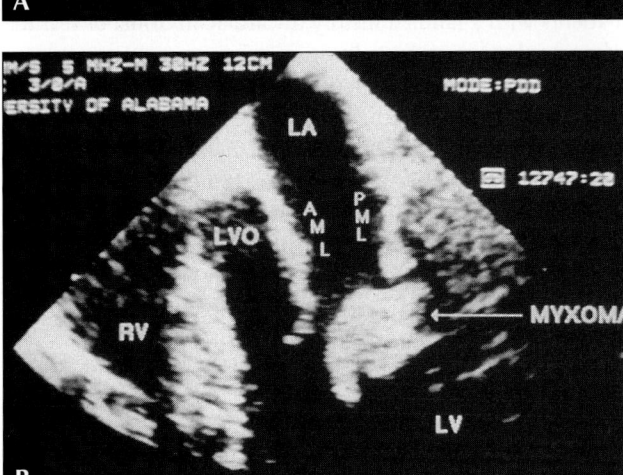

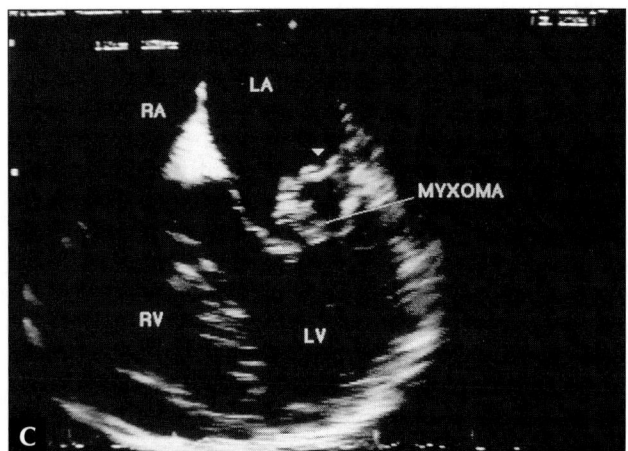

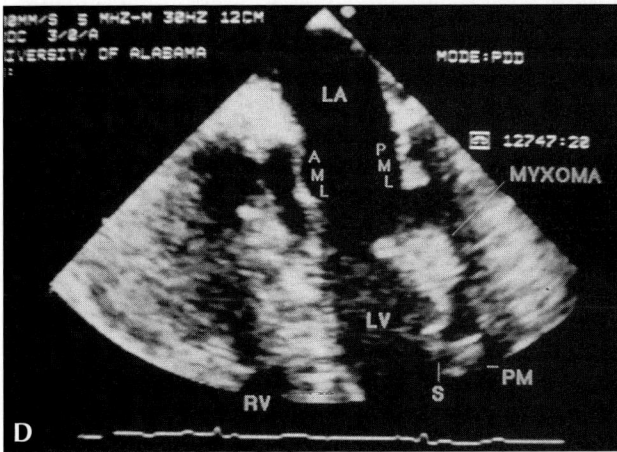

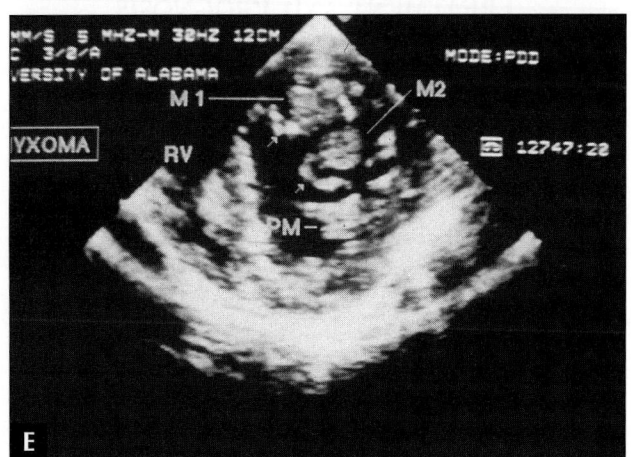

FIGURE 3 Transesophageal echocardiogram in a patient with multicentric left ventricular myxomas mimicking a left atrial tumor. In systole (A), a large tumor mass is seen within the left atrium (LA) behind the closed position of the mitral leaflets imaged in the four-chamber plane. In diastole (B), the mass has moved from LA into the left ventricle (LV), mimicking the motion pattern of a left atrial tumor. Intermittently, especially during the transesophageal study in the awake state, the mass was also visualized in LA in diastole, suggesting intermittent trapping of the tumor in the left atrium. The *arrowhead* points to the thinner portion of the mass in contact with the LA free wall (C). There is no evidence in A, B, or C to suggest (LV) attachment of the tumor. In (D), the attachment of the tumor to a papillary muscle (PM) head in LV by a long stalk (S) is clearly delineated. The long stalk makes it possible for the tumor to prolapse into LA in systole and move back into LV in diastole as well as for trapping in LA to occur. In the transgastric LV short-axis view (E), two separate tumors (M, M_2) with their stalks (*arrows*) are seen in the vicinity of the papillary muscles. AML—anterior mitral leaflet; PML—posterior mitral leaflet; RA—right atrium; RV—right ventricle. (*From* Samdarshi and coworkers [24]; with permission.)

Type of tumor	Treatment	Prognosis
Benign primary tumor	Usually surgical excision (lipomatous hypertrophy of atrial septum is benign and does not need any treatment)	Excellent; recurrence rare
Malignant primary tumor	Surgery not effective in the majority of patients because of extensive cardiac involvement or metastases; partial resection plus chemotherapy or radiotherapy may prolong survival in a few patients	Generally poor
Metastatic-secondary tumors	Surgery only palliative; almost always associated with widespread metastatic involvement of other organs	Poor

Table 8. Treatment and prognosis of cardiac tumors

secondary valve obstruction, and cardiac tumor size than two-dimensional echocardiography [14].

Angiography

Cardiac catheterization and selective angiocardiography are not necessary in all cases of cardiac tumors, especially with the advent of transesophageal echocardiography and magnetic resonance imaging. Cardiac tumors that are amenable to surgery frequently can be diagnosed by those two noninvasive techniques. In some cases, however, cardiac catheterization may allow visualization of the vascular supply of the tumor and identify the source of its blood supply and its relationship to the coronary arteries. The major risk of angiography is embolization resulting from dislodgement of tumor fragment or associated thrombus [15]. Therefore, its use before surgery is becoming increasingly less common, except perhaps for the sole purpose of assessing the coronary anatomy.

Treatment and Prognosis

Benign Tumors

Operative excision is the treatment of choice for most benign tumors (Table 8) and in many cases results in complete cure. Despite the histologically benign nature of these cardiac tumors, they are potentially lethal because of clinical manifestations of valvular obstruction, embolization, cardiac-rhythm disturbances, conduction defects, or sudden death. It is not uncommon for patients to die or experience a major complication while awaiting surgery. It is therefore mandatory to carry out the operation promptly after the diagnosis has been established [16]. Open heart surgery with cardiopulmonary bypass is required in most cases. This procedure allows for adequate inspection and removal of all tumor fragments. The dislodgement of tumor fragments represents a major risk during surgery and may result in embolization. Because early surgery is curative, patients with recurrent unexplained, albeit nonspecific cardiac symptoms should undergo echocardiographic evaluation. The high sensitivity of this technique permits adequate screening in most patients provided that the technical quality is adequate for diagnosis.

Numerous reports have documented complete cure of left and right atrial myxomas during a follow-up of up to 22 years [16,17••]. Causes of recurrent atrial myxomas include incomplete resection of the original tumor with regrowth or intracardiac implantation from the original tumor. Castells and coworkers [18••] reported a low recurrence rate of 4.7%. Patients with a familial history of cardiac myxoma or features of a complex myxoma syndrome may have tumor recurrence in 12% to 22% of cases as opposed to 1% of cases with sporadic atrial myxoma. Echocardiographic follow-up is important for detecting recurrent tumors in such patients. Following resection of myxoma, it is generally recommended that all patients have periodic follow-up by two-dimensional echocardiography for detection of recurrence. Although no criteria have been established, echocardiographic follow-up every 2 to 5 years is reasonable depending on patient symptomatology; suspected complex myxoma requires closer follow-up.

Other benign tumors also have been excised with a high degree of success. These includes rhabdomyoma, hamartoma, fibroma hemangioma, and papillary fibroelastomas (Table 8).

Malignant Tumors

Surgery is not an effective treatment for the great majority of primary malignant tumors of the heart, either because of the large mass of cardiac tissue involved or the presence of metastases. A major role for surgery in such cases is to establish the diagnosis and to explore the possibility of a curable benign tumor. Survival times from 1 to 3 years have been reported following partial resection with additional chemotherapy or radiation therapy. Lymphosarcoma of the heart frequently responds to chemotherapy, radiation therapy, or both [19]. Most reports indicate a failure to alter the course of cardiac sarcomas even with various combinations of surgery, chemotherapy, and radiation therapy. Surgery for metastatic cardiac tumors is largely palliative; surgically placed pericardial windows are commonly used to treat large pericardial effusions and cardiac tamponade.

References and Recommended Reading

Recently published papers of particular interest have been highlighted as:
- Of interest
- •• Of outstanding interest

1. Fine G: Primary tumors of the pericardium and heart. *Cardiovasc Clin* 1973, 5:207–238.
2. Prichard RW: Tumors of the heart: review of the subject and report of 150 cases. *Arch Pathol* 1951, 51:98–128.

3. Bulkley BH, Hutchins GM: Atrial myxomas: a fifty year review. *Am Heart J* 1979, 97:639–643.

4. Peters MN, Hall RJ, Cooley DA, *et al.*: The clinical syndrome of atrial myxoma. *JAMA* 1974, 230:695–701.

5. McDevitt HO, Bodomer WF: Protean clinical manifestations of primary tumors of the heart. *Am J Med* 1972, 52:1–8.

6. Farah MG: Familial cardiac myxoma. A study of relatives of patients with myxoma. *Chest* 1994, 105:65–68.

7. McCarthy PM, Piehler JM, Schaff HV, *et al.*: The significance of multiple recurrences and "complex" cardiac myxomas. *Thorac Cardiovasc Surg* 1986, 91:389–396.

8. Carney JA: Difference between nonfamilial and familial cardiac myxomas. *Am J Surg Pathol* 1983, 9:53–55.

9. Harvey WP: Clinical aspects of cardiac tumors. *Am J Cardiol* 1968, 21:328–343.

10. Roberts WC, Glancy DL, DeVita VT Jr: Heart in malignant lymphoma (Hodgkin's disease, lymphosarcoma, reticulum cell sarcoma and mycosis fungoides). A study of 196 autopsy cases. *Am J Cardiol* 1968, 22:149–153.

11. Panidis IP, Mintz GS, McAllister MO: Hemodynamic consequence of left atrial myxoma assessed by Doppler ultrasound. *Am Heart J* 1986, 111:927–931.

12.•• Ofili EO, Labovitz AJ: Transesophageal echocardiography in the evaluation of cardiac source of embolus and intracardiac masses. *J Invasive Cardiol* 1992, 4:349–358.

13. Jack CM, Cleland J, Geddes JS: Left atrial rhabdomyosarcoma and the use of digital gated computed tomography in its diagnosis. *Br Heart J* 1986, 55:305–307.

14. Freedberg RS, Kronzon I, Rumancik WM, Liebeskind D: The contribution of magnetic resonance imaging to the evaluation of intracardiac tumors diagnosed by echocardiography. *Circulation* 1988, 77:96–103.

15. Pindyck F, Pierce EC, Baron MG, Lukban SB: Embolization of left atrial myxoma after transeptal cardiac catheterization. *Am J Cardiol* 1972, 30:569–571.

16. Semb BK: Surgical considerations in the treatment of cardiac myxoma. *J Thorac Cardiovasc Surg* 1984, 87:251–259.

17.•• Bortolotti V, Maraglino G, Rubino M, *et al.*: Surgical excision of intracardiac myxomas: a 20 year follow up. *Ann Thorac Surg* 1990, 49:449–453.

18.•• Castells E, Ferran V, Octavio de Toledo MC, *et al.*: Cardiac myxomas: surgical treatment, long term results and recurrence. *J Cardiovasc Surg* 1993, 34:49–53.

19. Vergnon JM, Vincent M, Perinett M, *et al*: Chemotherapy of metastatic primary cardiac sarcomas. *Am Heart J* 1985, 110:682–684.

20. McAllister HA, Fenoglio JJ: Tumors of the cardiovascular system. In *Atlas of Tumor Pathology*. Washington, DC: Armed Forces Institute of Pathology; 1978.

21. Meller J, Teichholz LE, Pichard AD, *et al.*: Left ventricular myxoma: echocardiographic diagnosis and review of the literature. *Am J Med* 1977, 66:816–823.

22. Vidaillet HJ Jr, Seward JB, Fyke FE III, *et al.*: Syndrome myxoma: a subset of patients with cardiac myxoma associated with pigmented skin lesions and peripheral and endocrine neoplasms. *Br Heart J* 1987, 57:247–255.

23. Nanda NC, Mahan EF III: Transesophageal echocardiography. American Heart Association Council Clinical Cardiology Newsletter; Summer, 1990:3–22.

24. Samdarshi TE, Mahan EF III, Nanda NC, *et al.*: Transesophageal echocardiography diagnosis of multicentric left ventricular myxomas mimicking a left atrial tumor. *J Thorac Cardiovasc Surg* 1992, 103:471–474.

Nonpenetrating Cardiac Trauma

A. James Liedtke

> **Key Points**
> - Rapid deceleration impact injuries are a major cause of myocardial contusion.
> - A 12-lead electrocardiogram is the time-tested *sine qua non* of diagnosing myocardial contusion.
> - Current assessment of outcome statistics of cardiac complications secondary to myocardial contusion provides prospective clues to identifying high- and low-risk patients.
> - It is now possible to develop a triage algorithm for managing patients with myocardial contusion.
> - Direct injury to coronary arteries threatens myocardial perfusion and viability.
> - Therapeutic strategies for coronary artery disease may be applicable to lesions resulting from coronary trauma.

Cardiac injury secondary to severe, nonpenetrating, blunt chest-wall injury is a perilous, unpredictable consequence of deceleration impact injuries. It commonly occurs in motor vehicle accidents, is sometimes fatal, and is difficult to diagnose, particularly if accompanied by more obvious injuries of other organ systems. Parmley and coworkers [1], in one of the initial reviews on this topic, noted that cardiovascular involvement (most commonly contusion and rupture) in nonpenetrating trauma was not infrequent but was routinely unrecognized. Hospitals and trauma centers throughout the United States have dedicated increasingly greater staff and resources to the triage and management of trauma victims with suspected cardiac lesions.

Some trauma experts view this commitment as excessive. They argue that diagnostic and management systems be reevaluated to justify their cost. They further propose critically reviewing and possibly revamping utilization criteria for those triage algorithms, which necessitate intensive care facilities and expensive diagnostic and therapeutic procedures. This chapter focuses on two cardiac lesions: myocardial contusion and direct coronary artery trauma.

MYOCARDIAL CONTUSION

Diagnostic Criteria

Myocardial contusion has nonspecific diagnostic criteria and an uncertain clinical outcome, including major cardiac complications and, occasionally, cardiac death. One early view of this disorder (*ie*, that myocardial contusion is analogous to myocardial infarction) is probably flawed or incomplete and is not substantiated by recent literature. Evidence in 1973 [2] was biased by the more dramatic expressions of myocardial trauma and contusion. With a more complete database developed from recent observations, the spectrum of injury expression is more complete. The perspectives of morbidity and mortality are being adjusted; however, myocardial contusion lacks definitive diagnostic criteria.

TABLE 1 MECHANISM OF INJURY IN PATIENTS WITH SUSPECTED MYOCARDIAL CONTUSION FOLLOWING BLUNT CHEST TRAUMA

Mechanism	Patients, n
Car or truck accident	214
Pedestrian accident	30
Motorcycle accident	16
Fall	26
Other	26
Total (227 men; 85 women)	312

From McLean and coworkers [9••]; with permission.

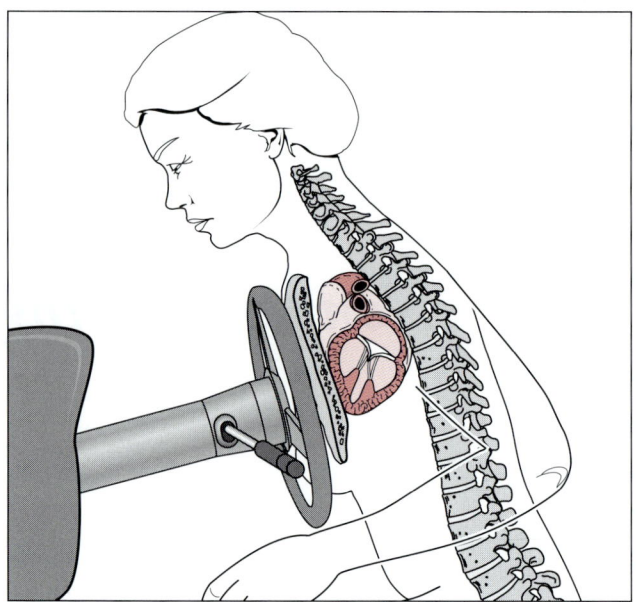

FIGURE 1 Typical impact injury to the anterior chest wall when the driver is thrust against the fixed steering column. Myocardial contusion results from high-speed deceleration accidents, most typically experienced by motor-vehicle and motorcycle crashes and auto–pedestrian accidents.

Myocardial infarction and myocardial contusion differ markedly with respect to the specificity of their diagnostic clues. Symptom presentation of chest-wall pain and thoracic tenderness in patients with trauma is nonspecific. Physical examination is only helpful in defining certain complications of major cardiac injury, such as pericardial tamponade, cardiac arrhythmias, primary or secondary valvular insufficiency, and heart failure. Historically, acquisition of serum enzymes (*ie*, serum glutamic-oxaloacetic transaminase and lactate dehydrogenase) leukocyte count, and sedimentation rate lacked specificity. Their modern replacements (creatine kinase [CK] isoenzymes) still do. The most reliable means of establishing the diagnosis is a 12-lead electrocardiogram, which remains the keystone of diagnosing myocardial contusion and is further enhanced as a predictive marker by the observed abnormalities in rhythm that occur early after injury.

Current literature encompasses a large population of patients studied with detailed workups [3–5,6••,7••,8•,9••, 10••]. It can be reviewed to determine which diagnostic maneuvers stand the test of time, what has been learned in terms of population outcome data to triage, and how to stratify patients as low-risk or more likely to suffer cardiac complications.

Myocardial contusion is an injury of the twentieth century. Most cases occur because of rapid deceleration events (before the era of air bags) secondary to motor-vehicle accidents or auto–pedestrian accidents [3,9••] (Table 1, Fig. 1). Representative diagnostic clinical criteria for patients with suspected myocardial contusion are listed in Table 2. These criteria reflect the lack of specific diagnostic signs, symptoms, and laboratory parameters while heightening awareness of the possible presence of cardiac injuries. This list includes mechanisms of injury at the scene of the accident, any symptoms and physical evidence if present, electrocardiographic findings suggestive of ischemia and infarction, conduction delays and dysrhythmias, and any other biochemical evidence suggestive for tissue injury of the heart muscle.

Updated outcome statistics of cardiac complications secondary to myocardial contusion confirm its reputation as a potentially life-threatening condition, both as a primary consequence of blunt chest-wall injury and as a disorder associated with other complications. For example, in traumatic thoracic aortic rupture, myocardial contusion worsens perioperative morbidity and

TABLE 2 REPRESENTATIVE DIAGNOSTIC CLINICAL CRITERIA OF PRESUMPTIVE MYOCARDIAL CONTUSION*

Study	Criteria
Foil and coworkers [6••]	Presence of chest pain, chest-wall contusion or tenderness, or sternal tenderness; a likely mechanism of injury such as rapid deceleration injury, bent or broken steering wheel, or a blow to the chest, dysrhythmias or ECG abnormalities (exclusive of sinus tachycardia)
Norton and coworkers [7••]	ECG pattern consistent with evolving or resolving pattern of acute injury; CK-MB isoenzyme fraction ≥5 % of the total CK concentration, or an elevated CK concentration with a "positive" MB fraction; an abnormal ECHO (hypokinesis, pericardial effusion, acute valvular injury; apical thrombus; wall thickening with edema or hemorrhage)
Miller and coworkers [3]	History of direct blows to the chest, broken steering-wheel accidents; likely mechanism of injury; physical evidence of anterior chest-wall injury, precordial bruising, fractured sternum, or anterior rib fractures
Ross and coworkers [4]	ECG and CK-MB isoenzyme assay monitored over the first 72 hours
	ECG criteria: arrhythmias, atrial or ventricular ectopy, conduction defects, any ischemic changes; CK-MB percentage >2.5%

*Exclusive of autopsy results.
CK—creatine kinase; ECG—electrocardiogram; ECHO—echocardiogram.

Table 3. Outcome statistics of patients with nonpenetrating blunt chest-wall injury

Study	Patients reviewed, n	Patients with presumed or suspected MC, n	Deaths secondary to MC, n	Other cardiac complications
Wisner and coworkers [12••]	3010	110	27*	19 Dysrhythmias (4 required treatment) 2 Cardiac rupture
Foil and coworkers [6••]	1936	524	0	23 Dysrhythmias (19 required treatment) 3 Myocardial infarctions 2 Pericardial effusions 4 Hemodynamic instability
Cachecho and coworkers [10••]	336	336	0	13 Atrial fibrillation (4 required treatment) 12 Supraventricular tachycardia/sinoatrial node dysfunction (7 required treatment) 24 Ventricular irritability (4 required treatment for ventricular tachycardia or ventricular bigeminy/trigeminy) 19 BBB or atrioventricular block 18 Ischemia 4 Congestive heart failure (all required treatment)
McLean and coworkers [9••]	312	312	35 (at least 4 had MC)	27 With ventricular ectopic score > 3, Including 17 ventricular tachycardia (2 required treatment) 14 Atrial fibrillation or sinus arrest or both (at least 5 treated) 11 New Q waves (4 died)
Dubrow and coworkers [5]	243	172	1 (MC not causal)	1 Ventricular ectopy 4 Ventricular tachycardia (2 required treatment) 3 Atrial ectopy 1 Atrial fibrillation 1 right BBB 1 Ischemia 1 Myocardial infarction
Miller and coworkers [3]	172	28	At least 3 (MC not necessarily causal in 2)	12 Dysrhythmia (4 required treatment) 4 Pericardial effusions
Norton and coworkers [7••]	88	27	0	2 Atrial dysrhythmia 6 Ventricular dysrhythmias (5 required treatment) 8 Conduction delays 3 Myocardial infarction (all required treatment) 3 Cardiogenic shock (all required treatment) 1 Apical thrombus (required treatment)
Ross and coworkers [4]	64	58	0	25 ECG changes with ST-T wave abnormalities 10 Ventricular ectopy 9 right BBB 3 Atrioventricular block 2 Atrial ectopy 3 Atrial fibrillation 4 Operative complications: ventricular ectopy, ventricular fibrillation, nodal rhythm, pulmonary edema

*Includes cardiac rupture, pericardial tear, coronary arterial injury.
BBB—bundle-branch block; ECG—electrocardiogram; MC—myocardial contusion.

mortality by promoting cardiac instability and cardiac arrest [11]. Deaths have also been reported [3,9••,12••] (Table 3). This complication is infrequent, however, and typically occurs with severe injury to other organ systems. Other complications are more frequent and include pericardial tears and effusions, nonlethal and lethal cardiac ruptures, acute myocardial infarction, transient myocardial ischemia, congestive heart failure, pulmonary edema and atrial thrombus, and cardiac dysrhythmias [3–5,6••,7••, 9••,10••,12••] (Table 3). Cardiac dysrhythmias include atrial ectopy, atrial fibrillation, sinoatrial nodal arrest, ventricular ectopy, ventricular tachycardia, ventricular fibrillation, nodal rhythm, atrioventricular conduction block, and intraventricular conduction delay. These rhythm disturbances sometimes require medical treatment or pacemaker insertion.

Updated statistics confirm that myocardial contusion is hazardous and requires careful diagnostic and electrical

Table 4A. Abbreviated Injury Scale scores for trauma to head/neck, face, and thorax Injury Severity Score regions (condensed 1985 revision for clinical practice)

AIS Score	Head/neck	Face	Thorax
1 (Minor)	Headache/dizziness 2° to head trauma C spine strain with no fracture or dislocation	Corneal abrasion Superficial tongue laceration Nasal or mandibular ramus* fracture Tooth fracture/avulsion or dislocation	Rib fracture* Thoracic spine strain Rib-cage contusion Sternal contusion
2 (Moderate)	Amnesia from accident Lethargic/stuporous/obtunded; can be roused by verbal stimuli Unconsciousness < 1 h Simple vault fracture Thyroid contusion Brachial plexus injury Dislocation or fracture spinous or transverse process of C spine Minor compression fracture (≤ 20%) C spine	Zygoma, orbit,* body,* or subcondylar mandible* fracture LeFort I fracture Scleral/corneal laceration	2–3 rib fractures Sternum fracture Dislocation or fracture spinous or transverse process T spine Minor compression fracture (≤ 20%) T spine
3 (Severe, not life-threatening)	Unconsciousness 1–6 h Unconsciousness < 1 h with neurologic deficit Fracture base of skull Comminuted compound or depressed vault fracture Cerebral contusion/subarachnoid hemorrhage Intimal tear/thrombosis carotid A Contusion larynx, pharynx Cervical cord contusion Dislocation or fracture of lamina body, pedicle or facet of C spine Compression fracture > 1 vertebra or > 20% anterior height	Optic nerve laceration LeFort II fracture	Lung contusion/laceration ≤ 1 lobe Unilateral hemo- or pneumothorax Diaphragm rupture ≥ 4 rib fractures* Intimal tear/minor laceration/ thrombosis subclavian or innominate artery Inhalation burn, minor Dislocation or fracture of lamina body, pedicle or facet of T spine Compression fracture ≥ 1 vertebra or > 20% height Cord contusion with transient neurologic signs
4 (Severe, life-threatening)	Unconsciousness 1–6 h with neurologic deficit Unconsciousness 6–24 h Appropriate response only to painful stimuli Fractured skull with depression > 2 cm, torn dura or tissue loss Intracranial hematoma ≤100 mL Incomplete cervical cord lesion Laryngeal crush Intimal tear/thrombosis carotid A with neurologic deficit	LeFort III fracture	Multilobar lung contusion or laceration Hemopneumomediastinum Bilateral hemopneumothorax Flail chest Myocardial contusion Tension pneumothorax Hemothorax > 1000 mL Tracheal fracture Intimal aortic tear Major laceration subclavian or innominate A Incomplete cord syndrome
5 (Critical)	Unconsciousness with inappropriate movement Unconscious > 24 h Brain stem injury Intracranial hematoma > 100 mL Complete cervical cord lesion C4 or below	—	Major aortic laceration Cardiac laceration Ruptured bronchus/trachea Flail chest/inhalational burn requiring mechanical support Laryngotracheal separation Multilobar lung laceration with tension pneumothorax hemopneumomediastinum, or > 1000 mL hemothorax Cord laceration or complete cord lesion
6 (Maximum injury)	Crush fracture, crush laceration brain stem Decapitation Cord crush/laceration or total transection with or without fracture C3 or above	—	Total severence aorta Chest massively crushed

From Civil and Schwab [16]; with permission. *Add AIS 1 if associated with hemothorax, pneumothorax, or hemopneumo. †AIS 1 to these fractures if open, displaced, or comminuted. AIS—Abbreviated Injury Scale; C—cervical; T—thoracic.

TABLE 4B ABBREVIATED INJURY SCALE SCORES FOR TRAUMA TO THE ABDOMEN, EXTREMITIES, AND EXTERNAL INJURY SEVERITY SCORE REGIONS (CONDENSED 1985 REVISION FOR CLINICAL PRACTICE)

AIS score	Abdomen	Extremities	External
1 (Minor)	Abrasion/contusion superficial laceration scrotum, vagina, vulva, perineum Lumbar spine strain Hematuria	Contusion elbow, shoulder, wrist, ankle Fracture/dislocation finger, toe Sprain A-C joint, shoulder, elbow, finger, wrist, hip, ankle, toe	Abrasions/contusions ≤ 25 cm on face/hand ≤ 50 cm on body Superficial lacerations ≤ 5 cm on face/hand ≤ 10 cm on body 1° burn up to 100% 2° or 3° burn/degloving injury < 10% total body
2 (Moderate)	Contusion/superficial laceration stomach, mesentery, SB, bladder, ureter, urethra Minor contusion/laceration kidney, liver, spleen pancreas Contusion duodenum/colon Dislocation or fracture spinous or transverse process L-spine Minor compression fracture (≤ 20%) L spine Nerve root injury	Fracture humerus,* radius,* ulna,* fibula, tibia,* clavicle, scapula, carpals metacarpals, calcaneus tarsals, metatarsals, pubic rami or simple pelvic fracture Dislocation elbow, hand, shoulder, A-C joint Major muscle/tendon laceration Intimal tear/minor laceration axillary, brachial, popliteal A; axillary, femoral, popliteal vein	Abrasions/contusions > 25 cm on face or hand > 50 cm on body Laceration > 5 cm on face or hand > 10 cm on body 2° or 3° burn or degloving injury 10%–19% of total body
3 (Severe, not life-threatening)	Superficial laceration duodenum/colon/rectum Perforation SB/mesentery/bladder ureter/urethra Major contusion/or minor laceration with major vessel involvement, or hemoperitoneum > 1000 mL of kidney/liver/spleen/panc Minor iliac artery or vein laceration Retroperitoneal hematoma Dislocation or fracture of lamina body, facet or pedicle of L spine Compression fracture > 1 vertebra or > 20% anterior height Cord contusion with transneurologic signs	Comminuted pelvic fracture Fractured femur Dislocation wrist/ankle/knee/hip Below knee or upper extremity amputation Rupture knee ligaments Sciatic nerve laceration Intimal tear/minor laceration femoral artery Major laceration ± thrombosis axillary or popliteal artery; axillary, popliteal, or femoral vein	2° or 3° burn or degloving injury 20%–29% of total body
4 (Severe, life-threatening)	Perforation stomach duodenum/colon/rectum Perforation with tissue loss stomach/bladder SB/ureter/urethra Major liver laceration Major iliac artery or vein laceration Incomplete cord syndrome Placental abruption	Pelvic crush fracture Traumatic above knee amputation/crush injury Major laceration femoral or brachial artery	2° or 3° burn or degloving injury 30%–39% total body
5 (Critical)	Major laceration with tissue loss or gross contamination of duodenum/colon/rectum Complex rupture liver, spleen/kidney/pancreas Complete cord lesion	Open pelvic crush fracture	2° or 3° burn or degloving injury 40%–89% total body
6 (Maximum injury)	Torso transection	—	2° or 3° burn or degloving injury ≥ 90% total body

From Civil and Schwab [16]; with permission. *Add AIS 1 to these fractures if open, displaced, or comminuted. ABS—Abbreviated Injury Scale; C—cervical; L—lumbar; S—small bowel; T—thoracic.

monitoring, dedicated professional staff, and the availability of sophisticated resources to conduct complex diagnostic and rapid therapeutic intervention; however, is this labor-intensive and costly triage algorithm mandatory for all patients with presumed myocardial contusion? Several reports agree on the markers defining a high-risk population of patients with myocardial contusion [3,7••,9••,10••]. Cardiac complications strongly correlate with the presence and severity of multiorgan injuries as defined by the Injury Severity Score (ISS) [13]. This score derives from the Abbreviated Injury Scale, which was created by the Committee on Medical Aspects of Automotive Injury of the American Medical Association [14], revised in 1985 [15], and subsequently rendered "user-easy" [16] (Tables 4A–C).

TABLE 4C CALCULATION OF INJURY SEVERITY SCORE*		
ISS body region	AIS score	Square of AIS score
Head/neck	_____	_____
Face	_____	_____
Thorax	_____	_____
Abdomen	_____	_____
Extremities	_____	_____
External	_____	_____

*From Civil and Schwab [16]; with permission.
ISS = sum of squares of 3 highest AIS scores.
ISS–Injury Severity Score; AIS–Abbreviated Injury Scale.

Using multivariant analysis, Norton and colleagues [7••] proposed that an abnormal electrocardiogram on admission and an ISS of 10 or higher were highly predictive of a myocardial contusion, and that in their absence the probability of contusion (1%) was virtually excluded. Probability estimates from their analysis are shown in Table 5. They further noted that because these two predictive markers are easily acquired in the emergency department, a patient population at high risk for myocardial contusion could be rapidly identified and triaged to the appropriate intensive care unit.

Cachecho and coworkers [10••] also observed a relationship between ISS and cardiac complications in a stable group of young patients with asymptomatic myocardial contusion. Increasing the ISS from 6.6 ± 6.1 to 23.5 ± 16.2 led to an increase in the occurrence of cardiac complications and dysrhythmias from 0% to 29%. Other important prognosticators were electrocardiogram abnormalities, which were either present on arrival at the emergency department or developed within the first 4 to 24 hours [3,6••]; an adverse clinical course including hemodynamic shock [3]; and the occurrence or presence of atrial fibrillation, which in one study [9••] was shown to be an increased risk factor for predicting cardiac deaths. Also important was the identity of patients at low risk for either the diagnosis of contusion or its complications. Foil and coworkers [6••] noted that a normal electrocardiogram on admission and the lack of development of cardiac dysrhythmias in the first 4 hours of observation virtually excluded significant cardiac sequelae, even in patients with physical findings of chest-wall contusion. They further proposed that these patients did not warrant hospitalization. These findings were again confirmed by Cachecho and coworkers [10••], who observed in their patients that a normal or only minimally abnormal electrocardiogram did not require sophisticated cardiac monitoring during hospitalization and that the hospital stay strongly correlate with ISS.

Dubrow and coworkers [5] defined their entrance criteria based on radionuclide angiography. This technique is insensitive to smaller lesions and is only diagnostic for those injuries with observably decreased global left ventricular ejection fraction or induced abnormalities in segmental wall motion. The ISS range was correspondingly higher (12.7 to 30.7) in three patient subgroups. Despite the higher absolute ISS values, mortality rates were lower than those predicted by their ISS ranking. This disparity was so wide (10% to 20% predicted vs. 0.58% observed) that the authors concluded that in stable patients, "myocardial contusion does not by itself increase the risk of complication, does not necessitate intensive care unit monitoring, should be devalued when computing ISS scores, may account for lengthy and often unnecessary hospitalization, and in patients at risk for complications may be (more easily) identified by ECG abnormalities on arrival to the Emergency Department." [5]

The merit of CK-MB isoenzyme analysis is contested. Fabian and coworkers [17] reported that in 140 of 1110 patients suffering nonpenetrating trauma and at increased risk for blunt cardiac injury, 56 had likely evidence for myocardial contusion as estimated either by increased CK-MB concentrations in blood or by abnormalities on the admission electrocardiogram. The authors cautioned, however, that elevated isoenzymes were transient and required careful sampling (at admission and every 6 hours for the first 24 hours). If these sampling times were missed, up to 75% of their patients with myocardial contusion would not have been so diagnosed. Other data, however, have not been confirmatory. In one study of 138 patients with severe injury, including possible myocardial contusion [10••], only 1.4% had positive isoenzymes compared with 32% who had diagnostic electrocardiographic changes. Another study [6••] found no significant association between CK isoenzyme changes and the occurrence of cardiac related complications, and a third [3] observed that combined findings of electrocardiogram abnormalities and elevated CK isoenzymes were of no higher predictive value in defining patients at higher risk than using the electrocardiogram alone. In a final report of 182 patients

TABLE 5 CALCULATION OF THE PROBABILITY OF MYOCARDIAL CONTUSION USING ISS AND ECG IN 88 PATIENTS			
Predictors of myocardial contusion		Probability of myocardial contusion	Patients with myocardial contusion, n
ISS >10	Abnormal ED ECG		
Yes	Yes	0.8656	9
No	Yes	0.3538	12
Yes	No	0.0396	4
No	No	0.0396	0

From Norton and coworkers [7••]; with permission.
ECG—electrocardiogram; ED—emergency department; ISS—Injury Severity Score.

with significant blunt chest wall trauma [18], the authors concluded that "CK-MB determinations in patients with suspected blunt myocardial injury were unjustifiably expensive and added confusion to an already vague clinical area." The problem of enzyme analysis is compounded in trauma cases by the presence of skeletal muscle injury, which almost always occurs in severe blunt chest-wall injury and lowers the CK-MB fraction (< 3%) relative to the total CK concentration in blood [19•].

Imaging Modalities

It is probably too early to cast final judgment on the newer imaging modalities being employed to diagnose myocardial contusion, but the available data are not encouraging for either radionuclide angiography or two-dimensional transthoracic echocardiography. This may relate to the size and severity of the contusion injury, which *a priori* must be at least moderate to large or severe to affect a motion abnormality visible by noninvasive testing. An association has been described among patients with positive radionuclear imaging and mortality [9••], but when a more complete population of trauma patients is surveyed, the sensitivity and specificity of this testing mode is reduced.

Radionuclide angiography

McLean and colleagues [8•] performed radionuclear angiography in 163 patients who suffered thoracic trauma. Only seven patients had abnormal studies; five of them died. Postmortem findings in four patients showed evidence of prior infarction in three and one new anterior infarction in the fourth. Another report [9••] noted that a radionuclear study performed 1 week after injury showed normal wall motion and ejection fractions in a patient with biventricular contusions who died late. A third study reported a positive relationship between the extent of blunt trauma estimated by ISS and cardiac-gated, blood-pool scintigraphy using labeled technetium-99m, but with much less accuracy than with using electrocardiographic abnormalities [10••].

The results of a small series of patients studied by coronary perfusion imaging using thallium-201 are more encouraging [20]. Approximately 70% of these patients with blunt chest trauma had scintigraphic defects related to areas of myocardial contusion, and all patients with these defects had either paroxysmal dysrhythmias or electrocardiogram abnormalities. Godbe and coworkers [21•] reported that thallium-201 imaging with single-photon emission computed tomography is useful in predicting those patients suffering severe chest-wall trauma at increased risk for developing cardiac dysrhythmias.

Transthoracic echocardiography

Mixed results have confounded the use of two-dimensional transthoracic echocardiography. In animal studies, the diagnosis of contused myocardium seemed well-suited to two-dimensional echocardiography using the criteria of (1) increased end-diastolic wall thickness, (2) increased echo brightness, and (3) impaired regional systolic function" [22]. The precision and merits of this tool, however, have not been generally confirmed in clinical trials. In 172 patients with either blunt chest trauma or suspected or proven myocardial contusion evidenced by other clinical or laboratory criteria, myocardial contusion by echocardiography criteria was not obvious in 49% [23], 74% [3], 81% [12••], and 86% [17] of cases. Another 7% to 15% of cases were either technically inadequate or nondiagnostic in quality. In those echocardiographic studies that were positive, myocardial contusion, wall-motion disorders, and small pericardial effusions were noted. It is presumed that as with radionuclear imaging, two-dimensional transthoracic echocardiography is only helpful in confirming large-sized contusions sufficient either to affect regional contractility or to produce other complications such as pericardial effusion. Conversely, it is inferred that the specificity and sensitivity of this procedure for smaller-sized injury is sufficiently reduced to jeopardize the accuracy of diagnosis.

Transesophageal echocardiography

Transesophageal echocardiography is a new imaging strategy in patients with blunt chest-wall trauma. The modality has a better signal-to-noise ratio and imaging capability than transthoracic echocardiography. Nineteen prospective patients with severe chest-wall injury were evaluated by transesophageal echocardiography [24•]. Patients were studied within 12 hours of trauma. No procedural complications were reported. Investigations were undertaken for widened mediastinum (> 8 cm on chest film), and a variety of lesions were noted, including tricuspid, mitral, and aortic insufficiency; pericardial effusions; myocardial contusions; and aortic hematoma. In 5 of 19 patients with hypokinetic motion abnormalities compatible with myocardial contusion, isoenzyme analysis was negative.

Transesophageal echocardiography was also successful in characterizing traumatic aortic transection in one patient suffering blunt chest-wall trauma [25•]. In addition, it was deemed critical in another patient for selecting medical over surgical treatment for trauma-induced mitral regurgitation with leaflet prolapse [26•].

Coronary Artery Trauma

In 1973, the question of coronary artery trauma in blunt chest-wall injury was speculative because of a deficiency in essential information and too few unequivocal cases with direct documentation of the diagnosis using coronary cineangiography [2]. This literature is still not available in large series comparable to those described for myocardial contusion. In 1979, Allen and Liedtke [27] listed five categories to characterize the case material:

1. Cardiac contusion (or myocardial infarction) in the absence of sustained injury to a major coronary artery,
2. Cardiac contusion (or myocardial infarction) associated with perfusion abnormalities of a major coronary artery,
3. Coronary artery fistula formation,
4. Coronary artery rupture, and
5. Animal experiments evaluating the effect of blunt trauma on the coronary vasculature.

It is difficult to separate myocardial infarction from myocardial contusion without mechanisms that specifically relate tissue injury with flow abnormalities in the major coronary vessels, particularly for contusions or infarctions in the presence of normal coronary arteries. In this instance, tissue damage may reflect primary myocardial injury, including trauma to the microcirculation; transient epicardial arterial spasm; or clot formation with secondary lysis, which cannot be adequately described by subsequent arteriography. Literature is limited to several case reports that detail the relationship between arterial damage and tissue necrosis. Chest injury has resulted from sporting accidents, accidents of childhood, and workplace events, as well as from traffic accidents [28,29•, 30–32,33•]. In almost every circumstance in which coronary trauma was established or suspected, there were electrocardiographic findings of acute myocardial infarction.

In contrast to recommendations developed for the early triage of patients with myocardial contusion, myocardial infarct occurred 3 and 15 days after the initial traumatic event in two patients in these reports [31,33•]. Either delayed vasomotor spasm or a hypercoagulopathy may contribute to the late clinical development of infarction. Accompanying these coronary injuries were examples of hypotension or shock, intraarterial clot formation, posttraumatic angina with an abnormal exercise tolerance evaluation, severe myocardial injury with depressed left ventricular ejection fraction and left ventricular aneurysm formation, tachyarrhythmias (nonsustained ventricular tachycardia), and complete heart block requiring temporary pacemaker insertion [29,30–32,33•]. This latter finding confirms previous observations of complete heart block noted in the setting of blunt chest-wall trauma [34].

Therapy

These coronary injuries are well-suited to the therapeutic strategies developed for managing acute myocardial infarction. For example, intracoronary urokinase was infused for 2 hours in a patient with left anterior descending coronary arterial thrombus that had occluded both the anterior descending artery and first diagonal branch of that perfusion system [29•]. Also, Lijoi and coworkers [33•] attempted percutaneous transluminal coronary angioplasty of a totally obstructed left anterior descending coronary artery and were initially successful. The vessel reoccluded at 24 hours, and the patient was subsequently managed with surgical revascularization. In a 6-year-old boy with complicated cardiac trauma from a crush injury, cardiac surgery was employed to excise a left ventricular aneurysm that extended from the coronary sulcus to the apex of the heart and was filled with thrombus [30]. The operation was successful, and symptoms of heart failure that had developed before surgery resolved.

Coronary artery rupture secondary to blunt chest-wall injury is life-threatening. Heyndricks and associates [35] reported a 62-year-old patient involved in a car accident who presented with acute inferior myocardial infarction and hypotension. The patient received several supportive maneuvers, including assisted ventilation, pacemaker insertion, resuscitation, and pericardiocentesis. Treatment was unsuccessful, and the patient died 9 hours after injury. Autopsy revealed 13 rib fractures and the presence of blood bilaterally in both pleural spaces. One bone splinter had perforated the left pleura, lacerated the pericardium, and torn the right coronary artery from its origin on the aorta. There was also a smaller, transverse tear of the intima of the left coronary

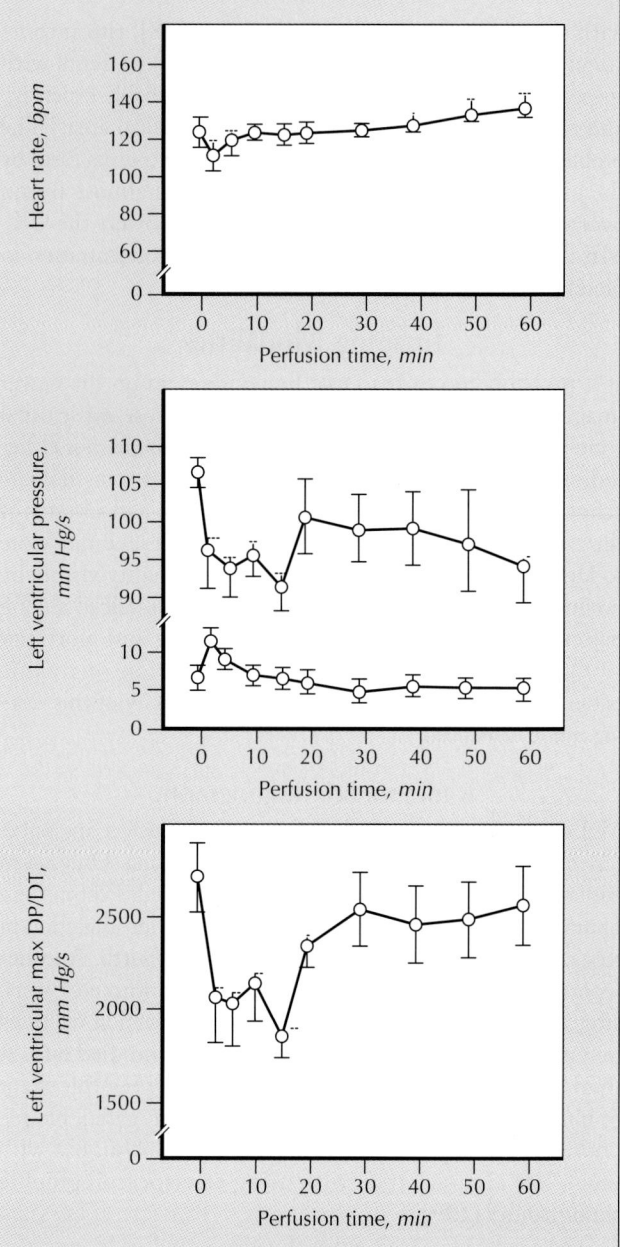

FIGURE 2 Changes in various parameters in global hemodynamic function in traumatized hearts. The major interval of mechanical dysfunction occurs early after the impact injury. **Middle panel**, bottom open circles represent left ventricular end-diastolic pressure; top circles represent left ventricular peak systolic pressure. Dots represent statistical significance by paired Student's t-test comparisons with pretrauma values: .—$P < 0.05$; ..—$P < 0.01$; ...—$P < 0.005$. Bars represent ± 1 SEM. Max DP/DT—maximum rate of pressure development during isovolumic contraction.

artery as well as a nonperforating tear of the aorta distal to the left subclavian artery. Histologic and histochemical examination confirmed the presence of an extensive, inferior myocardial infarction.

Consequences of Coronary Injury

In animal studies with controlled injuries to the coronary arteries, Sabbah and coworkers [36,37] described multiple coronary lesions by either microscopic examination or selective coronary arteriograms. They noted complete and partial obstructions to major coronary vessels, extravasation of blood from traumatic vascular wounds, accompanying extravascular hemorrhages, and a small arteriovenous fistula. Despite the angiographic severity of these lesions, which were evident by the third day after trauma, almost all findings resolved to near-normal or normal by 2 to 5 weeks of follow-up.

Even in the absence of demonstrable anatomic lesions, (*ie*, no spasm, thrombosis, hemorrhage, or laceration), functional consequences of direct coronary injury occur [38]. In this report, the epicardial-to-endocardial flow ratios measured by radioactive microspheres increase in absolute magnitude after injury and were accompanied by decreased coronary vascular resistance in the vascular bed distal to the impact site. Other coronary abnormalities included a reduction in reactive hyperemia reflective of decreased coronary flow reserve and concomitant declines in regional systolic shortening, left ventricular pressure development, and left ventricular maximum rate of pressure development during isovolumic contraction. Metabolically, myocardial oxygen consumption and lactate extraction were decreased.

One unifying interpretation of these data is that there is an adverse reflex pattern of coronary perfusion with distribution of flow away from the subendocardial zone. This flow is sufficient to decrease coronary oxygen delivery and mechanical performance and to alter glucose metabolism, suggestive of early myocardial ischemia (Figs. 2 and 3, Table 6). These data *in toto* suggest that the coronary vasculature is not immune from direct injury after blunt chest-wall trauma; that consequences of this trauma may be expressed in a variety of clinical conditions, including life-threatening myocardial infarction or contusion; and that even without anatomic obstruction, derangements in coronary flow, which are functionally adverse (particularly to the subendocardium) may occur with subsequent mechanical and metabolic sequelae.

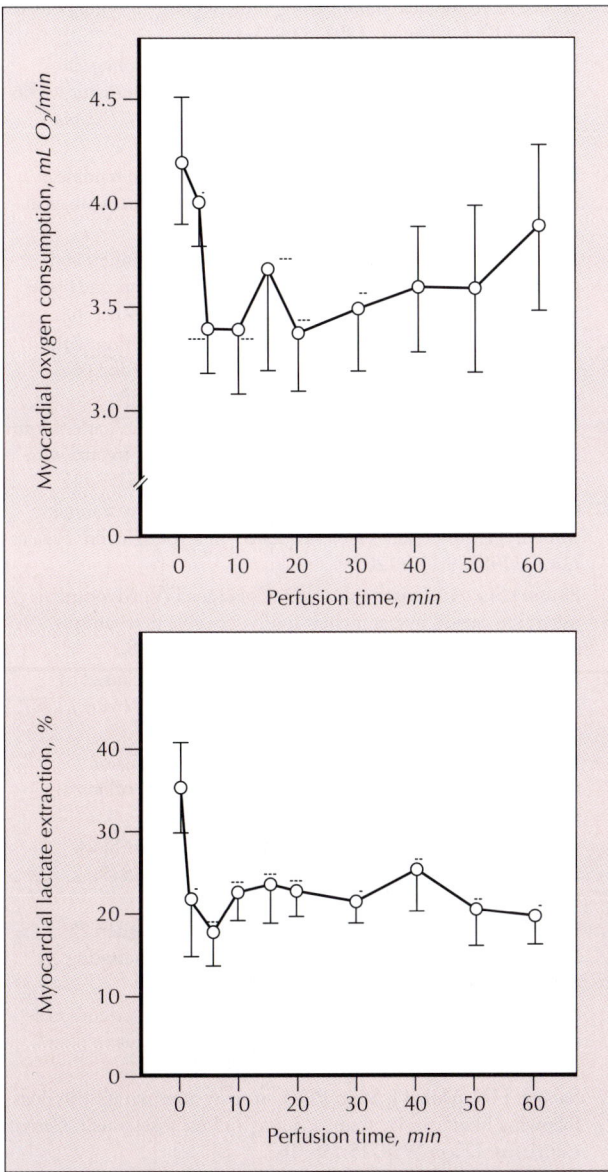

FIGURE 3 Changes in regional metabolism for oxygen consumption and lactate extraction in the perfusion distribution of the traumatized artery. The metabolic consequences of coronary injury, particularly for depressed lactate extraction, appear to last longer than for mechanical dysfunction. *Dots* represent statistical significance by paired Student's *t*-test comparisons with pretrauma values: .—$P < 0.05$; ..—$P < 0.01$; ...—$P < 0.005$. *Bars* represent ± 1 SEM.

TABLE 6 PERFUSION DATA IN FOUR TRAUMATIZED ANIMALS INJECTED WITH MICROSPHERE

	Epicardial/endocardial flow ratio		
	Impact	LAD	LCF
Pretrauma			
Mean	0.94	0.97	1.36
SEM	0.15	0.09	0.24
5 Min after trauma			
Mean	1.60	1.30	1.42
SEM	0.36	0.07	0.36
P	< 0.025	< 0.005	NS
55 Min after trauma			
Mean	1.54	1.25	1.17
SEM	0.26	0.06	0.16
P	< 0.005	< 0.001	NS

From Liedtke [38]; with permission.
Impact—LAD perfusion system directly beneath and around the impact site; LAD—left anterior perfusion system; LCF—left circumflex perfusion system; NS—not significant; *P*—statistical comparisons with pretrauma data; SEM—standard error of the mean.

References and Recommended Reading

Recently published papers of particular interest have been highlighted as:
• Of interest
•• Of outstanding interest

1. Parmley FF, Manion WC, Mattingly TW: Nonpenetrating traumatic injury of the heart. *Circulation* 1958, 18:371–396.
2. Liedtke AJ, DeMuth WE: Nonpenetrating cardiac injuries: a collective review. *Am Heart J* 1973, 86:687–697.
3. Miller FB, Shumate CR, Richardson JD: Myocardial contusion: when can the diagnosis be eliminated? *Arch Surg* 1989, 124:805–808.
4. Ross P, Degutis L, Baker CC: Cardiac contusion: the effect on operative management of the patient with trauma injuries. *Arch Surg* 1989, 124:506–507.
5. Dubrow TJ, Mihalka J, Eisenhauer DM, *et al.*: Myocardial contusion in the stable patient: what level of care is appropriate? *Surgery* 1989, 106:267–274.
6.•• Foil MB, Mackersie RC, Furst SR, *et al.*: The asymptomatic patient with suspected myocardial contusion. *Am J Surg* 1990, 160:638–643.
7.•• Norton MJ, Stanford GG, Weigelt JA: Early detection of myocardial contusion and its complications in patients with blunt trauma. *Am J Surg* 1990, 160:577–582.
8.• McLean RF, Devitt JH, Dubbin J, McLellan BA: Incidence of abnormal RNA studies and dysrhythmias in patients with blunt chest trauma. *J Trauma* 1991, 31:968–970.
9.•• McLean RF, Devitt JH, McLellan BA, *et al.*: Significance of myocardial contusion following blunt chest trauma. *J Trauma* 1992, 33:240–243.
10.•• Cachecho R, Grindlinger GA, Lee VW: The clinical significance of myocardial contusion. *J Trauma* 1992, 33:68–73.
11. Kram HB, Appel PL, Shoemaker WC: Increased incidence of cardiac contusion in patients with traumatic thoracic aortic rupture. *Ann Surg* 1988, 208:615–618.
12.•• Wisner DH, Reed WH, Riddick RS: Suspected myocardial contusion: triage and indications for monitoring. *Ann Surg* 1990, 212:82–86.
13. Copes WS, Champion HR, Sacco WJ, *et al.*: The Injury Severity Score revisited. *J Trauma* 1988, 28:69–77.
14. Committee on Medical Aspects of Automotive Safety: Rating the severity of tissue damage. 1. The Abbreviated Injury Scale. *JAMA* 1971, 215:277–280.
15. *The Abbreviated Injury Scale (AIS) 1985 revision*. Des Plaines, IL: American Association for Automotive Medicine; 1985.
16. Civil ID, Schwab CW: The Abbreviated Injury Scale, 1985 revision: a condensed chart for clinical use. *J Trauma* 1988, 28:87–90.
17. Fabian TC, Mangiante EC, Patterson CR, *et al.*: Myocardial contusion in blunt trauma: clinical characteristics, means of diagnosis, and implications for patient management. *J Trauma* 1988, 28:50–57.
18. Keller KD, Shatney CH: Creatine phosphokinase-MB assays in patients with suspected myocardial contusion: diagnostic test or test of diagnosis? *J Trauma* 1988, 28:58–63.
19.• Sobel BE, Jaffe AS: The value and limitations of cardiac enzymes in the recognition of acute myocardial infarction. *Heart Dis Stroke* 1993, 2:26–32.
20. Bodin L, Rouby J-J, Viars P: Myocardial contusion in patients with blunt chest trauma as evaluated by thallium-201 myocardial scintigraphy. *Chest* 1988, 94:72–76.
21.• Godbe D, Waxman K, Wang FW, *et al.*: Diagnosis of myocardial contusion: quantitative analysis of single photon emission computed tomographic scans. *Arch Surg* 1992, 127:888–892.
22. Pandian NG, Skorton DJ, Doty DB, Kerber RE: Immediate diagnosis of acute myocardial contusion by two-dimensional echocardiography: studies in a canine model of blunt chest trauma. *J Am Coll Cardiol* 1983, 2:488–496.
23. Reid CL, Kawanishi DT, Rahimtoola SH, Chandraratna PAN: Chest trauma: evaluation by two-dimensional echocardiography. *Am Heart J* 1987, 113:971–976.
24.• Shapiro MJ, Yanofsky SD, Trapp J, *et al.*: Cardiovascular evaluation in blunt thoracic trauma using transesophageal echocardiography (TEE). *J Trauma* 1991, 31:835–840.
25.• Brooks SW, Cmolik BL, Yong JC, *et al.*: Transesophageal echocardiographic examination of a patient with traumatic aortic transection from blunt chest trauma: a case report. *J Trauma* 1991, 31:841–845.
26.• Turabian M, Chan K-L: Rupture of mitral chordae tendineae resulting from blunt chest trauma: diagnosis by transesophageal echocardiography. *Can J Cardiol* 1990, 6:180–182.
27. Allen RP, Liedtke AJ: The role of coronary artery injury and perfusion in the development of cardiac contusion secondary to nonpenetrating chest trauma. *J Trauma* 1979, 19:153–156.
28. de Feyter PJ, Roos JP: Traumatic myocardial infarction with subsequent normal coronary arteriogram. *Eur J Cardiol* 1977, 6:25–31.
29.• Ledley GS, Yazdanfar S, Friedman O, Kotler MN: Acute thrombotic coronary occlusion secondary to chest trauma treated with intracoronary thrombolysis. *Am Heart J* 1992, 132:518–521.
30. Cizmarova E, Simkovic I, Zelenay J, Masura J: Post-traumatic coronary occlusion and its consequences in a young child. *Pediatr Cardiol* 1988, 9:117–120.
31. Foussas SG, Athanasopoulos GD, Cokkinos DV: Myocardial infarction caused by blunt chest injury: possible mechanisms involved—case reports. *Angiology* 1989, 40:313–318.
32. Pringle SD, Davidson KG: Myocardial infarction caused by coronary artery damage from blunt chest injury. *Br Heart J* 1987, 57:375–376.
33.• Lijoi A, Tallone M, Parodi E, *et al.*: Coronary occlusion secondary to blunt chest trauma: a first attempt at balloon angioplasty. *Tex Heart Inst J* 1992, 19:291–293.
34. Brennan JA, Field JM, Liedtke AJ: Reversible heart block following nonpenetrating chest trauma. *J Trauma* 1979, 19:784–788.
35. Heyndricks G, Vermeire P, Goffin Y, Van den Bogaert P: Rupture of the right coronary artery due to nonpenetrating chest trauma. *Chest* 1974, 65:577–579.
36. Sabbah HN, Stein PD, Hawkins ET, *et al.*: Extrinsic compression of the coronary arteries following cardiac trauma in dogs. *J Trauma* 1982, 22:937–943.
37. Sabbah HN, Mohyi J, Stein PD: Coronary arteriography in dogs following blunt cardiac trauma: a longitudinal assessment. *Cathet Cardiovasc Diagn* 1988, 15:155–163.
38. Liedtke AJ, Allen RP, Nellis SH: Effects of blunt cardiac trauma on coronary vasomotion, perfusion, myocardial mechanics, and metabolism. *J Trauma* 1980, 20:777–785.

Diseases of the Aorta

28

Gregg M. Yamada
Joseph S. Alpert

> ### Key Points
> - Seventy-five percent of arteriosclerotic aortic aneurysms involve the infrarenal abdominal aorta.
> - Thoracic aneurysms most commonly result from atherosclerosis; most involve the descending thoracic aorta.
> - Abdominal aortic aneurysms 4 cm or more in diameter and thoracic aortic aneurysms more than 6 to 7 cm in diameter require surgical repair.
> - Magnetic resonance imaging, computed tomography, and transesophageal echocardiography are highly sensitive and specific for the diagnosis of aortic dissection.
> - Untreated aortic dissections are associated with a high mortality.
> - Arteritis syndromes including Takayasu's arteritis, giant cell arteritis, and the seronegative spondyloarthropathies are associated with varying degrees of aortic involvement.
> - Most aortoiliac emboli are cardiac in origin.
> - Embolization of small cholesterol crystals may follow surgical or catheter manipulation, leading to the cholesterol emboli syndrome.

A complex array of diseases, either congenital or acquired, may affect the aorta (Table 1). This chapter reviews the pathogenesis, clinical manifestations, and therapy of the most common aortic processes, including arteriosclerotic aneurysms, dissection, arteritis, and thromboembolic disease.

ARTERIOSCLEROTIC AORTIC ANEURYSMS

Arteriosclerotic aortic aneurysms include both abdominal and thoracic aortic aneurysms.

Abdominal Aortic Aneurysms

Pathophysiology

Seventy-five percent of aortic aneurysms involve the abdominal aorta distal to the origin of the renal arteries. Approximately 25% occur within the thoracic aorta. Most of these aneurysms are fusiform and result from arteriosclerotic weakening of the elastic media; other causes of aortic aneurysms are listed in Table 2. Aneurysmal dilatation leads to increased aortic wall tension, which results in further enlargement of the aneurysm.

Presentation

Most patients who present with abdominal aortic aneurysms are asymptomatic. The diagnosis is suspected when routine physical examination reveals a pulsatile midepigastric mass or when aortic calcification is seen on abdominal radiographs (Fig. 1).

TABLE 1 DISEASES OF THE AORTA
Arteriosclerotic aortic aneurysms
Aortic dissection
Aortic arteritis
Takayasu's arteritis
Giant cell arteritis
Ankylosing spondylitis
Psoriatic arthritis
Reiter's syndrome
Aortic thromboembolic disease
Aortic bacterial infection (syphilis, tuberculosis)
Traumatic injuries of the aorta
Aortic tumors
Coarctation and pseudocoarctation of the aorta
Hypoplastic aortic syndromes

TABLE 2 CAUSES OF AORTIC ANEURYSMS
Acquired
Atherosclerosis
Cystic medial degeneration
Infection (syphilis, tuberculosis)
Aortitis (infectious)
Trauma
Congenital
Aortitis (noninfectious)
Aneurysms associated with coarctation and patent ductus arteriosus

Diagnosis

The diagnosis may be confirmed with computed tomography (CT), magnetic resonance imaging (MRI), angiography, or ultrasonography. Abdominal ultrasonography is the most practical and cost-effective method for determining and monitoring aneurysm size [1,2], although CT provides additional preoperative information, delineating possible suprarenal extension or other abdominal abnormalities [3,4].

Treatment and prognosis

Prognosis is related to the size of the aneurysm, with larger aneurysms (> 5 cm in diameter) expanding more rapidly and being more likely to rupture than smaller aneurysms [5,6,7••]. Aneurysm expansion rate is approximately 0.5 cm/y. Asymptomatic aneurysms 4 cm or more in diameter (or twice the diameter of the infrarenal aorta) should be surgically repaired [8••], and symptomatic or rapidly expanding aneurysms require immediate repair. The operative mortality rate for elective repair is approximately 3% to 5% [9].

Thoracic Aortic Aneurysms
Pathophysiology

Atherosclerosis is the most common cause of thoracic aortic aneurysms. Less common causes include annuloaortic ectasia, syphilis or other infections, and aortic valve disease. Arteriosclerotic thoracic aneurysms occur most frequently in the descending aorta and are typically fusiform, with the ascending aorta and the aortic arch less commonly involved. Patients with descending thoracic aortic aneurysms also may have associated abdominal aortic aneurysms [10]. Syphilitic aneurysms, which have a predilection for the ascending aorta, are often saccular.

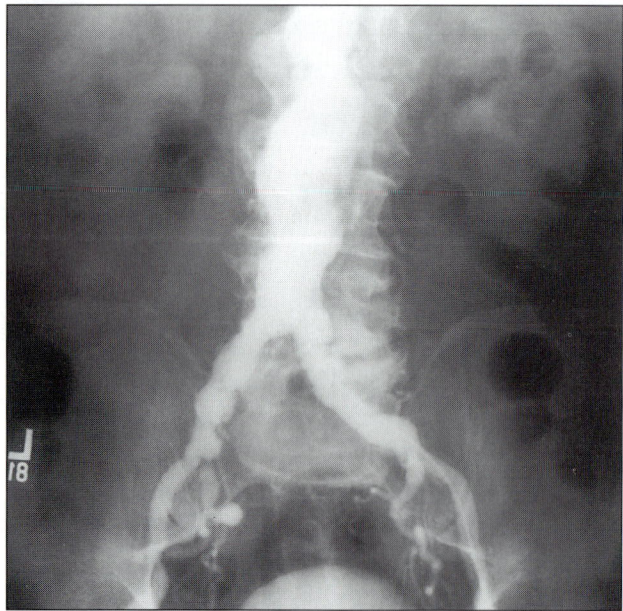

FIGURE 1 Abdominal aortogram demonstrating a fusiform infrarenal abdominal aortic aneurysm. (*From* Cipriano and coworkers [21]; with permission.)

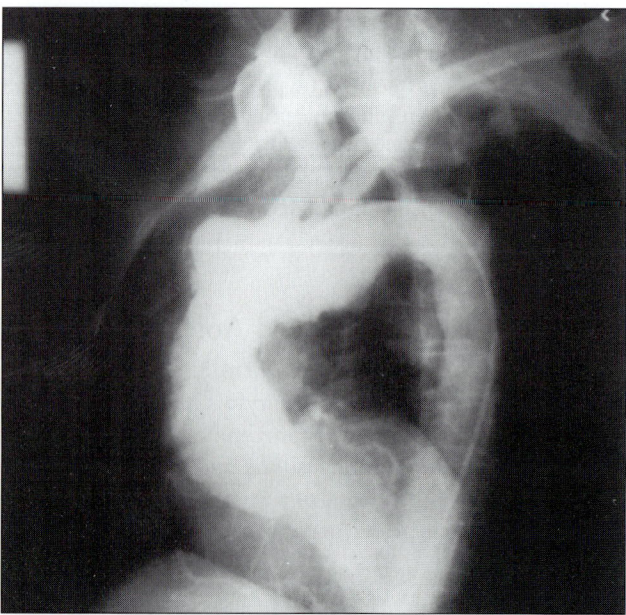

FIGURE 2 Thoracic aortogram demonstrating a saccular thoracic aortic aneurysm. (*From* Cipriano and coworkers [21]; with permission.)

TABLE 3 FACTORS PREDISPOSING TO AORTIC DISSECTION
Primary or secondary cystic medial degeneration combined with: Atherosclerosis   Hypertension   Advanced age   Aortic valve disease   Coarctation of the aorta   Aortic trauma, including iatrogenic trauma   Pregnancy

Aneurysms caused by cystic medial degeneration may involve the aortic sinuses and aortic valve, resulting in myocardial ischemia and valvular insufficiency.

Presentation

Descending aortic aneurysms are usually asymptomatic. In contrast, ascending aortic aneurysms are more likely to be symptomatic because of their impingement on adjacent thoracic structures. Patients may complain of a deep, aching anterior chest discomfort. Less common symptoms include dyspnea, cough, and hoarseness.

Palpable pulsations may be present along the anterior chest wall at either sternal border, the sternoclavicular borders, or the suprasternal notch. Aortic insufficiency and signs of Marfan's syndrome may be noted. Tracheal deviation, hoarseness, superior vena cava syndrome, and discrepant pulses and blood pressure also may be found.

Diagnosis

Thoracic aortic aneurysm may be suspected from routine posteroanterior and lateral radiographs, and it may be confirmed by angiography in patients requiring surgical resection (Fig. 2). Computed tomography, MRI, and transesophageal echocardiography (TEE) are sufficient to make the diagnosis, however, if surgery is not being considered.

Treatment and prognosis

Less information is available on the natural history of thoracic aortic aneurysms than for abdominal aneurysms. Symptomatic thoracic aneurysms are associated with a 5-year survival rate of 27%, compared with 58% in asymptomatic patients. Symptomatic thoracic aneurysms, or those over 6 to 7 cm in diameter in either the ascending or descending thoracic aorta, require prompt surgical attention [11]. Because of the high prevalence of associated cardiovascular disease (eg, coronary artery disease), patients must be carefully selected for surgery. Early surgical mortality is approximately 5% to 10% and most often results from myocardial infarction, congestive heart failure, stroke, renal failure, or sepsis [12].

AORTIC DISSECTION

Pathophysiology

Aortic dissection results from a sudden intimal rupture followed by the formation of a dissecting hematoma along or within the aortic media separating the intima from the adventitia. Two thirds of all aortic dissections occur in the ascending aorta 2 to 5 cm above the aortic valve. The descending aorta, just distal to the origin of the left subclavian artery, is the second most common site of aortic dissection.

Cystic degenerative changes of the elastic and smooth muscle elements of the aortic media predispose the patient to the development of aortic dissection [13]; other factors associated with aortic dissection are listed in Table 3. Aortic dissection is more common in men, and hypertension is present in most patients with descending aortic dissection. Aortic dissection occurs in various connective tissue disorders associated with prominent, congenital cystic medial degeneration (eg, Marfan's syndrome, Ehlers-Danlos syndrome). An increased frequency of aortic dissection is also seen in patients with aortic coarctation, congenital bicuspid aortic valve, aortic stenosis, and pregnancy. Iatrogenic causes include cardiac catheterization, cardiac surgery, intraaortic balloon counterpulsation, cardiopulmonary bypass, and prosthetic valve surgery.

The most widely cited classification for aortic dissection is that of DeBakey [14], which uses the location of the intimal tear and the extent of the aortic dissection as points of classification (Table 4) [14]. Type I dissections arise just above the aortic valve and extend into the descending aorta. Type II dissections are localized within the ascending aorta. Type III dissections originate in the descending aorta just distal to the origin of the left subclavian artery and extend into the abdominal aorta (Fig. 3).

A simpler classification (ie, the DeBakey classification) identifies the DeBakey types I and II dissections as proximal or ascending (type A) dissections and DeBakey type III dissections as distal or descending (type B) dissections (Fig. 4) [15]. Acute aortic dissections are those present for less than 2 weeks.

TABLE 4 DeBAKEY CLASSIFICATION OF AORTIC DISSECTION

Classification	Description
I	Originates in the ascending aorta and propagates distal to the brachiocephalic artery
II	Originates in and is confined to the ascending aorta
III	Originates in the descending aorta near the ligamentum arteriosum
IIIA	Dissection does not extend below the diaphragm
IIIB	Dissection extends below the diaphragm

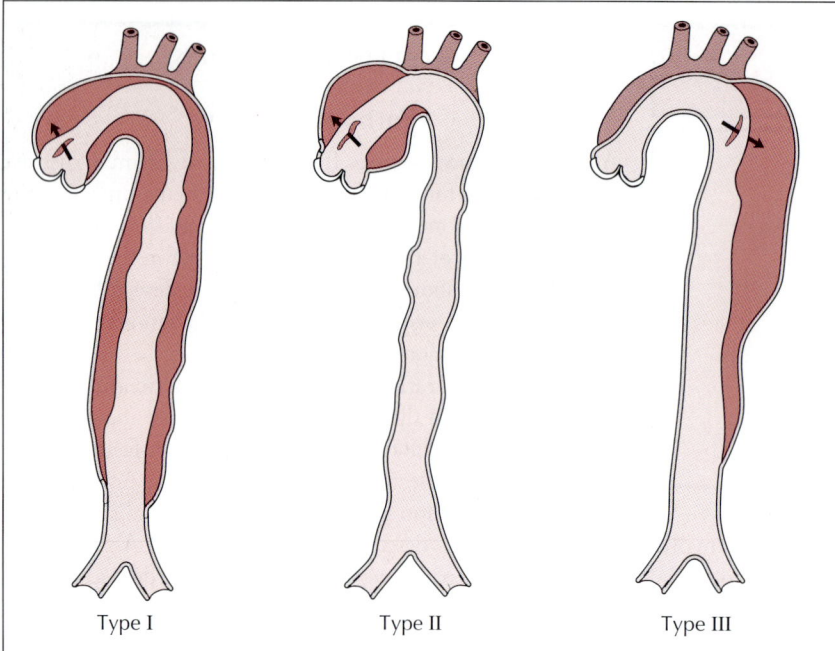

FIGURE 3 The DeBakey classification of aortic dissection. (*From* Eagle and DeSanctis [17••]; with permission.)

Presentation

Severe chest pain described as "stabbing," "ripping," or "tearing" in character is present in most patients. Unlike the presentation of myocardial ischemia, which often develops over several minutes, the intensity of the pain is extreme at onset. The site of dissection may be suggested by the location of the pain, but the pain commonly migrates into the neck, back, and extremities as the dissection extends along the aorta.

Aortic insufficiency, pulse abnormalities, neurologic deficits, and evidence of cardiac tamponade may be present in patients with ascending aortic dissection. Pulse deficits are less common in distal aortic dissections but if present may involve the femoral and left subclavian arteries. Although most patients present with hypertension, hypotension may signify aortic rupture, cardiac tamponade, or subclavian artery dissection.

Diagnosis

The diagnosis of aortic dissection may be suspected from the history and physical examination, and it be confirmed with echocardiography, CT, MRI, or angiography. Routine posteroanterior radiographs may reveal progressive mediastinal widening (Fig. 5). Separation of intimal calcification from the adventitial border by more than 1 cm is highly suggestive of dissection. Magnetic resonance imaging, CT, and TEE are each highly sensitive; MRI and CT are more specific studies [16••]. Echocardiography, CT, and MRI are each appropriate as initial, noninvasive screening studies for patients in whom clinical suspicion of acute dissection exists. TEE is most suitable in unstable patients, whereas either MRI or CT is more

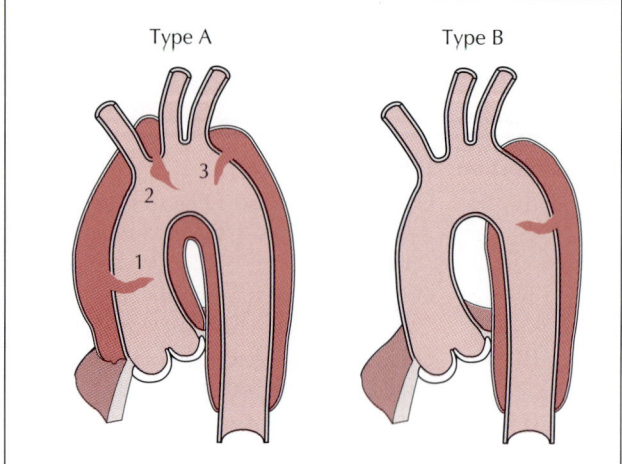

FIGURE 4 The DeBakey classification of aortic dissection. (*From* Miller and coworkers [22]; with permission.)

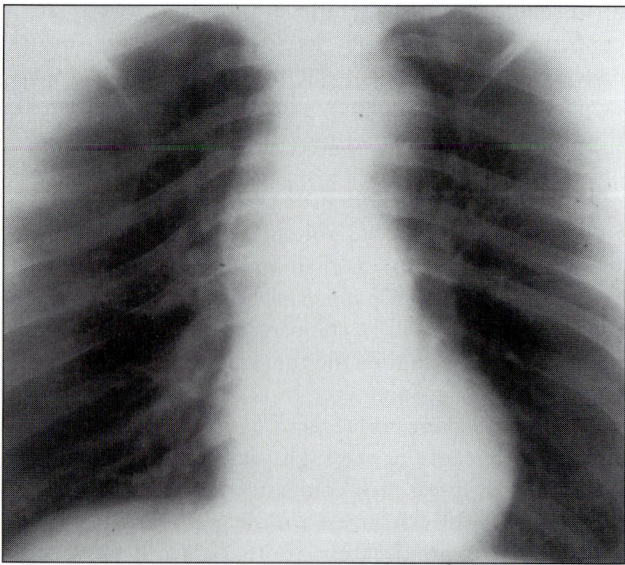

FIGURE 5 Posteroanterior chest radiograph demonstrating mediastinal widening caused by aortic dissection of the ascending aorta. (*From* Kidd and coworkers [23]; with permission.)

useful for monitoring chronic dissection [16••]. Transthoracic echocardiography allows the clinician to visualize proximal dissections, whereas TEE, CT, and MRI allow better visualization of distal dissections. Despite the utility of noninvasive assessment, aortic angiography is often necessary preoperatively, because it shows the site of intimal rupture, extent of dissection, involvement of major aortic branches, aortic valve competence, and coronary anatomy (Fig. 5) [17••].

Treatment and Prognosis

Acute type A (ascending) aortic dissections (Fig. 6) almost invariably require immediate surgical therapy. Acute type B (descending) aortic dissections and chronic dissections of any location are first managed medically; surgery is reserved for complications such as rupture, expansion, continued pain, or distal ischemia. Untreated aortic dissections are associated with a 21% mortality at 24 hours, a 37% mortality at 48 hours, a 74% mortality at 2 weeks, and a 90% mortality at 3 months [17••].

All patients with suspected aortic dissection require intensive monitoring for cardiac arrhythmias, hypotension, declining renal function, and other signs of systemic hypoperfusion before definitive diagnostic procedures are performed. The aim of medical therapy is to decrease both systemic arterial pressure and the rate of rise in aortic pressure. Analgesics and sedatives should be administered as needed. Intravenous β-blockers (*eg*, metoprolol) in combination with vasodilators (*eg*, sodium nitroprusside) should be administered to all patients with hypertension. Patients with hypotension require transfusion and emergent surgical correction [17••]. The surgical technique used depends on the location the of dissection.

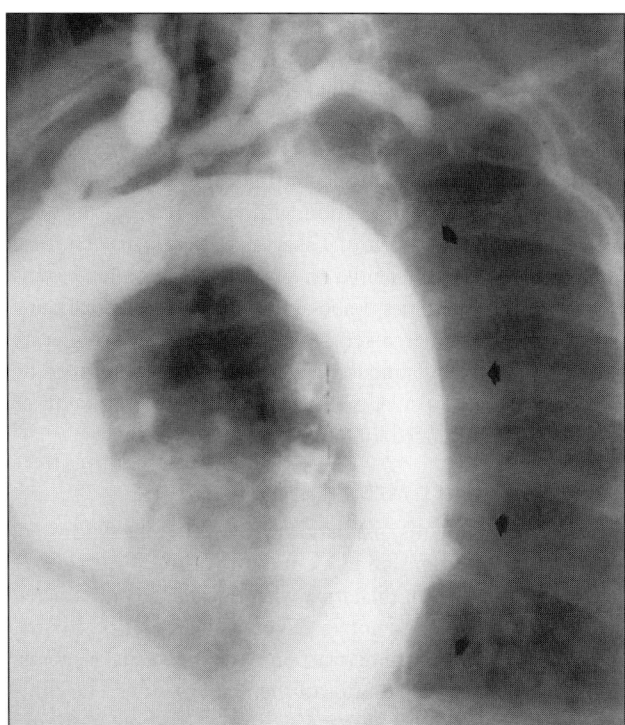

FIGURE 6 Ascending aortogram demonstrating type A aortic dissection. (*From* Cigarroa and coworkers [24]; with permission.)

AORTIC ARTERITIS

Aortitis results from a variety of vasculitic syndromes and is characterized by obstruction of the aorta and its branches with dilatation and aneurysm formation. Aortic arteritis includes Takayasu's arteritis, giant cell arteritis, and other arteritis syndromes with rare origins.

Takayasu's Arteritis

Pathophysiology

Takayasu's arteritis is a chronic vasculitis involving the aorta and its primary branches, and it affects adolescent and young women. Asian, African, Native American, and Hispanic women are affected more often than white women. The cause of Takayasu's arteritis is unknown, but an immunopathogenic mechanism is suspected. Prominent intimal proliferation and fibrosis are characteristic, with involvement of the media, adventitia, and vasa vasorum resulting in luminal narrowing and aneurysm formation. The subclavian, carotid, vertebral, and renal arteries are the most frequently affected.

Presentation

Fatigue, fever, malaise, weight loss, night sweats, and arthralgias predate ischemic manifestations. Pain and tenderness develop over the involved arteries, with diminished pulses, bruits, hypertension, heart failure, and retinopathy present on examination. Less common manifestations include coronary ischemia caused by ostial involvement of the coronary arteries, myocarditis, aortic regurgitation, and pulmonary hypertension.

Diagnosis

The diagnosis of Takayasu's arteritis is suspected in any woman younger than 40 years of age who develops bruits with diminished or discrepant peripheral pulses and blood pressures. The characteristic vascular abnormalities on angiography (*ie*, luminal irregularity, narrowing, dilatation, and aneurysm) are confirmatory. More comprehensive diagnostic criteria have been proposed [18]. Laboratory abnormalities are nonspecific and include an elevated erythrocyte sedimentation rate (ESR), anemia of chronic inflammation, and thrombocytosis.

Treatment and prognosis

The clinical course of Takayasu's arteritis varies, but slow progression is typical. Steroids are effective in alleviating symptoms and arresting disease progression; and cyclophosphamide is helpful in patients unresponsive to steroids. Renovascular hypertension is responsive to angiotensin-converting enzyme inhibitors and should be treated aggressively. The role of ASA or chronic anticoagulation in decreasing ischemic symptoms is not established [18].

Giant Cell Arteritis

Giant cell (or temporal) arteritis is a vasculitis affecting medium-sized arteries, typically those of the head and neck.

The aorta and its primary branches are involved less commonly. White women over 50 years of age are most often affected.

Patchy or segmental granulomatous arterial inflammation is present. The etiology of giant cell arteritis is unknown, but an autoimmune mechanism is possibly responsible. Symptoms may develop gradually and include fatigue, headache, polymyalgia rheumatics, jaw claudication, and visual loss. Aortic arch involvement similar to that of Takayasu's arteritis may be seen, and patients are usually febrile on examination, with tenderness over the temporal arteries. Laboratory studies reveal a markedly elevated ESR, decreased serum albumin level, and moderate anemia of chronic inflammation. The diagnosis is confirmed by temporal artery biopsy. Corticosteroids are the treatment of choice and are continued for 1 to 2 years.

Other Arteritis Syndromes

Ankylosing spondylitis, psoriatic arthritis, Reiter's syndrome, and Behçet's syndrome are rare causes of aortitis. Typical findings include aortic root dilatation with thickened and retracted aortic valve leaflets and aortic valvular insufficiency. Histopathologic changes reveal destruction of elastic medial elements with an obliterative endarteritis of the vasa vasorum. The clinical course varies, and treatment is directed at the underlying disease process. Aortic valve replacement may be required.

AORTIC THROMBOEMBOLIC DISEASE

Aortic thromboembolic disease includes aortic and atheromatous emboli.

Aortic Embolism

Pathophysiology

Acute aortoiliac occlusion may result from thromboembolic disease or, less commonly, acute thrombosis. Most aortoiliac emboli originate from the left heart, with only a minority arising from a thrombus overlying an arteriosclerotic aortic plaque. Predisposing factors for aortic thromboembolism are listed in Table 5.

Presentation

Acute, severe lower extremity pain with numbness, paresthesias, and weakness in the ischemic distribution is typical. The lower extremities are cold, pale, and cyanotic, with diminished or absent pulses.

Diagnosis

Clinical presentation is suggestive of the diagnosis, and angiography is confirmatory. Transesophageal echocardiography is useful in identifying cardiac sources of emboli [19].

Treatment and prognosis

Transfemoral artery catheter embolectomy is the procedure of choice and is performed by cardiovascular specialists. All patients are initially heparinized, and chronic anticoagulation is usually required.

Atheromatous Emboli (Cholesterol Emboli Syndrome)

Pathogenesis

Embolization of small cholesterol crystals into distal arterial beds may follow manipulation of an atherosclerotic segment of the aorta during surgery or catheterization. Spontaneous embolization is less common.

Presentation

Clinical presentation may include livedo reticularis, ecchymotic and gangrenous extremities, renal failure, hypertension, pancreatitis, abdominal pain, and neurologic deficits [20].

Diagnosis

Diagnosis is suspected clinically and is confirmed by demonstrating intra-arterial cholesterol crystals in muscle or skin.

Treatment and prognosis

Treatment for cholesterol microembolism is supportive, with prevention of necrosis and infection being the mainstays of therapy. Anticoagulation may exacerbate further embolization, and its use is controversial.

REFERENCES AND RECOMMENDED READING

Recently published papers of particular interest have been highlighted as:

•• Of outstanding interest

1. Littooy FN, Steffan G, Greisler HP, et al.: Use of sequential B-mode ultrasonography to manage abdominal aortic aneurysms. *Arch Surg* 1989, 124:419–421.
2. Shapira OM, Pasik S, Wassermann JP, et al.: Ultrasound screening for abdominal aortic aneurysms in patients with peripheral vascular disease. *J Cardiovasc Surg* 1990, 31:170–172.
3. Gomes MN, Choyke PL: Pre-operative evaluation of abdominal aortic aneurysms: ultrasound or computed tomography. *J Cardiovasc Surg* 1987, 28:159–166.
4. Pillari G, Chang JB, Zito J, et al.: Computed tomography of abdominal aortic aneurysm. *Arch Surg* 1988, 123:727–732.
5. Sterpetti AV, Schultz RD, Feldhaus RJ, et al.: Abdominal aortic aneurysm in elderly patients: selective management based on clinical status and aneurysmal expansion rate. *Am J Surg* 1985, 150:772–776.

TABLE 5 FACTORS PREDISPOSING TO AORTIC THROMBOEMBOLISM
Myocardial infarction with mural thrombus
Ventricular aneurysm
Prosthetic valves
Atrial fibrillation
Cardiomyopathy
Endocarditis (bacteria, marantic)
Paradoxic embolism (patent foramen ovale or atrial septal defect)
Atrial myxoma
Idiopathic origin

6. Naevoid MP, Ballad DJ, Hailed J: Prognosis of abdominal aortic aneurysms: a population-based study. *N Engl J Med* 1989, 321:1009–1014.

7.•• Ernest CB: Abdominal aortic aneurysm. *N Engl J Med* 1993, 328:1167–1172.

8.•• Hollier LH, Taylor LM, Ochsner J: Recommended indications for operative treatment of abdominal aortic aneurysms: report of a subcommittee of the joint council of the Society for Vascular Surgery and the North American Chapter of the International Society for Cardiovascular Surgery. *J Vasc Surg* 1992, 15:1046–1056.

9. Sullivan CA, Rohrer MJ, Cutler BS: Clinical management of the symptomatic but unruptured abdominal aortic aneurysm. *J Vasc Surg* 1990, 11:799–803.

10. Crawford ES, Cohen ES: Aortic aneurysm. A multifocal disease. *Arch Surg* 1982, 117:1393–1400.

11. Crawford ES, Crawford JL, Hazim SJ, *et al.*: Thoracoabdominal aortic aneurysms: preoperative and intraoperative factors determining immediate and long-term results of operations in 605 patients. *J Vasc Surg* 1986, 3:389–404.

12. Moreno-Cabral CE, Miller C, Mitchell S, *et al.*: Degenerative and atherosclerotic aneurysms of the thoracic aorta. *J Thorac Cardiovasc Surg* 1984, 88:1020–1032.

13. Dale JR, Pape LA, Cohn LH, *et al.*: Dissection of the aorta: pathogenesis, diagnosis, and treatment. *Prog Cardiovasc Dis* 1980, 23:237–242.

14. DeBakey ME, McCollum CH, Crawford ES, *et al.*: Dissection and dissecting aneurysms of the aorta: twenty year follow-up of five hundred twenty seven patients treated surgically. *Surgery* 1982, 92:1118–1134.

15. Erbel R, Delert H, Meyer J, *et al.*: Effect of medical and surgical therapy on aortic dissection evaluated by transesophageal echocardiography: implications for prognosis and therapy. *Circulation* 1993, 87:1604–1615.

16.•• Nienaber CA, von Kodolitsch Y, Nicolas V, *et al.*: The diagnosis of thoracic aortic dissection by noninvasive imaging procedures. *N Engl J Med* 1993, 328:1–9.

17.•• Eagle KA, DeSanctis RW: Aortic dissection. In *Current Problems in Cardiology.* Chicago: Year Book Medical Publishers, 1989:227–278.

18. Ishikawa K: Diagnostic approach and proposed criteria for the clinical diagnosis of Takayasu's arteriopathy. *J Am Coll Cardiol* 1988, 12:964–972.

19. Karalis DG, Krishnaswamy D, Victor MF, *et al.*: Recognition and embolic potential of intraaortic atherosclerotic debris. *J Am Coll Cardiol* 1991, 17:73–78.

20. Hendel RC, Cuenoud HF, Giansiracusa DF, Alpert JS: Multiple cholesterol emboli syndrome: bowel infarction after retrograde angiography. *Arch Intern Med* 1989, 2371–2374.

21. Ciprano PR, Alonso DR, Baltaxe HA, Gay WA: Multiple Aortic aneurysms in relapsing polychondritis. *Am J Cardiol* 1976, 37:1097–1102.

22. Miller DC, Stinson EB, Oyer PE, *et al.*: Operative treatment of aortic dissections: experience with 125 patients over a sixteen-year period. *J Thorac Cardiovasc Surg* 1979, 78:365–369.

23. Kidd JN, Reul GJ, Cooley DA, *et al.*: Surgical treatment of aneurysms of the ascending aorta. *Circulation* 1976, 54(suppl 3):111–119.

24. Cigarroa JE, Isselbacher EM, DeSanctis RW, Eagle KA: Diagnostic imaging in the evaluation of suspected aortic dissection: old standards and new directions. *N Engl J Med* 1993, 328:35–43.

Selected Bibliography

Baron JF: Dipyridamole-thallium scintigraphy and gated radionuclide angiography to assess cardiac risk before abdominal aortic surgery. *N Engl J Med* 1994, 330:663–339.

Debeider A, Thomas M, Marrinan M: Traumatic rupture of the thoracic aorta diagnosed by transesophageal echocardiography. *Br Heart J* 1993, 70:393–394.

Geva T, Hornberger LK, Sanders SP, *et al.*: Echocardiographic predictors of left ventricular outflow tract obstruction after repair of interrupted aortic arch. *J Am Coll Cardiol* 1993, 22:1953–1960.

Roman MJ, Rosen SE, Kramerfox R, Devereux RB: Prognostic significance of the pattern of aortic root dilatation in the marfan syndrome. *J Am Coll Cardiol* 1993, 22:1470–1476.

Diseases of Peripheral Arteries and Veins 29

John A. Spittell, Jr.
Peter C. Spittell

> ### Key Points
> - In addition to evaluating peripheral arterial pulsations, elevation-dependency tests provide confirmation of occlusive arterial disease in an extremity and a rough estimation of the degree of any ischemia.
> - The most sensitive indicator of occlusive arterial disease in a lower extremity is an abnormal ankle:brachial index 1 minute after standard exercise.
> - Arteriography is not necessary for the diagnosis of atherosclerotic occlusive peripheral arterial disease; it is indicated when restoration of pulsatile flow is planned.
> - In the nondiabetic person with only intermittent claudication, restoration of pulsatile flow is elective.
> - Features that suggest an uncommon type of occlusive peripheral arterial disease include a young person, involvement of the upper extremity and/or digits, and presentation as acute ischemia without prior symptoms of occlusive peripheral arterial disease.
> - Atheroembolism (blue toes and livedo reticularis) may occur spontaneously from an atherosclerotic aorta or aneurysm, with the initiation of anticoagulant therapy, or follow arterial interventions or surgery.
> - When venous thromboembolism recurs in the face of adequate anticoagulant effect, a secondary cause should be strongly suspected.
> - Chronic indurated cellulitis (*ie*, lipodermatosclerosis), a complication of inadequately controlled chronic venous insufficiency, may mimic infection but can be relieved by good elastic support to the affected limb.

When symptomatic, diseases of peripheral arteries and veins cause pain, swelling, changes in skin color, or ulceration of the extremities or digits. The ease with which arterial and venous circulation of the extremities can be evaluated by physical examination and noninvasive methodology makes clinical diagnosis an office or bedside exercise in many cases.

DISEASES OF PERIPHERAL ARTERIES

Peripheral arterial disease is common and can present as either an acute or a chronic disorder, the latter being more common. Because occlusive and aneurysmal diseases are principally atherosclerotic in origin, they are the most frequently encountered disorders, but the less common types present the generalist with interesting diagnostic problems. Although the abnormalities presented by peripheral arterial disorders usually can be identified by a careful patient history and physical examination, noninvasive diagnostic studies are readily available to provide objective confirmation of clinical findings.

Occlusive Peripheral Arterial Disease

Occlusive peripheral arterial disease can be chronic or acute. The lower extremities are much more frequently involved than the upper extremities. Acute arterial occlusion can be thrombotic or embolic. Chronic occlusive arterial disease is most often caused by atherosclerosis, but thromboangiitis obliterans (Buerger's disease), giant cell arteritis, trauma, and external arterial compression (entrapment), although less common, are important for the clinician to keep in mind [1••,2].

Diagnosis

A useful way to think of occlusive peripheral arterial disease is the Fontaine classification (Table 1). The classic feature of symptomatic occlusive arterial disease in the lower extremities is intermittent claudication, which is characterized by aching, cramping, or tiredness that occurs with walking and is relieved by standing still. It may be mimicked by musculoskeletal disorders, chiefly pseudoclaudication from lumbar spinal stenosis (Table 2). When more severe ischemia develops, the patient experiences pain at rest (ischemic rest pain) and, with even minor trauma, ischemic ulceration (Fig. 1, Table 3) occurs.

Reduced or absent pulsation of the extremity arteries is the classic physical finding in occlusive arterial disease. Arterial narrowing upstream may cause audible systolic bruits over large arteries, and when the lumen becomes more narrowed (usually > 80%) creating a gradient in diastole, the bruit may extend into diastole. A useful clinical estimate of the degree of ischemia can be obtained by observing development of pallor on elevation of the extremity and then the time required for return of color to the skin and the superficial veins to fill on dependency of the extremity or extremities after elevation (Table 4). In the upper extremity, the

TABLE 1 FONTAINE CLASSIFICATION

Stage	Clinical feature
1	Silent
2	Intermittent claudication
3	Rest ischemia
4	Ulceration or gangrene

From Fontaine and coworkers [11]; with permission.

TABLE 2 CONDITIONS CONFUSED WITH INTERMITTENT CLAUDICATION

Site of claudication	Confused conditions
Foot	Foot strain
	Tight shoes
	Plantar neuroma
Calf	Muscle strain
	Flat feet
	Osteoarthritis of knee
Thigh	Sciatica
	Pseudoclaudication caused by spinal stenosis
Hip	Osteoarthritis of hip
	Pseudoclaudication caused by spinal stenosis

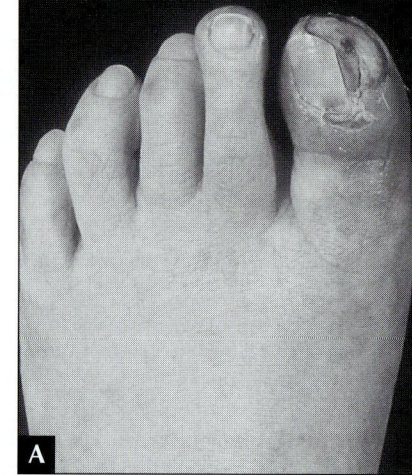

FIGURE 1 A, Ischemic ulceration, first toe. B, Ischemic ulceration, second toe and medial aspect of ankle.

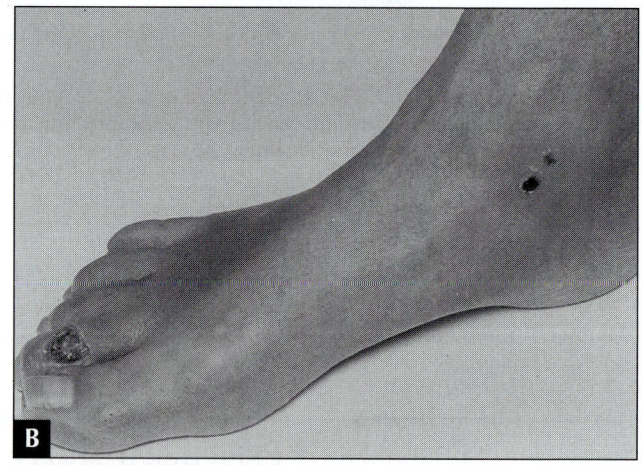

TABLE 3 CHARACTERISTICS OF ISCHEMIC AND VENOUS STASIS ULCERATION

	Ischemic	Venous stasis
Location	Toe, heel, foot	Medial distal leg
Pain	Severe	Only when infected
Surrounding skin	± inflamed	Stasis pigmentation
Ulcer edge	Discrete	Shaggy
Ulcer base	Pale, eschar	Healthy

TABLE 4 OFFICE ESTIMATION OF THE DEGREE OF ISCHEMIA			
Degree	Elevation pallor, sec*	CR, sec†	VFT, sec‡
None	None in 60	10	15
Moderate	Pallor in 30–60	15–20	20–30
Severe	Pallor in < 30	40+	40+

*Elevation of extremity at an angle of 60° above level.
†Color return (CR) to skin of foot on dependency after elevation.
‡Superficial venous filling time (VFT) on dependency after elevation.

Allen test (Fig. 2) to evaluate circulation in the hand and the thoracic outlet maneuvers (Fig. 3) are useful when occlusive arterial disease is present.

When taken with the patient supine using a standard blood pressure cuff and a handheld continuous-wave Doppler, the systolic brachial and ankle blood pressures provide an objective measure of lower extremity arterial circulation. Normally, the systolic blood pressure at the ankle exceeds that at the brachial level. When these pressures are determined before and after standard exercise (Table 5), functional as well as semiquantitative assessment of the occlusive arterial disease can be made. Arteriography is usually not needed unless restoration of pulsatile flow is being considered or some unusual type of occlusive arterial disease is suspected.

Differential diagnosis

As noted, arteriosclerosis is by far the most common cause of occlusive peripheral arterial disease. Uncommon types of occlusive arterial disease are suggested by their occurrence in young persons, acute (often digital) ischemia, or associated systemic symptoms.

Arteriosclerosis is more common in men over 40 years of age, particularly those with the risk factors of tobacco use, hyperlipidemia, or diabetes mellitus. It affects large- and medium-sized extremity arteries as well as the coronary and cerebral arteries.

Less common types of occlusive peripheral arterial disease include thromboangiitis obliterans (Buerger's disease), traumatic (repetitive, blunt-type) occlusive arterial disease in the hand, occlusive disease caused by compression of a peripheral artery (popliteal artery entrapment [Table 6] and thoracic outlet compression of the subclavian artery), and the arteritides (giant cell arteritis and connective tissue disorders). In connective tissue disorders, the occlusive disease is usually digital. Giant cell (temporal, cranial) arteritis affects persons over 60 years of age whose dominant symptoms are headache and those of a systemic illness, whereas Takayasu's arteritis typically affects the branches of the aortic arch in young women.

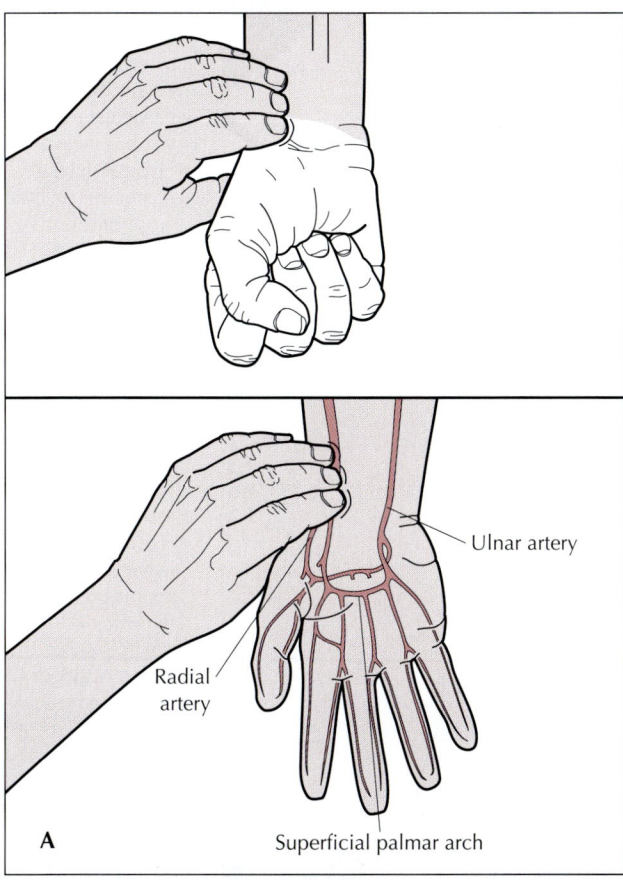

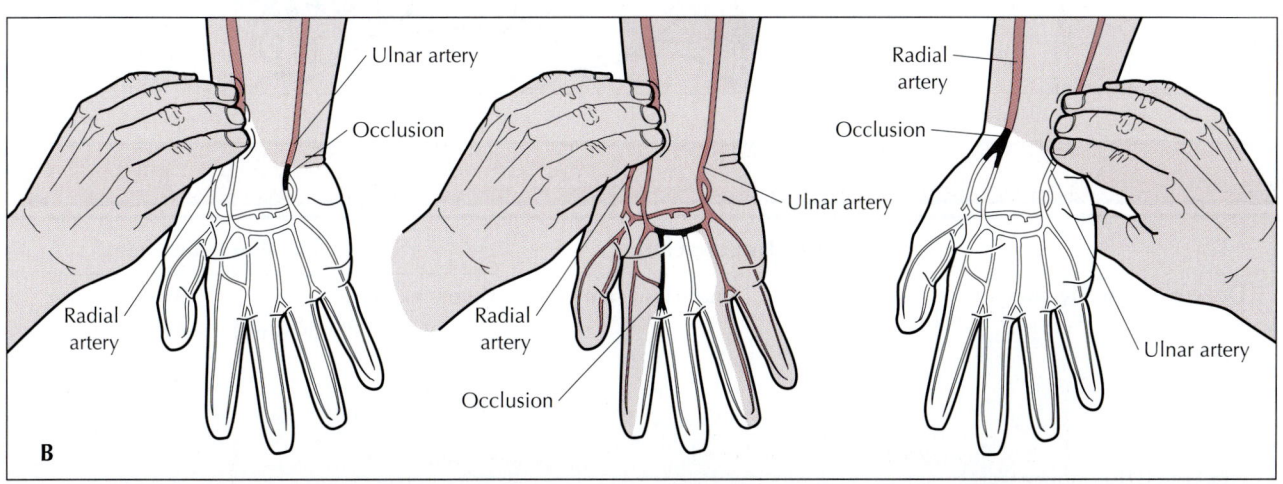

FIGURE 2 Allen test. **A,** Normal (negative) result, indicating patency of ulnar artery and superficial palmar arch. **B,** Abnormal (positive) results caused by occlusion of ulnar artery (*left*), superficial palmar arch (*bottom center*), and radial artery (*right*). (*From* Spittell [13]; with permission.)

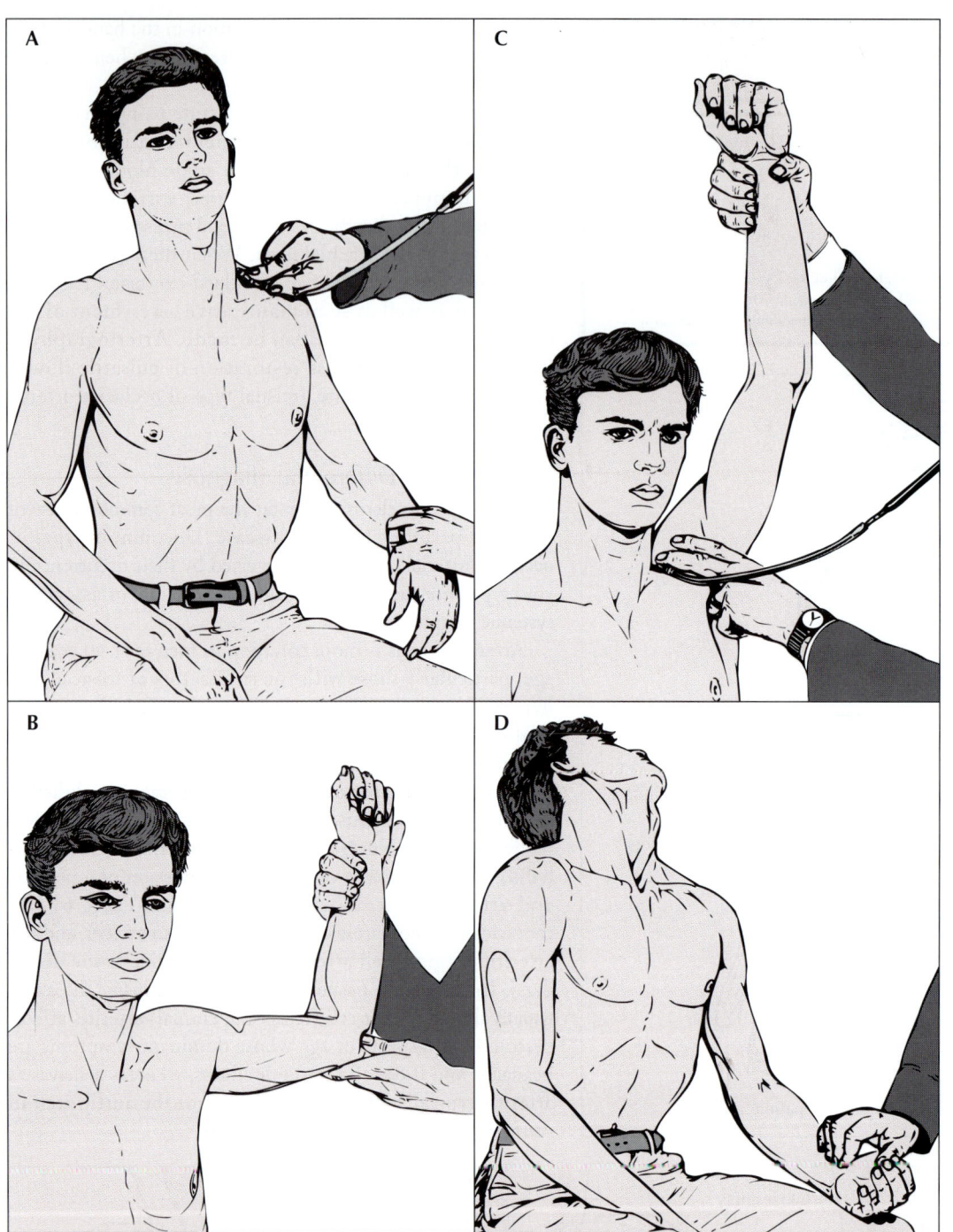

FIGURE 3 A, Costoclavicular maneuver, active. Auscultation over subclavian artery, above or below midportion of clavicle, may reveal systolic bruit as artery is compressed. Radial pulse and bruit over subclavian artery disappear when complete compression of subclavian artery occurs. **B,** Costoclavicular maneuver, passive. **C,** Hyperabduction maneuver. Axillary artery may be completely or incompletely compressed. In the latter case, bruit may be heard above or below the clavicle or, on occasion, deep in the axilla. **D,** Scalene or Adson maneuver. This test is used in both cervical rib or anomalous first thoracic rib syndrome and scalenus anticus syndrome. Auscultation over subclavian artery being tested may reveal bruit when the artery is partially compressed. (*From* Fairbairn and coworkers [14]; with permission.)

TABLE 5 NONINVASIVE LABORATORY ASSESSMENT OF ARTERIAL INSUFFICIENCY OF LEGS

	Standard exercise		Systolic blood pressure index*	
Degree of insufficiency	Claudication	Duration, *min*	Before exercise	After exercise
Minimal	0	5	Normal to mildly abnormal	Abnormal
Mild	Present	5	> 0.8	> 0.5
Moderate	Present	< 5	< 0.8	< 0.5
Severe†	Present	< 3	< 0.5	< 0.15

From Spittell [12]; with permission.

*Systolic pressure index is obtained by dividing the systolic ankle blood pressure by the systolic brachial blood pressure, both measured with the patient supine (normal, 0.95 or greater).

†Often, the systolic ankle blood pressure is less than 50 mm Hg.

TABLE 6 CLINICAL FEATURES OF LESS COMMON TYPES OF OCCLUSIVE PERIPHERAL ARTERIAL DISEASE

Thromboangiitis obliterans (Buerger's disease)
Men affected more than women
Tobacco use
Age < 30 y
Small arteries upper and lower extremities involved
Claudication of arch or calf
Migratory superficial phlebitis common

Occlusive arterial disease of hands from repetitive blunt trauma
Often occupational—tools, "hammerhand"
Dominant hand
Tobacco use (predisposing factor)

Popliteal artery entrapment
Young men affected more than women
Symptoms unilateral
Calf pain with walking not running
Decreased or absent pedal pulses
Diagnosis by arteriography

Prognosis

Survival of persons with arteriosclerosis is shortened because of associated coronary and cerebral artery disease. The risk of limb loss for the person without diabetes whose only symptom is intermittent claudication is approximately 5% in 5 years; when the ischemia is more severe (ischemic pain at rest or ischemic ulcer), the risk is approximately 12% in 5 years [3]. When arteriosclerosis obliterans (ASO) is symptomatic in the person with diabetes, the prognosis for limb loss is approximately fourfold that of the person without diabetes [4].

In thromboangiitis obliterans, the risk of limb loss is greater than in ASO. It depends mainly on the severity of the ischemia at the time of diagnosis and whether the patient stops using tobacco permanently.

In chronic occlusive arterial disease caused by repetitive, blunt trauma to the hand, loss of digits can occur if the cause is not recognized and corrected (Fig. 4). Limb or digital loss can occur with arterial compression syndromes as a result of embolization from mural thrombus that develops in the poststenotic aneurysm because of chronic arterial compression. In occlusive arterial disease caused by arteritis, frequency of limb loss depends on the severity of ischemia at the time of diagnosis and how much control over the arteritis is achieved.

Management

Definitive management of chronic occlusive arterial disease should be individualized according to its etiology, severity, disability, and prognosis, but the physician should have all patients take general measures to protect the ischemic limb from trauma and avoid vasoconstrictive influences. These general measures include the following:

1. Stop tobacco use,
2. Avoid trauma,
3. Wear proper footwear,
4. Attend to regular foot care and hygiene,
5. Walk on a regular basis,
6. Avoid vasoconstriction, and
7. Control atherosclerosis risk factors.

For all persons, conservative measures are indicated; control of risk factors (hyperlipidemia, hypertension, and diabetes) is indicated to delay progression of the atherosclerosis. The importance of discontinuing tobacco use should be emphasized. Continued smoking increases the risk of limb loss tenfold [3]. A regular walking program may increase the walking distance, and a trial of pentoxifylline [5] may provide additional symptomatic relief of intermittent claudication. Careful attention to foot care and hygiene as well as selection of proper footwear is important. In the management of associated coronary and hypertension disease, drugs that may cause vasoconstriction (β-blockers and clonidine) are best avoided when alternative agents can be safely used.

In persons with traumatic occlusive disease, measures to protect the hand (regular use of gloves and avoiding blunt trauma) in addition to general measures are important to

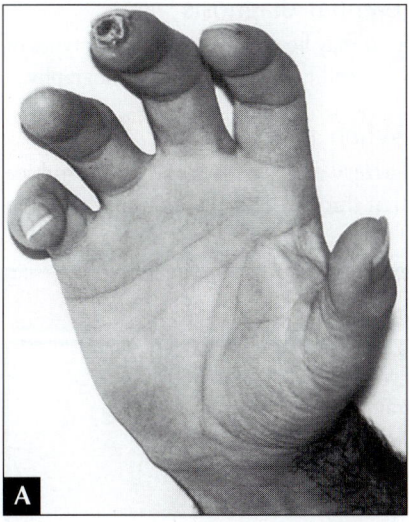
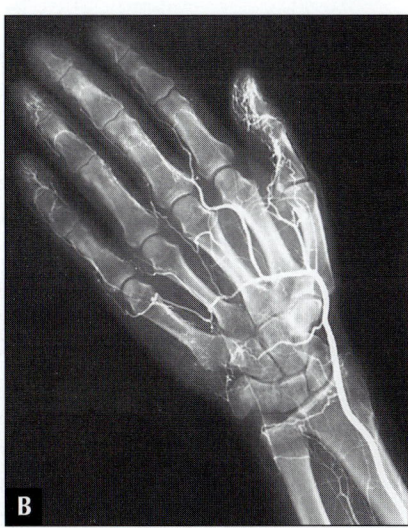

FIGURE 4 Right hand of a 42-year-old, right-handed millwright. **A,** Ischemic ulceration of the finger. **B,** Arteriogram showing a narrowed ulnar artery and occlusion of the ulnar portion of the superficial palmar arch.

prevent progression. If ischemic ulceration has already occurred, an α-blocking agent or sympathectomy can be used to hasten healing and provide longer-term protection of the ischemic digit [6]. When occlusive arterial disease is caused by arteritis, management should include therapy of the systemic process and general measures to protect the ischemic limb.

When to refer

In symptomatic arteriosclerosis obliterans, restoration of pulsatile flow by either arterial surgery or percutaneous angioplasty can be used to relieve disabling claudication in the nondiabetic person. It is also indicated (when feasible) for the management of ischemic rest pain, ischemic ulceration, and symptomatic occlusive arterial disease in persons with diabetes. The frequency of coronary artery disease as a comorbid condition must always be kept in mind during preoperative evaluation and risk stratification if restoration of pulsatile flow is planned for persons with atherosclerotic occlusive peripheral arterial disease [7•]. The appropriate management of arterial compression syndromes is surgical relief.

Acute Peripheral Arterial Occlusion

Acute occlusion of a peripheral artery can be thrombotic or embolic. Symptoms can be dramatic with one or all of the five *P*s (pain, pallor, paresthesia, paralysis, and pulseless) or may be more subtle (*eg*, abrupt onset of intermittent claudication or shortening of walking distance in a person with existing claudication). The distinction between embolic and thrombotic arterial occlusion is frequently inferential (Table 7) but may be important, as either type can be a clue to an otherwise occult systemic or cardiovascular disorder.

Differential diagnosis

The differential diagnosis of acute peripheral arterial occlusion includes arterial spasm from drugs (*eg*, ergotism) or associated with extensive, acute, deep venous thrombosis.

Management

Initial management of acute arterial occlusion should include protection of the ischemic limb (do not heat, cool, or elevate) and heparin therapy to protect the collateral circulation while the etiology is being determined. Definitive management options include surgical thromboembolectomy, thrombolytic therapy, or antithrombotic therapy. Factors influencing the choice of therapy include size of the artery occluded, condition of the limb, etiology of the occlusion, and the general and cardiac status of the patient.

Atheroembolism from proximal aortic or arterial atherosclerotic plaques or aneurysms is now being recognized with increasing frequency as a result of improving noninvasive imaging techniques, particularly transesophageal echocardiography [8]. Features suggestive of atheroembolism includes livedo reticularis, cyanotic digits, hypertension, renal insufficiency, transient eosinophilia, and an elevated sedimentation rate.

When to refer

Management is difficult unless the origin of the atheroembolic material can be surgically removed.

Peripheral Arterial Aneurysm

Like occlusive peripheral arterial disease, arterial aneurysms are most often atherosclerotic, more frequent in lower than in upper extremity arteries, and much more common in men than in women.

Diagnosis

Until an aneurysm becomes symptomatic as a result of complications (Table 8), the diagnosis depends on a careful physical examination or incidental recognition on radiography or ultrasonography performed for some other reason. Iliac artery aneurysms are usually associated with abdominal aortic aneurysms. Symptomatic iliac artery aneurysms may cause groin or perineal pain, iliac vein obstruction, or obstructive urologic symptoms [9].

Aneurysms of the femoral and popliteal arteries rarely occur in women. Popliteal aneurysms are bilateral approximately 50% of the time, and in over 40% of cases, they are associated with aneurysms elsewhere in the body, most often the abdominal area.

Differential diagnosis

Peripheral artery aneurysm may be confused with other types of mass, but differentiation is readily made with ultrasonography.

When to refer

Untreated peripheral artery aneurysms frequently produce complications, most often thromboembolic, that may threaten

TABLE 7 ACUTE ARTERIAL OCCLUSION
Conditions suggesting embolic arterial occlusion
Heart failure
Atrial fibrillation
Recent myocardial infarction
Proximal atherosclerosis
Proximal arterial aneurysm
Conditions suggesting thrombotic arterial occlusion
Symptomatic peripheral arterial disease
Acute arterial trauma
Myeloproliferative disease
Active arteritis
Acute aortic dissection

TABLE 8 COMPLICATIONS OF ANEURYSMS
Pressure on surrounding structures
Thrombosis
Distal embolization
Rupture
Infection

the limb, so elective surgical treatment before complications occur gives the best results. Arteriography before surgery is needed to evaluate the arterial circulation proximal and distal to the aneurysm.

DISEASES OF VEINS

Clinicians are appropriately most interested in acute deep venous thrombosis because of its embolic potential, but other disorders of veins (varicose veins and chronic venous insufficiency) are frequent causes of complications and morbidity, much of which can be prevented by proper management.

Venous Thrombosis

Both superficial and deep venous thrombosis are important clinical events from both the diagnostic and therapeutic aspects.

Diagnosis

Superficial thrombophlebitis, presenting as a reddened, tender nodule or cord in the course of a superficial vein, is readily diagnosed on physical examination. Deep venous thrombosis, however, is notorious for its variable clinical manifestations depending on the location and extent of the venous occlusion. Symptoms may include pain or swelling in the limb, and findings on physical examination may include tenderness over the involved vein and, when proximal to the calf, pitting edema distally and increased superficial (collateral) venous pattern.

The variability of clinical findings have made duplex ultrasonography the diagnostic procedure of choice in proximal deep vein thrombosis [10•], but when only calf veins are involved, contrast venography remains the diagnostic gold standard. Impedance plethysmography is a useful noninvasive diagnostic test for deep vein obstruction, particularly in cases of recurrent proximal deep venous thrombosis.

Differential diagnosis

Superficial thrombophlebitis is easily differentiated from acute lymphangitis, because the latter is accompanied by chills and high fever. Occasionally, nodular conditions (erythema nodosum or vasculitis) require biopsy to confidently differentiate them.

Deep venous thrombosis involves a much more complicated differential diagnosis that includes nonthrombotic (chronic) venous obstruction, sciatica, muscle strain or tear, and acute lymphangitis and cellulitis. Unless physical findings or noninvasive diagnostic studies permit confident differential diagnosis, contrast venography is necessary.

Management

Therapy of superficial thrombophlebitis is basically symptomatic: local warm moist packs, analgesics, and elevation of the extremity. If the process extends despite such treatment, a short course of oral anticoagulant therapy may be used to effect resolution.

Therapy for acute deep venous thrombosis continues to be heparin initially, followed by oral anticoagulant therapy for 3 or preferably 6 months. Thrombolytic therapy is usually reserved for acute, extensive, deep venous thrombosis (*eg*, axillary subclavian vein thrombosis or phlegmasia cerulea dolens [Fig. 5] in young persons to obtain rapid resolution and lessen the chances of venous valvular damage). Anticoagulant therapy must be instituted as soon as thrombolytic therapy ends so as to prevent rethrombosis. An algorithm for management of the patient with suspected deep venous thrombosis is shown in Figure 6.

Recurring superficial or deep venous thrombosis is an important clinical problem, both diagnostically and therapeutically. Causes that need to be considered are shown in Table 9. Oral anticoagulant therapy provides effective management of the primary types and coagulation disorders, but particularly in secondary types, recurrences may occur despite adequate oral anticoagulant therapy.

When to refer

Superficial phlebitis of a varicose vein is generally an indication for surgical removal.

Chronic Venous Insufficiency

An important and often neglected sequel of deep venous thrombosis is chronic deep venous insufficiency resulting from postphlebitic venous stasis. Regular use of properly fitted, adequate (30 to 40 mm Hg compression at the ankle) elastic stockings can prevent complications of chronic venous insufficiency.

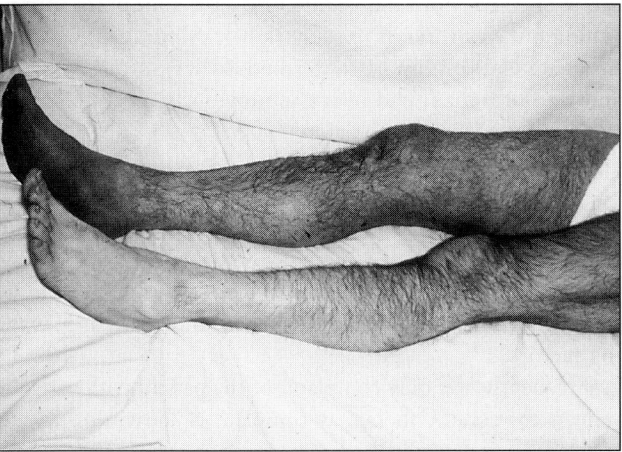

FIGURE 5 Phlegmasia cerulea dolens (extensive venous thrombosis of the whole right lower extremity).

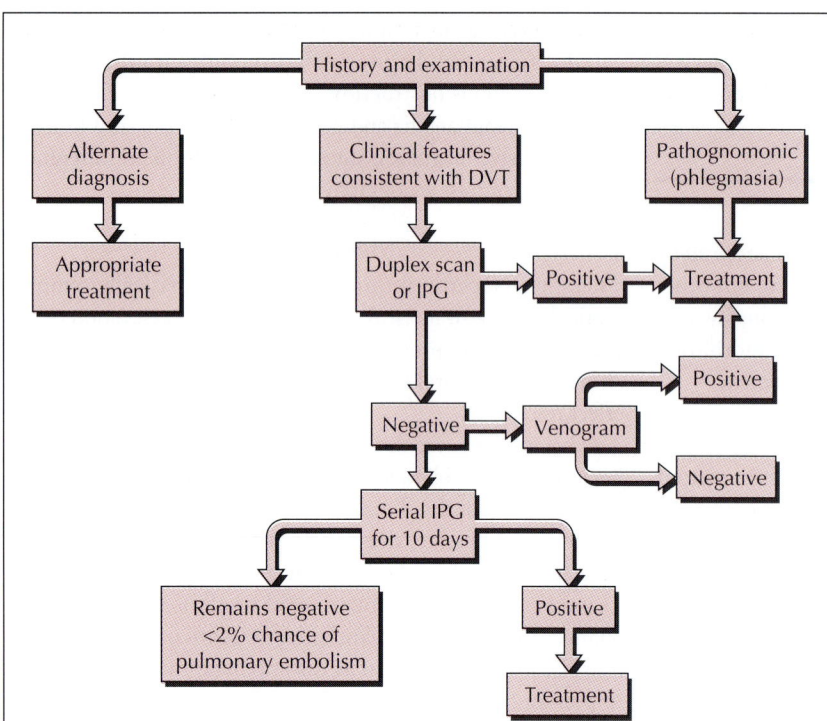

FIGURE 6 Algorithm for clinically suspected deep venous thrombosis (DVT). IPG—impedance plethysmography.

TABLE 9 RECURRENT VENOUS THROMBOSIS	

Primary (idiopathic)
 Familial
 Nonfamilial
 	
 Secondary
 Thromboangiitis obliterans
 Ulcerative bowel disease
 Myeloproliferative disease
 Connective tissue disease
 Oral contraceptives
 Neoplasms
	Coagulation Disorders
	 Hereditary
	   Antithrombin III deficiency
	   Protein C deficiency
	   Protein S deficiency
	   Dysfibrinoginemia
	 Acquired antiphospholipid
	   antibody syndromes
	   Circulating anticoagulant
	     with systemic lupus
	   Nonlupus types

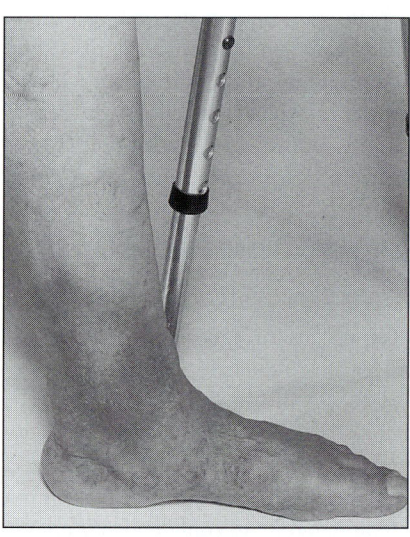

FIGURE 7 Chronic indurated cellulitis.

The generalist is likely to be consulted by the patient who develops chronic tender induration of the medial distal leg because of uncontrolled chronic deep venous insufficiency (Fig. 7). The reddened, tender, indurated features of this complication (termed *lipodermatosclerosis* or *chronic indurated cellulitis*) suggest infection, but the problem is chronic venous stasis and its management the use of adequate support (Fig. 8) when the patient is ambulatory. The process gradually recedes with use of good elastic support over a foam pad for a period of several weeks. When resolved, recurrence can be prevented by the regular, daily use of adequate elastic support when ambulatory.

Venous stasis ulceration (Fig. 9), when early and small (< 1.0 cm), often can be managed on an ambulatory basis with the same type of elastic support described for chronic indurated cellulitis applied over a sterile dressing. Larger stasis ulcers are best managed by rest and elevation with moist dressings (sterile normal saline or 0.25% aluminum subacetate) until clean and, if needed, skin grafting. After healing, adequate elastic support (described earlier), often with the addition of a foam pad over the previously ulcerated area, should be used when ambulatory.

Varicose Veins

Varicose veins are the most common venous disorder seen by the generalist. They may be primary or secondary to postphlebitic chronic deep venous insufficiency. Obesity, pregnancy, and right heart failure are aggravating factors.

Frequently, the only complaint of the patient with varicose veins is cosmetic. Others may complain of "heaviness" in the affected leg or dependent edema.

Distinction between primary and secondary varicose veins is important if surgical treatment is being considered. Associated chronic deep venous insufficiency can be identified by Doppler ultrasonography of deep veins if surgical treatment of the varicose veins is an option.

Management

Use of adequate elastic support is indicated for asymptomatic primary varicose veins and for those associated with chronic deep venous insufficiency. Sclerotherapy may be used for minor primary varicose veins and for cutaneous venous stars.

When to refer

Surgical treatment (stripping) is indicated for primary varicose veins causing symptoms or venous stasis that is not controlled with elastic support and when there is acute superficial varicose vein thrombophlebitis. Surgery is also indicated to remove large varicosities for cosmetic reasons.

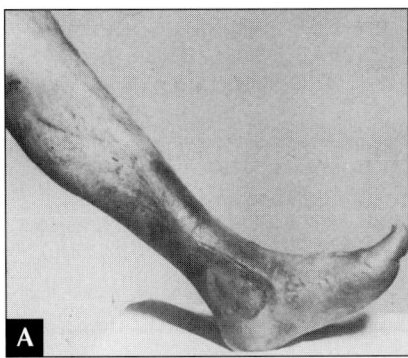
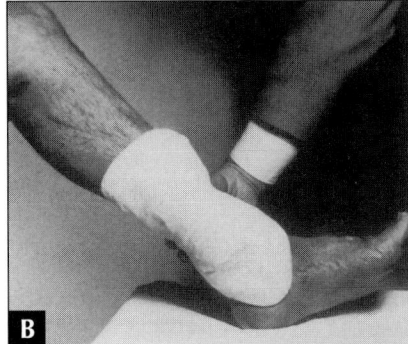
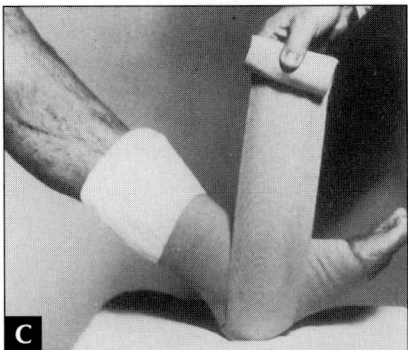
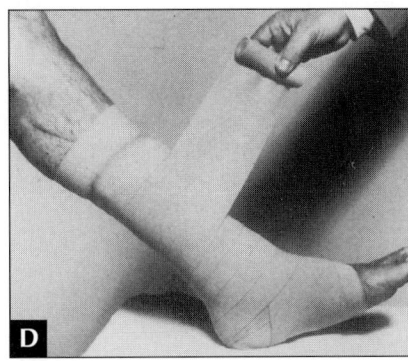

FIGURE 8 A–D, Application of foam pad under bandage for treatment of chronic indurated cellulitis or small venous stasis ulceration (*From* Juergens and Lofgren [16]; with permission.)

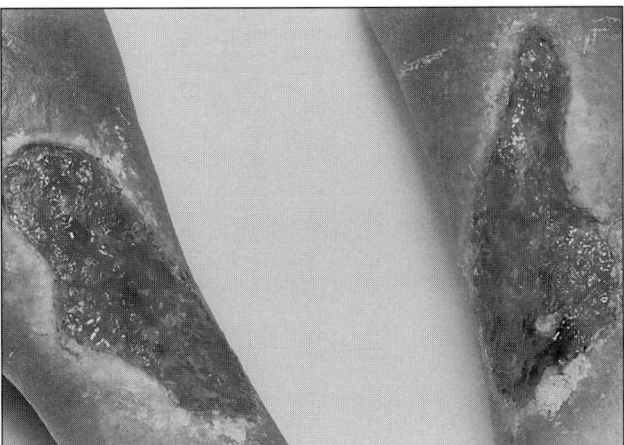

FIGURE 9 Large venous stasis ulcerations of both lower extremities.

References and Recommended Reading

Recently published papers of particular interest have been highlighted as:
- Of interest
- •• Of outstanding interest

1.•• Spittell JA Jr: Diagnosis and management of occlusive peripheral arterial disease. *Curr Probl Cardiol* 1990, 15:1–35.
2. Spittell JA Jr: Some uncommon types of occlusive peripheral arterial disease. *Curr Probl Cardiol* 1983, 8:3–35.
3. McDaniel MD, Cronenwett JL: Basic data related to natural history of intermittent claudication. *Ann Vasc Surg* 1989, 3:273–277.
4. Reiber GE, Pecoraro RE, Koepsell TD: Risk factors for amputation in patients with diabetes. *Ann Intern Med* 1992, 117:97–105.
5. Lindgarde F, Jehres R, Bjorkman H, *et al.*: Conservative drug treatments in patients with moderately severe chronic occlusive peripheral arterial disease. *Circulation* 1989, 80:1549–1556.
6. Spittell PC, Spittell JA Jr: Occlusive arterial disease of the hand due to repetitive blunt trauma. *Int J Cardiol* 1993, 38:281–292.
7.• Gersh BJ, Rihal CS, Rooke TW, Ballard DJ: Evaluation and management of patients with both peripheral vascular and coronary artery disease. *J Am Coll Cardiol* 1991, 18:203–214.
8. Tunick PA, Rosenzweig BP, Katz ES *et al*: High risk for vascular events in patients with protruding aortic atheromas: prospective study. *J Am Coll Card* 1994;23:1085–1090.
9. Lipoff O, Hoover EL, Diaz C, *et al.*: Initial report of a mycotic aneurysm of the common iliac artery with compression of the ipsilateral ureter and femoral vein. *Texas Heart Inst J* 1986, 13:321–324.
10.• Heliboer H, Bueller HR, Lansing AWA, *et al.*: A comparison of real-time compression ultrasonography with impedance plethysmography for the diagnosis of deep-vein thrombosis in symptomatic outpatients. *N Engl J Med* 1993, 329:1365–1369.
11. Fontaine R, Kreay R, Gaugloff JM, *et al.*: Long-term results of restorative arterial surgery in obstructive diseases of the arteries. *J Cardiovasc Surg* 1964, 5:463–472.
12. Spittell JA Jr: Recognition and management of chronic atherosclerotic occlusive peripheral arterial disease. *Mod Concepts Cardiovasc Dis* 1981, 50:19–23.
13. Spittell JA Jr: Occlusive peripheral arterial disease: guidelines for office management. *Postgrad Med* 1982, 71:137–151.
14. Fairbairn JF II: Clinical manifestations of peripheral vascular disease. In *Peripheral Vascular Diseases*, edn 5. Edited by Juergens JL, Spittell JA Jr, Fairbairn JF II. Philadelphia: WB Saunders; 1972:4–25.
15. Verstraete M. The diagnosis and treatment of deep-vein thrombosis. *N Engl J Med* 1993; 329:1418–1419.
16. Juergens JL, Lofgren KA: Chronic venous insufficiency. In *Peripheral Vascular Disease*, edn 5. Edited by Juergens JL, Spittel JA Jr, Fairbairn JF II. Philadelphia: WB Saunders; 1980:820.

Select Bibliography

Bergan JJ, Yao JST: *Venous Disorders*. Philadelphia: WB Saunders; 1991.

Spittell JA Jr: *Contemporary Issues in Peripheral Vascular Disease. Cardiovascular Clinics*. Philadelphia: FA Davis; 1992.

Young JR, Graor RA, Olin JO, Bartholemew JR: *Peripheral Vascular Diseases*. St. Louis: Mosby–Year Book; 1991.

Cerebrovascular Complications of Cardiac Disorders

Seemant Chaturvedi
Marc Fisher

> **Key Points**
> - Many cardiac conditions are associated with cerebral embolism.
> - Patent foramen ovale and aortic arch plaques are receiving increased attention as embolic sources.
> - Transesophageal echocardiography can increase the yield of embolism source detection.
> - Warfarin is effective in primary and secondary prevention in nonvalvular atrial fibrillation.
> - There is a small risk of brain hemorrhage with coronary artery thrombolysis.

The relationship between cardiac disorders and stroke has become increasingly evident. A wide variety of cardiac abnormalities are associated with an enhanced potential for stroke occurrence. In addition, diagnostic and therapeutic modalities used in cardiology can contribute to cerebral ischemia or hemorrhage. Further adding to the cardiac-cerebrovascular link is the possibility that many of the therapeutic approaches employed for the treatment of acute myocardial ischemia may be relevant for acute ischemic stroke.

CARDIAC SOURCES OF STROKE

Cardioembolic stroke has assumed increasing importance as diagnostic advances for detecting cardiac sources for emboli have progressed. Currently, a cardioembolic source for stroke is recognized in 15% to 20% of the approximately 500,000 new strokes per year that occur in the United States. This percentage is even higher in younger stroke patients (*ie*, those younger than 50 years of age). Potential cardiac sources of emboli are shown in Figure 1, and the frequency of emboli attributed to various sources is shown in Figure 2.

Formation of intracardiac thrombi related to stasis, endothelial disruption, valvular abnormalities, and right-to-left shunts are common mechanisms for embolization in these disparate conditions. These cardiac emboli typically lodge in an intracranial vessel equal to their diameter at right angles to a larger parent artery, causing a clinical stroke syndrome related to the region of ischemic injury (Fig. 3). Cardioembolic stroke is the most likely diagnosis in a stroke patient who has a recognized cardiac disorder, associated embolization, and the abrupt onset of neurologic deficits. Supportive evidence includes the presence of prior or concurrent emboli in other organs or cerebral vascular territories and angiographic demonstration of vascular branch occlusion. The presence of a potential cardiac source for emboli does not conclusively establish the diagnosis of cardioembolic stroke because other potential stroke sources, such as large artery atherosclerosis or small intracranial vessel disease, are also present in approximately 33% of such patients. Therefore, the clinical diagnosis of cardioembolic source remains an educated guess. In reviewing the various

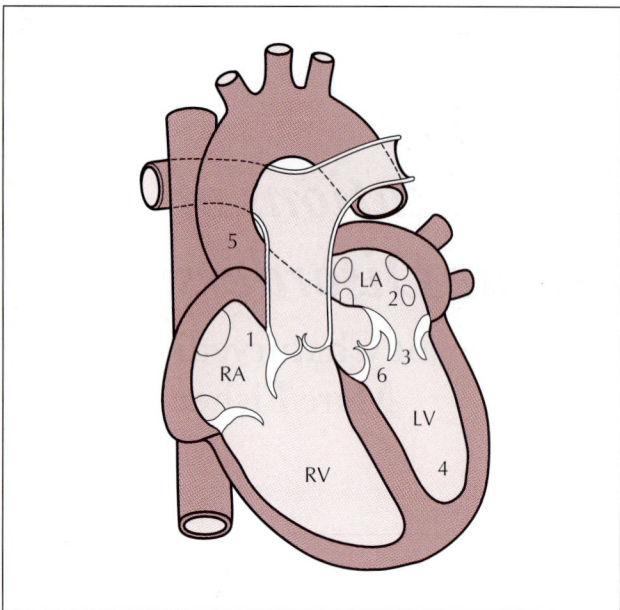

FIGURE 1 Sources of cardiogenic emboli: 1, paradoxical emboli (patent foramen ovale); 2, left atrium (LA) (atrial fibrillation, myxoma); 3, mitral valve (endocarditis, mitral valve prolapse, annulus calcification, prosthetic valve, other vegetations); 4, left ventricle (LV) (dyskinesia or akinesia, cardiomyopathy); 5, aorta (plaques); 6, aortic valve (endocarditis, prosthetic valve). RA—right atrium; RV—right ventricle.

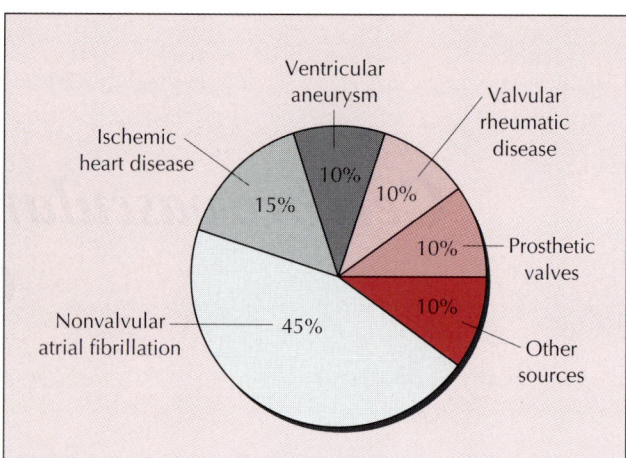

FIGURE 2 Sources of cardioembolism.

etiologies for cardioembolic stroke, it is helpful to consider high-risk and medium-risk sources (Table 1).

High-Risk Sources

Nonvalvular atrial fibrillation (NVAF) is the most common cardiac disorder that predisposes to stroke occurrence. It is common in the elderly, and the annual stroke risk in untreated patients is approximately 5% (range 3% to 8%). The Stroke Prevention in Atrial Fibrillation (SPAF) investigators attempted to define clinical and echocardiographic features that would be indicative of increased embolic risk. Clinically, recent congestive heart failure (within 3 months), hypertension, and previous thromboembolism noticeably augmented the likelihood of peripheral embolization [1•]. Echocardiographically, left ventricular dysfunction and a dilated left atrium constituted the main predictive factors [2•]. Younger patients (< 60 years) without clinical risk factors made up a distinctly lower risk group. Acute myocardial infarction (MI) is associated with stroke development in approximately 1% of cases. Patients with transmural anterior wall MI have the greatest risk for thrombus formation and stroke occurrence. Most emboli occur within 4 weeks after the MI. The risk lessens 4 weeks to 6 months after MI, although at later dates akinetic ventricular segments and left ventricular aneurysms assume greater importance.

Rheumatic valvular disease has decreased in developed countries but remains an important source for stroke in developing countries. Rheumatic mitral valve disease has the highest inci-

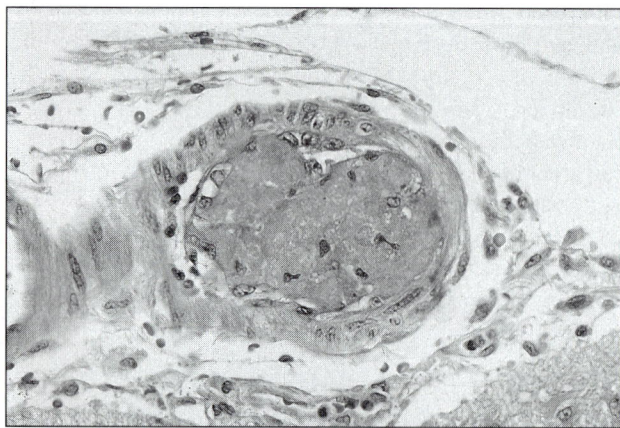

FIGURE 3 Embolus obstructing a cortical vessel.

TABLE 1 SOURCES OF CARDIOEMBOLIC STROKE
High-risk sources
Mechanical prosthetic valves
Mitral stenosis with atrial fibrillation
Atrial fibrillation
Left atrial thrombus
Sick sinus syndrome
Recent myocardial infarction (< 4 wk)
Left ventricular thrombus
Dilated cardiomyopathy
Akinetic segment
Myxoma
Infective endocarditis
Medium-risk sources
Mitral valve prolapse
Mitral annulus calcification
Mitral stenosis without atrial fibrillation
Patent foramen ovale
Nonbacterial thrombotic endocarditis
Hypokinetic segment
Myocardial infarction (> 4 wk, < 6 mo)

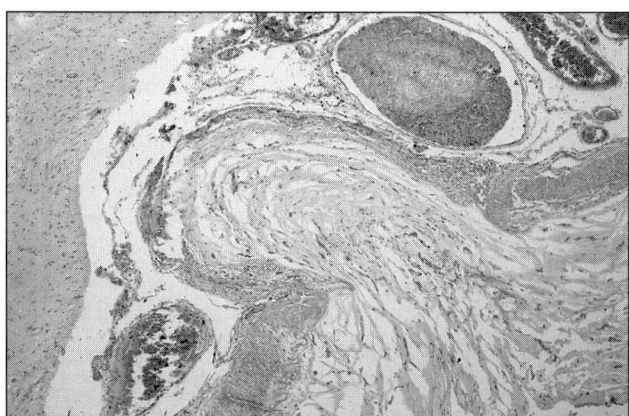

FIGURE 4 Myxomatous tissue within a cerebral vessel.

dence of systemic embolism among common forms of heart disease, and it is generally accepted that long-term anticoagulation is effective in lowering the frequency of systemic emboli.

Prosthetic cardiac valves remain an important source of cardiac stroke development, despite advances in valve design. Mechanical valves pose a greater embolic threat than do biologic valves.

Infective endocarditis is a significant source of cardioembolic stroke in both young patients and the elderly. In one series of 203 patients, brain ischemia occurred in 19% of patients [3]. Echocardiographically documented vegetations did not always correlate with stroke risk. Most strokes occurred at the time of presentation, and recurrent strokes were uncommon if the primary infection was controlled.

Patients with sick sinus syndrome also have a substantial risk for stroke, and it is unclear if cardiac pacing reduces this risk. In one report of 10 patients who developed ischemic strokes following pacemaker placement, the high-risk patients appeared to be those who converted to AF in the presence of a ventricular demand pacer [4].

Two less-common entities that can still have a high rate of embolization are dilated cardiomyopathy and left atrial myxoma. In dilated cardiomyopathy, globally impaired ventricular performance promotes stasis and thrombus formation. The annual rate of embolization has been estimated at 3.5% [5].

Atrial myxomas are the most common primary cardiac tumors, and they are often quite friable (Fig. 4). Myxoma-related stroke occurs most often in persons ranging from 30 to 60 years of age, and recurrent emboli before surgery are common (Fig. 5) [6]. Anticoagulation is not always successful in preventing reembolization.

Medium-Risk Sources

Mitral valve prolapse (MVP) is a common, although heterogeneous, condition. It is estimated to have a prevalence of 5% in the general population [7]. Studies of stroke in young adults have had widely differing figures, ranging from 2% to more than 30% of strokes attributable to MVP. Certain subgroups of patients are believed to be at increased risk for developing infective endocarditis or peripheral embolization, or both (*eg*, men older than 45 years of age with systolic murmurs and patients with myxomatous degeneration of the valve leaflets and chordae).

Nonbacterial thrombotic endocarditis, or marantic endocarditis, is believed to be the most common cause of stroke in the cancer patient, at least based on autopsy studies [8]. This condition is characterized by the deposition of small, sterile thrombi on valves and may be responsible for multiple focal deficits in patients with neoplasms.

Recently, two new sources for embolic stroke—one in the heart and the other in the thoracic aorta—have been recognized. Paradoxical emboli were thought to be a rare cause of stroke; however, several studies in younger stroke patients employing contrast echocardiography have demonstrated that a patent foramen ovale (PFO) is four to five times more common in stroke patients than in age-matched controls. The prevalence of PFO is highest in those stroke patients who have no other obvious source for their stroke. One study compared the echocardiograms of patients with stroke of determined origin with those of patients with cryptogenic stroke [9]. In both the younger (< 55 years) and older age groups, a PFO was significantly more common in patients with cryptogenic stroke (48% vs 4% and 38% vs 8%, respectively). The presence of a PFO in a patient with an otherwise unexplained stroke certainly suggests a relationship, but conclusively establishing that paradoxical embolization has occurred remains difficult. The presence of venous or cardiac thrombus would be supportive.

Elevation of the right heart pressure is another related factor to paradoxical embolization with PFO, and the patient should be carefully questioned for any Valsalva-like episode before stroke onset. The natural history of recurrent stroke in patients with PFO is uncertain. The most appropriate inter-

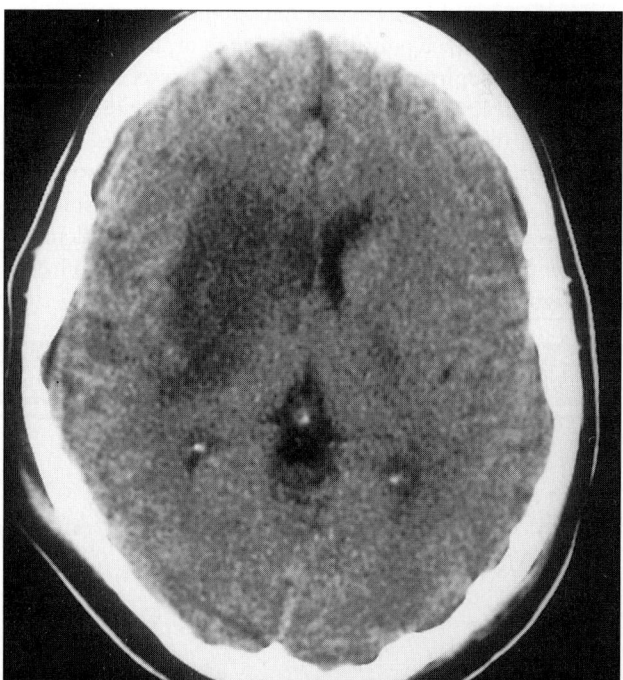

FIGURE 5 Computed tomography scan of a young woman with myxoma-related stroke.

vention is also uncertain because only anecdotal information is currently available, but we currently recommend antiplatelet agents as initial therapy unless there is documented venous thrombosis.

Ulcerated plaques in the aortic arch (AA) are the other recently recognized source of cerebral emboli that can be classified as a pericardiac disorder. Previously, isolated case reports suggested the potential relationship between ulcerated plaques in the AA and embolic stroke. A more comprehensive, recent study evaluated the autopsies of 500 patients with neurologic disease [10]. It was found that 26% of cerebrovascular disease patients had AA plaques, whereas it was present only in 5% of controls with other neurologic disorders. In stroke patients with no other recognized cause, 61% had an ulcerated AA, as compared with 22% of stroke patients with another potential source.

Transesophageal echocardiography can evaluate the AA and detect ulcerated plaques, providing a relatively simple method to detect this potential source for embolic stroke. Information concerning the natural history and best therapeutic approach for stroke related to ulcerated AA plaques is not currently available.

The capability to noninvasively detect cardiac sources for embolic stroke has been the main reason for enhanced recognition of the relationship between the two disorders. Transthoracic echocardiography (TTE) is widely employed as an initial screening procedure to detect valvular heart disease, dyskinetic segments, intracardiac thrombi and masses, and cardiomyopathies. The addition of contrast agents, such as agitated saline, is helpful for detecting right-to-left shunts. However, TTE is relatively insensitive, especially for detecting thrombi and left atrial appendage abnormalities and for evaluating the atrial septum. Several studies have compared the diagnostic acumen of TTE with transesophageal echocardiography (TEE), which provides visualization of those abnormalities. Transesophageal echocardiography detects potential cardiac sources for emboli significantly better than TTE. However, the significance of some TEE findings, such as spontaneous left atrial contrast, is uncertain. The best way to employ TEE in the evaluation of patients with ischemic stroke is continuing to evolve, but it should be considered in younger patients without an obvious stroke source, who have a nondiagnostic TTE.

STROKE PREVENTION

The substantial stroke risk associated with untreated NVAF prompted five large treatment trials, and the results are now available [11•,12,13•,14,15]. In both the SPAF study and the Danish Atrial Fibrillation, Aspirin, Anticoagulation (AFASAK) study, patients were randomly assigned to receive warfarin, aspirin, or placebo; however, because the trial designs were different, a direct comparison of warfarin with aspirin is not possible. In AFASAK, eligible NVAF patients were assigned randomly to one of the three treatment groups. In SPAF, warfarin-eligible patients were assigned to anticoagulation or placebo, whereas warfarin-ineligible patients were assigned to aspirin or placebo. Both studies did demonstrate a significant reduction of ischemic stroke and systemic emboli by warfarin as compared with placebo (Table 2). In SPAF, 325 mg/d of aspirin also significantly reduced end-point occurrence, but in AFASAK, 75 mg/d of aspirin had no effect. A third open-label study, the Boston Area Anticoagulation Trial for Atrial Fibrillation (BAATAF), compared warfarin with placebo. The incidence of ischemic stroke was very low in the warfarin group, 0.4% per year, significantly less than the 3.0% per year rate in the placebo group. A fourth study, the Canadian Atrial Fibrillation Study (CAFA), which was double blind, was terminated early, but a nonsignificant trend for benefit with warfarin was observed. The observed rate of major hemorrhagic side effects ranged from 0.8% to 2.5% per year in these studies. Finally, in the Veterans Affairs study of 571 men, warfarin was compared with placebo, and the cerebral infarction rate in the warfarin group was notably decreased (0.9% per year vs 4.3%).

Taken together, these studies strongly support the beneficial effects of warfarin in low doses (international normalized ratio [INR] of 2.0 to 3.0, prothrombin time ratio of 1.2 to 1.5) to reduce primary stroke risk in NVAF patients. The role of aspirin in primary stroke prevention in NVAF has not been established, but the initial SPAF results suggest that it may be useful when 325 mg every day is prescribed in patients younger than the age of 70 to 75 years. A direct comparison between warfarin and aspirin by the SPAF investigators is in progress, and the results should be forthcoming. Secondary stroke prevention in NVAF patients who have already suffered an initial stroke is another important consideration.

TABLE 2 COMPARISON OF STUDIES OF WARFARIN FOR ISCHEMIC STROKE AND SYSTEMIC EMBOLI

				Outcome events per year		
Study	Patients, n	Men, %	Mean age, y	Warfarin vs control, %/%	Aspirin vs control, %/%	Major bleeds per year, %
AFASAK	1007	64	74	2.2/5.5	4.7/5.5	0.8
SPAF	1330	71	67	2.3/7.4	3.6/6.3	1.5
BAATAF	420	72	68	0.4/3.0	—	0.8
CAFA	378	75	68	3.0/4.6	—	2.5
VA	525	100	67	0.9/4.3	—	1.3

AFASAK—The Danish Atrial Fibrillation, Aspirin, Anticoagulation Study; BAATAF—The Boston Area Anticoagulation Trial for Atrial Fibrillation Study; CAFA—The Canadian Atrial Fibrillation Study; SPAF—The Stroke Prevention in Atrial Fibrillation Study.

The recently completed European Atrial Fibrillation Trial demonstrated the efficacy of warfarin in this setting as well, with a decrease in the annual stroke incidence from 12% in the placebo group to 4% in the warfarin group [16••].

Therapy with a low-to-moderate dose of warfarin is indicated in patients with AF who can tolerate this therapy. Patients who are not good candidates for anticoagulation or who do not wish to be placed on warfarin should consider aspirin (325 mg/d). Patients younger than 60 years of age with lone or paroxysmal AF should also consider aspirin use at this dosage [17•].

The role of warfarin and aspirin for primary stroke prevention in other cardiac disorders has not been as well studied. Warfarin is widely used in patients with rheumatic valvular disease and prosthetic cardiac valves.

Patients with acute anterior MI and documented ventricular thrombi are also at high risk, and anticoagulants are frequently employed. There have been reports of up to a 55% reduction in the cerebral infarction rate in MI patients treated with long-term warfarin after the acute phase, but this area remains somewhat controversial [18].

Anticoagulants are frequently employed in dilated cardiomyopathy (especially when the ejection fraction is less than 15%), although the need for a clinical trial to study this issue has been raised. The role of anticoagulation in paradoxical embolization, marantic endocarditis, ventricular aneurysms, and other less-common disorders remains uncertain.

CEREBROVASCULAR COMPLICATIONS OF CARDIAC THERAPY

Thrombolytic therapy is commonly and effectively used to treat patients with acute MI. A dreaded complication of thrombolytic therapy is the development of intracerebral hemorrhage. This complication, which occurs in 0.75% of patients, has been carefully studied in all clinical trials, and it appears that independent predictors of possible intracranial hemorrhage include the following: 1) age older than 65 years, 2) body weight less than 70 kg, 3) hypertension on hospital admission, 4) and administration of alteplase [19].

Stroke is an uncommon but devastating complication of coronary artery bypass graft (CABG) surgery. The risk of stroke is between 1% and 5% depending on the study surveyed. The mechanisms causing CABG-related stroke could be either hemodynamic or cardioembolic, with the latter being the more common cause. Patients with a history of prior stroke have an increased risk of cerebral infarction during CABG surgery [20••]. Potential embolic sources (such as a calcified aorta, ventricular thrombus, arrhythmias, and air in the heart or bypass line) must be assiduously watched for, and marked decreases in blood pressure are another obvious situation to be avoided.

CONCLUSION

We believe that every patient with cerebral ischemia (either transient or with a completed stroke) should be evaluated by a neurologist, because many neurologic conditions can produce the same symptom complex. In addition, diagnostic and therapeutic advances are occurring at a rapid rate in cerebrovascular disease, and a stroke neurologist would be best apprised of the most recent developments.

In terms of cardiogenic embolism, technologic advances have contributed to the increasing recognition of the interconnection between cardiac disorders and stroke. Perhaps many of the currently cryptogenic stroke cases will eventually be assigned to the category of cardioembolic stroke. The similarity between ischemic injury in the heart and the brain implies that therapeutic advances in one area may be helpful and relevant to the other. The exchange of information between cardiologists and neurologists should remain of vital importance to both disciplines.

REFERENCES AND RECOMMENDED READING

Recently published papers of particular interest have been highlighted as:
- Of interest
- •• Of outstanding interest

1.• The Stroke Prevention in Atrial Fibrillation Investigators: Predictors of thromboembolism in atrial fibrillation: I. Clinical features of patients at risk. *Ann Intern Med* 1992, 116:1–5.

2.• The Stroke Prevention in Atrial Fibrillation Investigators: Predictors of thromboembolism in atrial fibrillation: II. Echocardiographic features of patients at risk. *Ann Intern Med* 1992, 116:6–12.

3. Hart R, Foster J, Luther M, Kanter M: Stroke in infective endocarditis. *Stroke* 1990, 21:695–700.

4. Fisher M, Kase C, Stelle B, Mills R: Ischemic stroke after cardiac pacemaker implantation in sick sinus syndrome. *Stroke* 1988, 19:712–715.

5. Falk R: A plea for a clinical trial of anticoagulation in dilated cardiomyopathy. *Am J Cardiol* 1990, 65:914–915.

6. Knepper L, Biller J, Adams H, Bruno A: Neurologic manifestations of atrial myxoma. *Stroke* 1988, 19:1435–1440.

7. Cerebral Embolism Task Force: Cardiogenic brain embolism. *Arch Neurol* 1989, 46:727–743.

8. Rogers L, Cho E, Kempin S, Posner J: Cerebral infarction from non-bacterial thrombotic endocarditis. *Am J Med* 1987, 83:746–756.

9. DiTullio M, Sacco R, Gopal A, *et al.*: Patent foramen ovale as a risk factor of cryptogenic stroke. *Ann Intern Med* 1992, 117:461–465.

10. Amarenco P, Duyckaerts C, Tzourio C, *et al.*: The prevalence of ulcerated plaques in the aortic arch in patients with stroke. *N Engl J Med* 1992, 326:221–225.

11.• Stroke Prevention in Atrial Fibrillation Investigators: Stroke prevention in atrial fibrillation study. *Circulation* 1991, 84:527–539.

12. Petersen P, Godtfredsen J, Boysen G, *et al.*: Placebo-controlled, randomised trial of warfarin and aspirin for prevention of thromboembolic complications in chronic atrial fibrillation: the Copenhagen AFASAK study. *Lancet* 1989, 1:175–179.

13.• The Boston Area Anticoagulation Trial for Atrial Fibrillation Investigators: The effect of low dose warfarin on the risk of stroke in patients with nonrheumatic atrial fibrillation. *N Engl J Med* 1990, 323:1505–1511.

14. Connolly S, Laupacis A, Gent M, *et al.*: Canadian Atrial Fibrillatin Anticoagulation (CAFA) study. *J Am Coll Cardiol* 1991, 18:349–355.

15. Ezekowitz M, Bridgers S, James K, *et al.*: Warfarin in the prevention of stroke associated with nonrheumatic atrial fibrillation. *N Engl J Med* 1992, 327:1406–1412.

16.•• European Atrial Fibrillation Trial Study Group: Secondary prevention in non-rheumatic atrial fibrillation after transient ischemic attack or minor stroke. *Lancet* 1993, 342:1255–1262.

17.• Albers G, Sherman D, Gress D, *et al.*: Stroke prevention in nonvalvular atrial fibrillation: a review of prospective randomized trials. *Ann Neurol* 1991, 30:511–518.

18. Smith P, Arnesen H, Holme I: The effect of warfarin on mortality and reinfarction after myocardial infarction. *N Engl J Med* 1990, 323:147–152.

19. Simoons M, Maggioni A, Knatterud G, *et al.*: Individual risk assessment for intracranial hemorrhage during thrombolytic therapy. *Lancet* 1993, 342:1523–1528.

20.•• Furlan A, Sila C, Chimowitz M, Jones S: Neurologic complications related to cardiac surgery. *Neurol Clin* 1992, 10:145–166.

SELECT BIBLIOGRAPHY

Kanter M, Sherman D: Embolic stroke of cardiac origin. In *Current Therapy in Neurologic Disease*, edn 3. Edited by Johnson R. Philadelphia: BC Decker; 1990:181–186.

Koudstaal P: Cardioembolic stroke. In *Current Review of Cerebrovascular Disease*. Edited by Fisher M, Bogousslavsky J. Philadelphia: Current Medicine; 1993:41–47.

Sherman D: Prevention of cardioembolic stroke. In *Prevention of Stroke*. Edited by Norris J, Hachinski V. New York: Springer-Verlag; 1991:149–160.

Streifler J, Furlan A, Barnett H: Cardiogenic brain embolism: incidence, varieties, and treatment. In *Stroke*, edn 2. Edited by Barnett H, Mohr J, Stein B, Yatsu F. New York: Churchill Livingstone; 1992:967–994.

Rheumatic Diseases and the Heart 31

Deborah M. DeMarco
David F. Giansiracusa

> ### Key Points
> - Physicians must have an awareness of the resurgence of rheumatic fever and the importance of antibiotic prophylaxis.
> - Recognition of Lyme disease and spondyloarthropathies as a cause of bradycardia and conduction disturbances is important.
> - There is potential involvement of all components of the heart in patients with systemic lupus erythematosus, rheumatoid arthritis, and scleroderma.
> - Coronary artery thrombosis can be secondary to either phospholipid antibodies or vasculitis.
> - The high frequency of asymptomatic cardiac involvement in scleroderma indicates the need for cardiac evaluation in all newly diagnosed patients.

The heart can suffer involvement in a spectrum of rheumatic diseases (Table 1). Cardiac disease is usually the result of the primary inflammatory, metabolic, or infiltrative process or is secondary to other organ system disease. Although the pathophysiologic mechanisms of these rheumatic diseases are quite diverse, some or all of the components of the heart may be affected by each of these conditions.

ACUTE RHEUMATIC FEVER

Acute rheumatic fever (ARF) is a rare sequela of group A streptococcal infection of the upper respiratory tract. Its manifestations, as outlined in the Jones criteria (Table 2) [1], remain the means of diagnosis for the initial attack. Carditis is its principal cardiac manifestation and has decreased in incidence in adults from 65% to 30% since the 1940s, but it remains at 70% to 90% in children. In chronic rheumatic heart disease, carditis may result in scarring of the heart valves and subsequent valvular heart disease. In a few patients, severe carditis occurs with rapid onset of complications, possibly leading to death.

Often, carditis in ARF is asymptomatic and is diagnosed by detection of a new murmur during the physical examination. Other major criteria for diagnosis include the presence of cardiomegaly, congestive heart failure, and pericardial friction rub or other signs of pericardial effusion. The most common murmur associated with ARF is mitral regurgitation followed by aortic insufficiency. First-degree heart block may be seen on the electrocardiogram, but it is neither specific nor prognostically important. There is no characteristic electrocardiogram pattern for ARF.

Diagnosis

Establishing a definitive diagnosis of rheumatic fever is important not only for acute management of disease manifestations, but also because of the potential need for antibiotic prophylaxis. In addition to the Jones criteria (Table 2), the diagnosis depends on establishing an antecedent streptococcal infection by laboratory tests; an

Table 1 Sites of Involvement of Rheumatic Diseases and the Heart

Disease	Aortic root	Pericardium	Myocardium	Endocardium	Coronary arteries	Conduction abnormality	Arrhythmias
Acute rheumatic fever	—	Pericarditis	Cardiomyopathy	Valvulitis, chronic valvular disease	—	+	—
Lyme disease	—	Pericarditis	Cardiomyopathy	—	—	Atrioventricular block	Atrial and ventricular tachyarrhythmias
Systemic lupus erythematosus	Aortitis (rare)	Pericarditis (tamponade, constriction)	Myocarditis (rare)	Libman–Sacks syndrome, thrombosis (antiphospholipid antibody syndrome)	Vasculitis, accelerated atherosclerotic disease, thrombosis (antiphospholipid antibody syndrome), embolic antiphospholipid antibody syndrome	Atrioventricular block (neonatal)	Ventricular
Rheumatoid arthritis	Granulomatous vasculitis	Pericarditis, constriction	Granulomatous myocarditis, interstitial myocarditis	Valvulitis	Vasculitis, accelerated atherosclerotic disease	+	—
Systemic sclerosis (scleroderma)	—	Pericarditis	Myocardial fibrosis, cor pulmonale	—	Intimal hyperplasia	+	Supra and ventricular
Dermatomyositis and polymyositis	—	—	Myocarditis	—	Vasculitis	+	+
Vasculitis	—	Pericarditis	Myocardial infarction	—	Vasculitis	+	+
Spondyloarthropathies (ankylosing spondylitis, Reiter's syndrome)	Aortitis	—	—	Aortic regurgitation	—	+	—
Polychondritis	Aortitis	Pericarditis (rare)	—	Aortic and mitral valvulitis	Vasculitis	+	+
Marfan syndrome	Dilatation, dissection	—	—	Mitral valve prolapse, aortic insufficiency	—	—	—
Ehlers–Danlos syndrome	Dilatation	—	Ventricular and atrial septal defects	Aortic insufficiency, mitral prolapse, tricuspid prolapse, bicuspid aortic valves, pulmonary regurgitation	—	—	—
Amyloidosis	—	Constrictive pericarditis	Restrictive cardiomyopathy	Valvular disease (tricuspid, mitral)	Intraarterial deposition	+	+

TABLE 2 JONES CRITERIA (REVISED) FOR DIAGNOSIS OF INITIAL ATTACK OF RHEUMATIC FEVER
Major manifestations
Carditis
Polyarthritis
Chorea
Erythrema marginatum
Subcutaneous nodules
Minor manifestations
Clinical
Arthralgia
Fever
Laboratory
Elevated erythrocyte sedimentation rate
C-reactive protein
Leukocytosis
Prolonged P-R interval
Supporting evidence of streptococcal infection
Increased titer of antistreptococcal antibodies (antistreptolysin-O or others)
Positive throat culture for group A *Streptococcus*
Adapted from Shulman and coworkers [1]; with permission.

elevated titer of at least one antibody on the antistreptolysin-O assay, anti-DNAse B, or antihyaluronidase test can be detected in approximately 95% of patients with ARF [2•]. The rapid Streptozyme (Wampole Laboratories, Cranbury, NJ) slide test is not recommended because of its variable results.

Treatment

The current recommended treatment course is outlined in Table 3. All household members should have throat cultures taken, because reinfection may occur if the organism is not eradicated from the environment. Antiinflammatory medication is usually administered for arthritis, fever, and mild carditis, although it is not protective against the subsequent development of chronic rheumatic heart disease. Patients with severe carditis require prompt administration of corticosteroid therapy as an adjunct to their cardiac medications.

Secondary prophylaxis is recommended for patients who have had ARF (Table 3). Duration of prophylaxis remains controversial, but it can safely be discontinued if 1) the patient is older than 20 years of age; 2) the most recent attack occurred more than 5 years previously; 3) there was no carditis with the previous attack; and 4) there is no evidence of rheumatic heart disease [3•]. The likelihood of the patient's exposure to children and the patient's reliability are considerations.

LYME DISEASE

Lyme disease, a systemic illness caused by the spirochete *Borrelia burgdorferi*, has cardiac manifestations in 4% to 10% of untreated patients. The cardiac complications usually develop 4 to 8 weeks after exposure to an infected tick, but they can occur as early as 4 days after the onset of the initial illness [4]. Sometimes, they may predate the initial antibody response.

The most common cardiac abnormalities (Table 1) include atrioventricular block, myopericarditis, and left ventricular dysfunction, but cardiomyopathy and atrial and ventricular tachycardias have been reported [4]. Almost all patients with atrioventricular conduction disturbances manifest first-degree block at some time during their course; high-grade block occurs in up to 50% of patients, and symptomatic complete heart block, in approximately 8% [4]. The block is usually at or above the level of the atrioventricular node, predicting a benign prognosis, but more sinister conduction disturbances may occur. Temporary cardiac pacing is frequently needed by patients who have severe heart block with hemodynamic instability. Permanent pacemaker insertion is rarely indicated. The block generally resolves completely with antibiotic treatment, and the long-term prognosis is excellent (Table 4) [5].

SYSTEMIC LUPUS ERYTHEMATOSUS

Cardiovascular involvement occurs in 29% to 66% of patients with systemic lupus erythematosus (SLE) (Table 1) [6]. Autopsy and even echocardiographic studies may document significant findings in the heart without clinically apparent disease.

Pericardial disease is the most common cardiac manifestation of SLE, documented at autopsy in approximately 80% of patients but seen as symptomatic disease in 8% to 50% of patients. It usually presents in association with SLE disease activity in other organs.

Patients with symptomatic pericarditis generally present with anterior or substernal chest pain that is characteristically pleuritic and relieved by leaning forward. The pain may be associated with dyspnea or arrhythmias. A pericardial friction rub may be heard on auscultation. A chest roentgenogram may reveal an enlarged cardiac silhouette. Transient electrocardiographic changes (ST-segment elevation and PR-interval depression) may be seen. Echocardiography may reveal pericardial effusions or pericardial thickening. Life-threatening complications of pericarditis include cardiac tamponade and

TABLE 3 TREATMENT RECOMMENDATIONS FOR ACUTE RHEUMATIC FEVER

Drug	Dosage
Acute treatment	
Penicillin	250 mg four times daily for 10 days
Erythromycin	250 mg four times daily for 10 days
Prophylaxis	
Penicillin G benzathine	1.2×10^6 U intramuscularly every 4 weeks
Penicillin V	250 mg orally twice daily
Sulfadiazine	0.5 g orally once daily
Erythromycin	250 mg orally twice daily

Table 4. Antibiotic therapy for Lyme disease

Stage-symptoms	Regimen*	Length, d
Early Lyme disease	Doxycycline, 100 mg b.i.d. or amoxicillin, 500 mg t.i.d. or erythromycin, 250 mg q.i.d.	10–21
Neurologic symptoms		
Bell's palsy only	Doxycycline, 100 mg b.i.d. or amoxicillin, 500 mg t.i.d.	21
Meningitis, encephalitis	Penicillin G, 20 million U/d IV or ceftriaxone, 2 g/d	14–21
Radiculoneuropathy		
Lyme carditis		
Mild (first-degree AV block, normal left ventricular function)	Doxycycline, 100 mg b.i.d.	30
Moderate to severe (high degree AV block)	Penicillin G, 20 million U/d IV or ceftriaxone, 2 q/d IV May require temporary pacemaker	14–21
Lyme arthritis	Doxycycline, 100 mg b.i.d. or amoxicillin, 500 mg q.i.d. plus probenecid, 500 mg q.i.d. or penicillin G, 20 million U/d IV or ceftriaxone, 2 g/d IV	30
Pregnancy		
Early-localized	Amoxicillin, 500 mg t.i.d.	21
Late-disseminated	Penicillin G, 20 million U/d IV or ceftriaxone 2 g/d IV	14–21

*Failures occur with all regimens.
AV—atrioventricular; b.i.d.—twice per day; IV—intravenous; q.i.d.—four times per day; t.i.d.—three times per day.

---

constriction, but both are rare. Pericardial fluid is usually exudative with high protein and normal to low glucose levels compared with serum.

Symptomatic pericarditis can often be successfully treated with nonsteroidal antiinflammatory drugs such as indomethacin, 50 mg three times daily, and, occasionally, oral corticosteroids at low dosages (15 to 30 mg/d). Hemodynamically compromising effusions require pericardial aspiration and high-dose intravenous corticosteroids.

Myocardial involvement in SLE should be categorized as primary or secondary. Primary myocarditis is rare, occurring clinically in 2.1% to 14% of patients with SLE. Patients present with unexplained tachycardia, congestive heart failure (rarely), ventricular arrhythmias, conduction defects, electrocardiogram abnormalities (including ST-T wave changes), and cardiomegaly without evidence of valvular or pericardial disease. Endocardial biopsy specimens may confirm histologically the presence of myocarditis.

Secondary causes of myocardial dysfunction in SLE include systemic hypertension, valvular disease, pulmonary disease, coronary artery ischemia, drug toxicity, and amyloidosis. These secondary causes are often clinically more important than true lupus myocarditis.

Treatment of SLE patients with carditis includes distinguishing primary from secondary disorders and appropriately treating any secondary cardiac insult. Antiinflammatory and immunosuppressive therapy should be reserved for active lupus carditis.

Coronary artery involvement in SLE includes embolic events, thromboses [7], vasculitis, and premature atherosclerosis. The treatment of the SLE patient with acute myocardial ischemia initially should be similar to that of patients with atherosclerotic coronary artery disease. However, the etiology of the ischemia must be determined by arteriography because coronary arteritis must be treated with corticosteroids and immunosuppressant agents.

The most characteristic cardiac manifestation of SLE is nonbacterial verrucous endocarditis, so-called Libman-Sacks endocarditis, which occurs on the ventricular surface of the mitral valve. A similar lesion involving the aortic valve has also been described, as well as a necrotizing valvulitis secondary to vasculitis of the smaller vessels supplying the valve. Libman-Sacks lesions rarely produce significant valvular dysfunction. However, hemodynamically significant aortic and mitral insufficiency may occur. Valve replacements may be required, but the associated mortality has been as high as 25%. Rarely, lesional material of Libman-Sacks endocarditis may dislodge and embolize.

Conduction abnormalities and arrhythmias owing to SLE are not usually clinically significant and should be managed the same way as in patients without SLE. If acute conduction disease is suspected clinically to be secondary to myocarditis or arteritis, a short trial of corticosteroids should be initiated in the hemodynamically compromised patient [6].

The infants of mothers with SLE also may suffer cardiac disease, most commonly in the form of neonatal heart block. This syndrome in infants is referred to as permanent neonatal lupus and is associated with maternal anti–Ro (SSA) antibodies.

RHEUMATOID ARTHRITIS

Rheumatoid arthritis may involve all structures of the heart as the result of granulomatous proliferation or vasculitis

(Table 1) [8]. Echocardiography can detect pericarditis and valvular disease, whereas endocardial biopsies can diagnose myocardial involvement [9].

Pericarditis, the most common of the rheumatoid cardiac manifestations with an incidence of approximately 50% by autopsy studies, rarely causes impairment of left ventricular function. However, constrictive pericarditis or a large pericardial effusion may compromise cardiac output and require pericardial aspiration or pericardiectomy.

Pericardial effusions generally respond to administration of 30 to 40 mg/d of prednisone over a several-week period. Pericardiocentesis should be performed early if tamponade is suspected or if there is a question of septic or suppurative pericarditis. In cases of constrictive pericarditis, pericardiectomy is the only effective therapy.

The myocardium may be affected by granulomatous inflammation, interstitial myocarditis, and coronary artery vasculitis. Cardiac conduction abnormalities, including complete heart block, may develop as a result of rheumatoid nodules. The heart block tends to occur in patients with severe, erosive, nodular-forming disease and is generally permanent. Coronary arteritis and amyloidosis are less common causes of heart block.

Arteritis in the rheumatoid patient may affect the coronary arteries and aorta, resulting in myocardial infarction, dilatation of the aortic root, and aortic valvular insufficiency, respectively.

Endocardial involvement is generally a result of granulomatous inflammation that may affect all four valves. Aortic valvular insufficiency is well documented. Mitral and tricuspid disease so severe as to cause symptoms is very rare.

SCLERODERMA

Systemic sclerosis (scleroderma) is a generalized disorder of connective tissue characterized by fibrosis and vascular obliteration. Cardiac involvement (Table 1) may be primary or secondary to involvement of other organ systems and, together with renal disease, is the leading cause of early death [10]. Cardiac disease in systemic sclerosis may also be secondary to other organ system involvement, such as malignant hypertension, uremia, and cor pulmonale as a result of severe pulmonary hypertension or severe interstitial lung disease.

Pericardial disease, although common at autopsy, is not often recognized clinically. Pericardial involvement presents most commonly as an indolent chronic pericardial effusion of variable size in an asymptomatic patient or in one who may have nonspecific findings such as chest pain, dyspnea, and cardiomegaly or symptoms of congestive heart failure. Chronic pericardial effusions may be a premonitory indicator of the development of renal failure within 6 months. Less commonly, pericardial disease may occur as an acute inflammatory process with dyspnea, chest pain, fever, and pericardial friction rub.

Asymptomatic pericardial disease usually does not predict a poor clinical course in contrast to symptomatic involvement. Pericardial tamponade may occur but is thought to be uncommon. Constrictive and restrictive pericarditis have been reported but appear to be extremely rare.

Involvement of the myocardium, specifically focal myocardial fibrosis, has been found in autopsied scleroderma patients, but clinically evident disease occurs much less frequently. Vasospasm of the coronary microvasculature may be the primary etiology [11]. In patients with the CREST (calcinosis, Raynaud's disease, esophageal dysfunction, sclerodactyly, telangiectasia) variant of scleroderma, resting right ventricular function is abnormal more commonly than in generalized scleroderma (systemic sclerosis) and is usually secondary to pulmonary vascular disease.

Conduction and electrocardiogram abnormalities in systemic sclerosis are common and diverse. The electrocardiogram is normal in approximately 50% of patients. Only 10% of patients had electrocardiogram infarct patterns, most commonly in the septal region. Low-voltage and nonspecific ST segment abnormalities are the most common electrocardiogram disturbances. Ventricular conduction abnormalities occur in approximately 2% to 5% of systemic sclerosis patients. Infarcts and conduction disease also are thought to be caused by diffuse myocardial fibrosis. These abnormalities may lead to complete heart block or asystole. Thus, myocardial fibrosis and thallium perfusion abnormalities are common in patients with systemic sclerosis, but global left ventricular function is usually maintained. Ventricular arrhythmias are the primary cause of sudden death in up to 60% of patients.

Diagnosis

Because of the frequency of subclinical cardiac involvement and the high cardiac mortality in patients with systemic sclerosis, baseline cardiac evaluation should be performed in all newly diagnosed patients, including ambulatory 24-hour electrocardiogram monitoring, electrocardiograms, and radionucleotide imaging (thallium perfusion scans). If patients have symptoms suggestive of coronary artery disease, cardiac catheterization should be considered to evaluate for coexistent atherosclerosis.

Treatment

Treatment of cardiac manifestations of systemic sclerosis and CREST remains somewhat empiric but should be directed at the specific symptoms or problems. Angiotensin-converting enzyme inhibitors or calcium channel blockers should be used to manage hypertension. Angina resulting from coronary vasospasm may respond to calcium channel blockers. Angina secondary to coronary artery disease should be treated as it is for non–systemic sclerosis patients. Symptomatic pericardial effusions usually respond to nonsteroidal antiinflammatory agents, but corticosteroids are occasionally required. Drugs that can exacerbate underlying conduction disturbances should be avoided. Because of a possible increased mortality associated with use of antiarrhythmic agents, systemic sclerosis patients so treated should be monitored closely with repeated ambulatory electrocardiograms.

POLYMYOSITIS AND DERMATOMYOSITIS

Cardiac abnormalities in polymyositis and dermatomyositis (Table 1) have been identified in as many as 40% of patients, perhaps more commonly in dermatomyositis. Only approximately 15% of patients have symptomatic cardiac involvement. Some have suggested that cardiac disease is an important prognostic factor in polymyositis and dermatomyositis [12].

The electrocardiogram is abnormal in 25% to 100% of patients. The most common abnormalities are nonspecific ST-T wave changes, atrioventricular block, and axis deviation. Rarely, complete heart block requiring permanent pacemaker implantation may occur. Abnormal Q waves resembling myocardial infarction may occur without underlying coronary artery disease. Arrhythmias occur less frequently.

Congestive heart failure may occur either as a result of the disease or secondary to hypertension associated with long-term corticosteroid therapy. Myocarditis has been found at autopsy in some patients with histories of congestive heart failure as well as in patients who have not had congestive heart failure prior to death. Myocardial fibrosis has not been a common histologic finding.

Studies of coronary arteries have shown vasculitis, arteritis obliterans, and angiographically normal vessels despite ischemic changes on the electrocardiogram. Coexistent atherosclerotic disease also may be found.

The diagnostic evaluation of patients with polymyositis and dermatomyositis should include a baseline electrocardiogram, creatine phosphokinase with MB fraction, and echocardiogram. It is not clear if 24-hour ambulatory electrocardiogram monitoring should be performed as a screening study in all newly diagnosed patients or only those with symptoms of rhythm disturbances. Persistent elevation of creatine phosphokinase-MB despite normal skeletal muscle strength may indicate ongoing myocarditis and should prompt further noninvasive testing such as thallium perfusion scanning.

There are no controlled trials that specifically evaluate treatment of cardiac disease in polymyositis and dermatomyositis. High-dose prednisone (60 to 80 mg/d) is usually required for at least 6 weeks at diagnosis, with tapering as indicated by clinical examination and muscle enzyme testing. Management of congestive heart failure, in addition to the conventional measures, may also require use of high-dose corticosteroids.

VASCULITIS

The vasculitides are a group of disorders in which inflammation and necrosis of blood vessel walls result in organ system abnormalities caused by thrombosis and hemorrhage. Several forms of necrotizing systemic vasculitis may involve the heart. Kawasaki syndrome, which causes giant coronary artery aneurysms, occurs in children. Polyarteritis nodosa, Wegener's granulomatosis, and the Churg-Strauss syndrome may affect the heart and are discussed herein. Cardiac involvement in these disorders requires no special treatment.

Wegener's Granulomatosis

This relatively rare form of vasculitis shows cardiac involvement (Table 1) in up to 30% of untreated patients but in only 10% to 15% of those treated with cytotoxic agents. Coronary arteritis leading to myocardial infarction and pericarditis are the most common cardiac complications. Pericarditis often is symptomatic and may lead to tamponade. Any portion of the heart may be involved, leading to congestive heart failure, heart block, or arrhythmias, but these complications are much less common [13].

Polyarteritis

Polyarteritis is a necrotizing vasculitis involving small and medium-sized muscular arteries. Cardiac involvement (Table 1) is observed in nearly 60% of patients in autopsy series but is often clinically silent. Congestive heart failure, pericarditis, myocardial infarction, and conduction abnormalities are the most common manifestations. Congestive heart failure may be caused by hypertension, which is seen in greater than 50% of patients, or by coronary insufficiency.

Churg-Strauss Syndrome

Also called allergic granulomatous angiitis, Churg-Strauss syndrome usually occurs in patients with a history of asthma or allergic rhinitis. The heart is a primary target organ (Table 1). Cardiac granulomas are commonly found at autopsy [13]. Widespread myocardial damage may result from vasculitis affecting the coronary vessels. Cardiac disease may present as acute pericarditis, constrictive pericarditis, congestive heart failure, or myocardial infarction and accounts for approximately 50% of deaths of patients with Churg-Strauss syndrome. Electrocardiograms are abnormal in at least 50% of patients. Careful cardiovascular evaluation should be done early in patients with suspected Churg-Strauss syndrome because delayed treatment can lead to myocardial infarction and intractable congestive heart failure [13].

SPONDYLOARTHROPATHIES

The seronegative spondyloarthropathies are a group of disorders that include ankylosing spondylitis, Reiter's syndrome or reactive arthritis, psoriatic arthritis, and the arthritis of inflammatory bowel disease (ulcerative colitis and regional enteritis, or Crohn's disease).

Cardiac involvement (Table 1) occurs in approximately 5% of individuals with ankylosing spondylitis, generally in patients with longstanding disease [14]. Inflammation of the aortic valve and root and of the atrioventricular node may cause aortic regurgitation and conduction abnormalities that may also occur in patients with Reiter's syndrome. Aortic valve fibrosis and thickening may be appreciated by echocardiography. Fibrosis extending to the interventricular system may cause complete heart block or milder forms of atrioventricular conduction abnormalities in 5% to 10% of men with ankylosing spondylitis. HLA-B27 has also been associated with isolated aortic regurgitation and with aortic regurgitation associated with severe conduction abnormalities. Subtle abnormalities of diastolic function have been found frequently in patients with ankylosing spondylitis.

Heart block and aortitis have been reported in up to 10% of individuals with severe, longstanding Reiter's syndrome. Conduction defects, such as P-R interval prolongation, second-degree block with Wenckebach's phenomenon, and complete heart block, may occur early in Reiter's syndrome [15].

RELAPSING POLYCHONDRITIS

Polychondritis is an episodic disorder of cartilage associated with inflammatory arthritis, aortitis, and inflammation of the aortic and mitral valves. It affects predominately middle-aged, white individuals, although cardiac involvement is more common in men.

Cardiac involvement (Table 1) occurs in 20% to 40% of patients and is the second most common cause of death, beyond respiratory tract involvement. Abnormalities include aortic insufficiency and mitral insufficiency and, less commonly, pericarditis, abnormal electrocardiograms, paroxysmal atrial tachycardia, cardiac ischemia, and the conduction abnormalities, including complete heart block [16].

Because cardiac involvement may be asymptomatic, some authors suggest baseline electrocardiograms, chest roentgenograms, and echocardiograms in all patients with relapsing polychondritis. If valvular disease is detected, the echocardiogram can be useful for follow-up.

Corticosteroids have been the mainstay of therapy, but immunosuppressives also have been used for organ-threatening, corticosteroid-resistant disease activity. Successful valvuloplasty and valve replacements have been reported, but valve dehiscence may occur as a result of persistent inflammation [17].

CONNECTIVE TISSUE DISEASE, INCLUDING MARFAN SYNDROME AND EHLERS-DANLOS SYNDROME

Cardiovascular abnormalities associated with Marfan syndrome (Table 1) include aneurysmal dilatation of the ascending aorta, aortic valve insufficiency, coarctation of the aorta, mitral valve prolapse, mitral annulus calcification with mitral regurgitation, atrial and ventricular septal defects, tetralogy of Fallot, patent ductus arteriosus, and pulmonary artery aneurysms. Aneurysmal dilatation of the ascending aorta with rupture and aortic regurgitation are the causes of the shortened lifespan of 32 years in patients with Marfan syndrome. Annual echocardiographic monitoring is recommended until the aorta exceeds 50% of normal for body surface area, at which time echocardiographic monitoring should be done every 6 months. Management of aortic dilatation in Marfan syndrome includes β-blockade, specifically propranolol, and avoidance of vigorous activity. Pregnancy appears to be safe if aortic dilatation is not present. Surgical intervention with aortic grafting repair has proved beneficial when aortic dilatation reaches 6 cm [18].

Cardiovascular abnormalities in patients with Ehlers-Danlos syndrome (Table 1) include large artery aneurysms (the most serious manifestation of the syndrome), atrial septal defects, aortic valve insufficiency, ventricular papillary muscle dysfunction, dextrocardia, and conduction abnormalities. In patients with type IV Ehlers-Danlos syndrome, the so-called "vascular" or "ecchymotic" type, death generally occurs within the first two decades of life because of rupture of major arteries and gastrointestinal bleeding. Tetralogy of Fallot, peripheral pulmonary stenosis, bifid pulmonary artery, and dextrocardia also have been reported [19].

Mitral valve prolapse is a fairly common cardiac manifestation of both Marfan syndrome and Ehlers-Danlos syndrome. Therefore, patients with mitral valve prolapse should be evaluated clinically for these diseases.

AMYLOIDOSIS

The heart is a common site of amyloid deposition in both systemic and localized forms of amyloidosis (Table 5). Cardiac involvement is universally present in primary and myeloma-associated amyloidosis and is a major cause of death [20]. Amyloid also frequently affects the hearts of individuals with familial-hereditary amyloidosis but rarely occurs in those with secondary amyloidosis.

The primary manifestations of amyloid heart disease are cardiomegaly and low-output congestive heart failure. Cardiac

TABLE 5 COMPARISONS OF CARDIAC AMYLOIDOSIS IN PRIMARY AMYLOID VERSUS SENILE CARDIAC AMYLOID		
	Heart in primary amyloid (*n* = 21)	Senile cardiac amyloid (*n* = 26)
Cardiac amyloid deposits	Higher grade deposits, perifiber and mixed, frequent vascular involvement	Lower grade deposits, predominantly nodular distribution pattern, infrequent vascular involvement
Mean age of patients, y	57.6	83
Male-to-female ratio	1.6:1	5.5:1
Congestive heart failure, %	76	35
Pseudoinfarction electrocardiogram findings, %	45	Uncommon
Sudden death, %	33	19

Data from Smith and coworkers [20]; with permission.

amyloidosis also may present as constrictive pericarditis, restrictive cardiomyopathy, cardiac conduction disorders, and arrhythmias and may simulate ischemic heart disease with typical or atypical angina and "pseudoinfarct" electrocardiogram findings [20]. The diagnosis of amyloid heart disease should be considered in elderly individuals with heart disease of unknown etiology, particularly in those without atherosclerosis and valvular heart disease, and in patients in their fifth and sixth decades of life who have multisystem disease consistent with systemic amyloidosis and have the previously mentioned cardiac presentations.

Intractable heart failure may be the first manifestation and the cause of death in systemic amyloidosis. Amyloid is deposited diffusely in the myocardium but also may involve the pericardium, endocardium, and heart valves. The atrioventricular valves are more commonly involved than the pulmonary and aortic valves [20]. Murmurs are present occasionally.

Pericardial effusions are rare, but signs of constrictive pericarditis or restrictive myocardiopathy may develop. Pericardial involvement tends to occur in patients with high-grade amyloid deposits [20]. The demonstration of left ventricular diastolic pressures greater than those on the right helps to distinguish restrictive cardiomyopathy from constrictive pericarditis.

Ischemic heart disease secondary to amyloid deposition in intramyocardial arteries occurs in less than 2% of patients. Electrocardiograms may reveal the pattern of anteroseptal infarction in the absence of evidence of infarction at autopsy.

Amyloid deposits in the sinus node or fibrosis of the conduction system may cause rhythm disturbances in both patients with primary amyloid and senile cardiac amyloid [20]. Amyloid-induced neuropathy resulting in orthostatic hypotension may also cause dizziness, light-headedness, or syncope in the patient with amyloid heart disease.

Various invasive and noninvasive procedures are used to evaluate for cardiac amyloidosis. Echocardiograms may reveal thick-walled ventricles with normal or reduced-sized cavities. Left ventricular diastolic abnormalities are detectable by echocardiography even prior to development of clinically apparent amyloid heart disease. Ejection fractions may be normal despite significant heart failure, reflecting impaired cardiac relaxation (impaired diastolic function). Two-dimensional echocardiograms may reveal "granular sparkling." Diffuse uptake of 99m pyrophosphate may reflect the severity of myocardial Tc2 amyloid infiltration. Endomyocardial biopsy is the only definitive means of detecting amyloid deposits in the heart [20].

The median survival after diagnosis of primary or multiple myeloma-associated amyloid is approximately 12 months, with median survival of only 6 months from the onset of congestive heart failure in those with cardiac involvement. Of patients with primary amyloid, cardiac disease is reported to be the cause of death in 30% to 50% and is probably underreported [20]. The three variables of congestive heart failure, amount of weight loss, and presence of monoclonal light chains in urine predict poor outcome.

Although there is no specific therapy for amyloidosis, treatment of a predisposing disease may be useful. Alkylating agents have been used to treat primary amyloidosis, but they do not reverse the disease. Colchicine prevents acute febrile attacks in familial Mediterranean fever and retards amyloid deposition and further renal function deterioration in these individuals. Colchicine also may prolong survival in patients with primary amyloid.

Congestive heart failure secondary to amyloid heart disease should be treated with salt restriction and judicious use of diuretics. Hypovolemia should be avoided because ventricular filling may be compromised because of ventricular wall stiffening. Postural hypotension also may result from volume depletion secondary to decreased fluid intake or protein–osmotic diuresis, adrenal insufficiency, autonomic neuropathy, and low-output cardiac failure. Mineralocorticoids, elastic stockings, treatment of malabsorption, and fluid supplementation are supportive therapies. Great care should be used when treating with digitalis because of the risk of the development of conduction abnormalities and arrhythmias in patients with cardiac amyloid.

References and Recommended Reading

Recently published papers of particular interest have been highlighted as:
- Of interest

1. Shulman ST, Kaplan EL, Bisno AL, *et al.*: Jones criteria (revised) for guidance in the diagnosis of rheumatic fever. *Circulation* 1984, 69:203A–208A.
2.• Gaasch WH: Guidelines for the diagnosis of rheumatic fever. *JAMA* 1992, 268:2069–2073.
3.• Berrios X, del Campo E, Guzman B, *et al.*: Discontinuing rheumatic fever prophylaxis in selected adolescents and young adults. *Ann Intern Med* 1993, 118:401–406.
4. Cox J, Krajden M: Cardiovascular manifestations of Lyme disease. *Am Heart J* 1991, 122:1449–1455.
5. McAlister HF, Klementowicz PT, Andrews C, *et al.*: Lyme carditis: an important cause of reversible heart block. *Ann Intern Med* 1989, 110:339–345.
6. Mandell BF: Cardiovascular involvement in systemic lupus erythematosus. *Semin Arthritis Rheum* 1987, 17:126–141.
7. Lockshin MD: Antiphospholipid antibody syndrome. *Rheum Dis Clin North Am* 1994, 20:45–59.
8. Harris ED Jr: Clinical features of rheumatoid arthritis. In *Textbook of Rheumatology*, edn 4. Edited by Kelly WN, Harris ED Jr, Ruddy S, Sledge CB. Philadelphia: WB Saunders; 1993:898–900.
9. Maione S, Valentini G, Giunta A, *et al.*: Cardiac involvement in rheumatoid arthritis: An echocardiographic study. *Cardiology* 1993; 83:234–239.
10. Bulpitt KJ, Clements PJ, Lachenbruch PA, *et al.*: Early undifferentiated connective tissue disease III: outcome and prognostic indications in early scleroderma (systemic sclerosis). *Ann Intern Med* 1993, 118:602–609.
11. Janosik DL, Osborn TG, Moore TL, *et al.*: Heart disease in systemic sclerosis. *Semin Arthritis Rheum* 1989, 19:191–200.

12. Hochberg MC, Feldman D, Stevens MB: Adult onset polymyositis/dermatomyositis: an analysis of clinical and laboratory features and survival in 76 patients with a review of the literature. *Semin Arthritis Rheum* 1986, 15:168–178.
13. Specks U, DeRemee RA: Granulomatous vasculitis: Wegener's granulomatosis and Churg-Strauss syndrome. *Rheum Dis Clin North Am* 1990, 16:377–397.
14. Arnett FC: Seronegative spondyloarthropathies. *Bull Rheum Dis* 1987, 37:1–12.
15. Dier T, Rosencrance JG, Chillag SA: Cardiac conduction manifestations of Reiter's syndrome. *South Med J* 1991, 84:799–800.
16. Bowness P, Hawley IC, Morris T, *et al.*: Complete heart block and severe aortic incompetence in relapsing polychondritis: clinicopathologic findings. *Arthritis Rheum* 1991, 34:97–100.
17. Van Decker W, Panidis IP: Relapsing polychondritis and cardiac valvular involvement. *Ann Intern Med* 1988, 109:340–341.
18. Gott VL, Pyeritz RE, Magovern GJ, *et al.*: Surgical treatment of aneurysms of the ascending aorta in the Marfan syndrome: results of composite-graft repair in 50 patients. *N Engl J Med* 1986, 314:1070–1074.
19. Leier CV, Call TD, Fulkerson PK, *et al.*: The spectrum of cardiac defects in the Ehlers-Danlos syndrome. *Ann Intern Med* 1980, 92:171–178.
20. Smith JT, Kyle RA, Lie JT: Clinical significance of histopathologic patterns of cardiac amyloidosis. *Mayo Clin Proc* 1984, 59:574–555.

SELECT BIBLIOGRAPHY

Askari AD, Huetter TL: Cardiac abnormalities in polymyositis/dermatomyositis. *Semin Arthritis Rheum* 1982, 12:208–219.

Bergfeldt L: HLA-B27 associated rheumatic diseases with severe cardiac bradyarrhythmias. *Am J Med* 1983, 75:210–215.

Galve E, Ordi J, Barquinero J, *et al.*: Valvular heart disease in the primary antiphospholipid syndrome. *Ann Intern Med* 1992, 16:293–298.

Grant SCD, Levy RD, Venning MC, *et al.*: Wegener's granulomatosis and the heart. *Br Heart J* 1994, 71:82–86.

Khamashta MA, Hughes GRU: Antiphospholipid antibodies and valve disease in patients with systemic lupus erythematosus [letter]. *J Am Coll Cardiol* 1993, 22:1269–1270.

Renaldini E, Spandrio S, Cerudelli B, *et al.*: Cardiac involvement in Churg-Strauss syndrome: A follow-up of three cases. *Eur Heart J* 1993, 14:1712–1716.

Roldan CA, Crawford M: Reply [letter], *J Am Coll Cardiol* [letter]. 1993, 22:1269–1270.

Steers AC, Grodzicki RL, Kornblatt AN, *et al.*: The spirochete etiology of Lyme disease. *N Engl J Med* 1983, 308:733–740.

Veasy LG, Wiedmeier SE, Orsmond GS, *et al.*: Resurgence of acute rheumatic fever in the intermountain area of the United States. *N Engl J Med* 1987, 316:421–426.

The Aging Heart

32

J. V. Nixon

> **Key Points**
> - Morphological, physiological, and cellular changes in the cardiovascular system are associated with the normal aging process.
> - The prevalence of cardiovascular disease processes, including chronic ischemic heart disease, acute myocardial infarction, hypertension, arrhythmias, and valvular heart disease, changes with age.
> - Medical therapy should be focused on preservation of cardiac preload, heart rate, and contractility.
> - The value of surgical or interventional therapy must be assessed for age.

Clinical assessment of the older cardiovascular patient must incorporate a series of unique variables. Aging is accompanied by changes in the cardiovascular system [1]. Furthermore, lifestyle impacts the extent and rate of these cardiovascular changes. Thus, in the general aging population, the assessment of changes in cardiovascular function must encompass changes in lifestyle and disease prevalence as well as alterations caused by aging [2••].

CHANGES IN CARDIAC ANATOMY AND PHYSIOLOGY

Aging is associated with a gradual increase in cardiac weight, principally in left ventricular mass and wall thickness [3] (Table 1). Aortic root dilatation and left atrial enlargement have been demonstrated. Importantly, left ventricular volumes remain unchanged. Experimental studies have shown that an increase in collagen-tissue laydown with a diffuse development of fibrous tissue as well as an increase in myocardial cell size are associated with the age-related cardiac hypertrophy [4] (Fig. 1). These data generally agree with morphologic and biopsy studies in older patients [5]. In addition, several experimental studies have documented the myocardial cellular changes associated with aging (Table 2).

Details of functional changes in the aging cardiovasculature of humans are limited by the suitability of the population selected, the lifestyle of such a study population, and the utility of noninvasive diagnostic technologies with specific self-imposed limitations. Nevertheless, systolic function is maintained both at rest and during exercise [6] (Fig. 2). The response of heart rate to exercise is attenuated in the elderly. Thus, during exercise, the older heart compensates for the attenuated heart-rate response by increasing end-diastolic and stroke volumes to preserve cardiac output [6]. The increased left ventricular wall mass serves to maintain a normal wall stress in the presence of increased left ventricular volumes during exercise.

Although the altered diastolic function or compliance clearly shown in experimental studies is difficult to document accurately in humans by noninvasive methods, several noninvasive parameters of diastolic filling have consistently

TABLE 1 AGE-RELATED CHANGES IN CARDIAC ANATOMY

Experimental studies
Myocardial hypertrophy
Individual cellular enlargement
Increased collagen
Increased fibrous tissue

Human studies
Increased left ventricular mass
Increased interventricular septal and posterior left ventricular wall thickness
Left atrial enlargement
Aortic root dilatation

TABLE 2 AGE-RELATED CHANGES IN CARDIAC PHYSIOLOGY

Experimental studies
Prolonged calcium transient
Prolonged transmembrane potential
Prolonged contraction duration
Prolonged relaxation
Increased resting and dynamic stiffness
Diminished responses to digitalis glycosides, norepinephrine, and isoproterenol

Human studies
Increased left ventricular wall mass
Increased left ventricular stroke volume during exercise
Decreased diastolic stiffness
Decreased diastolic filling

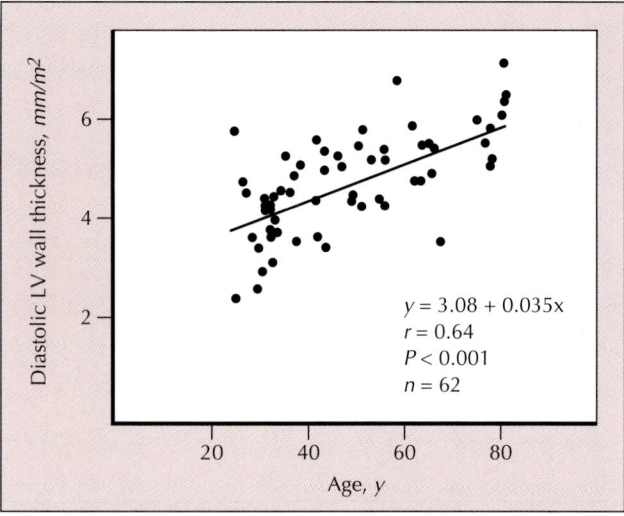

FIGURE 1 Linear regression plot showing the relation between increased age and increased diastolic left ventricular (LV) wall thickness in male participants in the Baltimore Longitudinal Aging Population. (*From* Gerstenblith and coworkers [3]; with permission.)

been shown to be altered with age [7•]. Both Doppler echocardiographic and radionuclide techniques show the reduction in early rapid diastolic filling and the increased dependence on atrial contraction seen with aging (Figs. 3, 4, and 5). These findings reflect the increased stiffness associated with the morphologic changes of the aging heart.

AGING AND CARDIOVASCULAR DISEASE

Table 3 summarizes the changes that occur in the cardiovascular system with aging. Any treatment algorithm in an older cardiovascular patient has many branches. In the older patient, prevalence of the disease process and any unique forms of presentation must be considered. The value of surgical or interventional therapy must be assessed for age. Furthermore, medical therapy is directed at the preservation of cardiac preload, heart rate, and contractility, emphasizing controlled afterload reduction as an option.

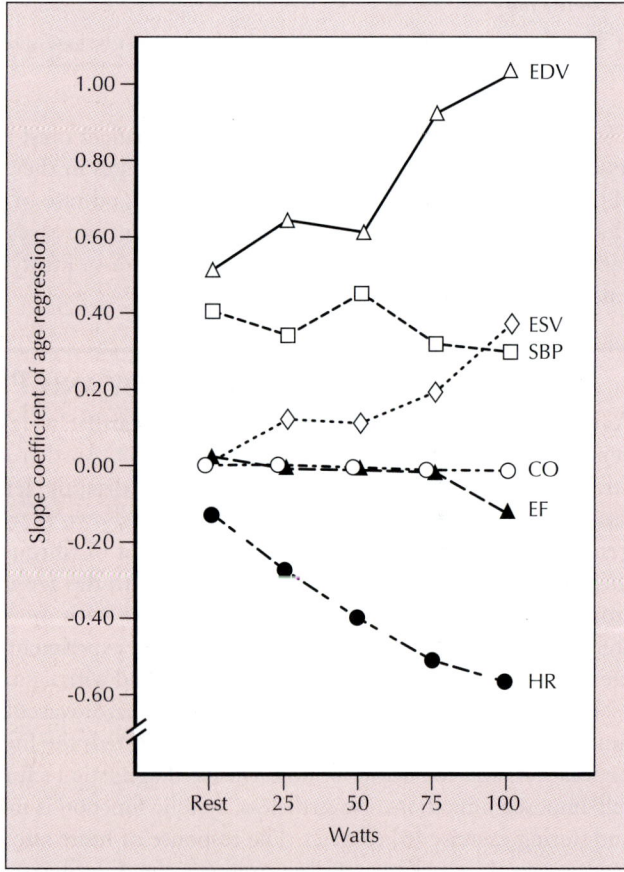

FIGURE 2 The slopes of the regression functions of age for end-diastolic volume (EDV), end-systolic volume (ESV), systolic blood pressure (SBP), cardiac output (CO), ejection fraction (EF), and heart rate (HR) at rest and increasing incremental workloads from 25 to 100 W during dynamic exercise in the Baltimore Longitudinal Aging Population. (*From* Rodeheffer and coworkers [6]; with permission.)

Chronic Ischemic Heart Disease

Prevalence

The prevalence of atherosclerotic heart disease increases significantly with age; more than 50% of people older than 65 years of age die from the effects of coronary artery disease [2••]. Furthermore, the prevalence of diagnosed coronary disease in this age group is only 30% to 50% of the prevalence of significant disease found at autopsy.

Thus, the recommendation of categories of therapeutic agents such as calcium channel–blocking agents, angiotensin-converting enzyme inhibitors, and α-adrenergic blocking agents occurs for the management of such common cardiovascular diseases in the older patient as ischemic heart disease, congestive heart failure, and hypertension (Table 4).

Diagnosis

Because of an age-related, altered lifestyle, including a decline in physical activity, presenting symptoms are often different

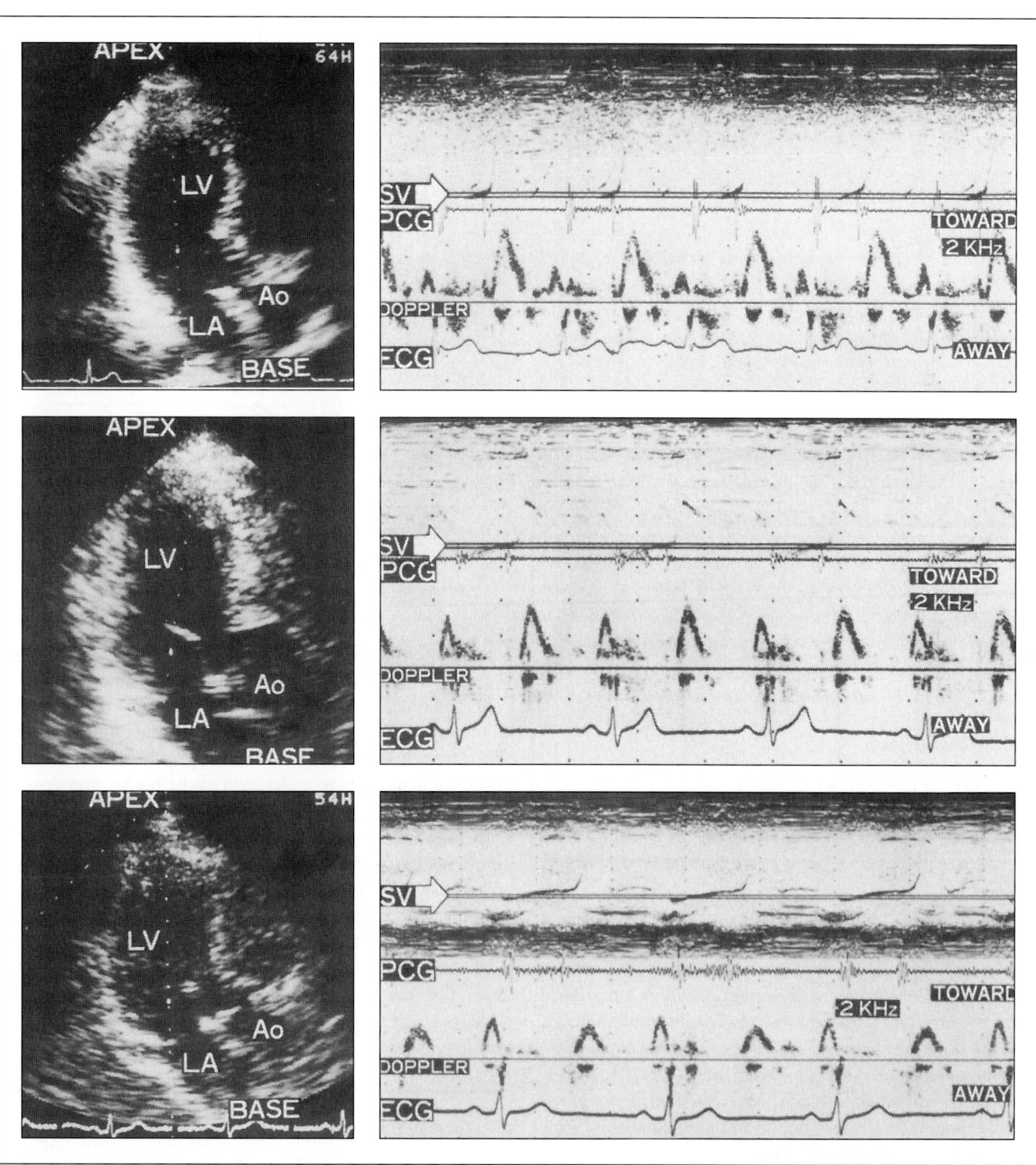

FIGURE 3 Changes in Doppler echocardiographic left ventricular (LV) diastolic filling patterns in normal subjects. **Top**, A 26-year-old man. **Middle**, A 48-year-old man. **Lower**, A 59-year-old man. Ao—aorta; ECG—electrocardiogram; LA—left atrium; PCE—phonocardiogram; SV—sample volume. (*From* Miyatake and coworkers [24]; with permission.)

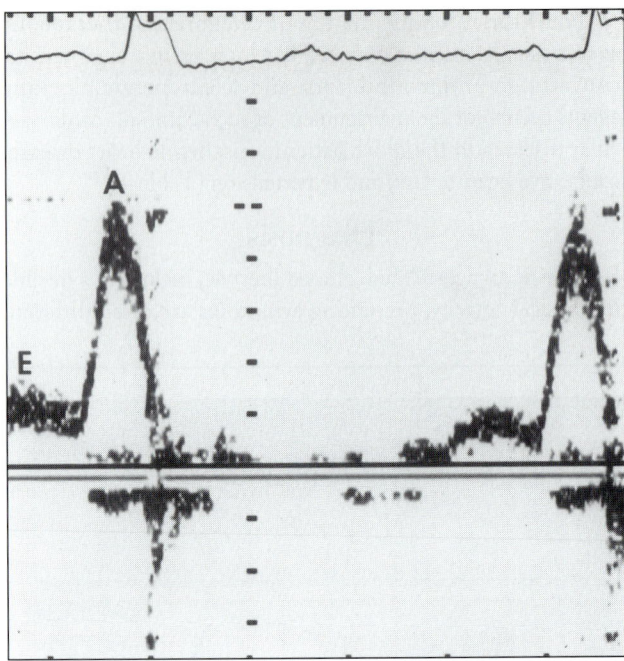

FIGURE 4 Doppler echocardiographic left ventricular diastolic filling pattern in an elderly patient with hypertension showing slow deceleration of the E wave, prolonged deceleration time, prominent A wave, and altered E:A ratio. (*From* Shah and Pai [25]; with permission.)

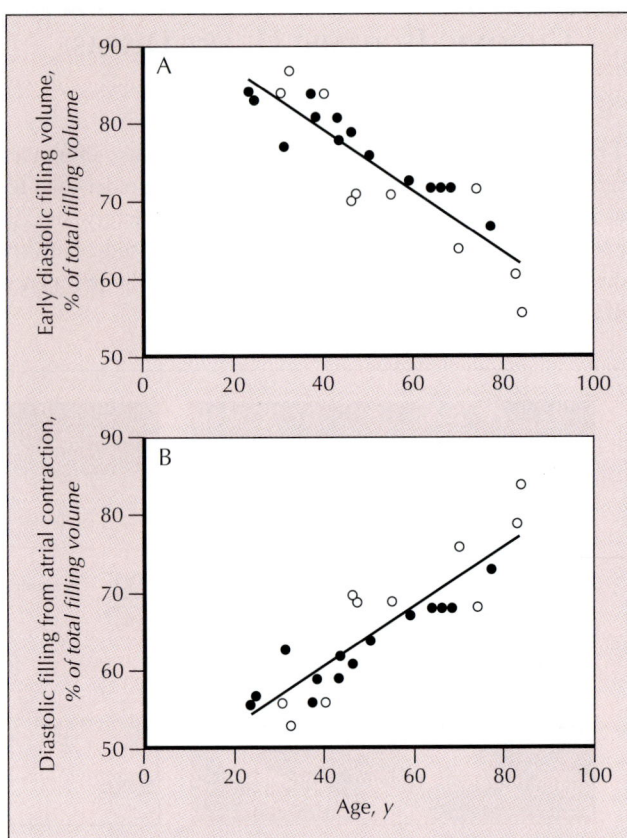

FIGURE 5 The relative contribution of early diastolic filling (**A**) and atrial contraction (**B**) to left ventricular filling as assessed by Doppler echocardiography in healthy men (*closed circles*) and women (*open circles*) ranging from 20 to 80 years of age. (*From* Lakatta [26]; with permission.)

TABLE 3 PHYSIOLOGIC IMPLICATIONS OF AGE-RELATED CHANGES IN CARDIOVASCULAR SYSTEM

Central effects
Preload	Attenuated
Contractility	Not attenuated
Heart rate	Attenuated at all levels of exercise
Afterload	Not attenuated

Peripheral effects

Decreased vascular distensibility

Decreased β-adrenergic responsiveness

than with younger patients. As a manifestation of systolic or diastolic dysfunction, dyspnea is a more prominent symptom than pain, which is usually a manifestation of physical exertion. Also, silent myocardial ischemia is more prevalent in older patients [8]. Added heart sounds and mitral regurgitation are normal variants related to age. Exercise stress testing may be of limited value in older patients because of their altered physical capability and the increased incidence of resting ST-segment electrocardiogram abnormalities. Thus, stress-imaging techniques, both stress echocardiography and stress thallium perfusion, and in particular pharmacologic stress-imaging technology, may be more productive in older patients [9].

Therapy

Appropriate management of risk factors, particularly hypertension therapy and smoking cessation, applies at all ages [2••]. All antiischemic agents, nitrates, β-blockers, and calcium antagonists are effective in older patients. Therapy is more favorably directed at afterload reduction, however, which is effectively performed by dihydropyridine calcium antagonists. Concomitant consideration of the higher prevalence of silent ischemia in these patients suggests the selection of controlled or sustained-release preparations or those with a prolonged intrinsic half-life to maintain constant therapeutic plasma levels. Percutaneous transluminal coronary angioplasty is a therapeutic option in older patients in whom low mortality rates persist regardless of age [10] (Table 5). Data from the Coronary Artery Surgery Study (CASS) show increased intraoperative mortality and morbidity rates in older patients after bypass surgery, yet long-term survival and pain relief are compatible with results in younger patients (Fig. 6) [11].

ACUTE MYOCARDIAL INFARCTION

Prevalence

The increased prevalence of coronary atherosclerosis was discussed in the previous section.

Table 4. Advantages and Disadvantages of Various Classes of Antihypertensive Agents in Elderly Patients

Clinical variables	Diuretic	α-Blocker	ACE inhibitor	β-blocker	Calcium antagonist
Volume depletion	+	–	–	–	–
Suppression of heart rate	–	–	–	+	±
Suppression of cardiac output	–	–	–	+	±
Regression of LVH	–	+	+	±	+
Suppression of VEA	–	–	–	+	+
Preservation of renal function	+	–	+	–	+
Regression of atherosclerosis	–	±	–	±	+
Improved lipid profile	–	±	±	±	±
Effective with low PRA	+	+	–	–	+

From Nixon [16•]; with permission.
+—variable associated with this class of drug; –—variable not associated with this class of drug; ±—variable associated with this class of drug in some cases, but not in others; ACE—angiotensin-converting enzyme; LVH—left ventricular hypertrophy; PRA—plasma renin activity; VEA—ventricular ectopic activity.

Table 5. Results of Coronary Angioplasty in the Elderly

	Older (> 65 y)*	Younger (< 65 y)†
Total series		
Primary success	98 (81%)	412 (80%)
Mean CSA stenosis	92 → 35	87 → 15
Gradient, mm Hg	41 → 8	57 → 15
Last 200 cases	43	157
Primary success	40 (93%)	142 (90%)
Major complications		
Emergency CABG	5 (4.1%)	24 (4.7%)
MI (Q wave)	3 (2.5%)	15 (2.9%)
Death	1 (0.8%)	0

From Raisner and coworkers [10]; with permission.
*n=121.
†n=518.
CABG—coronary artery bypass surgery; CSA—cross-sectional area; MI—myocardial infarction.

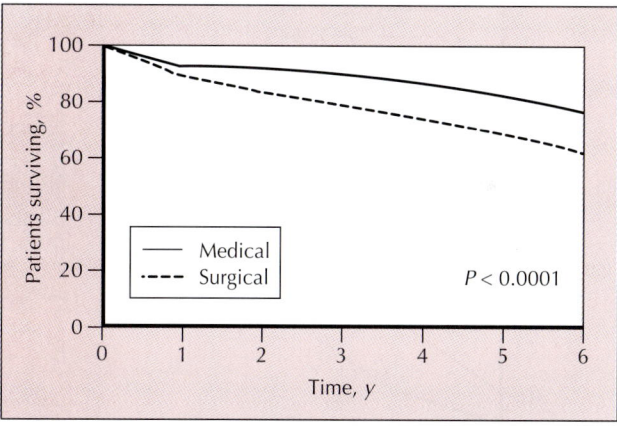

Figure 6 Cumulative 6-year survival in surgical and medical groups among 1491 patients 65 years of age or older from the Coronary Artery Surgery Study (CASS) registry. Survival is adjusted for left ventricular wall motion, congestive heart failure, number of diseased vessels, and associated medical diseases, and age at angiography. (*From* Gersch and coworkers [11]; with permission.)

Diagnosis

The diagnostic methods used in younger patients are equally accurate in older patients. Presenting symptoms may be altered by age. Older patients with acute myocardial infarction may present more often with dyspnea or arrhythmias rather than chest pain (Table 6).

Therapy

Mortality and morbidity rates are higher in older patients [2••]. These higher rates may be age-related, caused by the higher prevalence of ischemic heart disease, or they may be caused by the greater frequency of concomitant diseases, particularly hypertension. Results vary among trials of thrombolytic therapies in older patients with acute myocardial infarction, although recent data show lower mortality rates in the treated groups. Contraindications to thrombolytic therapy increase with age. Secondary prophylactic therapy with β-blockers is equally effective in older as in younger postmyocardial infarction patients [12].

Hypertension

Prevalence

The prevalence of both systolic and diastolic hypertension in the elderly is not as high as previously thought [13]. Nevertheless, systolic and diastolic hypertension remain significant independent cardiovascular risk factors for both mortality and morbidity (Fig. 7) [14]. Furthermore, the prevalence of associated left ventricular hypertrophy

TABLE 6 PRESENTING SYMPTOMS OF ACUTE MYOCARDIAL INFARCTION IN ELDERLY PATIENTS

Symptoms	Patients, %		
	65–74 y	75–84 y	> 85 y
Chest pain	78	60	38
Dyspnea	41	44	43
Sweating	34	23	14
Syncope	3	18	18
Confusion	3	8	19
Stroke	2	7	7

From Reeder and Gersch [27]; with permission.

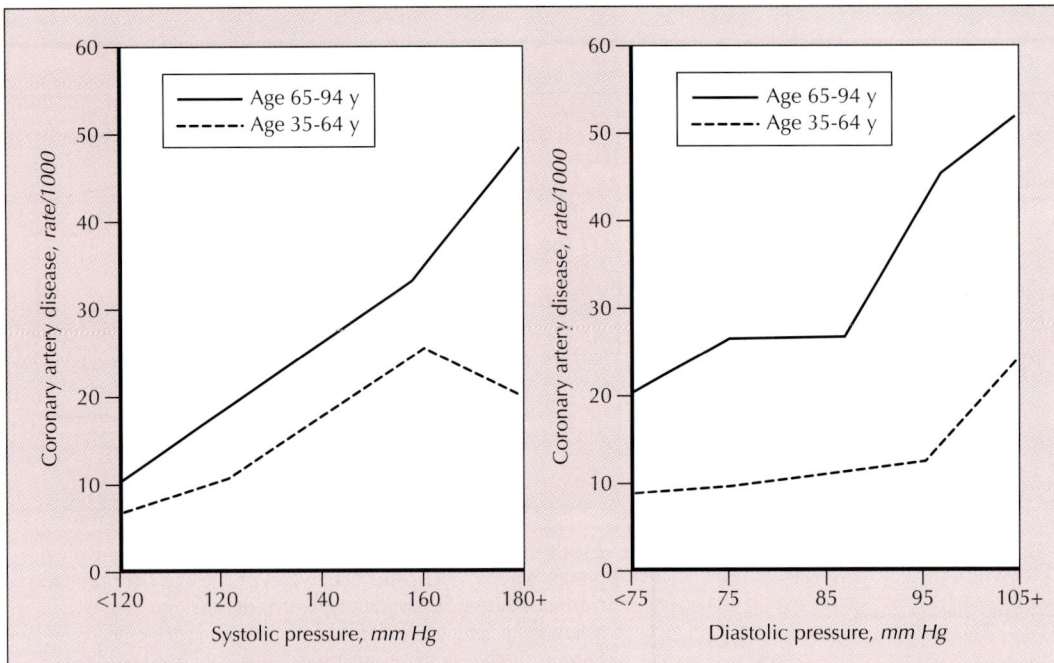

FIGURE 7
Biennial rate of coronary artery disease according to blood pressure and relation to age for men in the Framingham Study. (*From* Levy and coworkers [28]; with permission.)

compounds substantially the cardiovascular risk [15]. Identification of pseudohypertension in this age group also significantly reduces the frequency of the diagnosis of hypertension [16•] (Fig. 8).

Diagnosis

Recent data provide suitable endpoints above or below which the mortality and morbidity risk of the disease significantly increases. Recently, the Systolic Hypertension in the Elderly Program (SHEP) showed that morbidity rates are reduced when patients older than 60 years with isolated systolic hypertension above 160 mm Hg are treated with diuretics [17] (Fig. 9). Also, Cruickshank and coworkers [18] report increased coronary events when diastolic pressures are lowered below a J point of 85 to 90 mm Hg (Fig. 10).

Therapy

Recommended nonpharmacologic modalities include dietary modifications, weight loss, consistent exercise, sodium restrictions, and reduction in alcohol consumption [19]. Pharmacologic therapy may be more favorably directed in the older patient by maintaining cardiac preload, heart rate, and contractility, and by emphasizing the suitability of afterload reduction. Also, both contraindications to and the adverse effects of all medications are more frequent in older patients. Furthermore, certain therapies are better suited to the older patient. Diuretics effectively reduce morbidity rates in older patients with systolic hypertension [15]. Their less desirable characteristics include their primary physiologic effect on cardiac preload and their potential for precipitating hypokalemic arrhyth-

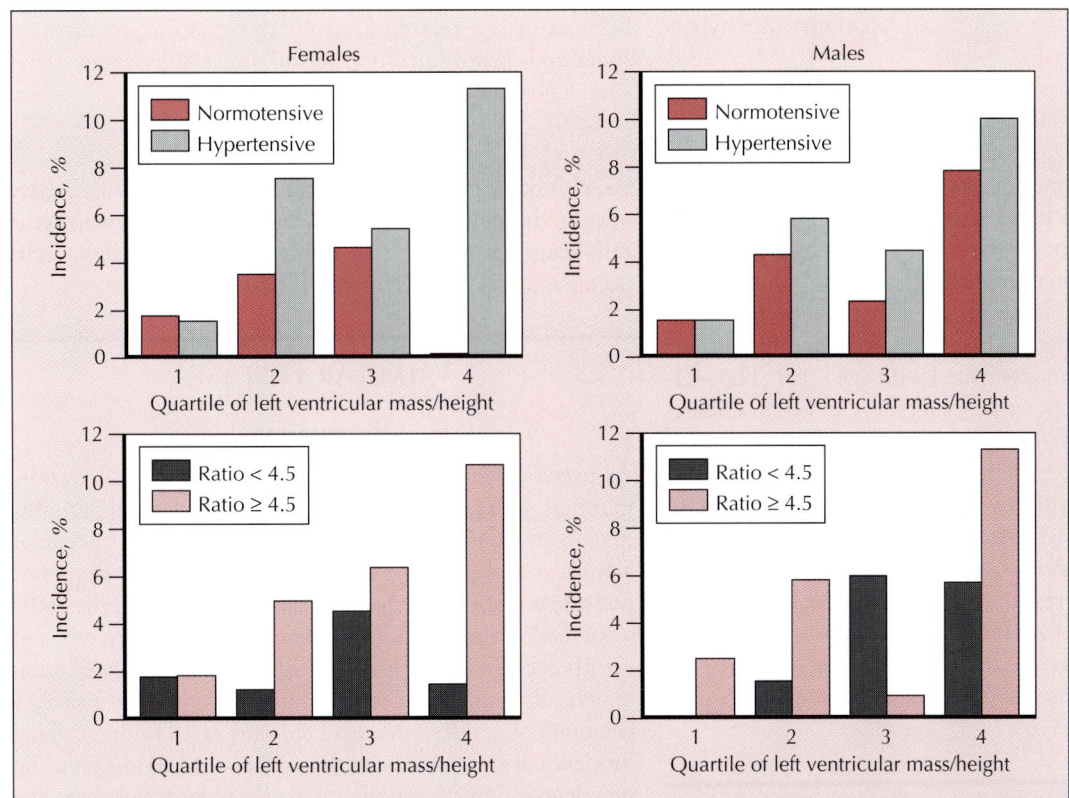

FIGURE 8 Four-year incidence (per 100 subjects) of initial coronary disease events according to gender-specific quartiles of left ventricular mass/height in women (*left panels*) and men (*right panels*). **Top,** Rates stratified by hypertension status. **Bottom,** Rates stratified by ratio of total/high density lipoprotein cholesterol. (*From* Levy and coworkers [15]; with permission.)

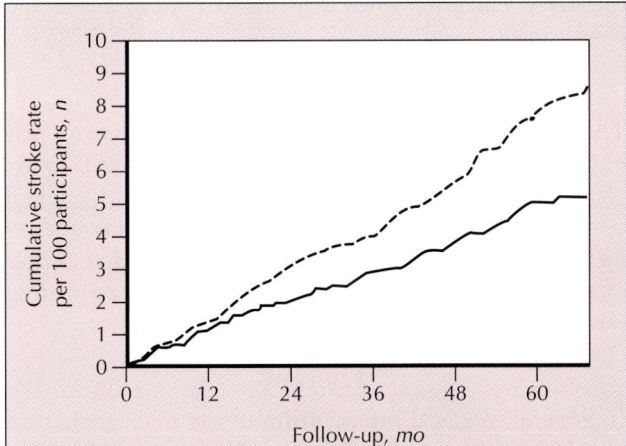

FIGURE 9 Cumulative fatal plus nonfatal stroke rate per 100 participants in the active treatment (*solid line*) and placebo (*broken line*) groups during the Systolic Hypertension in the Elderly Program (SHEP). (*From* SHEP Cooperative Research Group [17]; with permission.)

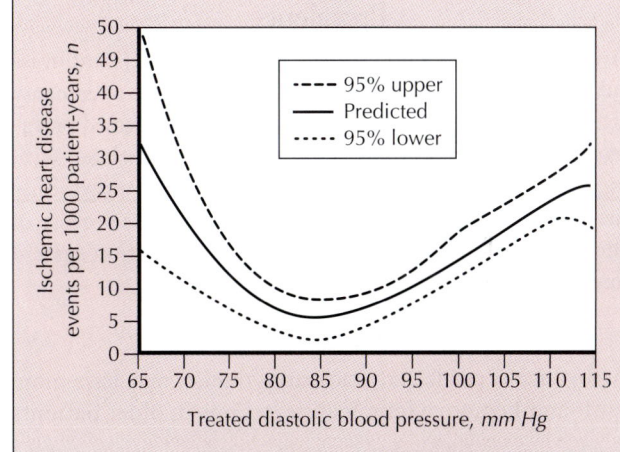

FIGURE 10 Results of studies that stratified cardiac events by treated diastolic blood pressure. Ischemic heart disease events combine mortality and morbidity. (*From* Farnett and coworkers [29]; with permission.)

The Aging Heart

mias, particularly in the presence of left ventricular hypertrophy [16•].

The negative inotropic and chronotropic effects of β-blockers reduce their suitability in older patients, as does their tendency to suppress conduction system activity. Nevertheless, β-blockers are the optimal form of secondary prophylaxis after myocardial infarction in all age groups [11]. Also, the incidence of postural hypotension after application of primary vasodilators is higher in the elderly [9].

The dose response to an angiotensin-converting enzyme inhibitor may be lower in an older patient, because plasma renin activity levels are attenuated with age [16•]. The incidence of adverse effects, such as coughing, and contraindications are higher in older patients. Nevertheless, recent studies show these compounds to be effective secondary agents in older patients with mild hypertension [19]. Calcium antagonists, particularly dihydropyridenes, are the vasodilator of choice in patients with low renin activity. These compounds effectively induce regression of left ventricular hypertrophy. Furthermore, calcium antagonists may suppress ventricular arrhythmias in patients with left ventricular hypertrophy, improve abnormal diastolic function, and potentially regress atherosclerotic plaques [16•, 19] (Table 4).

ARRHYTHMIAS

Prevalence

Arrhythmias occur with greater frequency in older cardiovascular patients because of their increased prevalence of coronary artery disease and hypertension; however, this increased prevalence of arrhythmias does not appear to be associated with increased mortality or morbidity [2••]. Also, bradyarrhythmias may occur with greater frequency in older patients because of the increased prevalence of nodal and conduction system disease [2••].

Diagnosis

Arrhythmias, particularly tachyarrhythmias, may have more profound hemodynamic manifestations in older patients because of age-related diastolic dysfunction, requiring a sustained diastolic filling period and a significant atrial contraction.

Therapy

As with other forms of cardiovascular therapy, the frequency of contraindications to and the adverse effects of antiarrhythmic drugs are greater in an older population. Sequential pacing is useful in older patients [2••].

VALVULAR DISEASE

Prevalence

As previously discussed, added heart sounds and systolic murmurs such as mitral regurgitation are normal variant findings in an elderly population. The cause and prevalence of valvular pathology in the elderly relates primarily to degenerative disease. Senile degeneration and calcification of the aortic valve renders aortic stenosis a disease of the sixth, seventh, and eighth decades [20] (Fig. 11). Although aortic regurgitation may result from a congenitally bicuspid valve, it is mainly a condition of middle rather than old age [21]. The diminishing incidence of rheumatic heart disease has resulted in a reducing prevalence of mitral stenosis among the older population. The prevalence of coexisting coronary artery disease is higher in this age population, which may impact both diagnosis and management.

Diagnosis

The clinical characteristics of different valvular diseases may be altered or suppressed by the presence of age-related characteristics that are normal variants. The clinical suspicion of coexistent valvular pathology in an older patient warrants careful assessment by Doppler echocardiography, which is capable of accurately quantifying valvular stenosis and estimating valvular regurgitation [22].

Therapy

In general, surgical intervention in the management of valvular heart disease is only affected by an increased intra operative surgical risk and any concomitant age-related conditions such as coronary artery disease [2••,21]. The outcome after valve replacement for aortic stenosis and mitral stenosis does not appear to be impacted by age [21] (Fig. 12). Balloon aortic valvuloplasty is a therapeutic option in older patients with significant aortic stenosis; however, restenosis rates of up to 80% within 2 years leave questions of therapeutic efficacy [23]. Balloon mitral valvuloplasty appears to be a therapeutic option for a younger mitral stenosis patient as confirmed by experience and limitations imposed by a preoperative echocardiographic scoring system [21,22]. Clinical indications for valvular replacement in aortic regurgitation and mitral regurgitation also do not appear to be affected by age [21]; however, the same reservations regarding age-related concomitant diseases do apply.

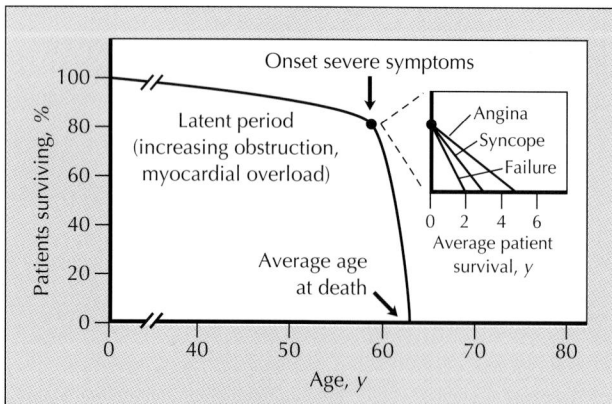

FIGURE 11 The natural history of aortic stenosis. (*From* Ross and Braunwald [30]; with permission.)

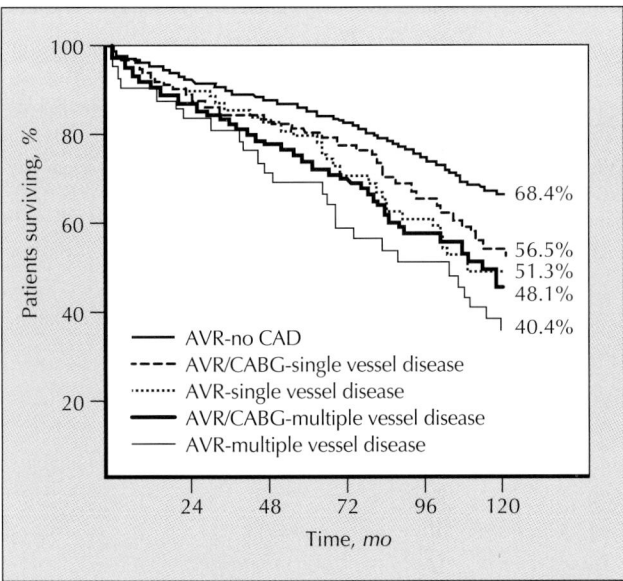

FIGURE 12 Late survival for patients undergoing isolated aortic valve replacement (AVR) and AVR plus coronary artery bypass grafting (CABG), grouped according to no coronary artery disease (CAD), single-vessel CAD, and multiple-vessel CAD. (*From* Lytle and coworkers [31]; with permission.)

References and Recommended Reading

Recently published papers of particular interest have been highlighted as:

- Of interest
- •• Of outstanding interest

1. Nixon JV: Effects of aging on the heart. *Choices Cardiol* 1993, 7:119–120.
2. •• Weisfeldt ML, Lakatta EG, Gerstenblith G: Aging and the heart. In *Heart Disease*, edn 4. Edited by Braunwald E. Philadelphia: WB Saunders; 1992:1656–1669.
3. Gerstenblith G, Fredrickson J, Yin FCP, *et al.*: Echocardiographic assessment of a normal adult aging population. *Circulation* 1977, 56:273.
4. Lakatta EG: Alterations in the cardiovascular system that occur with advancing age. *Fed Proc* 1979, 38:163.
5. Unverforth DV, Fetter JK, Unverforth BJ, *et al.*: Human myocardial histologic characteristics in congestive heart failure. *Circulation* 1983, 68:1194.
6. Rodeheffer RJ, Gerstenblith G, Becker LC, *et al.*: Exercise cardiac output Is maintained with advancing age in healthy human subjects: cardiac dilatation and increased stroke volumes compensate for diminished heart rate. *Circulation* 1984, 69:203.
7. • Nixon JV, Burns CA: Cardiac effects of aging and diastolic dysfunction in the elderly. In *Heart Failure and Left Ventricular Diastolic Dysfunction*, edn 1. Edited by Gaasch WH, LeWinter M. Philadelphia: Lea & Febiger; 1994:427–435.
8. Miller PF, Sheps DS, Bragdon EE, *et al.*: Aging and pain perception in ischemic heart disease. *Am Heart J* 1990, 120:22.
9. Lam JYT, Chaitman BR, Glaenzer M: Safety and diagnostic accuracy of dipyridamole-thallium imaging in the elderly. *J Am Coll Cardiol* 1988, 11:585.
10. Raisner AE, Hust RG, Lewis JM, *et al.*: Transluminal coronary angioplasty in the elderly. *Am J Cardiol* 1986, 57:29.
11. Gersch BJ, Krenmal RA, Schaff HV, *et al.*: Comparison of coronary artery bypass surgery and medical therapy in patients 65 years of age or older. *N Engl J Med* 1985, 313:217.
12. Norwegian Multicenter Study Group: Timolol-induced reduction in mortality and reinfarction in patients surviving acute myocardial infarction. *N Engl J Med* 1981, 304:801.
13. Hypertension Detection and Follow-up Program Cooperative Group: Five year findings of the Hypertension Detection and Follow-Up Program. Mortality by race, sex, and age. *JAMA* 1979, 242:2572.
14. Kannel WB, Gordon T, Schwartz MJ: Systolic versus diastolic blood pressure and risk for coronary heart disease: the Framingham Study. *Am J Cardiol* 1971, 27:335.
15. Levy D, Garrison RJ, Savage DD, *et al.*: Left ventricular mass and incidence of coronary heart disease in an elderly cohort. *Ann Intern Med* 1989, 110:101.
16. • Nixon JV: Treating hypertension in the elderly: a physiological basis for selections of therapy. *Cardiol Elderly* 1993, 1:441–446.
17. SHEP Cooperative Research Group: Prevention of stroke by antihypertensive drug treatment in older persons with isolated systolic hypertension: final results in the systolic hypertension in the elderly program (SHEP). *JAMA* 1991, 265:3255.
18. Cruickshank JM, Thorp JM, Zacharias FJ: Benefits and potential harm of lowering high blood pressure. *Lancet* 1987, i:581.
19. Applegate WB: Hypertension in elderly patients. *Ann Intern Med* 1989, 110:901.
20. Carabello BA: Timing of surgery in mitral and aortic stenosis. *Cardiovasc Clin* 1991, 9:229.
21. Braunwald E: Valvular heart disease. In *Heart Disease*, edn 4. Edited by Braunwald E. Philadelphia: WB Saunders; 1992:1007.
22. Feigenbaum H: Echocardiography. In *Heart Disease*, edn 4. Edited by Braunwald E. Philadelphia: WB Saunders; 1992:81.
23. Safian RD, Kentz RE, Berman AD: Aortic valvuloplasty. *Cardiovasc Clin* 1991, 9:289.
24. Miyatake K, Okamoto M, Kinoshiter N, *et al.*: Augmentation of atrial contribution to left ventricular inflow with aging as assessed by intracardiac Doppler flowmetry. *Am J Cardiol* 1984, 53:586.
25. Shah PM, Pai RG: Diastolic heart failure. *Curr Probl Cardiol* 1992, 12:821.
26. Lakatta EG: The aging heart. *Ann Intern Med* 1990, 113:456.
27. Reeder GS, Gersch BJ: Acute myocardial infarction. In *Stein's Internal Medicine*. Edited by Stein JH. St. Louis: Mosby–Year Book; 1993.

28. Levy D, Wilson PWF, Anderson KM, *et al.*: Stratifying the patient at risk from coronary disease: new insights from the Framingham Study. *Am Heart J* 1990, 119:712.
29. Farnett L, Mulrow CD, Linn WD, *et al.*: The J-curve phenomenon and the treatment of hypertension: is there a point beyond which pressure reduction is dangerous? *JAMA* 1991, 265:489.
30. Ross J Jr, Braunwald E: Aortic stenosis. *Circulation* 1968, 38(suppl 5):61.
31. Lytle BW, Cosgrove DM, Gill CC, *et al.*: Aortic valve replacement combined with myocardial revascularization: late results and determinants of risk for 471 in-hospital survivors. *J Thorac Cardiovasc Surg* 1988, 95:402.

SELECT BIBLIOGRAPHY

Wenger NK: Cardiovascular disease in the elderly. In *Current Problems in Cardiology*. Edited by O'Rourke RA. St. Louis: Mosby–Year Book; 1992:10.

Wiesfeldt ML, Lakatta EG, Gerstenblith G: Aging and the heart. In *Heart Disease*, edn 4. Edited by Braunwald E. Philadelphia: WB Saunders; 1992:1656–1669.

Pregnancy and the Heart

Brad S. Burlew
Howard R. Horn
Jay M. Sullivan

> ### Key Points
> - Pregnancy imposes a hemodynamic burden on the cardiovascular system.
> - Severe valvular stenotic lesions are poorly tolerated; regurgitant lesions have better outcomes.
> - Mitral valve prolapse is rarely a problem.
> - Anticoagulation worsens the outcome during pregnancy.
> - Pulmonary hypertension is associated with a very poor outcome.
> - With careful medical care and appropriate hemodynamic monitoring, most patients with cardiac disease can be safely carried through pregnancy and delivery.

Pregnancy is a condition that places temporary but significant hemodynamic stresses on the woman with underlying cardiac disease. The risk of complications from these stresses depends on the nature of the maternal cardiac abnormality; ranging from negligible risk with mitral valve prolapse to a very high likelihood of maternal and fetal death in patients with advanced pulmonary hypertension. Skillful management of the gravid patient with cardiac disease depends on an understanding of the normal clinical findings associated with the gravid state, the recognition of cardiac disease in the pregnant woman, and an understanding of the likely response of a specific disorder to the hemodynamic changes.

Fortunately, the prevalence of heart disease in the reproductive female population is fairly low (between 0.4% and 4.1%) [1,2]. Worldwide, rheumatic heart disease accounts for up to 90% of the cardiac disorders seen in pregnant women. Mitral stenosis is the most common lesion, occurring in approximately 90% of women with rheumatic heart disease. In the United States, Canada, and Western Europe, rheumatic heart disease now accounts for a diminishing portion (approximately 45% to 75%) of all cases of heart disease [2–4]. Congenital heart disease accounts for much of the remainder, with patients with surgically corrected congenital heart disease and those with prosthetic valves forming a relatively new category of pregnant women with heart disorders.

SIGNS AND SYMPTOMS ASSOCIATED WITH PREGNANCY

The signs and symptoms of pregnancy are a consequence of the normal physiologic changes that occur. These changes include an increase in maternal total blood volume, which reaches maximal values of 50% above baseline (nongravid) values. Plasma volume increases more than the red blood cell mass, which increases by only approximately 10%, resulting in a relative hemodilution [1]. This accounts for the physiologic anemia of pregnancy (Fig. 1).

Resting cardiac output also increases during pregnancy approximately 40% to 50% above that of the nongravid state (Fig. 2) [5]. Increased cardiac output is initially mediated through an increased stroke volume; the stroke volume then

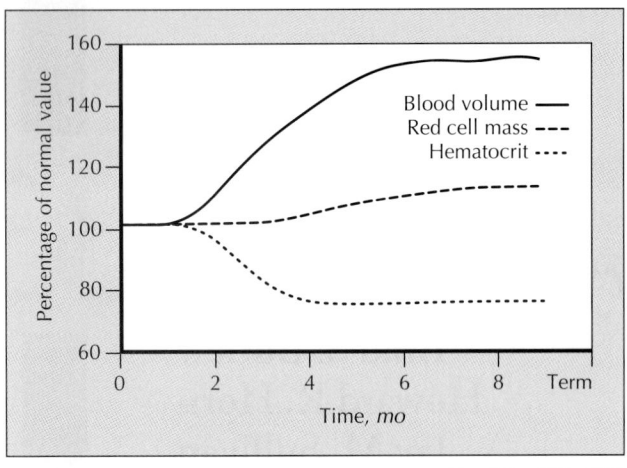

FIGURE 1 Hematologic effects of pregnancy.

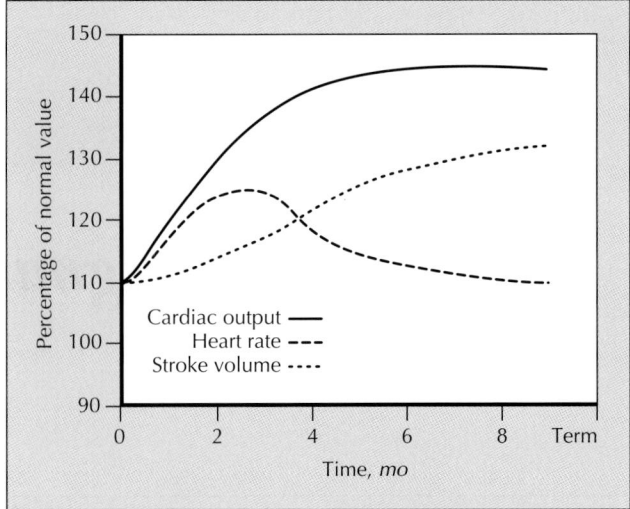

FIGURE 2 Hemodynamic effects of pregnancy.

returns toward the normal range while the heart rate progressively increases. The gravid uterus occasionally compresses the inferior vena cava in the recumbent and standing positions, reducing venous return and cardiac output (Fig. 3) [6].

Regional perfusion of various vascular beds within the body also changes during pregnancy (Fig. 4); increased blood flow to the uterus is observed, particularly during the third trimester. Renal perfusion is increased by approximately 30%. Blood flow to the hands also increases. The breasts often visibly enlarge, and auscultatory souffles are frequently heard, possibly secondary to increased blood flow. The overall effect of these changes in regional perfusion is lower peripheral vascular resistance at term than in the nongravid state [7].

As pregnancy progresses, variations occur in cardiac output, stroke volume, and regional perfusion patterns. As the uterus enlarges, alterations occur in venous return to the central circulation as well. These changes are associated with the development of symptoms and signs that may mimic heart disease. For example, exertional dyspnea normally occurs in over 50% of pregnant women. Orthopnea, paroxysmal nocturnal dyspnea, dizziness, and easy fatigability are quite common. Syncope and presyncope may occur in the normal gravid woman, presumably caused by compression of the inferior vena cava by the uterus. Patients also may experience chest discomfort, mimicking angina pectoris.

On physical examination, normal patients may have prominent neck veins, inspiratory rales, ventricular (S_3) gallops, cardiomegaly, and peripheral edema. Murmurs, particularly systolic flow murmurs with an intensity of up to grade 2 (out of 6), are often heard (Fig. 5). Although diastolic murmurs are unusual in pregnancy, a diastolic murmur over the pulmonic area similar to the Graham Steell murmur is sometimes heard. This murmur, which is believed to be related to a physiologic dilatation of the pulmonary artery, vanishes soon after delivery [1]. A diastolic flow murmur arising from the tricuspid valve is occasionally heard; it likewise disappears after delivery. Venous sounds such as venous hums and mammary souffles also can be heard [8].

ACQUIRED VALVULAR HEART DISEASE

Worldwide, mitral stenosis is the most frequently observed acquired valvular lesion in reproductive women. It also poses one of the most substantial risks to the survival of the mother and the fetus. Depending on the degree of stenosis, a pressure gradient develops across the valve, resulting in elevated pressures in the left atrium and the pulmonary veins. Factors that increase the left atrial pressure are those that increase the diastolic mitral valvular flow rate through an increase in cardiac output or heart rate (which dimin-

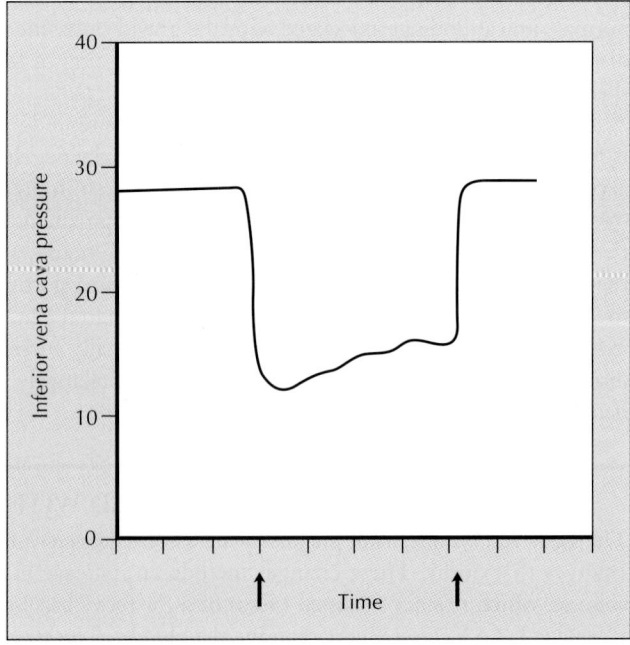

FIGURE 3 Hemodynamic effect of the gravid uterus. The uterus is lifted between the *arrows*. (*From* Kerr [6]; with permission.)

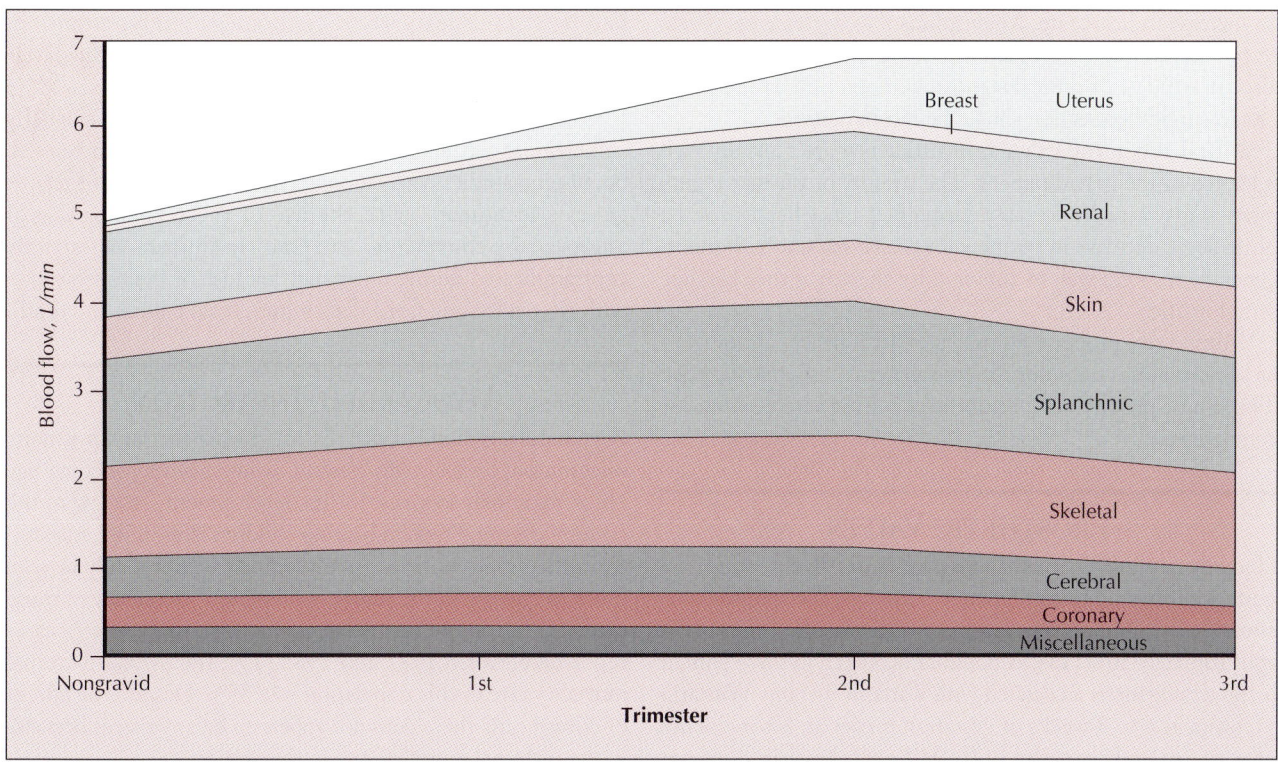

FIGURE 4 Regional blood flow in pregnancy.

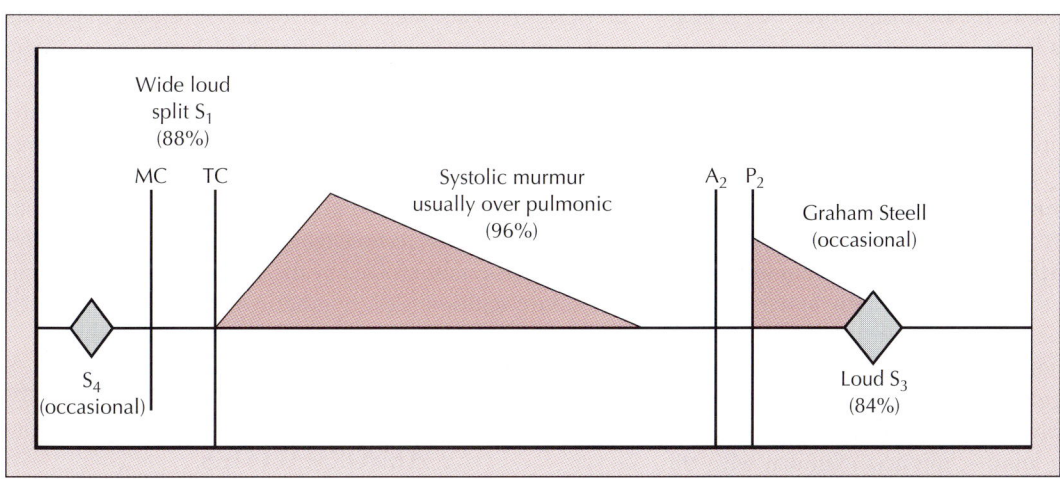

FIGURE 5 Auscultatory findings during pregnancy. A_2—aortic second sound; P_2—pulmonic second sound; S_1—first heart sound; S_3—third heart sound; S_4—fourth heart sound. (*Adapted from* Cutforth and MacDonald [25]; with permission.)

ishes the duration of diastole, increasing the diastolic transvalvular gradient).

Because of the normal physiologic increases in cardiac output during pregnancy and delivery, left atrial pressures tend to be more severely elevated in the gravid state as the diastolic flow across the stenotic mitral valve increases. The elevation in left atrial pressure can result in pulmonary edema and hypoxemia. Clinically, patients develop dyspnea, tachypnea, orthopnea, and paroxysmal nocturnal dyspnea, which are also symptoms often experienced by the normal gravid woman. Frank pulmonary edema and hemoptysis can occur in the third trimester and in the immediate postpartum period. Even patients who appear to be doing well can decompensate suddenly with the onset of rapid atrial tachycardia. Symptomatic tachycardias therefore must be treated promptly and effectively with digoxin and perhaps β-blockade, because pulmonary edema frequently ensues. Patients with refractory symptomatic atrial fibrillation should have cardioversion. Infection and even mild hyperthyroidism also need to be treated promptly in this setting, because these disorders can similarly trigger tachycardia and subsequent pulmonary edema. At parturition, monitoring of the patient's volume status with a pulmonary artery catheter is recommended [1,9,10].

Aortic stenosis appears to affect pregnancy adversely, with a 17% overall maternal mortality rate [11]. Patients with severe aortic stenosis are preload dependent with a fixed stroke volume. Any increase in cardiac output is mediated through an increase in heart rate. Medications that decrease heart rate or preload should be avoided if possible. Vasodilators should also be avoided. If critical stenosis is diagnosed before pregnancy, surgical correction should be recommended.

Mitral and aortic valvular insufficiency are typically well tolerated in the gravid patient. The severity of valvular regurgitation may actually decrease during pregnancy because of the physiologic decrease in peripheral vascular resistance. Patients generally respond well to conservative therapy if they become symptomatic.

Mitral valve prolapse unassociated with other cardiovascular abnormalities does not increase maternal or fetal risk [12]. The use of prophylactic antibiotics in this setting remains controversial.

PROSTHETIC VALVES

Hemodynamically, patients with prosthetic valves tend to fare quite well throughout pregnancy, although the spontaneous abortion rate in patients receiving anticoagulant therapy is approximately 50% [13]. A dominant concern in these patient is the teratogenesis associated with warfarin therapy. Warfarin exposure at 6 to 9 weeks of gestation carries an 8% incidence of warfarin embryopathy [14]. Although heparin does not cross the placenta, prolonged intravenous therapy is associated with maternal complications, including development of heparin-induced osteopenia. In view of these issues, widely followed recommendations for anticoagulation during pregnancy consist of the administration of intravenous heparin during the first trimester and use of oral warfarin therapy during the second and third trimesters [15]. During the last weeks of pregnancy, intravenous heparin is again administered, because late exposure to warfarin is clearly associated with increased peripartum hemorrhage.

Although this protocol was designed to minimize risk to the fetus and the mother, the use of intravenous heparin does not appear to result in a significantly better outcome [16]. Because of this, pregnancy in patients requiring systemic anticoagulation is probably best avoided. Management of the anticoagulated pregnant patient with a prosthetic valve is probably best accomplished in consultation with a cardiologist or another physician familiar with this problem.

PERIPARTUM CARDIOMYOPATHY

Peripartum cardiomyopathy is a disease of unknown etiology associated with development of congestive heart failure during the final month of pregnancy or during the 5 months after delivery. This disorder occurs initially in people who have not previously had heart disease and in whom other explanations for congestive failure are not apparent. It is more common among blacks, is more likely to occur in a woman of 30 years of age or older, who is pregnant with twins or who has toxemia, and is more likely to occur during a third or subsequent pregnancy. If the patient has ever acquired peripartum cardiomyopathy, it is likely to return in subsequent pregnancies, particularly if the patient had persistent postpartum cardiomegaly. Hypertension, myocarditis, and dietary factors may play roles in the development of peripartum cardiomyopathy [17•,18].

Standard therapy with digoxin and diuretics is usually sufficient. If needed, hydralazine and nitrates also can be used, because no studies have demonstrated the induction of teratogenesis in humans with the use of these agents. Use of angiotensin-converting enzyme inhibitors is strictly contraindicated during pregnancy because of their association with neonatal craniofacial deformities, renal failure, and death.

MYOCARDIAL INFARCTION

Fortunately, ischemic heart disease during pregnancy is quite uncommon, undoubtedly because women of reproductive age are at extremely low risk for its development. In view of the current US trend toward bearing children later in life, myocardial infarction among pregnant women will probably be seen more frequently in the future. The present frequency of myocardial infarction in pregnancy is very low, with only 70 cases reported between 1922 and 1985 [19]; the overall maternal mortality rate in this population was 35%. Despite the advent of critical care, there does not appear to be any recent decrease in the maternal mortality rate in this setting.

Current management recommendations include efforts to reduce cardiac workload, such as bed rest, parenteral nitrate therapy, and conduction anesthesia during delivery. It was previously recommended that oxytocin not be used in patients with ischemic heart disease. Currently, however, synthetic oxytocin, which does not contain arginine vasopressin, is available; in appropriate doses, it is unlikely to increase coronary vasoconstriction. With the intravenous bolus administration of 5 to 12 U, oxytocin does produce a 30% decrease in mean arterial pressure and a 50% increase in cardiac output among healthy patients undergoing tocolysis. These hemodynamic effects can be avoided by the administration of oxytocin as a dilute solution [20]. Synthetic oxytocin has been used successfully in pregnant patients after myocardial infarction.

SELECTED DEVELOPMENTAL ABNORMALITIES

Primary pulmonary hypertension is associated with high fetal and maternal mortality rates. Generally, cardiac abnormalities associated with pulmonary hypertension (with or without right-to-left communication) are associated with a maternal mortality rate of approximately 50% [8]. Avoidance or interruption of pregnancy is indicated. Congenital heart disease in the pregnant woman usually poses some hazard to the mother. These patients are best treated in conjunction with a specialist familiar with these abnormalities. Genetic counseling also may be appropriate.

Other developmental abnormalities include Marfan syndrome and hypertrophic cardiomyopathy. With its connective tissue abnormality, Marfan syndrome is associated with a high incidence of aneurysmal dilatation of the aortic root. In one study [21], dissection or rupture of the aortic root occurred in 50% of affected pregnant women, although the overall frequency of these events is probably much lower. Serial echocardiography has been recommended to monitor the progression of dilatation or the development of dissection of the aortic root. The risk of sudden death is believed to be proportional to the diameter of the aortic root [21]. Nonetheless, undetected dissections have occurred despite close echocardiographic monitoring; the availability of endoscopic echocardiography may improve sensitivity in this regard. Meticulous control of blood pressure with β-blockade is an approach we have used for this condition.

Hypertrophic obstructive cardiomyopathy is usually associated with uneventful pregnancies. The outflow obstruction is dynamic and dependent on factors such as blood pressure and ventricular preload, both of which should be maintained if possible. During pregnancy, patients should be encouraged to lie preferentially in the lateral decubitus positions. This maneuver relieves inferior vena caval obstruction, preserving ventricular preload. Because of the likelihood of marked worsening of the dynamic outflow obstruction, β-sympathomimetic tocolytic agents are strictly contraindicated in this disorder.

Regional anesthesia, with its risk of hypotension, should also be avoided [22].

Conclusions

With careful medical care and appropriate hemodynamic monitoring, most patients with cardiac disease can be safely carried through pregnancy and delivery [23]. Unfortunately, termination of the pregnancy is still sometimes indicated. In patients with severe congestive failure, termination should be considered during early pregnancy, because continuation of the pregnancy is likely to result in an unacceptable outcome for both the mother and fetus. Similarly, therapeutic abortion should be considered in patients with primary or secondary pulmonary hypertension (with or without right-to-left communications) and in those with cyanotic congenital heart disease. These clinical conditions can be associated with maternal mortality rates in excess of 50%. Termination of the pregnancy during the first or second trimester presents a more favorable risk to the patient [24].

References and Recommended Reading

Recently published papers of particular interest have been highlighted as:

- Of interest

1. Conradsson T, Werkö L: Management of heart disease in pregnancy. *Prog Cardiovasc Dis* 1974, 16:407–419.
2. McFaul PB, Dornan JC, Lamki H, Boyle D: Pregnancy complicated by maternal heart disease: a review of 519 women. *Br J Obstet Gynaecol* 1988, 95:861–867.
3. Szekely P, Snaith L: *Heart Disease and Pregnancy*. London: Churchill Livingstone; 1974:53.
4. Shime J, Mocarski EJM, Hastings D, *et al.*: Congenital heart disease in pregnancy: short and long term implications. *Am J Obstet Gynecol* 1987, 156:313–322.
5. Robson SC, Hunter S, Boys RJ, Dunlop W: Serial study of factors influencing changes in cardiac output during pregnancy. *Am J Physiol* 1989, 256:H1060–H1065.
6. Kerr MG: The mechanical effects of the gravid uterus in late pregnancy. *J Obstet Gynaecol Br Comm* 1965, 72:513–529.
7. Metcalf J, Ueland K: Maternal cardiovascular adjustment to pregnancy. *Prog Cardiovasc Dis* 1974, 16:363–374.
8. McAnulty JH, Metcalfe J, Ueland K: General guidelines in the management of cardiac disease. *Clin Obstet Gynecol* 1981, 24:773–789.
9. Lang RM, Borow KM: Pregnancy and heart disease. *Clin Perinatol* 1985, 12:551–569.
10. Ueland K, Hansen JM: Maternal cardiovascular dynamics II: posture and uterine contractions. *Am J Obstet Gynecol* 1969, 103:1–7.
11. Arias F, Pineda J: Aortic stenosis and pregnancy. *J Reprod Med* 1978, 20:229–232.
12. Tang LCH, Chan SYW, Wong VCW, Ma H: Pregnancy in patients with mitral valve prolapse. *Int J Gynaecol Obstet* 1985, 23:217–221.
13. Vitali E, Donnatelli F, Quaini E, *et al.*: Pregnancy in patients with mechanical prosthetic heart valves. *J Cardiovasc Surg* 1986, 27:221–227.
14. Pauli RM, Hall JG, Wilson KM: Risks of anticoagulation during pregnancy. *Am Heart J* 1980, 100:761–762.
15. Hirsch J, Cade JF, O'Sullivan EF: Clinical experience with anticoagulation therapy during pregnancy. *BMJ* 1970, 1:270–275.
16. Hall JG, Pauli RM, Wilson KM: Maternal and fetal sequelae of anticoagulation during pregnancy. *Am J Med* 1980, 68:122–140.
17.• Homans D: Peripartum cardiomyopathy. *N Engl J Med* 1985, 312:1432–1437.
18. O'Connell JB, Costanzo-Nordin MR, Subramanian R, *et al.*: Peripartum cardiomyopathy: clinical, hemodynamic, histologic and prognostic characteristics. *J Am Coll Cardiol* 1986, 8:52–56.
19. Hankins GDV, Wendel GD, Leveno KJ, Stoneham J: Myocardial infarction during pregnancy: a review. *Obstet Gynecol* 1985, 65:139–146.
20. Weis FR, Markello R, Mo B, Bochiecho P: Cardiovascular effects of oxytocin. *Obstet Gynecol* 1975, 46:211–214.
21. Pyeritz RE: Maternal and fetal complications of pregnancy in the Marfan syndrome. *Am J Med* 1981, 71:784–790.
22. Shah DM, Sunderji SG: Hypertrophic cardiomyopathy and pregnancy: report of a maternal mortality and review of literature. *Obstet Gynecol Surv* 1985, 40:444–448.
23. Whittemore R, Hobbins JC, Engle MA: Pregnancy and its outcome on women with and without surgical treatment of congenital heart disease. *Am J Cardiol* 1982, 50:641–651.
24. Elkayam U, Gleicher N: Cardiac problems in pregnancy. *JAMA* 1984, 251:2838–2839.
25. Cutforth R, MacDonald CB: Heart sounds and murmurs during pregnancy. *Am Heart J* 1966, 71:741–747.

The Transplanted Heart

Charles K. Moore
John B. O'Connell

> **Key Points**
> - Heart transplantation is now firmly established as a treatment option for some patients with end-stage heart disease.
> - Five-year survival rates following heart transplantation in many centers now exceed 70%.
> - Exercise testing with measurement of peak oxygen consumption is a useful adjunct in assessing the need for transplantation.
> - The most common maintenance immunosuppression regimen following heart transplantation uses cyclosporine, azathioprine, and prednisone in combination.
> - The leading cause of death beyond the first year after transplantation is accelerated coronary artery disease, a process believed to represent a form of "chronic rejection."

The presence of this chapter in a textbook of general internal medicine indicates the successful role now played by heart transplantation in the treatment of advanced heart disease. Following its highly publicized beginnings in the late 1960s, the procedure suffered from relatively poor survival rates, limiting application of heart transplantation to just a few centers worldwide through the 1970s. Advancements such as the development of the transvenous endomyocardial biopsy, and especially the introduction of the immunosuppressant cyclosporine in 1981, dramatically improved success rates and led to rapid increases in the use of cardiac transplantation throughout the United States.

CURRENT RESULTS

Centers performing heart transplantation proliferated rapidly in the first half of the 1980s after the introduction of cyclosporine (Fig. 1*A*) [1]. Both the number of active centers and the total number of heart transplantations performed yearly (both worldwide and in the United States), however, have now leveled off (Fig. 1*B*) (United Network for Organ Sharing Scientific Registry, Unpublished data) [1]. Heart transplantation currently is strictly limited by the availability of donor hearts.

The dramatic improvement in survival after heart transplantation over the last 25 years is clearly evident in Figure 2 [2]. Many centers now achieve 1-year actuarial survival rates exceeding 90%. Five-year actuarial survival rates now surpass 70%, and individual heart transplant recipients have survived more than 20 years (United Network for Organ Sharing Scientific Registry, Unpublished data). Equally important, heart transplantation dramatically improves functional status. One year after transplant, 86% of recipients are in New York Heart Association (NYHA) class I [3], and 50% are employed full-time [4].

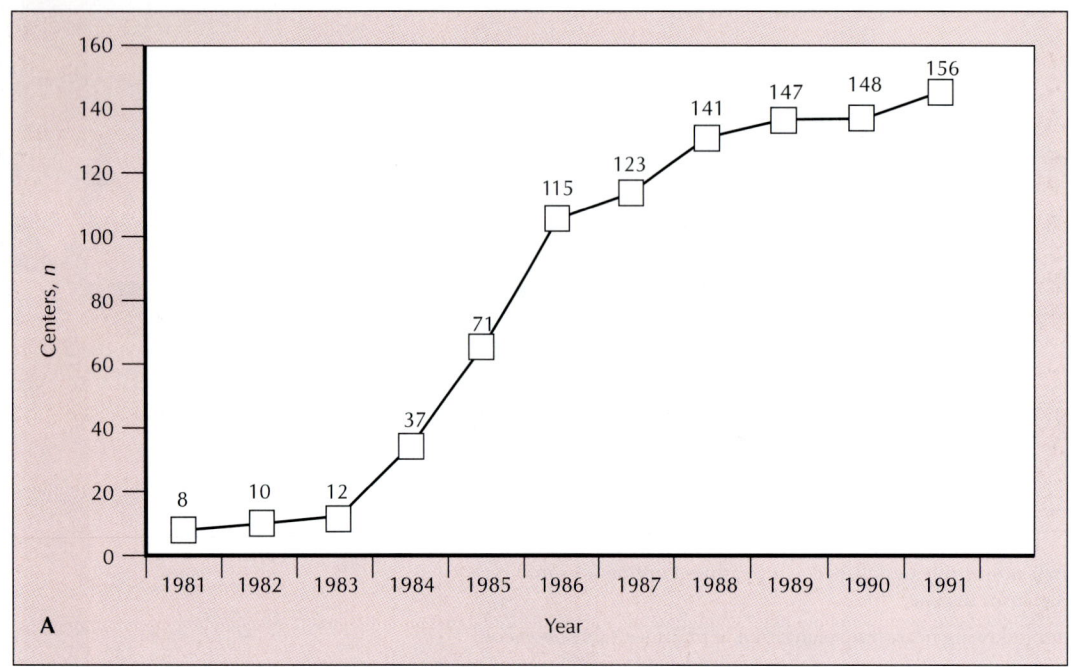
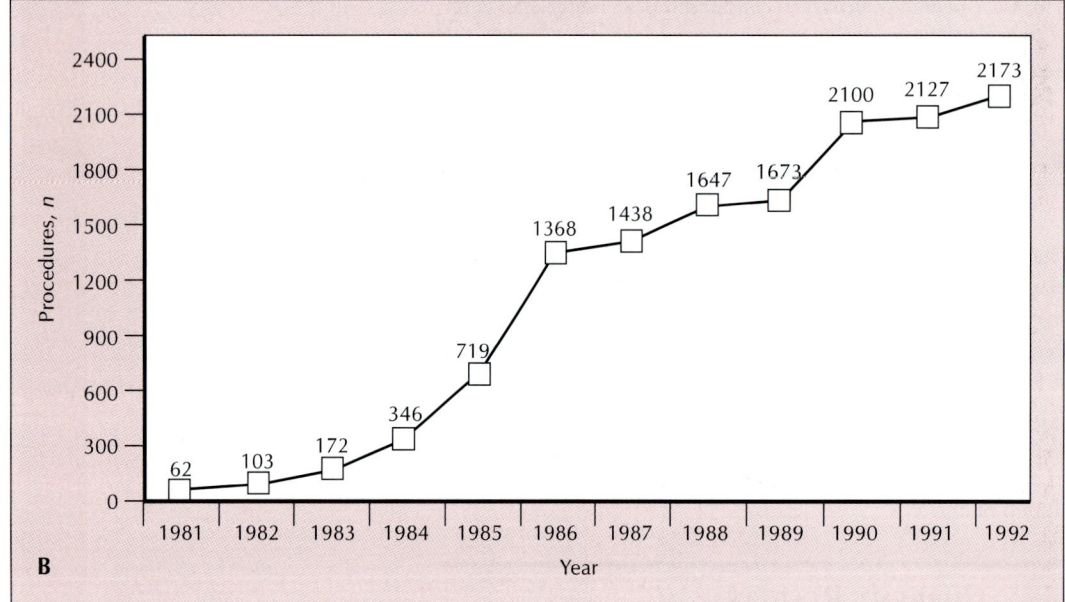

FIGURE 1 **A**, Number of heart transplant centers in the United States by year. (*From* O'Connell and coworkers [1]; with permission.) **B**, Number of heart transplants performed in the United States by year. (*From* O'Connell and coworkers [1] and United Network for Organ Sharing Scientific Registry [Unpublished data]; with permission.)

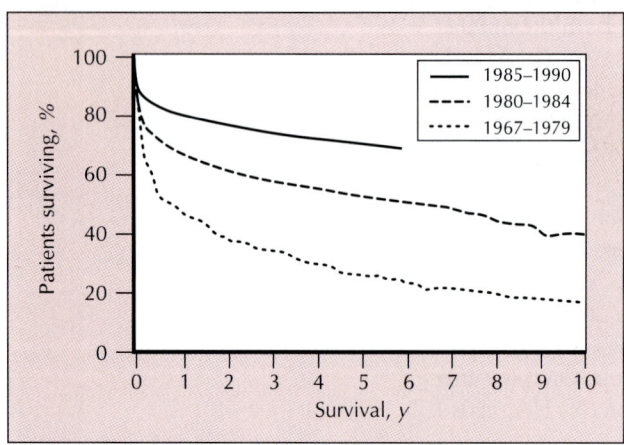

FIGURE 2 Actuarial survival associated with heart transplantation during three successive periods. (*From* Kriett and Kaye [2]; with permission.)

Recipient Selection

The improvement in survival rates after heart transplantation combined with an increasing prevalence of congestive heart failure has led to a marked increase in the number of patients likely to benefit from transplantation. Unfortunately, the supply of donor hearts has stagnated in recent years (as noted previously). As a result, the number of patients awaiting transplantation continues to escalate (Fig. 3). In 1991, more than 800 patients died awaiting heart transplantation. Over 300 patients are added to the waiting list each month, and only 150 receive transplants (Fig. 3). While efforts to expand the number of donor organs continue, the importance of selecting patients most likely to benefit from transplantation is obvious.

Indications

Any cardiac condition associated with substantial morbidity and mortality not amenable to any other form of therapy may be an indication for heart transplantation. Dilated cardiomyopathy remains the most common indication, but severe coronary artery disease or "ischemic cardiomyopathy" is a close second (Fig. 4) [5]. Other possible indications are shown in Table 1. Although the causes of heart disease may vary, severe symptoms (NYHA functional class III to IV) or a poor expected 12-month survival should be present. In the last decade, 71% of heart transplant recipients have been in NYHA class IV and 25% in class III [3]. The determination of prognosis in patients with advanced heart disease is difficult at best, with numerous factors playing a role (Table 2). Poor left ventricular systolic function (low ejection fraction) alone is not sufficient for transplant candidacy, because usually only those patients with associated advanced symptoms of heart failure or life-threatening arrhythmias carry a 6- to 12-month mortality risk great enough to warrant immediate transplant consideration.

Exercise testing with measurement of oxygen consumption by expired gas analysis is a useful adjunct in assessing the need

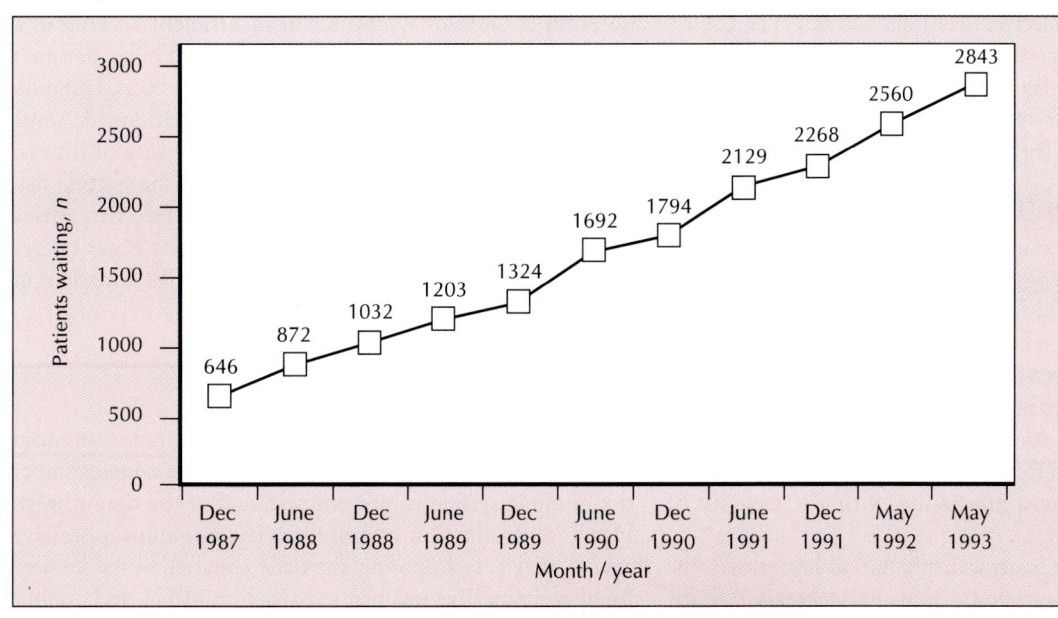

Figure 3 United Network for Organ Sharing National Heart Transplant Waiting List. (*From* O'Connell and coworkers [1] and United Network for Organ Sharing Scientific Registry [Unpublished data]; with permission.)

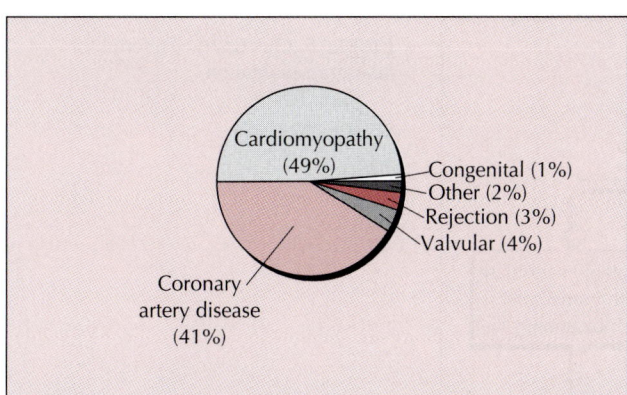

Figure 4 Causes of heart disease in heart transplant recipients. (*From* Kaye [5]; with permission.)

Table 1 Causes of Heart Disease in Transplant Candidates

End-stage cardiomyopathy
    Idiopathic dilated
    Ischemic
    Infiltrative, restrictive (*eg*, amyloidosis, sarcoidosis)
    Valvular
    Hypertrophic
Myocarditis
Refractory angina, ischemia not amenable to surgery or angioplasty
Inoperable primary cardiac tumors
Refractory life-threatening arrhythmias not controllable with implantable cardioverter defibrillator
Uncorrectable congenital heart disease
Refractory heart transplant rejection

Table 2. Adverse prognostic factors in heart failure

Low left ventricular ejection fraction
Advanced NYHA functional class
Presence of an ventricular S_3 gallop
Reduced serum sodium
Elevated plasma catecholamine levels
Increased pulmonary capillary wedge pressure
Reduced cardiac index
Low peak exercise oxygen consumption
Ventricular tachycardia
Antiarrhythmic drug use

NYHA—New York Heart Association.

---

for transplantation. Not only does it provide an objective confirmation of the subjective determination of NYHA functional class, peak exercise oxygen consumption (pVO$_2$) has also been shown to predict 12-month survival in patients with severe left ventricular systolic dysfunction and resultant congestive heart failure [6•].

Contraindications

Although a transplant candidate's present level of symptoms and cardiovascular prognosis are critical to the selection process, expected morbidity and mortality *after* heart transplantation must also be addressed. Patients with end-stage heart disease and irreversible, uncontrollable, or untreatable comorbid conditions are not suitable candidates for transplantation (Table 3). Coexisting medical problems independently affect posttransplantation morbidity and mortality adversely, or they may do so in combination with the toxicity of immunosuppressive drugs.

As experience with heart transplantation has grown, the number of absolute contraindications has decreased. Some patients with diabetes mellitus now routinely undergo transplantation and appear to have similar morbidity and mortality rates to patients without diabetes in the first year after transplantation [7]. The upper age limit has steadily increased to the degree that most transplantation programs now consider selecting patients of up to 65 years of age (or even older in highly select patients).

The Selection Process

Patients with NYHA class III or IV symptoms caused by heart disease not amenable to other treatment modalities and no absolute contraindication should be referred to a heart transplant center for consideration. Such patients will undergo an extensive evaluation directed at identifying and assessing all of the factors noted previously (Table 4). A committee of physicians and other health-care personnel generally makes a decision on each candidate. Some patients will be found to be unacceptable because of one or more contraindications, whereas others may have transplantation deferred because of symptoms of insufficient severity or a relatively favorable prognosis (Fig. 5). Those patients deemed acceptable and in imminent need of transplantation will be actively "listed" on a computerized, nationwide waiting list. Organs are allocated based on severity of illness, blood group, body size, and finally, time on the waiting list. Severity of illness is generally limited to two categories (Table 5). Waiting time for a suitable donor heart ranges from as little as 1 day to 1 year or more, with a median of approximately 6 months [8].

MANAGEMENT

At the time of transplantation, the recipient trades advanced heart disease for another significant problem—suppression of the immune system to prevent rejection of the donor heart. Despite introduction of more specific immunosuppressive agents such as cyclosporine, the toxic potential of the modern immunosuppressive regimen remains formidable, and optimal

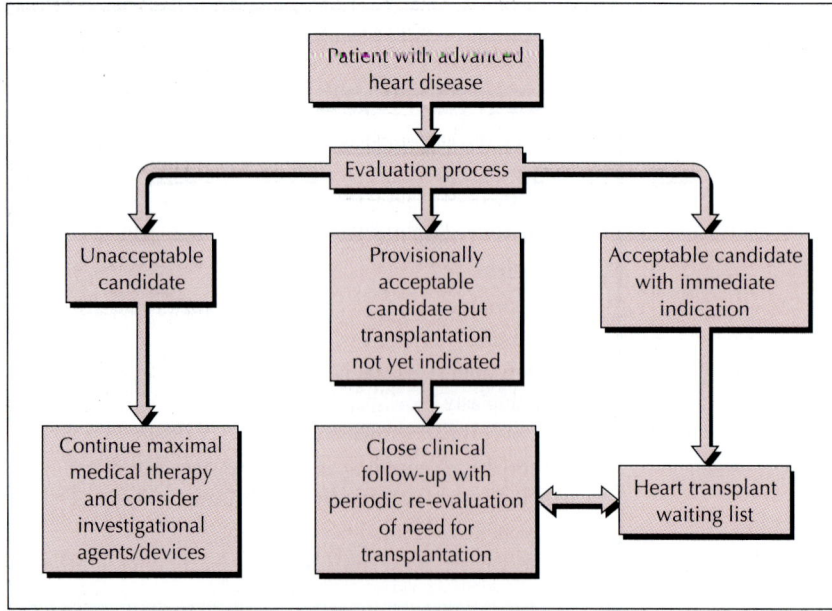

FIGURE 5 Outcomes of referral for heart transplantation.

TABLE 3 CONTRAINDICATIONS FOR HEART TRANSPLANTATION

Irreversibly elevated pulmonary vascular resistance
Systemic illness associated with poor prognosis
Active malignancy
Uncontrolled infection
Insulin-dependent diabetes mellitus with end-organ damage
Severe peripheral or cerebrovascular disease
Morbid obesity
Irreversible major organ dysfunction (pulmonary, hepatic, renal)
Recent pulmonary infarction
Active gastrointestinal hemorrhaging
Psychosocial instability

TABLE 5 HEART TRANSPLANT RECIPIENT STATUS CRITERIA

Status 1
Patients requiring cardiac or pulmonary assistance with one or more of the following devices:
  Total artificial heart
  Left and/or right ventricular assist systems
  Intraaortic balloon pump
  Ventilator
Or, patients meeting both of the following criteria:
  In an intensive care unit
  Requires inotropic agents to maintain adequate cardiac output
Or, patients less than 6 months old

Status 2
All other waiting patients who do not meet Status 1 criteria

From United Network for Organ Sharing Scientific Registry [Unpublished data]

TABLE 4 MEDICAL EVALUATION BEFORE CARDIAC TRANSPLANTATION

History and physical (complete)

Hematologic profile
Complete blood count, chemistries, BUN, Cr, ALT, AST, ALP, GGT, total and direct bilirubin, prothrombin time, partial thromboplastin time

Stool occult blood testing

Serologic assays
Hepatitis A, B, C; syphilis; human immunodeficiency virus; cytomegalovirus; Epstein-Barr virus; *Toxoplasma gondii*; varicella

Histocompatibility testing
Blood type and antibody screen
Panel-reactive antibody screen
HLA typing

Urine profile
Urinalysis
Creatinine clearance (24-h collection)

Radiologic testing
Chest radiography
Radionuclide ventriculography
Abdominal ultrasonography
Carotid and peripheral Doppler studies*

Ventilatory testing
Complete pulmonary function studies
Exercise capacity testing (pVO_2)

Cardiologic evaluation
Electrocardiogram
Echocardiogram
Right heart catheterization
Left heart catheterization*
Coronary angiogram*
Endomyocardial biopsy*
Radionuclide ventriculogram*

Consultation
Social services
Dentistry
Psychiatry*
Dental

From Olinde and coworkers [19]; with permission.
*As indicated.
ALP—alkaline phosphatase; ALT—alanine aminotransferase; AST—aspartate aminotransferase; BUN—blood urea nitrogen; Cr—creatinine; GGT—gamma-glutamyl transferase; HLA—human lymphocyte antigen.

posttransplantation care requires constant vigilance for potential complications.

Normal Allograft Physiology

The surgical technique of orthotopic heart transplantation is simplified by anastomosing a residual cuff of the recipient's right and left atrial tissue to the donor atria rather than separately anastomosing two venae cava and four pulmonary veins (Fig. 6). As a result, two sinus nodes are present postoperatively. Atrial activity from the recipient sinus node can often be seen on the electrocardiogram dissociated from the sinus rhythm of the donor heart. This recipient atrial activity is electrically isolated from the donor heart by the suture line.

Another unique feature of the donor heart is denervation. All transplanted hearts remain denervated for at least 1 year and are partially denervated thereafter. Without the normally dominant inhibitory parasympathetic influence, resting heart rate in the transplant recipient frequently exceeds 90 bpm. Denervation also modifies the response of the donor heart to exercise. Without direct sympathetic innervation, the tachycardic response to exercise depends on circulating catecholamines, an

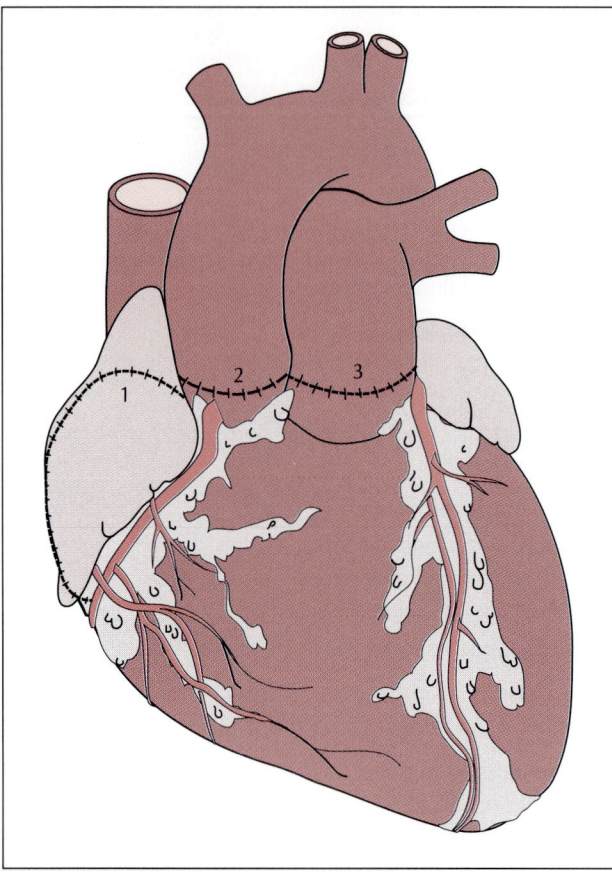

FIGURE 6 Anterior view after orthotopic heart transplantation demonstrates right atrial (1), aortic (2), and pulmonary arterial (3) suture lines. The left atrial suture line is hidden behind the heart in this view.

inherently slower mechanism. Thus, transplant recipients require a longer warm-up and cool-down phase during exercise. Despite these differences in physiology, heart transplant recipients are generally capable of achieving normal exercise tolerance; some even participate in competitive athletics.

Rejection

The incidence of acute allograft rejection and death resulting from transplant rejection is greatest early after transplantation and diminishes gradually with time (Fig. 7) [9]. The transvenous right ventricular endomyocardial biopsy technique allows unprecedented surveillance for rejection on a repetitive outpatient basis. Consequently, most episodes of acute rejection are diagnosed before significant symptoms develop or the systolic function of the allograft decreases. Signs and symptoms that may suggest acute allograft rejection are shown in Table 6. Suspicion of acute rejection is a medical emergency and warrants immediate consultation with the transplant center. Treatment options for acute rejection are numerous, but "pulse" therapy with intravenous methylprednisolone (eg, 1 g of methylprednisolone intravenously four times a day for 3 days) or oral prednisone remains the most common therapy for episodes of sufficient severity to warrant a significant augmentation in immunosuppressive treatment. For more severe or corticosteroid-resistant rejection episodes, potent

polyclonal and monoclonal antilymphocyte antibody preparations are available (eg, antithymocyte globulin and muromonab-CD3).

Maintenance Immunosuppression

The majority of heart transplant centers now practice "triple therapy" maintenance immunosuppressive therapy, using cyclosporine, azathioprine, and corticosteroids. Use of several agents allows a total level of immunosuppression sufficient to keep rejection at bay yet avoid significant toxicity from any single agent (Fig. 8). Each immunosuppressant carries a unique toxicity profile (Table 7). Morbidity secondary to chronic corticosteroid administration can be especially problematic, prompting many programs to wean steroid doses gradually to a minimal level or even discontinue therapy with these agents entirely in some patients.

In addition to the intrinsic toxicity of immunosuppressive drugs, significant interactions with other commonly prescribed medications pose a real threat to the heart transplant recipient. The metabolism of cyclosporine in particular can be dramatically affected, leading to either elevated blood levels and toxicity (eg, renal failure) or decreased blood levels and transplant rejection (Table 8). Other drugs to be used only with caution include nonsteroidal antiinflammatory drugs, which exacerbate nephrotoxicity from cyclosporine, and allopurinol, which dramatically impairs metabolism of azathioprine, therefore requiring a three- or fourfold dose reduction. Recipients are routinely advised to contact the heart transplant center before starting therapy with *any* new drugs.

Infections

Suppression of the immune system to prevent rejection also enhances susceptibility of the transplant recipient to a variety of infectious agents. Before cyclosporine was available, infections accounted for over 50% of all deaths in heart transplant recipients [10]. With cyclosporine-based immunosuppressive

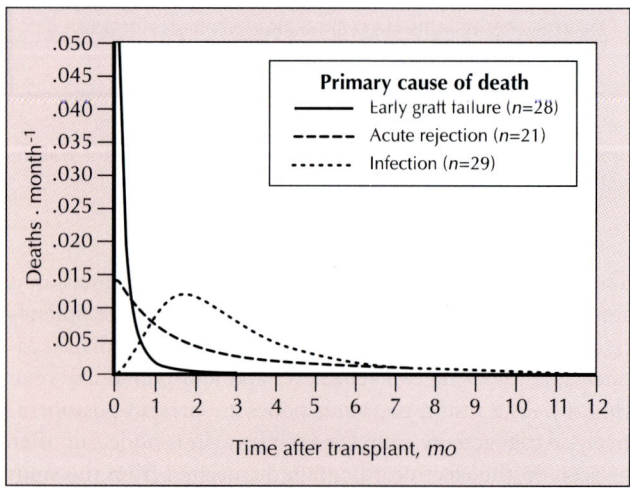

FIGURE 7 Instantaneous risk of death from early graft failure, acute rejection, and infection for 914 patients in the Transplant Cardiologists Research Database. (*From* Bourge and coworkers [9]; with permission.)

Table 6 Signs and Symptoms of Acute Cardiac Allograft Rejection*	
Signs	**Symptoms**
Relative hypotension	Dyspnea
Elevated jugular venous pressure	Fatigue
Ventricular S_3 gallop	Orthopnea
Rales	
Peripheral edema	
Low-grade fever	
Arrhythmias	

*Rejection commonly occurs without any signs or symptoms however.

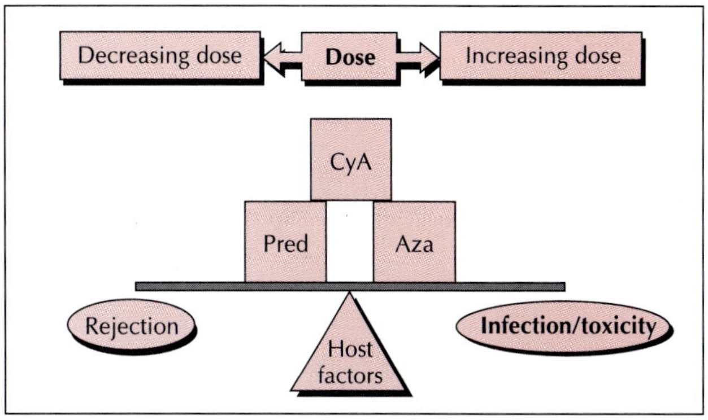

Figure 8 Adjusting the doses of immunosuppressive drugs requires a balance between insufficient (leading to rejection) and excessive (resulting in infection or toxicity) immunosuppression. Aza—azathioprine; CyA—cyclosporine; Pred—prednisone.

Table 7 Side Effects and Toxicity of Immunosuppressants	
Corticosteroids	**Cyclosporine**
Cushing's syndrome	Hypertension
Osteoporosis	Renal insufficiency
Myopathy	Hirsutism
Cataracts	Tremor
Peptic ulcer disease	Gingival hyperplasia
Impaired wound healing	Elevated LFT results
Hyperlipidemia	Seizures
Glucose intolerance	Headache
Hypertension	Hypomagnesemia
Osteonecrosis	Photosensitivity
Emotional lability	Paresthesias
Acne	
Azathioprine	
Leukopenia	
Anemia	
Thrombocytopenia	
Pancreatitis	
Nausea	
Elevated LFT results	

LFT—liver function test.

Table 8 Common Drug Interactions with Cyclosporine
Increases cyclosporine blood levels
Erythromycin
Ketoconazole
Fluconazole
Itraconazole
Diltiazem
Verapamil
Nicardipine
Metoclopramide
Decreases cyclosporine blood levels
Carbamazepine
Phenobarbital
Phenytoin
Rifampin

regimens, the infectious mortality rate is now less than 15% [11]. Deaths from infection peak at 1 to 3 months after transplantation, with a steady decline thereafter [2].

Bacterial pathogens account for the majority of severe infections, but viral, fungal, and protozoal agents each play an important role (Fig. 9) [12•]. The single most common severe infection is bacterial pneumonia (usually resulting from *Pneumococcus* infection in outpatients) [12•].

The majority of serious viral illnesses that arise after heart transplantation are caused by cytomegalovirus [12•], which is commonly associated with asymptomatic infection but can also result in life-threatening pneumonitis, hepatitis, or enteritis. "Cytomegalovirus syndrome" is a mononucleosis-like illness with fever, fatigue, and leukopenia. Patients who are seronegative before transplantation and then receive a heart from a seropositive donor are at highest risk for cytomegalovirus disease. Most programs use prophylactic therapy with intravenous ganciclovir, high-dose oral acyclovir, hyperimmune intravenous immunoglobulin, or some combination for at-risk patients during the first 3 to 4 months after transplantation (when the incidence of cytomegalovirus infection is greatest).

Infection with *Pneumocystis carinii* accounts for most protozoal infections and almost always induces pneumonitis [12•]. The incidence of *Pneumocystis* infections seems to vary by location, but many programs administer oral trimethoprim-sulfamethoxazole prophylaxis during the first 9 to 12 months after transplantation and at other times when patients are heavily immunosuppressed.

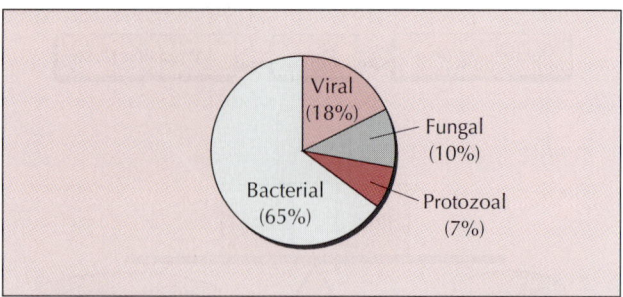

FIGURE 9 Distribution of pathogens causing severe infections in heart transplant recipients. (*From* Dummer [12•]; with permission.)

Accelerated Coronary Artery Disease

The donor heart is susceptible to a process involving accelerated intimal proliferation throughout the coronary vessels that can lead to myocardial ischemia and even infarction. The most widely accepted hypothesis proposes that the vasculature of the donor heart stimulates an immune response that culminates in myointimal thickening. As a result, this process has also been labeled *chronic rejection*. Coronary angiography has shown that this vascular abnormality can be seen in approximately 25% of recipients by 2 years after transplantation (Fig. 10) [13]; beyond the first year after transplantation, it is the leading cause of death [14]. Because of denervation of the donor heart, most patients with advanced allograft vasculopathy do not experience angina but may present with signs and symptoms of congestive heart failure. Because of the limited sensitivity and specificity of noninvasive studies in this population, most transplant programs perform yearly coronary angiography to screen for this process. At present, treatment options are limited, because the diffuse coronary lesions are rarely amenable to coronary artery bypass surgery or percutaneous transluminal coronary angioplasty. Some patients may be candidates for repeat transplantation.

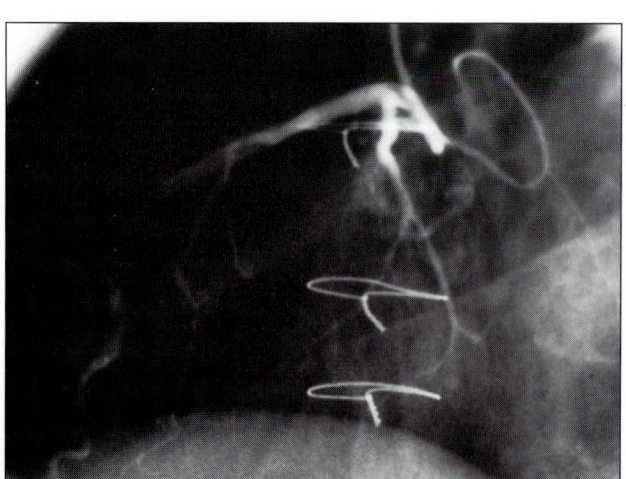

FIGURE 10 Angiography of the left coronary artery of a transplanted heart with accelerated coronary artery disease demonstrates rapid tapering of the lumen with loss of small distal vessels.

Other Complications

A myriad of other complications may strike the heart transplant recipient (Table 9) [15•]. Arterial hypertension is particularly common, with over 90% of patients receiving immunosuppressive maintenance "triple-therapy" requiring antihypertensive therapy by 6 months [16]. Corticosteroids, and especially cyclosporine, have been implicated as causative agents. Hemodynamic studies have shown elevated systemic vascular resistance with normal cardiac output [16]. Calcium channel blockers are very effective therapeutically, as are many other agents.

An increased incidence of malignancy is a well-recognized complication of chronic immunosuppression. Lymphoproliferative disorders can be especially lethal and may occur either early or late after transplantation. Therefore, regular assessment of transplant recipients should include careful examination for lymphadenopathy. Heavy immunosuppression, particularly with potent antilymphocyte-antibody preparations, is associated with an increased incidence of lymphoproliferative disease [17]. Some of these malignancies will respond to a reduction in immunosuppressive therapy alone [18]. Skin cancers are also a major problem, especially in patients who have had excessive exposure to the sun. Squamous cell carcinomas predominate and can be life-threatening if not detected early and aggressively treated [14].

ROLE OF THE GENERALIST

Despite a relatively favorable expected quality of life and survival after heart transplantation, regular and thorough general medical care is critical in minimizing complications. Most transplant programs encourage continued participation by the patient's primary-care provider, especially when the frequency of visits to the transplant center for biopsies diminishes. Close communication between the primary-care physician and the transplant team allows many problems to be appropriately handled close to the patient's home, obviating travel to the sometimes distant transplant center.

TABLE 9 COMPLICATIONS FOLLOWING HEART TRANSPLANTATION
Acute rejection
Infection
Accelerated coronary artery disease
Systemic hypertension
Malignancy
Chronic renal insufficiency
Gout
Hyperlipidemia
Osteoporosis
Osteonecrosis
Obesity
Glucose intolerance

References and Recommended Reading

Recently published papers of particular interest have been highlighted as:
• Of interest

1. O'Connell J, Gunnar R, Evans R, *et al*.: Task Force 1: Organization of heart transplantation in the US. *J Am Coll Cardiol* 1993, 22:8–14.
2. Kriett J, Kaye M: The Registry of the International Society for Heart and Lung Transplantation: Eighth Official Report—1991. *J Heart Lung Transplant* 1991, 10:491–498.
3. Kaye M: The Registry of the International Society for Heart and Lung Transplantation: Tenth Official Report—1993. *J Heart Lung Transplant* 1993, 12:541–548.
4. Young J, Winters W, Bourge R, *et al*.: Task Force 4: Function of the heart transplant recipient. *J Am Coll Cardiol* 1993, 22:31–41.
5. Kaye M: The Registry of the International Society for Heart and Lung Transplantation: Ninth Official Report—1992. *J Heart Lung Transplant* 1992, 11:599–606.
6. • Mancini D, Eisen H, Kussmaul W, *et al*.: Value of peak exercise oxygen consumption for optimal timing of cardiac transplantation in ambulatory patients with heart failure. *Circulation* 1991, 83:778–786.
7. Ladowski J, Kormos R, Uretsky B, *et al*.: Heart transplantation in diabetic recipients. *Transplantation* 1990, 49:303–305.
8. United Network of Organ Sharing: *Annual Report of the U.S. Scientific Registry for Organ Transplantation and the Organ Procurement and Transplantation Network*. Publication number ES-1, D-12. Rockville, MD: US Department of Health and Human Services; 1990.
9. Bourge R, Naftel D, Costanzo-Nordin M, *et al*.: Pretransplantation risk factors for death after heart transplantation: a multiinstitutional study. *J Heart Lung Transplant* 1993, 12:549–562.
10. Pennock J, Oyer P, Reitz B, *et al*.: Cardiac transplantation in perspective for the future. *J Thorac Cardiovasc Surg* 1982, 83:168–177.
11. Hofflin J, Potasmon I, Baldwin J, *et al*.: Infectious complications in heart transplant recipients receiving cyclosporine and corticosteroids. *Ann Intern Med* 1987, 106:209–216.
12. • Dummer J: Infectious complications of transplantation. *Cardiovasc Clin* 1990, 20:163–178.
13. Olivari M, Homans D, Wilson R, *et al*.: Coronary artery disease in cardiac transplant patients receiving triple-drug immunosuppressive therapy. *Circulation* 1989, 80:111–115.
14. Miller L, Schlant R, Kobashigawa J, *et al*.: Task Force 5: Complications. *J Am Coll Cardiol* 1993, 22:41–54.
15. • Miller L: Long-term complications of cardiac transplantation. *Prog Cardiovasc Dis* 1991, 33:229–282.
16. Olivari M, Antolick A, Ring W: Arterial hypertension in heart transplant recipients treated with triple-drug immunosuppressive therapy. *J Heart Transplant* 1989, 8:34–39.
17. Swinnen L, Costanzo-Nordin M, Fisher S, *et al*.: Increased incidence of lymphoproliferative disorder after immunosuppression with the monoclonal antibody OKT3 in cardiac transplant recipients. *N Engl J Med* 1990, 323:1723–1728.
18. Penn I: Cancers after cyclosporine therapy. *Transplant Proc* 1988, 20:276–279.
19. Olinde KD, Moore CK, O'Connell JB: The selection of recipients for cardiac transplantation. *Develop Cardiol* 1993, 3:1–12.

Selected Bibliography

Miller L, Naftel D, Bourge R, *et al*.: Infection after heart transplantation: a multiinstitutional study. *J Heart Lung Transplant* 1994, 13:381–383.

Olson L, Rodeheffer R: Management of patients after cardiac transplantation. *Mayo Clin Proc* 1992, 67:775–784.

Stevenson L: Advanced congestive heart failure. Inpatient treatment and selection for cardiac transplantation. *Postgrad Med* 1993, 94:97–112.

Young J: Cardiac allograft arteriopathy: an ischemic burden of a different sort. *Am J Cardiol* 1992, 70:9F–13F.

PULMONARY AND CRITICAL CARE MEDICINE III

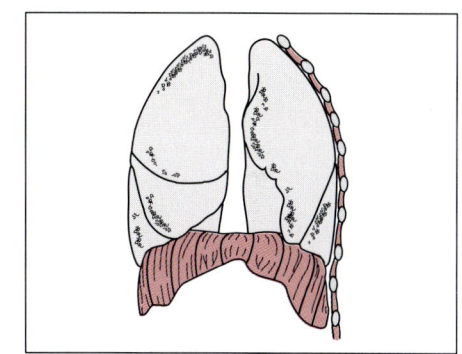

Section Editor
Roger C. Bone

From smoking cessation to the increasing incidence of pneumonia to new research on acute respiratory distress syndrome, the physician specializing in pulmonary and critical care medicine is confronted with numerous patient care challenges. Pulmonary and critical care medicine is highly dependent on machinery and technology—not only to sustain life, but also to measure the patient's vital body functions. Yet, it also relies on the physician's ability to intuit problems and seek innovative solutions when faced with complex cases.

Fittingly, this section of *Current Practice of Medicine* leads off with a chapter on diagnosis. A recurring theme throughout these ten chapters is the absolute necessity of performing proper diagnostic procedures. For example, chapter 2 discusses the diagnostic distinction between asthma and chronic obstructive pulmonary disease.

The seriousness of pulmonary medicine and critical care is another theme emphasized throughout these chapters. Whether a patient suffers from bronchogenic carcinoma, nosocomial pneumonia, or toxic fume exposure, proper care and any chance for recovery demands early diagnosis and aggressive treatment. Even then, success often is limited.

Finally, these chapters demonstrate the scope of pulmonary and critical care medicine. Some dangers are personal and preventable, such as those caused by smoking. Some are work related, such as those pulmonary diseases associated with miners. Of course, pulmonary and critical care complications often mark the end of the road for the patient with other serious and progressively worsening diseases.

I believe the following chapters will be an excellent resource for the reader, and I extend my thanks to all of the contributors.

Pulmonary Diagnostic Studies

Robert L. Rosen

> ### *Key Points*
> - Spirometry is useful in the diagnosis and monitoring of obstructive lung disease.
> - Measurement of lung volumes and diffusion capacity are used to evaluate restrictive lung disease.
> - Pulmonary vascular abnormalities can be diagnosed using a combination of ventilation/perfusion lung scans and contrast angiography.
> - Although lung biopsy obtained by thoracoscopy or thoracotomy may be required to diagnose structural lung abnormalities, many infectious and inflammatory lung processes can be diagnosed bronchoscopically using bronchoalveolar lavage and transbronchial biopsy.

Diagnostic studies of both physiologic and structural parameters are often useful for evaluating patients with pulmonary-related symptoms. Physiologic measures of air flow, lung volume, gas exchange, and exercise capabilities can confirm the lung as the site of disease, separate obstructive from restrictive lung disease, and define the degree of dysfunction. Information regarding structural and histologic abnormalities can be obtained from radiologic and biopsy procedures.

PULMONARY FUNCTION TESTS

Spirometry

Spirometry is the measurement of expired gas volumes from total lung capacity measured against time, and can be an office-based procedure [1•]. Useful spirometric measurements include the forced vital capacity (FVC), the forced expiratory volume in 1 second (FEV_1), and the forced expiratory flow rate during the midportion of the FVC ($FEF_{25\%-75\%}$) (Fig. 1). An isolated reduction in $FEF_{25\%-75\%}$ may reflect airflow obstruction localized primarily in the small airways. The key determination, however, is the ratio of FEV_1/FVC. A reduced $FEV_1/FVC\%$ is diagnostic of airflow obstruction, but other parameters are necessary to differentiate the various clinical components of obstructive lung disease. These include bronchitis, emphysema, and hyperreactive airway disease (Table 1). Inhaled bronchodilators can be administered at the time of spirometry to patients with obstruction. A greater than 15% increase in either FVC or FEV_1 indicates a reversible component.

Lung Volume Determinations

These are useful for assessing restrictive lung diseases. Reduced FVC in the absence of airflow obstruction may imply restrictive lung disease, but that must be confirmed by reduced lung volumes. The primary measurement is of the functional residual capacity, which represents the resting volume of the chest. Functional residual capacity is a consequence of the balance of the chest wall forces that tend to expand the thoracic cavity with the countering collapsing elastic forces of the lung. Other

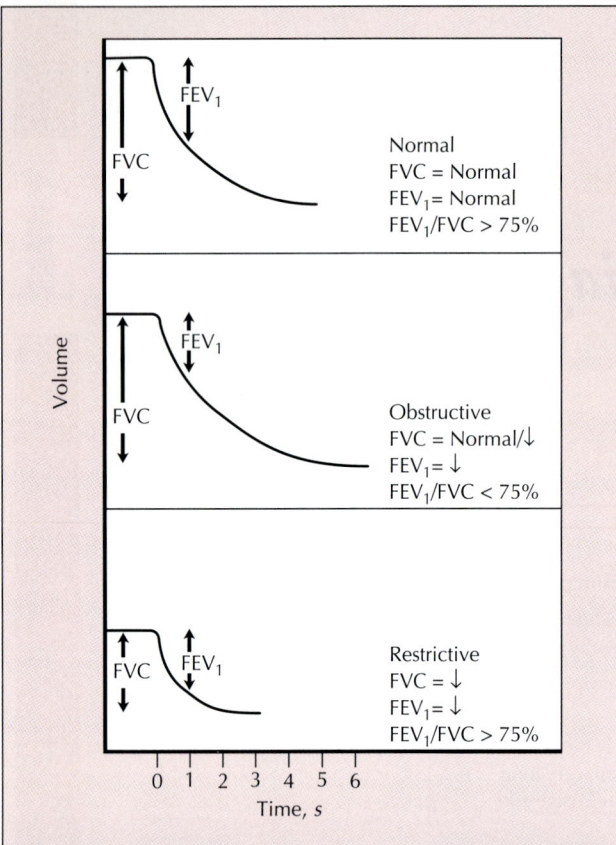

FIGURE 1 Spirometry measures expired gas volumes from total lung capacity against time. FEV_1—forced expiratory volume in 1 second; FVC—forced vital capacity.

TABLE 1 DIAGNOSTIC FINDINGS IN CHRONIC OBSTRUCTIVE LUNG DISEASE
Chronic bronchitis
Reduced FEV_1/FVC
History of productive cough
Emphysema
Reduced FEV_1/FVC
Reduced DLCO
Bullae present on chest x-ray or CT
Hyperreactive airway disease
Reduced FEV_1/FVC
Response to bronchodilator
Positive methacholine challenge test
FEV_1—forced expiratory volume in 1 second; FVC—forced vital capacity; DLCO—single-breath diffusing capacity; CT—computed tomography.

lung volumes can be derived by means of inspiratory and expiratory maneuvers performed from the measured functional residual capacity. Determinations of total lung capacity, functional residual capacity, and residual volume provide the most useful information. Restrictive lung disease is defined by a reduced total lung capacity, and lung volume patterns allow distinctions to be made among the various types of restrictive lung diseases: parenchymal, pleural, neuromuscular, and chest wall. In addition, lung volumes provide information about the degree of air trapping (increased residual volume) and hyperinflation (increased functional residual capacity) in patients with severe obstructive lung disease (Fig. 2).

Diffusing Capacity of the Lungs

The diffusing capacity of the lung, measured as milliliters of gas transferred per millimeter of mercury driving pressure per minute, reflects the ability of the lung to transfer gas from alveoli to the blood. The diffusability of carbon monoxide is measured rather than oxygen, for technical reasons, but the measurement is useful because factors that limit the transfer of carbon monoxide affect oxygen in a similar manner. The diffusing capacity is reduced by factors that reduce alveolar-capillary surface area, increase the thickness of the interstitium, or reduce lung perfusion. Reduced measurements not related to lung disease can also occur in patients with anemia because of the reduced ability of the blood to take up and carry carbon monoxide. Diffusing capacity may be increased under conditions that increase the amount of blood in the chest, either intravascularly or extravascularly (Table 2).

Arterial Blood Gases

Determinations of arterial blood gases complete the standard physiologic evaluation of the respiratory system. Alterations in ventilation are documented by deviations of the arterial partial pressure of carbon dioxide ($PaCO_2$) from the normal level of 40 torr (36 to 44 torr), with the $PaCO_2$ inversely proportional to the level of ventilation. Thus, hypoventilation is associated with an elevated $PaCO_2$ level and hyperventilation with a reduced level. Correlations of the $PaCO_2$ level with the arterial pH can define whether the ventilatory change is acute or chronic. Measuring the partial pressure of oxygen (PaO_2) provides useful information about the ability of the lung to transfer oxygen to the blood.

INHALATION CHALLENGE TESTS

A methacholine challenge test can be used for diagnosing intermittent obstructive lung disease that cannot be documented by standard spirometry [2]. Using this test, bronchospasm is induced by having the patient inhale the acetylcholine analogue, methacholine. Methacholine challenge is unnecessary and is contraindicated for patients with known obstructive lung disease, but it can provide useful diagnostic information about patients with intermittent dyspnea or unexplained cough. The test is performed by having a patient inhale sequentially higher concentrations of methacholine until a 20% reduction in FEV_1 occurs or a maximal cumulative dose of approximately 200 mg is reached. If airflow obstruction is induced, a diagnosis of hyperresponsive airway disease can be made. Similar inhalation challenges can be performed with inhaled occupational or environmental substances that a patient feels may be the cause of breathing problems. Standards for these challenges are not well documented, however.

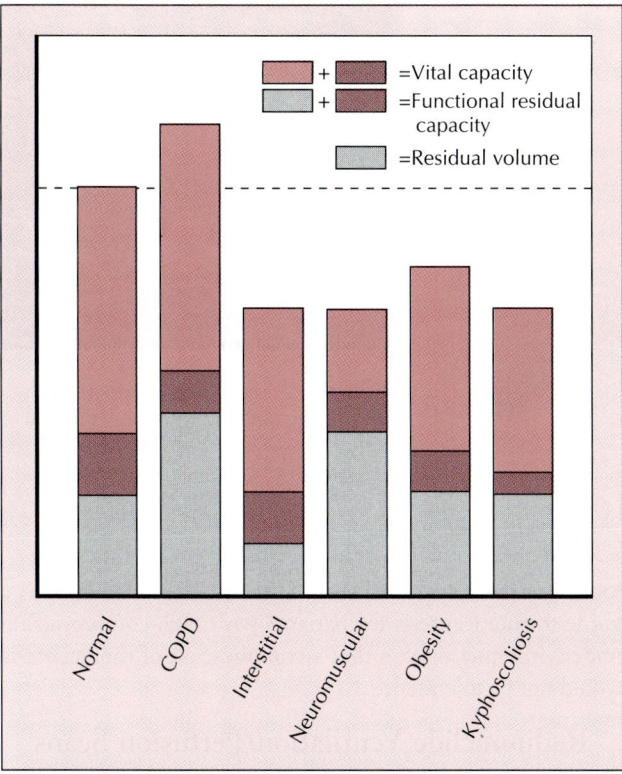

FIGURE 2 Relative lung volumes in normal and disease states. COPD—chronic obstructive pulmonary disease.

EXERCISE TESTING

By providing physiologic measurements of cardiovascular and ventilatory function, cardiopulmonary exercise testing can assess factors contributing to a patient's dyspnea or exercise limitation [3•]. Measurements of heart rate, respiratory rate, blood pressure, tidal volume, minute ventilation, oxygen uptake, carbon dioxide production, and arterial blood gases in response to given levels of work can help to distinguish whether a patient's complaints of dyspnea, fatigue, or exercise limitation are related to cardiac dysfunction, pulmonary limitation, or deconditioning. At peak exercise, normal patients, deconditioned patients, and patients with cardiac disease will be able to achieve greater than 85% of predicted maximal heart rate, whereas patients with lung disease will be limited before they reach maximal heart rate. In a failing heart, stroke volume cannot be increased easily, and the heart compensates by increasing rate disproportionately. The heart rate of patients with cardiac limitation will increase more rapidly than normal in response to a given level of exercise. Pulmonary dysfunction is characterized by ventilatory limitation, with a decreased breathing reserve at peak exercise, an inability to decrease dead space ventilation, and oxyhemoglobin desaturation [3•].

Exercise testing is also clinically useful for diagnosing exercise-induced asthma and for determining an oxygen prescription for patients with exercise-induced hypoxemia (Table 3).

IMAGING TECHNIQUES

A wide array of imaging techniques is available to evaluate patients with pulmonary disease. Conventional chest radiographs, contrast radiography, ultrasound techniques, radionuclide studies, and computed tomography (CT) are all used in the diagnosis of chest diseases (Figs. 3 and 4).

Chest Roentgenography

Chest roentgenography, with the standard posterior-anterior and lateral views, remains the initial imaging technique for evaluating pulmonary pathology. Pulmonary parenchymal, vascular, and pleural processes can usually be identified. Variations of the standard technique include rib detail films for evaluating fractures, lateral decubitus radiographs for distinguishing pleural lesions or loculated fluid from free-flowing

TABLE 2 ALTERATIONS IN DIFFUSING CAPACITY OF THE LUNG
Decreased diffusing capacity
Reduced alveolar-capillary surface area
Emphysema
Lung resection
Increased interstitial thickness
Fibrosis
Alveolitis
Granulomatous disease (sarcoid, fungal, mycobacterial)
Lymphangitic carcinomatosis
Pulmonary edema
Decreased perfusion
Thromboembolic disease
Anemia
Increased diffusing capacity
Asthma
Mitral stenosis
Polycythemia
Alveolar hemorrhage

TABLE 3 CARDIOPULMONARY EXERCISE TESTING
Indications
Dyspnea
Diseased exercise tolerance
Oxygen prescriptions
Determination of disability
Determination of anaerobic threshold for athletic training
Contraindications
Unstable angina or recent myocardial infarction
Pulmonary hypertension
Complications
Cardiac arrhythmia
Myocardial infarction
Musculoskeletal injury
Vascular injury related to arterial line placement

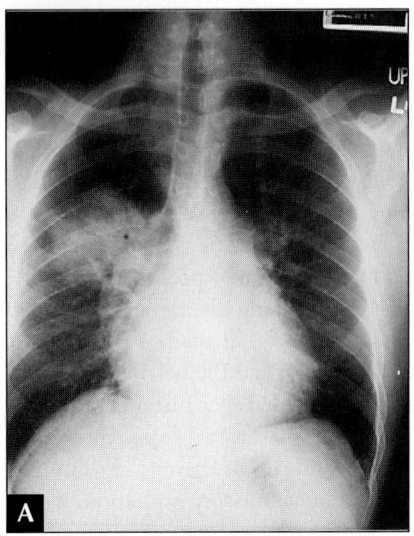 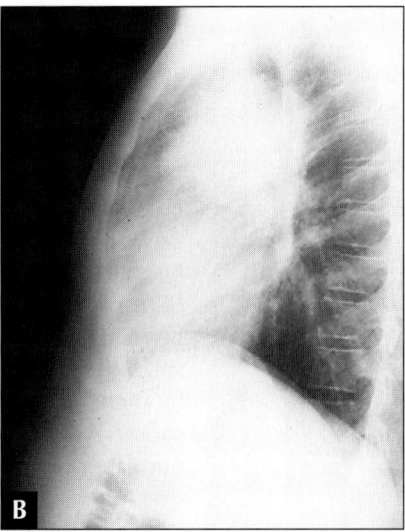 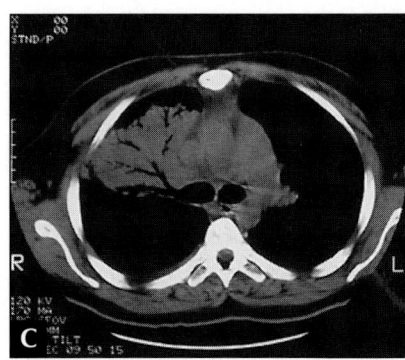

FIGURE 3 Consolidating pneumonia involving the anterior segment of the right upper lobe as visualized by **A**, posterior-anterior, **B**, lateral chest radiographs, and **C**, computed tomography.

effusions, and apical lordotic or oblique films for visualizing or localizing abnormalities that are not clearly defined by the conventional frontal and lateral views.

Contrast radiographic procedures include pulmonary angiography and bronchography. Angiography remains the gold standard for diagnosing pulmonary embolism and arteriovenous malformations (Fig. 5).

Ultrasound

Ultrasound of the chest is used to identify and localize pleural fluid in patients with very small amounts of fluid or loculated pockets of effusion. Ultrasound is also used as a guide to thoracentesis for patients with such compromising underlying lung disease that a complication of thoracentesis would not be tolerated.

Radionuclide Ventilation/Perfusion Scans

Radionuclide ventilation/perfusion scans are used for patients with a suspected pulmonary embolism (Fig. 6) [4]. Perfusion scanning is commonly performed using macroaggregates of human serum albumin radiolabeled with technetium-99m, whereas ventilation scanning is performed after inhalation of

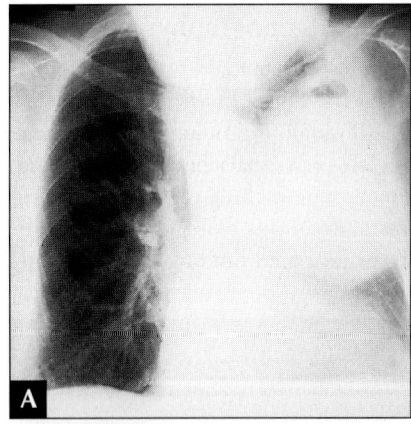

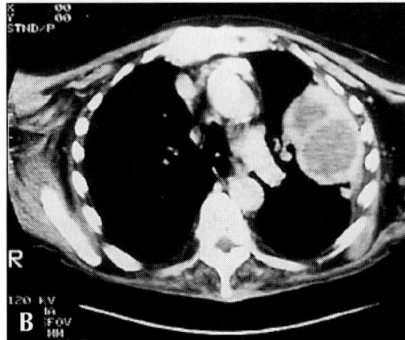

FIGURE 4 Left upper lobe lung abscess as seen on **A**, standard chest radiograph and **B**, computed tomography.

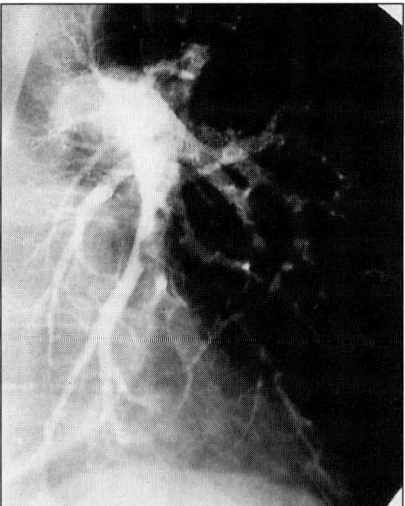

FIGURE 5 Pulmonary angiogram showing intravascular filling defect diagnostic of pulmonary thromboembolism.

FIGURE 6 Perfusion lung scan showing multiple defects consistent with pulmonary emboli. ANT—anterior; Llat—left lateral; LPO—left posterior oblique; POST—posterior; Rlat—right lateral; RPO—right posterior oblique.

xenon-133. In a patient with a normal chest radiograph and no history of pulmonary disease, finding multiple segmental perfusion defects without corresponding ventilation defects is more than 90% diagnostic of pulmonary embolism; likewise, finding no perfusion defects reduces the likelihood of clinically significant pulmonary embolic disease to almost zero. Many ventilation/perfusion scans have patterns intermediate between these diagnostic patterns, however, and other studies will be necessary to confirm or rule out the diagnosis. Perfusion scans are also useful for evaluating a right-to-left shunt, which may occur with pulmonary arteriovenous malformations or intracardiac shunts. In these cases, the patient will have a normal lung scan, but radiolabeled albumin that bypasses the capillary bed of the lung will be seen in other regions of the body, such as the brain or kidneys. If resectional surgery of the lung is planned, a quantitative perfusion scan can assess the impact of removal of part of the lung and its vascular bed before surgery is performed [4].

Conventional and Computed Tomography

Conventional tomography provides definition of coin lesions, showing border irregularities that may occur in malignancies and patterns of calcification that may imply a benign process.

Computed tomography has essentially replaced conventional tomography for thoracic imaging because of its ability to allow recognition of different tissue densities (including fat), calcification, and subtle differences in the densities of adjacent structures [5]. It also provides cross-sectional images, thus allowing better visualization of structures that are superimposed on conventional radiographs. These factors have improved the ability to visualize mediastinal and hilar structures as well as pleural and chest wall lesions. High-resolution CT (1- to 2-mm sections as contrasted with the standard 10-mm CT sections) has added a new dimension to this imaging technique. High-resolution CT has proved extremely useful for diagnosing bronchiectasis, essentially replacing contrast bronchography. It can also aid in detecting and characterizing diffuse parenchymal diseases and can help to define the extent of such diseases. Varying patterns and predilections for lung regions can aid in the differential diagnosis of diffuse lung disease [5].

DIAGNOSTIC PROCEDURES

Sputum Examination

Evaluating a simple expectorated or induced sputum sample can yield very useful information for diagnosing infectious or malignant pulmonary pathology. Centrally located endobronchial carcinoma can often be diagnosed from sputum cytology. Mycobacterial and fungal disease can also be diagnosed if organisms can be identified on smear or by culture. Bacterial infections can be more difficult to diagnose from sputum evaluation because of contamination from oral secretions; however, careful examination of a Gram stain of sputum, looking at areas with heavy concentrations of leukocytes and a predominant organism, can provide presumptive information about the diagnosis of a bacterial process.

Bronchoscopy

Fiberoptic bronchoscopy, which has virtually replaced rigid bronchoscopy, allows direct visualization of the proximal tracheobronchial tree and sampling of pulmonary secretions and tissue (Table 4) [6•,7•]. Using topical anesthesia, a flexible fiberoptic scope can be passed transnasally or orally over the vocal cords and into the trachea. Direct inspection of the airways to the level of fourth-order bronchi can be done. Through a small channel in the bronchoscope, fluid can be instilled and bronchial secretions withdrawn (Table 5) [6•,7•].

TABLE 4 DIAGNOSTIC BRONCHOSCOPY INDICATIONS

Indications
Cough without obvious etiology
Hemoptysis
Abnormal chest x-ray
Carcinoma
    Bronchogenic
    Metastatic
Diffuse lung disease
    Infectious
    Inflammatory
Poorly responsive pneumonia
Intrathoracic lymphadenopathy
Esophageal and mediastinal masses
Tracheobronchial obstruction
Persistent pneumothorax
Thoracic trauma
Foreign body
Contraindications
Inability to ventilate or oxygenate patient
Severe bronchospasm
Bleeding diathesis precludes brushing or biopsy
Complications
Fever, hoarseness
Drug reaction and anaphylaxis related to anesthetic
Hypotension and bradycardia related to vasovagal response
Bleeding and pneumothorax related to biopsy or brushing
Transient hypoxemia related to lavage
Death (<1%)

TABLE 5 BRONCHOSCOPICALLY OBTAINED SPECIMENS

Infectious
Bronchial washings
Bronchoalveolar lavage
Protected catheter brushes
Transbronchial lung biopsy
Neoplastic
Bronchial washings
Bronchoalveolar lavage
Brushings
Perbronchial needle aspiration
Bronchial/transbronchial lung biopsy
Inflammatory
Bronchoalveolar lavage (differential cell counts)
Transbronchial lung biopsy

Table 6 Thoracentesis
Indications
Undiagnosed pleural effusion
Suspected infected effusion (empyema)
Relief of respiratory compromise
Contraindications
Bleeding diathesis
Insufficient fluid
Single lung
Insufficient pulmonary reserve to transiently tolerate a pneumothorax
Complications
Pain (20%)
Persistent cough (10%)
Subcutaneous hematoma
Pneumothorax (10%)
Splenic laceration
Hepatic laceration
Hemothorax
Hemoptysis

Bronchoalveolar lavage, which provides a sampling of alveolar and distal bronchiolar secretions, consists of wedging the bronchoscope into a distal airway and instilling aliquots (usually 20 mL) of normal saline, up to a total of 100 to 200 mL. Bronchoalveolar lavage is well tolerated by patients and provides specimens for evaluating opportunistic infections and inflammatory lung processes [8]. Small brushes passed through the bronchoscope can obtain scrapings of bronchial mucosa for cytologic examination. Perbronchial needle aspirations can also obtain material for cytologic evaluation. Small bronchial and alveolar (transbronchial) biopsies provide tissue specimens for histologic examination to evaluate structural abnormalities.

Thoracentesis

Thoracentesis, whereby a needle is inserted into the pleural space, should be performed whenever an undiagnosed pleural effusion is present (Table 6). Abnormal fluid in the pleural space can be transudate, exudate, blood, pus, or chyle. The direct evaluation of pleural fluid by chemical and cytologic means is the most expedient approach to diagnosis. An undiagnosed exudate is often secondary to metastatic neoplasm, and cytologic examination of the fluid can often be diagnostic. Performing a closed pleural (parietal) biopsy if the initial fluid cytology is negative can provide further diagnostic material. In as many as 30% of malignant effusions, however, the diagnosis cannot be made without using a more invasive procedure. A closed pleural biopsy is also indicated for evaluating a presumed tuberculous effusion to obtain material for histologic evaluation of granulomas and material for culture, but for most other pleural processes it does not add significant information.

Thoracoscopy

Thoracoscopy has recently had a resurgence in popularity [8,9•]. A video thoracoscope can be introduced into the pleural space with the patient under local or general anesthesia and the lung collapsed. Under direct visualization, biopsies can be made of lesions on the parietal or visceral pleural surfaces. In addition, the procedure can be used to perform biopsies of lung parenchyma, as well as hilar, mediastinal, and esophageal masses. The procedure can be performed with minimal morbidity, resulting in reduced postoperative pain and length of stay compared with use of standard thoracotomy [9•,10•].

Open-Lung Biopsy

Open-lung biopsy remains the gold standard for the structural evaluation of thoracic disease. Lung masses that remain undiagnosed by other means can be both diagnosed and, in the case of primary neoplasm, definitively removed. Diffuse parenchymal disease that is not granulomatous or neoplastic often requires the larger specimen provided by open-lung biopsy for diagnosis. Inflammatory processes involving bronchioles, alveoli, or blood vessels usually cannot be confirmed histologically from the small samples obtained by bronchoscopic transbronchial biopsy. Although open-lung biopsy requires general anesthesia and a postprocedure chest tube, the associated mortality is minimal and the procedure is well tolerated by most patients.

References and Recommended Reading

Recently published papers of particular interest have been highlighted as:
- • Of interest
- •• Of outstanding interest

1. • Crapo RO. Pulmonary-function testing. *N Engl J Med* 1994, 331:25–30.
2. Irwin RS, Pratter MR: The clinical value of pharmacologic bronchoprovocation challenge. *Med Clin North Am* 1990, 74:767–778.
3. Sue DY, Wasserman K: Impact of integrative cardiopulmonary exercise testing on clinical decision making. *Chest* 1991, 99:981–992.
4. Kramer EL, Divgi CR: Pulmonary applications of nuclear medicine. *Clin Chest Med* 1991, 12:55–75.
5. Muller NL, Miller RR: Computed tomography of chronic diffuse infiltrative lung disease. *Am Rev Respir Dis* 1990, 142:1206–1215, 1440–1448.
6. • Prakash UBS, Offord KP, Stubbs SE: Bronchoscopy in North America: the ACCP Survey. *Chest* 1991, 100:1668–1675.
7. • Prakash UBS, Stubbs SE: The bronchoscopy survey: some reflections. *Chest* 1991, 100:1660–1667.
8. Goldstein RA, Rohatgi PK, Bergofsky EH: Clinical role of bronchoalveolar lavage in adults with pulmonary disease. *Am Rev Respir Dis* 1990, 142:481–486.
9. • Mack MJ, Aronoff RJ, Acuff TE, *et al*.: Present role of thoracoscopy in the diagnosis and treatment of diseases of the chest. *Ann Thorac Surg* 1992, 54:403–408.
10. • Loddenkemper R, Boutin C: Thoracoscopy: present diagnostic and therapeutic indications. *Eur Respir J* 1993, 6:1544–1555.

Obstructive Diseases

Gregory R. Owens

> ### Key Points
> - It is critical to differentiate asthma from chronic obstructive pulmonary disease (COPD) by patient history, pulmonary function testing, and chest radiography.
> - Every physician should be well versed in the now-standardized techniques of smoking cessation.
> - Algorithms for the management of COPD are currently gaining popularity.
> - Inhaled medications, especially the anticholinergics, are the drugs of choice in patients with COPD.
> - Antibiotic therapy successfully shortens the course of exacerbations of COPD.
> - Oxygen therapy is the only intervention shown to decrease mortality in patients with COPD.

Numerous diseases cause airflow obstruction, including bronchiectasis, cystic fibrosis, asthma, and chronic obstructive pulmonary disease (COPD). The latter two are the dominant clinical entities in the United States. Asthma is defined pathophysiologically as a disease of airway hyperresponsiveness. The two entities that comprise COPD—chronic bronchitis and emphysema—are defined very differently. Chronic bronchitis is defined by symptoms: the presence of a chronic productive cough on most days for 2 successive years. Emphysema is defined pathologically by the presence of enlarged airspaces and the frank destruction of alveolar walls. In the early 1960s there was a tendency to lump together all these disease states. However, more recent information concerning the pathophysiology of asthma has led to the belief that asthma should be considered as a separate disease, and that the term *COPD* should be reserved for patients who have only chronic bronchitis and emphysema. Indeed, a recent official statement of the American Thoracic Society defined COPD as "a disorder characterized by abnormal tests of expiratory flow over periods of several months of observation"[1]. This chapter focuses only on patients with COPD.

SIGNIFICANCE OF THE PROBLEM

Although there has been much emphasis recently on the appropriate management of patients with asthma, it is important to recognize that COPD is in several ways a more serious disease. While deaths caused by asthma have increased recently, reaching a total of 4000 deaths in 1989, COPD caused approximately 85,000 deaths in the same year (Table 1) and is the fifth leading cause of death in the United States [2]. Likewise, while more than 7 million people in the United States have asthma, most recent estimates indicate that over 13 million Americans have COPD. Finally, the economic costs of COPD are staggering. In 1985, COPD was the reason for over 10 million visits to physicians and for approximately 2 million hospitalizations.

Cause of death	1985	1986	1987	1988	1989
Diseases of the heart	771,169	765,490	760,353	765,156	733,867
Malignant neoplasms	461,563	469,376	476,927	485,048	496,152
Cerebrovascular disease	153,050	149,643	149,835	150,517	145,551
Accidents and adverse effects	93,457	95,277	95,020	97,100	95,028
Chronic obstructive pulmonary diseases	74,662	75,559	78,380	82,853	84,344
Pneumonia and influenza	67,615	69,812	89,225	77,652	76,550

TABLE 1 LEADING CAUSES OF DEATH OVER A FIVE-YEAR PERIOD

From National Center for Health Statistics [2]; with permission.

ETIOLOGY

There is little doubt about the cause of COPD; cigarette smoking is thought to be the cause in at least 85% to 90% of all the cases of COPD in the United States. Interestingly, the relationship between smoking and COPD was first suggested only in the 1950s. Before then, mechanical stresses and recurrent pulmonary infections had been thought to cause airflow obstruction.

The role of other factors in the genesis of COPD is considerably less certain. These factors include occupational exposures to agents (such as coal dust and potash), recurrent childhood respiratory infections, cigarette smoking, and air pollution. Likewise, the role of genetic factors, such as atopy, is uncertain, with the exception of the entity α-1-antiprotease deficiency. In patients with this disease, the lack of the neutralizing enzyme, which provides approximately 90% of all inhibitory capacity against proteolytic enzymes, allows the unchecked development of autodigestion of the lung, resulting ultimately in emphysema [3].

CAUSES OF AIRFLOW OBSTRUCTION

The causes of airflow obstruction differ greatly between patients with asthma and those with COPD (Fig. 1). Although for many years the cause of obstruction in patients with asthma was attributed to bronchospasm, it is clearly secondary to an influx of inflammatory cells, especially neutrophils and eosinophils, and the associated edema and swelling. The role of airway inflammation in patients with COPD is almost certainly considerably less important, with other factors causing airflow obstruction and the associated symptom of dyspnea. Patients with chronic bronchitis develop shortness of breath from physical obstruction of the airway lumen by secretions. These patients have Goblet cell metaplasia with hypersecretion of mucus and obstruction of the bronchioles. In addition, and probably more importantly, mucus gland hyperplasia develops in the larger airways. This pathologic finding is well correlated with the presence and severity of the symptoms of chronic bronchitis.

Patients with emphysema develop symptoms for yet a different reason. Because of the destruction of the pulmonary parenchyma, which normally tethers open the airways, any form of positive pressure in the lungs will cause almost immediate collapse of the airways, creating a classical appearance of the flow volume loop (see following).

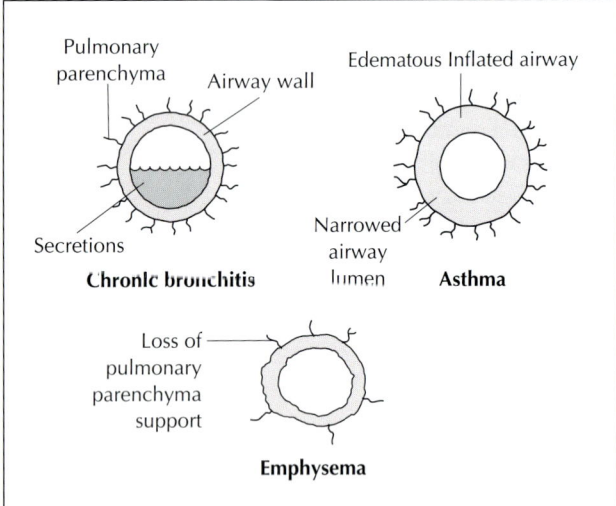

FIGURE 1 Physical or mechanical causes of airflow obstruction. In patients with chronic bronchitis, the airway and supporting structures are normal, and airflow obstruction is caused by physical blockage of the airway lumen by secretions. In patients with asthma, secretions are not present but the airway lumen is narrowed by an edematous, inflamed airway. In patients with emphysema, the airway itself is relatively normal, but the supporting structures of the lung that normally tether open the airway are lost.

DIAGNOSIS

Pulmonary Function Testing

Although some patients with chronic bronchitis may have normal pulmonary function (known as *simple chronic bronchitis*), the primary functional abnormality seen in patients with COPD is a slowing of expiratory flow. This is characterized on pulmonary function testing by a decrease in the forced expiratory volume in 1 second (FEV_1) (Fig. 2). A different graphic representation of the spirometric information, the flow volume loop, offers a vivid display of the dramatic airway collapse that occurs in patients with emphysema (Fig. 3).

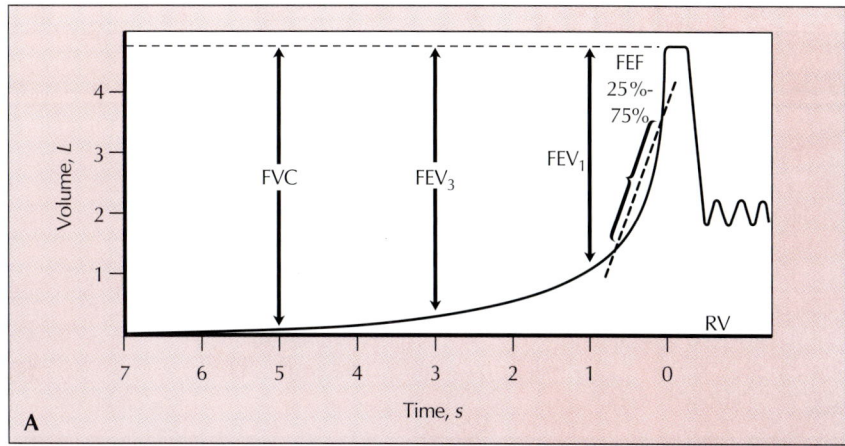
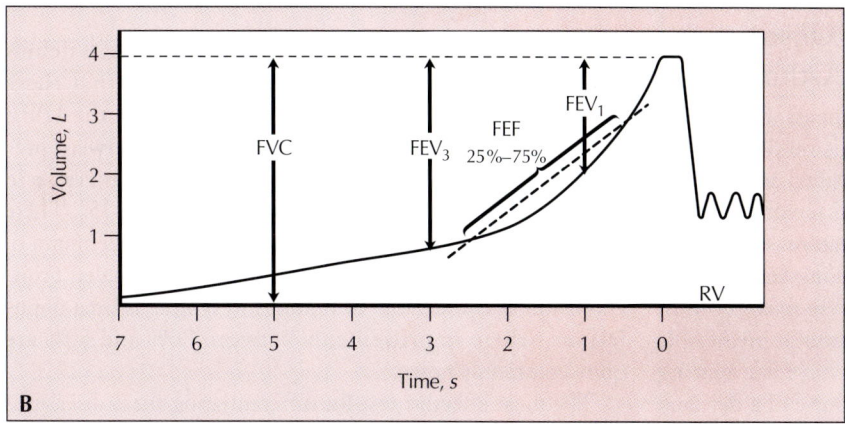

FIGURE 2 **A**, Appearance of a normal spirometric tracing, sometimes called a volume time tracing. Notice that the amount of air expired in 1 second (FEV_1) is approximately 4 L. **B**, Appearance of a spirometric maneuver in a patient with chronic obstructive pulmonary disease. Notice the slowing of expiratory flow. The FEV_1 is approximately 2 L. FVC—forced vital capacity; FEV_3—forced expiratory volume in 3 seconds; $FEF_{25\%-75\%}$—forced expiratory flow, mid–expiratory phase; RV—residual volume.

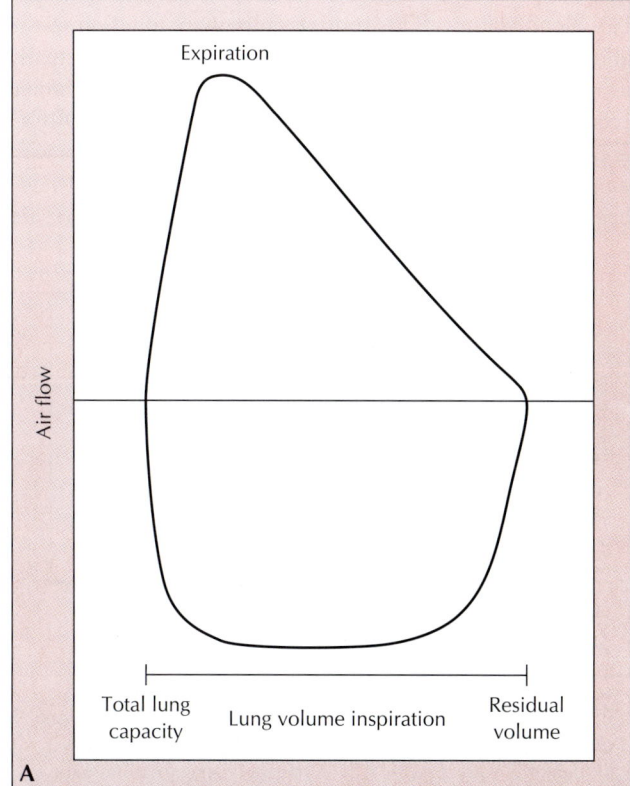
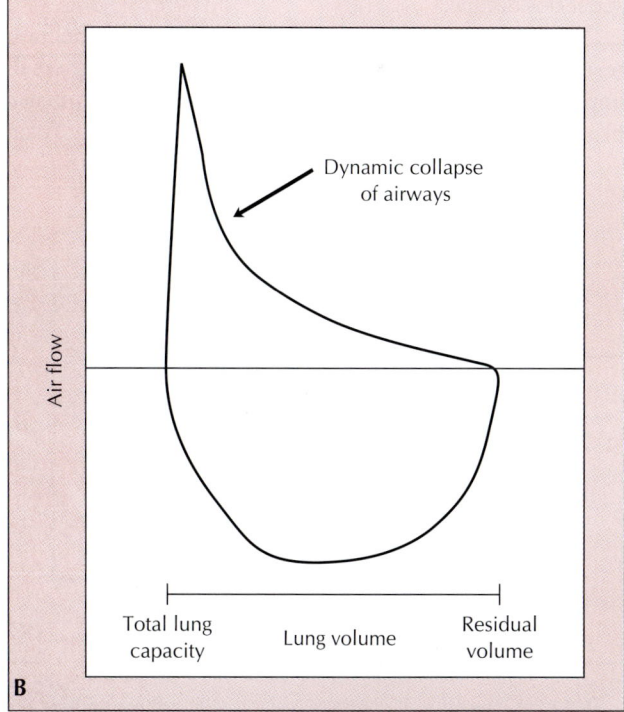

FIGURE 3 **A**, Appearance of a normal flow volume loop. Note the very rapid initial expiratory flow followed by a gradual decrease in airflow as the patient's pulmonary function approaches residual volume. **B**, Flow volume loop in patients with emphysema. Although initial peak flows are relatively preserved, after reaching peak flow there is a dramatic decrease in airflow obstruction caused by dynamic collapse of the airways.

Obstructive Diseases

TABLE 2 FEATURES DIFFERENTIATING CHRONIC OBSTRUCTIVE PULMONARY DISEASE FROM ASTHMA		
Features	COPD	Asthma
Airflow obstruction	Constant	Variable
Course	Progressive	Variable
Response to bronchodilators	Variable	Usually large
Airway reactivity	Variable	Universal
Diffusing capacity	Decreased	Normal to high
Response to exercise	Arterial desaturation	Arterial desaturation

From Owens [4]; with permission.
COPD—chronic obstructive pulmonary disease.

Differential Diagnosis: Chronic Obstructive Pulmonary Disease Versus Asthma

It is important to attempt to differentiate patients with asthma from those with COPD. Although there is no doubt some overlap in characteristics (sometimes described as *asthmatic bronchitis*), there are a series of features that separate the two diseases (Table 2) [4]. Two of the major features that differentiate the two entities are the short- and long-term clinical courses. Patients with COPD have relatively fixed levels of pulmonary function, and their symptoms occur at predictable levels of exertion. Patients with asthma have fluctuating pulmonary function, even throughout the course of a day, and their symptoms vary from day to day (Fig. 4). In the long-term setting, patients with COPD have an accelerated decline in pulmonary function with aging compared with normal patients (Fig. 5). In general, patients with asthma do not suffer this decline.

There are also differences noted on pulmonary function testing. First, patients with COPD have relatively small improvements in pulmonary function when given an inhaled bronchodilator. Indeed, the concept of relatively fixed pulmonary function is described in the most recent definition of COPD. However, there is no doubt that these patients do respond to inhaled β-agonists. In the IPPB Study, 965 participants with severe COPD underwent pre- and postbronchodilator spirometry. The mean increase in FEV_1 noted in that study was approximately 15% [5]. There were a few individuals who actually had improvements of over 30% in their FEV_1. This response to an inhaled bronchodilator is comparable to findings in typical asthma populations, where improvements between 20% and 50% are quite commonly noted.

The most effective test for differentiating these diseases is the single-breath carbon monoxide diffusing capacity (DLCO), which is primarily a measure of capillary surface area and capillary blood volume. This routine pulmonary function test is abnormally low in patients with emphysema, but is actually supranormal in patients with asthma. Patients with only chronic bronchitis have normal DLCO values. The decrease in DLCO is caused by the parenchymal destruction found in patients with emphysema. Patients with asthma have a high DLCO value because of hyperinflation pulling open capillary beds that are

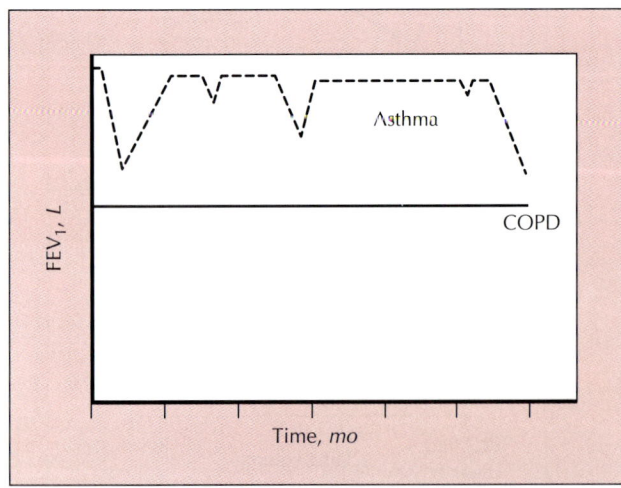

FIGURE 4 The clinical course of patients with asthma and chronic obstructive pulmonary disease (COPD). Note that airflow obstruction is relatively constant over a duration of months in patients with COPD, but fluctuates considerably in patients with poorly controlled asthma.

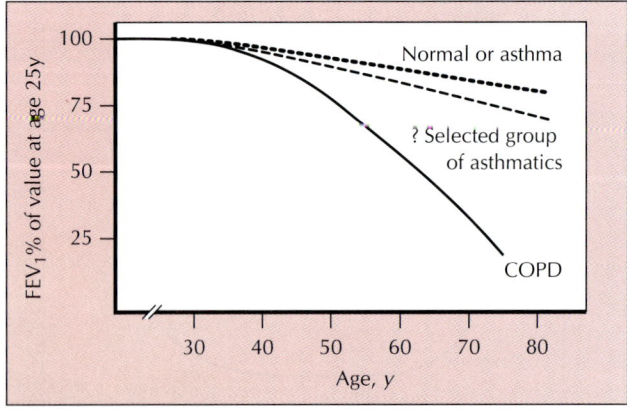

FIGURE 5 Long-term clinical course of patients with asthma and chronic obstructive pulmonary disease (COPD). It is generally thought that patients with asthma have a change in pulmonary function with aging that is comparable to normal nonsmoking individuals. Questions have been raised whether a select group of asthmatics have decreases in pulmonary function that are excessive for their age. However, patients with COPD have a much more dramatic decline in pulmonary function over time.

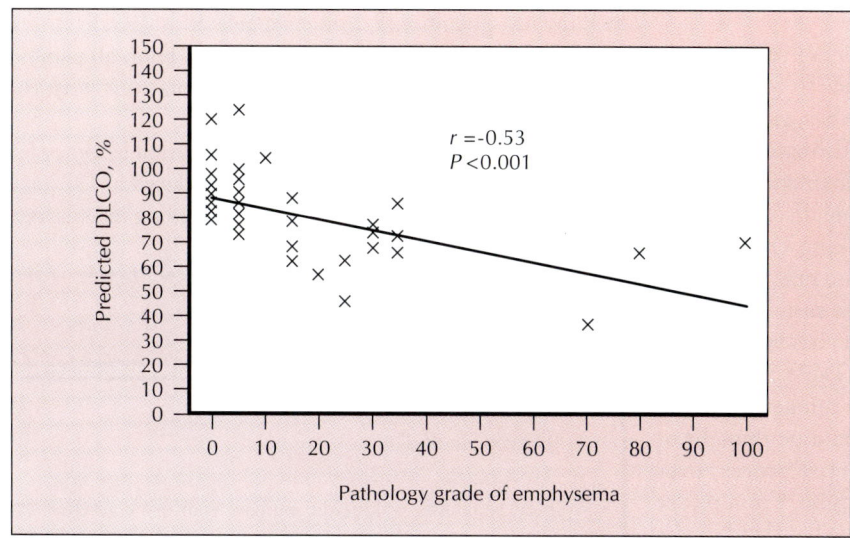

FIGURE 6 Relationship of single-breath carbon monoxide diffusing capacity (DLCO) and the pathologic grade of emphysema. There is a relatively strong inverse correlation between the value for the percent-predicted DLCO and the pathologic grade of emphysema found in lung resection specimens. (*From* Morrison, *et al.* [6]; with permission.)

then filled with blood. Not only does the DLCO value differentiate these diseases of airflow obstruction, but it actually quantitates the degree of emphysema present (Fig. 6) [6].

Patients with asthma and COPD respond differently to exercise and to inhalation challenge testing. Approximately 90% of patients with asthma will develop bronchoconstriction after or during a bout of exercise, especially in cold temperatures. Patients with COPD have no change in pulmonary function with exercise, but have a tendency to develop arterial desaturation with exercise. This desaturation is noted almost exclusively in patients with emphysema.

The final difference noted between the two groups is the response to methacholine challenge. Patients with asthma respond vigorously and uniformly to the inhalation of this drug. Indeed, airway hyperresponsiveness defines the disease. The degree of hyperresponsiveness correlates well with the severity of the disease and the amount of medication required to control the patient's symptoms. Recent information from the Lung Health Study indicates that airway hyperresponsiveness is not universally present in patients with COPD and the degree of hyperresponsiveness is considerably less than that seen in patients with COPD [7•].

MANAGEMENT

The management of patients with COPD is somewhat controversial because of the insidious onset of the disease (many people do not even know they have it), the relative lack of reversibility of pulmonary function abnormalities, and the conflicting results of pharmacologic studies found in the literature. The management of patients with COPD may be categorized into four components: 1) identification that a smoker has COPD, 2) smoking cessation, 3) the prevention of infectious complications, and 4) attempts to reverse, at least partially, decrements in lung function.

Identification of Smokers

Surprisingly, many smokers are unaware of the deleterious effects that cigarette smoking has on their pulmonary function. Although the smoker may recognize that his or her early-morning cough is secondary to smoking ("smoker's cough"), he or she may be unaware that the gradually progressive nature of shortness of breath during exercise is caused by the gradual development of COPD. It is quite typical for a patient who is developing COPD to decrease the amount or duration of daily tasks in order to minimize the sensation of dyspnea. The gradually developing shortness of breath is usually ascribed to the aging process. Thus, it is of utmost importance that the physician attempt to identify the development of COPD at a time when interventions may make the greatest difference, *ie*, early in the disease rather than later, when irreversible processes have developed (Fig. 7).

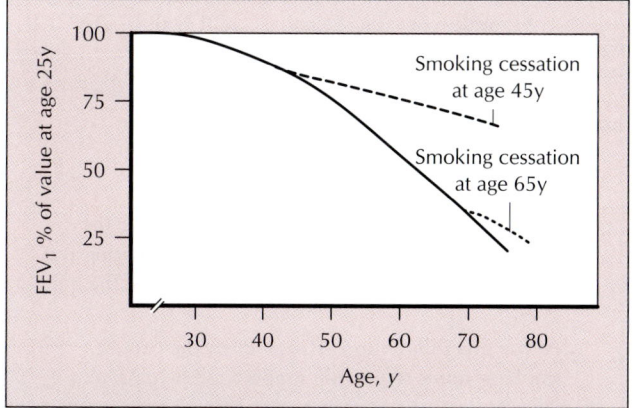

FIGURE 7 Effect of smoking cessation at 45 and 65 years of age. It is generally thought that the decline in pulmonary function seen in patients after smoking cessation is the same as that seen in nonsmokers, although smokers may start from a lower baseline. FEV_1—forced expiratory volume in 1 second.

First, every smoker must be identified. It has recently been suggested that smoking status be identified as a vital sign and recorded with the vital signs to allow for unequivocal identification of the smoker [8]. Second, all smokers with respiratory symptoms, especially shortness of breath, should undergo pulmonary function testing with spirometry to identify those individuals with decrements in lung function who are highly likely to go on to develop progressive symptoms.

Smoking Cessation

Because smoking underlies the vast majority of patients who develop COPD, every effort should be made to convince the smoker to consider smoking cessation. The behavioral science underpinning smoking cessation and the pharmacologic therapy of nicotine addiction have advanced dramatically in the past decade. Physicians who have become discouraged in their previous attempts to induce smoking cessation in patients should become re-energized because new approaches have yielded much better results than those seen in the past. The behavioral process of smoking cessation has been divided into four relatively well-defined stages (Table 3) [9]. The physician's goal is to gradually move the smoker from one stage to the next. Smoking cessation should be thought of not as a point in time but rather as an active process over time, much like the treatment of hypertension. From recent clinical trials, the National Cancer Institute has developed a manual that contains a standardized approach to smoking cessation, based on the four "A's" of physician intervention (Table 4) [10]. This approach, together with nicotine replacement therapy, has resulted in substantial improvements in cessation rates in smokers.

Most studies of nicotine replacement with nicotine polycrilex (nicotine chewing gum), along with behavioral modification programs, have found that between 20% and 35% of smokers have been able to successfully quit smoking for at least 3 months after their quit date [11•]. With the recent release of transdermal nicotine replacement, enthusiasm about the success of smoking cessation has been rekindled, with some studies showing success rates as high as 61% at 6 weeks (Fig. 8) [12•]. Thus, there is encouraging new information that a strategy combining nicotine replacement and behavioral modification is a much more successful approach to breaking the smoking habit than either approach alone. Indeed, nicotine replacement without behavioral modification is no more effective than placebo in inducing smoking cessation.

Prevention of Infectious Diseases

Another relatively noncontroversial area in the management of patients with COPD is the importance of vaccination against influenza and pneumococcal pneumonia. Influenza vaccines have been given for years and have lead to a decrease in influenza pneumonia, influenza-related hospitalizations, and influenza-related deaths in the elderly. Thus, all patients with COPD should receive annual vaccinations with the appropriate influenza virus of that year.

The importance of pneumococcal vaccination is somewhat less certain. Although the vaccine was introduced in 1977 and a large body of information is available regarding its effective-

Table 3 Behavioral Stages of Smoking Cessation

Stage	Behavior
Precontemplation	The patient is not thinking seriously about smoking cessation.
Contemplation	The patient is seriously pondering quitting smoking.
Action phase	The patient is actively involved in doing those things which will lead to smoking cessation.
Maintenance	The patient has achieved smoking cessation and is avoiding relapse.

From DiClemente, *et al.* [9]; with permission.

Table 4 The Physician's Four A's to Smoking Cessation

1. **Ask** about smoking at every opportunity.
    a. "Do you smoke?"
    b. "How much?"
    c. "How soon after waking do you have your first cigarette?"
    d. "Are you interested in stopping smoking?"
    e. "Have you ever tried to stop before?" If so, "What happened?"
2. **Advise** all smokers to stop.
    a. State your advice clearly. For example: "As your physician, I must advise you to stop smoking now."
    b. Personalize the message to quit. Refer to the patient's clinical condition, smoking, history, family history, personal interests, or social roles.
3. **Assist** the patient in stopping.
    a. Set a quit date. Help the patient pick a date within the next 4 weeks; acknowledge that no time is ideal.
    b. Provide self-help materials. The smoking cessation coordinator or support staff member can review the materials with the patient if desired (Call 1-800-4-CANCER for NCI's *Quit for Good* materials).
    c. Consider prescribing nicotine gum, especially for highly addicted patients (those who smoke one pack a day or more or who smoke their first cigarette within 30 minutes of waking).
    d. Consider signing a stop-smoking contract with the patient.
    e. If the patient is not willing to quit now:
        • Provide motivating literature (Call 1-800-4-CANCER for NCI's *Why Do you Smoke?* pamphlet).
        • Ask again at the next visit.
4. **Arrange** follow-up visits.
    a. Set a follow-up visit within 1 to 2 weeks after the quit date.
    b. Have a member of the office staff call or write the patient within 7 days after initial visit, reinforcing the decision to stop and reminding the patient of the quit date.
    c. At the first follow-up visit, ask about the patient's smoking status to provide support and help prevent relapse. Relapse is common; if it happens, encourage the patient to try again immediately.
    d. Set a second follow-up visit in 1 to 2 months. For patients who have relapsed, discuss the circumstances of the relapse and other special concerns.

From National Cancer Institute (NCI) [10]; with permission.

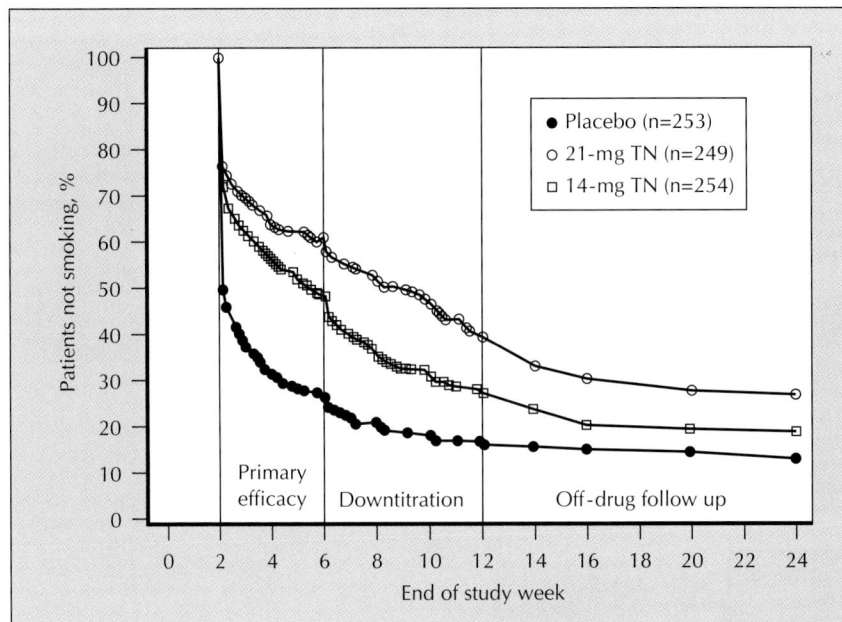

FIGURE 8 Effect of transdermal nicotine (TN) on smoking cessation rates. The first 2 weeks of study were not considered in the analysis of efficacy. Note the smoking cessation rate of 61% at 6 weeks and 42% at 3 months in the high-dose transdermal nicotine group. (*From* Transdermal Nicotine Study Group [12•]; with permission.)

ness, there are conflicting reports in the literature. Early studies suggested that normal individuals and patients with COPD develop adequate antibody titers, which led to the suggestion that all patients with COPD should receive the vaccine. More recent studies have questioned the development of adequate antibody titers and have noted that the pneumococcus is not as common a cause of pneumonia as it once was. Although there are uncertainties, most experts believe that the pneumococcal vaccine should be given to all patients with COPD because of its safety, low cost, and probable efficacy.

Bronchodilator Therapy

If the COPD patient has been identified, smoking cessation attempted, and vaccination given, attention must be turned to the relief of dyspnea with bronchodilators. This is an area of great controversy with much conflicting information and many strongly held beliefs that may not stand the scrutiny of time. The traditional approach to patients with COPD was to treat with a sustained release theophylline preparation and an inhaled β-agonist (sympathomimetic), as was done for patients with asthma. However, there has been a shift in the management of patients with COPD (Fig. 9); the anticholinergic bronchodilator ipratropium bromide has gradually become the accepted initial therapy of patients with COPD [13••]. There are several reasons for this change. First, numerous studies comparing the bronchodilator efficacy of ipratropium to both theophylline and the β-agonists have shown that in conventional doses ipratropium is a more potent bronchodilator than either of the other agents (Figs. 10 and 11) [14,15]. Second, there has been a delayed recognition of the toxicity of theophylline, and to a considerably less extent, the β-agonists. Thus, the most potent agent, ipratropium bromide, is also the most safe. Ipratropium may have an additional beneficial effect by reducing sputum production without affecting mucus viscosity. Finally, there may be a small subgroup of patients with COPD who respond only to anticholinergic agents.

If the patient's symptoms are not adequately controlled, the β-agonists are the next drug class to be considered. Although these agents have been widely used for over 20 years, there is no unanimity about whether these agents should be used on a fixed-dose regimen or what the appropriate dose should be. Because of the relative safety of these agents (hypokalemia and a worsening of arrhythmias) and the usual improvement in symptoms, most experts suggest that a fixed-dose routine should be used, unlike current asthma therapy which favors the "as needed" use of β-agonists [16].

Few areas are as controversial as the debate over the use of theophylline, especially in patients with COPD. The primary question raised in the past few years is whether the drug has any effect that cannot be provided by another agent. Four long-term, double-blind, placebo controlled trials have been performed in patients with COPD. All four of the studies noted that the use of theophylline was associated with a 10% to 15% improvement in FEV_1. However, only one of the four studies showed that theophylline decreased dyspnea and the only study that evaluated exercise tolerance found no change. Perhaps the major beneficial feature of theophylline compared with inhaled bronchodilators is its sustained duration of action, which has been shown to effectively decrease nocturnal declines in pulmonary function and to reduce respiratory symptoms in the morning [17].

The role of corticosteroid therapy in patients with COPD is also controversial. Most clinical trials indicate that approximately 10% to 15% of patients with COPD will respond to oral or inhaled corticosteroids [18]. Unfortunately, it is impossible to predict reliably which patient will respond, although some studies have suggested that the patients most likely to respond are those with asthma-like clinical components such as wheezing or sputum or blood eosinophilia.

Antibiotics have traditionally been given to patients with exacerbations of COPD, although for many years there were no scientific data to support this empirical practice. A recent large, blinded clinical trial of this problem fortunately has

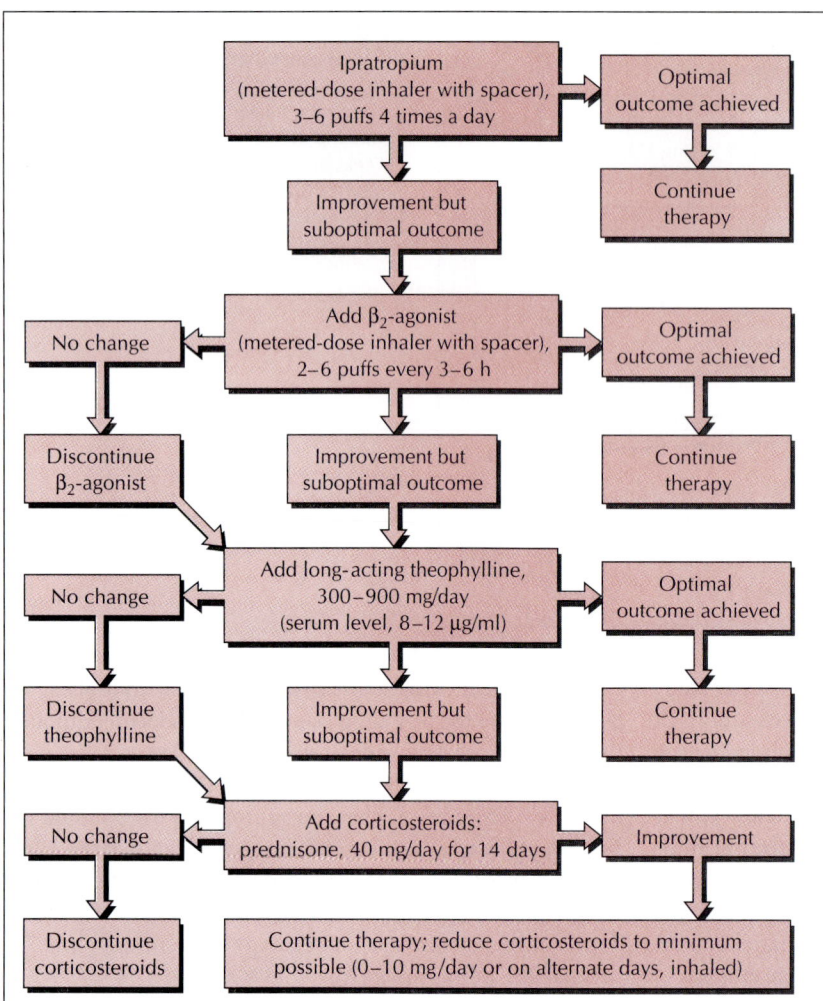

FIGURE 9 Algorithm of the approach to bronchodilator therapy in patients with clinically significant chronic obstructive pulmonary disease. Note that anticholinergic bronchodilators are now considered to be the drugs of choice in these patients. (*From* Ferguson and Cherniack [13••]; with permission.)

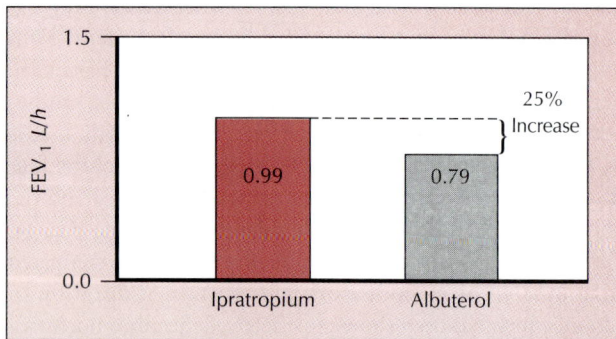

FIGURE 10 Comparison of the bronchodilator efficacy of anticholinergic versus β-agonist bronchodilators in patients with chronic obstructive pulmonary disease. Note that the anticholinergic bronchodilator is the considerably more potent bronchodilator. FEV_1—forced expiratory volume in 1 second. (*From* Braun, *et al.* [14]; with permission.)

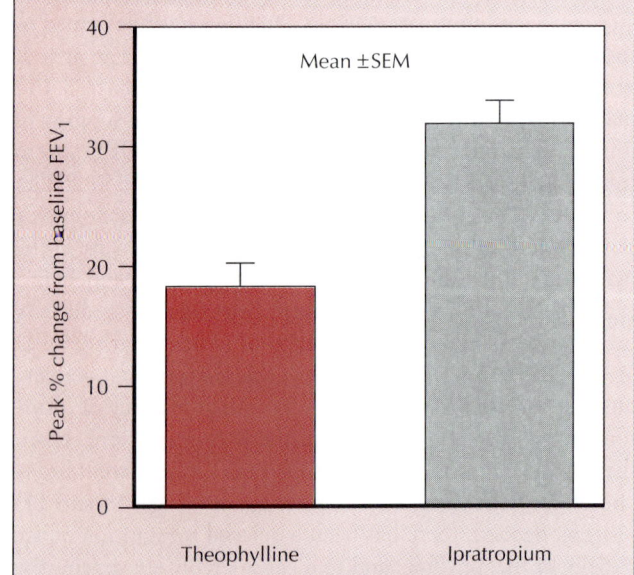

FIGURE 11 Comparison of the bronchodilator efficacy of theophylline and ipratropium in patients with chronic obstructive pulmonary disease. Note that the improvement in pulmonary function seen with the anticholinergic bronchodilator is approximately 80% greater. FEV_1—forced expiratory volume in 1 second; SEM—standard error of the mean. (*From* Bleecker and Britt [15]; with permission.)

TABLE 5 OUTCOME OF EXACERBATIONS OF CHRONIC OBSTRUCTIVE PULMONARY DISEASE		
Exacerbations	Placebo group % (n)	Antibiotic group % (n)
Success	55.0 (99)	68.1 (124)
No resolution	23.3 (42)	18.7 (34)
Deterioration	18.9 (34)	9.9 (18)
Other	2.9 (5)	3.2 (6)
From Anthonisen, *et al.* [19]; with permission.		

found that empiricism was correct (Table 5) [19]. The study showed that antibiotic therapy with ampicillin, tetracycline, or erythromycin given to patients with an exacerbation of their COPD led to a more rapid improvement in pulmonary function, a shortened clinical course, and a decrease in the likelihood of hospitalization or progression of symptoms.

Oxygen Therapy

The provision of supplemental oxygen to hypoxemic patients with COPD is the only intervention shown to decrease mortality in these patients (Fig. 12). Both the Medical Research Council (MRC) trial in Great Britain and the Nocturnal Oxygen Therapy (NOT) trial in the United States showed that the provision of oxygen for 15 hours a day in the MRC trial or 24 hours a day in the NOT trial was associated with a decrease in mortality [20•]. In both trials, the patients enrolled had values of their arterial oxygen tension of less than 55 mm Hg. Recently, it has been suggested that patients with COPD who do not meet conventional criteria for oxygen therapy may have an improvement in exercise tolerance and a decrease in dyspnea when treated with supplemental oxygen [22].

Because oxygen therapy has become widely used, several attempts have been made to compare the conventional nasal cannula approach to other delivery systems to determine the optimal delivery system. One of the important recent discoveries has been the delivery of oxygen via a transtracheal catheter (Fig. 13). After a minor surgical procedure for its placement, a transtracheal catheter has been shown to decrease oxygen flow requirements (by approximately 50%), to decrease dyspnea, to increase exercise tolerance (presumably by flushing CO_2 from the upper airway and decreasing the anatomic dead space), and to decrease the rate of hospitalization [23].

Rehabilitation

The importance of exercise training or pulmonary rehabilitation has grown in recent years, probably because of a series of studies that documented improvement in patients undergoing this form of therapy. Improvement in quality of life, an increase in maximal oxygen consumption, and a decrease in hospitalization rate have been demonstrated. Although many previous studies have trained patients at inappropriately low exercise levels, one of the more recent discoveries indicates that the COPD patients can train at nearly maximal levels, unlike normal individuals who train usually at 60% of their maximal exercise level [24•].

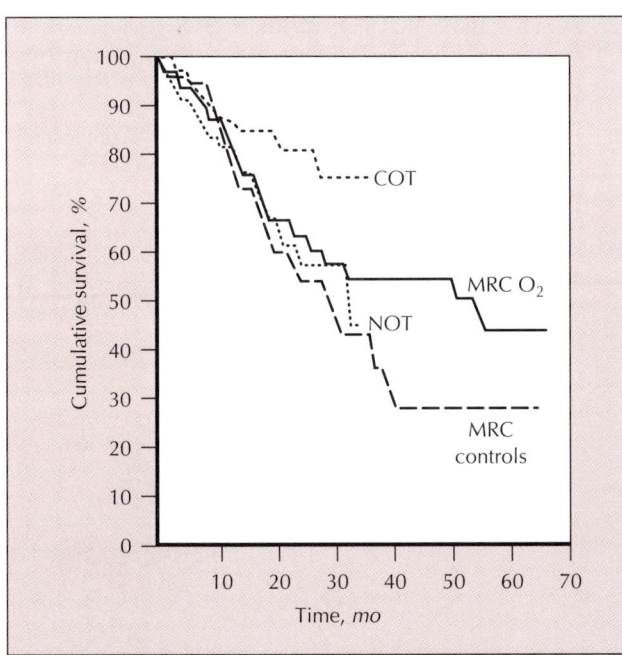

FIGURE 12 Survival of patients (men younger than 70 years) receiving long-term oxygen therapy and control subjects—the Medical Research Council (MRC) and Nocturnal Oxygen Therapy (NOT) trials. Survival of those in the MRC control group receiving no oxygen had clearly the worst survival. Survival of those in the NOT group receiving oxygen 12 hours per day was similar to that in the MRC group receiving 15 hours of oxygen per day (MRC O_2). Clearly the best survival, however, was that in the continuous oxygen therapy (COT) group, in which patients received oxygen for more than 19 hours per day. (*From* Flenley [21]; with permission.)

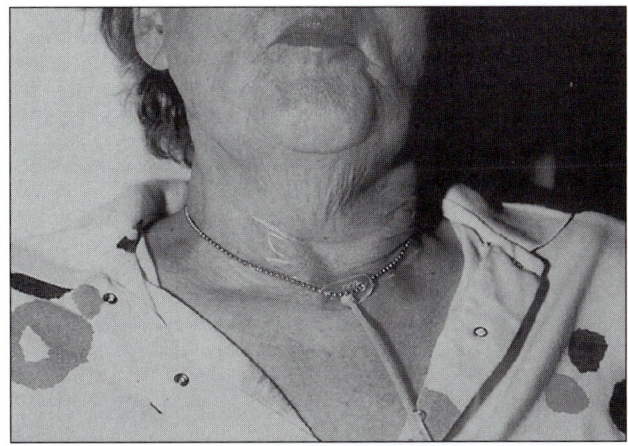

FIGURE 13 Photograph of a patient after insertion of a transtracheal catheter. The oxygen delivery system used is unobtrusive.

References and Recommended Reading

Recently published papers of particular interest have been highlighted as:
- Of interest
- •• Of outstanding interest

1. American Thoracic Society: Standards for the diagnosis and care of patients with COPD and asthma. *Am Rev Respir Dis* 1987, 136: 225–244.
2. National Center for Health Statistics: *Vital Statistics of the United States. Vol. 11.* Mortality, Part A for data years 1985–89, *Public Health Service.* Washington, U.S. Government Printing Office:
3. Eriksson S: Alpha$_1$-antitrypsin deficiency: Lessons learned from the bedside to the gene and back again. Historic Perspectives. *Chest* 1989, 95:181–189.
4. Owens G: Physiologic comparisons of obstructive pulmonary diseases. *J Resp Dis* 1990, 11:S23–S29.
5. Anthonisen NR, Wright EC, IPPB Trial Group: Response to inhaled bronchodilators in COPD. *Chest* 1987, 91:36S–39S.
6. Morrison NJ, Abboud RT, Ramadan F, *et al.*: Comparison of single breath carbon monoxide diffusing capacity and pressure-volume curves in detecting emphysema. *Am Rev Respir Dis* 1989, 139:1179–1187.
7. • Tashkin DP, Altose MD, Bleecker ER, *et al.*: The Lung Health Study: Airway responsiveness to inhaled methacholine in smokers with mild to moderate airflow limitation. *Am Rev Respir Dis* 1992, 145:301–310.
8. Fiore MC: The new vital sign: Assessing and documenting smoking status. *JAMA* 1991, 266:3183–3184.
9. DiClemente CC, Prochaska JO, Fairhurst SK, *et al.*: The process of smoking cessation: An analysis of precontemplation, contemplation, and preparation stages of change. *J Consult Clin Psychol* 1991, 59:295–304.
10. Glynn T, Manley M: *How to Help Your Patients Stop Smoking: A National Cancer Institute Manual for Physicians.* Bethesda, MD: National Cancer Institute, 1991.
11. • Schwartz JL: Methods of smoking cessation. Philadelphia: WB Saunders; 1992:457–476. [Medical Clinics of North America, 76.] 1992, 76:451–476.
12. • Transdermal Nicotine Study Group: Transdermal nicotine for smoking cessation. Six-month results from two multicenter controlled clinical trials. *JAMA* 1991, 266:3133–3138.
13. •• Ferguson GT, Cherniack RM: Management of chronic obstructive pulmonary disease. *N Engl J Med* 1993, 328:1017–1022.
14. Braun SR, Levy SF, Grossman J: Comparison of ipratropium bromide and albuterol in chronic obstructive pulmonary disease: A three-center study. *Am J Med* 1991, 91:28S–32S.
15. Bleecker ER, Britt EJ: Acute bronchodilating effects of ipratropium bromide and theophylline in chronic obstructive pulmonary disease. *Am J Med* 1991, 91:24S–27S.
16. Sears MR, Taylor DR, Print CG, *et al.*: Regular inhaled beta-agonist treatment in bronchial asthma. *Lancet* 1990, 336:1391–1396.
17. Martin RJ, Pak J: Overnight theophylline concentrations and effects on sleep and lung function in chronic obstructive pulmonary disease. *Am Rev Respir Dis* 1992, 145:540–544.
18. James AL, Finucane KE, Ryan G, *et al.*: Bronchial responsiveness, lung mechanics, gas transfer, and corticosteroid response in patients with chronic airflow obstruction. *Thorax* 1988, 43:916–922.
19. Anthonisen NR, Manfreda J, Warren CPW, *et al.*: Antibiotic therapy in exacerbations of chronic obstructive pulmonary disease. *Ann Intern Med* 1987, 106:196–204.
20. • Boyars MC, Deatrick SW: Meeting the challenges of home oxygen therapy. *J Respir Dis* 1992, 13:364–374.
21. Flenley DC: Oxygen therapy in the treatment of COPD. In *Chronic Obstructive Pulmonary Disease*, edn 1. Edited by Cherniack NS. Philadelphia: WB Saunders, 1991:468–476.
22. Dean NC, Brown JK, Himelman RB, *et al.*: Oxygen may improve dyspnea and endurance in patients with chronic obstructive pulmonary disease and only mild hypoxemia. *Am Rev Respir Dis* 1992, 146:941–945.
23. Hoffman LA, Wesmiller SW, Sciurba FC, *et al.*: Nasal cannula and transtracheal oxygen delivery. A comparison of patient response after 6 months of each technique. *Am Rev Respir Dis* 1992, 145:827–831.
24. • Casaburi P, Patessio P, Ioli F, *et al.*: Reductions in exercise lactic acidosis and ventilation as a result of exercise training in patients with obstructive lung disease. *Am Rev Respir Dis* 1991, 143:9–18.

Neoplasms of the Lung

Samuel Louie
Glen Lillington

Key Points
- Bronchogenic carcinoma is the most common cause of cancer-related deaths in both men and women in the United States.
- Tobacco smoking is the main etiologic factor, but exposure to other toxic substances plays a role in some cases.
- In most instances, the tumor is already incurable at the time the diagnosis is first established.
- Although the 5-year survival rate with therapy is only 10% to 15% overall, it may be as high as 70% to 80% in tumors presenting as a small solitary pulmonary nodule that are treated promptly. Early recognition of such cases mainly depends on the vigilance and timely intervention by the primary care physician.
- For purposes of management, bronchogenic carcinomas are divided into two groups: small cell carcinomas and non–small cell carcinomas. Small cell carcinomas are treated with radiation and/or chemotherapy, with surgical resection only in rare cases. Non–small cell carcinomas are treated surgically where possible; chemotherapy or radiation therapy has very limited efficacy.
- At present, the most effective measure for control of bronchogenic carcinoma is prevention, primarily by reducing tobacco smoking.

BRONCHOGENIC CARCINOMA

Bronchogenic carcinoma refers not to a single lung neoplasm but to a group of aggressive malignant tumors of the lower respiratory tract. It is the most common cause of cancer-related death for both women and men in the United States [1••]. During the past 10 years, the annual incidence and mortality rate of lung cancer has increased more than that of any other major malignancy. In 1950, there were 18,318 deaths from lung cancer in the United States. In 1993, more than 170,000 new cases were diagnosed, and nearly 150,000 of those patients were expected to die as a result of this disease. Diagnosis at an early stage of lung cancer is a diagnostic and therapeutic challenge for the general physician. The challenge is difficult because of the prevalence of bronchogenic carcinoma, the lack of specific signs and symptoms, and the generally poor 5-year survival rate, despite advances in surgery, chemotherapy, and radiotherapy in the past decade.

Etiology

Tobacco smoking is the most important of the recognized causes of bronchogenic carcinoma; only 12% of cases occur in nonsmokers. Tobacco smoke alone contains more than 40 known mutagens, tumor promoters, and carcinogens [2•]. Prolonged cigarette smoking is associated with a 20-fold increased risk for developing bronchogenic carcinoma; the risk correlates directly with the duration of smoking and the number of cigarettes consumed daily (Table 1). The risk decreases after 10 to 15 years of smoking cessation. Even "second-hand" or passive exposure to tobacco smoke increases the risk of developing bronchogenic carcinoma by 40% to 70%.

Table 1 Relation of smoking to lung cancer	
Smoking/category	Deaths from lung cancer/100,000
Pipe or cigar	60
Mixed	80
Cigarettes only	140
1–14 Cigarettes/d	80
15–24 Cigarettes/d	130
≤25 Cigarettes/d	260

From Doll and Peto [3].

Environmental risk factors include exposure to ionizing radiation (including soil radon) and exposure to asbestos, arsenic, chromium, nickel, and a number of other industrial substances. Asbestos inhalation is the most important industrial hazard and is associated with a 100-fold risk in smokers. Other risk factors include air pollution, localized or diffuse lung scarring, chronic obstructive pulmonary disease, and possibly vitamin A, vitamin E, and β-carotene deficiencies. Sixty years is the average age of onset. Bronchogenic carcinoma is rare in patients younger than 40 years of age.

Classification

Bronchogenic carcinomas are classified pathologically into four major cell types [1••], all of which are strongly associated with cigarette smoking, except for bronchogenic adenocarcinoma. Although each of the four carcinomas have fairly distinctive clinical and radiologic characteristics (Table 2), determination of the exact pathologic type requires biopsy of the primary lung tumor or of the peripheral organs involved by metastatic spread. Special stains or electron microscopy may be required to identify specific cell types.

Squamous cell

Squamous cell bronchogenic carcinoma comprises 30% of all cases. The tumor is often centrally located in the main bronchus or the proximal portion of the lobar bronchus, frequently leading to partial or complete bronchial obstruction. Typical histologic features include intracytoplasmic keratin and intercellular bridging. Sputum cytologic examinations are often positive, and the tumor can generally be directly visualized at bronchoscopy. With optimal therapy, the 5-year survival rate in patients with this tumor is approximately 35%.

Adenocarcinoma

Adenocarcinoma of the lung comprises 35% of bronchogenic carcinoma cases. The tumor is commonly a peripheral solitary nodule or mass. The pathologic characteristic is glandular formations with intracellular and intraluminal mucin. Sputum cytologic examination is often negative, and bronchoscopy frequently fails to demonstrate the tumor. Bronchogenic carcinomas arising in parenchymal scars are most often adenocarcinomas. Patients with small (stage I) adenocarcinomas have the best prognosis after surgery of all bronchogenic carcinomas.

Bronchioloalveolar tumor, or alveolar cell carcinoma, which comprises approximately 5% of bronchogenic carcinomas, is a subgroup of adenocarcinoma of the lung. It is the most common lung cancer in young adults. Tumor cells arise in the terminal portion of the bronchial tree and alveoli and grow along the alveolar walls and airways without disturbing the alveolar architecture. Growth is often slow. If the tumor is unifocal, small, and nonmucinous, prognosis after surgical removal is excellent. However, the mucinous tumors may be multifocal or even diffuse; these cases have a poor prognosis.

Large cell

Large cell bronchogenic carcinoma comprises approximately 15% of cases and often presents as a large, lobulated parenchymal mass that is cavitated. Hemoptysis is common. The tumor is undifferentiated and has no squamous or glandular characteristics. Patients with these tumors have the poorest prognosis of all non–small cell carcinomas of the lung.

Small cell

Small cell bronchogenic carcinoma comprises 20% to 25% of cases and traditionally is considered neuroendocrine in origin. With therapy, the 5-year survival rate is less than 5%. In terms of clinical management, small cell carcinomas are managed differently than non–small cell bronchogenic carcinomas (*ie*, squamous cell, large cell, and adenocarcinoma).

Clinical Manifestations

Symptoms and signs of bronchogenic carcinoma may be absent at the time of diagnosis in 10% to 20% of cases. Key signs and symptoms such as cough, dyspnea, wheezing, and hemoptysis are nonspecific and are often absent in early stages of lung cancer. Hemoptysis, change in pattern of cough, unexplained chest pain, recurrent pneumonia, unintentional weight loss with anorexia, or hoarseness in a two-pack-per-day smoker older than 40 years should prompt the taking of a thorough history and a physical examination with a chest roentgenogram.

Table 2 Clinical features of bronchogenic carcinoma			
Cell type	Incidence, %	Radiologic findings	5-y survival, %
Adenocarcinoma	35	Peripheral mass, solitary nodule	27
Squamous cell	30	Hilar mass, atelectasis or postobstructive pneumonia	37
Large cell	15	Large peripheral mass	27
Small cell	20	Hilar mass, adenopathy	<1

TABLE 3 PARANEOPLASTIC SYNDROMES OF BRONCHOGENIC CARCINOMA

Syndrome	Nature	Tumor	Mechanism
Inappropriate antidiuretic hormone (SIADH)	Hyponatremia	Small cell	Antidiuretic hormone
Cushing syndrome	Hypercortisolism	Small cell	ACTH-like hormone
Hypercalcemia	Elevated blood calcium	Squamous cell	PTH-like hormone
Gyecomastia	Gonadotrophic hormone	Large cell	Ectopic gonadotropin
Eaton-Lambert syndrome	Myasthenic state	Small cell	IgG antibodies
Peripheral neuropathy	Motor and sensory loss	All types	Unknown
Cerebellar degeneration	Ataxia	All types	Autoantibodies

ACTH—adrenocorticotropic hormone; PTH—parathyroid hormone; SIADH—syndrome of inappropriate antidiuretic hormone.

Recurrent episodes of pneumonia in the same area of lung may be a presenting feature. Chest pain is a late symptom, often indicating pleural involvement, direct invasion of the chest wall, mediastinum or diaphragm, or metastatic deposits in bones. Tumor encroachment on mediastinal structures can cause hoarseness, hemidiaphragmatic palsy, dysphagia, dyspnea, chylothorax, or signs of superior vena caval obstruction. Arm pain and Horner syndrome may be manifestations of Pancoast's tumor in which an apical bronchogenic carcinoma directly invades the brachial plexus. Swelling of the face and arms, with distended veins, may result from tumorous obstruction of the superior vena cava. Metastatic involvement of distant organs may cause hepatic insufficiency, neurologic deficits, seizures, and adrenal insufficiency. Systemic manifestations include weight loss, weakness, and anorexia. The presence of such symptoms is a poor prognostic sign. Paraneoplastic syndromes (Table 3), especially with small cell carcinoma, can develop in 15% to 20% of cases. These clinical syndromes may be caused by ectopic production of hormones by the bronchogenic carcinoma; however, the mechanism by which the tumor produces some clinical manifestations is unknown. On occasion, the paraneoplastic syndrome is the presenting manifestation of the underlying tumor.

Physical findings vary, depending on cell type and spread of disease. Evidence of metastatic spread to regional lymph nodes, liver, bone, skin, adrenal glands, or brain occurs more commonly than is appreciated. Palpable lymph nodes, pathologic bone fractures, seizures, and signs and symptoms of adrenal insufficiency may be clues to an underlying bronchogenic carcinoma.

At the time of diagnosis, only 20% of bronchogenic carcinomas are localized to the thorax, and 25% have metastases to regional lymph nodes. More than half of cases have metastases to distant organs, occurring most commonly with small cell carcinoma and adenocarcinoma. Endobronchial tumors, (*eg*, squamous cell carcinoma, small cell carcinoma) may obstruct a segmental or subsegmental bronchus and cause distal atelectasis. A persistent and localized wheeze or dullness to percussion with decreased breath sounds are encountered often in these cases. In contrast, peripheral tumors (*eg*, adenocarcinoma, large cell carcinoma) often present with few physical findings. Acanthosis nigricans may be associated with adenocarcinoma. Unexplained clubbing or deep vein thrombophlebitis may be early manifestations of occult bronchogenic carcinoma.

Radiologic Manifestations

In approximately 10% to 20% of cases, the possibility that bronchogenic carcinoma is present is first considered when an abnormality is discovered by standard chest roentgenography in an asymptomatic patient. Such abnormalities are usually solitary pulmonary nodules or lung masses (Figs. 1 and 2). On occasion, lung masses reach astonishingly large sizes without manifesting pulmonary signs or symptoms.

Other radiologic changes commonly seen with bronchogenic carcinomas include unilateral hilar enlargement

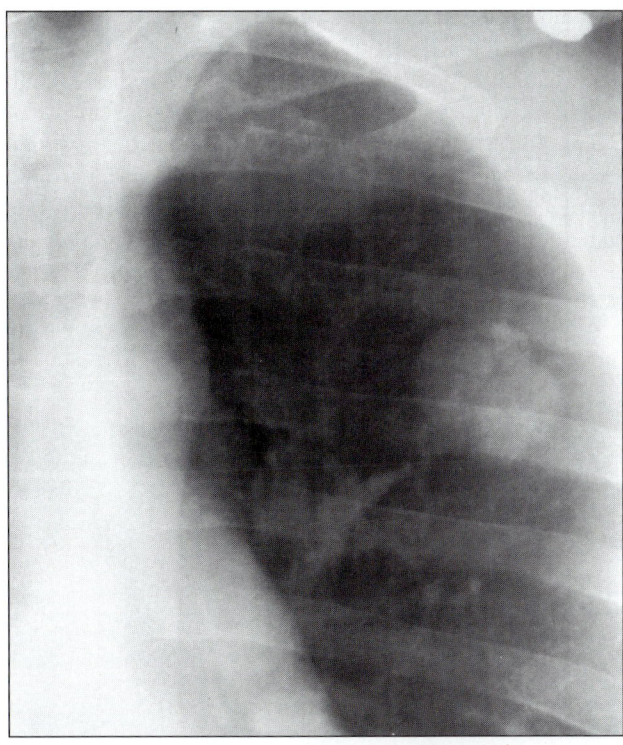

FIGURE 1 Posteroanterior chest roentgenogram showing a 3-cm solitary pulmonary nodule in the left upper lung field. Spherical lesions greater than 3 cm in diameter are usually referred to as masses rather than as nodules.

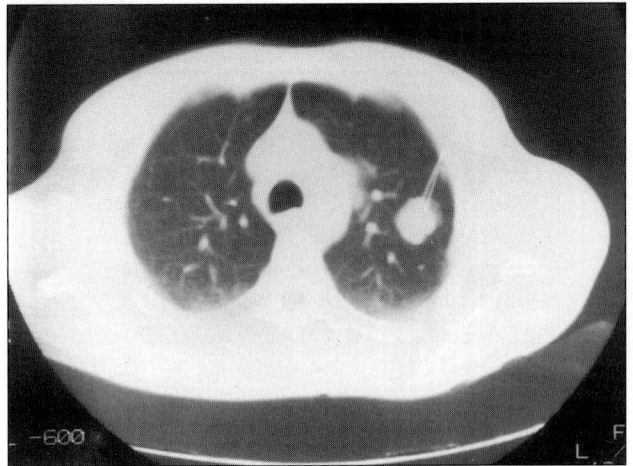

FIGURE 2 Computed tomography scan of the patient in Figure 1. The nodule is seen in the left upper lobe. The border is smooth but lobulated. A transthoracic aspiration biopsy needle has been inserted into the lesion.

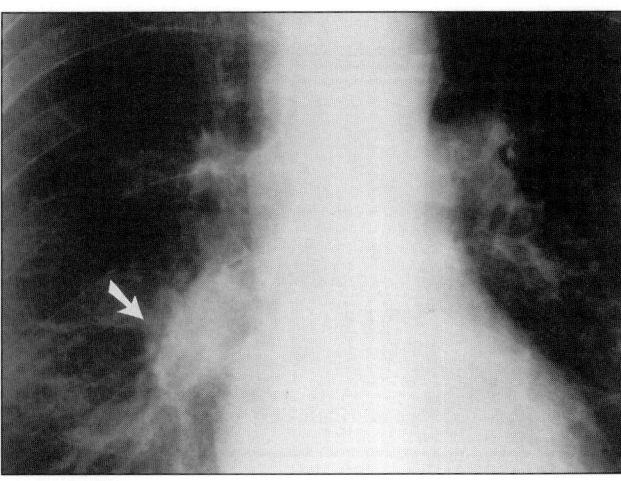

FIGURE 3 Portion of a posteroanterior roentgenogram showing unilateral hilar enlargement in the right lung (*arrow*) caused by tumor in the hilar lymph nodes. The primary lung tumor is posterior to the hilum and is poorly seen in this projection.

(Fig. 3), segmental or lobar atelectasis (Fig. 4), atelectasis of an entire lung, recurrent pneumonia in the same area of the lung, and one or more poorly defined areas of alveolar filling [4]. The apical tumor (Pancoast's syndrome, superior sulcus tumor) may appear as a small pleural cap, which often escapes scrutiny. Enlargement of the upper mediastinum is commonly caused by malignant lymphadenopathy from metastasis of the primary tumor. Pleural effusions are most common with adenocarcinoma and occur in 10% to 20% of patients with lung cancer.

A computed tomography (CT) scan of the chest is indicated in virtually all cases of suspected bronchogenic carcinoma. It clarifies the presence, size, position, and anatomic nature of abnormalities, and helps determine if there is direct involvement of the chest wall or mediastinum by tumor extension. Most importantly, CT helps identify the presence and location of enlarged hilar and mediastinal lymph nodes (Fig. 5), which aids in planning surgery. Mediastinal lymph nodes less than 1 cm in diameter are often benign, but nodes greater than 1.5 cm in diameter have a high probability of malignancy. However, not all enlarged lymph nodes are malignant, and not all malignant lymph nodes are enlarged. Nodal biopsy is necessary with nodes measuring between 1 and 1.5 cm during staging procedures. Magnetic resonance imaging (MRI) is about as effective as CT in examining hilar and mediastinal nodes, but may be superior in detecting mediastinal or chest wall involvement. Either CT or MRI can be used to detect metastases to brain, liver, or adrenal glands. The new technique of positron emission tomography (PET) scanning is probably the most sensitive and specific imaging test for the detection of malignant involvement of mediastinal nodes and metastases in other organs [5].

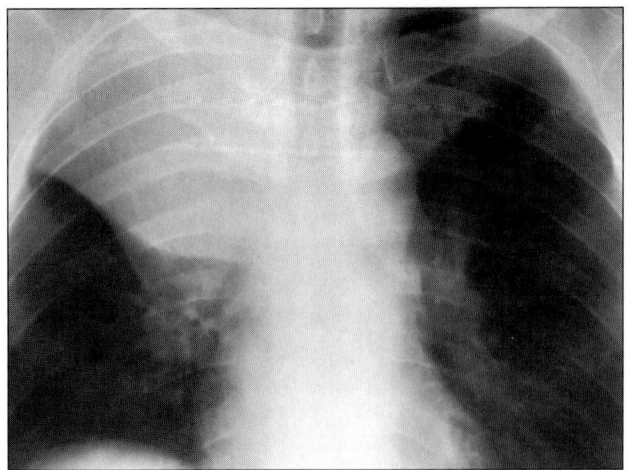

FIGURE 4 Posteroanterior chest roentgenogram showing atelectasis of the right upper lobe caused by obstruction of the right upper lobe bronchus by tumor. The sharply defined interface of the opacified lobe is caused by the horizontal fissure, which is rotated upward by the loss of volume.

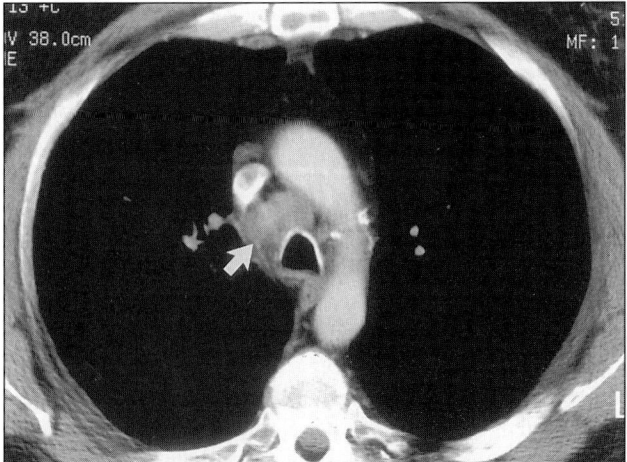

FIGURE 5 Computed tomography scan just above the level of the carina. Lymphadenopathy caused by tumor is seen in the left hilum (*short arrow*). Because no other areas of node involvement were detected in "cuts" at other levels, this tumor is potentially resectable.

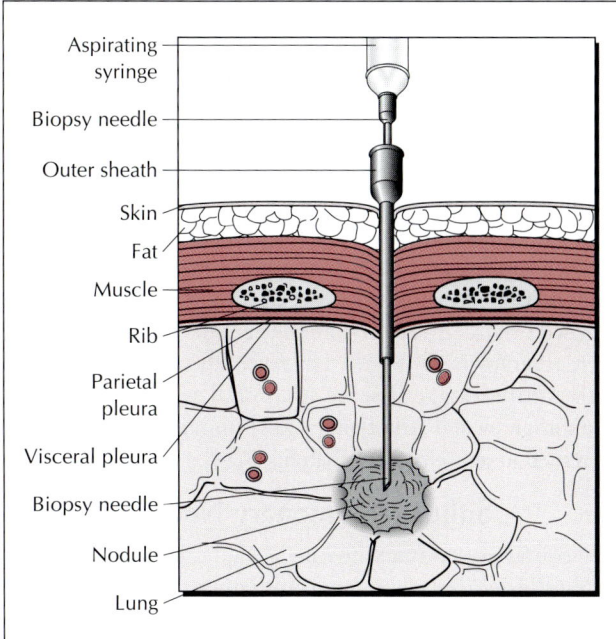

FIGURE 6 Diagram of the transthoracic needle aspiration biopsy technique. An outer sheath crosses the pleural space into the lung. The biopsy needle is passed through the sheath into the lung, where it impales the nodule. Use of the sheath allows multiple specimens to be obtained.

Diagnostic Tests

When a patient presents with symptoms, signs, or radiologic changes suggestive of bronchogenic carcinoma, it is necessary to obtain pathologic confirmation of the diagnosis to allow optimal choice of therapy. Sputum cytology may show malignant cells in 60% to 70% of patients with bronchogenic carcinoma with an abnormal chest radiograph, but this does not indicate the site of the lesion in the lung. False-positive results are not uncommon.

Bronchoscopy is indicated in most cases to determine the presence, location, and histologic cell type of the suspected lesion. A biopsy or brushing can be performed on central tumors with a very high diagnostic yield. Bronchoscopy may provide staging information, *eg*, primary tumors less than 2 cm from the carina (stage III) are usually unresectable. A biopsy on peripheral tumors beyond the visual range of the bronchoscope can sometimes be performed under fluoroscopic guidance, particularly if the lesion is greater than 2 cm in diameter. In cases of occult lung cancer (*ie*, positive sputum cytology with a normal chest radiograph), multiple bronchoscopic biopsies of all abnormal-appearing areas may identify an *in situ* carcinoma. Bronchoscopy is safe; complications are uncommon and usually minor.

Transthoracic needle aspiration biopsy of lesions situated in the lung (Fig. 6) is about 90% sensitive in cases of bronchogenic carcinoma and may determine that the nodule is benign. However, pneumothorax is a complication in 15% to 20% of cases.

Thoracentesis should always be done when pleural fluid is present. Malignant pleural effusions are exudative and frequently bloody. Cytologic examination of pleural fluid is usually sufficient, but needle biopsy of the parietal pleura may be required. Malignant cells in pleural fluid are a contraindication to resective surgery.

Mediastinoscopy allows sampling of mediastinal paratracheal lymph nodes to determine tumor spread and, thus, may play an important role when CT findings are not definitive and surgical resection is contemplated. Nodal involvement with tumor usually contraindicates attempts to resect the primary tumor. Video-assisted thoracoscopy can be used for biopsy or even for resection of very peripheral (subpleural) tumors. For resection of most malignant tumors, however, a standard thoracotomy is required.

Staging

Staging of bronchogenic carcinoma determines the size, location, and extent of the primary lung tumor; the presence and extent of lymph node involvement; and the presence of distant metastases. [6•,7].

Staging provides a guide to therapeutic options and prognostic information (Table 4).

Therapy

Prevention and risk avoidance, particularly smoking cessation, are the best means for reducing morbidity and mortality of bronchogenic carcinomas. Treatment results for the carcinomas are discouraging; the overall 5-year survival rate with treatment is 10% to 15%. Most patients with bronchogenic carcinoma are obviously incurable at the time of first contact with the physician. The use of chest roentgenograms to screen for early lung cancers has limited use [4,8].

The three primary therapeutic techniques available include resective surgery, combination chemotherapy, and radiotherapy. Referral to a specialist is required. Surgical resection of the tumor carries a mortality of 3% to 10%, but offers the only chance for cure [9]. Surgery is eventually used

Stage	Tumor location	5-y survival
I	Confined to lung	40% to 80%, with surgical resection
II	Hilar involvement	10% to 20%, with surgical resection
IIIA	Locally extensive intrathoracic involvement	10%, with surgical resection
IIIB	Locally extensive intrathoracic involvement	5%, no surgical resection indicated
IV	Metastases to other organs	1%, no surgical resection indicated

TABLE 4 STAGES OF BRONCHOGENIC CARCINOMA

in less than 30% of cases. If the patient has chronic obstructive pulmonary disease, complete pulmonary function testing, arterial blood gas analysis, and lung perfusion scanning are necessary to determine if tumor resection is feasible [9,10]. If the calculated postoperative forced expiratory volume in 1 second is less than 0.8 L, pneumonectomy or lobectomy may cripple the patient by causing chronic respiratory failure and ventilator dependence. The presence of coexisting medical problems may also preclude resective surgery. The risk of death from thoracotomy is increased in patients with chronic obstructive pulmonary disease (*eg*, $PaCO_2$ under 65 mmHg and $PaCO_2$ over 45 mmHG) and coronary heart disease. It is now possible to resect some cases of bronchogenic carcinoma by video-assisted thoracoscopy (VAT) without a formal thoracotomy [11].

Chemotherapy significantly improves the quality and duration of life in many patients with small cell carcinoma, but has a limited role in other forms of bronchogenic carcinoma [12]. Radiotherapy can provide significant palliation in all forms of bronchogenic carcinoma, both for the primary tumor and for local and distant metastases, and occasionally may be used in curative doses. Endobronchial laser therapy may provide palliation in some patients with central endobronchial obstructions unresponsive to conventional therapy. This may be combined with brachytherapy, which is the endobronchial placement of interstitial radiation adjacent to the tumor.

Because small cell bronchogenic carcinoma behaves differently from other bronchogenic carcinomas and has such a different prognosis, for purposes of therapeutic planning it is considered separately from non–small cell carcinomas (*ie*, squamous cell, adenocarcinoma, large cell).

Non–Small Cell Bronchogenic Carcinoma

Formal staging of the tumor is the first step in the management process. This includes the use of CT in most cases and mediastinoscopy in some cases. A patient with stage I and stage II tumors is managed by prompt surgical excision, unless the general condition of the patient contraindicates the thoracotomy with resection or if the patient declines surgery. Complete pulmonary function testing may be required to determine the feasibility of lung resection [9,10]. If surgery is not performed, palliative radiotherapy is indicated. No dramatic survival benefit has been shown with combination chemotherapy.

Patients with stage IIIA tumors are sometimes managed by surgical resection. Reports are conflicting on whether the addition of chemotherapy, radiotherapy, or both increases survival in patients with these tumors [13•]. In patients with stage IIIB and stage IV tumors, the standard treatment is palliative radiotherapy to the primary tumor, to symptomatic metastatic deposits, or to both. The role of combination chemotherapy is controversial [13•].

Small Cell Bronchogenic Carcinoma

Small cell bronchogenic carcinoma is, in most cases, disseminated at the time of first presentation. Metastases that contraindicate surgery are considered to be present, even if not clinically detectable [14]. A staging system that distinguishes patients with limited-stage disease (absence of tumor in contralateral lung and distant metastases) from those with extensive-stage disease is useful prognostically. Head CT scan, bone marrow biopsy, and radionuclide scans can help determine stage in small cell carcinoma. Bony metastases are most common in small cell carcinoma. Chemotherapy with combinations of cytotoxic agents (*eg*, cisplatin, vincristine, etoposide, cyclophosphamide, doxorubicin) produces a 50% complete remission rate in limited-stage disease and a 20% complete remission rate in extensive-stage disease. Remission is always followed by recurrence. The 5-year survival rate without chemotherapy is 1% to 5%. However, about 10% of patients with limited-stage disease are cured with combination chemotherapy and radiotherapy [12]. In rare instances, surgical resection of the tumor is helpful [9,14].

Solitary Pulmonary Nodule

The solitary pulmonary nodule is a spherical, well-circumscribed lesion less than 3 cm in diameter. Approximately 20% to 40% of such lesions are neoplasms (usually bronchogenic carcinoma); less commonly, such lesions are a solitary metastasis from an extrapulmonary primary tumor, for example, in the breast or colon. Most benign nodules are healed infectious granulomas and are often calcified. Patients with malignancies presenting in this fashion have a 5-year survival rate of 70% to 80% after surgical resection [15•]. Appropriate management of these lesions is critically important; they should never be ignored.

The standard management strategy is to regard all nodules as malignant and to resect them promptly, unless benignity is established by 1) the presence of a benign pattern of intranodular calcification; 2) stability, defined as lack of growth in size over a 2-year period, determined by a retrospective review of previous chest roentgenograms; or 3) a biopsy obtained by bronchoscopy or needle aspiration showing definitive evidence that the nodule is benign [15•]. The prospective determination of stability by serial chest roentgenograms, the wait-and-watch approach, has merit in limited circumstances. In rare instances, high-resolution CT of the nodule indicates that the nodule is benign with a high degree of certainty [16].

Pancoast's Syndrome

Bronchogenic carcinoma arising at the apex of the lung and growing upward into the base of the neck presents problems in diagnosis and management. The primary tumor may be small and difficult to identify on the chest roentgenogram. The combination of preoperative radiation and resective surgery is sometimes curative.

Superior Vena Cava Syndrome

Obstruction of the superior vena cava by metastatic tumor creates a striking clinical picture of swelling, cyanosis, and venous distension in the head, neck, and arms. This condition is an oncologic emergency and occurs most often with small cell carcinoma and squamous cell carcinoma. Radiotherapy is the treatment of choice with non–small cell carcinoma, whereas combination chemotherapy is favored in cases of small cell carcinoma.

OTHER PRIMARY LUNG TUMORS

Benign Tumors

There are a number of relatively rare benign tumors of the tracheobronchial tree or lung parenchyma [17]. The bronchial tumors present with hemoptysis or bronchial obstruction, and the parenchymal tumors present as asymptomatic nodules or masses discovered by chest roentgenography. The growth rate is almost always slow.

The hamartoma is the most common benign tumor. In 50% of cases, the diagnosis can be established by high-resolution CT [16]. Other tumors, all rare, include plasma cell granuloma, chondroma, fibroma, lipoma, leiomyoma, hemangioma, granular cell myoblastoma, histiocytoma, and benign "sugar" tumor.

Malignant Tumors

Bronchial carcinoid tumor may cause central airway obstruction or, in 20% of cases, appear as a peripheral nodule. Although the tumor (*eg*, breast, colon, renal carcinoma) grows slowly, it is malignant and should be resected if feasible [18]. Other tracheobronchial malignancies include cylindroma (*ie*, adenoid cystic carcinoma) and mucoepidermoid carcinoma. Laser therapy is often helpful in cases that are not resectable. Malignant mesothelioma is discussed in Chapter 8 of this section.

METASTATIC LUNG TUMORS

Metastases to the lung are usually hematogenous [19]. Although a metastatic deposit from an extrapulmonary primary tumor may appear as a solitary pulmonary nodule, the lesions are usually multiple, spherical, smoothly circumscribed, and vary in size. The steady increase in size and number of nodules is virtually pathognomonic, even in the uncommon cases in which the primary site of the tumor is occult. In some instances, the metastatic process is lymphogenous, with deposits in the intraseptal lymphatics, which gives rise to a reticular pattern on chest roentgenogram (lymphangitic carcinomatosis).

The pathologic nature of lung nodules may be confirmed by bronchoscopic or transthoracic needle aspiration biopsy. Because metastases from certain organs (*eg*, thyroid, breast, prostate) may respond well to therapy, it is usually advisable to identify the nature of the primary tumor.

ROLE OF THE GENERALIST

In most cases of bronchogenic carcinoma, the generalist physician is the first to detect the clinical changes that suggest the presence of a tumor. These may include persistent cough, hemoptysis, dyspnea, chest pain, or evidence of metastatic spread. Prompt initiation of an appropriate diagnostic workup by the generalist may allow identification of the tumor at a stage when the lesion is still potentially curable. The cure rate is highest when the tumor presents as an asymptomatic radiologic abnormality. Although the use of serial screening chest roentgenograms for individuals with risk factors such as smoking has been downplayed in the past, there is recent evidence to suggest that this may be advisable [8], and it is requested by many patients. An annual roentgenographic examination for persons at special risk seems reasonable.

Because proof of the presence of bronchogenic carcinoma ordinarily requires specialized biopsy procedures, referral to a pulmonologist or thoracic surgeon should be carried out at an early stage of the investigation.

REFERENCES AND RECOMMENDED READING

Recently published papers of particular interest have been highlighted as:
- Of interest
- •• Of outstanding interest

1. •• Symposium on intrathoracic neoplasms: *Mayo Clin Proc* 1993, 68:168–188, 273–296, 371–392, 475–498, 593–611, 680–690, 795–817, 880–891.
2. • Beckett WS: Epidemiology and etiology of lung cancer. *Clin Chest Med* 1993, 14:1–15.
3. Doll R, Peto R: Mortality in relation to smoking: 20 years observation on male British doctors. *BMJ* 1976, 2:1525–1536.
4. White CS, Templeton PA: Radiologic manifestations of bronchogenic cancer. *Clin Chest Med* 1993, 14:55–67.
5. Wahl RL, Quint LE, Greenough RL, *et al.*: Staging of mediastinal non-small cell lung cancer with FDG, PET, CT, and fusion images: preliminary prospective evaluation. *Radiology* 1994, 191:371–377.
6. • Mountain CF: Lung cancer staging classification. *Clin Chest Med* 1993, 14:43–51.
7. Armstrong P, Vincent JM: Review: Staging non-small cell lung cancer. *Clin Radiol* 1993, 46:1–10.
8. Smart CR: Annual screening using chest x-ray examination for the diagnosis of lung cancer. *Cancer* 1993, 72:2295–2298.
9. Shields TW: Surgical therapy for carcinoma of the lung. *Clin Chest Med* 1993, 14:121–148.
10. Marshall MC, Olsen GN: The physiological evaluation of the lung resection candidate. *Clin Chest Med* 1993, 14:305–320.
11. McKenna RJ, Jr: Lobectomy by video-assisted thoracic surgery with mediastinal node sampling for lung cancer. *J Thorac Cardiovasc Surg* 1994, 107:879–882.
12. Ihde DC: Chemotherapy of lung cancer. *N Engl J Med* 1992, 327:1434–1441.
13. • Masters GA, Vokes EE, Douglas IS, White Sk: Should non–small cell carcinoma of the lung be treated with chemotherapy? *Am J Respir Crit Care Med* 1994, 151:1285–1290.
14. Ginsburg RJ: Surgery and small cell lung cancer: an overview. *Lung Cancer* 1989, 5:232–236.
15. • Lillington GA: Management of solitary pulmonary nodules. *Dis Mon* 1991, 37:269–318.
16. Zwirewich CV, Vedal S, Miller RR, *et al.*: Solitary pulmonary nodule: high-resolution CT and radiologic-pathologic correlation. *Radiology* 1991, 179:469–476.
17. Lillington GA: Benign tumors. In *Textbook of Respiratory Medicine*, edn 2. Edited by Murray JA, Nadel J, Philadelphia: WB Saunders, 1994.
18. Davila DG, Dunn WF, Tazelaar HD, *et al.*: Bronchial carcinoid tumor. *Mayo Clin Proc* 1993, 68:795–803.
19. Whitesell PL, Peters SG: Pulmonary manifestations of extrathoracic malignant lesions. *Mayo Clin Proc* 1993, 68:483–491.

SELECT BIBLIOGRAPHY

Carr DT, Holoye DY, Hong WK: Bronchogenic carcinoma. In: *Textbook of Respiratory Medicine*, edn 2. Edited by Murray JA, Nadel J. Philadelphia: WB Saunders, 1994

Dewan NA, Gupta NC, Redepenning LS, *et al.*: Diagnostic efficacy of PET-FDG imaging in solitary pulmonary nodules. *Chest* 1993, 104:997–1002.

Hillers TK, Sauve MD, Guyatt GH: Analysis of published studies on the detection of extrathoracic metastases in patients presumed to have operable non-small cell lung cancer. *Thorax* 1994, 49:14–19.

Moore EH, Templeton PA: Imaging the advancing frontier of lung cancer operability. *Semin Respir Med* 1992, 13:293–308.

Infectious Lung Diseases
Michael S. Niederman

> ### *Key Points*
> - Empiric therapy of community-acquired pneumonia is often required, because as many as 50% of all patients have no identified etiologic pathogen, in spite of extensive diagnostic testing.
> - Risk factors for mortality from community-acquired pneumonia include a respiratory rate greater than 30 breaths per minute, a diastolic blood pressure less than 60 mm Hg, and evidence of dehydration with a blood urea nitrogen level greater than 20 mg/dL.
> - The approach to empiric therapy of community-acquired pneumonia involves an assessment of the presence of advanced age, comorbid illness, need for hospitalization, and severity of illness on initial presentation.
> - Clinical features are not always reliable for helping to predict the microbial etiology of community-acquired pneumonia.
> - Nosocomial pneumonia is the most common hospital-acquired infection to lead to patient mortality.
> - The bacteriology of early-onset and late-onset nosocomial pneumonia differ, and resistant gram-negative organisms are a particular concern for late-onset pneumonia.
> - Preventive strategies for community-acquired pneumonia exist and are effective, whereas preventive strategies for nosocomial pneumonia are still being tried and are of limited proven value.

Pneumonia is the sixth leading cause of death in the United States and the number one cause of death from infectious diseases. Whether arising in the community or in the hospital, pneumonia occurs when infectious pathogens (bacteria, viruses, fungi, mycobacteria, parasites) overcome existing host defenses. Pneumonia may be the result of impaired host defenses, as a consequence of comorbid illness or therapeutic interventions, or the result of exposure to a virulent infectious agent. Thus, many patients who develop respiratory infections have an underlying illness that has placed them at risk [1]. Pneumonia is particularly common among those who have pre-existing heart or lung disease, are of advanced age, or are already critically ill. When host defenses are normal, pneumonia can occur because of the presence of an excessively large number of organisms or because of exposure to a particularly virulent pathogen.

Acute bronchitis can occur in patients with or without underlying lung disease, whereas chronic bronchitis usually occurs in smokers and is frequently complicated by acute bronchial infection. Although acute bronchitis rarely leads to mortality, it is an important factor leading to respiratory decline in patients with chronic obstructive lung disease. It is also an important source of morbidity and a common precipitant of hospitalization.

BRONCHITIS

Acute infection of the bronchial tree, without parenchymal lung involvement, characterizes bronchitis, an infection occurring in the presence or absence of pre-existing lung disease (*see* Chapter 2, Obstructive Diseases). Patients with chronic bronchitis are particularly susceptible to acute bronchitic episodes, which often lead to a decline in respiratory status.

Clinical Features

The previously healthy patient with acute bronchitis presents with cough and sputum, often accompanied by dyspnea and wheezing. It is the most common cause of hemoptysis, although the quantity of expectorated blood is usually small to moderate. Other symptoms of acute bronchitis include burning chest pain and wheezing.

In the setting of chronic bronchitis, an acute bronchitic exacerbation is associated with 1) a change in sputum volume and color, 2) purulent secretions, and 3) increasing dyspnea. The severity of an exacerbation can be graded by how many of these three cardinal symptoms are present. When all three are present, the patient is particularly likely to benefit from antimicrobial therapy.

Many episodes of bronchitis follow upper respiratory illness; thus, the patient can also have malaise, fatigue, anorexia, chills, and myalgias. Physical examination is nonspecific, often revealing rhonchi, wheezes, or rales. The primary method for distinguishing bronchitis from pneumonia is by chest radiograph; no (new) infiltrate is present with bronchitis. In the patient with chronic bronchitis, there is a broad differential diagnosis of acute exacerbation:

- Bacterial bronchitis: *Haemophilus influenzae* (nontypeable), pneumococcus, *M. catarrhalis*, others
- Atypical pathogen bronchitis: *Mycoplasma pneumoniae*
- Viral bronchitis
- Pneumonia
- Chemical bronchitis
- Allergic tracheobronchitis
- Pulmonary embolism
- Congestive heart failure
- Pneumothorax

Diagnosis

Laboratory testing is not specific for bronchitis, but can be useful to differentiate the diagnosis from other processes. A sputum Gram stain may help to distinguish bacterial from viral infection and to identify the most likely pathogen, if the exacerbation is bacterial (Fig. 1). With a bacterial exacerbation, the sputum Gram stain will have numerous neutrophils and more than 8 to 18 organisms per high-power field [2].

Sputum culture is less valuable than Gram stain, because it may not point to the predominant pathogen and cannot be used to distinguish colonization from infection. Although normal nonsmokers usually have sterile lower respiratory tract secretions, smokers and those with chronic bronchitis often do not. Patients with chronic bronchitis are commonly colonized by *H. influenzae* (nontypeable), *M. catarrhalis*, or *S. pneumoniae*, and these same three pathogens are common causes of acute bacterial bronchitis. Other organisms causing acute bronchitis include viruses, *M. pneumoniae*, *H. parainfluenzae*, and occasionally enteric gram-negative bacilli.

Therapy and Prevention

A number of supportive measures are used for treating and preventing acute bronchitis, including smoking cessation, bronchodilators, corticosteroids, and vaccinations (see Chapter 2). Antibiotics are also widely used, even though as many as half of all exacerbations are nonbacterial. Reasons for using antibiotics include the following: 1) it is often clinically impossible to distinguish bacterial from nonbacterial exacerbations; 2) viral bronchitis can be complicated by secondary bacterial infection; and 3) several well-controlled studies show that antibiotic therapy leads to a more frequent and rapid resolution of symptoms and restoration of peak flow rates than when no antibiotics are administered [3•].

When antibiotics are chosen, they should be continued for 10 to 14 days, although no clear consensus for optimal duration exists. Ideally the antibiotic chosen should be active against pneumococcus, *H. influenzae*, and *M. catarrhalis*. It should also be free of serious side effects and easily taken. Effective older antibiotics include amoxicillin, trimethoprim/sulfamethoxazole, erythromycin, and tetracyclines, although each has gaps in its antimicrobial spectrum. Notably, amoxicillin can be inactivated by the beta-lactamases produced by some species of *H. influenzae* and most species of *M. catarrhalis*. Erythromycin is often poorly tolerated and has no activity against *H. influenzae*. Newer antimicrobials that avoid some of these problems include beta lactam/beta-lactamase inhibitor combinations and the newer macrolides (clarithromycin and azithromycin), which extend macrolide activity to *H. influenzae* and are better tolerated than erythromycin. The quinolones can also be used for bronchitic infection, but do not have absolute reliability against pneumococcus but should still be effective in this setting. Some of the newer agents are more convenient than the older preparations and can be administered once or twice a day.

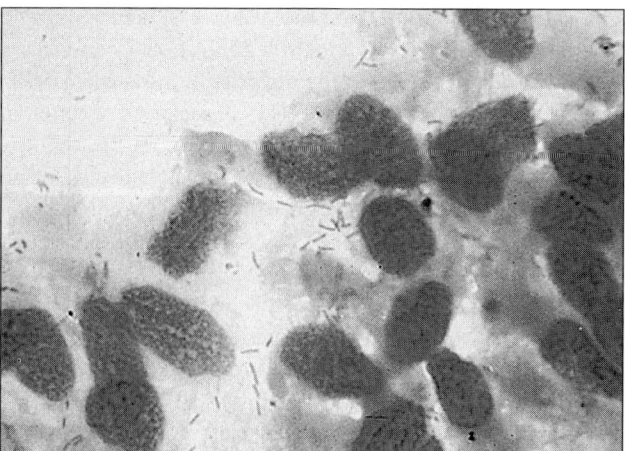

FIGURE 1 Sputum Gram stain from a patient with an acute exacerbation of chronic bronchitis. Numerous neutrophils and very few contaminating squamous epithelial cells are present. A predominant bacterial flora of *Haemophilus influenzae* is demonstrated.

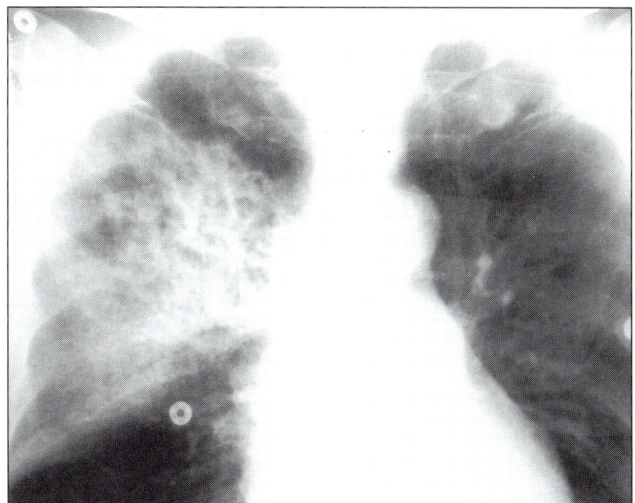

FIGURE 2 Chest radiograph from a patient with bacteremic pneumococcal pneumonia. The radiograph demonstrates a mixture of bronchopneumonia and alveolar infiltration in the right lung in a lobar distribution.

TABLE 1 PATHOGENS IN COMMUNITY-ACQUIRED, MILD PNEUMONIA IN OUTPATIENT THERAPY
Patient younger than 60 years of age with no comorbidity
Streptococcus pneumoniae
Mycoplasma pneumoniae
Respiratory tract viruses
Chlamydia pneumoniae
Haemophilus influenzae (especially in smokers)
Others: *Legionella* spp., *Staphylococcus aureus*, *Pneumocystis carinii*, gram-negative bacilli
Unusual organisms: *Mycobacterium tuberculosis*, endemic fungi
Patient older than 60 years of age with and/or without comorbid illness
S. pneumoniae
H. influenzae
Aerobic gram-negative bacilli
Oropharyngeal anaerobes
S. aureus
Respiratory tract viruses
Others: *Legionella* spp., *Moraxella catarrhalis*
Unusual organisms: *M. tuberculosis*, endemic fungi, *P. carinii*
Pathogens are listed in descending order of frequency.

COMMUNITY-ACQUIRED PNEUMONIA

Up to 6 million cases of pneumonia and influenza occur annually in the United States. The majority of these infections arise in the community, with approximately 20% requiring hospitalization. Patients with community-acquired pneumonia (CAP) who do not require hospitalization have a low mortality rate, in the range of 1% to 5%. When hospitalization is required for this infection, the mortality rate may be as high as 20% to 25%, in spite of the availability of potent antimicrobials. This observation underscores the fact that pneumonia frequently preys on patients who are debilitated, chronically ill, and not able to overcome infection [4•,5•].

Clinical Features

When CAP is present, patients may have a variety of respiratory and nonrespiratory symptoms. The "typical" pneumonia syndrome is characterized by the abrupt onset of fever, chills, pleuritic chest pain, toxicity, productive cough, and a lobar infiltrate on chest radiograph (Fig. 2). This presentation is classically seen with infection due to pneumococcus and other bacterial pathogens. In contrast, the "atypical" pneumonia syndrome is characterized by the gradual onset of a low-grade fever (often after an upper respiratory tract infection), a nonproductive cough, the absence of toxicity, and an interstitial lung infiltrate on chest radiograph. This pattern is seen in some patients with pneumonia caused by *Mycoplasma pneumoniae*, *Chlamydia pneumoniae*, and viral infection.

A number of studies have shown that the above-mentioned patterns of clinical symptoms are not very useful for predicting the etiologic pathogens for CAP [6]. This limitation is probably a result of the following factors: 1) elderly patients with pneumonia often present with indistinct clinical features and without respiratory symptoms, even when bacteria such as pneumococcus are responsible; 2) *Legionella* species cause a clinical syndrome with features of both typical and atypical pneumonia; and 3) many patients with CAP have no identifiable etiologic pathogen, and thus it is impossible, in many patients, to validate the accuracy of clinical features in predicting the responsible organism.

Etiologic Pathogens

Many carefully done studies have been unable to identify an etiologic pathogen in as many as 50% of all patients with CAP, particularly if sputum cultures alone (which cannot distinguish colonization from pneumonia) are used to define the responsible pathogen [4•,5•]. The most commonly identified pathogen for CAP is *Streptococcus pneumoniae* for all patient populations, regardless of age or severity of illness. In identifying the next most likely pathogens, a number of considerations, all of which influence the bacteriologic spectrum of pneumonia, should be taken into account. These factors include patient age (> or < 60 years), the presence of comorbidity, and the severity of illness [7••].

In young patients without comorbid illness, the most likely pathogens for CAP are *S. pneumoniae*, *M. pneumoniae*, viruses, and *C. pneumoniae* (Table 1). In this population, infection from *Legionella* species become a consideration only if the pneumonia is severe, and *Haemophilus influenzae* infection is a consideration if the patient is a smoker (even in the absence of chronic lung disease). Among the elderly (including those in nursing homes) and those with comorbidity, infection with *S. pneumoniae*, *H. influenzae*, anaerobes, *Staphylococcus aureus*, and enteric gram-negative bacilli should be considered (Table 1). If the patient is ill enough to require hospitalization (*see* below discussion) all of the above organisms should be considered. In fact, several studies of severe CAP have demonstrated that the most common pathogens for this infection are *S. pneumoniae*, *Legionella pneumophila*, and enteric gram-negative bacilli. If the patient has recently received antibiotics, has been on long-term corticosteroids, or has structural lung disease (bronchiectasis, cystic fibrosis) and then develops a moderate to severe pneumonia, *Pseudomonas aeruginosa* must be suspected as a possible pathogen (Table 2). In all patients with CAP, unusual pathogens should be considered, particularly if the patient is not responding to seemingly appropriate therapy. These unusual pathogens include *Mycobacterium tuberculosis*, *Pneumocystis carinii* (which may be the first manifestation of AIDS), and endemic fungi (histoplasmosis, coccidiodomycosis, blastomycosis).

Severity of Illness and Need for Hospitalization

There are no established guidelines for when to admit patients with CAP to the hospital. Hospitalization should be considered if the patient requires therapy that cannot be given at home, such as intravenous antibiotics, intravenous hydration, supplemental oxygen, and hemodynamic and ventilatory support [8•]. In addition, hospitalization might be useful if the patient has factors predicting an increased risk of mortality or a complicated course of illness (Table 3). If the patient is unable to reliably come for medical follow-up or does not have a stable social situation to assure compliance with therapy, hospitalization may be useful. Among patients older than 65 years of age, hospitalization should be considered for those who have an associated serious illness.

In the last few years, a number of studies have reported an entity termed *severe CAP*, but there is no uniform definition of this illness [9••,10••]. The presence of severe pneumonia usually necessitates admission to the intensive care unit, and is characterized by having at least one of the following:

- Respiratory rate > 30/min
- Respiratory failure: PaO_2/FiO_2 ratio < 250, or acute respiratory acidosis
- Need for mechanical ventilation
- Rapid deterioration on chest radiograph (infiltrate increases by > 50% in 48 hours after admission)
- Shock
- Need for vasopressors
- Urine output < 20 mL/hour
- Severe sepsis with end organ dysfunction

Diagnosis

When pneumonia is suspected, the physician should attempt to answer the following questions: 1) Are the symptoms caused by pneumonia or caused by another disease process

TABLE 2 COMMUNITY-ACQUIRED PNEUMONIA PATHOGENS IN HOSPITALIZED PATIENTS

Not maximally severe pneumonia
Streptococcus pneumoniae
Haemophilus influenzae
Polymicrobial (including anaerobes)
Aerobic gram-negative bacilli
Legionella spp.
Staphylococcus aureus
Chlamydia pneumoniae
Respiratory tract viruses
Other: *Mycoplasma pneumoniae*, *Moraxella catarrhalis*
Unusual organisms: *Mycobacterium tuberculosis*, endemic fungi, *Pneumocystis carinii*

Severe pneumonia (often treated in the intensive care unit)
S. pneumoniae
Legionella spp.
Aerobic gram-negative bacilli (including *Pseudomonas aeruginosa*)
M. pneumoniae
Respiratory tract viruses
Others: *H. influenzae*
Unusual organisms: *M. tuberculosis*, endemic fungi, *P. carinii*

Pathogens are listed in descending order of frequency.

TABLE 3 REASONS TO CONSIDER HOSPITALIZATION FOR PATIENTS WITH COMMUNITY-ACQUIRED PNEUMONIA

Patient older than 65 years of age plus comorbid illness
    Comorbid illnesses: chronic lung disease, chronic heart disease, diabetes mellitus, chronic renal failure, underlying cause for recurrent aspiration (certain neurologic illnesses), postsplenectomy
Abnormal physiology
    Respiratory rate >30/min
    Diastolic blood pressure <60 mm Hg
    Systolic blood pressure <90 mm Hg
    Temperature >101°F
    Confusion
Serious laboratory abnormalities
    White blood cell count <4000 or >30,000
    Blood urea nitrogen >20 mg/dl
    PaO_2 <60 mm Hg on room air
    $PaCO_2$ >50 mm Hg
    Multilobar infiltrate on chest radiograph
    Acute coagulopathy
Unstable social situation
Unable to take oral therapy
Immunosuppression (recent chemotherapy or >15 mg/day prednisone-equivalent corticosteroids)
Needed therapy cannot be given at home
    Oxygen therapy
    Intravenous hydration
    Hemodynamic or ventilatory support

PaO_2—arterial partial pressure of oxygen; $PaCO_2$—arterial partial pressure of carbon dioxide.

that mimics pneumonia? 2) How ill is the patient, what complications are present, and is hospitalization needed? 3) What is the likely etiologic pathogen, and what tests are needed to establish the appropriate choice of antibiotics?

To determine if symptoms are caused by pneumonia, a chest radiograph should be obtained. Securing a radiograph may be a particularly useful procedure in the elderly because it will determine if a pulmonary process is responsible for such nonspecific symptoms as failure to thrive, worsening of an underlying illness, confusion, falling, or fever. In the elderly, the most sensitive indicator of the presence of respiratory infection is tachypnea, with a respiratory rate greater than 20/min; the presence of this finding should prompt the immediate ordering of a chest radiograph.

The findings on the chest radiograph may be useful in the differential diagnosis of nonspecific symptoms and may help to determine the presence of nonpneumonic processes, such as bronchitis (normal radiograph with associated cough, sputum, and dyspnea), congestive heart failure, lung mass, or pulmonary infarction. The finding of a posterior upper lobe infiltrate should prompt consideration of tuberculosis; the finding of a cavitary infiltrate may suggest aspiration pneumonia or an obstructing endobronchial lesion; and the finding of a pleural effusion mandates a diagnostic thoracentesis to rule out associated empyema (*see* Chapter 8, Diseases of the Pleura). Finally, the radiograph can be used to define the severity of illness; for example, a severe case of pneumonia is likely if the infiltrate is multilobar or rapidly progressive or has a pattern compatible with the diagnosis of adult respiratory distress syndrome.

The remaining steps of the diagnostic approach should be dictated by practical issues: 1) the availability of specific diagnostic tests and the presence of respiratory secretions for examination; and 2) an assessment of the the severity of illness, with more aggressive testing reserved for those who are severely ill. If the patient is ill enough to be hospitalized, sputum can be collected for a Gram stain (a good sample will have > 25 neutrophils and < 10 squamous cells per low-power field) in order to identify the most likely etiologic pathogen, although the usefulness of this test has been questioned [7••]. Sputum culture may be helpful if drug-resistant organisms are suspected (pneumonia that developed while the patient was taking antibiotics) or if unusual pathogens (*M. tuberculosis*, endemic fungi) are suspected. Extensive serologic testing and collection of secretions for viral cultures are rarely needed in individual cases and are more useful for epidemiologic purposes or for investigation of the patient who is not responding appropriately to empirical therapy. Hospitalized patients should have two sets of blood cultures collected, and any pleural fluid should be sampled to rule out empyema.

Therapy

Hospitalized patients and outpatients can be treated empirically, according to the recommendations in Table 4. In both patient groups, it is impossible to determine how long therapy should be given, but most patients are treated for at least 10 to 14 days, although some of the newer antimicrobials may allow for shorter courses of therapy. Even with appropriate therapy, clinical improvement may not be evident for 48 to 72 hours.

TABLE 4 EMPIRICAL THERAPY OF PATIENTS WITH COMMUNITY-ACQUIRED PNEUMONIA

Outpatient therapy
Patient younger than 60 years of age with no comorbidity
    Erythromycin
    or New macrolides: clarithromycin, azithromycin
    or Tetracyclines*
Patient greater than age 60 with/without comorbid illness
    Second-generation cephalosporin
    or Beta lactam/beta-lactamase inhibitor combination
    or Trimethoprim/sulfamethoxazole
    or Quinolone plus clindamycin
    or Quinolone plus penicillin

Inpatient therapy
Not maximally severe pneumonia
    Second- or third-generation cephalosporin
    or Beta lactam/beta-lactamase inhibitor combination
    ± Macrolide
Severe pneumonia
    Macrolide ± Rifampin (if *Legionella* spp. likely)
    plus†
    Third-generation cephalosporin with anti-Pseudomonal activity
    or Imipenem/cilastatin
    or Ciprofloxacin

*Many *Streptococcus pneumoniae* are resistant and this antimicrobial should only be used if the patient is allergic to or intolerant of macrolides.
†Consider initial dual anti-Pseudomonal therapy.

Radiographic resolution of CAP is much slower, requiring weeks to months, particularly if the patient has bacteremia or a serious coexisting illness, or is of advanced age or an alcoholic. If the patient with suspected CAP is not responding to empirical therapy, several considerations are pertinent: 1) Is the infection caused by a pathogen that is resistant to or not covered by the antibiotic regimen? 2) Does the patient have HIV infection, or is the pneumonia caused by a nonbacterial pathogen? 3) Is the disease process a noninfectious one, such as congestive heart failure, pulmonary embolus with infarction, or inflammatory lung disease (*eg*, bronchiolitis obliterans and organizing pneumonia or Wegener's granulomatosis)? 4) Is there an extrapulmonary complication of pneumonia, such as empyema, endocarditis, or meningitis?

Prevention

Because CAP and influenza occur in specific populations that are known to be at risk, immunization with pneumococcal and influenza vaccine should be considered for individuals with the indications listed below:
- Elderly: > age 65 years
- Chronic heart or lung disease
- Splenectomy or splenic dysfunction*
- Immunosuppressive illness interfering with cell-mediated immunity

Multiple myeloma
Hodgkin's disease
AIDS*
- Alcoholism
- Renal failure
- Diabetes
- Residence in a chronic care facility

*Known risk factor for pneumococcal infection, influenza vaccine may not be needed.

Influenza vaccine should be given yearly in the fall, and pneumococcal vaccine should be given when an at-risk condition is identified. Pneumococcal vaccine may need to be repeated as often as every 6 years, especially in the elderly and those with chronic medical illness, but there are no firm guidelines for revaccination at the current time.

NOSOCOMIAL PNEUMONIA

Nosocomial pneumonia accounts for approximately 500,000 episodes of pneumonia annually. It is the number one cause of death from nosocomial infections: among mechanically ventilated patients, the mortality rate may be as high as 50% to 70% [11]. Although many critically ill patients die with pneumonia, several studies have documented that nosocomial pneumonia has an attributable mortality of its own; thus, critically ill medical patients may be dying not only with this infection, but because of it [12••]. Among the elderly residents of nursing homes, pneumonia is a common infection and the infection most likely to lead to death.

When a patient has been in the hospital for 48 to 72 hours and then develops a parenchymal respiratory infection, nosocomial pneumonia is present. This form of pneumonia can arise in the intensive care unit or on a medical or surgical floor. Patients are at risk for the infection because of the nature of their underlying medical illnesses or because of specific therapeutic interventions. In the hospital setting, these two factors often lead to impairment of lung host defenses, while the patient simultaneously is exposed to a large number of potentially pathogenic bacteria. The risk factors for nosocomial pneumonia are summarized in Table 5 [11].

Pathologic Pathogens

Unlike CAP, nosocomial pneumonia is most commonly the result of enteric gram-negative bacilli or *S. aureus*. In general, early-onset pneumonias (within the first week of hospitalization) are due to *S. aureus*, anaerobes, or enteric gram-negative bacilli, while the late-onset pneumonias are due to enteric gram-negative bacilli [13]. If the patient has been mechanically ventilated for a prolonged period or has received corticosteroids or multiple broad-spectrum antimicrobials, *P. aeruginosa* is the most likely pathogen. Nosocomial pneumonia can occasionally be the result of infection with pneumococcus, *H. influenzae*, or viral agents, with these organisms being more commonly present in patients who are not severely ill. Up to 40% of patients who have nosocomial pneumonia and are mechanically ventilated have polymicrobial infections, with multiple pathogens acting simultaneously to cause the infections [14].

Diagnosis

The recognition of nosocomial pneumonia, especially in the mechanically ventilated patient, is difficult and clinical features are nonspecific. Most clinicians diagnose the infection by the finding of a new or progressive lung infiltrate plus fever, leukocytosis, purulent sputum, and potential pathogens in the sputum. This clinical definition is overly sensitive, and many patients who satisfy these criteria will have other disease processes present, such as atelectasis, congestive heart failure, or adult respiratory disease syndrome. Because of the nonspecificity of the clinical presentation of pneumonia, some have advocated the use of invasive diagnostic methods involving quantitative sampling of lung secretions with bronchoalveolar lavage or a bronchoscopically directed, protected specimen brush. The accuracy of these methods varies widely in reported series, and the ability of these techniques to improve patient outcome is uncertain. For this reason, these methods cannot be viewed as the standard care at the present time [15].

Therapy

Once the clinical diagnosis of pneumonia is made, antimicrobial therapy is necessary. Although initial therapy is usually empirical,

TABLE 5 RISK FACTORS FOR NOSOCOMIAL PNEUMONIA

Altered immune function
Due to underlying illness
  Acute lung injury
  Hemorrhagic shock
  Intra-abdominal infection
  Sepsis
  Chronic medical diseases: diabetes, congestive heart failure, chronic lung disease, renal insufficiency, malnutrition, malignancy, obesity
Due to therapeutic interventions
  Endotracheal intubation
  General anesthesia
  General surgery
  Immunosuppressives
  Oxygen
  Sedatives and other common medications
  Lack of enteral feeding
Increased exposure to bacteria
  Endotracheal intubation
  Elevation of gastric pH: enteral feeding into the stomach, antacids, H_2-antagonists
  Positioning patient supine (increased aspiration risk)
  Nasogastric tube
  Systemic antibiotics leading to bacterial overgrowth
  Respiratory therapy equipment: nebulizers, tubing with condensate from humidification

TABLE 6 ANTIBIOTIC THERAPY OF NOSOCOMIAL PNEUMONIA
Treatment of most common pathogens
Second- or third-generation cephalosporin
or β-lactam/β-lactamase inhibitor combination
or Ciprofloxacin ± clindamycin
or Imipenem/cilastatin
or Aminoglycoside plus clindamycin
Anti-Pseudomonal antibiotics (combination therapy)
Anti-Pseudomonal penicillins: azlocillin, mezlocillin, piperacillin
Anti-Pseudomonal cephalosporins: ceftazidime or cefoperazone
Imipenem
Aztreonam
Ciprofloxacin
Aminoglycosides
Methicillin-resistant *Staphylococcus aureus*
Vancomycin

antibiotic choices can be adjusted when the results of sputum culture and sensitivity are obtained. In an intubated patient, sputum culture usually reveals the responsible pathogen, but it may also demonstrate other colonizing pathogens as well. Initial, empiric antibiotics should be directed at the pathogens most likely to be present in the sputum sample and thought to be etiologic, realizing that many cases of nosocomial pneumonia, unlike CAP, are polymicrobial.

The antibiotics that can be used for nosocomial pneumonia are listed in Table 6, but there are several controversies relevant to therapeutic decisions that should be noted. Some patients may be adequately treated with a single agent, while others require combination therapy. There is no firm consensus about the adequacy of monotherapy, but it may be adequate if an appropriate single agent can be found that covers all likely pathogens. However, patients with suspected bacteremia caused by *P. aeruginosa* or any pneumonia due to *P. aeruginosa* should receive combination therapy in order to reduce mortality and prevent the emergence of resistance during therapy.

There is no strict recommendation for how long a patient should be treated for nosocomial pneumonia. Some data indicate safe early transition from intravenous to oral therapy with the quinolones, if the responsible organism is susceptible, because these agents are well-absorbed and penetrate respiratory secretions well.

Prevention

No proven strategies for reducing the risk of nosocomial pneumonia have been found, although prophylactic antibiotics have been tried, with no observed reduction in mortality rates. Simple strategies directed at pathogenetic principles may be useful. These include the use of nutritional support, preferably via the enteral route and with a feeding tube advanced beyond the stomach; positioning the patient in the semi-erect posture in order to minimize the risk of gastric aspiration; careful selection of intestinal bleeding prophylaxis; mobilization of respiratory secretions by a variety of methods, including the use of rotational bed therapy; and careful handling of respiratory therapy equipment [16].

References and Recommended Reading

Recently published papers of particular interest have been highlighted as:
- Of interest
- • Of outstanding interest

1. Skerrett SJ, Niederman MS, Fein AM: Respiratory infections and acute lung injury in systemic illness. *Clin Chest Med* 1989, 10:469–502.
2. Chosdosh S: Treatment of chronic bronchitis: state of the art. *Am J Med* 1991, 6A:87S–92S.
3.• Anthonisen NR, Manfreda J, Warren CPW, *et al.*: Antibiotic therapy in exacerbations of chronic obstructive pulmonary disease. *Ann Intern Med* 1987, 106:196–204.
4.• Marrie TJ, Durant H, Yates L: Community-acquired pneumonia requiring hospitalization: a 5-year prospective study. *Rev Infect Dis* 1989, 11:586–599.
5.• Fang GD, Fine M, Orloff J, *et al.*: New and emerging etiologies for community-acquired pneumonia with implications for therapy: a prospective multicenter study of 359 cases. *Medicine* 1990, 69:307–316.
6. Farr BM, Kaiser DL, Harrison BDW, *et al.*: Prediction of microbial aetiology at admission to hospital for pneumonia from the presenting clinical features. *Thorax* 1989, 44:1031–1035.
7.•• Niederman MS, Bass JB, Campbell GD, *et al.*: Guidelines for the initial management of adults with community-acquired pneumonia: diagnosis, assessment of severity, and initial antimicrobial therapy. *Am Rev Respir Dis* 1993, 148:1418–1426.
8.• Fine MJ, Smith DN, Singer DE: Hospitalization decision in patients with community-acquired pneumonia: a prospective cohort study. *Am J Med* 1990, 89:713–721.
9.•• Torres A, Serra-Batlles J, Ferrer A, *et al.*: Severe community-acquired pneumonia: epidemiology and prognostic factors. *Am Rev Respir Dis* 1991, 144:312–318.
10.•• Farr BM, Soman AJ, Fisch MJ: Predicting death in patients hospitalized for community-acquired pneumonia. *Ann Intern Med* 1991, 115:428–436.
11. Niederman MS, Craven DE, Fein AM, *et al.*: Pneumonia in the critically ill hospitalized patient. *Chest* 1990, 97:170–179.
12.•• Fagon JY, Chastre J, Hance AJ, *et al.*: Nosocomial pneumonia in ventilated patients: a cohort study evaluating attributable mortality and hospital stay. *Am J Med* 1993, 94:281–288.
13. Rello J, Ausina V, Castella J, *et al.*: Nosocomial respiratory tract infections in multiple trauma patients: influence of level of consciousness with implications for therapy. *Chest* 1992, 102:525–529.
14. Fagon J, Chastre J, Domart Y, *et al.*: Nosocomial pneumonia in patients receiving continuous mechanical ventilation: prospective analysis of 52 episodes with use of a protected specimen brush and quantitative culture techniques. *Am Rev Respir Dis* 1989, 139:877–884.
15. Niederman MS: Diagnosing nosocomial pneumonia: to brush or not to brush. *J Intens Care Med* 1991, 6:151–152.
16. Levine SA, Niederman MS: The impact of tracheal intubation on host defenses and risks for nosocomial pneumonia. *Clin Chest Med* 1991, 12:523–543.

SELECT BIBLIOGRAPHY

Cockerill FR, Muller SR, Anhalt JP, *et al*.: Prevention of infection in critically ill patients by selective decontamination of the digestive tract. *Ann Intern Med* 1992, 117:545–553.

deBoisblanc BP, Castro M, Everret B, *et al*.: Effect of air-supported, continuous, postural oscillation on the risk of early ICU pneumonia in nontraumatic critical illness. *Chest* 1993, 103:1543–1547.

Fein AM, Feinsilver SH, Niederman MS: Atypical manifestations of pneumonia in the elderly. *Clin Chest Med* 1991, 12:319–336.

Niederman MS: Gram-negative colonization of the respiratory tract: pathogenesis and clinical consequences. *Semin Respir Infect* 1990, 5:173–184.

Selective Decontamination of the Digestive Tract Trialists' Collaborative Group: Meta-analysis of the randomized controlled trials of selective decontamination of the digestive tract. *Br Med J* 1993, 307:525–532.

Disorders of the Pulmonary Circulation

Lewis J. Rubin

> **Key Points**
> - There are many causes of pulmonary hypertension, and establishing the etiology is crucial for optimal management.
> - A methodic approach to diagnosis, using a carefully performed history and physical examination, and a series of noninvasive and invasive tests will usually lead to a definitive diagnosis.
> - Initial therapy should be directed at treating the underlying condition, when one exists.
> - Vasodilator therapy should be reserved for conditions in which significant pulmonary vasoconstriction is known to be present, and should be guided by hemodynamic evidence of responsiveness and tolerance.
> - The diagnosis of pulmonary embolism rests on the demonstration of thrombus in the lung, through noninvasive (lung scan) or invasive (angiogram) tests.
> - Most patients with acute pulmonary embolism can be treated with heparin; however, patients with massive pulmonary embolism may be treated with thrombolytic agents.

Unlike many other disorders affecting the cardiorespiratory system, disorders of the pulmonary circulation are often difficult to diagnose and are frequently even more challenging to treat. This difficulty is largely the result of the nonspecific nature of the signs and symptoms of patients with pulmonary vascular diseases, as well as the absence of uniquely sensitive or specific noninvasive diagnostic tests for many disorders of the lung circulation. Furthermore, our lack of understanding of the pathogenesis of many pulmonary vascular diseases and the incomplete elucidation of the physiologic mechanisms governing the maintenance of normal pulmonary vasomotor tone have, until recently, hampered the development of effective therapies. Pulmonary vascular disease is a major determinant of mortality in patients with chronic respiratory disease, and pulmonary thromboembolism causes approximately 150,000 deaths per year. Primary pulmonary hypertension, although rare, is a potentially fatal disorder that typically attacks individuals in the prime of life. This chapter provides an overview of disorders of the pulmonary circulation and outlines an approach to their diagnosis and treatment.

PULMONARY HYPERTENSION

The normal pulmonary circulation is a low-resistance circuit that is capable of both dilation of existing vessels and recruitment of unused vasculature to accommodate marked increases in blood flow without increasing perfusion pressure. Additionally, the lung circulation has the capacity to vasoconstrict in response to local disturbances in alveolar ventilation, primarily through hypoxic pulmonary vasoconstriction, to optimize gas exchange by matching regional ventilation to perfusion. Many disorders can cause elevations in pulmonary artery pressure,

Table 1. Classification of Pulmonary Hypertension by Etiology

I. **Diseases affecting the air passages of the lung and alveoli**
  A. Chronic obstructive lung disease
  B. Cystic fibrosis
  C. Infiltrative or granulomatous diseases
    1. Sarcoidosis
    2. Idiopathic pulmonary fibrosis
    3. Connective tissue diseases
    4. Radiation fibrosis
    5. Pneumoconiosis
  D. Upper airway obstruction
  E. Congenital developmental defects
  F. Adult respiratory distress syndrome

II. **Diseases affecting thoracic cage movement**
  A. Kyphoscoliosis
  B. Neuromuscular weakness
  C. Sleep apnea syndrome
  D. Idiopathic hypoventilation
  E. Pleural fibrosis

III. **Diseases directly affecting the pulmonary vasculature**
  A. Primary pulmonary hypertension
  B. Granulomatous pulmonary hypertension
  C. Toxin-induced pulmonary vascular disease
    1. Anorexic agents
    2. Intravenous drug use
    3. L-tryptophan
    4. Cocaine
  D. Sickle cell disease
  E. Thromboembolic disease
  F. Pulmonary vasculitis
  G. Pulmonary veno-occlusive disease
  H. Congenital heart disease
  I. Chronic portal hypertension
  J. Human immunodeficiency virus infection

IV. **Diseases affecting the pulmonary vasculature by extrinsic compression**
  A. Mediastinal tumors
  B. Aneurysms
  C. Granulomata
  D. Mediastinal fibrosis

V. **Left ventricular dysfunction and left atrial hypertension**

---

either by directly affecting the pulmonary vasculature or by indirectly altering the structure or function of the lung. The result of increased pulmonary artery pressure is an increased afterload to the normally thin-walled right ventricle. This condition leads to right ventricular hypertrophy and, ultimately, to right ventricular failure as the right ventricle loses its ability to maintain flow against increased upstream resistance. Although no uniform definition for pulmonary hypertension exists, it is generally considered to be present when the mean pulmonary artery pressure exceeds 25 mm Hg at rest or 35 mm Hg with exercise [1].

Diagnosis

Most patients with chronic pulmonary hypertension present with nonspecific symptoms that are indicative of the presence and extent of impaired right ventricular function. For example, dyspnea on exertion is the commonest presenting complaint and is usually the result of the inability of the right ventricle to increase cardiac output appropriately with activity. Chest pain, similar in quality and location to typical angina pectoris, is a more ominous sign, being indicative of right ventricular ischemia. Syncope, occurring most often with exertion or immediately after exertion, results when a major compromise to cardiac output occurs during activity. The presence of hepatomegaly, ascites, and pedal edema are indicative of right ventricular volume overload and failure. Less common presenting complaints include hoarseness, which results from compression of the recurrent laryngeal nerve by enlarged main pulmonary arteries; hemoptysis from rupture of atherosclerotic pulmonary vessels; arrhythmias; and seizures. Because all of these symptoms are nonspecific, it is not surprising that a correct diagnosis of pulmonary hypertension is often delayed for months or years after the onset of symptoms.

Differential Diagnosis

Once pulmonary vascular disease has been considered as the cause of a patient's symptoms, a methodic and comprehensive evaluation should be initiated, both to confirm the presence and severity of pulmonary vascular and right ventricular disease and to establish its cause. Pulmonary hypertension is not a disease *per se*, but rather a hemodynamic abnormality common to many conditions. Because the approach to therapy is dependent on the etiology, a diagnosis of pulmonary hypertension should establish its cause before a therapeutic course is begun. A classification of the causes of pulmonary hypertension is shown in Table 1. A diagnosis of primary pulmonary hypertension (PPH) requires the clinical exclusion of all other etiologies of pulmonary vascular disease.

Obtaining a careful history and performing a meticulous physical examination may provide important clues about the pathogenesis of pulmonary hypertension. For example, a history of daytime somnolence may suggest sleep-disordered breathing and pulmonary hypertension, resulting from frequent nocturnal episodes of hypoxemia and hypercapnia. A history of Raynaud's phenomenon is suggestive of a connective tissue disorder or PPH. A history of intravenous or inhaled drug use suggests pulmonary vascular disease caused by chronic granulomatous vasculitis, resulting from talc or other foreign materials that often contaminate illicit drugs; cocaine-induced pulmonary vasoconstriction; or HIV-associated pulmonary vascular disease. The use of anorexic agents has also been implicated in a potentially reversible form of pulmonary hypertension, presumably by promoting vasoconstriction through their amphetamine-related pharmacologic effects. A family history of pulmonary hypertension should raise the possibility of familial PPH or a hereditary prothrombotic state with chronic, recurrent thromboembolism.

Physical examination may disclose many important diagnostic and prognostic features: skin changes of systemic sclerosis or vasculitis would lead one to suspect a connective tissue disease as the cause. The auscultation of rales could be indicative of chronic interstitial lung disease, left ventricular failure, or other causes of left atrial pressure overload. Bruits audible over the chest, indicative of flow through partially occluded large pulmonary arteries, may occur in patients with chronic thrombotic pulmonary hypertension. Neck vein distention with prominent CV waves are commonly seen in many forms of pulmonary hypertension and are indicative of right atrial pressure overload and tricuspid regurgitation, respectively. Palpation of the precordium often discloses a right ventricular heave and, occasionally, a palpable pulmonic component to the second heart sound or a systolic thrill of tricuspid insufficiency. Patients with severe chronic obstructive lung disease may have a palpable right ventricular impulse in the subxiphoid region as a result of lung hyperinflation. Cardiac auscultation may disclose an accentuated pulmonic component to the second heart sound, a right-sided fourth heart sound and the holosystolic murmur of tricuspid insufficiency (both heard best at the parasternal region on inspiration), or the diastolic murmur of pulmonic insufficiency. Fixed splitting of the second heart sound suggests the presence of pulmonary hypertension resulting from an atrial septal defect with a right-to-left shunt (Eisenmenger syndrome). Ascites may suggest right ventricular failure, particularly if tender hepatomegaly and hepatojugular reflux are also present. Clubbing does not occur in PPH, and its presence is suggestive of Eisenmenger syndrome, chronic respiratory disease, or cirrhosis with portal-pulmonary hypertension. Peripheral cyanosis may be seen in hypoxemic lung disease or in any process in which cardiac output is markedly reduced and peripheral oxygen extraction is increased; central cyanosis generally implies the presence of a significant right-to-left shunt. Peripheral edema indicates the presence of right ventricular failure in patients with pulmonary hypertension.

The diagnostic approach subsequent to a physical examination should include tests to confirm the clinical suspicion and cause of pulmonary vascular disease. Liver function tests may disclose abnormalities suggestive of chronic cirrhosis or hepatic dysfunction due to passive congestion. An elevated hematocrit value may be an early clue to chronic hypoxemia due to chronic respiratory disease or an unsuspected right-to-left shunt. Serologic studies may suggest the presence of a connective tissue disease, particularly when the results are positive in high titers.

An electrocardiogram usually demonstrates evidence of right ventricular hypertrophy in patients with significant pulmonary hypertension (Fig. 1), including a QRS axis greater than 110°, a prominent R wave in the right precordial leads, and peaked P waves in the inferior and right precordial leads (P pulmonale). The presence of ST-segment depression in leads V_1 through V_3 is consistent with right ventricular strain and implies severe right ventricular pressure overload. The findings on the electrocardiogram are nonspecific, in that different etiologies for right ventricular overload cannot be differentiated. Nevertheless, it is a useful, inexpensive, and noninvasive screening tool in patients with suspected pulmonary vascular disease.

A chest radiograph can demonstrate evidence of right ventricular and proximal pulmonary vascular enlargement, as well as provide useful information about underlying parenchymal lung disease (Fig. 2). The presence of Kerley B lines with right ventricular enlargement is suggestive of either left ventricular disease or pulmonary veno-occlusive disease.

Pulmonary function testing may provide clues to the presence of unsuspected parenchymal lung disease; lung function test results are usually normal or demonstrate a mild restrictive defect in patients with PPH, whereas the presence and severity of pulmonary hypertension correlate with the severity of impairment in lung function in patients with parenchymal lung

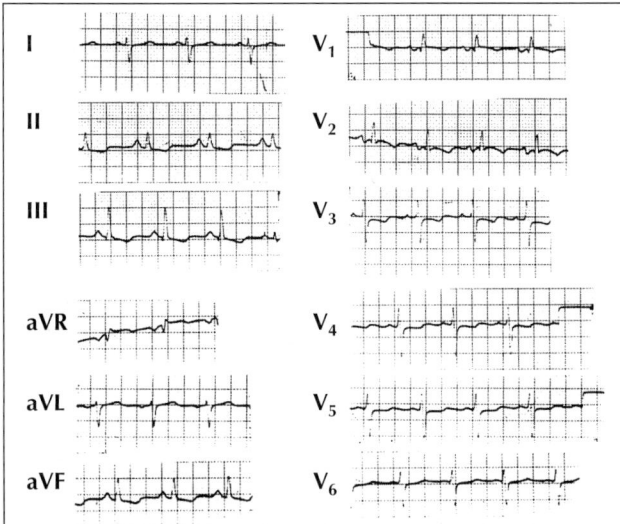

FIGURE 1 Electrocardiogram from a patient with primary pulmonary hypertension that demonstrates right axis deviation and right ventricular hypertrophy with a strain pattern.

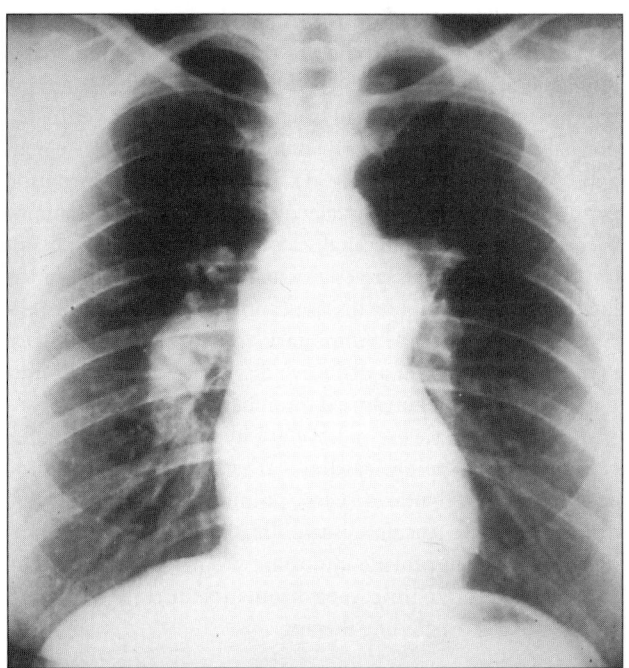

FIGURE 2 Chest radiograph from a patient with primary pulmonary hypertension that demonstrates enlarged main pulmonary arteries.

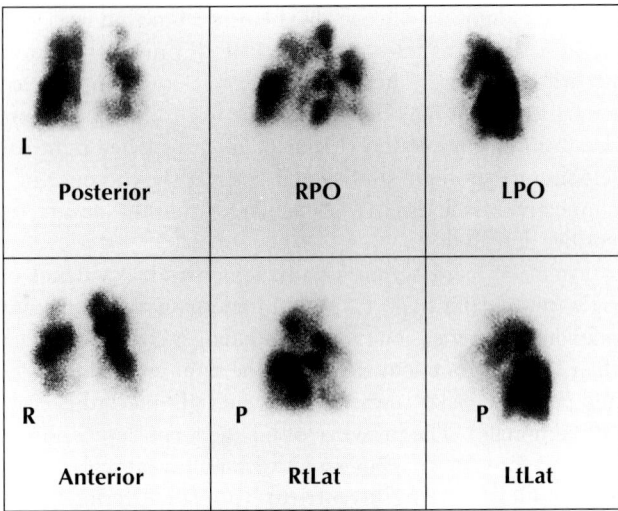

FIGURE 3 Perfusion lung scan from a patient with chronic thromboembolic pulmonary vascular disease that demonstrates multiple perfusion defects, which have a "moth-eaten" appearance. RPO—right posterior oblique; LPO—left posterior oblique; RtLat—right lateral; LtLat—left lateral.

disease. Arterial blood gas analysis with the patient breathing ambient air may be helpful in establishing a diagnosis and in indicating the need for supplemental oxygen as an initial component to therapy. Pulmonary hypertension is usually present in patients with parenchymal lung disease when the arterial partial pressure of oxygen decreases below 55 mm Hg.

Chronic thromboembolic pulmonary hypertension is a particularly important condition to consider in a patient presenting with signs of pulmonary vascular disease because specific and successful therapy is available. Accordingly, a ventilation-perfusion lung scan should be performed if unexplained pulmonary hypertension is present or if the hemodynamic abnormalities appear to be out of proportion to the severity of parenchymal lung disease. Patients with chronic thromboembolic disease typically manifest segmental or large areas that are ventilated normally but perfused poorly, if at all, giving a "moth-eaten" appearance on the scan (Fig. 3). In contrast, the ventilation perfusion scan in PPH is usually qualitatively normal. Scanning over the kidneys or brain can disclose the presence of a right to left shunt because tracer activity is normally seen only in the lung. If thromboembolic disease cannot be excluded from the results of a lung scan, pulmonary arteriography should be performed to establish a definitive diagnosis and to determine the site and extent of organized thrombus.

Patients with severe pulmonary hypertension should be referred for complete cardiac catheterization to exclude congenital or valvular disease, pulmonary veno-occlusive disease, or left ventricular disease. In addition, baseline hemodynamic data can provide important prognostic information. Finally, hemodynamic measurements during a trial of vasodilators aid in guiding therapy.

Therapy

An algorithm for the treatment of pulmonary hypertension is presented in Figure 4. Initial therapy for pulmonary hypertension should be directed at treating the underlying condition, when one exists. For example, patients with chronic obstructive pulmonary disease and pulmonary hypertension often experience considerable improvement from treatments aimed at improving airflow and gas exchange, such as bronchodilators, mucolytics, and corticosteroids. Supplemental oxygen therapy improves survival in patients with hypoxemic obstructive lung disease [2] and often reduces the severity of pulmonary hypertension in other lung diseases associated with hypoxemia. Supplemental oxygen is recommended for patients with an arterial PO_2 of less than 55 mm Hg at rest or with activity, or less than 59 mm Hg if P pulmonale, a hematocrit value of greater than 55%, or edema, are present. Patients should be encouraged to use supplemental oxygen for at least 18 hours a day, because even brief periods of hypoxemia may provide a sufficient stimulus for hypoxic pulmonary vasoconstriction and chronic vascular remodeling to persist.

Thromboendarterectomy should be considered for patients with chronic thrombotic pulmonary hypertension, because this procedure results in marked improvement in hemodynamics when the clot is surgically approachable [3]. Interruption of the inferior vena cava using a transvenous filter is also advised for such patients, regardless of whether their pulmonary vascular disease can be treated surgically.

Patients with severe pulmonary hypertension are at risk for pulmonary thromboembolism, even when this is not the cause of their vascular disease. Because the hypertensive pulmonary vascular bed has little capability to adapt to the stress of even a small degree of additional vascular occlusion produced by clot, an acute embolism can be a life-threatening event in this setting. Thus, patients with either PPH or chronic thromboembolic pulmonary hypertension should receive long-term oral anticoagulant therapy; in doses adjusted to achieve a moderate prolongation of the prothrombin time (approximately 1.3 to 1.5 times that of control). Patients with other forms of pulmonary hypertension may also benefit from anticoagulant therapy; however, no data are available on these other conditions. Accordingly, the risks and benefits should be weighed when anticoagulant therapy is considered, particularly in patients with secondary forms of pulmonary hypertension.

The rationale for vasodilator therapy for pulmonary hypertension is based on the premise that pulmonary vasoconstriction may be an early and potentially reversible component in some conditions. This rationale is supported by the pathologic demonstration of medial hypertrophy, suggestive of the presence of a vasoconstrictive stimulus, in some patients with PPH and secondary forms of pulmonary hypertension. Many systemic vasodilators (notably the calcium channel blocking agents) have been shown to produce significant and sustained improvement in pulmonary hemodynamics and regression of right ventricular hypertrophy in some patients [4]; however, not all patients with pulmonary hypertension should be considered candidates for vasodilator therapy, and serious adverse effects can occur in unresponsive patients. Centers with expertise in vasodilator testing and management are usually the best places for patients to be evaluated for this form of therapy.

The most widely used vasodilators to treat pulmonary hypertension are the calcium channel blockers nifedipine and diltiazem, both of which are commercially available in sustained-release forms. The optimal dose varies, although doses higher than those generally used to treat systemic hypertension or angina pectoris are apparently required in pulmonary hypertension. Side effects include systemic hypotension, worsening hypoxemia, and worsening right ventricular failure. These effects are the result of the negative inotropic properties of the calcium channel blockers. Peripheral edema may occur either from the latter properties or from the salt- and water-retaining properties of these drugs.

Diuretics are useful in the management of right ventricular failure, although they should be used cautiously because excessive diuresis can reduce right ventricular preload and output. Furosemide, 40 to 120 mg/d, is often sufficient to maintain a compensated state. When signs of right ventricular failure persist after increasing doses of furosemide, more potent agents, such as metolazone or bumetanide, can be added. Serum electrolyte levels must be monitored in patients taking these potent diuretics because potassium or magnesium supplementation may be necessary. Cardiac glycosides have no role in the treatment of pulmonary hypertensive disorders unless coexistent left ventricular failure is present.

Patients with pulmonary hypertension that is refractory to the approaches outlined earlier may be referred for more aggressive therapy, including continuous-infusion prostacyclin or transplantation. Prostacyclin, which is still under investigation at the time of this writing, is a potent, short-acting vasodilator that has been infused continuously by use of a portable infusion pump connected to a long-term intravenous catheter in patients with severe PPH [5•]. Although some patients have improved sufficiently with continuous prostacyclin therapy to justify long-term treatment, at present, it is most widely used as a bridge to transplantation.

Lung transplantation is the surgical treatment of choice for surgical management of nonthrombotic pulmonary hypertension that is refractory to medical therapy. Marked hemodynamic improvement has been demonstrated in patients with severe pulmonary hypertension who underwent single lung transplantation [6•], demonstrating the remarkable capacity of the right ventricle to recover when it is presented with a low-resistance downstream circuit for its outflow, even when overt right ventricular failure was present preoperatively. Unfortunately, the limited supply of donor organs has limited the utility of lung transplantation. Additionally, patients who undergo transplantation are at risk for rejection and opportunistic infections. The 3-year survival of patients undergoing

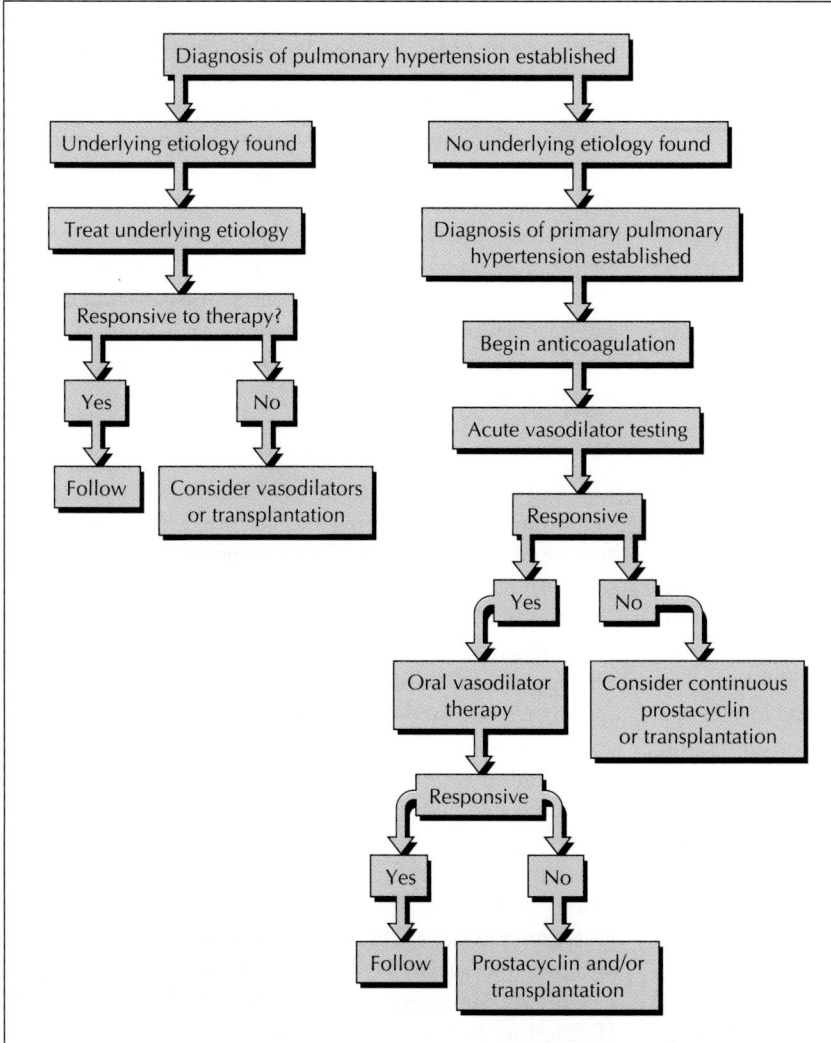

FIGURE 4 Algorithm for the management of pulmonary hypertension.

lung transplantation is currently approximately 65% to 75%. Patients with pulmonary hypertension with complex congenital heart defects that cannot be surgically corrected usually require combined heart-lung transplantation.

Prognosis and Natural History

Whether it occurs as a primary or secondary process, pulmonary hypertension is a serious condition, not only robbing those affected of their strength and physical stamina but also shortening their lives. Patients with pulmonary hypertension complicating chronic respiratory disease have a poorer prognosis than those with comparable ventilatory impairments who do not have concomitant pulmonary vascular disease [7]. Not surprisingly, those with the most severe pulmonary hypertension have the shortest survival. In PPH, the degree of pulmonary artery pressure elevation and the state of right ventricle function, assessed by measurements of right atrial pressure and cardiac index, predict survival [8•]. These data are useful in determining whether individual patients may be candidates for invasive therapies (*see* Fig. 4).

In contrast to pulmonary hypertension secondary to parenchymal lung disease, the natural history of PPH and pulmonary vascular disease occurring in patients with connective tissue disease is variable but can be rapidly progressive. There do not appear to be any demographic or epidemiologic characteristics that predict a rapid, downhill course, although patients who present with signs of right ventricular failure or a markedly reduced cardiac output are most likely to fare poorly.

PULMONARY THROMBOEMBOLISM

Pulmonary thromboembolism is estimated to cause over 150,000 deaths per year in the United States, but its diagnosis is often elusive, and its management evokes confusion among many practitioners. Recent studies from both the United States and Canada have provided considerable useful information regarding the approach to diagnosis and management, and a consensus has recently been published that should facilitate a logical approach in most patients [9•].

More than 80% of pulmonary emboli arise from the venous system of the lower extremities. Other sources include the upper extremities; the jugular or subclavian veins, particularly when these structures have been inserted with indwelling catheters; and the right ventricle. Although most patients who experience a pulmonary thromboembolic event have risk factors for its development, pulmonary emboli can occur in patients are seen with no apparent predisposition. The major risk factors for the development of pulmonary thromboembolism include age, immobilization, recent surgery, pregnancy, or underlying cardiopulmonary disease. Less commonly, patients are seen with a prothrombotic state caused by a circulating "lupus anticoagulant," anticardiolipin antibodies, antithrombin III or protein C or S deficiencies, or Trousseau's syndrome (recurrent, migratory thrombophlebitis in the setting of malignancy).

Diagnosis

The commonest clinical manifestations of pulmonary embolism include dyspnea, pleuritic chest pain, and tachypnea, and more than 97% of patients present with one or more of these complaints [10]. Routine laboratory testing is often nondiagnostic in this setting: electrocardiography typically shows nonspecific ST-T wave changes and sinus tachycardia, and chest radiographic results may be normal or may show atelectasis, pulmonary infiltrates, or pleural effusions. Similarly, arterial blood gas analysis may demonstrate an increased alveolar-arterial oxygen gradient; however, this result is not specific for pulmonary thromboembolism. In addition, a normal arterial PO_2 does not exclude this diagnosis, because a PaO_2 of greater than 80 mm Hg is present in more than 15% to 25% of patients with pulmonary embolism without underlying cardiopulmonary disease. Thus, a high degree of clinical sensitivity followed by a meticulous evaluation is necessary in the management of a patient with suspected pulmonary embolism.

The ventilation-perfusion scan is the most useful noninvasive test to diagnose or exclude pulmonary embolism. A high-probability scan, defined as one or more segmental or lobar mismatched defects, is indicative of pulmonary embolism in over 85% of patients, whereas normal or near-normal results virtually exclude the diagnosis of pulmonary embolism [11]. Patients with intermediate or indeterminate scan results have pulmonary embolism demonstrated in 20% to 30% of subsequent diagnostic studies. Patients with underlying cardiopulmonary disease are likelier to have a nondiagnostic lung scan result because of the presence of pre-existent mismatching of ventilation and perfusion.

Pulmonary arteriography remains the gold standard for the diagnosis of pulmonary embolism, with a false-negative rate of less than 2% and a mortality rate of less than 0.5%. However, angiography may not be available to all physicians; noninvasive studies of the lower extremities, such as impedance plethysmography or B-mode imaging, are useful in patients with suspected pulmonary embolism, particularly when proximal deep venous thrombus is present. An algorithm for the diagnostic approach to suspected pulmonary embolism is shown in Figure 5.

Therapy

The treatment of uncomplicated pulmonary embolism is largely directed at preventing a recurrence, which may be fatal, by using the anticoagulants heparin and warfarin. Heparin is administered intravenously by continuous infusion in doses adjusted to achieve a prolongation of the activated partial thromboplastin time of approximately twice that of control. Therapy is usually continued for 7 to 10 days. Warfarin therapy can be initiated concomitantly because it often takes several days to achieve an adequate prolongation of the prothrombin time with oral warfarin. Most patients with uncomplicated pulmonary embolism should be treated with warfarin for 3 to 6 months, whereas patients with massive or recurrent pulmonary embolism should be treated for longer periods or for life. Careful monitoring of the degree of anticoagulation and the avoidance of drugs, which may interfere with the anticoagulant activity of these agents, is imperative.

Patients who experience a massive pulmonary embolism (defined as hemodynamic compromise or two or more

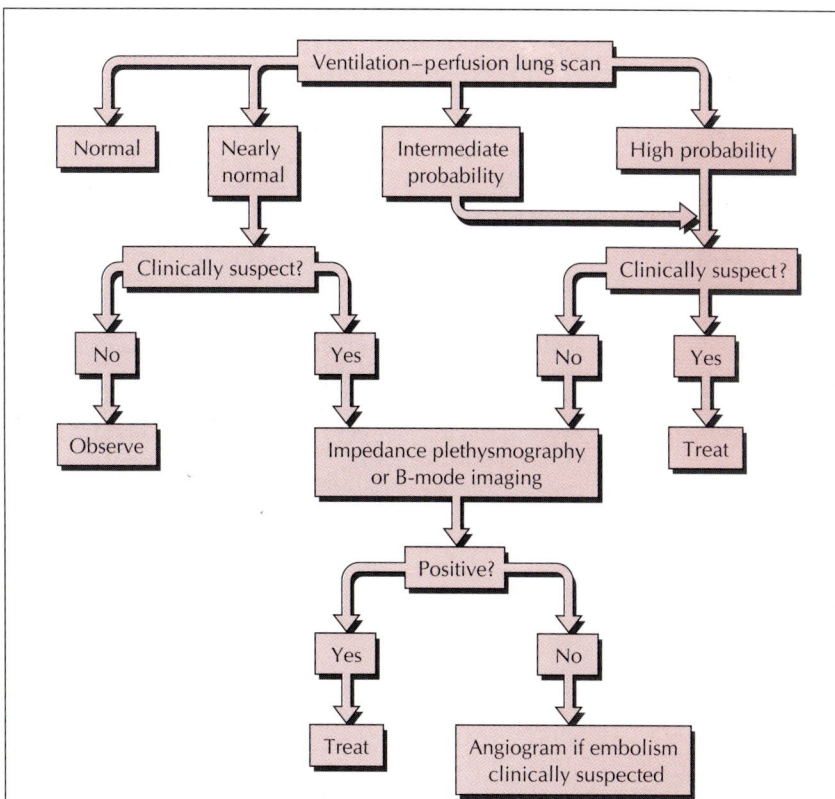

FIGURE 5 Algorithm for the diagnosis of pulmonary embolism. IPG—impedance plethysmograph.

obstructed lobar vessels or their equivalent) may benefit from intravenous thrombolytic therapy with streptokinase, urokinase, or recombinant tissue plasminogen activator [12]. The goal of therapy is to dissolve fresh clot by creating a systemic lytic state. Thrombolytic therapy with urokinase or streptokinase is generally continued for 12 to 72 hours, depending on the agent used and the extent of thrombosis, and is followed by a conventional course of heparin and warfarin. Patients who are receiving thrombolytic agents should be monitored carefully for signs of spontaneous hemorrhage, and invasive procedures or vascular punctures should be performed only when absolutely necessary because of the increased risk of bleeding. At present, no one thrombolytic agent exists that is clearly superior, and the choice of agent should be guided by the physician's experience and familiarity with the agent. Although streptokinase is less expensive, the incidence of allergic reactions, usually manifested by fever and hypotension, is more common with this agent. Tissue plasminogen activator is more expensive but has the advantage of exerting a thrombolytic effect after a brief (2-hour) infusion.

Patients with a pulmonary embolism who have an absolute contraindication to anticoagulation, a recurrence despite adequate anticoagulation, or a life-threatening complication of anticoagulation despite therapeutic prolongation of coagulation tests may be candidates for inferior vena cava interruption [13]. Numerous devices are in use for this indication, but filters that can be inserted percutaneously are the most widely employed. Filter patency is usually well preserved, and catheter migration is rare in the devices now available. Patients with chronic pulmonary hypertension due to pulmonary thromboembolism should have a filter inserted in addition to long-term therapy with anticoagulants. These patients should be referred to specialized centers for further treatment, including consideration for thromboendarterectomy.

In patients who are at increased risk for the development of pulmonary thromboembolism (individuals who are undergoing major surgery or those who are immobilized or confined to bed for prolonged periods of time), prophylactic measures can markedly reduce the risk of thromboembolic events. Heparin, in doses of 5000 U administered subcutaneously every 8 to 12 hours, reduces the incidence of deep venous thrombosis and thromboembolism and is associated with a low incidence of adverse effects. External pneumatic compression devices are a suitable alternative in patients who are not candidates for low-dose heparin therapy. These measures should be instituted before surgery so that the maximal benefit can be achieved. Early ambulation should also be encouraged.

REFERENCES AND RECOMMENDED READING

Recently published papers of particular interest have been highlighted as:
- Of interest
- Of outstanding interest

1. Rich S, Dantzker DR, Ayres SM, *et al.*: Primary pulmonary hypertension: a national prospective study. *Ann Intern Med* 1987, 107:216–223.
2. Nocturnal Oxygen Therapy Trial Group: Continuous or nocturnal oxygen therapy in hypoxemic chronic obstructive lung disease: a clinical trial. *Ann Intern Med* 1980, 93:391–398.

3. Moser KM, Daily PO, Peterson K, *et al.*: Thromboendarterectomy for chronic, major vessel thromboembolic pulmonary hypertension: immediate and long-term results in 42 patients. *Ann Intern Med* 1987, 107:560–565.

4. Rich S, Brundage BH: High dose calcium blocking therapy for primary pulmonary hypertension: evidence for long-term reduction in pulmonary arterial pressure and regression of right ventricular hypertrophy. *Circulation* 1987, 76:135–141.

5.• Rubin LJ, Mendoza J, Hood M, *et al.*: Treatment of primary pulmonary hypertension with continuous intravenous prostacyclin (epoprostenol). *Ann Intern Med* 1990, 112:485–491.

6.• Pasque MK, Trulock EP, Kaiser LR, *et al.*: Single-lung transplantation for pulmonary hypertension. *Circulation* 1991, 84:2275–2279.

7. Traver GA, Cline MG, Burrows B: Predictors of mortality in chronic obstructive pulmonary disease. *Am Rev Respir Dis* 1979, 119:895–902.

8.• D'Alonzo GE, Barst RJ, Ayres SM, *et al.*: Survival in patients with primary pulmonary hypertension: results from a national prospective registry. *Ann Intern Med* 1991, 115:343–349.

9.• Stein PD, Hull RD, Saltzman HA, *et al.*: Strategy for diagnosis of patients with suspected acute pulmonary embolism. *Chest* 1993, 103:1553–1559.

10. Stein PD, Terrin ML, Hales CA, *et al.*: Clinical, laboratory, roentgenographic and electrocardiographic findings in patients with acute pulmonary embolism and no preexisting cardiac or pulmonary disease. *Chest* 1991, 100:598–603.

11. Hull RD, Hirsh J, Carter CJ, *et al.*: Pulmonary angiography, ventilation lung scanning, and venography for clinically suspected pulmonary embolism with abnormal perfusion lung scan. *Ann Intern Med* 1983, 98:891–899.

12. Marder VJ, Sherry S: Thrombolytic therapy: current status: Parts 1 and 2. *N Engl J Med* 1988, 318:1512–1520; 1585–1595.

13. Goldhaber SZ, Buring JE, Lipnick RJ, *et al.*: Interruption of the inferior vena cava by clip or filter. *Am J Med* 1984, 76:512–517.

Interstitial Lung Disease

Om P. Sharma
Takateru Izumi

> **Key Points**
> - Dyspnea and dry cough are symptoms of interstitial lung disease.
> - Finger clubbing and end-inspiratory rales suggest idiopathic pulmonary fibrosis.
> - Evidence of multisystem involvement (*eg*, lungs, eyes, joints, skin, liver, spleen) suggest collagen vascular disease, sarcoidosis, or vasculitides.
> - Lung biopsy should be performed before the end-stage fibrosis masks identifying features.
> - High-resolution computed tomography supports the diagnosis and monitors disease activity.
> - Corticosteroids and cytotoxic agents are used as treatment initially; in severe, progressive disease, lung transplantation should be considered.

Interstitial lung disease comprises a number of clinical disorders that affect the alveolar walls and pulmonary interstitium. These disorders include bacterial, fungal, viral, protozoal, and parasitic infections; collagen vascular disorders (*eg*, systemic lupus erythematosus, rheumatoid arthritis, progressive systemic sclerosis, ankylosing spondylitis, mixed connective tissue disease); hypersensitivity lung disease or extrinsic allergic alveolitis; inorganic pneumoconioses; drug-induced and iatrogenic syndromes; and disorders of unknown origin (*eg*, sarcoidosis, idiopathic pulmonary fibrosis, eosinophilic granuloma and alveolar proteinosis, and bronchiolitis obliterans organizing pneumonitis [BOOP]). Many of these diseases are benign and self-limiting; others are chronic, progressive, and irreversible. The lung involvement may be one manifestation of a multisystem process, or it may be the only organ affected (Fig. 1). All interstitial lung diseases, however, have certain common clinical, radiologic, and physiologic features that should be recognized [1•,2–4].

CLINICAL FEATURES

Many patients with interstitial pulmonary disease are asymptomatic. Dyspnea is the most frequent symptom. At first, dyspnea appears only on exercise, then it progresses to breathlessness at rest. A dry cough, particularly on exertion, is frequently present. Fever, chills, and weight loss are the main symptoms in interstitial pulmonary infections. Dyspnea, associated with fever, and cough in an immunosuppressed host is often due to *Pneumocystis carinii* pneumonitis, cytomegalovirus infection, miliary tuberculosis, or fungal infection. Fever, chest tightness, cough, and dyspnea that occur 4 to 6 hours after exposure to an organic dust most likely indicate hypersensitivity pneumonitis. Severe dyspnea with significant weight loss but without fever occurs in lymphangitic carcinomatosis. Tachypnea is often present. Auscultation of the lungs may reveal localized or diffuse, end-inspiratory crackles or rales in patients with idiopathic pulmonary fibrosis, hypersensitivity pneumonitis, and asbestosis. Rhonchi or wheezing may be present in some patients with hypersensitivity pneumonitis. Clubbing of the fingers occurs and is common in patients with idiopathic pulmonary fibrosis and asbestosis (Fig. 2*A*). Erythema nodosum, uveitis, and parotid enlargement are important features of sarcoidosis (*see* Fig. 2*B*). Multiorgan involvement is a feature of sarcoidosis, collagen vascular diseases, histiocytosis X, and neurofibromatosis (Table 1).

History

A thorough occupational history is of paramount importance in revealing the diagnosis (Table 2). History of past or recent exposure to infection, inhalation of inorganic or mineral particles, occupational and nonoccupational (hobbies, drugs, pets) exposure to organic dust and antigens, irradiation, drugs, oxygen, or chronic aspiration should be discussed. Many interstitial lung diseases are common in smokers, including histiocytosis X, alveolar proteinosis, amiodarone toxicity, idiopathic pulmonary fibrosis, asbestosis, and calcified pleural plaques. In nonsmokers, sarcoidosis and hypersensitivity pneumonitis are common. The patient's country of origin and recent travel history may supply a critical clue. For example, a diffuse nodular–interstitial roentgenographic pattern suggests tropical eosinophilia in an Indian patient but suggests pulmonary schistosomiasis in an Egyptian patient.

Chest Roentgenographic Changes

The chest roentgenogram is abnormal in 90% to 95% of the patients with interstitial lung disease. It is often the first abnormality to be recognized. Although radiographic features may not provide the definitive diagnosis, certain roentgenographic patterns are highly suggestive of certain disorders

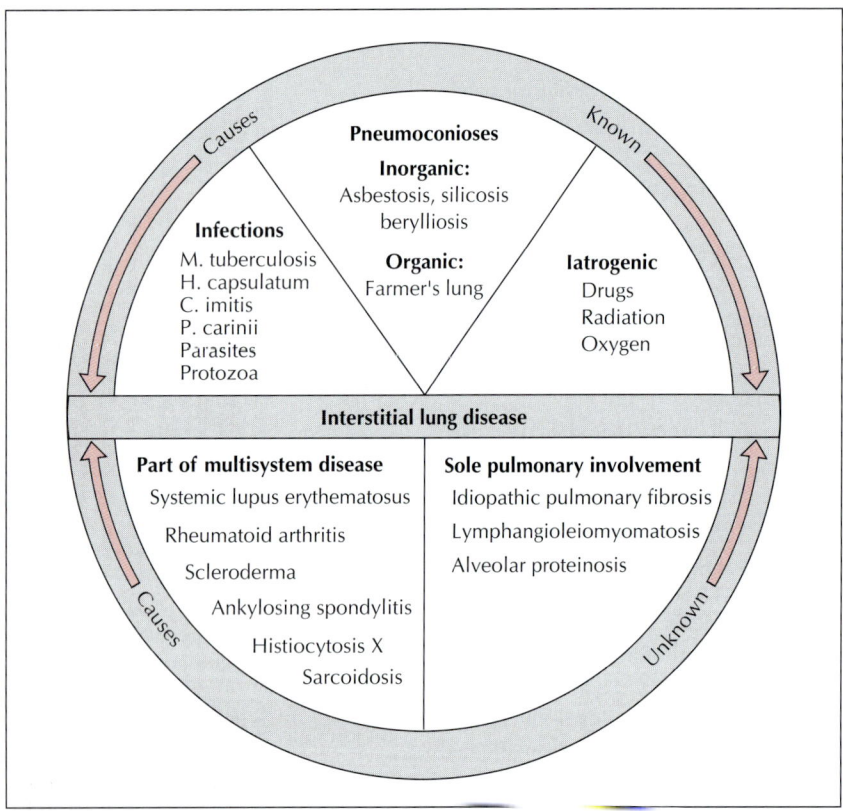

FIGURE 1 Causes of interstitial lung disease: a clinical classification.

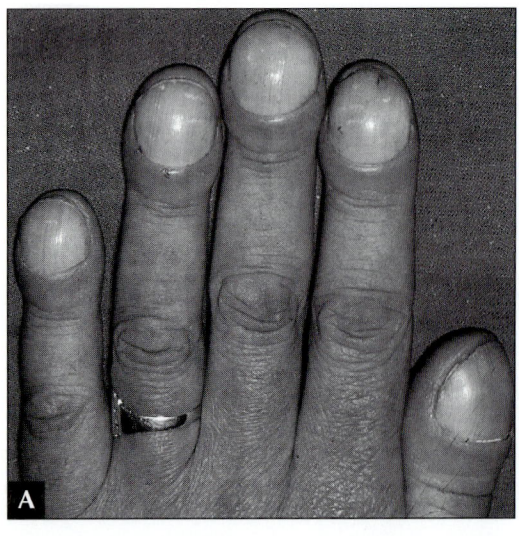

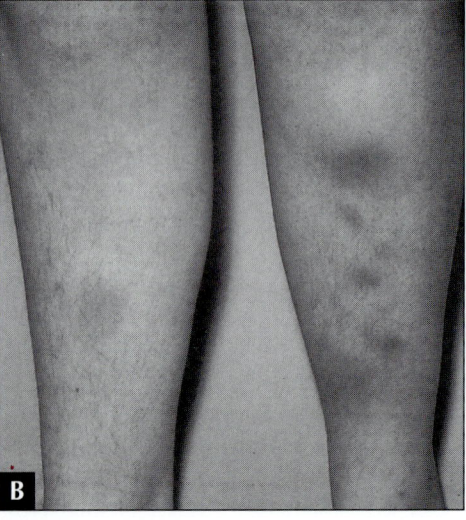

FIGURE 2 A, Finger clubbing occurs in approximately 60% of patients with idiopathic pulmonary fibrosis. **B**, Erythema nodosum consists of red, tender lumps on shins. When it occurs with bilateral hilar adenopathy, this syndrome is typical of acute sarcoidosis. (*See* Color Plate.)

TABLE 1 Differential diagnosis of diffuse interstitial lung disease

Disease	History	Clinical features	Laboratory test	Chest radiographic features	Lung histology
Sarcoidosis	Multisystem involvement	Dyspnea; red-eye, erythema nodosum	Hypercalcemia, Kveim test positive hyperglobulinemia, high SACE	Bilateral hilar adenopathy with or without pulmonary infiltrate	Noncaseating granuloma
Extrinsic allergic alveolitis	Exposure to an organic dust	Fever, cough, chest tightness	Precipitin antibodies in serum	Upper lung fields commonly affected	Cellular infiltration, granulomas
Rheumatoid disease	Arthritis, morning stiffness	Multisystem involvement, dyspnea	Rheumatoid factor positive	Diffuse lung involvement, pleural effusion	Necrobiotic nodules, vasculitis
Progressive systemic sclerosis	Raynaud's phenomenon, dysphagia	Progressive dyspnea		Lower lung fields	Fibrosis
Systemic lupus erythematosus	Multisystemic involvement	Dyspnea, cough, hemoptysis	Lupus erythematous cells and antinuclear antibodies	Bibasilar linear shadows, vanishing lungs	Vasculitis
Drug-induced lung disease	Relevant drug intake	Fever, chest tightness, dyspnea	Eosinophilia in some cases	Diffuse infiltration	Cellular infiltrate, granulomas, vasculitis
Pneumoconiosis	Exposure to dust (silica, asbestos, beryllium)	Dyspnea; may be asymptomatic	Not helpful	Upper lung fields commonly affected in silicosis, eggshell calcification; diffuse reticulonodular infiltrates in asbestosis, pleural calcification; diffuse interstitial infiltrate	Asbestos bodies; beryllium in tissue
Miliary tuberculosis	History of tuberculosis contact	Fever, weight loss, cough	Tuberculin test may be positive; sputum urine, and bone marrow cultures may show acid-fast bacilli	Miliary nodular infiltrate	Caseating granulomas, acid-fast bacilli present
Lymphangitic carcinoma	Smoking history	Dyspnea, fever, weight loss	Sputum, transbronchial lung biopsy	Diffuse interstitial infiltration	Carcinoma
Histiocytosis X	Smoking, dyspnea	None	Langerhans' cells in bronchoalveolar lavage	Honeycombing, pneumothorax	Histiocytosis X bodies
Idiopathic pulmonary fibrosis	Flu-like illness	Dyspnea, fingerclubbing, basilar rales	Lung biopsy	Diffuse interstitial infiltrate, honeycombing	Cellular infiltration, fibrosis

SACE—serum angiotensin-converting enzyme.

TABLE 2 Questions about occupational/environmental history

Where do you live?
How long have you lived in your present home?
Did respiratory symptoms appear after you moved into your new home?
Is there anything unusual about your home (air conditioner, water cooler, sauna, old shower curtain)?
What is the general environment of your home (urban, suburban, garden, type of trees)?
What are your hobbies (pets, painting, cooking, carpentry, photography)?
Is there any relationship between your symptoms and your work or home?
Are you better on weekends and vacations away from home?
Are you ill when you are at work?
Have others at work or at home had similar symptoms?

Table 3. Chest Roentgenographic Changes in Interstitial Lung Disease

Hilar adenopathy	Upper lobe involvement	Diffuse involvement and pneumothorax
Sarcoidosis (B,U)	Tuberculosis (typical and atypical)	Histiocytosis X
Lymphoma (B,U)	Histoplasmosis	Lymphangioleiomyomatosis
Pneumoconiosis (B)	Coccidioidomycosis	Neurofibromatosis
Bronchogenic carcinoma (B,U)	Allergic bronchopulmonary aspergillosis	Sarcoidosis
Tuberculosis (B,U)	Sarcoidosis	Idiopathic pulmonary fibrosis
Coccidioidomycosis (B,U)	Hypersensitivity pneumonitis	Marfan's syndrome
Histoplasmosis (B,U)	Histiocytosis X	
Phenytoin-induced disease (B)	Progressive massive fibrosis (sarcoidosis, coal worker's pneumoconiosis)	
Talc granulomatosis (B,U)	Ankylosing spondylitis	
Brucellosis (B)	*Pneumocystis carinii* pneumonitis	
Infectious mononucleosis (B)	Radiation pneumonitis	
Amyloidosis (B,U)	Marfan's syndrome	
	Cystic fibrosis	

B—bilateral; U—unilateral.

(Table 3). In general, roentgenographic shadows described as "ground glass haziness," linear, nodular, and reticulonodular are suggestive of active disease, whereas honeycombing represents the end-stage fibrosis (Fig. 3).

Laboratory and Immunologic Tests

Laboratory and immunologic tests help little in establishing the cause and nature of interstitial lung disease. Only tests that seem directly relevant to a clinical situation should be administered (Table 4).

Lung Function Tests

As a result of the inflammation and fibrosis of the alveolar walls and the vicinal structures, the lungs become stiff and have a greatly decreased lung compliance (Fig. 4). Lung volumes are reduced, the diffusing capacity is impaired, and the alveolar–arterial oxygen difference is widened. Large airway function generally remains normal, but small airway dysfunction is often present. In some interstitial diseases, particularly in hypersensitivity pneumonitis and sarcoidosis, airway obstruction may be prominent.

Disease Activity

Chest roentgenograms and lung function tests may indicate the extent of functional abnormalities. However, it is difficult to assess the activity of inflammation except by repeated lung biopsies. Three methods have been proposed to evaluate the intensity of inflammation: 1) bronchoalveolar lavage, 2) gallium scanning, and 3) conventional and high-resolution computed tomography (CT) scans. Indications for these tests are not clearly defined, and their value in day-to-day management of interstitial disease is uncertain [5,6•,7].

Histologic Diagnosis

In most cases, the lung biopsy should be performed early in the disease, particularly in the young and middle-aged patient, before end-stage fibrosis obliterates any identifying hallmarks. Biopsy tissue obtained transbronchially or by open thoracotomy is submitted for bacteriologic, fungal, immunologic, and electron microscopic studies.

Important Interstitial Diseases

In the differential diagnosis of interstitial pulmonary disorders, sarcoidosis, collagen vascular disorders, and idiopathic pulmonary fibrosis are the most common, causing about two thirds of all cases. Also to be considered are hypersensitivity pneumonitis, drug-induced pulmonary disease, pulmonary infiltration with eosinophilia (PIE) syndrome, histiocystosis X, pulmonary alveolar proteinosis, and pulmonary vasculitis.

Sarcoidosis

Sarcoidosis is a multisystem granulomatous disorder of unknown cause that most commonly affects young adults. Although the disease presents to clinicians of different disciplines (Fig. 5), the lungs are the most commonly affected organs. Approximately 20% to 50% of patients may have symptoms of dyspnea, cough, and chest discomfort. Irrita-

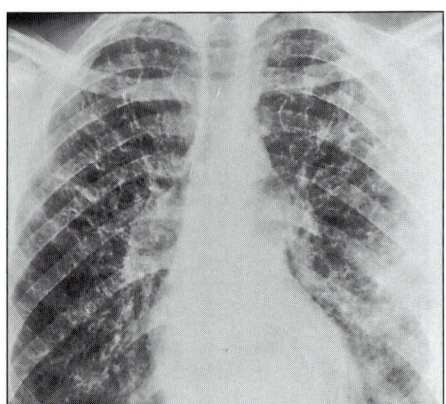

Figure 3 Postero-anterior chest roentgenogram showing honeycombing in a patient with advanced idiopathic interstitial fibrosis.

TABLE 4 COMMONLY USED LABORATORY AND IMMUNOLOGIC TESTS

Test	Finding	Disease
Complete blood count	Leukopenia	Sarcoidosis
		Brucellosis
		Tuberculosis
	Eosinophilia	Drug-induced disease
		Vasculitis
		Parasites
Sedimentation rate	Elevated	Collagen vascular diseases
		Lymphangitic carcinomatosis
Sputum and body fluids	Acid-fast fungi	Disseminated tuberculosis
		Histoplasmosis
		Coccidioidomyosis
Kveim-Siltzbach test	Positive	Sarcoidosis
Angiotensin-converting enzyme	Elevated	Sarcoidosis
Antineutrophil cytoplasmic antibody	Positive	Wegener's granulomatosis
Serum alkaline phosphatase	Elevated	Granulomatous diseases
Serum calcium	Elevated	Carcinomatosis
		Sarcoidosis
Serum lactic dehydrogenase	Elevated	*Pneumocystis carinii* pneumonia
		Alveolar proteinosis
Lymphocyte transformation	Positive	Berylliosis
Precipitin antibody (IgG)	Present	Hypersensitivity pneumonitis

tion, photophobia, and loss of usual acuity result from the acute uveitis. A form of sarcoidosis with ocular involvement, parotid enlargement, and cranial nerve palsy is called Heerfordt's syndrome. Occasionally, chronic skin lesions, polyuria, polydipsia, facial palsy, arthritis, heart block, and neurologic lesions are the presenting features.

There are four stages of intrathoracic changes:
- Bilateral hilar adenopathy (Fig. 6*A*)
- Bilateral hilar adenopathy accompanied by diffuse pulmonary infiltration (Fig. 6*B*)
- Interstitial infiltration or fibrosis without hilar adenopathy (Fig. 6*C*)
- Bullae, cysts, and emphysematous changes (Fig. 6*D*)

Once clinical suspicion is aroused, a biopsy of the affected organ should be performed for histologic confirmation. The basic histologic lesion in sarcoidosis is a discrete round granuloma made up of densely packed epithelioid cells, a few multinucleated giant cells, and a scanty layer of lymphocytes. A granulomatous response similar to that of sarcoidosis is found in many other conditions, and the clinician should correlate the clinical, laboratory, and histologic findings to arrive at the most likely diagnosis.

Corticosteroids are used if patients have dyspnea and abnormal pulmonary function. Other indications for therapy include ocular involvement, myocardial sarcoidosis, central nervous system disease, hypercalcemia, hypersplenism, and disfiguring skin lesions. Prednisone (20 to 40 mg/d) for 2 to 3 months, then a gradually reduced dosage to about 5 to 10 mg/d, is an effective regimen. Chloroquine, immunosuppressive drugs, and radiation have also been used with varying success [8].

Hypersensitivity Pneumonitis

Hypersensitivity pneumonitis, or extrinsic allergic alveolitis, is caused by repeated inhalation of organic dusts and protein particles of animal and plant origin (*see also* Chapter 4, Allergy & Immunology section). Farmer's lung is the most common type of hypersensitivity pneumonitis. There are three clinically distinct presentations (acute, subacute, and chronic), but only acute and chronic syndromes are discernible.

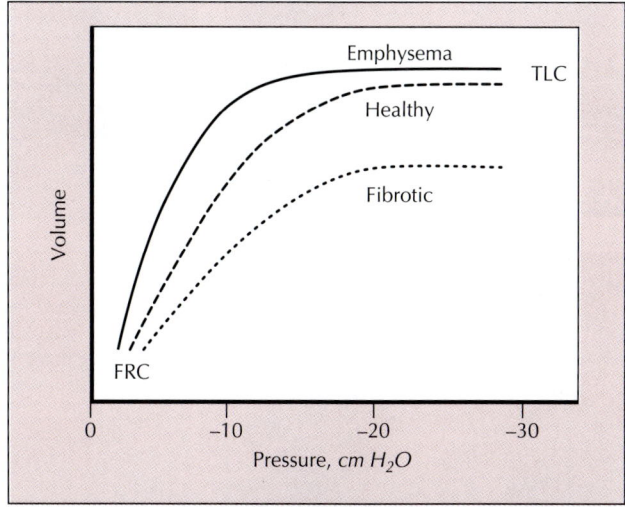

FIGURE 4 Lung function testing in fibrotic lung reflects lung stiffness. Lung compliance is reduced, unlike emphysema in which lung compliance is increased. TLC—total lung capacity; FRC—functional residual capacity.

FIGURE 5 Multisystem involvement in sarcoidosis.

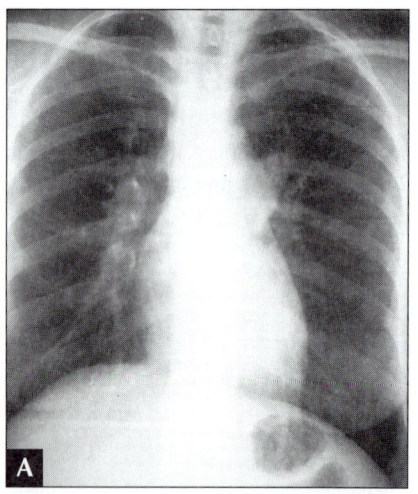
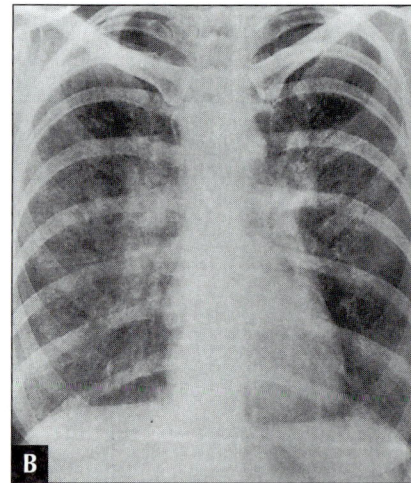
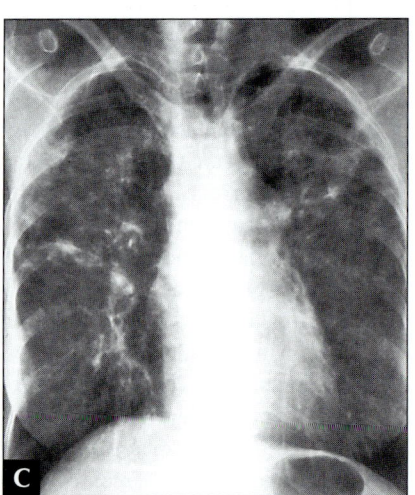
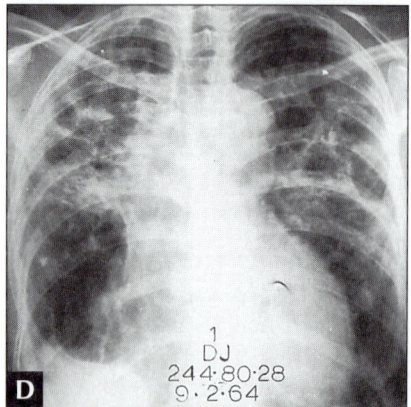

FIGURE 6 Sarcoidosis. **A**, Bilateral hilar adenopathy (stage I). **B**, Bilateral hilar adenopathy with early nodules interstitial disease (stage II). **C**, Interstitial infiltrate is increased (stage III). **D**, Marked progression of disease with loss of volume of the right upper lung field. The disease involves predominantly the upper lung fields (stage IV).

Table 5. Comparison of Sarcoidosis and Hypersensitivity Pneumonitis

Features	Sarcoidosis	Hypersensitivity pneumonitis
Age, y	20–50	Any
Symptoms	Asymptomatic; dyspnea, fever, weight loss	Fever, dyspnea, weight loss, chest tightness
Multisystem involvement	Eyes, skin, liver, spleen, peripheral lymph nodes	None
Chest radiograph	Bilateral hilar adenopathy with or without pulmonary infiltration	No adenopathy, widespread infiltration
Pleural involvement	Rare	Absent
Delayed hypersensitivity	Depressed	Normal
Precipitin antibodies (IgG)	Absent	Present
Serum angiotensin-converting enzyme	Elevated in two thirds of patients	Rarely elevated
Bronchoalveolar lavage	T-lymphocyte (helper) predominance	T-lymphocyte (suppressor) predominance
Kveim test	Positive	Negative
Inhalational challenge	Not applicable	Positive
Treatment	Corticosteroids, chloroquine, immunosuppressive drugs	Prevention, corticosteroids

Symptoms of acute hypersensitivity pneumonitis include cough, fever, chest tightness, and malaise. These symptoms appear 4 to 8 hours after the most recent exposure to the offending antigen. This symptom complex may be mistaken for an episode of viral or mycoplasma pneumonia. In the chronic stage, the patient complains of only progressive dyspnea with or without cough. Ultimately, chronic irreversible pulmonary fibrosis may lead to polycythemia and cor pulmonale. Chest x-ray films and skin tests are of limited help in the diagnosis. Precipitating (IgG) antibodies are present in as many as 90% of the patients.

The most important step in diagnosis is the recognition of environmental or occupational exposure (*see* Table 2). The best treatment is avoidance of the antigenic exposure. In severe cases, administration of corticosteroids for 2 to 4 weeks resolves clinical, functional, and radiologic findings. In chronic forms of the disease, corticosteroids may delay the onset of further damage caused by continuing fibrosis. Hypersensitivity pneumonitis should be differentiated from sarcoidosis because both diseases produce noncaseating pulmonary granulomas (Table 5) [9•].

Collagen Vascular Disorders

The connective tissue disorders constitute a heterogenous group of acquired disorders characterized by acute, chronic inflammation of synovial and serosal membranes, small blood vessels, and a high frequency of visceral involvement that includes the lungs, heart, and kidneys. Although lungs are frequently involved in all connective tissue disorders, including rheumatoid arthritis, systemic lupus erythematosus, scleroderma, polymyositis–dermatomyositis complex, ankylosing spondylitis, and mixed connective tissue disease, the incidence and pattern of the pulmonary disease vary significantly (Fig. 7). Rarely, lung involvement appears long before the other systemic manifestations of the disease. The lung changes lead to restrictive pulmonary impairment. Except for chest pain associated with pleural inflammation, the most common symptom of lung affliction is dyspnea, which occasionally may occur even when the chest x-ray and lung function tests are normal.

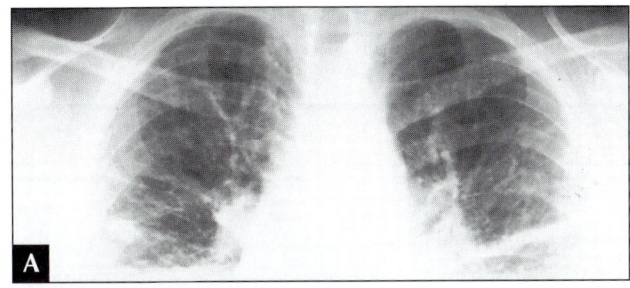
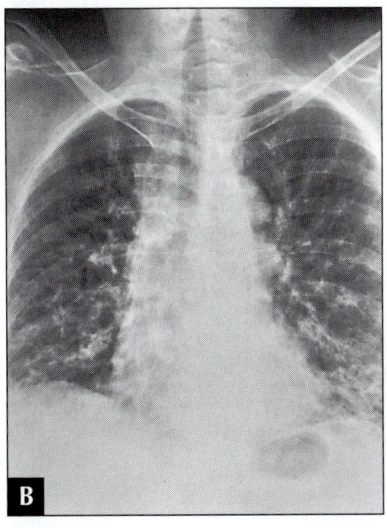

Figure 7 Collagen vascular disease. **A**, In lung involvement due to systemic lupus erythematosus, the chest roentgenogram shows small lungs with bilateral, linear basal atelectatic areas that are sometimes associated with small pleural effusions. **B**, In rheumatoid lung disease, diffuse interstitial involvement is prominent.

In general, treatment is successful in early stages of the disease when inflammation is cellular rather than fibrotic. Prednisone (1.0 mg/kg) is effective in treating systemic lupus erythematosus, dermatomyositis–polymyositis, and rheumatoid disease. Scleroderma lung disease is usually unresponsive to therapy. Cyclophosphamide, azathioprine, methotrexate, and penicillamine have also been tried when steroids fail [10].

Drug-Induced Pulmonary Disease

A high index of suspicion and a meticulous clinical history are required to recognize drug-induced lung disease, because the clinical, physiologic, and radiographic features are nonspecific and the patients taking the offending drugs and chemicals often have other complex illnesses (Table 6). Furthermore, the pathologic changes are not always pathognomonic. Nevertheless, the lung biopsy is almost always needed to exclude opportunistic infections and other interstitial disorders [11,12].

Pulmonary Infiltration with Eosinophilia Syndrome

Pulmonary infiltration with eosinophilia (PIE) syndrome is the association of pulmonary infiltrates and systemic eosinophilia. The patient usually has fever, cough, and chest roentgenographic abnormality. There are many causes of PIE syndrome (Table 7). Many of these disorders are benign and do not need treatment. Corticosteroids are often used to suppress symptoms [13].

Histiocytosis X

Histiocytosis X (Langerhans' cell granuloma; pulmonary eosinophilic granuloma) is characterized by an abnormal collection of histiocytes or Langerhans' cells in the lung. The disease primarily affects young and middle-aged smokers. Cough, dyspnea, and chest discomfort are common symptoms. Spontaneous pneumothorax occurs in approximately 25% to 30% of patients. A small number of patients have bone lesions and diabetes insipidus. If a chest roentgenogram shows interstitial disease with or without honeycombing involving the upper lung fields and pneumothorax, the most likely diagnosis in histiocytosis X (Fig. 8) [14].

Pulmonary Alveolar Proteinosis

Pulmonary alveolar proteinosis is an alveolar filling disease with little interstitial involvement. Adults in the third to sixth decades of life are most likely affected. Chest roentgenographs show bilateral alveolar space densities. Serum lactate dehydrogenase (LDH) levels are usually high. The alveolar–arterial oxygen difference is wide, indicating severe ventilation-perfusion abnormality and shunting (Fig. 9) [15].

Pulmonary Vasculitis and Alveolar Hemorrhage Syndrome

Pulmonary vasculitis is defined as necrotizing inflammation of vessel walls. Patients usually have complex multisystemic disease. The diagnosis is often based on characteristic histopathologic features. Wegener's granulomatosis, Churg-Strauss disease, polyarteritis nodosa, bronchocentric granulomatosis, and lymphomatoid granulomatosis are the important entities [16]. Many of these vasculitides have hemoptysis as the initial clinical manifestation [17•]. In patient's with diffuse interstitial disease and hemoptysis, Goodpasture's syndrome and idiopathic pulmonary hemosiderosis should be considered. Alveolar hemorrhage is rare in other collagen vascular disease [18].

TABLE 6 DRUGS AND AGENTS THAT CAUSE LUNG DISEASE

Antibiotics	Cardiac medications	Chemotherapeutic drugs
Nitrofurantoin	Amiodarone	Bleomycin
Sulfonamides	Procainamide	Busulfan
Penicillins	Tocainide	Mitomycin C
Cephalosporins	Propranolol	Nitrosourea carmustine
Isoniazid	Hydralazine	Methotrexate
Tetracycline	**Illicit drugs**	Cyclophosphamide
Hydrochlorothiazide	Heroin	Chlorambucil
Anti-inflammatory agents	Methadone	Melphalan
Aspirin	Propoxyphene	Vinblastine
Nonsteroidal anti-inflammatory agents	**Toxic gases**	Azathioprine
Penicillamine	O_2	**Miscellaneous agents**
Gold	SO_2	Radiation
Corticosteroids	NO_2	Talc
		Tryptophan
		Tocolytics
		Diphenylhydantoin
		Methysergide
		Lymphangiography dye

TABLE 7 DIFFERENTIAL DIAGNOSIS OF PULMONARY INFILTRATION WITH EOSINOPHILIA

Disease	History	Clinical features	Laboratory test	Chest radiographic features	Challenge test	Lung histology
Allergic bronchopulmonary aspergillosis	Atopic host with asthma	Fever, episodic wheezing, sputum plugs	Elevated serum IgE, precipitating antibody to Aspergillus, types I and III responses on skin tests	Transient infiltrates, central bronchiectasis	Immediate bronchospasm followed by a late reaction 4–6 hours later	Not applicable
Tropical eosinophilia	Native of India and Southeast Asia	Fever, night sweats, nocturnal wheezing, and cough	Filarial skin test positive; filarial complement-fixation test positive	Miliary infiltrate	Not applicable	Eosinophilic infiltrate with giant cells and granulomata
Tuberculosis	History of contact tuberculosis	Fever, cough, weight loss	Tuberculin test can be positive; sputum, urine, and bone marrow culture may show acid-fast bacilli	Cavity, soft infiltrate, hilar adenopathy, and miliary infiltrate	Not applicable	Caseating granulomata
Coccidioidomycosis	Recent travel or residence in endemic area	Asymptomatic but fever, chills, cough, and erythema nodosum may occur	Coccidioidin skin test positive, coccidioidin complement-fixation and precipitin tests positive	Hilar adenopathy, infiltration	Not applicable	Granulomatous lesion with necrosis
Histoplasmosis	Recent travel or residence in endemic area	Asymptomatic but fever, chills, cough, and erythema nodosum may occur	Histoplasmin skin test positive; complement-fixation test may be helpful	Hilar adenopathy, cavity, localized or diffuse infiltrate and calcification	Not applicable	Granulomatous lesion with necrosis
Brucellosis	Farm worker, drinking raw milk, working in slaughterhouse	Fever, weight loss, night sweats	Brucella skin test positive; complement-fixation antibodies; blood cultures positive	Nonspecific changes	Not applicable	Granulomatous lesion
Parasites	Endemic area	Fever, anemia	Stool examination may show ova	Nonspecific changes	Not applicable	Nonspecific cellular response
Drug induced pulmonary infiltration with eosinophilia	Nitrofurantoin, penicillin, methotrexate, dilantin	Fever, chest tightness, dyspnea	Eosinophilia		May produce Arthus reaction	Cellular infiltrate
Sarcoidosis	Occurs frequently in young black women	Dyspnea, fever, iritis, skin lesions	Hypercalcemia, hypergammaglobulinemia, positive Kveim test, high serum angiotensin-converting enzyme	Bilateral hilar adenopathy with or without infiltration	Not applicable	Noncaseating granuloma
Wegener's granulomatosis and polyarteritis	Respiratory infections and multisystemic involvement	Fever, malaise, weight loss, asthmatic episodes	Eosinophilia, raised sedimentation rate, hyperglobinemia, ANCA positive	Infiltrates, cavity formation, single or multiple nodules	Not applicable	Necrotic lesions surrounded by giant cells, lymphocytes, plasma cells, eosinophils
Histiocytosis X	Mostly children and young adults	Fever, malaise, bone pains, diabetes insipidus, cough	Occasional anemia	Nodular and diffuse lesions, honeycombing, pneumothorax	Not applicable	Aggregates of mature eosinophils and mononuclear cells, histiocytosis X bodies
Loffler's syndrome		Fever, dry-cough lasting less than a month	Nonspecific tests	Transient infiltrate	Not applicable	Eosinophilic infiltrate
Chronic eosinophilic pneumonia	Mostly adults	Fever, cough, night sweats, weight loss, persistent weakness	Nonspecific tests	Peripherally located infiltrate	Not applicable	Eosinophilic monocytic, and histiocytic infiltrate in alveoli and interstitial tissues

ANCA—antineutrophil cytoplasm antibodies.

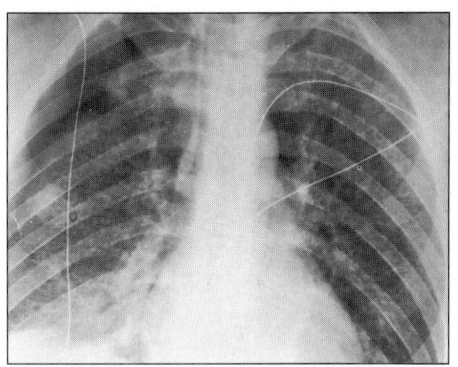

FIGURE 8 Chest radiograph showing diffuse honeycombing and pneumothorax in a patient with eosinophilic pneumonia.

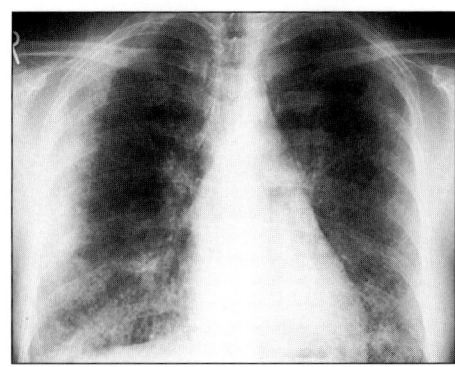

FIGURE 9 Pulmonary alveolar proteinosis, an alveolar filling process, produces ground glass, patchy opacities on a chest radiograph.

Idiopathic Pulmonary Fibrosis

The diagnosis of idiopathic pulmonary fibrosis (cryptogenic fibrosing alveolitis) is one of exclusion. Patients are usually in the fourth to sixth decade of life, men and women are equally affected, and there is no racial predisposition for the disease. The diagnosis is confirmed by lung biopsy. In early idiopathic pulmonary fibrosis, the alveolar spaces are filled with alveolar macrophages, and the alveolar walls are infiltrated by inflammatory cells, including plasma cells, lymphocytes, eosinophils, and neutrophils. This early stage leads to pulmonary fibrosis and honeycombing.

Corticosteroids are the primary form of therapy. Although cytotoxic agents have been effective in some patients who are resistant to steroids, well-controlled studies have not been performed. In selected instances, lung transplantation should be considered [1•,3].

REFERENCES AND RECOMMENDED READING

Recently published papers of particular interest have been highlighted as:
- Of interest

1.• DePaso WJ, Winterbaur RH: Interstitial lung disease. *Dis Mon* 1991, 37:63–133.
2. Crystal RG, Bitterman PB, Rennard ST, *et al.*: Interstitial lung diseases of unknown cause: disorders characterized by chronic inflammation of the lower respiratory tract. *N Engl J Med* 1984, 310:154–160.
3. Olson J, Colby T: Hamman-Rich syndrome visited. *Mayo Clin Proc* 1990, 65:1538–1548.
4. Epler GR, Colby TV, McLoud TC, *et al.*: Bronchiolitis obliterans organizing pneumonia. *N Engl J Med* 1985, 312:152–158.
5. Klech H, Pohl W: Use of bronchoalveolar lavage in sarcoidosis and other interstitial lung disorders. In *Sarcoidosis and Other Granulomatous Disorders. Lung Biology in Health and Disease*, vol 73. Edited by James DG. New York: Dekker; 1994:456–504.
6.• Muller NL, Miller RR: Computed tomography of chronic diffuse interstitial lung diseases. I, II. *Am Rev Respir Dis* 1990, 142:1206–1215, 1440–1448.
7. James DG, Rizzato G, Sharma OP: Bronchopulmonary lavage (BAL): a window of the lungs. *Sarcoidosis* 1992, 9:3–14.
8. Sharma OP: Sarcoidosis. *Dis Mon* 1990, 36:471–535.
9.• Sharma OP: Hypersensitivity pneumonitis. *Dis Mon* 1991, 37:411–471.
10. Wiedman HP, Matthay RA: Pulmonary manifestations of the collagen vascular disease. *Clin Chest Med* 1989, 10:677–722.
11. Kramer MS, Leventhal JM, Hulchison TA, *et al.*: Algorithm for the operational assessment of adverse drug reactions. *JAMA* 1979, 242–623.
12. Sharma OP, Kalkat G: Drug induced clinical syndromes mimicking sarcoidosis. *Sarcoidosis* 1991, 8:3–5.
13. Jederlinic PJ, Sicilian L, Gaensler EA: Chronic eosinophilic pneumonia: a report of 19 cases and a review of the literature. *Medicine* 1988, 67:154–162.
14. Hance AJ, Cadrenal J, Soler P, Basset F: Pulmonary and extrapulmonary Langerhan's granulomatosis. *Semin Respir Med* 1988, 9:349–368.
15. Prakash UBS, Barham SS, Carpenter HA, *et al.*: Pulmonary alveolar lipoproteinosis: experience with 34 cases and a review. *Mayo Clin Proc* 1987, 62:499–518.
16. Cordier JF, Valeyer D, Guillevin L, *et al.*: Pulmonary Wegener's granulomatosis: a clinical and imaging study of 77 cases. *Chest* 1990, 97:906–912.
17.• DeRemee R: Wegener's granulomatous. In *Sarcoidosis and Other Granulomatous Disorders. Lung Biology in Health and Disease*, vol 73. New York: Dekker; 1994:657–680.
18. Leatherman JW, Davies SF, Hoidal JR: Alveolar hemorrhage syndromes. Diffuse microvascular lung hemorrhage in immune and idiopathic disorders. *Medicine* 1984, 63:343–361.

SELECT BIBLIOGRAPHY

DePaso WJ, Winterbauer RH: Interstitial lung disease. *Dis Mon* 1991, 37:63–133.

Gauldie J, Jordana M, Cox G. Cytokines and pulmonary fibrosis. *Thorax* 1993, 48:931–935.

Lalancette M, Carrier G, Laviolette M, *et al.*: Farmer's lung long-term outcome and lack of predictive value of Bronchoalveolar lavage fibrosing factors. *Am Rev Respir Dis* 1993, 148:218–221.

Laurent GJ, Coker RK, McAnulty RJ. TGF-beta antibodies: a novel treatment for pulmonary fibrosis. *Thorax* 1993, 48:953–954.

Occupational and Environmental Lung Diseases

Guillermo A. do Pico

Keith C. Meyer

> ### *Key Points*
> - Occupational and environmental exposures continue to be a leading cause of lung disease and disability.
> - Pneumoconiosis—chronic, progressive, and mostly irreversible—should be included in the differential diagnosis of interstitial lung diseases.
> - Occupational asthma will not improve with pharmacologic therapy unless causative exposure ceases.
> - Toxic inhalations can be fatal; affected patients may require life-support measures, but the majority tend to recover almost completely.
> - Occupational lung diseases are preventable, and early recognition can lead to recovery without disability.

Occupational and environmental exposures continue to be a leading cause of lung disease and disability. The pulmonary effects of occupational and environmental exposures are summarized in Table 1. (Occupation-associated infectious diseases and cancers are discussed elsewhere in this book.) The pneumoconioses, caused by inorganic dusts, are chronic, progressive, and mostly irreversible and need to be included in the differential diagnosis of diffuse interstitial lung diseases. Occupational asthma is acute, recurrent, and completely or partially reversible with proper therapy. It is important to identify the occupational origin, because this asthma does not improve with pharmacologic therapy unless causative exposure ceases. Toxic inhalations can be fatal or require life-support measures. Recovery tends to be almost complete in the majority of cases, but in some cases there is residual disabling lung disease.

OCCUPATIONAL ASTHMA

Occupational asthma (OA) is characterized by variable airflow limitation or airway hyperresponsiveness caused by conditions that exist in a particular occupational environment [1••] (*see also* Bardana, Occupational Asthma, in the Allergy & Immunology volume). Occupational asthma is characterized clinically by cough, wheezing, chest tightness, and dyspnea, which develop during, immediately after, or several hours after work. The *allergic form* of OA manifests after a sensitization latency period of months to years and is associated with specific and nonspecific bronchial hyperreactivity. *Nonallergic irritant-induced* OA develops after a worksite exposure to an irritant gas, vapor, aerosol, mist, or fume with persistent nonspecific bronchial hyperreactivity (Fig. 1) [2•]. *Reactive airways dysfunction syndrome* (RADS) [3] is an abrupt onset of a recurrent and persistent asthma-like syndrome (cough, wheezing, dyspnea, airways obstruction) in a previously well person, occurring within 12 hours of an exposure to a high concentration of an irritant gas, fume, or vapor. After the initial episode, the patient continues to have symptoms of bronchial irritability in

Table 1 Occupational and Environmental Exposure Effects
Systemic
Asphyxia, *eg*, carbon monoxide, cyanide
Neurotoxic, *eg*, pesticides, hydrogen sulfide
Febrile syndrome, *eg*, organic dust, metal fumes
Granulomas, *eg*, Beryllium
Local
Airways
Bronchitis, acute or chronic
Asthma
Asthma-like disease
Bronchiolitis
Alveoli
Pneumoconiosis (inorganic dusts)
Fibrosis, *eg*, silicosis
Granulomas, *eg*, berylliosis
Deposits, *eg*, iron
Alveolitis
Allergic alveolitis, *eg*, farmers' lung
Toxic, *eg*, endotoxin
Chemical, *eg*, plastics
Edema
Chemical, *eg*, nitrogen oxides
Pleura
Asbestos-related disease
Fibrosis
Hyaline plaques
Effusion

response to many environmental stimuli (*eg*, cold air, smoke, traffic exhaust fumes, hairsprays, perfumes, bleaches, and so forth). Numerous occupations are associated with exposure to agents that induce OA [1••,2•,3,4••].

Diagnosis

The diagnosis of OA may not be readily apparent. The following clues may suggest the diagnosis:
- Adult onset asthma
- A latency period of months or years (onset can be dramatic in RADS)
- A close temporal relationship to workplace exposure with symptoms manifesting during work, soon after work, or several hours after work

Additionally, late asthmatic reactions manifested as nocturnal asthma are not often recognized by the worker or the physician as work related. Symptoms may become more severe during the week, but some cases are worse at the beginning of the work week.

Improvement usually occurs when off work. Initially, symptoms of cough and chest tightness improve overnight but gradually require longer off-work periods, weekends, vacations, or laid-off periods. Eventually, continuous symptoms aggravated by work exposures may appear. Because disease progresses if exposures continue, typical asthma attacks temporally related to work become less recognizable by the patient or the physician. The expected response to pharmacologic treatment of asthma may not occur if occupational exposure is not avoided or corrected. A small proportion of workers who are sensitized to a specific antigen develop asthma, whereas irritant-induced OA affects a larger proportion of workers. Many agents, such as toluene diisocyanate (TDI), can act as a sensitizer at very small doses in a few susceptible persons and cause severe chemical tracheobronchitis at high concentrations in all human subjects exposed to it.

Physical and radiologic examinations do not help differentiate OA from other forms of asthma. However, pulmonary function tests can support the diagnosis of OA if airflow obstruction (reduced forced expiratory volume in 1 second [FEV_1], FEV_1/forced vital capacity [FVC], forced expiratory flow [$FEF_{25\%-75\%}$]) and hyperinflation (increased residual volume/total lung capacity), which improves after cessation of exposure, are found. In some cases, asthma persists for years after employees have left their jobs. Provocation testing of airflow obstruction should be carried out if spirometry is normal at the time the patient is seen. Nonspecific airway hyperreactivity (AHR) in the asthmatic range caused by methacholine or histamine challenge supports the diagnosis. However, its absence does not exclude the diagnosis if the patient has not been exposed recently or is receiving treatment.

Other diagnostic approaches include at-work challenge by detecting changes in spirometry before and after a work-shift or a work-week exposure or by serial peak expiratory flow rate (PEFR) measurements. Serial PEFR measurements with a portable flow meter can provide valuable information if the physician is aware of its limitations. Measurements should be done frequently (every 2 hours), for 2 to 3 weeks at work and for at least 10 days while the patient is out of the workplace environment [1••,2•]. Such testing requires training of a reliable patient and visual interpretation by an experienced specialist (no arithmetic analysis exists). The sensitivity and specificity are approximately 70% to 80%. Serial quantitative measurements of nonspecific AHR by methacholine challenge may be a useful addition to serial PEFR. Work exposure simulation can be undertaken. However, such testing could affect technical staff, and a special facility is required for testing.

Specific-agent-inhalation challenge is considered by some the "gold standard" for diagnosis of OA [1••]. A negative test does not necessarily rule out the diagnosis but is evidence against it if the worker is still employed. It is debatable if specific challenges are always necessary; in actuality, these are seldom performed. There is no standardization for such testing, they are costly, and they can be dangerous. However, they may be valuable for 1) medicolegal purposes; 2) identification of the precise etiologic agent; 3) investigation of a previously unreported inducer; and 4) delineation of the types of the response (*eg*, early, late, or dual) [2•]. Special testing other than routine pulmonary function testing should be performed by an experienced specialist because of problems with selection of proper antigen, dosing, delivery systems, reproduction of complex interactions, loss of sensitization, antigen preparation, and the possibility of life-threatening reactions.

Blood or sputum eosinophilia, if present, suggests allergic asthma. Skin tests for assessment of immediate-type sensitivity to worksite antigens should be performed and interpreted by a specialist aware of the limitations and dangers. Antigen preparations are not standardized. Identification of specific antibodies by radioallergosorbent test (RAST) or enzyme-linked immunosorbent assay (ELISA), although sensitive, are not always reliable because of false-positive and false-negative results.

When to Refer

Patients should be referred to a specialist with experience in OA whenever feasible. In some instances, the primary physician can easily make the clinical diagnosis if the typical clinical and physiologic characteristics are present as described previously, particularly if the worker was exposed to a well-known causative agent. Simple use of serial peak flow measurements in a trustworthy patient over several weeks could be valuable. Unfortunately, many cases of OA are complex and its diagnosis requires additional experience. Patients should be referred to an asthma specialist (pulmonologist or allergist) if any of the following factors are involved:
- If cause is not clear
- If clinical features are not characteristic
- If the suspected agent is not a previously identified cause
- If no improvement occurs after discontinuing the suspected exposure
- If workers' compensation is involved (unless the primary physician is experienced in disability evaluation)

Prognosis

The prognosis is relatively variable. Many patients fail to recover after cessation of exposure (up to 60% to 90%). However, the disease tends to stabilize approximately 2 years after exposure ceases. The patient should be considered totally disabled to work where the offending agent may be present but not necessarily disabled for other types of employment. Work environment modification should be attempted if feasible.

Treatment

Pharmacologic therapy [4••] will fail unless the causative agent is removed from the working environment or the worker changes jobs. Personal protective devices may reduce irritant-induced asthma-like symptoms but should not be recommended to the highly sensitized person. If the patient will not or cannot avoid the exposure, the severity of the reactions can be reduced by personal protection or through the use of inhaled cromolyn or corticosteroids.

PNEUMOCONIOSIS

Chronic inhalation of high concentrations of inorganic dusts, usually in occupational settings, can cause a form of diffuse interstitial lung disease with structural alteration of lung parenchyma, which is referred to as a *pneumoconiosis*. Numerous occupations are potentially associated with the inhalation of significant amounts of inorganic dusts that can cause diffuse parenchymal lung disease (Table 2). Prolonged dust exposure and a latency period of 2 to 3 decades usually pass before the development of clinically evident disease (Fig. 2). In general, airborne particles ranging from 0.2 to 10.0 μm in diameter can be deposited in the lower respiratory tract, whereas larger particles tend to be deposited in the upper airway [5]. However, asbestos fibers that are thin (3 to 5 μm diameter) but up to 150 μm in length have aerodynamic qualities that allow deep penetration into the lower respiratory tract. The total dust burden and adequacy of clearance mechanisms are important determinants of disease, and usually 20 or more years of workplace exposure are required for a pneumoconiosis to appear [6•]. However, with substances such as beryllium compounds, relatively brief exposure periods may cause lung inflammation.

Fibrosis caused by inorganic dust exposure primarily involves alveolar walls of the lower respiratory tract. Asbestosis and silicosis are currently encountered less frequently than in the early and mid-20th century because of improved industrial hygiene with decreased exposure levels, but these disorders are still the most frequently encountered pneumoconioses. Asbestos inhalation can cause other forms of lung disease, which are encountered more frequently than asbestos-related pulmonary fibrosis [7•], including benign pleural effusion, pleural plaque, rounded atelectasis, and mesothelioma.

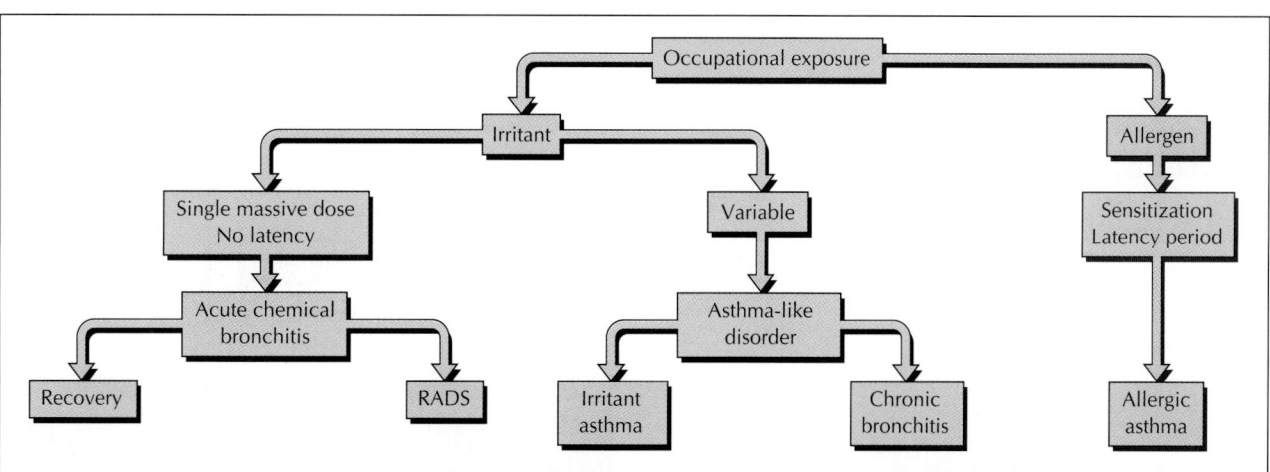

FIGURE 1 Occupational bronchial diseases development via an allergic or irritant mechanism. RADS—reactive airways dysfunction syndrome.

TABLE 2 OCCUPATIONAL EXPOSURE CAUSING PNEUMOCONIOSES	
Type of pneumoconiosis	Exposure settings
Asbestosis	Construction
	Insulators
	Sheet-metal workers
	Boilermakers
	Factory workers
	Textiles
	Friction products
	Shipyard workers
Silicosis	Underground mines
	Foundries
	Factories
	Pottery
	Enamel
	Bricks
	Sand-blasting
	Glass-making
Coal-workers' pneumoconiosis	Underground coal mines
	Drillers
	Continuous miner-operators
	Roof bolters
	Surface coal mines
	Drillers
Hard metal disease	Tungsten carbide production
	Manufacture
	Fabrication
	Finishing
Berylliosis	Beryllium production
	Processing
	Fabrication

Diagnosis

Several observations are of key importance in the diagnosis of pneumoconiosis. Because exposure to inorganic dusts may have occurred in the distant past and have ceased decades before overt lung disease becomes manifest, a detailed and complete occupational and environmental exposure history is of paramount importance in evaluating a patient with interstitial lung disease that may be linked to inorganic dust exposure. Patients usually present with progressive dyspnea, although radiographic changes may be detected in routine screening examinations of asymptomatic individuals. Adventitial sounds heard during chest auscultation or clubbing of the digits may or may not be present, depending on the type of pneumoconiosis [8]. Pulmonary function testing tends to reveal a restrictive ventilatory defect but can vary greatly; interpretation may be difficult if coexistent airways obstruction caused by tobacco smoking is present. Plain chest radiography may reveal nodular densities in the mid- to upper lung fields or reticular or reticulonodular patterns in the lower lung fields. The presence or absence of some manifestations of disease determined by physical examination, pulmonary function testing, or chest radiography may give important clues as to the presence and type of pneumoconiosis (Table 3). High-resolution computed chest tomography may be helpful in addition to other testing. It may be highly suggestive of a particular entity, and it may, for example, facilitate differentiation of asbestosis from idiopathic pulmonary fibrosis [9]. Although the diagnosis of pneumoconiosis can ultimately be made with a biopsy of lung tissue in most instances, lung biopsy is infrequently required to establish the diagnosis. The diagnosis of asbestosis, for example, can be made on the basis of clinical findings (Table 4) with a reasonable degree of reliability [10].

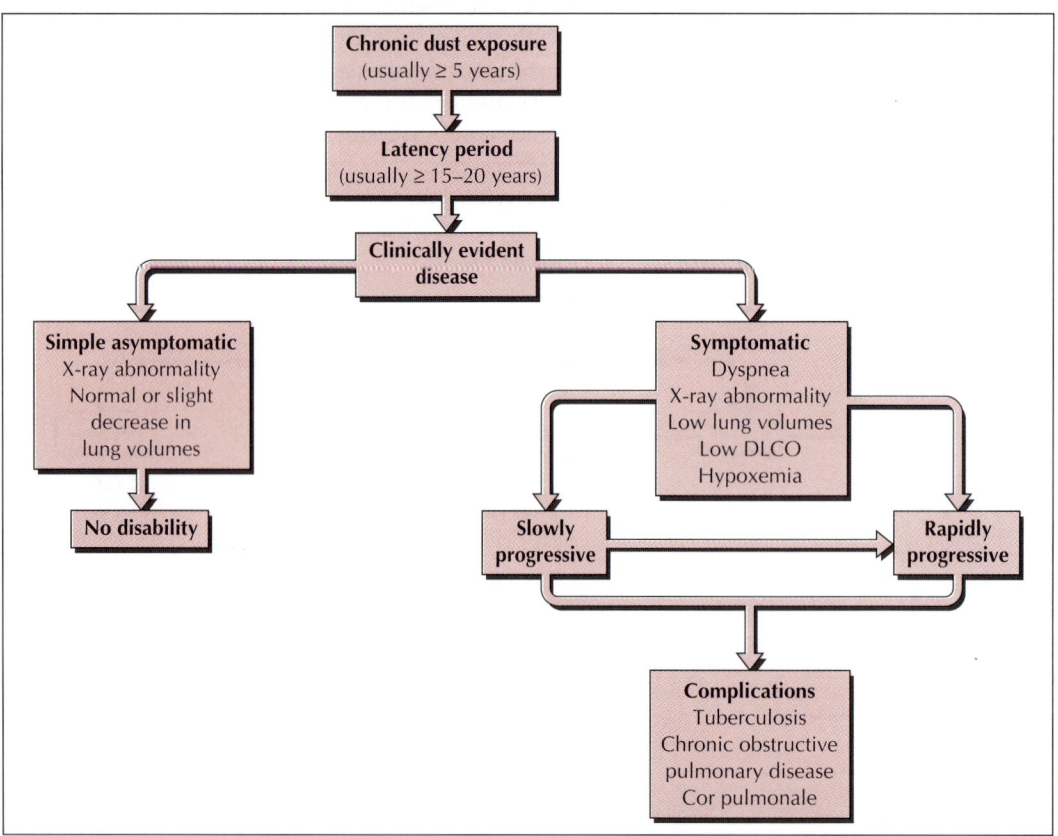

FIGURE 2
Disease progression due to inorganic dust-induced pulmonary interstitial fibrosis. DLCO—single-breath carbon dioxide diffusing capacity.

TABLE 3 DIFFERENTIAL DIAGNOSIS OF SELECTED PNEUMOCONIOSES			
Observation	Asbestosis	Silicosis	Berylliosis
History	Exposure	Exposure	Exposure
Physical examination	Rales Clubbing	No rales	No/few rales
Radiology			
Roentgenogram	Small irregular opacities Lower lung field Pleural plaques	Well-circumscribed nodules Upper lung field Massive fibrosis	Miliary pattern Upper or mid lung field Hilar adenopathy
Computed tomography	Subpleural lines Pleural plaques	Dense nodules	Ill-defined nodules Adenopathy
Pulmonary function	Restriction Late obstruction	Restriction	Restriction Late obstruction

Prognosis

Pulmonary impairment is progressive in many patients with pneumoconiosis, although lung function can be fairly stable in some, and the rate of deterioration varies considerably for a given disease entity. The disease may stabilize after cessation of exposure in coal workers' pneumoconiosis or chronic beryllium disease. Silicosis may be complicated by pulmonary tuberculosis, and simple silicosis may progress to massive fibrosis.

Treatment

Treatment with antiinflammatory or other agents has been generally unsuccessful in preventing progression of disease for patients with asbestosis or silicosis [6•]. Therefore, industrial hygiene measures with avoidance of exposure to dusts in the workplace or other settings and public education are of utmost importance to prevent the development of pneumoconioses. In certain instances, such as chronic beryllium disease, granulomatous pulmonary inflammation may stabilize or regress with cessation of exposure or immunosuppressive therapy. Patients with more severe disease with evidence of hypoxemia should receive supplemental oxygen therapy. Single lung transplantation is an option for selected patients with progressive disease and impending respiratory failure.

TABLE 4 CRITERIA FOR THE DIAGNOSIS OF ASBESTOSIS

Necessary findings
Reliable history of exposure
Appropriate time interval between exposure and identification of disease

Findings of additional value
Small irregular opacities on chest radiograph
Restrictive ventilatory impairment with forced vital capacity below lower limit of normal
Diffusing capacity for carbon monoxide below lower limit of normal
Bilateral late or pan inspiratory crackles at the posterior lung bases not cleared by cough

From Murphy and coworkers [10]; with permission.

INHALATION INJURY

Toxic gases, mists, fumes, and smoke are capable of inducing acute lung injury or systemic toxicity by acting as irritants, asphyxiants, or neurotoxins (Table 5). Pesticides, such as malathion, can cause respiratory failure and death through respiratory muscle paralysis via its anticholinesterase effect and hemorrhagic pulmonary edema via its irritant effect (Fig. 3). Massive toxic inhalations occur during fires and accidents or during the transportation or the repair of equip-

TABLE 5 CLASSIFICATION OF TOXIC INHALANTS

Irritants
Acrolein, aldehydes *eg*, burning plastics
Ammonia, *eg*, transportation accidents, leaks in fertilizer tanks, refrigeration
Chlorine, *eg*, transportation accidents, water sewage treatment
Hydrogen sulfide, *eg*, in septic tanks
Methylisocyanate, *eg*, pesticide production (Bhopal, India), plastic industries
Nitrogen oxides, *eg*, farm silos, explosives, ice-rink resurfacing
Phosgene, *eg*, fires, paint stripping
Sulfur dioxide, *eg*, paper mills, refrigeration

Asphyxiants
Simple: (interfere with oxygen delivery) *eg*, carbon monoxide, smoke in fires *eg*, methane, CO_2 in manure pits
Chemical: (interfere with cell respiration) *eg*, hydrogen cyanide from burning plastics *eg*, hydrogen sulfide, methane in manure pit

Neurotoxins
Insecticides: *eg*, Organophosphate (malathion)
Herbicides: *eg*, paraquat (also, lung fibrosis)
Fumigants: *eg*, methylbromide
Warfare gases: *eg*, anticholinesterase

Febrile syndrome inducers
Oxides of zinc fumes, *eg*, welding galvanized steel (metal fume fever)
Pyrolysis products of fluorocarbons (Teflon) (polymer fume fever)

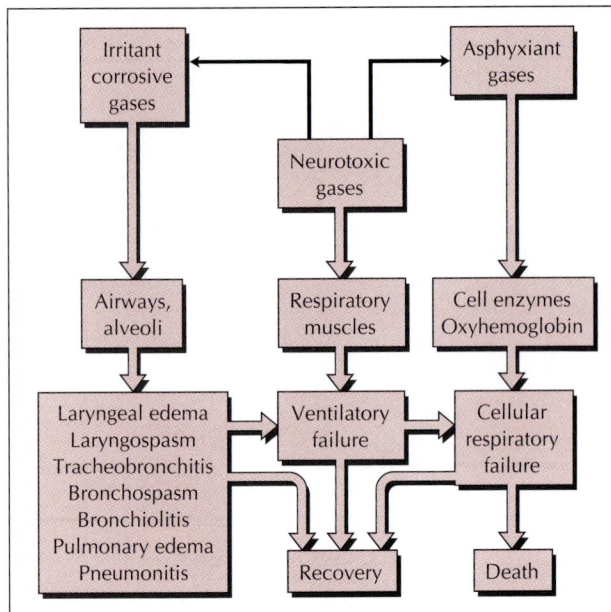

FIGURE 3 Effects of massive inhalation of toxic fumes. Some gases have asphyxiant and irritant effects, *eg*, nitrogen dioxide. Neurotoxic gases can also have irritant or asphyxiant effects, *eg*, hydrogen sulfide. (*From* do Pico [11••]; with permission.)

ment used in the storage, circulation, or processing of these chemicals. Firefighters, industrial workers using these toxic chemicals, and the general population present near the accidents are at risk for inhalation injury.

Clinical Manifestations and Course of Toxic Fume Inhalation

Irritant-corrosive gases

Massive irritant toxic fume exposure can cause inflammation and burns with edema, ulcerations, necrosis, hemorrhage in the airways, and hemorrhagic pulmonary edema (Table 6) [11••,12•]. Eyes and exposed skin are also commonly involved. After an acute massive toxic exposure the patient may die rapidly from asphyxia, have symptoms and signs of upper airway irritation, or develop pulmonary edema (Fig. 4). The physician should be aware that, as observed in near-drowning, pulmonary edema and acute respiratory distress syndrome (ARDS) may develop gradually over 24 to 72 hours after exposure and even after a deceptive period of initial improvement.

Airways obstruction and pulmonary infection are frequent after severe injury to airway epithelium due to impaired defense mechanisms, airway plugging by secretions and cellular debris, and bronchospasm. Currently, most patients are expected to survive and recover with little or no residual dysfunction. However, in some cases, long-term sequelae such as chronic bronchitis, airflow obstruction, bronchial hyperreactivity, asthma-like disease (*see* irritant occupational asthma and reactive airways disease syndrome), bronchiolitis obliterans, or residual psychophysiologic dyspnea without lung disease can occur.

Asphyxiants

Asphyxiants impair oxygen binding to hemoglobin (*eg*, carbon monoxide or nitrogen dioxide causing tissue hypoxia) or cause direct injury to cell enzymes (*eg*, hydrogen sulfide, hydrogen cyanide) [13•, 14, 15••, 16••]. Carbon monoxide poisoning is associated with fires, faulty indoor heaters, and internal combustion engines. There is no direct correlation between carboxyhemoglobin levels and severity of symptoms. At carboxyhemoglobin levels of greater than 20%, there may be severe headache, palpitations, tachypnea, tachycardia, weakness, impaired mentation, syncope, seizures, and coma [13•]. Smokers' baseline carboxyhemoglobin levels may be as high as 13%. Neurologic deterioration from ischemic brain injury can manifest 3 to 30 days

TABLE 6 EXAMPLES OF IRRITANT GASES

Gas	Water solubility	Predominant site of injury	Usual onset of symptoms	Comments
Acrylic aldehyde	Soluble	Airway—alveoli	Minutes	Very irritating
Ammonia	Soluble	Upper airway*	Immediate	Alkali burns, corneal burns
Chlorine	Slightly soluble	Airway—alveoli	Minutes to hours	Acid burns, strong oxidant
Hydrogen sulfide	Soluble	Airway—alveoli	Minutes to hours	Alkali irritation, central nervous system, asphyxiant
Methylisocyanate		Airway—alveoli	Minutes to hours	Highly reactive, methemoglobin, carboxyhemoglobin
Nickel carbonyl	Insoluble	Alveoli	Hours	Volatile liquid, cerebral edema
Nitrogen dioxide	Insoluble	Alveoli—bronchioles	Hours	Acid burns, delayed symptoms, mild irritation, strong oxidant
Ozone	Slightly soluble	Airway	Minutes to hours	Strong oxidant
Phosgene	Insoluble	Alveoli—bronchioles	Hours	Acid burns, delayed symptoms, mild irritation
Sulfur dioxide	Very soluble	Upper airway*	Immediate	Acid burns, corneal burns

*Alveolar injury as pulmonary edema or hemorrhagic alveolitis has been reported at very high concentrations, usually hours or days after exposure.

after apparent recovery from the exposure. The prognosis is worse in those who have had a period of unconsciousness, have prior cardiac disease, or are older than 60 years of age.

Thermal injury

In smoke inhalation the main causes of death and lung injury are toxic irritant gases and carbon monoxide poisoning [13•]. However, dry heat may damage the upper airways, and steam may damage the entire respiratory tract. In addition, combustion of synthetic materials may produce neurotoxins, such as cyanide and highly irritant acrolein. Soot particles, although perhaps not toxic themselves, may absorb acid toxins and impair lung defense.

Treatment of Toxic, Smoke, or Thermal Injury

The management approach to toxic, smoke, or thermal injury is summarized in Figures 5 and 6 [11••,12•, 13•, 14, 15••, 16••]. Deposits of injurious agents should be neutralized by removing clothing, showering under water, and irrigating acid and alkaline burns affecting the skin and eyes. If carbon monoxide exposure is suspected, 100% oxygen should be initiated by non-rebreather mask, and arterial blood gas levels, carboxyhemoglobin levels, and directly measured oxygen saturation (not calculated) should be obtained. The administration of oxygen, particularly if ambient atmospheric pressure is increased, can facilitate clearance of carbon monoxide by reducing the half-life of carboxyhemoglobin. The half-life elimination of carbon monoxide can be reduced from 5 hours to 90 minutes breathing 100% oxygen at 1 atm and to 25 minutes at 3 atm (hyperbaric). The efficacy of the specific therapy for cyanide poisoning has been questioned. Cyanide blood levels cannot be measured rapidly enough to be helpful (Fig. 6). Some patients do not require treatment but should be observed for 48 to 72 hours. Clear indications for hospitalization are severe respiratory distress, laryngospasm, severe hypoxemia, and pulmonary edema. Other less severe findings have less predictive value but suggestions are given in Figure 5.

The goal of therapy is to establish and maintain an adequate airway, ventilation, gas exchange, and hemodynamics when they are compromised. Fluid overload must be avoided and oxygen saturation should be maintained at above 90%. In severe cases of ARDS, mechanical ventilation is life saving and allows spontaneous healing and recovery. It has not been clearly established if other therapeutic modalities (eg, corticosteroids, prophylactic antibiotics) alter the course of the disease. If the patient is not intubated, close observation of the state of consciousness, voice quality, and secretion clearance should be continued, and laryngoscopy should be performed if necessary. If the patient is intubated, an endotracheal airway should be maintained until the face, neck, and upper airway edema are adequately resolved. If pulmonary edema or lower airways obstruction does not develop, extubation is feasible when the airway edema resolves; adequate oxygenation is maintained with less than 40% FIO_2 (forced inspiration of oxygen), and the patient is alert. If intubated, pulmonary toilet should be aggressively maintained with frequent suctioning,

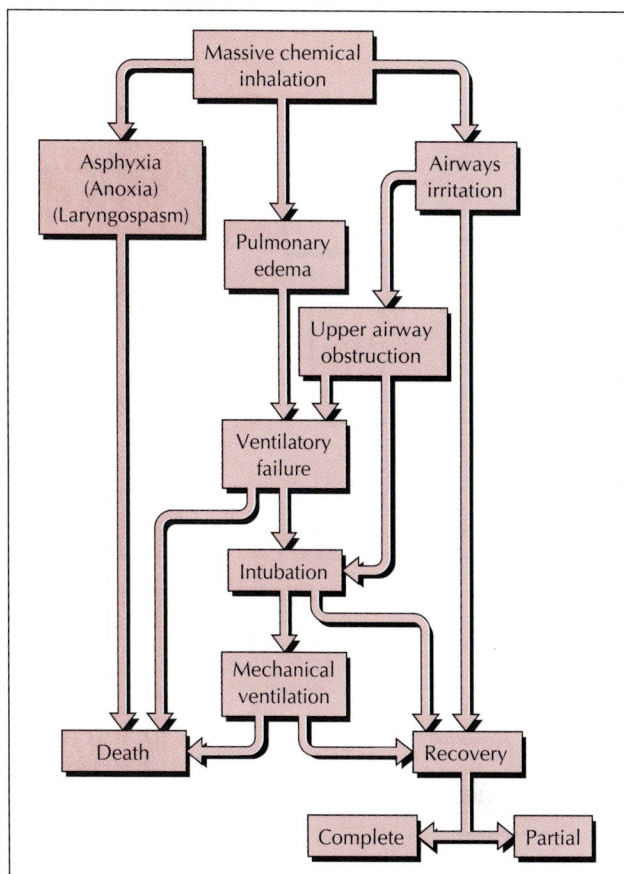

FIGURE 4 Potential clinical course after massive exposure to an irritant chemical. (*Modified from* do Pico [11••]; with permission.)

changes of position, and bronchodilatation. Patients must be observed for complications such as atelectasis or pneumonia and have frequent chest radiographs and sputum smears.

Endotracheal intubation is favored over tracheostomy if the airway must be secured or mechanical ventilatory assistance is required. Early intubation is recommended because, as edema increases, it becomes more difficult to cannulate the airway [11••,12•, 13•, 14, 15••, 16••]. Tracheostomy through burn tissue is not advisable because of the increased risk for infection, necrosis, and residual stenosis [16••]. Therapeutic bronchoscopy to remove debris and soot may be needed if there is severe airway obstruction or atelectasis that does not respond to other therapy. Antibiotics are indicated if there is evidence of infection but are not indicated for prophylaxis [11••,12•, 13•, 14, 15••, 16••].

The use of corticosteroid therapy is highly controversial and is not indicated in patients with large cutaneous burns and smoke inhalation. Increased mortality and infectious complications are associated with parenteral corticosteroid administration [11••,15••,16••]. However, corticosteroids may be helpful in very symptomatic persons after an exposure to nitrogen dioxide, sulfur dioxide, ammonia, or phosgene [11••,12•]. Corticosteroids are of questionable value but are widely used after inhalation injury by hydrochloride, ozone, or chlorine [11••], and they have no proven benefit in treating noncardiogenic pulmonary edema or ARDS.

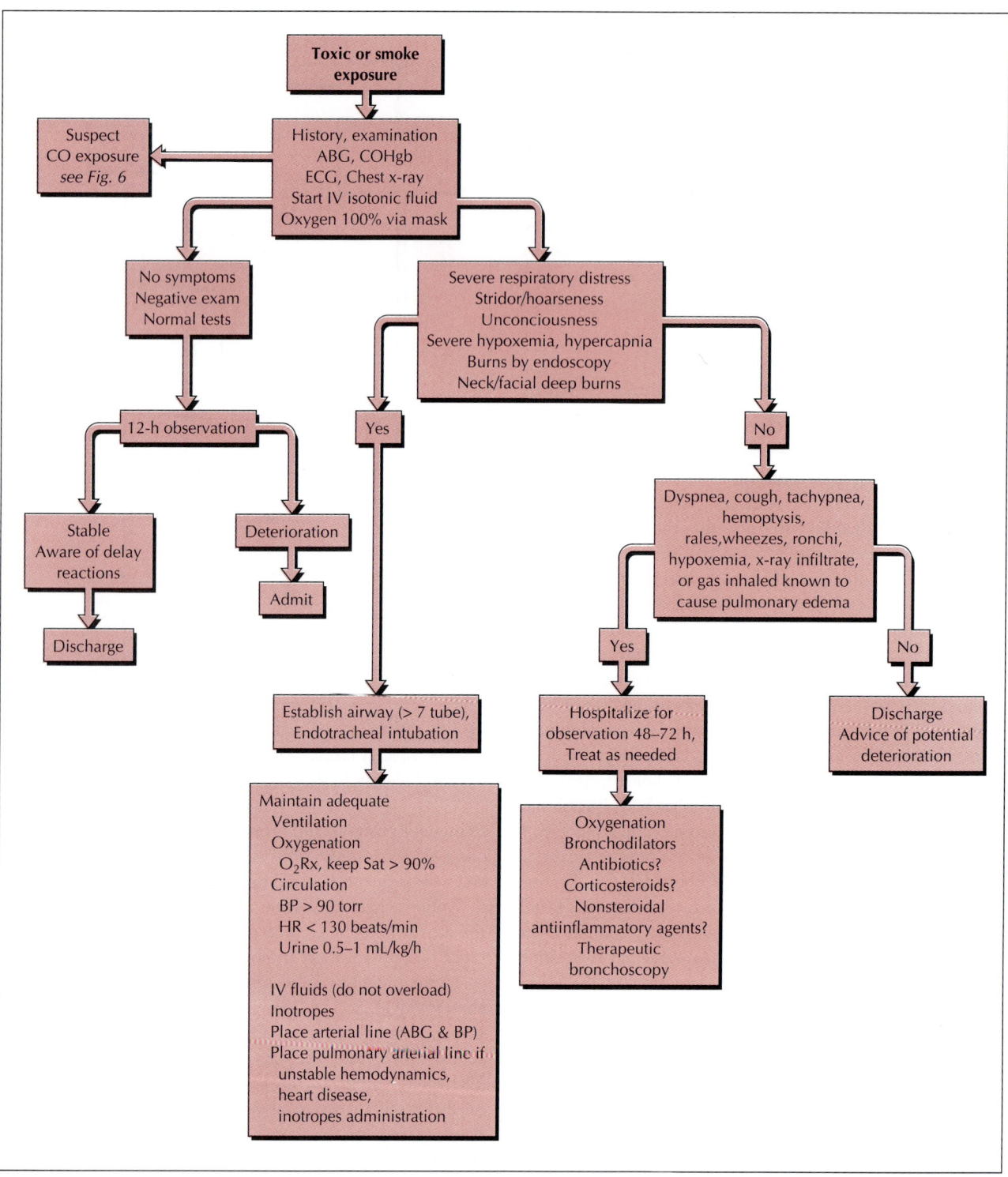

FIGURE 5 Management approach to toxic smoke or thermal exposure. CO—carbon monoxide; ABG—arterial blood gases; COHgb—carboxyhemoglobin; BP—blood pressure; ECG—electrocardiogram; HR—heart rate; IV—intravenous; O_2Rx—oxygen therapy.

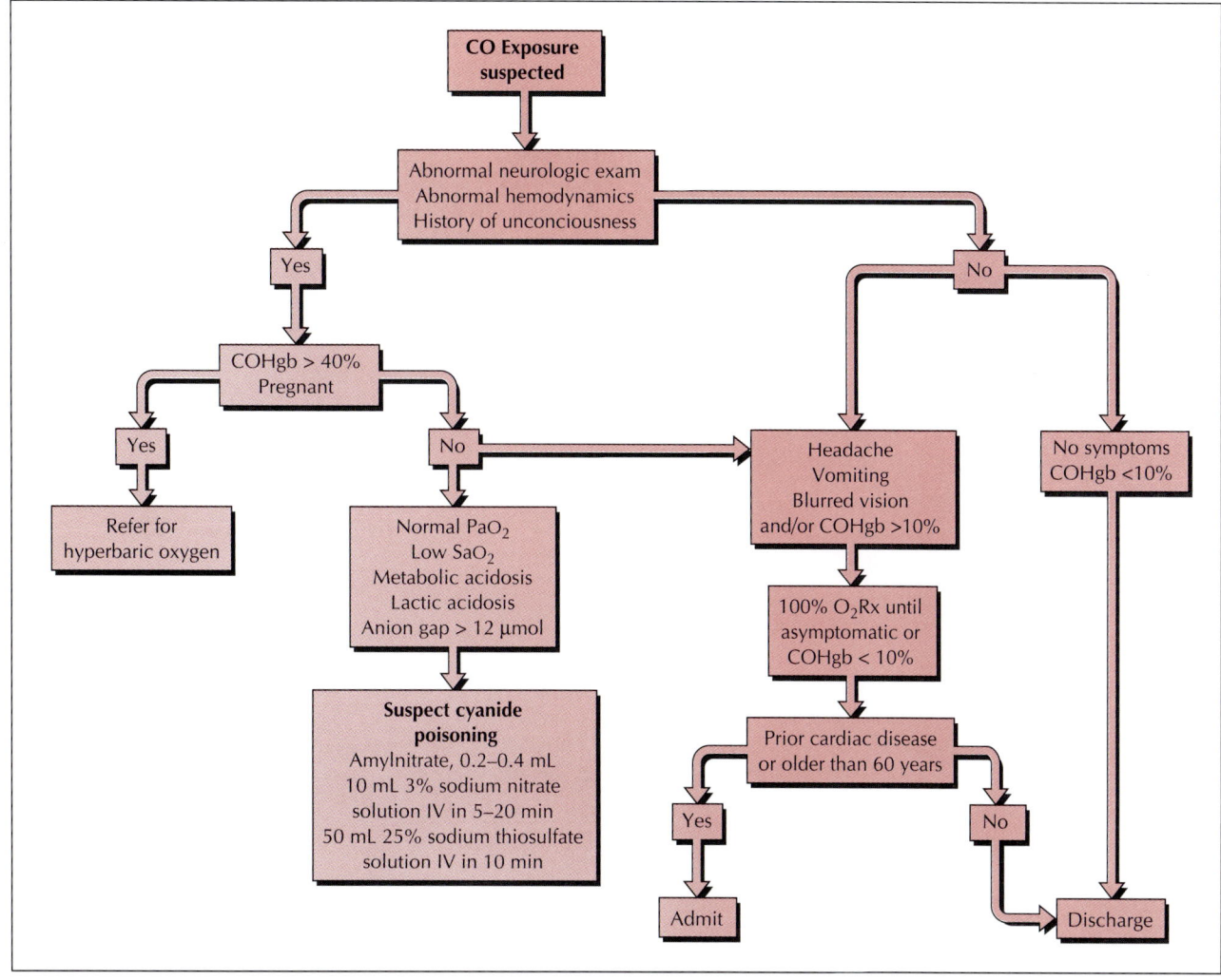

FIGURE 6 Management approach to suspected carbon monoxide poisoning from smoke inhalation. CO—carbon monoxide; COHgb—carboxyhemoglobin; PaO$_2$—arterial partial pressure of oxygen; SaO$_2$—arterial oxygen saturation; O$_2$Rx—oxygen therapy; IV—intravenous.

References and Recommended Reading

Recently published papers of particular interest are highlighted as:
- Of interest
- Of outstanding interest

1.•• Bernstein IL, Chan-Yeung M, Malo J, Bernstein DI: *Asthma in the Workplace.* New York: Marcel Dekker; 1993.
2.• Alberts WM, Brooks SM: Advances in occupational asthma. *Clin Chest Med* 1992, 13:281–302.
3. Brooks SM, Weiss MA, Bernstein IL: Reactive airways dysfunction syndrome (RADS). *Chest* 1985, 88:376–384.
4.•• International consensus report on diagnosis and treatment of asthma. Bethesda, MD: National Heart, Lung, and Blood Institute, NIH Publ. No. 92-3091, 1992.
5. Muir DCF: Particle deposition. In *The Lung: Scientific Foundations*, edn. 1. Edited by Crystal RG, West JB. New York: Raven Press; 1992:1839–1843.
6.• Rom WN, Crystal RG: Consequences of chronic inorganic dust exposure. In *The Lung: Scientific Foundations*, edn. 1. Edited by Crystal RG, West JB. New York: Raven Press; 1992:1885–1897.
7.• Rom WN: Cellular and molecular basis of the asbestos-related diseases. *Am Rev Respir Dis* 1991, 143:408–422.
8. DeRemee RA: *Clinical Profiles of Diffuse Interstitial Pulmonary Disease*, edn. 1. Mount Kisco: Futura; 1990:99–114.
9. Al-Jarad N, Strickland B, Pearson MC, *et al.*: High resolution computed tomographic assessment of asbestosis and cryptogenic fibrosing alveolitis: A comparative study. *Thorax* 1992, 47:645–650.
10. Murphy RL, Becklake MR, Brooks SM, *et al.*: The diagnosis of nonmalignant diseases related to asbestos. *Am Rev Respir Dis* 1986, 134:363–368.

11.•• do Pico GA: Toxic fume inhalation. In *Comprehensive Textbook in Pulmonary Medicine*. Edited by Bone R, George R. St. Louis: CV Mosby; 1993:N.5.1–N.5.15
12.• Weiss SM, Lakshminarayan S: Acute inhalation injury. *Clin Chest Med* 1994, 15:103–116.
13.• Rorison DG, McPherson SJ: Acute toxic inhalations. *Emerg Med Clin North Am* 1992, 10:409–435.
14. Langford RM, Armstrong RF: Algorithm for managing injury from smoke inhalation. *Br Med J* 1989, 299:902–905.
15.•• do Pico GA: Toxic gas inhalations. *Clin Resp Med* 1994, 1:84–92.
16.•• Haponik E. Clinical smoke inhalation. In *Occupational Medicine: State of the Art Reviews.*, vol. 8. Edited by DJ Shusterman. Philadelphia: Hanley & Belfus; 1993:430–468.

Select Bibliography

Bardana EJ Jr, Montanaro A, O'Hollaren MT: *Occupational Asthma*, edn. 1. Philadelphia: Hanley & Belfus; 1992.

Epler GR: Occupational lung diseases. *Clin Chest Med* 1992, 13:179–382.

Morgan WKC, Seaton A: *Occupational Lung Diseases*, edn. 2. Philadelphia: WB Saunders; 1984.

Rom WN, Ed.:*Environmental and Occupational Medicine*, edn. 2. Boston: Little, Brown, & Co; 1994.

Rosenstock L: Occupational pulmonary disease. *Occupational Medicine: State of the Art Reviews* 1987, 2:213–428.

Diseases of the Pleura

Steven A. Sahn

> ### Key Points
> - Pleural fluid analysis is the most effective test in establishing the diagnosis of patients with pleurisy.
> - The differential diagnosis can be narrowed to empyema, esophageal rupture, rheumatoid pleurisy, malignancy, lupus pleuritis, or tuberculous pleurisy when the pleural fluid pH is less than 7.30.
> - Primary spontaneous pneumothorax occurs in tall, thin, male smokers who have no clinical lung disease.
> - The most common cause of secondary spontaneous pneumothorax is chronic obstructive pulmonary disease, which should always be treated with chest tube drainage because of its threat to life.
> - Radiologic features suggesting a malignant effusion are massive size, bilateral effusions with a normal heart, interstitial lung disease with effusions, and absence of contralateral shift with a large effusion.
> - A malignant effusion with pH less than 7.30 predicts short survival, ease of diagnosis, and failure of chemical pleurodesis.
> - Talc pleurodesis is the most effective palliation for symptomatic, recurrent malignant effusions.

PLEURISY AND PLEURAL EFFUSIONS

The pleural space, which is bounded by the visceral and parietal pleura, is usually affected by primary disease of the thorax but, at times, may be targeted by a systemic illness or extrathoracic localized disease. The patient may or may not have pleuritic chest pain, a pleural effusion, or pleural air as a marker of pleural involvement. The purpose of this chapter is to review the state of the art relating to the pathophysiology, clinical manifestations, and management of patients with pleurisy and pleural effusions, pneumothorax, and malignant pleural effusions.

Pleurisy signifies pleural inflammation with or without pleural effusion. Pleurisy most commonly results from extension of localized disease of the lung (pneumonia), mediastinum (esophageal rupture), pericardium (pericarditis), or abdomen (subphrenic abscess) or from systemic disease. Patients with pleurisy usually have an associated pleural effusion; the presence or absence of pleural fluid helps narrow the differential diagnosis. Patients with viral pleurisy, rheumatoid pleurisy, and sarcoid often present with chest pain without a pleural effusion; in contrast, patients with bacterial pneumonia, lupus pleuritis, or postcardiac injury syndrome usually have an associated pleural effusion [1].

Stimulation of the visceral pleura and lung usually does not produce pain because only a scanty nerve supply of efferent twigs of sympathetic and vagal origin exists in the lung distal to the bronchi. In contrast, the parietal pleura is a highly sensitive surface, extensively supplied with sensory afferents from intercostal sympathetic, phrenic, and vagus nerves.

Injury to the costal parietal pleura produces sharp, localized pain at the site of inflammation. Peripheral diaphragmatic pleural inflammation results in localized pain, but, in addition, tends to extend over a greater area of the chest wall, back, or abdomen. Inflammation of the central portion of the diaphragmatic pleura results in referred pain to the ipsilateral posterior neck, shoulder, and trapezius muscle. Stimulation of the mediastinal parietal pleura over the pericardium may also refer pain to the neck. The pain is referred because most of the sensory fibers of the phrenic nerve enter at the C4 level of the spinal cord, which is the usual entry point of sensation from the shoulder [2•].

Clinical Features

Pleuritic chest pain may be minimal or severe and has been described as stabbing, shooting, or a "stitch" in the side. It is exacerbated by deep breathing, coughing, or sneezing and may be relieved by manual pressure against the chest wall that causes splinting; this maneuver, however, does not differentiate pleural inflammation from other causes of pleuritic-like pain caused by rib fractures or myositis.

Dyspnea is a frequent complaint and can result from voluntary and involuntary restriction in respiration imposed by the pain and accompanying large effusion or by underlying acute or chronic lung disease.

A pleural friction rub confirms the diagnosis of pleurisy. The description by Hippocrates—"the lung...squeaks like a leather strap"—is difficult to improve upon. A pleural friction rub, which is often evanescent, is usually audible during both phases of respiration, but is best heard at or near the end of inspiration. In contrast to a pericardial rub, the pleural friction rub disappears with breath holding. It is most frequently appreciated over the lateral and posterior regions of the thorax, where lung movement is greatest, and it may only be heard at these sites when the patient is encouraged to take a deep breath. Applying firm pressure to the stethoscope increases the intensity of the rub and eliminates a false friction rub caused when the stethoscope slides over the skin.

Differential Diagnosis

The symptoms associated with pleurisy are nonspecific, and the documentation of a pleural friction rub simply confirms pleural inflammation. The remaining history, physical findings, and pertinent laboratory tests enable the clinician to narrow the differential diagnosis of pleurisy. The clinical features of common disorders that cause pleurisy are shown in Table 1. The chest radiograph may establish the diagnosis of pneumothorax or suggest bacterial pneumonia (lobar consolidation with effusion), esophageal rupture (left pleural effusion with mediastinal and subcutaneous emphysema), or disease originating below the diaphragm (normal chest radiograph with the exception of pleural fluid).

Pleural fluid analysis is the most helpful diagnostic test in establishing the presumptive or definitive diagnosis of patients with pleurisy. Thoracentesis should be performed as soon as the presence of a reasonably sized pleural effusion is documented (*ie*, a distance of at least 1 cm from the inside of the chest wall to the fluid line on a lateral decubitus radiograph). Small or loculated pleural effusions can be aspirated with the help of ultrasonography. Essentially all patients with pleurisy have exudative effusions. Bloody effusions suggest pulmonary embolism, postcardiac injury syndrome, malignancy, uremic pleural effusion, pleural endometriosis, or benign asbestos pleural effusion. Pus aspirated from the pleural space establishes the diagnosis of empyema. An increased pleural fluid amylase (greater than the concomitant serum amylase) is found with pancreatitis, esophageal rupture, and malignancy. An elevated nucleated cell count with a neutrophil predominance is seen in bacterial pneumonia, esophageal rupture, pancreatitis, and subphrenic abscess. A low nucleated cell count with a lymphocyte predominance is seen in tuberculous pleurisy and malignant effusions. The differential diagnosis can be narrowed to empyema, esophageal rupture, rheumatoid pleurisy, lupus pleuritis, malignancy, or tuberculous pleurisy when the pH is less than 7.30 and when the pleural fluid/serum glucose ratio is less than 0.5 [1,3].

Treatment

The treatment and course of pleurisy will vary with the underlying disease. Drainage of the pleural space is necessary in empyema and in most patients with pneumothorax and malignancy. Patients with lupus pleuritis and postcardiac injury syndrome respond rapidly to corticosteroids. Most patients with pleuritic pain from any cause obtain relief from nonsteroidal antiinflammatory drugs. With appropriate and prompt treatment, most patients with pleurisy have successful outcomes; it is uncommon for patients with malignant pleural effusions to manifest pleuritic chest pain.

PNEUMOTHORAX

Classification

Pneumothorax (*ie*, air in the pleural space) can be classified as spontaneous (without trauma or obvious cause), traumatic (direct or indirect chest trauma), or iatrogenic. Primary spontaneous pneumothorax (PSP) occurs in individuals without clinical lung disease, while secondary spontaneous pneumothoraces (SSP) occur as complications of preexisting lung disease. A traumatic pneumothorax occurs from direct or indirect chest trauma. Iatrogenic pneumothorax results from a diagnostic or therapeutic misadventure.

Primary Spontaneous Pneumothorax

Causes

PSP are most commonly seen in tall, thin males when an apical subpleural bleb ruptures [4]. Subpleural blebs may result from congenital abnormalities, small airway inflammation, or disturbances of collateral ventilation [5]. More than 90% of patients with PSP are smokers or ex-smokers [6].

Clinical and physiologic features

Chest pain and dyspnea are the two prominent symptoms and usually occur while the patient is at rest. The physical examination may be unremarkable in patients with a small pneumothorax. In patients with a large pneumothorax, there may be decreased chest movement, decreased fremitus, hyper-resonance, and diminished or absent breath sounds on the ipsilateral side. A marked tachycardia (> 135) should alert the clinician to the possibility of a tension pneumothorax.

The physiologic consequences of a pneumothorax are decreases in vital capacity and arterial oxygen tension. In SSP, hypercapnia may develop [7]. The increased alveolar–arterial oxygen difference is due to low V/Q areas and shunts [8].

Diagnosis

The diagnosis of PSP depends on demonstration of the visceral pleural line on a chest radiograph (Fig. 1). In problematic cases, an expiratory film should be obtained with the patient in the erect position or the lateral decubitus position with the suspected side up. The expiratory technique provides a smaller surface of visceral pleura in contact with air because lung volume is reduced while pleural gas volume remains constant.

Treatment and prevention of recurrence

The major treatment decision in PSP is whether or not to remove the air from the pleural space. Because patients with PSP have no clinical lung disease, a more conservative approach can be taken if the pneumothorax is small and the leak has ceased. In general, if the patient's symptoms have resolved and the pneumothorax is thought to be less than 15%, observation is warranted. The pneumothorax gas should be reabsorbed in approximately 12 days, as it is estimated that 1.25% of the volume of the pneumothorax is absorbed daily [9]. The recurrence rate approaches 50% and increases with each subsequent pneumothorax.

Treatment options for PSP that are greater than 15% include supplemental oxygen, catheter aspiration, tube thoracostomy, or tube thoracostomy with instillation of a sclerosing agent. Pleural air is absorbed more rapidly when patients are given oxygen supplementation, as the net gradient for gas absorption from pleural space to blood will increase [10]. Catheter aspiration will be successful only if the air leak has stopped; its only advantage is decreasing the resolution time of the pneumothorax. Standard chest tube drainage results in rapid resolution of the pneumothorax; small catheters may be equally successful if the air leak is not large. The tube or catheter can be removed 24 to 48 hours after the lung is fully expanded and the air leak has ceased. Chest tube drainage does not appear to decrease the rate of recurrence [11]. Recent data suggest that intrapleural minocycline might have similar efficacy to tetracycline hydrochloride (now unavailable); however, talc slurry through a chest tube [12] and talc poudrage via a thoracoscope [13] is more efficacious. Recurrent pneumothorax is effectively treated by pleurectomy and pleural abrasion through the thoracoscope.

Recently, laser therapy with thoracoscopy has been advocated in the initial treatment and recurrence of spontaneous pneumothorax [14,15]. This treatment needs to be evaluated with a larger number of patients, especially regarding recurrence.

Secondary Spontaneous Pneumothorax
Causes

In contrast to the benign nature of PSP, SSP may be life-threatening because patients with SSP have underlying lung disease. There are multiple causes of SSP (Table 2); however, the most common etiology is chronic obstructive pulmonary disease [7]. Other frequent causes include cystic fibrosis and interstitial lung disease, especially pulmonary histiocytosis and stage IV sarcoidosis.

Clinical features and diagnosis

The two major symptoms of SSP, dyspnea and chest pain, are the same as those found with PSP; however, the presentation may be more dramatic. Shortness of breath is universal and some patients may have cardiovascular compromise. The finding of hypercapnia with pneumothorax signifies underlying lung disease, usually chronic obstructive pulmonary disease [7].

Occasionally it is difficult to differentiate between a pneumothorax and a bullous lesion. The visceral pleural line with pneumothorax usually follows the configuration of the chest wall, while a bullous lesion may have a concave relationship to the chest wall. Computed tomography may help differentiate problematic cases.

Treatment and prevention of recurrence

As recurrence rates of patients with SSP are similar to those with PSP and as, in the setting of lung disease, pneumothorax may be life-threatening, preventing recurrence should be of primary concern. Virtually all patients with SSP should be treated with tube drainage. Even with tube thoracostomy, lung expansion takes longer and the air leak persists longer in patients with SSP than in those with PSP. Options to prevent recurrence include intrapleural doxycycline or minocycline, insufflation of talc, talc slurry through a chest tube, laser therapy, and pleural abrasion by thoracoscopy or thoracotomy.

MALIGNANT PLEURAL EFFUSIONS

Epidemiology and Significance

There are approximately 250,000 new cases of malignant pleural effusions in the United States yearly. The diagnosis of a malignant effusion is established by demonstrating exfoliated malignant cells in pleural fluid; or finding these cells in pleural tissue obtained by percutaneous pleural biopsy, thoracoscopy, or thoracotomy; or by discovering these cells at autopsy. The two malignancies that most commonly metastasize to the pleura are lung and breast cancer (Table 3) [16•]. Malignant effusions frequently are the first manifestation and diagnostic source of the malignancy; they signal incurability, often represent the initial manifestation of recurrent tumor (particularly in lung and breast carcinoma and lymphoma), and portend a poor prognosis [17].

Paramalignant Effusions

A number of patients have a pleural effusion associated with a known malignancy even though malignant cells cannot be

TABLE 1 CLINICAL FEATURES OF DISEASES THAT CAUSE PLEURISY

Diagnosis	Clinical findings	Chest radiograph	Pleural fluid characteristics	Course and comments
Infection				
Viral pleurisy	Abrupt pleuritic pain, constitutional symptoms, WBC<10,000/μL	Small pleural effusion (10%–20%), infiltrate (20%)	Serous exudate, low WBC, PMNs, or mononuclears	Effusions transient; pleuritic pain may persist for several days
Bacterial pneumonia	Acute pleuritic pain, fever, chills, purulent sputum, WBC>15,000/μL	Alveolar infiltrate, small-to-large free-flowing or loculated effusion	PMN-predominant exudate, WBC>10,000/μL, may evolve into empyema ((↓)pH, (↓)glucose, (↑)LDH)	Uncomplicated effusion resolves in days with antibiotics; empyema requires drainage; pleuritic pain may be transient and tends to persist longer in empyema
Tuberculosis pleurisy	Abrupt or insidious onset, cough, pleuritic pain (75%), fever, pleuritic pain precedes cough	Small-to-moderate unilateral pleural effusion, coexisting parenchymal disease (33%)	Serous exudate (protein>5 g/dL), WBC<5000/μL, 80–90% lymphocytes, acute—may be PMN predominant, >5% mesothelial cells or eosinophilia makes tuberculosis unlikely, low glucose and pH (20%)	Pleuritic pain resolves in 2–4 months with or without treatment
Spontaneous esophageal rupture	Vomiting, severe chest pain, fever, hematemesis, dyspnea, subcutaneous emphysema	Left pleural effusion, widened mediastinum, mediastinal and subcutaneous air, pneumothorax	Turbid to purulent exudate; (↑) amylase, pH 6.00, squamous epithelial cells	Anaerobic empyema; contrast study of esophagus confirms diagnosis; surgical repair within 24 hours associated with survival of 90%
Immunologic				
Lupus pleuritis	Known SLE, pleuritic pain (> 85%), dyspnea, cough, pleural rub, fever	Unilateral or bilateral small to moderate effusions, alveolar infiltrates, atelectasis, large cardiac silhouette (30%)	Serous to serosanguineous exudate, WBC 5000/μL, PMN predominant early, pH and glucose low (20%), +LE cells, PF/S ANA>1	Rapid response to corticosteroids
Rheumatoid pleurisy	Males; within 10 y of onset of disease, subcutaneous nodules, moderate-to-severe arthritis, pleuritic pain, dyspnea; asymptomatic chest radiograph	Small-to-moderate unilateral pleural effusion, up to 33% have other manifestations of rheumatoid lung	Straw-colored, turbid, "debris;" low glucose and pH, LDH>1000 U/L, (↓) complement, RF≥1:320	Variable; spontaneous resolution over months; recurrences common; "dry" pleurisy; marked pleural fibrosis possible
Postcardiac injury syndrome	Pleuritic pain (>90%), fever, pleural and pericardial rub dyspnea, 3 wk (days to months) after cardiac surgery or myocardial infarction, (↑) ESR	Small-to-moderate left or bilateral pleural effusion, infiltrates on left	Bloody (70%) exudate; PMN predominant, normal pH and glucose	Resolves spontaneously or with NSAID or corticosteroids
Sarcoidosis	Pleuritic or nonpleuritic chest pain, dyspnea, asymptomatic, stage 2 or 3	Small-to-moderate unilateral pleural effusion, hilar and mediastinal adenopathy and interstitial disease	Straw-colored exudate, low WBC, >90% lymphocytes	Spontaneous resolution or with corticosteroids; "dry" pleurisy

Continued on next page

Table 1 Clinical features of diseases that cause pleurisy (Continued)

Diagnosis	Clinical findings	Chest radiograph	Pleural fluid characteristics	Course and comments
Diseases that originate below the diaphragm				
Pancreatitis	Abdominal symptoms, pleuritic pain and dyspnea in alcoholic	Small-to-moderate left pleural effusion, elevated diaphragm, basilar infiltrates	Serous-to-bloody exudate, WBC>10,000/µL, PMN predominant, (↑) amylase	Effusion and pleuritic pain resolve as pancreatitis subsides; no resolution in 2 wk suggests abscess or pseudocyst
Subphrenic abscess	Post-intraabdominal surgery, chest or abdominal symptoms, pleuritic pain, fever	Small-to-moderate unilateral pleural effusion, basilar infiltrates, elevated diaphragm	Turbid exudate, (↑) WBC, PMN predominant, pH>7.20, glucose—50 mg/dL	Diagnosis suggested by routine chest or abdominal films; abdominal CT most sensitive; drainage and antibiotics
Other				
Pneumothorax	Young, thin, tall male; COPD, interstitial lung disease; acute chest pain (>90%), may be pleuritic, dyspnea	Detection of visceral pleural line, small effusion (10%)	Sanguineous exudate because of ruptured vessels	Chest pain may be transient but may progress if air leak continues
Pulmonary embolism	Predisposing factor, acute dyspnea, pleuritic pain, hemoptysis	Small unilateral effusion, present on admission (90%), reaches maximum size early	Bloody exudate, PMN predominant found only in a third	Effusion regresses over several days without consolidation; resolves slower with radiographic infarction
Benign asbestos pleural effusion	Males >50 y, within 20 y of first asbestos exposure, pleuritic pain (20%), dyspnea	Small-to-moderate unilateral pleural effusion, other manifestations uncommon	Serous-to-bloody exudate, PMN or mononuclear predominant, may have eosinophilia	Pleural effusion resolves over several months; recurrence ipsilateral or contralateral
Uremic pleural effusion	Fever, chest pain (30%), transient pleural and pericardial friction rub in patient with uremia for months to years	Small-to-large unilateral pleural effusion, cardiomegaly; minimal pulmonary congestion	Serous-to-bloody exudate, low WBC, predominantly lymphocytes	Resolves with continued dialysis; some develop progressive pleural fibrosis (20%)

WBC—white blood cell count; SLE—systemic lupus erythematosus; ESR—erythrocyte sedimentation rate; PMN—polymorphonuclear leukocyte; COPD—chronic obstructive pulmonary disease; LDH—lactic dehydrogenase; NSAID—nonsteroidal antiinflammatory drug; CT—computed tomography.

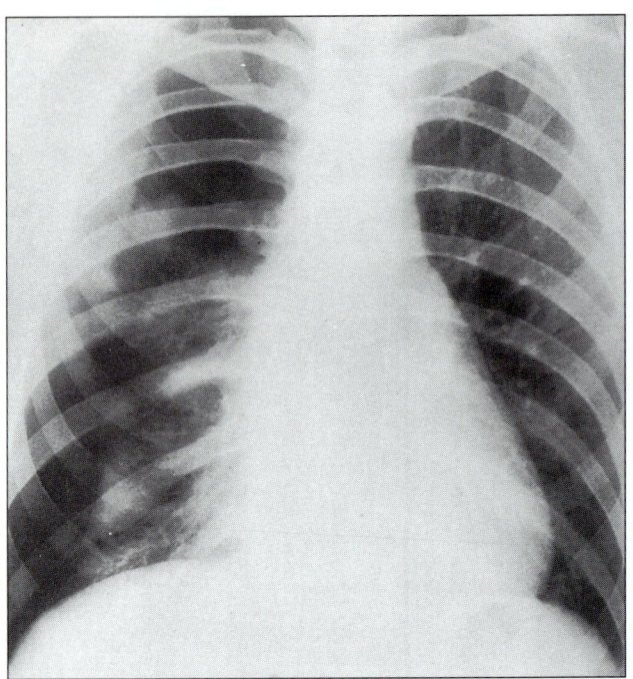

FIGURE 1 An erect posteroanterior view of a 56-year-old man with a large spontaneous pneumothorax on the right. The visceral pleural line is easily seen inferiorly as well as the collapsed lung with its crowded bronchovascular markings.

demonstrated in pleural fluid or tissue. These fluids should be classified as paramalignant effusions and are caused by local effect of the tumor, systemic effect of the tumor, and complications of therapy (Table 4) [16•].

Clinical Features

Patients with carcinomatous pleurisy most commonly present with symptoms attributable to a large pleural effusion, dyspnea on exertion, and cough [17]. The presence and degree of dyspnea are dependent on the volume of fluid and the patient's underlying pulmonary status. Approximately one fourth of patients with carcinoma of the pleura have chest pain as a presenting symptom, whereas more than two thirds of patients with mesothelioma experience chest pain. Patients with advanced carcinoma of the pleura may have substantial weight loss and appear chronically ill; however, some patients may be relatively asymptomatic at the time of initial diagnosis [17].

Diagnosis
Chest radiography

A malignant pleural effusion may be discovered initially on a routine chest radiograph (Fig. 2). Radiologic features suggesting pleural effusion due to malignancy include a massive pleural effusion, bilateral pleural effusions with a normal heart size, interstitial lung disease and effusions

TABLE 2 DISEASES ASSOCIATED WITH SECONDARY SPONTANEOUS PNEUMOTHORAX

Diseases	Comments
Disease of the airways	
COPD	Most common cause of SSP
Cystic fibrosis	Usually in adolescents and adults
Asthma	Associated with status asthmaticus
Interstitial lung disease	
Pulmonary histiocytosis X	Pneumothorax may be presenting problem; often recurrent
Sarcoidosis	Usually stage IV sarcoidosis
Idiopathic pulmonary fibrosis	Pneumothorax much less common than in pulmonary histiocytosis
Tuberous sclerosis	Usually found in women
Other types	Risk of pneumothorax increases with advanced stage of disease
Infection	
Necrotizing pneumonia	Gram-negative aerobes, anaerobes
Tuberculosis	Usually active
Atypical mycobacteria	Usually active
Pneumocystis pneumonia	Pneumothorax associated with aerosolized pentamidine when *Pneumocystis carinii* infection develops
Malignancy	
Lung cancer	Two most common tumors presenting as pneumothorax; incidence of
Sarcomas	pneumothorax due to metastatic malignancy <1% of all SSP
Others	
Lymphangioleiomyomatosis	Pneumothorax occurs in up to 80% of patients during course of disease
Endometriosis	Catamenial pneumothorax most common form of thoracic endometriosis
Marfan syndrome	Incidence of pneumothorax 4%–11% with recurrence common
Pulmonary infarction	Rare complication of infected infarction

COPD—chronic obstructive pulmonary disease; SSP—secondary spontaneous pneumothorax.

Table 3. Common causes of malignant pleural effusions

Malignancy	Comments
Lung cancer	Most common cause of a malignant effusion; 10% of all lung cancers; adenocarcinoma most common cell type; ipsilateral to primary lesion
Breast cancer	Second most common cause of a malignant effusion; ipsilateral or contralateral to primary lesion
Lymphoma	Non-Hodgkin's: direct pleural involvement
	Hodgkin's: lymphatic obstruction
Ovarian cancer	3% of all ovarian cancers; associated with ascites; short survival from diagnosis of pleural metastasis
Gastric cancer	3% of all gastric cancers; short survival from diagnosis of pleural metastasis

(lymphangitic carcinomatosis), and multiple pulmonary nodules and effusions. If contralateral mediastinal shift with a large effusion (> 1500 mL) is absent, malignancy is likely and the following diagnoses should be considered: 1) lung cancer of the ipsilateral mainstem bronchus causing atelectasis, 2) fixed mediastinum due to malignant lymph nodes, 3) malignant mesothelioma, and 4) extensive tumor infiltration of the ipsilateral lung (Fig. 3) [16•].

Pleural fluid analysis

Malignant pleural fluid may be serous, serosanguinous, or grossly bloody. An erythrocyte count greater than 100,000/µL in the absence of trauma should heighten the suspicion of malignancy. Malignant effusions are relatively noninflammatory; the nucleated cell count is modest (usually 2500–4000 cells/µL). The cellular population usually consists of lymphocytes, macrophages, and mesothelial cells, with lymphocytes often predominating (in the 50%–70% range). Malignant cells in pleural fluid are rare in some patients, whereas in others they constitute virtually the complete population of cells. Polymorphonuclear leukocytes usually constitute < 25% of the cell population. Pleural fluid eosinophilia is common in bloody pleural effusions, but is inexplicably uncommon in bloody malignant pleural effusions [18].

The pleural fluid is exudative in approximately 80% of cases; however, 2% to 19% of patients have malignant transudates due to atelectasis from bronchial obstruction, the early stages of mediastinal lymph node involvement, or concomitant disease (such as congestive heart failure) [17,19]. In general, transudative malignant effusions have been present

Table 4. Paramalignant pleural effusions

Etiology	Comments
Local effects of tumor	
Lymphatic obstruction	Predominant mechanism of pleural fluid accumulation in paramalignant and malignant effusions; most common cause of paramalignant effusion
Bronchial obstruction causing pneumonia	Parapneumonic effusion; does not exclude operability or curability in lung cancer; squamous cell most common cause
Bronchial obstruction causing atelectasis	Transudate; does not exclude operability or curability in lung cancer; squamous cell most common cause
Chylothorax	Disruption of thoracic duct; chyle in pleural space; lymphoma most common cause
Superior vena cava syndrome	Transudate; due to acute increase in systemic venous pressure; small cell lung cancer most common cause
Pneumothorax	Serosanguineous exudate; sarcoma as well as carcinoma causal
Systemic effects of tumor	
Pulmonary embolism	Hypercoagulable state; adenocarcinoma
Low plasma oncotic pressure	Serum albumin<1.5 g/dL; associated with anasarca
Results of therapy	
Radiation therapy	
Pleuritis	Same time course as radiation pneumonitis; exudate with tendency to loculation; may last for months
Mediastinal fibrosis	1–2 y after radiation: lymphatic obstruction, constrictive pericarditis, superior vena cava syndrome
Drug therapy	
Methotrexate	Pleuritis, pleural thickening, or effusion occurs with low- or high-dose therapy

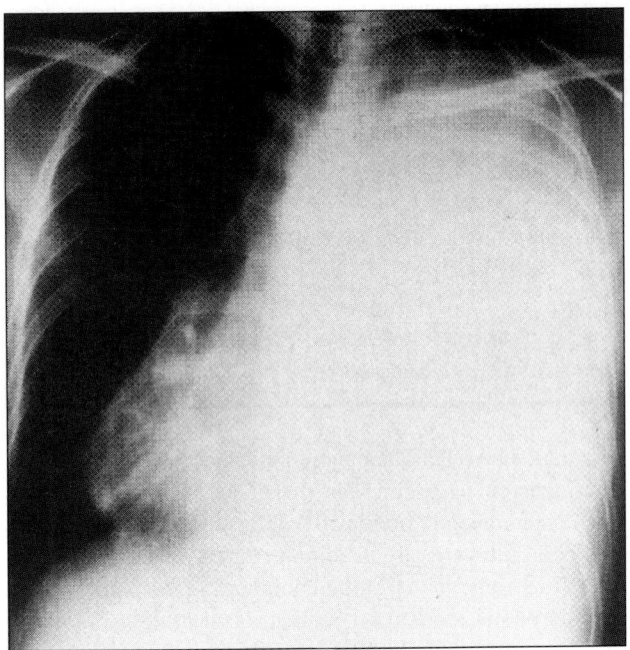

FIGURE 2 A massive pleural effusion in a 63-year-old woman with metastatic cervical carcinoma to the pleura. Note the contralateral mediastinal shift implying the absence of an ipsilateral endobronchial lesion or a fixed mediastinum.

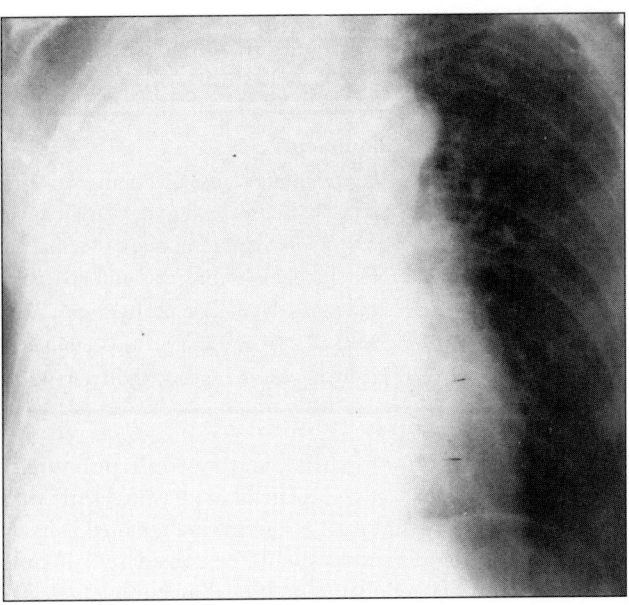

FIGURE 3 Complete opacification of the right hemithorax in a 70-year-old man with a history of asbestos exposure. Note the absence of expected contralateral shift in this patient with a malignant mesothelioma. The opacification of the right hemithorax represents mostly tumor encasing the lung resulting in a "fixing" of the lung and mediastinum.

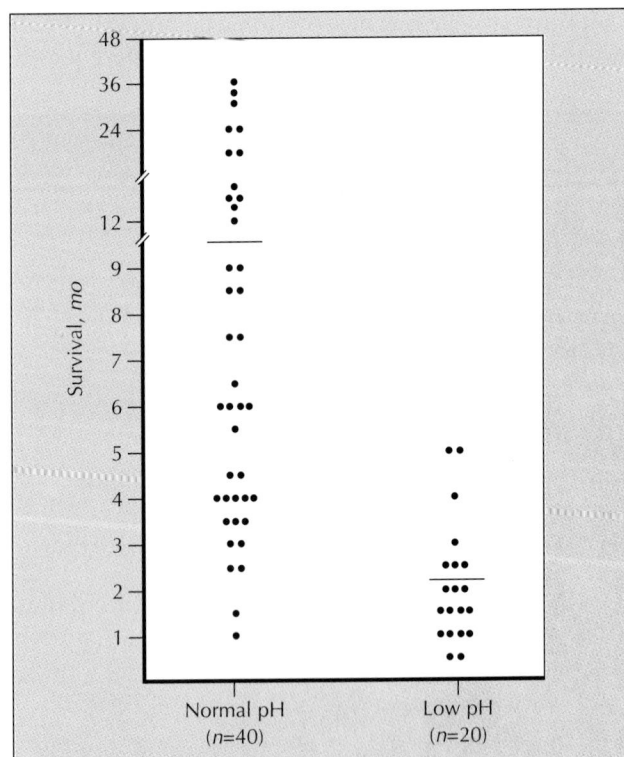

FIGURE 4 Survival in months from time of occurrence of malignant pleural effusion in patients with normal and low pH effusions. The horizontal lines represent the means of the groups. Patients with low pH malignant pleural effusions had a very short survival from initial thoracentesis. The mean survival in the low pH group was 2.1 months (range, 2 weeks–5 months) compared with 9.8 months (range, 1–36 months) in the normal pH group ($P<0.001$). (From Sahn, Good [20]; with permission.)

for less than 6 weeks at the time the initial thoracentesis is accomplished. Approximately 30% of patients with malignant pleural effusions have a low pH (< 7.30) and low glucose (pleural fluid/serum ratio < 0.5). Findings of pleural fluid acidosis and a low glucose concentration portend a short survival (Fig. 4), an easy diagnosis, and a poor response to chemical pleurodesis [20]. Approximately 10% of malignant pleural effusions have high amylase concentrations. The finding of a high level of salivary-like isoamylase in a patient who does not have esophageal perforation essentially establishes the diagnosis of malignancy, most commonly adenocarcinoma of the lung [21].

Cytology

Cytology is a more sensitive test for the diagnosis of malignant pleural effusion than percutaneous pleural biopsy because pleural metastases tend to be focal and the latter is a blind sampling procedure. The yield of either procedure increases as the disease becomes more advanced.

The diagnostic options for the patient with suspected malignancy and negative pleural fluid and pleural tissue studies include repeat testing in several weeks, thoracoscopy, and open pleural biopsy. The urgency of establishing the diagnosis of incurable malignancy depends on the clinical situation.

Treatment

When a malignant pleural effusion is diagnosed, palliative therapy should be contemplated, taking into account the patient's general condition, symptoms, and expected survival. Management options are listed in Table 5. Asymptomatic patients need not be treated; the majority will develop progressive pleural effusions that will evoke symptoms and

Table 5. Management of malignant and paramalignant pleural effusions

Option	Comments
Observation	Patient is asymptomatic; most effusions will progress and require therapy
Therapeutic thoracentesis	Prompt relief of symptoms; recurrence rate variable; recommended for patient with pleural fluid pH<7.30, trapped or collapsed lung
Chemotherapy	May be effective in lymphoma, small cell lung cancer, and breast cancer
Radiotherapy	Mediastinal radiation may be effective in lymphoma and with lymphomatous chylothorax
Chest tube drainage only	Usually not effective
Chest tube drainage with chemical pleurodesis	Effective agents include talc, doxycycline, minocycline, bleomycin, and *C. parvum*
Pleuroperitoneal shunt	When other options are not indicated; may be useful for chylothorax
Pleural abrasion and partial pleurectomy	Virtually 100% effective; can be done with thoracoscopy

require therapy, but some will reach a steady state of pleural fluid formation and removal and will remain asymptomatic. In the debilitated patient in whom a short survival is expected (based on general health, extent of disease, and biochemical characteristics of the pleural fluid), periodic outpatient therapeutic thoracentesis usually is preferable to hospitalization for tube thoracotomy and chemical pleurodesis. Pleural abrasion and pleurectomy are virtually always effective in producing pleural symphysis and controlling a malignant pleural effusion; however, the therapy requires either thoracoscopy or thoracotomy, which is associated with some morbidity and, in the case of thoracotomy, mortality.

The most effective method, short of pleurectomy and abrasion, for controlling a symptomatic malignant pleural effusion is chest tube drainage with instillation of a sclerosing agent [22••]. Doxycycline, 500 mg, and minocycline, 300 mg, have been successful in controlling malignant pleural effusions in 72% and 86%, respectively, of a small number of patients. Pain and fever have been the most frequent adverse effects. Often more than a single instillation of doxycycline has been required for success. Bleomycin has had a complete response rate of approximately 55% and has similar adverse effects as the tetracycline-class agents. The major drawback of bleomycin is its expense; a usual 1 U/kg dose costs more than $1000. Talc, taken mainly by insufflation through a thoracoscope, has proven to be efficacious with complete response rates of 90%. Although talc is inexpensive (less than $1), administration involves thoracoscopy and, in most cases, general anesthesia and an operating department, and therefore is a costly undertaking. Recent evidence suggests that talc slurry through a chest tube may be as effective as insufflation and may become the preferred route of administration [23].

The technique for intrapleural instillation of a sclerosing agent is critical for a good result. The pleural space needs to be drained as completely as possible so that the instilled agent is not diluted and the pleural surfaces remain in close contact during the time of the inflammatory insult. This is best accomplished by tube thoracostomy. Radiolabeled tetracycline has demonstrated rapid and complete dispersion in the pleural space without patient repositioning [24]. A follow-up clinical study also supported the concept that rotation is unnecessary after chemical instillation [25]. The chest tube can usually be removed when drainage is less than 150 mL/day. If a large volume of drainage persists, a repeat dose of the pleurodesis agent should be instilled.

A further option available for the patient with an intractable symptomatic effusion who cannot undergo pleurodesis is a pleuroperitoneal shunt. This allows for the one-way flow of fluid from the pleural space to the peritoneal cavity. The shunt may be of particular value in chylothorax, so that nutrients and lymphocytes can be recirculated [26].

Conclusion

The presence of a pleural effusion provides an opportunity for the internist to localize the dysfunctional organ system. With systematic analysis of the pleural fluid obtained at thoracentesis in conjunction with the patient's history, physical examination, and ancillary laboratory tests, a diagnosis, either definitive or presumptive, should be obtained in 75% to 80% of patients. In the remaining patients who are undiagnosed after initial thoracentesis, continued surveillance and possibly repeat thoracentesis usually will result in the correct diagnosis.

Most patients with a pleural effusion do not require specific therapy directed to the pleural space because the effusion will resolve with appropriate treatment of the underlying disease. Pneumothorax, empyema, and malignant pleural effusions, however, will usually require direct pleural manipulation.

References and Recommended Reading

Recently published papers of particular interest have been highlighted as:
- Of interest
- •• Of outstanding interest

1. Sahn SA: The state of the art: the pleura. *Am Rev Respir Dis* 1988, 138:184–234.
2.• Sahn SA, Heffner JE: Approach to the patient with pleurisy. In *Textbook of Internal Medicine*. edn 2. Edited by Kelley WN. Philadelphia: JB Lippincott; 1992:1887–1890.

3. Good JT Jr, Kaplan RL, Maulitz RM, *et al.*: The diagnostic value of pleural fluid pH. *Chest* 1980, 78:55–59.

4. Gobbel WG Jr, Rhea WG Jr, Nelson IA, Daniel RA Jr: Spontaneous pneumothorax. *J Thorac Cardiovasc Surg* 1963, 46:331–345.

5. Ohata M, Suzuki H: Pathogenesis of spontaneous pneumothorax. *Chest* 1980, 77:771–776.

6. Jansveld CAF, Dijkman JH: Primary spontaneous pneumothorax and smoking. *Br Med J* 1975, 4:559–560.

7. Dines DE, Clagett OT, Payne WS: Spontaneous pneumothorax in emphysema. *Mayo Clin Proc* 1970, 45:481–487.

8. Norris RM, Jones JG, Bishop JM: Respiratory gas exchange in patients with spontaneous pneumothorax. *Thorax* 1968, 23:427–433.

9. Kircher LT Jr, Swartzel RL: Spontaneous pneumothorax and its treatment. *JAMA* 1954, 155:24–29.

10. Chadaha TS, Cohn MA: Non-invasive treatment of pneumothorax with oxygen inhalation. *Respiration* 1983, 44:147–152.

11. Sermetis MG: The management of spontaneous pneumothorax. *Chest* 1970, 57:65–68.

12. Almind M, Lange P, Viskum: Spontaneous pneumothorax: comparison of simple drainage, talc pleurodesis, and tetracycline pleurodesis. *Thorax* 1989, 44:627–630.

13. Verschoof AC, Ten Velde GPM, Greve LH, Wouters EFM: Thoracoscopic pleurodesis in the management of spontaneous pneumothorax. *Respiration* 1988, 53:197–200.

14. Torre M, Belloni P: Nd:YAG laser pleurodesis through thoracoscopy: new curative therapy in spontaneous pneumothorax. *Ann Thorac Surg* 1989, 47:887–889.

15. Wakabayashi A, Brenner M, Wilson AF, *et al.*: Thorascopic treatment of spontaneous pneumothorax using carbon dioxide laser. *Ann Thorac Surg* 1990, 50:786–790.

16.• Sahn SA: Pleural malignancies. In *Pulmonary and Critical Care Medicine*. Edited by Bone RC, Dantzker DR, George RB, *et al.* Mosby-Year Book: St. Louis; 1993:1–12.

17. Chernow B, Sahn SA: Carcinomatous involvement of the pleura: an analysis of 96 patients. *Am J Med* 1977, 63:695–702.

18. Adelman M, Albelda SM, Gottlieb J, Haponik EF: Diagnostic utility of pleural fluid eosinophilia. *Am J Med* 1984, 77:915–920.

19. Clarkson B: Relationship between cell type, glucose concentration, and response to treatment in neoplastic effusions. *Cancer* 1964, 17:914–920.

20. Sahn SA, Good JT Jr: Pleural fluid pH in malignant effusions: diagnostic, prognostic, and therapeutic implications. *Ann Intern Med* 1988, 108:345–349.

21. Kramer MR, Saldana MJ, Cepero RJ, Pitchenik AE: High amylase levels in neoplasm-related pleural effusion. *Ann Intern Med* 1989, 110:567–569.

22.•• Walker PB, Vaughan LM, Sahn SA: Chemical pleurodesis for the treatment of malignant pleural effusions. *Ann Intern Med* 1994, 120:56–64.

23. Kennedy L, Rusch V, Strange C, *et al.*: Pleurodesis using talc slurry. *Chest* In press.

24. Lorch DG, Gordon L, Wooten S, *et al.*: The effect of patient positioning on the distribution of tetracycline in the pleural space during pleurodesis. *Chest* 1988, 93:527–529.

25. Dryzer SR, Allen ML, Strange C, Sahn SA: A comparison of rotation and nonrotation in tetracycline pleurodesis. *Chest* 1993, 104:1763–1766.

26. Milsom JW, Kron IG, Rheuban KS, Rodgers BM: Chylothorax: an assessment of current surgical management. *J Thorac Cardiovasc Surg* 1985, 89:221–227.

Disorders of the Control of Breathing

Neil V. Waravdekar
Clifford W. Zwillich

> ### Key Points
> - Hypoventilation may arise from a low respiratory drive, increased impediment to breathing, or a combination of both. Treatment should be directed at relieving the underlying cause.
> - Cheyne-Stokes respirations often require no treatment; however, oxygen therapy may decrease the amount of periodic breathing observed.
> - Obstructive sleep apnea can be a deadly disease and should be considered in patients with snoring, excessive daytime sleepiness, and witnessed apnea.
> - Sleep polysomnography is the gold standard for diagnosis of sleep apnea.
> - Nasal continuous positive airway pressure is an effective, noninvasive means of treating obstructive sleep apnea.

Disorders of the control of breathing are most frequently manifested by the presence of hypoventilation, cyclic breathing patterns, or sleep apnea. In the following chapter, the pathogenesis, diagnosis, and treatment of these entities will be considered.

VENTILATORY CONTROL SYSTEM

The control of ventilation is achieved by a delicate and intricate system that possesses the innate ability to maintain arterial partial pressure of oxygen (PaO_2) and arterial partial pressure of carbon dioxide ($PaCO_2$) within a narrow range, despite fluctuations in carbon dioxide production and oxygen consumption. This remarkable system is able to compensate for elevations in metabolic rate, as seen in exercise, with little or no variance in PaO_2 or $PaCO_2$ levels in the healthy individual.

The ventilatory control system has three components: sensors, a central controller, and effectors (Fig. 1) [1]. The primary *sensors* are the chemoreceptors, of which the carotid body senses PaO_2 and hydrogen ion concentration (H^+), and the medullary chemoreceptors sense $PaCO_2$ and H^+. Stimulation of the respiratory center by $PaCO_2$ or H^+ elevation or lowered PaO_2 results in increased alveolar ventilation, which lowers the $PaCO_2$ and increases the PaO_2. Other sensors also send input to the respiratory center, including the cerebral cortex, which is responsible for voluntary control of respiration. The central *controller* is the respiratory center, which is located in the brain stem and receives the afferent sensory input, processes it, and sends efferent impulses to the respiratory musculature (*eg*, diaphragm, intercostal muscles, abdominal muscles), which are the *effectors*. The cumulative effect of this system is that the arterial blood gases are closely regulated in a narrow range, and necessary adjustments are made to the system to accomplish this with a low expenditure of energy [2]. The elegance of this system is appreciated when it falters and derangements of PO_2 and PCO_2 occur.

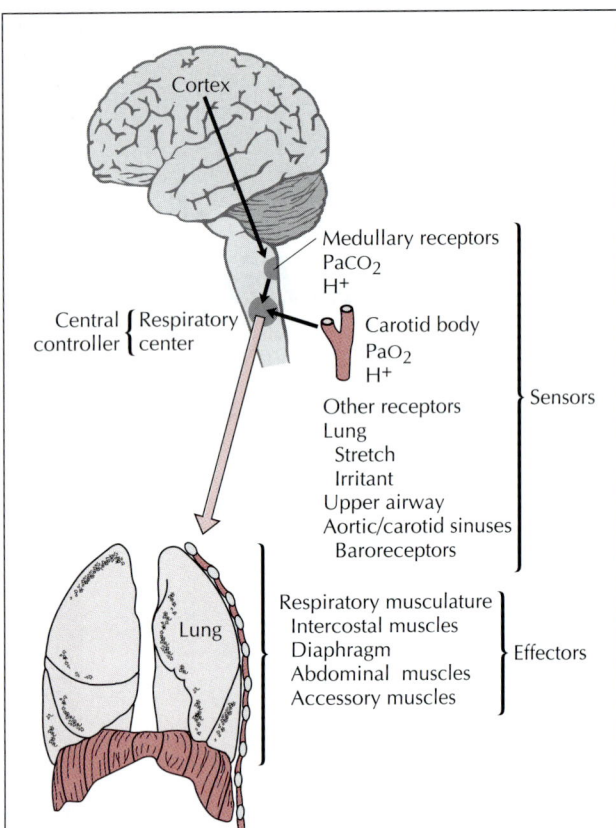

FIGURE 1 Integrative features of the ventilatory control system. (*From* Zwillich [11•]; with permission.)

Hypoventilation

The hallmark of hypoventilation is an elevation of alveolar pressure of carbon dioxide ($PaCO_2$), and hence, of PCO_2. In addition, an obligatory decrease in the PaO_2 occurs. Central to the appreciation of this concept is an understanding of the alveolar ventilation and alveolar gas equations [3]. An inverse relationship exists between alveolar ventilation and PCO_2 such that as alveolar ventilation decreases, PCO_2 increases; thus, hypoventilation occurs when alveolar ventilation is inadequate to remove the carbon dioxide that has been produced by the body.

$$PCO_2 \approx \frac{CO_2 \text{ production (K)}}{\text{Alveolar ventilation}}$$

The alveolar gas equation shows that a direct relationship exists such that 1) as alveolar ventilation decreases and $PaCO_2$ increases, with inspired PO_2 remaining constant, the alveolar PO_2 decreases; and 2) the low PAO_2 can be abolished by increasing the inspired PO_2.

$$PAO_2 = PIO_2 - \frac{PaPA_2}{R}$$

Where $PACO_2$ is alveolar PO_2, PIO_2 is inspired PO_2, R is the respiratory exchange ratio, which is 1. In summary, a decrease of alveolar ventilation by half can cause the $PaCO_2$ to double, and hence, the PaO_2 will be decreased. If the concentration of inspired oxygen is increased, the hypoxemia can be overcome but the hypercapnia will remain (Fig. 2).

Causes

Table 1 lists the causes of hypoventilation. Abnormalities of the respiratory control system may result in depression of the central respiratory drive. Drugs that diminish the drive frequently cause this problem. Central alveolar hypoventilation represents a relatively rare cause of hypercapnia and hypoxemia wherein a central nervous system lesion produces underbreathing as a result of an attenuation of the respiratory drive [4]. Families of people who have an inherited attenuation of the respiratory drive have also been described [5]. Hypothyroidism lowers respiratory drive and is a frequently overlooked cause of hypoventilation. This deficit is reversible with treatment with thyroid hormone [6]. Alternatively, some individuals hypoventilate for unknown reasons (idiopathic alveolar hypoventilation).

An increase in the impediment to breathing, as produced by neuromuscular, chest wall, and airway abnormalities, can cause hypoventilation. Asthma produces hypoventilation only when the forced expiratory volume in 1 second (FEV_1) is decreased to below 20% of normal, as is seen in severe exacerbations [7]. In chronic obstructive pulmonary disease, a FEV_1 of less than 35% or 1.0 L results in carbon dioxide retention [8]. Hypocalcemia, hypophosphatemia, and hypomagnesemia are metabolic derangements that can lead to hypoventilation.

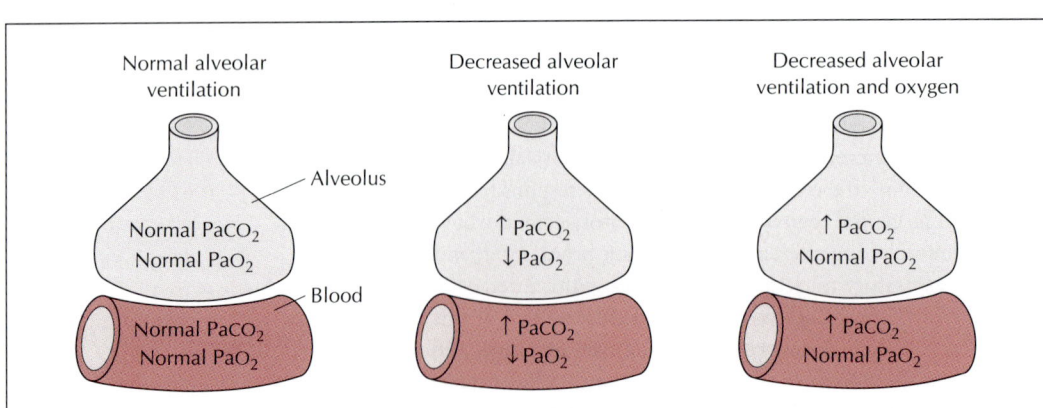

FIGURE 2 Carbon dioxide and oxygen tensions in normal and hypoventilated alveoli and the response to supplemental oxygen.

Table 1 Causes of hypoventilation
Low respiratory drive
Respiratory control abnormality
Depression by drugs (*eg*, morphine, barbiturates, benzodiazepines, anesthetics)
Central alveolar hypoventilation (brain stem disease) (*eg*, encephalitis, trauma, hemorrhage, tumor, stroke)
Familial attenuation of respiratory drive
Idiopathic alveolar hypoventilation
Hypothyroidism
Increased respiratory impediment
Effector (neuromuscular) abnormality
Anterior horn cell disease (*eg*, polio)
Disease of nerves to respiratory muscles (Guillain-Barré, diphtheria, phrenic nerve damage)
Myoneural junction disease (*eg*, myasthenia gravis, anticholinesterase poisoning, curare-like drugs, botulism)
Myopathy (*eg*, muscular dystrophy, other muscle diseases)
Chest wall abnormality
Crushed thoracic cage
Thoracoplasty
Kyphoscoliosis
Airway abnormality
Upper airway obstruction (*eg*, goiter, epiglottitis, tracheal stenosis)
Obstructive lung disease (*eg*, asthma, chronic obstructive pulmonary disease)
Metabolic abnormality
Hypocalcemia
Hypophosphatemia
Hypomagnesemia
Combined low drive and increased impediment
Obesity hypoventilation syndrome
Some chronic obstructive pulmonary disease

Table 2 Clinical features of hypoventilation
Central nervous system
Headache
Somnolence
Decreased cognitive ability
Constricted pupils
Diaphoresis
Asterixis
Coma
Cardiovascular system
Tachycardia
Arrhythmia
Cor pulmonale (late)
Polycythemia

Obesity hypoventilation syndrome is seen in a small number of obese patients and is a reflection of the combination of low respiratory drive and the impediment to respiration created by the body habitus [9]. This combined disorder is also seen in some chronic obstructive pulmonary disease patients.

Clinical Features

Clinical features of hypoventilation are manifested primarily in central nervous system and cardiovascular effects (Table 2). Headache, excessive sleepiness, decreased cognitive function, pupillary constriction, or even coma can result from the elevated carbon dioxide and decreased oxygen. These abnormalities in blood gases cause an increase in brain perfusion, which leads to an increase in intracranial pressure. Diaphoresis resulting from increased sympathetic discharge is often present, and evidence of metabolic encephalopathy may be found with a sign such as asterixis. Hypercapnia and hypoxemia can cause tachycardia, arrhythmia, or cor pulmonale, which results from pulmonary hypertension induced by pulmonary vasoconstriction. Thus, patients with chronic hypoventilation may have an elevated jugular venous pressure, hepatomegaly, or evidence of right ventricular hypertrophy. Polycythemia as a result of chronic hypoxemia may also be seen.

Diagnosis

Diagnosis of hypoventilation lies primarily in the arterial blood gas, which should show elevation of $PaCO_2$ and usually decreased PaO_2. Further evaluation consists of establishing which component of the ventilatory system is in error—the sensors, the central controller, or the effectors. Sleep polysomnography may be helpful in elucidating a cause because hypoventilation is frequently more pronounced during sleep. Assessment of $PaCO_2$ during voluntary hyperventilation is also helpful: if the patient is able to lower the $PaCO_2$ more than 10 mm Hg, a respiratory control center abnormality may be present [10].

Treatment

Treatment of hypoventilation is primarily aimed at alleviating the underlying cause and must be individualized. Resuscitation of the hypoventilating patient is the initial concern. The hypoxemia should be rapidly corrected, and subsequently, the hypercapnia should be addressed. The goals of treatment are increasing the respiratory drive and decreasing the impediment to breathing (Fig. 3) [11•]. If decreased respiratory drive is the cause, measures that reverse this abnormality, such as oxygen therapy, removal of suppressant drugs (*eg*, opiates, barbiturates, and anesthetics), addition of respiratory stimulant drugs (*eg*, progesterone [12]), mechanical ventilation, or phrenic nerve stimulation may be beneficial. If an impediment to breathing exists, bronchodilators, weight loss, or mechanical devices in the form of nocturnal assisted ventilation or continuous positive airway pressure may be useful.

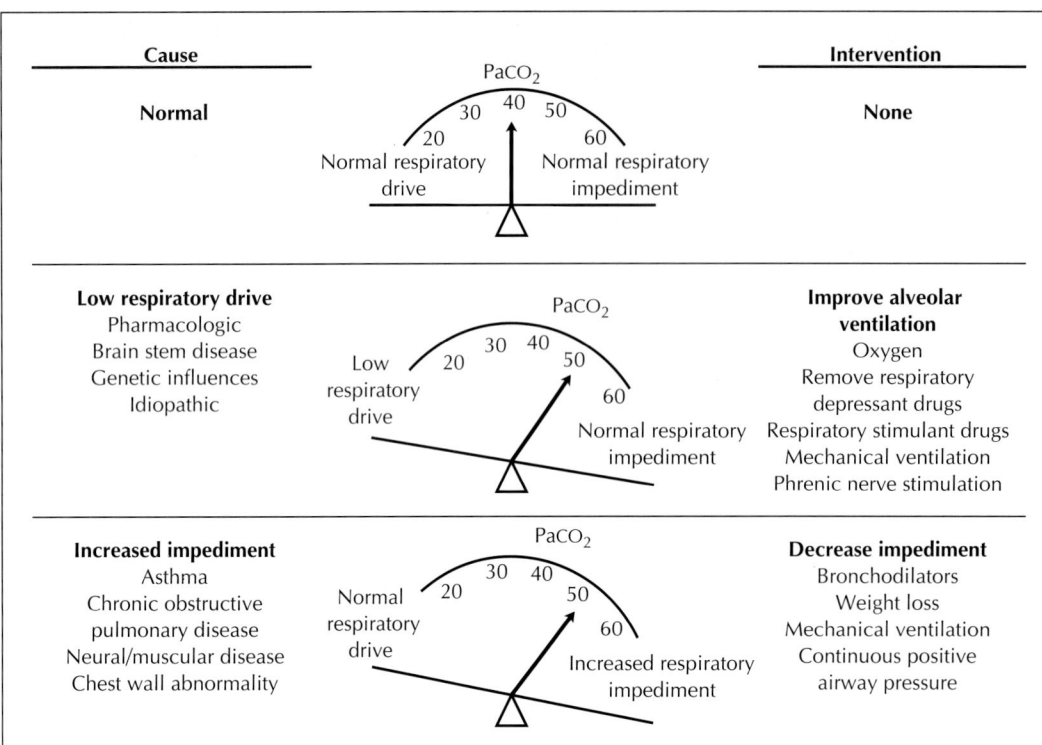

FIGURE 3
Treatment of hypoventilation. COPD—chronic obstructive pulmonary disease. (*From* Zwillich [11•]; with permission.)

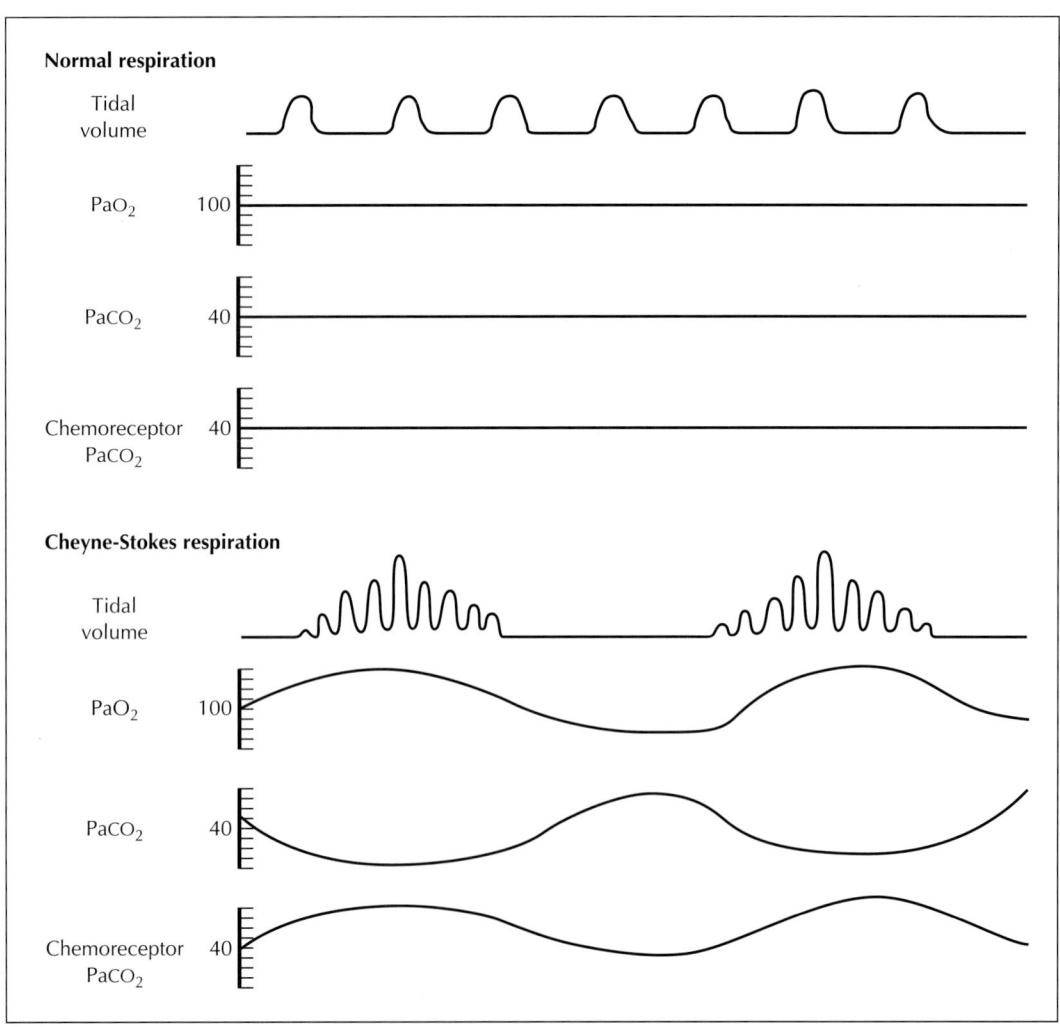

FIGURE 4
Normal and Cheyne-Stokes respirations. Diagrams generated by continuously monitored arterial blood gases and airflow measurement at the mouth/nose.

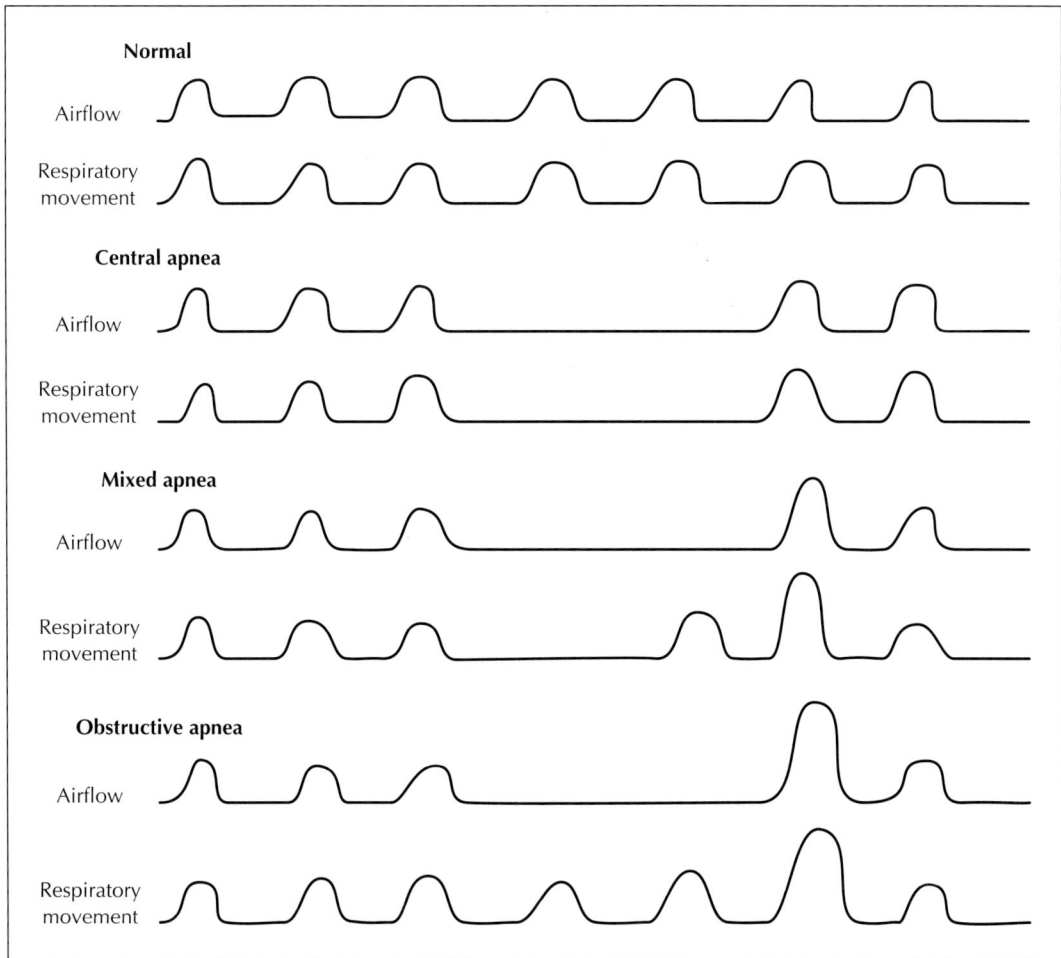

FIGURE 5 Airflow and respiratory movement in normal respiration, central apnea, mixed apnea, and obstructive apnea. Tracings generated by measuring airflow with a transducer at the mouth/nose and a monitoring device placed on the chest to assess respiratory movement.

DISORDERED BREATHING PATTERNS

Normal breathing consists of the rhythmic and orderly cycle of inspiration followed by expiration. At rest, the tidal volume and respiratory rate are fairly constant.

Cheyne-Stokes respiration is a cyclic breathing pattern in which crescendo increases are followed by decrescendo decreases in tidal volume with interspersed periods of apnea (Fig. 4). This breathing pattern is caused by alternating overcorrection and undercorrection of the P_{CO_2} [13•]. Just before the hyperapneic phase, $PaCO_2$ is elevated as a result of preceding apnea, and this phenomenon is sensed by the carotid body. A resultant increase in alveolar ventilation and a subsequent decrease in $PaCO_2$ then occur. With heart failure and decreased cardiac output, the transit time between the lungs and the carotid body is increased, resulting in a delay between the $PaCO_2$ sensed by the chemoreceptor and the $PaCO_2$ of the recently ventilated blood in the lungs. The chemoreceptor senses a $PaCO_2$ other than the actual $PaCO_2$ at that instant, and the ventilatory system continually overventilates and then underventilates. Thus, the abnormal respiratory pattern is born [14•].

Cheyne-Stokes respirations in the child can be a variant of normal; however, in the adult, congestive heart failure, uremia, drug effects, central nervous system damage, and high altitude can produce this pattern.

Treatment of Cheyne-Stokes respiration is directed at the underlying cause. Often no treatment is needed. Oxygen, if administered, can decrease or eliminate the amount of periodic breathing. Diuretics, hemodialysis, and withdrawal of pharmacologic agents may help, depending on the cause of the problem.

OBSTRUCTIVE SLEEP APNEA

Sleep apnea has gained widespread publicity in the media, and frequently patients present to the office with a magazine article, wondering if sleep apnea is the cause of their problems. Apnea is a cessation of respiration for a period of greater than 10 seconds.

During sleep, three forms of apnea have been described: central, mixed, and obstructive (Fig. 5). In *central* sleep apnea, the airway remains patent while an absence of respiratory effort and airflow occurs. (This topic is discussed in a subsequent section.) *Mixed* apnea begins with a central apnea and develops into an obstructive apnea; its clinical features and treatment are quite similar to those of obstructive apnea. *Obstructive* sleep apnea (OSA) occurs as a result of pharyngeal collapse when the dilating neural input to the airway diminishes as a result of sleep onset. Hence, the patient shows respiratory movements without airflow [15].

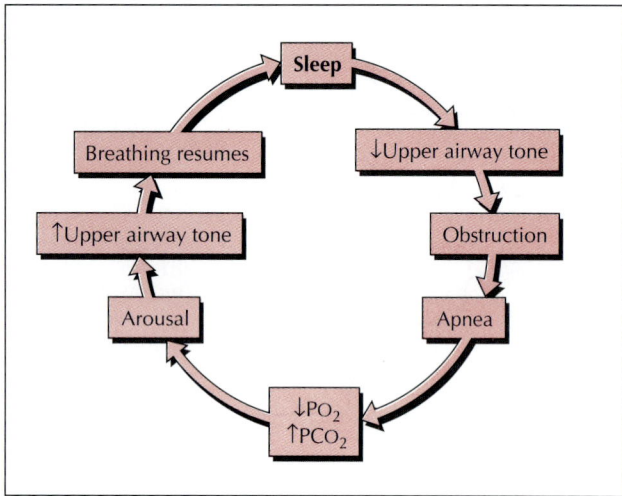

FIGURE 6 Cycle of events in sleep apneic patients. ↑—increase; ↓—decrease.

Complications of OSA include sleepiness, systemic hypertension, coronary artery disease, stroke, cardiac arrhythmia, and pulmonary hypertension [17,18•]. The sleepiness is a danger in itself because patients can fall asleep while driving motor vehicles or operating machinery, thereby injuring themselves and others.

Diagnosis

Diagnosis of OSA lies in clinical identification and then confirmatory testing. Loud snoring and witnessed apneas have been reported to be suggestive of OSA [19]. Sleep disruption results in excessive daytime sleepiness, and morning headaches may be a manifestation of hypercapnia. These patients are frequently obese and may have a short neck, small chin, or large tongue. The nocturnal polysomnogram is the gold standard in the evaluation of such patients. During sleep electroencephalography, eye movements, air flow, respiratory movement, oxyhemoglobin saturation, and muscle tone are recorded and subsequently evaluated to determine the degree to which sleep apnea exists (Fig. 7) [20]. More than 10 apneic events per hour of sleep are usually present in symptomatic patients.

Clinical Features

Clinical features of OSA are primarily related to its effects on the patient's sleep cycle. With each apneic event, arousal from sleep occurs before the resumption of breathing (Fig. 6). During the apneic period, significant hypoxemia and hypercapnia can occur. The net effect of this process is that sleep is disturbed hundreds of times each night. It is easy to understand why these patients awaken from sleep unrefreshed and have excessive daytime somnolence [16]. Snoring results from attempts to breathe against a partially occluded pharynx and may be so loud that the bed partners of these patients move to another room. Most of these patients are overweight men.

Treatment

Treatment of OSA involves various therapeutic modalities. Weight loss in the obese patient is an ideal but sometimes impractical solution. Continuous positive airway pressure in the form of a nasal mask can be used to overcome the pharyngeal obstruction and restore normal respiration during sleep [21]. This form of therapy is effective even in patients who have an open mouth during sleep because the positive pressure causes the soft palate to occlude the oral airway, and thus none of the positive pressure is lost (Fig. 8). Surgical interventions, such as reconstruction of the pharynx (uvulopalatopharyngo-

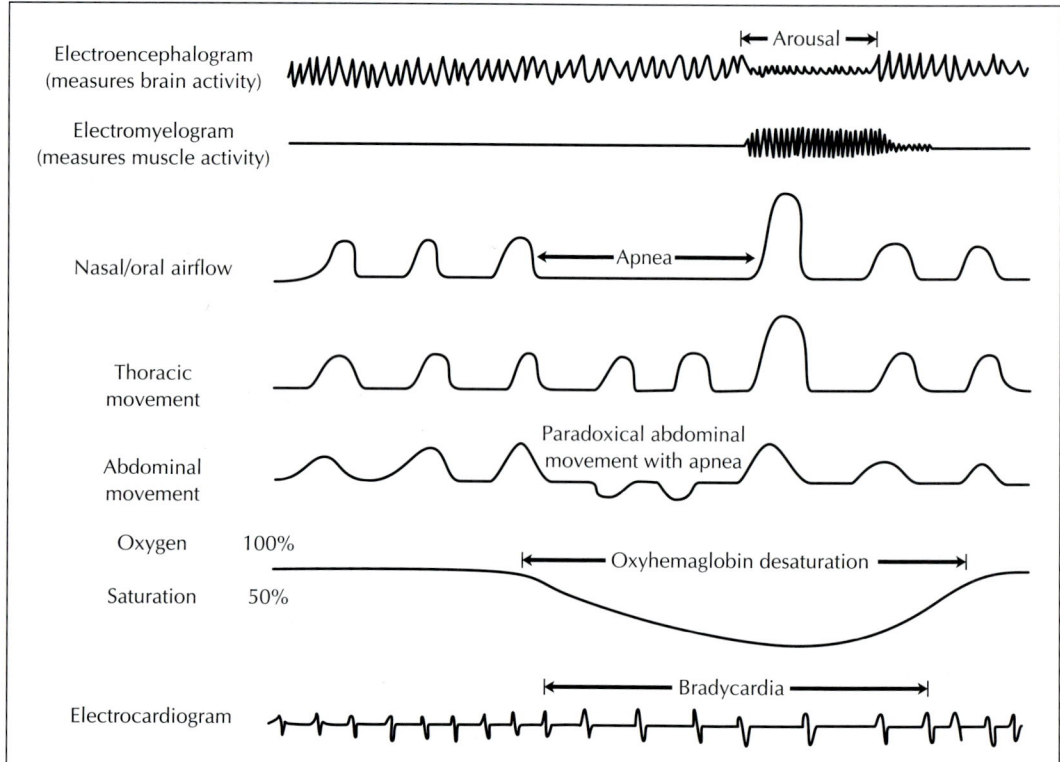

FIGURE 7 Sleep polysomnogram tracing showing an obstructive apnea. Polysomnograms are measured in patients in a sleep laboratory. Surface electrodes are placed on the patient's head (electroencephalogram), muscle (electromyogram), and chest (electrocardiogram). Oxygen sensors are attached to the skin. Airflow is measured at the mouth and nose.

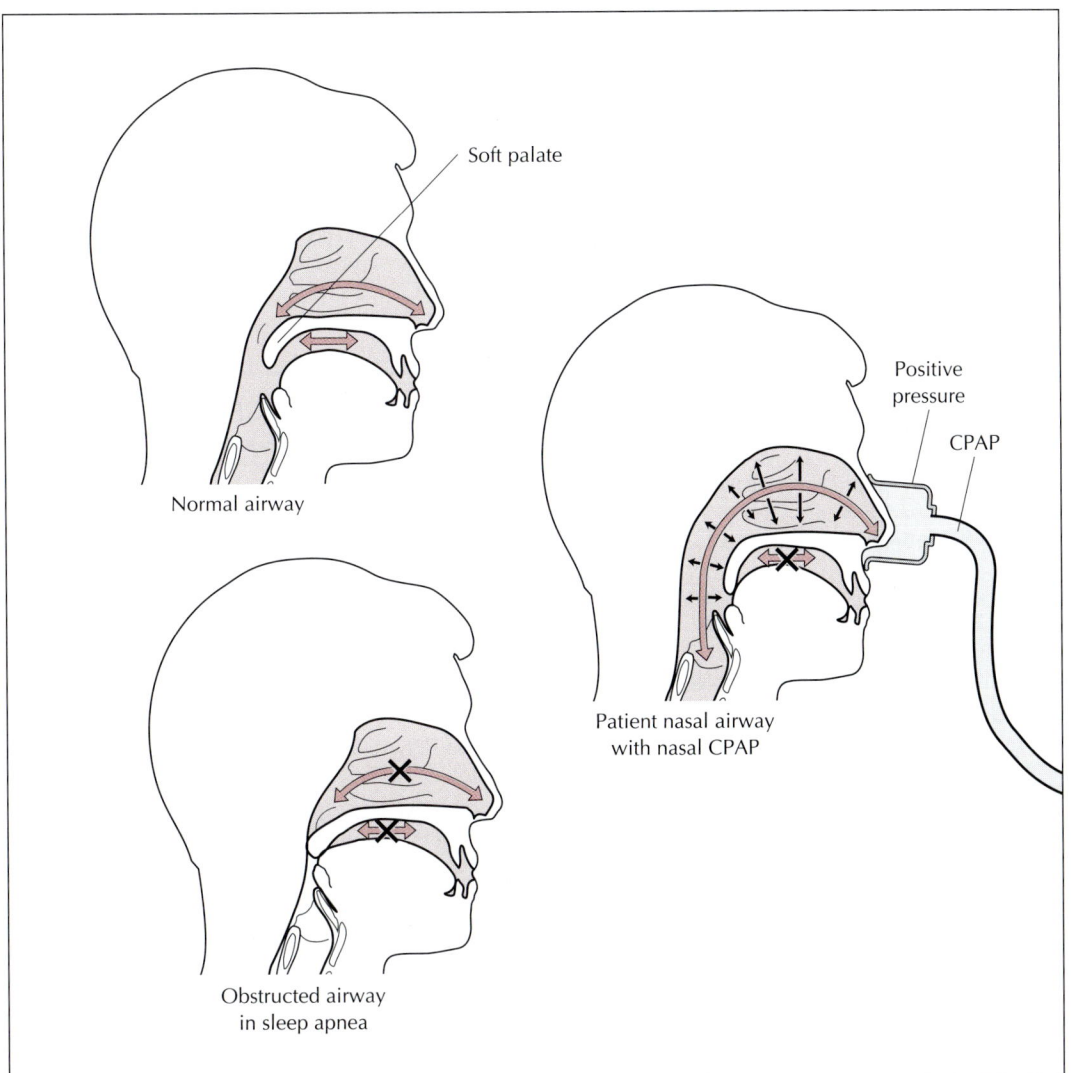

FIGURE 8
Normal upper airway, obstructed airway, and patient nasal airway treated by continuous positive airway pressure (CPAP).

plasty) and tracheostomy, have been used. Patients with OSA should refrain from using any depressant drugs, such as sedative-hypnotics and alcohol, because these agents cause worsening of the pharyngeal obstruction.

CENTRAL SLEEP APNEA

Central sleep apnea is present when air flow stops without airway obstruction. It results from interruption of the central respiratory drive. Only a fraction of patients with sleep apnea have central apneas, and the primary causes of this disorder are neural disorders and congestive heart failure. Insomnia and nocturnal awakenings are the predominant clinical features, rather than excessive daytime sleepiness, snoring, and obesity. Nocturnal polysomnograms in central sleep apnea show the apneas without obstruction or respiratory movement.

Treatment consists of determining an underlying cause, such as congestive heart failure, and treating it. Acetazolamide administration has been used in patients with central sleep apnea as a central stimulant [22]. Oxygen therapy is useful to some patients with central sleep apnea who have episodes of oxyhemoglobin desaturation. Nasal continuous positive airway pressure can be useful in some individuals who snore and resemble OSA patients. Phrenic nerve stimulation has also been reported to be of some benefit.

REFERENCES AND RECOMMENDED READING

Recently published papers of particular interest have been highlighted as:
- Of interest
- • Of outstanding interest

1. West J: Control of ventilation. In *Respiratory Physiology*, edn 4. Baltimore: Williams and Wilkins; 1990:115–129.
2. Berger A, Mitchell R, Severinghaus J: Regulation of respiration. *N Engl J Med* 1977, 297:91–97.
3. West J: Gas exchange. In *Pulmonary Pathophysiology*, edn 4. Baltimore: Williams and Wilkins; 1992:18–40.
4. Colice G, Bernat J: Neurologic disorders and respiration. *Clin Chest Med* 1989, 10:521–543.
5. Moore G, Zwillich C, Battaglia J, *et al.*: Respiratory failure associated with familial depression of ventilatory response to hypoxia and hypercapnia. *N Engl J Med* 1976, 295:861–865.
6. Zwillich C, Pierson D, Hofeldt F, *et al.*: Ventilatory control in myxedema and hypothyroidism. *N Engl J Med* 1975, 292:662–665.
7. McFadden E, Lyons H: Arterial blood gas tensions in asthma. *N Engl J Med* 1968, 278:1027–1032.

8. Lane D, Howell J, Giblin B: Relation between airways obstruction and CO2 tension in chronic obstructive airways disease. *BMJ* 1968, 3:707–709.

9. Luce J: Respiratory complications of obesity. *Chest* 1980, 78:626–631.

10. Zwillich C: The control of breathing in clinical practice: Its significance and assessment. *Semin Respir Med* 1983, 4:247–257.

11.• Zwillich C: Diseases of ventilatory control. In *Textbook of Internal Medicine* edn 2. Edited by Kelley W. Philadelphia: J B Lippincott; 1992:1790–1794.

12. Zwillich C, Natalino M, Sutton F, Weil J: Effects of progesterone in chemosensitivity in normal man. *J Lab Clin Med* 1978, 92:262–269.

13.• Kryger M: Abnormal control of breathing and sleep disorders. In *Introduction to Respiratory Medicine*, edn 2. Edited by Kryger M. New York: Churchill Livingstone; 1990:109–131.

14.• Hanley P, Zuberi N, Gray R: Pathogenesis of Cheyne-Stokes respirations in patients with congestive heart failure: relationship of arterial PCO_2. *Chest* 1993, 104:1079–1084.

15. Sullivan C, Issa F: Obstructive sleep apnea. *Clin Chest Med* 1985, 6:633–650.

16. Coleman R, Roffwarg H, Kennedy S, *et al.*: Sleep-wake disorders based on polysomnographic diagnosis: A national cooperative study. *JAMA* 1982, 247:997–1003.

17. Partinen M, Jamieson A. Guilleminault C: Long-term outcome for obstructive sleep apnea patients: Mortality. *Chest* 1988, 94:1200–1204.

18.• Parish J, Shepard J: Cardiovascular effects of sleep disorders. *Chest* 1990, 97:1220–1226.

19. Fein A, Niederman M, Sklarek H, *et al.*: Can clinical findings predict a positive sleep study? *Am Rev Respir Dis* 1986, 133:A55.

20. Iber C, O'Brien C, Shulter J, *et al.*: Single night studies in obstructive sleep apnea. *Sleep* 1991, 14:383–385.

21. Sullivan C, Issa F, Berthon-Jones M, *et al.*: Reversal of obstructive sleep apnoea by continuous positive airway pressure applied through the nares. *Lancet* 1981, 1:862–865.

22 White D, Zwillich C, Pickett C, *et al.*: Central sleep apnea: improvement with acetazolamide therapy. *Arch Int Med* 1982, 142:1816–1819.

SELECT BIBLIOGRAPHY

Baum G, Wolinsky E, eds: *Textbook of Pulmonary Diseases*, edn 5. Boston: Little, Brown and Company; 1994.

Guilleminault C, Partinen M, eds: *Obstructive Sleep Apnea Syndrome: Clinical Research and Treatment*. New York: Raven Press; 1990.

Kryger M: Symposium on Sleep Disorders. *Clin Chest Med* 1985, 6:553–718.

Murray J, Nadel J, eds: *Textbook of Respiratory Medicine*. Philadelphia: WB Saunders; 1988.

Wiegand L, Zwillich C: Obstructive sleep apnea. *Dis Mon* 1994, 40:197–252.

Wilson J, Braunwald E, Isselbacher K, *et al.*, eds: *Harrison's Principles of Internal Medicine*, edn 13. New York: McGraw-Hill; 1994.

Critical Care 10
Susan K. Pingleton

Key Points
- Acute respiratory failure is classified by arterial blood gases into hypoxemic or hypercapnic respiratory failure.
- The adult respiratory distress syndrome or noncardiogenic pulmonary edema is a form of hypoxemic respiratory failure caused by pulmonary capillary leak from a wide variety of clinical disorders such as sepsis that result in lung injury.
- Management of acute respiratory distress syndrome usually requires mechanical ventilation and therapy of the underlying causes of lung injury.
- Hypercapnic respiratory failure occurs in patients with asthma and chronic obstructive pulmonary disease as well as in patients with normal lungs but with neuromuscular disease.
- Multiple system organ failure is the acquired dysfunction of at least two organ systems in critically ill patients.

Acute respiratory failure (ARF) is a common critical illness affecting hundreds of thousands of patients each year. Hospital admission and intensive care unit (ICU) care is often required for adequate care of the patient with ARF. Acute respiratory failure can be caused by one of many disease states, including chronic obstructive lung disease (COPD), asthma, the adult respiratory distress syndrome (ARDS), and neuromuscular diseases. The clinician should be knowledgeable about the specific disease causing ARF because therapeutic objectives differ for each disease. Acute respiratory failure in the patient with COPD requires different therapeutic approaches than ARF in the patient with ARDS. This chapter provides basic approaches to ARF from diseases causing acute hypercapnic respiratory failure (*ie*, asthma, COPD) as well as acute hypoxemic respiratory failure (*ie*, ARDS). The indications and use of mechanical ventilation in the therapy of ARF are addressed. Complications of critical illness are also discussed.

ACUTE RESPIRATORY FAILURE

Acute respiratory failure is defined as an abnormality of the lung's gas-exchange function, with resultant disturbances in the exchange of oxygen or carbon dioxide between the alveolus and the pulmonary capillaries [1•]. The diagnosis and classification of respiratory failure are made by measurement of arterial blood gases. Acute respiratory failure is diagnosed when the arterial partial pressure of oxygen (PaO_2) is less than 50 mm Hg on room air (inspired oxygen concentration [FIO_2] of 0.21) or when the arterial partial pressure of carbon dioxide ($PaCO_2$) greater than 50 mm Hg on room air. Respiratory failure is classified into either hypoxemia respiratory failure, when the primary abnormality is a decreased oxygen tension, or hypercapnic respiratory failure, when an elevated $PaCO_2$ occurs in addition to hypoxemia (Table 1) [2].

TABLE 1 COMMON ETIOLOGIES OF ACUTE RESPIRATORY FAILURE

Hypoxemic respiratory failure (low PaO_2, normal or low $PaCO_2$)
Adult respiratory distress syndrome
Cardiogenic pulmonary edema

Hypercapnic respiratory failure (low PaO_2, high $PaCO_2$)
Neuromuscular disease
Asthma
Chronic obstructive pulmonary disease

PaO_2—arterial partial pressure of oxygen; $PaCO_2$—arterial partial pressure of carbon dioxide.

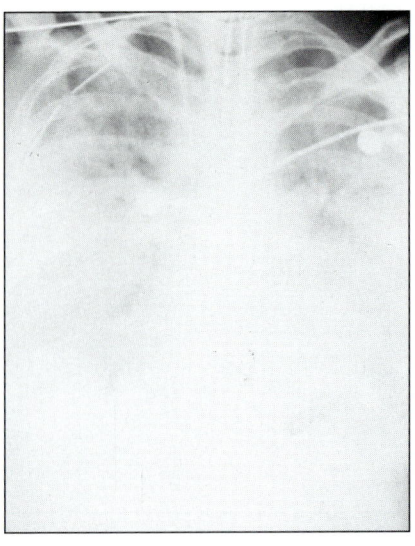

FIGURE 1 Chest radiograph of patient with adult respiratory distress syndrome. The radiograph shows diffuse bilateral alveolar infiltrates and normal cardiac silhouette.

Hypoxemic Respiratory Failure

Acute hypoxemic respiratory failure is characterized by severe hypoxemia that is relatively refractory to oxygen therapy. It is caused by any process that results in alveolar collapse or filling.

Adult respiratory distress syndrome

The adult respiratory distress syndrome (ARDS, or noncardiogenic pulmonary edema) is a form of ARF that occurs in a wide variety of medical, surgical, obstetric and gynecologic, and trauma patients [3]. Adult respiratory distress syndrome is caused by a complex inflammatory cascade that follows a severe systemic or pulmonary injury, resulting in a "leak" of fluid and protein from the pulmonary capillary into the interstitium (and eventually alveolar spaces). It results in a constellation of findings, including severe hypoxemia, diffuse infiltrates on chest x-ray, and decreased respiratory compliance (Fig. 1). In contrast, cardiogenic pulmonary edema, which may present clinically very similarly, is caused by an elevation of cardiac pressures causing pulmonary edema.

Adult respiratory distress syndrome is characteristically associated with a wide variety of clinical disorders that result in lung insult and subsequent lung injury [4•]. Sepsis is the disorder most frequently associated with ARDS; approximately 25% of patients with sepsis develop ARDS [5]. Other causes include hypovolemic shock, acid aspiration, multiple blood transfusion, pancreatitis, and fat emboli.

Clinical Presentation
In the alert patient, the presentation of ARDS (Table 2) is characterized by marked dyspnea and tachypnea with a respiratory rate greater than 30 breaths/min [4•]. Physical examination of the cardiopulmonary system is usually unremarkable in the absence of cardiogenic pulmonary edema. Specifically, abnormal heart sounds or inspiratory crackles are rarely found in patients with ARDS, but these commonly occur in patients with cardiogenic pulmonary edema. Gas exchange is severely altered in ARDS, and severe hypoxemia refractory to oxygen therapy is found commonly. Other characteristic diagnostic features of ARDS include diminished lung compliance and normal pulmonary vascular pressure. In ARDS, compliance decreases and a "stiff" lung results. Normal compliance is greater than 40 mL/cm H_2O but is often less than 20 mL/cm H_2O in ARDS. Bedside pulmonary artery catheterization with the Swan-Ganz catheter is helpful in determining whether the left heart plays a role in the pulmonary edema. The measurement of the pulmonary artery occlusion pressure (wedge) pressure estimates the left ventricular end-diastolic filling pressure. A wedge pressure less than 16 mm Hg in the setting of acute hypoxemic respiratory failure and diffuse alveolar infiltrates strongly suggests ARDS.

Treatment
The majority of treatment in ARDS is supportive, but the underlying cause of lung failure must be searched for and

TABLE 2 CRITERIA FOR THE DIAGNOSIS OF ACUTE RESPIRATORY DISTRESS SYNDROME

Clinical presentation
Tachypnea
Dyspnea

Clinical setting
Direct lung insult (*eg*, aspiration, inhalation, infection)
or
Systemic process with potential for lung injury (*eg*, sepsis, hypovolemic shock)

Radiologic appearance
Five-lobe alveolar infiltrate

Lung mechanics
Diminished lung compliance (< 40 mL/cm H_2O)

Gas exchange
Severe hypoxemia refractory to oxygen therapy

Normal pulmonary vascular pressure

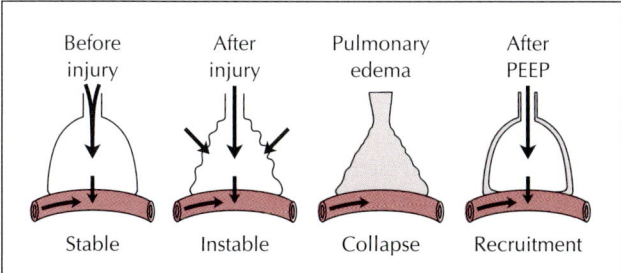

FIGURE 2. Mechanism of positive end-expiratory pressure (PEEP). The application of positive pressure to an injured, collapsed alveolus results in stabilization and, at times, re-expansion of the alveolus, resulting in physiologic and gas exchange improvement.

treated aggressively. The diagnosis and treatment of sepsis are particularly important in this context [6,7]. Initial therapy for all patients includes supplemental oxygen in the highest concentration available, often 100% oxygen. As hypoxemia in ARDS is most often severe and unresponsive to oxygen therapy, elective intubation is required. Ventilator management of ARDS should begin with an FIO_2 of 1.0, tidal volumes of 6 to 7 mL/kg and a respiratory rate of 20 to 28 breaths/min. During the initial phase of ventilatory management, sedation, and often muscle relaxation may be required to minimize oxygen consumption and airway pressures. Positive end-expiratory pressure (PEEP) is begun in ventilated patients who fail to oxygenate adequately with conventional ventilation. The addition of pressure at the end of expiratory phase is made to recruit distal alveoli that have been lost secondary to collapse and/or filling with exudate (Fig. 2). Ventilatory management should be directed at achieving the least possible PEEP that achieves 90% saturation on an FIO_2 of less than 0.6. Circulatory management is directed at reduction of pulmonary capillary wedge pressure to the least level consistent with adequate cardiac output, usually a wedge pressure of less than 16 cm H_2O after subtraction of PEEP. Other supportive therapies include airway maintenance and treatment of any secondary nosocomial infection.

Hypercapnic Respiratory Failure

Hypercapnic respiratory failure is caused by alveolar hypoventilation with decreased elimination of CO_2. Hypoxia also results because the rate of replenishment of alveolar oxygen decreases below the rate of oxygen removal by the pulmonary circulation. Hypercapnic respiratory failure can be subclassified into those disease states occurring in normal lungs and those occurring in abnormal lungs [1•]. Common causes of hypercapnic respiratory failure in abnormal lungs are asthma and COPD, where an increased dead-space ventilation is the primary pathophysiologic mechanism. Hypercapnic respiratory failure occurring in normal lungs is represented by neuromuscular diseases. In these instances, the lungs are normal, but the ventilation is decreased by weak respiratory muscles or inadequate neurologic drive to the muscles.

Acute severe asthma

The hallmark of acute severe asthma is marked obstruction to expiration airflow [8•]. The initial event is contraction of bronchial smooth muscle as a result of an immunologically mediated process, direct stimulation of irritant receptors within the airways, or both. The increased resistance to airflow occurs primarily during expiration, which leads to air trapping and hyperinflation. This airway obstruction, with resulting diaphragmatic muscle fatigue and wasted ventilation, results in carbon dioxide retention.

Clinical presentation

Clinically, acute severe asthma is evaluated by the history, physical examination, and laboratory evaluation of arterial blood gases and pulmonary function tests [9]. Historical features include a history of severe asthma as well as failure to respond to usual asthma medicines. A history of previous hospitalization or frequent emergency room visits are signals of severe disease. Patients requiring the use of corticosteroids as well as those with "brittle" asthma are also at high risk for acute severe asthma.

Evaluation of the patient begins with a general survey of his or her appearance [10]. Use of the accessory muscles and paradoxical thoracoabdominal motion suggests severe disease, as does diaphoresis with extreme dyspnea and the inability to speak more than a few words. Vital signs of respiratory rate greater than 30 breaths/min, heart rate greater than 120 breaths/min, and pulsus paradoxus greater than 18 mm Hg are markers of severe disease. The patient is often hypertensive and tachycardic, and may be unable to lie supine. Absence of audible wheezing in a severely dyspneic patient with asthma suggests insufficient airflow and indicates very severe obstruction. Wheezing may actually appear with treatment in this instance as airflow improves. Arterial blood gases can stage the severity of severe asthma (Table 3). A PaO_2 level less than 60 mm Hg with a $PaCO_2$ level greater than 40 mm Hg suggests severe asthma. Simple spirometry is an important diagnostic aid. Peak flow rates or forced expiratory volume in 1 second (FEV_1) less than 30%, or the failure of the peak flow rates to improve at least 10% with therapy suggest severe disease.

Causes of the exacerbation of asthma should be sought. In adults, exacerbations are commonly caused by infections of the

TABLE 3 CLASSIFICATION OF ASTHMA SEVERITY BY ARTERIAL BLOOD GASES

Stage No.	$PaCO_2$	PaO_2	pH
1	N	N	N
2	↓	N	↑
3	↓	N	↑
4	N	↓↓	N
5	↑	↓↓	↓

$PaCO_2$—arterial partial pressure of carbon dioxide; PaO_2—arterial partial pressure of oxygen; N—normal; ↓—decreased; ↑—increased; ↓↓—markedly decreased.

upper or lower respiratory tract (acute bronchitis commonly), medicine noncompliance, recent steroid taper, pneumothorax, stress, and exposure to known airway irritants. A significant number of exacerbations involve no known insult.

Treatment

After stabilization of vital signs, initial treatment of severe acute asthma includes inhaled β_2-agonists and intravenous corticosteroids [11•]. β_2 selective agents should be given frequently by inhalation every 20 minutes for the first hour. Commonly used agents include albuterol, metaproterenol, pirbuterol, and terbutaline. Subcutaneous β-agonists include epinephrine, which should be avoided in older asthmatics (> 40 years) and anyone with a history of heart disease. Intravenous corticosteroids should be used early in patients with severe asthma. The optimal dose is not known, but doses up of 80 to 125 mg of methylprednisolone every 6 to 8 hours have been recommended. Inhaled steroids are not useful in the treatment of severe asthma, but have a key role in chronic asthma.

Other potential therapy includes anticholinergics, *ie*, inhaled ipratropium bromide. Given the safety and lack of significant side effects associated with ipratropium, it is a reasonable adjunct, especially in patients who have a limited clinical response to β-agonists and corticosteroids. Little objective evidence exists that methylxanthine therapy adds any significant benefit to patients with acute asthma. Additionally, an increase in toxic side effects, including nausea and palpitations, can occur in this setting. In patients treated chronically with methylxanthines who present with acute asthma, it is reasonable to obtain a serum theophylline level, and, if subtherapeutic, to administer aminophylline to a safe therapeutic range. Antibiotics may be useful in patients with acute bronchitis and should be administered to patients with pneumonia.

Supplement oxygen is generally provided by nasal cannula. Oxygenation can be monitored by pulse oximetry and oxygen flow rates titrated to maintain oxygen saturation greater than 90%. In severely obstructed patients, frequent arterial blood gas determinations, in addition to oximetry, are important to document progressive increases in arterial CO_2 that would indicate impending ventilatory failure. Endotracheal intubation and mechanical ventilation may be indicated when progressive hypercapnia or hypoxemia occurs despite maximal medical therapy.

Prognosis

Death from asthma is rare, but it can occur [12]. Features that characterize patients at increased risk for asthma-associated death include age over 55 years, history of ICU admission, intubation, or respiratory acidosis, hospitalization for asthma in the prior year, recent withdrawal from systemic steroids, or psychological or psychosocial problems [13]. One apparent factor in many deaths is delay in initiating appropriate treatment for worsening asthma.

Acute respiratory failure due to neuromuscular disease

Hypercapnic respiratory failure in patients with normal lungs most commonly occurs in association with neuromuscular disease [14]. These patients have abnormal function of the respiratory muscles, the thoracic cage, or the respiratory center, which is responsible for respiratory drive. The causes are listed in Table 4.

Acute respiratory failure in neuromuscular disease is usually precipitated by several factors. Aspiration should be suspected in patients with bulbar involvement, whereas microatelectasis and lower respiratory tract infections are common among all patients with generalized weakness. Pulmonary hypertension and right-sided heart failure should be anticipated in chronically hypoxemic patients. Intercurrent illnesses, such as urinary tract sepsis, pulmonary embolus, or ischemic heart disease may occur. Patients with myasthenia gravis may experience cholinergic crises.

Diagnosis of respiratory muscle weakness is made using the vital capacity (VC) obtained from spirometry [15]. The VC averages approximately 50 mL/kg in normal adults; impaired secretion clearance occurs at a VC level of less than 30 mL/kg, and ventilatory failure occurs at a VC level of approximately 10 mL/kg. Characteristically patients with neuromuscular respiratory failure have a forced vital capacity (FVC) less than 4 to 5 mL/kg body weight, a progressive inability to handle oral secretions, and a cough. An FVC value of less than 1 L in this situation indicates the possible need for mechanical ventilation. Compromised patients are at risk for lobar atelectasis and pneumonia, which can result in hypoxia, hypercapnia, and respiratory failure.

Respiratory failure in patients with neuromuscular disease usually can be treated adequately with supplemental oxygen, coupled with frequent positioning and periodic hyperinflations, or the delivery of PEEP via face mask to improve atelectasis [15]. However, intubation and mechanical ventilation are usually called for if lung volumes and muscle strength have declined to previously mentioned levels. Tracheostomy is indicated for any patient who requires intubation for more than a few weeks.

MULTIPLE ORGAN DYSFUNCTION

Multiple system organ failure (MSOF) refers to the severe acquired dysfunction of at least two organ systems lasting for more than 24 hours in critically ill patients (Table 5) [16]. The

TABLE 4 DISEASE OF NEUROMUSCULAR FUNCTION LEADING TO ACUTE RESPIRATORY FAILURE

Level	Example
Upper motor neuron	Quadriplegia
Lower motor neuron	Poliomyelitis
	Amyotrophic lateral sclerosis
Peripheral neurons	Guillain-Barré syndrome
Myoneural junction	Myasthenia gravis
	Botulism
Respiratory muscles	Muscular dystrophy
	Polymyositis

TABLE 5 CRITERIA FOR ORGAN SYSTEM FAILURE

If the patient has one or more of the following during a 24-hour period, organ system failure exists on that day

Cardiovascular failure
Heart rate ≤ 54 beats/min
Mean arterial pressure ≤ 49 mm Hg
Systolic blood pressure ≤ 60 mm Hg
Ventricular tachycardia and/or fibrillation
Serum pH ≤ 7.24 with $PaCO_2$ ≤ 40 mm Hg

Respiratory failure
Respiratory rate ≤ 5 breaths/min or > 49 breaths/min
$PaCO_2$ ≥ 50 mm Hg
Alveolar-arterial oxygen gradient ≥ 350 mm Hg
Ventilator dependent

Renal failure
Urine output ≤ 479 mL/24 h or ≤ 15 mL/8 h
Serum BUN ≥ 100 mg/100 mL
Serum creatinine ≥ 3.5 mg/100 mL

Hematologic failure
White blood cell count ≤ 1,000 μL
Platelets ≤ 20,000 μL
Hematocrit ≤ 20%

Neurologic
Glasgow coma score ≤ 6 (in absence of sedation)

$PaCO_2$—arterial partial pressure of carbon dioxide; BUN—blood urea nitrogen.

---

most common etiology is shock, most often septic shock. Other causes include pancreatitis, thermal injury, trauma, connective tissue diseases, and liver failure. Each of these processes can activate the host's defense responses, leading to a common final pathway of humorally mediated end-organ damage and failure. The lung is the most common organ to fail in MSOF; ARDS is the most typical pulmonary lesion [7]. Acute renal failure, secondary to acute tubular necrosis, is the renal lesion commonly seen with MSOF. Encephalopathy, mild cardiac depression, bone marrow insufficiency, and liver dysfunction also occur in MSOF, although less commonly. Prognosis of MSOF simply relates to the number of organs involved. As a general guideline, if three of more organ systems have failed for more than 3 days, the patient has an extremely high mortality and is unlikely to survive.

Multiple therapies for MSOF have been evaluated, including corticosteroids and anti-inflammatory drugs such as anti-endotoxin antibodies. Because limited beneficial data are available, prevention of MSOF is essential. Shock should be treated aggressively to avoid tissue hypoxemia and end-organ failure. Organ-specific therapy such as mechanical ventilation, renal dialysis, and nutritional support are indicated while reversible precipitants of MSOF are treated.

SEPTIC SHOCK

Sepsis is defined as the systemic response of a host to infectious organisms or their toxins and is usually signaled by simple abnormalities in the vital signs such as tachycardia, tachypnea, and fever or hypothermia, all occurring on a background of clinically significant infection. The term sepsis syndrome implies progression of simple sepsis to include evidence of end-organ dysfunction or injury [4]. Septic shock is the extreme of sepsis syndrome, in which increasing end-organ dysfunction (lung, kidneys, liver) is associated with reduced blood pressure, usually defined as a systolic pressure of less than 90 mm Hg or a decrease of more than 40 mm Hg from baseline.

The etiology of sepsis is multiple [6]. Organisms that can cause sepsis include not only gram-negative rods, but also gram-negative cocci, gram-positive organisms, mycobacteria, rickettsia, protozoans, viruses, and fungi. Gram-negative rods elaborate endotoxin as part of their cell wall (Fig. 3). Gram-

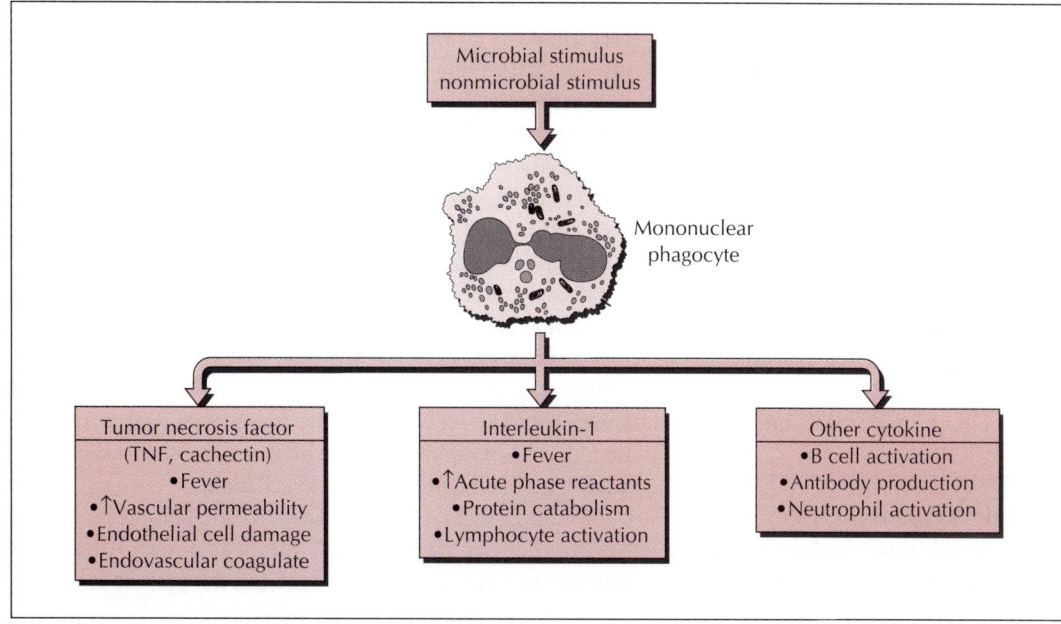

FIGURE 3. In the sepsis syndrome, gram-negative bacterial endotoxins do not act as direct "toxins" but rather as stimuli to host phagocytic cells that mediate the diverse manifestations of sepsis. Among the cytokines produced, tumor necrosis factor (TNF) is probably the most important mediator, directly or indirectly, of many of the major features of sepsis.

positive cocci elaborate a number of toxins, including that responsible for toxic shock syndrome. Other processes such as pancreatitis or burns can cause a syndrome indistinguishable from sepsis, likely through activation of host mechanisms similar to the response to infection.

Clinical Presentation

Patients with sepsis are generally tachycardiac, tachypneic, warm well-perfused, with good capillary refill, bounding pulses, and a wide pulse pressure due mainly to reduction of diastolic pressure. In untreated sepsis, the systolic pressure also drops. Altered mentation and oliguria are not uncommon. In addition, signs of focal infection in lungs, urinary tract, abdomen, central nervous system, joints, and soft-tissue must be sought so as to identify a potential source for sepsis.

Increased blood urea nitrogen and creatinine often accompany sepsis, first with low urinary sodium, then with inappropriately high urine sodium after tubular ischemia has occurred. Early sepsis is accompanied by a respiratory alkalosis. Later, a concomitant anion gap acidosis develops. Hypoxemia occurs when sepsis is caused by pneumonia or complicated by ARDS. Leukocytosis, leukopenia, hypoglycemia, and hyperglycemia are also seen. Disseminated intravascular coagulation and thrombocytopenia are the most common coagulation abnormalities of sepsis.

Treatment

The source of infection must be identified and treated early with antibiotics and surgical drainage when appropriate. Antibiotics are chosen based on Gram stain or culture results of relevant body fluids. Broad coverage of the category of probable pathogenic organisms, based on the clinical and Gram stain data, should be instituted until culture results return, usually 24 to 48 hours later. When all Gram stain and culture data are negative, but the sepsis persists despite appropriate management, noninfectious causes of sepsis syndrome such as thermal injuries, occult liver disease, and pancreatitis should be considered.

Supportive therapy includes aggressive fluid resuscitation. Large volumes of fluid may be required in early septic shock. The quantity and type of fluid used may vary among patients. Crystalloids are most commonly used; packed red blood cells are preferred for volume replacement up to a hematocrit level of 40. When patients do not respond to volume therapy, positive inotropes are administered. Dopamine, dobutamine, and occasionally norepinephrine and phenylephrine are used. Further supportive therapy should include control of fever, treatment of electrolyte disorders, and the coagulopathy of sepsis. Nutritional support is important. Other therapies such as monoclonal anti-endotoxin antibodies have been studied, but without overwhelming demonstration of efficacy at this time.

MECHANICAL VENTILATION

Conventional mechanical ventilation involves the use of positive-pressure devices that inflate the lungs by pushing gas into the upper airways [16]. Indications are multiple, but most commonly relate to progressive hypercapnia or hypoxemia. Acute respiratory acidosis is the primary reason to intubate and ventilate patients, not the absolute level of $PaCO_2$. Other reasons to intubate patients include depressed mental status with a risk for aspiration or trauma to the head and neck region.

Mechanical ventilators produce respiratory flows by generating positive pressures at the airway opening that are cycled with time. Ventilators are of two types: 1) pressure-cycled ventilators, which deliver a preset pressure terminating the breath after a given time or flow rate; and 2) volume-cycled ventilators, which deliver a preset volume. The tidal volume in a pressure-cycled ventilator is determined by respiratory system mechanics. Pressure-cycled ventilation has become more widely used in the ICU with the advent of pressure support ventilation.

Initiation of mechanical ventilation requires choices for several ventilator settings [16]. The first decision is the mode of ventilation. Assist-control ventilation is selected most commonly. The patient can initiate the mechanical breath by generating a small negative intrathoracic pressure (assisted ventilation) or the ventilator will automatically deliver lung inflations at a preset rate if the patient has no spontaneous efforts (controlled ventilation). In synchronized intermittent mandatory ventilation, the machine-delivered breaths are triggered by the patient's inspiratory effort up to a preset rate. Any breaths over this preset rate will be unassisted. Pressure support ventilation may be used as a primary mode of ventilation, but is more commonly used as an adjunct to other modes. In this mode, the patient receives a preset pressure trigger by an inspiratory effort. The breath is terminated when the inspiratory flow, which is determined by the respiratory systemic mechanics, decreases below a given level. The tidal volume is determined by the patient's respiratory system mechanics, such as lung and chest wall compliance.

Mechanical ventilators are commonly set to deliver inflation volumes (tidal volume) of 10 to 15 mL/kg ideal body weight. These volumes can cause overventilation with respiratory alkalosis and the risk of barotrauma. In patients with disease of low lung compliance as determined by high inflation pressures (ie, ARDS), much lower tidal volumes, 5 to 6 mL/kg, should be used. The rate of lung inflation is commonly set between 12 and 16 breaths/min, but nonsedated patients often "overbreathe" and trigger the ventilator at their intrinsic respiratory rate. The inspiratory-expiratory time ratio (I:E) is usually set at 1:3. This allows sufficient time for exhalation and the prevention of air trapping. In patients with slow emptying of air from the lung (eg, obstruction to expiratory airflow, COPD), the I:E ratio may need to be increased further to avoid the development of intrinsic PEEP. The FIO_2 levels should be set high initially, and is usually set at 1.0. It is then decreased rapidly with the goal of using the lowest possible FIO_2 to maintain adequate oxygenation.

Weaning from mechanical ventilation should be undertaken when whatever caused the need for ventilation is improved or eliminated so as enabling the patient to sustain spontaneous ventilation. Various weaning criteria substantiate the patient's ability to breath spontaneously. Methods of weaning include "T-piece" or "tube" weaning, whereby a T-shaped tube is inserted into the ventilator circuit and the patient breathes unassisted for a defined period. Intermittent mandatory ventilation allows the patient to breathe spontaneously with a backup level of ventilation that is progressively reduced in increments until there is no input from the ventilator. Pressure support ventilation allows the delivery of tidal breaths at preset pressures that are reduced as the patient is able to take over more respiratory effort. Limited data are available to conclusively define that one weaning technique is superior to the others. Pressure support ventilation is frequently used in patients with respiratory failure.

MANAGEMENT OF COMPLICATIONS OF ACUTE RESPIRATORY FAILURE

Survival from ARF that requires intubation and mechanical ventilation more often depends on the number and severity of complications related to life support and monitoring interventions than to the actual hypoxemia or hypercapnia. Multiple complications can occur (Table 6) [17]. Pulmonary complications of mechanical ventilation include pulmonary barotrauma. Barotrauma is defined as the presence of extra-alveolar air in abnormal locations. Clinical manifestations include pneumomediastinum, pneumothorax, and pneumoperitoneum. Risk factors include high tidal volumes, high airway pressures, and PEEP. Symptoms are unlikely to be specific, and the diagnosis is usually made by radiograph. Standard methods to reduce the frequency of barotrauma include measures to decrease alveolar inflation and pressures, tidal volumes, and PEEP. Tube thoracostomy is appropriate therapy for pneumothorax.

Complications related to airway management can occur during intubation, as well as during or after mechanical ventilation. If intubation is prolonged, sequelae can include cardiac arrest, seizures, gastric distention, and right mainstem intubation. Complications of endotracheal intubation result from injury to the hypopharynx, larynx, and trachea, and are related to the tube and the cuff. Virtually all patients with intubation for 2 or more days have laryngeal edema, ulceration, and hemorrhage. Stridor occurs in less than 5% of intubated patients. Hoarseness occurs in 75% of patients, but usually resolves in 1 month. Paranasal sinusitis may occur in 24% of intubated patients, especially those intubated with nasal tubes. Various factors are implicated in airway injury, and daily management of the intubated patients is directed at minimizing the likelihood of complications. The duration of "safe" endotracheal intubation before reversion to tracheostomy is not known. If extubation is unlikely after 7 to 10 days of treatment, tracheostomy is considered.

Gastrointestinal complications include gastrointestinal bleeding caused by acute gastric ulceration [17]. The primary mechanisms of ulceration are tissue acidosis or ischemia, which result in impaired mucosal handling of the hydrogen ion already present. The clinical diagnosis of gastrointestinal hemorrhage is made by the appearance of hematemesis, melena, bright red blood via the nasogastric tube, or signs of hypovolemic shock. Severe gastrointestinal bleeding occurs in approximately 5% of medical ICU patients. Bleeding occurs more commonly in prolonged ventilation, especially in patients with ARDS in whom it can be a sign of the MSOF syndrome. Therapy of stress ulceration should correct conditions favoring its development, such as hypoperfusion and acidosis. Prophylactic measures have centered on neutralizing gastric acidity with antacids or decreasing gastric acid secretion with histamine-receptor blockage such as cimetidine or ranitidine. Sucralfate provides protection without reducing levels of gastric acid. Nutrition is also an effective prophylaxis. All therapies except for sucralfate are associated with gastric colonization with the potential for transmission of gastric organisms into the airways with the development of nosocomial pneumonia.

Nosocomial pneumonia is a frequent complication in ventilated patients with respiratory failure [17]. Gram-negative bacilli represent more than 50% of the organisms responsible. Despite exogenous sources for these organisms (invasive monitoring devices, respiratory therapy equipment), most infections result from endogenous sources. The primary pathogenic mechanism of nosocomial lung infection relates to oropharyngeal colonization, with subsequent aspiration and resultant tracheobronchial colonization by gram-negative organisms. In addition, gastric colonization can be a source of organisms found in the airway. The clinical diagnosis of nosocomial pneumonia is very difficult, particularly in patients

TABLE 6 COMPLICATIONS OF ACUTE RESPIRATORY FAILURE

Pulmonary
Barotrauma
Pulmonary emboli
Airway complications

Gastrointestinal
Gastrointestinal hemorrhage
Diarrhea

Cardiovascular
Complications associated with pulmonary artery catheter
Ischemia
Arrhythmias

Nutrition
Malnutrition
Nutritionally associated hypercapnia

Infection
Sepsis
Nosocomial pneumonia

Renal
Acute renal failure

with radiographic infiltrates already present and other potential causes of fever and leukocytosis. For this reason, new techniques such as quantitative cultures of the protected specimen brush or bronchoalveolar lavage fluid are used. Both techniques attempt to bypass upper airway contamination to obtain lower airway secretions for a more acute diagnosis. General strategies aimed at the prevention of nosocomial pneumonia include efforts to improve host-defense mechanisms, as well as measures directed at decreasing airway colonization and bacterial inoculation into the lower airway. Empiric antibiotics are often administered in the setting of clinically suspected nosocomial pneumonia in the ventilated patient, but antibiotics may be ineffective and may increase the rate of serious gram-negative infection. Serious consideration should be given to obtaining quantitative cultures.

The development of renal failure in patients with respiratory failure is an ominous prognostic sign [17]. An early response to oliguria or new increases in blood urea nitrogen and creatinine levels should occur immediately. Common causes of acute renal failure in the ICU include hypoperfusion with prerenal azotemia, acute tubular necrosis, and tubular dysfunction after nephrotoxic drug administration. Obstructive uropathy must always be excluded. Renal ultrasound is an excellent screening test for this possibility. Every patient with renal dysfunction in the ICU should have a careful review of medication history. Therapy of acute renal failure should be directed at its apparent cause.

References and Recommended Reading

Recently published papers of particular interest have been highlighted as:
- Of interest
- •• Of outstanding interest

1.• Ladner A, Pingleton SK: Acute respiratory failure. In *Cardiac and Pulmonary Management*. Edited by Khan MG. Philadelphia: Lea & Febiger; 1993:813–840.
2. Balk R, Bone RC: Classification of acute respiratory failure. *Med Clin North Am* 1983, 67:551–556.
3. Murray JF, Matthay MA, Luce JM: An expanded definition of the adult respiratory distress syndrome. *Am Rev Respir Dis* 1988, 138:720–725.
4.• Marinelli WA, Ingbar DH: Diagnosis and management of acute lung injury. *Clin Chest Med* 1994, 15:517–546.
5. Bone RC: Pathogenesis of sepsis. *Ann Intern Med* 1991, 115:451–456.
6. Martin MA, Silverman HF: Gram-negative sepsis and the adult respiratory distress syndrome. *Clin Infect Dis* 1992, 14:1213–1228.
7. Suchyta MR, Clemmen TP: The adult respiratory distress syndrome: a report of survival and modifying factors. *Chest* 1992, 101:1074–1081.
8.• Leatherman J: Life-threatening asthma. *Clin Chest Med* 1994, 15:453–479.
9. Pingleton SK, Stites S, Wesselius L: Asthma. In *Cardiac and Pulmonary Management*. Edited by Khan MG. Philadelphia: Lea & Febiger; 1993:550–565.
10. British Thoracic Society: Guidelines for management of asthma in adults: acute severe asthma. *Brit Med J* 1990, 301:797–800.
11.• Braman SS, Kaemmerlen JT: Intensive care of status asthmaticus. *JAMA* 1990, 264:366–368.
12. Westerman DE, Benatar SR, Potgieter PD, *et al.*: Identification of the high-risk asthmatic patient: experience with 39 patients undergoing ventilation for status asthmaticus. *Am J Med* 1979, 66:565–572.
13. Weiss KB, Wagener DK: Changing patterns of asthma mortality: identifying target populations at high risk. *JAMA* 1990, 264:1683–1687.
14.• Bergofsky EH: Respiratory failure in disorders of the thoracic cage. *Am Rev Respir Dis* 1979, 119:643–658.
15. Hund EF, Borel CO, Cronblath DR, *et al.*: Intensive management and treatment of severe Guillain-Barré syndrome. *Crit Care Med* 1993, 21:433–446.
16. Matuschak GM: Multiple systems organ failure: clinical expression, pathogenesis, and therapy. In *Principles of Critical Care*. Edited by Hall JB, Schmidt GA, Wood LDH. New York: McGraw-Hill; 1992:613–636.
17. Pingleton SK: Complications of acute respiratory failure. *Am Rev Respir Dis* 1987, 137:1463–1485.

Select Bibliography

Curtis JR, Hudson LD: Emergent assessment and management of acute respiratory failure in COPD. *Clin Chest Med* 1994, 15(3):481–500.

Leatherman J: Life-threatening asthma. *Clin Chest Med* 1994, 15(3):453–479.

Marinelli WA, Ingbar DH: Diagnosis and management of acute lung injury. *Clin Chest Med* 1994, 15(3):517–546.

Morris AH: Adult respiratory distress syndrome and new modes of mechanical ventilation: reducing the complications of high volume and high pressure. *New Horizons* 1994, 2(1):19–33.

ENDOCRINOLOGY AND METABOLIC DISEASE

IV

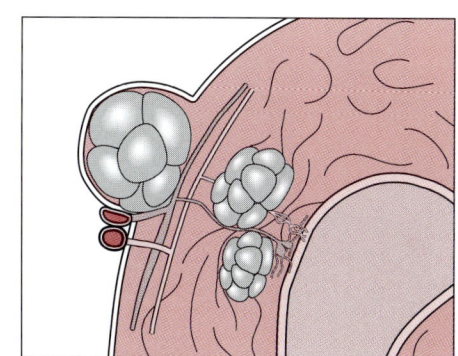

Section Editor
Stanley G. Korenman

Endocrinology can be thought of as the science of biological communication using hormones as chemical mediators of information transfer. This encompasses study of the molecular and cell biology of signalling, signal transduction, and genetic defects underlying endocrine disorders, in addition to classical endocrine physiology. Some clinicians might find the complexity of the new biology confusing, especially if they have no background in basic research.

In this section of *Current Practice of Medicine*, we deal with the clinical endocrine-related problems facing primary care physicians and endocrinologists, with the goal of helping them with the diagnosis and management of their patients. The authors describe the impact of new developments without dwelling excessively on the underlying scientific base of these advances. New procedures such as octreotide scanning and n-telopeptide assessment are described, as well as the potential impact of new treatments, such as alendronate.

Several chapters focus on presenting complaints rather than on specific endocrine organs. For example, chapters topic include vaginal bleeding, secondary amenorrhea, male reproductive problems, hypertension, and abnormal calcium concentrations. Focus also is placed on the rapidly growing geriatric population, with a chapter on special presentations of endocrine disorders on the elderly.

The authors have made an effort to provide practical, cost-effective, and definitive methods of investigating possible endocrine problems using well-reasoned algorithms when appropriate.

This text will be updated regularly. We welcome comments from readers as to content and approach. I may be reached at skorenma@med1.medsch.ucla.edu and am very interested in having a dialogue with colleagues on the front lines.

Neuroendocrinology
Myron Miller

...mon clinical entities, occurring most often
...blished by appropriate diagnostic studies.
...ected by hormonal replacement therapy.
...ten results from central nervous system
...ny common drugs.
...mia requires careful monitoring of serum
...e disturbances may be the presenting
...rs requires intervention by a team
...nologist, psychiatrist, and nutritionist.

...the many clinical disorders of the neuroen-
...alance and disorders of eating. Each disor-
...take (*ie*, water and food). The associated
...mary structural or functional alteration in
...lved in neuroendocrine regulation or may
...alterations resulting from systemic events

...ay arise as a result of disordered synthesis,
...antidiuretic hormone (vasopressin) or as a
...such as the kidney or gastrointestinal tract.
...res of dehydration, plasma volume deple-
...excretion rarely presents with edema, but
...emia is common.

...g, anorexia nervosa and bulimia, are not
...function but produce a variety of neuroen-
...the weight loss and associated nutritional
...cal manifestation of the neuroendocrine
...tion to the underlying eating disorder.

...Y WATER BALANCE

...Body Water

...and tonicity of the extracellular fluid compartment in the normal individual is maintained in a narrow range through the actions of the neurohypophysial
antidiuretic hormone, the cardiac atrial natriuretic hormone, thirst perception, and
the excretory function of the kidney. Antidiuretic hormone is regulated by plasma
tonicity, plasma volume, and blood pressure; through its action on the kidney, it

TABLE 1 DIFFERENTIAL DIAGNOSIS OF HYPOTONIC POLYURIA

Antidiuretic hormone-deficiency states	Antidiuretic hormone-resistant states	Primary polydipsia
Idiopathic and familial diabetes insipidus	Hereditary nephrogenic diabetes insipidus	Psychogenic
Head trauma	Spontaneous nephrogenic diabetes insipidus	Hypothalamic disease
Neurosurgical procedures	Acquired antidiuretic hormone resistance	Drug-induced
Tumor (primary and metastatic)	Renal tubular disease	**Osmotic diuresis**
Cerebral anoxia	Potassium deficiency	Glucose (Diabetes mellitus)
Granulomatous disease of hypothalamus	Hypercalcemia	Sodium
Histiocytosis	Drug-induced	Chronic renal disease
Sarcoidosis	Lithium	Diuretic-induced
Tuberculosis	Demethylchlortetacycline	Excessive intake
Pregnancy (vasopressinase production)		Mannitol
Hypothalamic osmoreceptor failure		
Central autonomic insufficiency		

results in water reabsorption. Atrial natriuretic hormone secretion is increased primarily in response to increase in intraatrial pressure and acts on the kidney to increase sodium excretion. Thirst perception is affected by plasma tonicity and intravascular volume with resultant change in water-seeking behavior. The ability of the kidney to respond to antidiuretic hormone and to atrial natriuretic hormone is influenced by renal blood flow, glomerular filtration rate, and the integrity of tubular function. Alterations in any of these components can result in derangement of extracellular fluid volume or plasma tonicity and is usually reflected by changes in serum sodium concentration [1•].

Diabetes Insipidus

The hypotonic polyuria characteristic of diabetes insipidus is a consequence of inadequate antidiuretic hormone action on the distal tubule and collecting duct of the kidney, either as a consequence of impaired antidiuretic hormone synthesis or release from the neurohypophysial system (central or hypothalamic diabetes insipidus) or as a consequence of impaired ability of the kidney to respond to the hormone (nephrogenic diabetes insipidus).

Causes of diabetes insipidus

Impaired ability to synthesize or release antidiuretic hormone can be the consequence of many disorders affecting the central nervous system (Table 1). In childhood and early adult years, idiopathic hypothalamic failure is common and in a small percentage of cases, may result from a defective gene for vasopressin that is inherited in an autosomal dominant fashion [2]. During pregnancy, a transient form may develop that has been attributed to high circulating levels of vasopressinase produced by the placenta with resultant degradation and inactivation of vasopressin in the blood [3]. The presence of diabetes insipidus must always raise the possibility of tumor or granulomatous disease involving the hypothalamus or posterior pituitary. Head trauma or surgery in the area of the hypothalamus or pituitary can result in sudden onset of diabetes insipidus, which may be transient or partial in 50% to 60% of cases and accompanied by defects in anterior pituitary function [4].

Failure of hypothalamic osmoreceptors to stimulate antidiuretic hormone release can result in diabetes insipidus, even though there may be adequate amounts of antidiuretic hormone in the neurons of the supraoptic and paraventricular nuclei. When there is an accompanying defect in thirst perception, the patient is at high risk of development of severe volume depletion and hypernatremia. Rarely recognized is the antidiuretic hormone deficiency that can accompany central autonomic insufficiency (multisystem atrophy, Shy-Drager syndrome) and clinically manifests by recumbent polyuria or a nocturnal polyuria. This disorder is most common in the elderly [5].

Nephrogenic diabetes insipidus may be congenital or acquired. The congenital form is rare, usually inherited, most commonly affects males, and has been linked to a defect in the renal vasopressin receptor resulting from an abnormal gene for the vasopressin receptor located on the X chromosome [6]. Acquired nephrogenic diabetes insipidus is more common and can occur as a result of the factors listed in Table 1.

High urine solute excretion can result in an obligatory renal water loss with polyuria and consequent increased thirst and polydipsia. This occurs most commonly with uncontrolled diabetes mellitus with glycosuria. Increased urinary sodium excretion can produce an osmotic diuresis and result from chronic renal disease, increased sodium intake, or the use of diuretic agents.

Diagnosis

Impaired ability of the kidney to conserve water results in polyuria, increased thirst, and polydipsia. The urine is pale and can range in amount from 2 to 3 L to as high as 25 L per 24 hours. Urinary frequency and nocturia may be as frequent as every 30 to 60 minutes. Cold fluids are usually the preferred means of quenching thirst but fluid intake rarely is adequate to offset urinary losses. Thus, the patient is usually mildly dehydrated, which may be reflected by hypernatremia, increased plasma osmolality, and elevation of the serum blood urea nitrogen and creatinine, whereas the urine remains dilute as reflected by urine osmolality. If access to fluids is impeded, severe dehydration with weakness, fever, dry mucous membranes, tachycardia, and orthostatic hypotension can rapidly develop.

Table 2. Response to Water Deprivation Test

Clinical condition	Maximum Uosm at plateau, mOsm/kg	Change in Uosm after vasopressin, %	Posm at plateau, mOsm/kg
Normal	764±212*	<5	289±7
Partial DI	438±116	>9	294±4
Severe DI	168±59	>50	306±12
Nephrogenic DI	<150	<45	302–320
Primary polydipsia	696±190	<5	>288
High-set osmoreceptor	>600	<5	>295

*Values are mean ± SD.
DI—diabetes insipidus.
Adapted from Miller *et al.* [7]; with permission.

In the majority of patients, the classification into central or nephrogenic diabetes insipidus, as well as the level of severity, can be determined by means of a structured dehydration test (Table 2) [7,8].

The intravenous infusion of hypertonic saline can be used to recognize the patient with a high-set osmoreceptor who fails to release antidiuretic hormone at normal levels of plasma osmolality and whose intact thirst perception prevents plasma osmolality from rising to a value high enough to trigger antidiuretic hormone release, so long as there is access to fluids. In this circumstance, infusion of 5% saline to achieve plasma osmolality above normal (*ie*, in excess of 294 mOsm/kg) will result in antidiuresis characterized by a sudden fall in free water clearance and rise in urine osmolality [8].

Measurement of vasopressin in blood or urine along with simultaneous plasma osmolality following water deprivation or hypertonic saline infusion may be of use in some patients (Fig. 1) [9]. Inadequate rise in plasma vasopressin is characteristic of central diabetes insipidus whereas elevated values are seen in nephrogenic diabetes insipidus.

A clinical disorder that may be difficult to differentiate from diabetes insipidus is primary polydipsia, the condition resulting from chronic overingestion of fluids. These patients often have a history of emotional disturbances including psychosis. The disorder can also be a manifestation of central nervous system dysfunction with increased thirst perception. Typically, polyuria and polydipsia are erratic and may not be accompanied by nocturia. Serum sodium or plasma osmolality may be low during episodes of polyuria, pointing to excessive fluid ingestion as the causative mechanism. A sufficiently long period of water deprivation will result in a normal response to this test procedure (Table 2).

Recent studies have shown that T_1-weighted magnetic resonance imaging may be helpful in establishing a diagnosis of diabetes insipidus. In normal subjects, the neurohypophysis is seen as a hyperintense signal whereas this signal is absent in the patient with central diabetes insipidus [10].

Treatment

When a diagnosis of central diabetes insipidus has been established, treatment is based on providing hormone replacement (Table 3). When the onset of diabetes insipidus has been acute, such as may occur following head trauma or surgery in the area of the pituitary or hypothalamus, treatment may be initiated with aqueous vasopressin given subcutaneously in doses of 5 to 10 U every 3 to 6 hours. The short duration of action of aqueous vasopressin allows recognition of return of endogenous neurohypophysial function, as may often occur in this group of patients. Acute diabetes insipidus is now usually treated with the vasopressin analog desmopressin acetate,

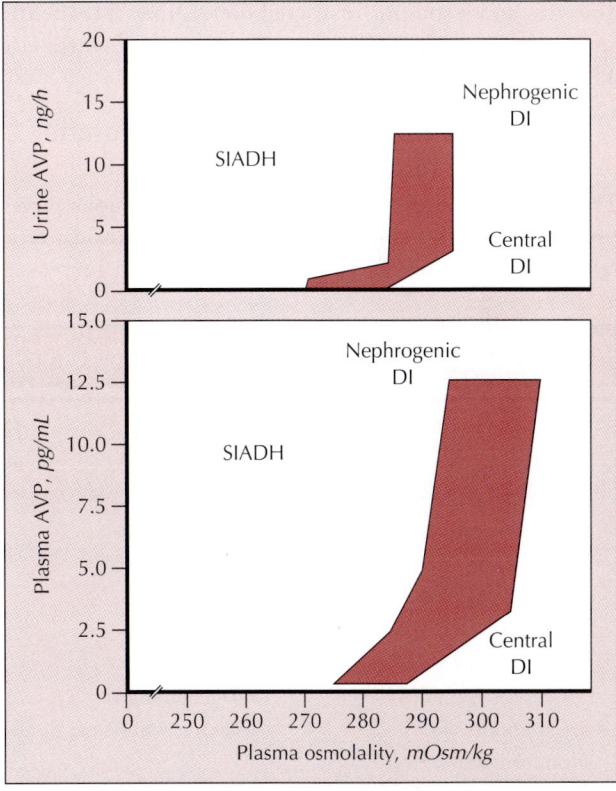

Figure 1 Relationship of plasma and urinary arginine vasopressin (AVP) to plasma osmolality in healthy subjects. The shaded areas include values from the water-loaded state, normal hydration, and dehydrated state. Regions shown are those in which values usually occur in patients with diabetes insipidus (DI), nephrogenic DI, and syndrome of inappropriate antidiuretic hormone secretion (SIADH). *From* Miller [23]; with permission.

which has enhanced and prolonged antidiuretic activity and is devoid of pressor activity [11]. The onset of antidiuresis is evident in 15 to 30 minutes. Attention must be paid to the type and volume of fluid being given to avoid volume overload or hyponatremia when desmopressin acetate is used. Thus, serum sodium or osmolality measurement serves as a useful guide to assessment of volume status. Each dose of desmopressin acetate is given only when there is return of polyuria as evidence that diabetes insipidus is still present.

The majority of patients with persistent or established diabetes insipidus achieve control of polydipsia and polyuria with two daily doses given at 12-hour intervals. Daily monitoring of body weight and periodic measurement of serum sodium are helpful means of assuring that fluid intake is appropriate. Patients with partial degrees of antidiuretic hormone deficiency may respond to treatment with several orally administered nonhormonal drugs that have the ability to stimulate antidiuretic hormone release or to enhance antidiuretic hormone action on the kidney (Table 3) [12].

The patient with nephrogenic diabetes insipidus will not respond to hormone replacement therapy. However, reduction in urine volume can be achieved by producing sodium depletion with associated decrease in intravascular volume and resultant increased renal tubular water and sodium reabsorption. This can be accomplished by administration of thiazide diuretics and a sodium-restricted diet. Other therapeutic approaches include amiloride or prostaglandin synthetase inhibitors (Table 3).

Syndrome of Inappropriate Antidiuretic Hormone Secretion

The syndrome of inappropriate antidiuretic hormone secretion (SIADH) is a consequence of increased antidiuretic hormone action on the kidney resulting from increased hormone in the circulation or enhanced renal tubular responsiveness to antidiuretic hormone that leads to water retention and hyponatremia. The excessive hormone action is the result of nonphysiologic stimuli for antidiuretic hormone release or of altered sensitivity of the renal vasopressin receptor.

Causes

In the middle-aged person, SIADH most commonly results from autonomous release of antidiuretic hormone from tumors where it is produced and released, with small cell carcinoma of the lung accounting for 80% of such patients. Other malignancies and inflammatory diseases of the lung that can lead to SIADH are listed in Table 4.

Almost any central nervous system disorder—including vascular, traumatic, infectious, inflammatory, and neoplastic—can result in increased antidiuretic hormone release with consequent SIADH [13]. This category of cause is especially common in the elderly, where the syndrome of inappropriate antidiuretic hormone secretion may be present in as many as 8% of community-residing persons and in more than 20% of hospitalized or nursing home patients. Drugs are another common cause of SIADH in which there is a special predilection for the elderly [12]. Exposure to general anesthetics can lead to SIADH in the postoperative period. This circumstance appears to be most common in premenopausal women who may experience sudden onset of severe hyponatremia leading to hypoxic encephalopathy, permanent brain damage, and death [14]. The obstetric patient who is given large amounts of oxytocin can experience water intoxication and hyponatremia as a result of the intrinsic antidiuretic activity of this hormone.

Diagnosis

The cardinal features of SIADH are dilutional hyponatremia with urine osmolality inappropriately concentrated and usually

Table 3 Treatment of diabetes insipidus

Agent	Dose	Duration of action, h	Indication
Hormonal replacement			
Aqueous vasopressin	5–10 units, sc	3–6	Short-term treatment of acute onset DI
Lysine vasopressin (Lypressin)	2–4 units, in	4–6	Short or long-term treatment of established DI
DDAVP (Desmopressin)	5–20 µg, in	12–24	Short-term treatment of acute onset DI and
	2–4 µg, sc	12–24	long-term treatment of established DI
ADH releaser/enhancer			
Chlorpropamide	200–500 mg/d	–	Long-term treatment of established partial DI
Clofibrate	500 mg/4 times per d	–	Long-term treatment of established partial DI
Nonhormonal action			
Thiazide diuretic			
Hydrochlorothiazide	50–100 mg/d	–	Long-term treatment of nephrogenic DI
Chlorthalidone	50 mg/d	–	Long-term treatment of nephrogenic DI
Prostaglandin inhibitor			
Indomethacin	1.5–3 mg/kg body weight, 2–3 times/d	–	Long-term treatment of nephrogenic DI
Amiloride	10 mg/2 times per d	–	Long-term treatment of nephrogenic DI

DI—diabetes insipidus; in—intranasal; sc—subcutaneous.

Table 4. Causes of Syndrome of Inappropriate Antidiuretic Hormone Secretion

Malignancy with ectopic hormone production
Small cell carcinoma of lung
Pancreatic carcinoma
Thymoma
Lymphosarcoma, reticulum cell sarcoma, Hodgkin's disease

Pulmonary disease
Pneumonia
Lung abscess
Tuberculosis

Central nervous system disorders
Trauma
Tumor
Infectious
Vascular
Acute intermittent porphyria
Lupus erythematosus

Drugs
Chlorpropamide
Vincristine
Vinblastine
Cyclophosphamide
Carbamazepine
Thiazide diuretics
Narcotics
General anesthetics
Tricyclic and serotonin uptake inhibitor antidepressants
Oxytocin

Other
Hypothyroidism
Positive pressure breathing

From Miller [8]; with permission.

---

greater than that of plasma, urinary sodium excretion greater than 20 mEq/L, and absence of edema [13]. Symptoms range from asymptomatic to mild in patients with minimal hyponatremia to weakness, lethargy, and confusion in patients with greater hyponatremia—generally less than 130 mEq/L. In patients with severe hyponatremia, often 115 mEq/L or less, further central nervous system symptoms may develop including convulsions and coma. Death may result from acute cerebral edema.

Routine laboratory measurements may provide support for the presence of dilutional hyponatremia such as low levels of serum blood urea nitrogen, creatinine, albumin, and uric acid. Serum osmolality is reduced whereas urine osmolality remains inappropriately concentrated.

The diagnosis of SIADH requires the exclusion of disorders that may have associated impairment in water excretion such as congestive heart failure, renal or hepatic disease, adrenal insufficiency, and hypothyroidism. Clinical evaluation must include history of drug use and be directed toward the possibility of underlying processes such as central nervous system, malignant, or infectious disease.

Additional support for the diagnosis of SIADH may be gained from an oral water load test in which administration of 20 mL/kg body weight of water will, in normal persons, result in excretion of greater than 80% of the load in the ensuing 5 hours along with dilution of the urine to less than 100 mOsm/kg (Table 5) [1]. Patients who fail to excrete the water load in a normal fashion and who have no other apparent cause of impaired water excretion can be considered to have SIADH. The test should not be done until the patient is free of symptoms of hyponatremia and the serum sodium before giving the water load is at least 125 mEq/L.

Measurement of plasma and urinary vasopressin may be of value in establishing the diagnosis in some patients (Fig. 1). Levels of vasopressin must be interpreted in relationship to the simultaneous serum osmolality, which should reveal failure of vasopressin levels to fully suppress in the presence of hypo-osmolality.

Treatment

The approach to management of the hyponatremia resulting from SIADH is dependent upon the symptomatic state of the individual and the rapidity with which the symptoms have developed (Table 6) [15,16•]. The onset over a period of 24 to 48 hours of confusion, stupor, or convulsions requires prompt implementation of therapy with the objective to increase serum sodium to approximately 125 mEq/L at the rate of 1 to 2 mEq/L per hour. This can be achieved by the intravenous administration of 75 to 150 mL of 3% saline solution per hour for 4 to 6 hours with frequent monitoring of serum sodium concentration. Correction beyond a level of approximately 125 mEq/L may be dangerous and lead to central pontine myelinolysis, a disorder that can lead to permanent brain damage or death. The risk is reduced if the rise in serum sodium does not exceed 12 mEq/L and is less than 125 mEq/L in the first 24 hours of therapy. Restoration of serum sodium to normal

---

Table 5. Response to Oral Water Load Test, 20 mL/kg Body Weight

Clinical condition	Minimum Uosm, mOsm/kg	Water load excreted in 5 h, %	Posm prior to water load, mOsm/kg
Normal	<100	>80	284–292
SIADH	>100	<80	<284*
Low set osmoreceptor	<100	>80	>284

*Posm may be normal if treated by fluid restriction prior to test.
SIADH—syndrome of inappropriate antidiuretic hormone secretion.
From Miller [8]; with permission.

TABLE 6 MANAGEMENT OF HYPONATREMIA RESULTING FROM SIADH		
Treatment modality	Mechanism of action	Potential adverse complications
Acute		
IV 3% saline solution 300–500 mL over 4–6 h, followed by 100 mL/h	Elevation of serum sodium Reduction of cerebral edema	Cerebral pontine myelinolysis Congestive heart failure
IV furosemide, 1 mg/kg body weight	Increased free water excretion in excess of sodium excretion	Hypokalemia, hypomagnesemia
Chronic		
Correction of underlying cause	Removal of stimulus for water retention	—
Water restriction, 800–1000 mL/24 h	Reduction of extracellular body water	Thirst stimulation
Butorphanol, 4 mg 2 times per day	Inhibition of ADH secretion	CNS effects: confusion, hallucination
Lithium carbonate, 600–1200 mg/d	Inhibition of ADH action via adenylate cyclase-cyclic AMP	CNS effects: confusion, dysarthria
Demeclocycline, 600–1200 mg/d	Inhibition of ADH action via adenylate cyclase-cyclic AMP	Azotemia, photosensitivity Nephrotoxicity in patients with hepatic disease or congestive heart failure
ADH inhibitors (not yet clinically available)	Competitive antagonism at renal V2 receptor	None known

ADH—antidiuretic hormone; CNS—central nervous system; SIADH—syndrome of inappropriate antidiuretic hormone.
From Miller [15]; with permission.

should not be undertaken within the first 48 hours of treatment. In patients with severe central nervous system symptoms and serum sodium of less than 105 mEq/L, simultaneous administration of intravenous furosemide in a dose of 1 mg/kg body weight may be of benefit. In this circumstance, monitoring for the possibility of diuretic-induced hypokalemia and hypomagnesemia will be necessary. After serum sodium has reached the desired level, further intravenous fluid should be in the form of 0.9% saline with monitoring of total fluid intake to avoid recurrence of hyponatremia.

Chronic hyponatremia, especially when asymptomatic or with mild symptoms (*ie*, lethargy and fatigue) can be treated more conservatively. If possible, identifiable causative factors should be addressed, such as cessation of a drug, treatment of infection, evacuation of a subdural hematoma, recovery from a cerebrovascular event, or treatment of hypothyroidism or glucocorticoid deficiency. The primary therapy of chronic SIADH is fluid restriction, which may need to be as low as 800 to 1000 mL per 24 hours and which may be difficult to sustain, especially if thirst is stimulated. In this circumstance, the tetracycline antibiotic demeclocycline in doses of 600 to 1200 mg daily can increase renal water by inhibiting the action of antidiuretic hormone on the kidney [17]. Onset of action usually is evident in 5 to 14 days and is recognized by a drop in urine osmolality and a corresponding increase in serum sodium concentration. If used chronically, renal function must be monitored because the drug can cause asymptomatic azotemia, which is reversible with discontinuation of demeclocycline.

DISORDERS OF EATING

Patients with either anorexia nervosa or bulimia may be seen by the internist or endocrinologist because of the neuroendocrine disturbances associated with these disorders and their consequent clinical expression, the most common of which is amenorrhea [18].

Anorexia Nervosa
Clinical features

This disorder most commonly affects late-adolescent and young-adult females in whom the frequency may be from 1% to 3%. Characteristically, there is self-induced starvation in pathologic pursuit of thinness, an accompanying distortion of body image, in which individuals perceive themselves as fat, abnormal food-related behaviors and, ultimately, amenorrhea, which may be primary or secondary (Table 7). Although little is understood regarding causation, it is clear that multiple psychologic factors are involved and that the severe weight loss itself leads to many physiologic derangements that aid in perpetuating the syndrome.

The severest stage of anorexia nervosa, in which body weight is less than 75% of ideal weight, may be accompanied by weakness in addition to amenorrhea and by clinical findings of hypothermia, hypotension, bradycardia, cardiac arrhythmia, parotid enlargement, pericardial effusion, and pancreatitis. If weight loss occurs before the onset of the pubertal growth spurt,

TABLE 7 DIAGNOSTIC CRITERIA FOR ANOREXIA NERVOSA
Onset before age 25 y
Weight loss of at least 25% of original body weight
Fixed and distorted attitude toward eating and weight
Absence of medical illness able to account for weight loss
Absence of a primary psychiatric disorder
Presence of amenorrhea, lanugo body hair, bradycardia, physical overactivity

TABLE 8 HORMONAL DISTURBANCES IN ANOREXIA NERVOSA
Hypothalamic-pituitary-gonadal axis
↓ Follicle-stimulating hormone
↓ Luteinizing hormone
Normal response to luteinizing hormone releasing hormone
Normal prolactin
↓ Estrogen (estradiol and estrone)
Growth hormone-somatomedin axis
↑ Basal growth hormone
↓ Growth hormone response to hypoglycemia or L-dopa
↑ Growth hormone response to glucose load
↓ Somatomedin C
Hypothalamic-pituitary-adrenal axis
Normal adrenocorticotropic hormone with blunted response to corticotropin releasing hormone
↑ Cortisol
Normal cortisol diurnal pattern but at higher levels
Impaired cortisol suppression following dexamethasone
Hypothalamic-pituitary-thyroid axis
Normal thyroid stimulating hormone
Delayed thyroid stimulating hormone response to thyrotropin releasing hormone
↓ T_4
↓ T_3
↑ rT_3
Posterior pituitary
↓ Vasopressin response to osmotic stimuli
↓ Renal response to vasopressin
↑—increased; ↓—decreased.

there may be impaired growth with short stature. Prolonged postpubertal period amenorrhea can lead to severe osteoporosis with bone pain and vertebral, rib, and femoral fractures. Laboratory abnormalities may include hypoglycemia, hypokalemia, hypophosphatemia, liver function abnormalities, coagulopathies, and vitamin and trace-mineral deficiencies.

Hormonal features

A number of hormonal disturbances are common in patients with anorexia nervosa (Table 8). Amenorrhea is a reflection of hypothalamic dysfunction with hypogonadotropic hypogonadism and accompanying hypoestrogenism. Thyroid function tests are consistent with those seen in the "sick euthyroid" syndrome with low-normal serum thyroxine, low triiodothyronine, increased reverse triiodothyronine, and normal basal thyroid-stimulating hormone, which may respond slowly to thyrotropin-releasing hormone stimulation.

Management

Most of the symptoms, laboratory and hormonal characteristics of anorexia nervosa, are reversible with weight gain [19]. However, restoration of body weight is difficult to achieve or sustain and the disorder has a high level of mortality. Hospitalization may be required for the patient whose weight is less than 75% of ideal.

Patients with lesser degrees of weight loss can be managed as outpatients with both medical and psychiatric support. Behavioral and family therapy appear to be the most effective approaches. Hormonal therapy with estrogen replacement should be initiated if there is evidence of osteoporosis. Although a large number of psychoactive drugs have been used, including antidepressants and benzodiazopines, there is no evidence that they have significant beneficial effects.

Bulimia Nervosa
Clinical features

Bulimia nervosa can be considered as a different clinical expression of the same underlying eating disorder that results in anorexia nervosa (*ie*, a pathologic fear of being fat). In bulimia, there is intermittent binge eating followed by purging through self-induced vomiting or laxative use. During binge episodes, huge amounts of food may be ingested with caloric intake as high as 50,000 calories a day. Episodes of gorging can be several times during a day, lasting from 1 to 8 hours. Subsequently, vomiting is induced by activating the gag reflex. Many patients will also use laxatives, diuretics, fasting, and exercise as a means of reducing weight. In contrast to anorexia nervosa, extreme weight loss does not usually occur and amenorrhea is much less frequently seen although irregular menses are common. However, bulimia may also be present in patients with anorexia nervosa. The patient with bulimia often has features of depression and may attempt suicide. Other dysfunctional behavior is common in bulimia and includes alcohol and drug abuse, stealing, and sexual promiscuity. A variety of symptoms, signs, and laboratory findings occurring in a young female should raise the possibility of bulimia (Table 9) [20].

Management

In mild cases of recent onset, patients with bulimia may respond to counseling regarding risks and to advice on normalization of diet. Cognitive-behavioral psychotherapy appears to be effective in reducing the frequency of binge episodes. Several studies suggest that antidepressant therapy may be of short-term benefit [21]. Treatment with tricyclics such as nortriptyline or desipramine in standard antidepressant doses may produce improvement in 4 weeks. There is evidence that altered function of the neurotransmitter serotonin may play a role in the abnormal eating behavior as well as in the accompanying depression. Thus, antidepressants that modulate central serotonin activity, such as fluoxetene, have been of benefit [22].

When to refer

Aggressive intervention in anorexia nervosa calls for an experienced multidisciplinary team of internist, psychiatrist, nutritionist, and nurse. Hyperalimentation may be necessary as an initial life saving measure as is correction of hypokalemia. Meals should be small but frequent. The goal of hospital care is to increase weight to 80 to 85% of ideal and at the same time provide intensive psychiatric care.

Table 9 Clinical features common in bulimia
Symptoms
Swelling of hands and feet
Abdominal fullness or bloating
Fatigue or weakness
Puffy cheeks
Tooth sensitivity
Depression
Irregular menses
Signs
Superficial ulcerations or calluses on dorsum of hands
Hypertrophy of salivary glands
Dental erosion
Orthostatic hypotension
Laboratory findings
Hypokalemia
Metabolic alkalosis
Impaired dexamethasone suppression of cortisol
Increased serum prolactin

In response to intensive treatment, appropriately 50% of patients achieve sustained normal weight and may start menses. However, the long-term prognosis for normal physical and mental health remains poor with strong likelihood of recurrent psychiatric and eating disturbances.

As with anorexia nervosa, severe cases of bulimia require intervention by an experienced psychiatrist or psychologist. The long-term outlook for patients with bulimia appears to be poorer than for those with anorexia nervosa.

References and Recommended Reading

Recently published papers of particular interest have been highlighted as:
- Of interest
- Of outstanding interest

1.• Miller M: Diseases of the posterior pituitary. In *Neuroendocrinology*. Edited by Nemeroff CB. Boca Raton: CRC Press; 1992:513–540.
2. Repaske DR, Phillips JA III, Kirby LT *et al.*: Molecular analysis of autosomal dominant neurohypophyseal diabetes insipidus. *J Clin Endocrinol Metab* 1990, 70:752–757.
3. Hughes JM, Barron WM, Vance ML: Recurrent diabetes insipidus associated with pregnancy: pathophysiology and therapy. *Obstet Gynecol* 1989, 73:462–464.
4. Moses AM: Clinical and laboratory observations in the adult with diabetes insipidus and related syndromes. *Frontiers Horm Res* 1985, 13:156–175.
5. Mathias CJ, Fosbraey P, daCosta DF, *et al.*: The effect of desmopressin on nocturnal polyuria, overnight weight loss, and morning postural hypotension in patients with autonomic failure. *Br Med J* 1986, 293:353–354.
6. Lightman SL: Molecular insights into diabetes insipidus. *N Engl J Med* 1993, 328:1562–1563.
7. Miller M, Dalakos T, Moses AM, *et al.*: Recognition of partial defects in antidiuretic hormone secretion. *Ann Intern Med* 1970, 73:721–729.
8. Miller M: Disorders of water metabolism. In *Endocrine Pathophysiology*, edn 3. Edited by Hershman JM. Philadelphia: Lea and Febiger; 1988:299–323.
9. Zerbe RL, Robertson GL: A comparison of plasma vasopressin measurement with a standard indirect test in the differential diagnosis of polyuria. *N Engl J Med* 1981, 305:1539–1546.
10. Moses AM, Clayton B, Hochhauser L: Use of T_1-weighted MR imaging to differentiate between primary polydipsia and central diabetes insipidus. *Am J Neuroradiol* 1992, 13:1273–1277.
11. Cobb WE, Spare S, Reichlin S: Neurogenic diabetes insipidus: management with dDAVP (1-desamino-8-D-arginine vasopressin). *Ann Intern Med* 1978, 88:183–188.
12. Miller M, Moses AM: Drug-induced states of impaired water excretion. *Kidney Int* 1976, 10:96–103.
13. Bartter FC, Schwartz WB: The syndrome of inappropriate secretion of antidiuretic hormone. *Am J Med* 1967, 42:790–806.
14. Ayus JC, Wheeler JM, Arieff AI: Postoperative hyponatremic encephalopathy in menstruant women. *Ann Intern Med* 1992, 117:891–897.
15. Miller M: Inappropriate ADH secretion. In *Current Therapy in Endocrinology and Metabolism*, edn 5. Edited by Bardin CW. Philadelphia: BC Decker Inc; 1994:186–189.
16.• Sterns RH: The management of symptomatic hyponatremia. *Sem Nephrology* 1990, 10:503–514.
17. Forrest JN, Cox M, Hong C, *et al.*: Superiority of demeclocycline over lithium in the treatment of chronic syndrome of inappropriate secretion of antidiuretic hormone. *N Engl J Med* 1978, 298:173–177.
18. Herzog DB, Copeland PM: Eating disorders. *N Engl J Med* 1985, 313:295–303.
19. Warren MP: Anorexia nervosa and other eating disorders. In *Principles and Practice of Endocrinology and Metabolism*. Edited by Becker KL. Philadelphia: JB Lippincott Co: 1990:1049–1054.
20. Mitchell JE, Seim HC, Colon E, *et al.*: Medical complications and medical management of bulimia. *Ann Intern Med* 1987, 107:71–77.
21. Pope HG, Hudson JI: Antidepressant drug therapy for bulimia: current status. *J Clin Psychiatry* 1986, 47:339–345.
22. Freeman CPL, Hampson M: Fluoxetine as a treatment for bulimia nervosa. *Int J Obes* 1987, 11(suppl 3):171–177.
23. Miller M: Assessment of hormonal disorders of water metabolism. *Clin Lab Med* 1984, 4:729–744.

Select Bibliography

Anderson AE: *Practical Comprehensive Treatment of Anorexia Nervosa and Bulimia*. Baltimore: Johns Hopkins University Press; 1985.

Baylis PH, Padfield PL: *The Posterior Pituitary: Hormone Secretion in Health and Disease*. New York: Marcel Dekker Inc; 1985.

Garfinkel PE, Garner DM: *The Role of Drug Treatments for Eating Disorders*. Monograph 1. New York: Brunner/Mazel; 1987.

Halmi KA: *Psychobiology and Treatment of Anorexia Nervosa and Bulimia Nervosa*. Washington, DC: American Psychopathological Association; 1992.

Robinson AG, DeRubertis FR: Disorders of sodium and water balance associated with adrenal, thyroid and pituitary disease. In *Diseases of the Kidney*, vol 3. Edited by Schrier RW, Gottschalk CW. Boston: Little, Brown; 1993.

Anterior Pituitary
Shlomo Melmed

> **Key Points**
> - Hypothalamic hormones regulate the secretion of anterior pituitary trophic hormones.
> - Functional pituitary tumors result in the clinical syndromes of hyperprolactinemia, acromegaly, or hypercortisolism (Cushing's Disease).
> - Pituitary failure is associated with hypogonadism, thyroid failure, growth disorders, and hypoadrenalism.
> - Magnetic resonance imaging is the most sensitive and precise imaging technique for diagnosing a pituitary mass.
> - Comprehensive management of pituitary tumors may include transsphenoidal surgical resection, pharmacologic agents, and/or irradiation.

Hypothalamic-releasing or -inhibiting hormones are secreted into the hypophysial–portal blood system and impinge on the anterior pituitary gland. Secretion of the pituitary trophic hormones is then regulated from specific cells that exhibit distinctive immunohistochemical characteristics (Fig. 1). The clinical manifestations of hypopituitarism depend on the degree of pituitary hormone deficiency, which may be isolated or may occur as a combined multiple hormone deficiency. The spectrum of hormone loss resulting from a destructive pituitary lesion initially results in loss of growth hormone, followed by loss of gonadotropin, thyroid-stimulating hormone, and finally corticotropin secretion. Causes are outlined in Table 1.

Each anterior pituitary cell, either singly or in combination, may give rise to pituitary adenomas that express pituitary hormones. Most nonfunctional tumors secrete gonadotropins or their α-subunit. Prolactin, growth hormone, and pro-opiomelanocortin-expressing adenomas account for most clinically functional adenomas that are removed surgically (Table 1).

HYPOTHALAMIC-PITUITARY TARGET HORMONE SYSTEMS

Hypothalamic–Pituitary Thyroid System

To test for pituitary thyroid-stimulating hormone reserve, thyrotropin releasing hormone (200 μg) is administered intravenously. Normally, there is a twofold to threefold increase in the thyroid-stimulating hormone level within 30 minutes after injection [1,2]. Hypothyroidism caused by thyroid failure or damage results in an exaggerated thyroid-stimulating hormone response, whereas a blunted response is seen with hyperthyroidism, exogenously administered thyroid hormone, and pituitary failure. Hypothyroidism of pituitary origin is characterized by low basal thyroid-stimulating hormone levels in the face of thyroid failure.

Hypothalamic–Pituitary Adrenal System

Testing for corticotropin reserve should be carefully supervised because it is potentially hazardous in patients with compromised adrenal function.

Insulin hypoglycemia

After intravenous insulin (0.05 to 0.1 U/kg) is administered, the blood sugar level should decrease to 50% of baseline within 30 minutes. A plasma cortisol response of 7 µg/dL above the baseline, a doubling of the baseline cortisol, or a peak value of at least 20 µg/dL indicates intact corticotropin reserve. Cortisol peaks approximately 30 to 45 minutes after hypoglycemia develops. Insulin-induced hypoglycemia is contraindicated in patients who have primary adrenal insufficiency or are elderly, suffer from ischemic heart disease, or are prone to cerebral seizures.

Metyrapone

Three grams of metyrapone are given orally at 11 PM with a snack. Metyrapone blocks the conversion of 11-deoxycortisol to cortisol, blocking the major negative feedback inhibitor of corticotropin secretion. The resultant release of corticotropin from negative feedback inhibition stimulates production of compound S. Serum compound S (11-deoxycortisol) and cortisol are measured at 8 AM the following morning. In patients with a normal pituitary–adrenal axis, compound S levels are more than 8 µg/dL. Plasma cortisol levels should be less than 5 µg/dL for the test to be valid. Metyrapone may not be readily available for testing.

Cortrosyn stimulation test

As an indirect, but accurate, test of pituitary corticotropin reserve, adrenal cortisol reserve is evaluated. Synthetic corticotropin 1–24 (Cortrosyn 250 µg, Organon, West Orange, NJ) given intravenously or intramuscularly results in a doubling of serum cortisol levels (*ie*, an increase of at least 7 µg/dL) or peak levels of more than 20 µg/dL within 60 minutes. A blunted cortisol response indicates either impaired pituitary corticotropin reserve or primary adrenal failure.

Corticotropin releasing factor

Corticotropin releasing factor administered intravenously (1 µg/kg) directly stimulates corticotropin release. Subsequent serum cortisol responses are measured during the subsequent 60 minutes. A blunted response to corticotropin-releasing factor is indicative of pituitary failure, whereas patients harboring a corticotroph cell adenoma causing Cushing's disease often have an exaggerated corticotropin response to corticotropin releasing factor. Patients with ectopic corticotropin-secreting tumors do not usually demonstrate a further increase in corticotropin levels in response to corticotropin releasing factor.

Test for corticotropin hypersecretion

One milligram of dexamethasone is given at bedtime, and cortisol level is measured at 8 AM to rule out corticotropin hypersecretion associated with Cushing's disease. A normal response is a cortisol level less than 5 µg/dL.

Hypothalamic–Pituitary Gonadal System

Hypothalamic gonadotropin releasing hormone regulates the secretion of both pituitary luteinizing hormone and follicle-stimulating hormone and is secreted in pulses every 60 to 120 minutes. In women, luteinizing hormone regulates ovulation and maintenance of the corpus luteum; in men, luteinizing hormone controls testosterone synthesis and secretion by the testicular Leydig cell. Follicle-stimulating hormone regulates ovarian follicular development and maturation and stimulates ovarian estro-

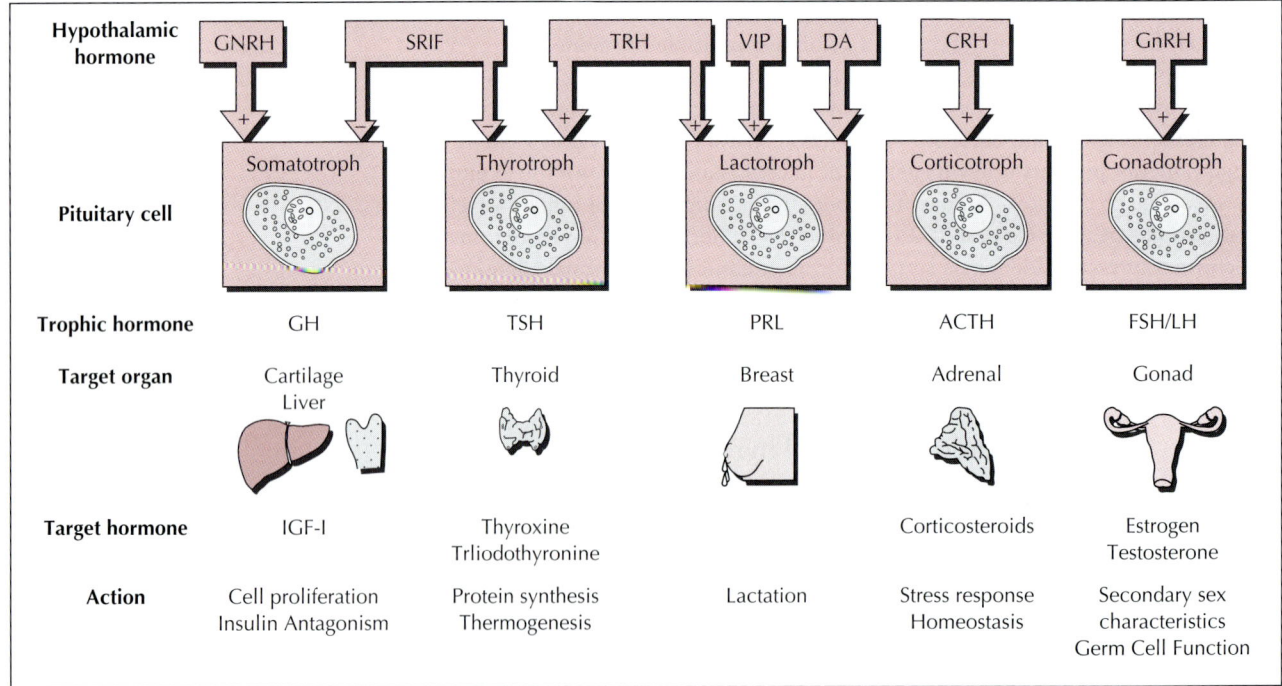

FIGURE 1 Hypothalamic–pituitary axis. ACTH—adrenocorticotropic hormone; CRH—corticotropin releasing hormone; DA—dopamine; FSH—follicle-stimulating hormone; GH—growth hormone; GH-RH—growth hormone releasing hormone; Gn-RH—gonadotropin releasing hormone; IGF-I—insulin-like growth factor I; LH—luteinizing hormone; PRL—prolactin; SRIF—somatostatin; TRH—thyrotropin releasing hormone; TSH—thyroid-stimulating hormone; VIP—vasoactive intestinal polypeptide.

gens in women. In men, follicle-stimulating hormone is responsible for development of seminiferous tubules and stimulates spermatogenesis. Feedback regulation of gonadotropin secretion is complex, with both positive and negative components mediated by steroids, polypeptide inhibitory hormones (inhibins), or stimulatory hormones (activins) of gonadal origin.

Gonadotropins

Concurrent measurement of serum gonadotropin and gonadal steroid concentrations provides an accurate assessment of gonadotropin deficiency. Circulating testosterone or estradiol levels are low with pituitary gonadotropin deficiency. Serum luteinizing hormone and follicle-stimulating hormone levels are measured in three pooled serum samples drawn 20 minutes apart to compensate for the neurosecretory pulses of pituitary gonadotropin release.

Gonadotropin releasing hormone

Administering 100 μg of gonadotropin releasing hormone results in luteinizing hormone levels peaking within 30 minutes and follicle-stimulating hormone levels plateauing after 1 hour. Normal responses vary according to stage of menstrual cycle, age, and sex of the patient. Luteinizing hormone levels usually increase about threefold, whereas follicle-stimulating hormone increase is more blunted. Absent response to gonadotropin releasing hormone does not reliably distinguish pituitary from hypothalamic causes of hypogonadism, and a normal response does not exclude the presence of pituitary hypogonadism.

TABLE 1 CAUSES OF HYPOPITUITARISM, CONGENITAL OR ACQUIRED

Congenital	**Physical agents**
Septo-optic dysplasia	Trauma
Hypogonadotropic hypogonadism	Ionizing radiation
	Stalk section
Prader-Willi syndrome	Surgery
Laurence-Moon-Biedl syndrome	**Infiltrations**
Isolated growth hormone deficiency	Hemochromatosis
	Metastatic carcinoma
Basal encephalocele	Amyloidosis
Vascular	**Tumors**
Pituitary apoplexy	Hypothalamic
Sheehan's syndrome	Craniopharyngioma
Arteritides and aneurysm	Glioma
Inflammatory	Germinoma
Lymphocytic hypophysitis	Meningioma
Histiocytosis	Hamartoma
Sarcoidosis	Leukemia and lymphoma
Tuberculosis	**Pituitary**
	Funcitoning or nonfunctioning macroadenomas
	Empty sella

Hypothalamic–Pituitary Growth Hormone System

Somatostatin and growth hormone–releasing hormone participate in a dual control system. Growth hormone–releasing hormone stimulates the release of growth hormone from the somatotrophs, whereas somatostatin inhibits the secretion of pituitary growth hormone. Growth hormone, quantitatively the main hormone secreted by the pituitary, mediates linear growth. Peak secretory bursts occur between 11 PM and 2 AM. Physical exercise, emotional stress, and nutritional status regulate growth hormone secretion at the level of the hypothalamus.

Growth hormone induces hepatic insulin-like growth factor I (IGF-I) production. IGF-I mediates most of the growth-promoting actions of growth hormone, and it suppresses growth hormone secretion. IGF-I is also produced by extrahepatic tissues and may play a role in local tissue growth. IGF-I is bound to several circulating binding proteins. Insulin-like growth factor binding protein (IGFBP)-3 is the main reservoir for circulating IGF-I is growth hormone-dependent, and is, therefore, increased in acromegaly and decreased in hypopituitarism. Smaller IGFBPs may regulate IGF-I action by determining IGF-I access to tissues.

Testing for growth hormone reserve

Intravenous administration of insulin (0.05 to 0.1 U/kg) should reduce blood glucose to at least 40 mg/dL, or to 50% of the patient's initial blood glucose levels. Growth hormone peak response (> 7 ng/mL) occurs between 60 and 90 minutes afterward. For the growth hormone–releasing hormone test, intravenous growth hormone–releasing hormone (1 μg/kg) directly tests somatotroph secretory capacity. Growth hormone levels peak within the first hour, and patients with hypopituitarism do not respond to growth hormone releasing hormone. A growth hormone response after repeated growth hormone releasing hormone stimulation may be indicative of a hypothalamic disorder, with defective synthesis of endogenous growth hormone releasing hormone. A blunted growth hormone response to growth hormone releasing hormone is also associated with obesity and type II diabetes. Arginine, L-dopa, and clonidine hydrochloride are additional pharmacologic stimuli of growth hormone.

Testing for growth hormone hypersecretion

Growth hormone normally is suppressed to less than 1 ng/mL within 60 minutes of ingesting 75 g of oral glucose. Paradoxic growth hormone responses to glucose occur in approximately 75% of patients with acromegaly.

Measuring basal IGF-I levels is useful in screening growth hormone excess, because IGF-I levels do not fluctuate rapidly and reflect integrated growth hormone secretion over time. Levels above 2.2 U/mL usually indicate acromegaly or gigantism. IGF-I levels are not useful in screening for hypopituitarism, because levels may overlap with normals.

Hypothalamic–Pituitary Prolactin System

The primary hypothalamic prolactin inhibitory factor is dopamine. Dopamine antagonists, such as metoclopramide, enhance prolactin secretion, as do drugs that attenuate hypothalamic dopamine, including the phenothiazines. Prolactin

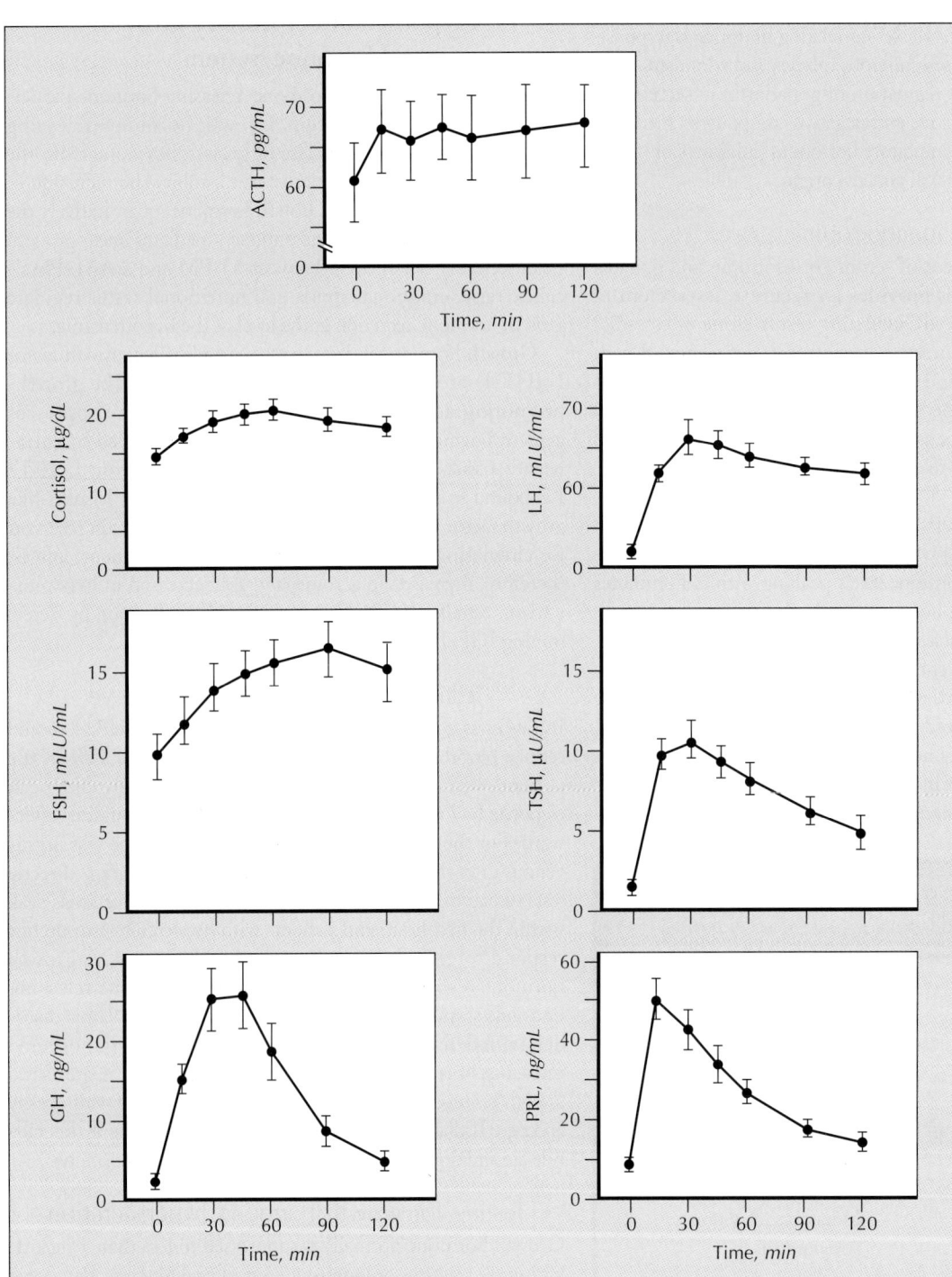

FIGURE 2 Basal (zero time) samples are initially drawn for each hormone measurement. All four hypothalamic releasing hormones are administered intravenously sequentially over 60 seconds, followed by venous sampling for specific hormone radioimmunoassay at the indicated times. ACTH—adrenocorticotropic hormone; FSH—follicle-stimulating hormone; GH—growth hormone; LH—luteinizing hormone; PRL—prolactin; TSH—thyroid-stimulating hormone. (*Adapted from* Cohen *et al* [2]; with permission.)

has a high degree of homology with growth hormone and placental lactogen and is stimulated by estrogen, an important peripheral regulator of prolactin secretion.

Testing for prolactin reserve

Intravenous administration of thyrotropin releasing hormone (200 μg) elicits a threefold to fivefold peak prolactin response after 10 to 20 minutes.

Testing for prolactin hypersecretion

A basal prolactin level greater than 200 ng/mL strongly suggests the presence of a prolactin-secreting adenoma.

Quadruple bolus testing

All four hypothalamic releasing hormones may be administered simultaneously, providing efficient and precise method for comprehensive testing of anterior pituitary reserve function (Fig. 2 and Table 2).

CLINICAL SYNDROMES: SYMPTOMS AND DIAGNOSIS

Clinical features associated with hypo- or hyperfunction of the anterior pituitary gland depend on the specific trophic hormones whose secretion is disordered.

Hypopituitarism

Deficiency of growth hormone

Growth retardation with short stature, fasting hypoglycemia, and occasionally, delayed puberty occur during infancy and childhood. Adults may manifest central adiposity, muscle weakness, psychologic depression, and hyperlipidemia.

Deficiency of gonadotropins

During childhood, central hypogonadism results in pubertal failure. Breast development is delayed, and pubic and axillary hair do not grow, although some sexual hair growth occurs if the corticotropin–adrenal axis is intact and stimulates adrenal androgen production. In girls, primary amenorrhea is present; in boys, small testes and phallus and sparse body hair are evident. Isolated gonadotropin deficiency results in tall adolescents with eunuchoid proportions, (*ie*, upper-to-lower segment ratio is less than 1). In postpubertal women, features of hypogonadism include secondary amenorrhea, breast atrophy, and loss of pubic and axillary hair. Men manifest testicular atrophy, decrease in body hair, decreased libido, impotence, and infertility.

Thyroid-stimulating hormone deficiency

Deficiency of thyroid-stimulating hormone secretion causes thyroid failure. The lack of thyroid hormone secretion results in lethargy, cold intolerance, constipation, bradycardia, and hoarseness. Low circulating levels of thyroid-stimulating hormone in the presence of low thyroid hormone levels distinguish thyroid stimulating hormone deficient patients from those with primary hypothyroidism.

Corticotropin deficiency

Corticotropin deficiency causes adrenal failure with features including orthostatic hypotension, weakness, hypothermia, nausea, vomiting, dehydration, lethargy, coma, and even death. Hypokalemia is usually not present because of the maintenance of mineralocorticoid secretion by the intact renin–angiotensin system.

Vasopressin deficiency

Vasopressin deficiency occurs with posterior pituitary lesions, resulting in diminished release of vasopressin and resultant diabetes insipidus.

Diagnosis

Hypopituitarism should be suspected in all patients who have previously undergone pituitary surgery, irradiation, or recent pregnancy [3]. Decreased pituitary reserves should also be suspected in patients with hypogonadism, infertility, and unexplained hypothyroidism. The absence of an elevated pituitary trophic hormone in the face of adrenal, thyroid, or gonadal failure confirms the diagnosis. Biochemical testing for these patients involves dynamic assessment of growth hormone and gonadotropin secretion. Attenuation of thyroid and adrenal pituitary reserves, however, usually only occurs later in the development of frank pituitary failure. Once the diagnosis has been confirmed, a magnetic resonance imaging (MRI) scan is helpful in excluding the presence of a pituitary or sellar mass that would impinge on normal pituitary tissue.

Treatment of hypopituitarism is outlined in Table 3. Although growth hormone replacement in adult hypopituitary patients is experimental, the availability of recombinant human growth hormone has allowed investigation of the following potential adult applications:

Hypopituitarism
Aging
Obesity
Catabolic states
Wound healing
Osteoporosis
Ovulation induction
Immune rescue

Pituitary Tumors

Local neurologic effects of pituitary tumors

Most patients with pituitary tumors larger than 1 cm in diameter experience severe headache, probably as a result of pressure on the diaphragma sella by the tumor mass (Fig. 3) [4]. The optic chiasm, which lies above the pituitary sella turcica, is frequently compressed by the encroaching tumor, causing initial loss of red perception, bitemporal hemianopsia, or a superior bitemporal defect. Hypothalamic invasion by pituitary tumors can result in diabetes insipidus, sleep or appetite disorders, and changes in autonomic function. Cavernous sinus invasion leads to cranial nerve palsies with ptosis, ophthalmoplegia, or diplopia; hemorrhage into the tumor may

TABLE 2 ADMINISTRATION OF HYPOTHALAMIC RELEASING HORMONES AS A COMBINED ANTERIOR PITUITARY FUNCTION TEST

Hypothalamic hormone	Radioimmunoassay of pituitary hormone	Venous sampling time after infusion, *min*
TRH 200 µg	TSH	15, 30
	PRL	10, 15
CRF 1 µg/kg	ACTH	10, 45, 60
GH-RH 1 µg/kg	GH	45, 60
Gn-RH 100 µg	FSH	45, 60, 90
	LH	15, 30

ACTH—corticotropin; CRF—corticotropin releasing factor; FSH—follicle-stimulating hormone; GH—growth hormone; GH-RH—growth hormone releasing hormone; Gn-RH—gonadotropin releasing hormone; LH—luteinizing hormone; PRL—prolactin; TRH—thyrotropin releasing hormone; TSH—thyroid-stimulating hormone.

Table 3. Treatment of Hypopituitarism

Trophic hormone deficit	Replacement
Corticotropin	Hydrocortisone (20 mg AM; 10 mg PM)
	Cortisone acetate (25 mg AM; 12.5 mg PM)
Thyroid-stimulating hormone	L-thyroxine (0.1–0.15 mg daily)
Follicle-stimulating hormone/luteinizing hormone	Males:
	Testosterone enanthate (200 mg intramuscularly every 2 wk)
	Females:
	Ethinyl estradiol (0.02–0.05 mg)
	Conjugated estrogens (0.65–1.25 mg daily for 25 d)
	Estradiol skin patch (4–8 mg, twice weekly) with progesterone on days 16–25 to facilitate uterine shedding
	For fertility: Menopausal gonadotropins, human chorionic gonadotropins
Vasopressin	Intranasal desmopressin (0.05–0.1 mL twice daily)
Growth hormone	Replacement is experimental in adults

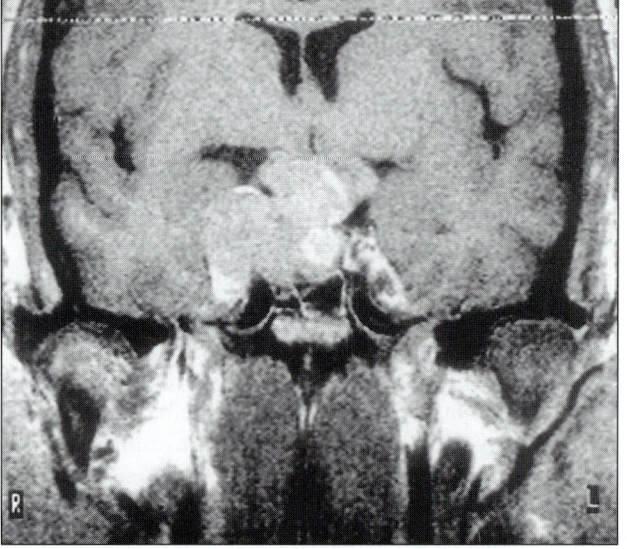

Figure 3 Magnetic resonance imaging scan of invasive pituitary macroadenoma impinging on local brain structures.

result in acute necrosis with severe headache, visual impairment, paralysis, lethargy, and coma.

Diagnosis

Either the local effects of the pituitary mass or the hormonal aberrations induced by adenomas lead to signs and symptoms. These may present initially with compression of adjacent neurologic structures with concurrent systemic effects resulting from excess peripheral hormonal action. Hypersecretion of a pituitary trophic hormone can cause acromegaly, amenorrhea–galactorrhea, impotence, or Cushing's disease (Table 4).

Diagnosis of pituitary adenomas has been aided by sophisticated MRI imaging procedures that detect microadenoma masses as small as 2 mm in diameter and provide the best visualization of the hypothalamus.

Growth Hormone-Secreting Pituitary Tumors

Increased growth hormone secretion may be caused by pituitary or extrapituitary tumors, and may manifest in different ways, depending on the age of the patient (Fig. 4) [5]. In children or adolescents whose epiphyseal growth centers have yet

Table 4. Pituitary Adenomas

Cell origin	Product	Clinical syndrome
Lactotroph	PRL	Hypogonadism, galactorrhea
Somatotroph	GH	Acromegaly
Corticotroph	ACTH	Cushing's disease
Mixed GH and PRL	GH, PRL	Acromegaly, hypogonadism
Plurihormonal	Any	Varies
Gonadotroph	FSH, LH, subunits	Hypogonadism or no effect
Thyrotroph	TSH	Hyperthyroidism
Null cell; oncocyte	None	Pituitary failure

ACTH—corticotropin; FSH—follicle-stimulating hormone; GH—growth hormone; LH—luteinizing hormone; PRL—prolactin; TSH—thyroid-stimulating hormone.

to fuse, gigantism may occur. In adults, excessive secretion of growth hormone results in acromegaly in which clinical features occur slowly. The clinical presentation reflects the effects of local tumor growth, peripheral tissue changes, and the metabolic and systemic effects of continuous growth hormone and IGF-I hypersecretion.

Extrapituitary causes of acromegaly are rare and include pancreatic islet-cell, lung, and intestinal carcinoid tumors [6].

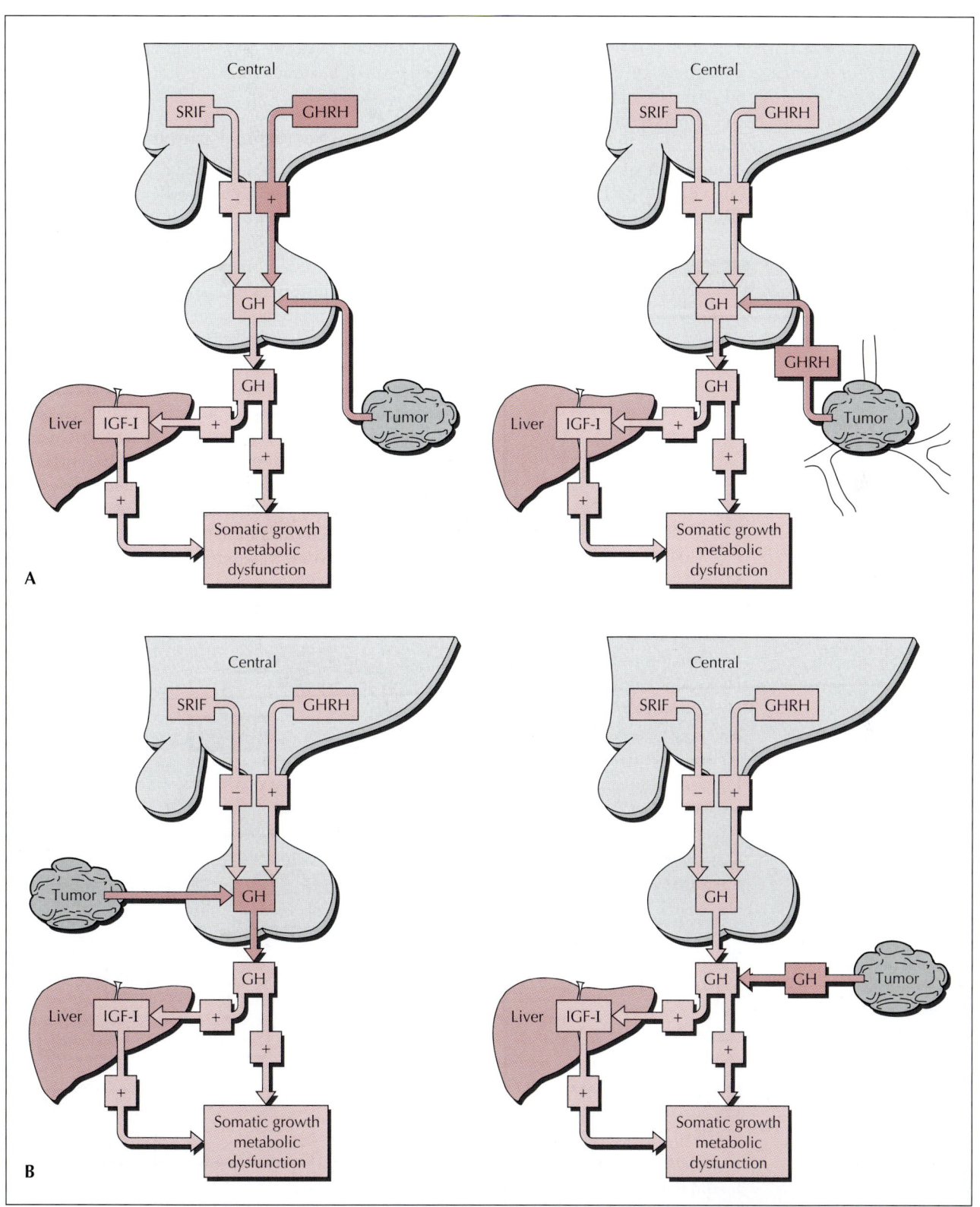

FIGURE 4 Central and peripheral causes of acromegaly. **A**, Excess GHRH secretion. **B**, Excess GH secretion. GH—growth hormone; GHRH—growth hormone releasing hormone; IGF-I—insulin-like growth factor I; SRIF—somatostatin. (*From* Melmed [5];with permission.)

Regardless of the tumor location, patients with acromegaly present with the classical clinical features of acromegaly, along with elevated circulating levels of growth hormone and growth hormone–releasing hormone (Table 5).

Diagnosis

Unrestrained growth hormone secretion is the hallmark of acromegaly. For a conclusive diagnosis, growth hormone levels are greater than 1 ng/mL after an oral glucose load. Biochemical evidence of IGF-I hypersecretion correlates well with a diagnosis of active acromegaly. Initial screening for acromegaly includes measurement of serum IGF-I concentration, because there are virtually no false-positive findings in adults (Fig. 5) [7]. When an elevated IGF-I level is detected, the patient should be evaluated further with a MRI scan of the anterior pituitary and a post-glucose growth hormone determination. If no pituitary mass is detected, further imaging is performed to locate an ectopic tumor source of growth hormone releasing hormone or growth hormone. Measurements of immunoreactive serum growth hormone releasing hormone levels may distinguish between growth hormone releasing hormone and growth hormone sources.

Prolactin-Secreting Pituitary Tumors

Prolactin-secreting pituitary tumors are diagnosed more often in women than in men, possibly as a result of the difference in clinical manifestations between women and men (Table 6) [8]. Microadenomas are more common in women, and macroadenomas are more frequent in men, possibly reflecting a different natural history in men and women. Only a small percentage of microadenomas in women develop into macroadenomas. Prolactinomas frequently cause menstrual disturbances; therefore, tumors in women are generally discovered earlier than in men. In men, decreased libido, impotence, and infertility are the presenting features. At diagnosis, macroadenomas may also have caused visual field abnormalities, hypothyroidism, and adrenal insufficiency.

Approximately 15% of women with amenorrhea have elevated levels of serum prolactin, and approximately one third of women with galactorrhea without amenorrhea have hyperprolactinemia. Of women presenting with both signs, more than three fourths have increased prolactin levels. Infertility

Table 5 Clinical Features of Acromegaly

Local tumor effects
- Pituitary enlargement
- Visual field defects
- Cranial nerve palsy
- Headache

Somatic

Acral enlargement	Thickening of soft tissue of hands and feet
Musculoskeletal	Prognathism
	Malocclusion
	Arthralgias
	Carpal tunnel syndrome
	Proximal myopathy
	Hypertrophy of frontal bones
Skin	Hyperhydrosis
	Skin tags
Colon	Polyps
Cardiovascular	Left ventricular or septal hypertrophy
	Hypertension
	Congestive heart failure
Sleep disturbances	Sleep apnea
	Narcolepsy
Visceromegaly	Tongue
	Thyroid
	Salivary gland

Endocrine–metabolic

Reproduction	Menstrual abnormalities
	Galactorrhea
	Decreased libido, impotence
Multiple endocrine Neoplasia (I)	Hyperparathyroidism
	Pancreatic islet cell tumors
Carbohydrate	Impaired glucose tolerance
	Insulin resistance
Lipids	Hypertriglyceridemia
Mineral	Hypercalciuria
	Urinary hydroxyproline

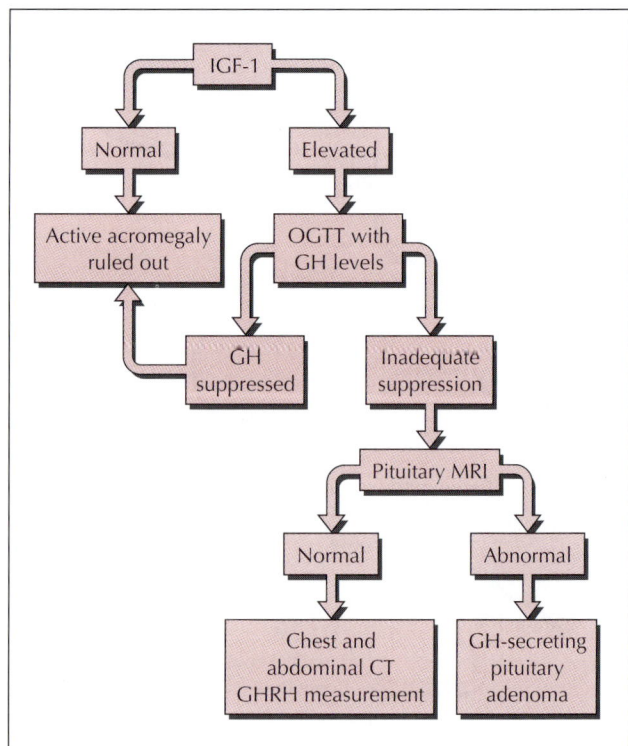

Figure 5 Diagnosis of acromegaly. GH—growth hormone; GH-RH—growth hormone releasing hormone; IGF-I—insulin-like growth factor I; OGTT—oral glucose tolerance test.

Table 6 Clinical features of patients with prolactin-secreting pituitary adenomas	
Women	**Men**
Amenorrhea	Headaches
Oligomenorrhea	Visual abnormalities
Galactorrhea	Decreased libido
Headaches	Impotence
Infertility	Infertility

Table 7 Causes of hyperprolactinemia

Physiologic
Pregnancy and lactation
Stress
Exercise
Chest wall trauma

Pathologic
Hypothalamic
  Inflammation
  Tumor
Pituitary
  Lactotroph microadenoma or macroadenoma
  Acromegaly
  Stalk section due to sellar mass
  Empty sella syndrome
Peripheral
  Hypothyroidism
  Chronic renal failure

Pharmacologic
Psychotropic agents
  Phenothiazines
  Tricyclic antidepressants
Opiates
Metoclopramide
Cimetidine
Antihypertensive
  Methyldopa
  Reserpine
Hormones
  Estrogens
  Thyrotropin-releasing hormone

occurs as the result of anovulation or an inadequate luteal phase in women and low sperm counts or impotence in men.

Elevated prolactin levels may suppress the cyclic release of gonadotropins and may interrupt the peripheral action of gonadotropins on the gonads. Women frequently present with estrogen deficiency and decreased vaginal secretions, causing dyspareunia and osteopenia. Hyperprolactinemia can also cause elevated androgen levels, leading to hirsutism and acne. In men, serum testosterone levels are depressed in at least two thirds of patients with prolactinomas. When the tumor is detected and treated early, testosterone levels ultimately increase. Irreversible damage to the pituitary gonadotrophs by an expanding tumor may, however, prevent the normalization of testosterone levels. Elevated prolactin levels may also attenuate the peripheral action of testosterone, perhaps by interfering with the conversion of testosterone to dihydrotestosterone.

Diagnosis

Diagnosis of prolactin-secreting pituitary adenoma involves measuring basal serum prolactin concentrations. When levels exceed 200 ng/mL (upper limit of normal is 25), a pituitary tumor is likely to be present. Prolactin levels below 200 ng/mL may be caused by a variety of secondary conditions (Table 7). To confirm the presence of a tumor, MRI scanning of the pituitary region should be used when persistent hyperprolactinemia is demonstrated.

There is no definitive test to determine whether elevated prolactin levels result from pituitary tumors or from other causes.

Gonadotropin-Secreting Pituitary Tumors

Gonadotropin-secreting pituitary tumors are usually nonfunctional and are associated with hypogonadism. Patients are usually asymptomatic or may seek care because of local pressure signs [9].

Most patients have increased circulating levels of glycoprotein hormone α subunits, which may only be demonstrable after thyrotropin releasing hormone administration. Gonadal function is usually suppressed with low or normal testosterone levels, or low or normal sperm counts. Rarely, excess production of luteinizing hormone alone by a tumor may result in increased levels of testosterone.

Diagnosis

The diagnosis is difficult in women because of the associated high gonadotropin levels usually found in postmenopausal women. Primary gonadal failure or menopause may cause secondary pituitary enlargement due to hyperplastic gonadotroph cells, further confounding the differential diagnosis.

Thyroid-Stimulating Hormone–Secreting Pituitary Tumors

The thyroid-stimulating hormone–secreting pituitary tumors are rare, often plurihormonal, and secrete growth hormone, prolactin, and α glycoprotein subunits in addition to thyroid-stimulating hormone. Thyroid-stimulating hormone–secreting tumors present with signs and symptoms of hyperthyroidism, and features include thyroid-stimulating hormone levels inappropriate to the elevated thyroid hormone levels. Approximately one third of patients with thyroid-stimulating hormone–secreting pituitary tumors have thyroid-stimulating hormone levels less than 10 U/L. Ultrasensitive thyroid-stimulating hormone radioimmunoassays should be used to discriminate between low and inappropriately "normal" circulating thyroid-stimulating hormone levels in patients with hyperthyroidism and suspected thyrotroph cell adenoma [10].

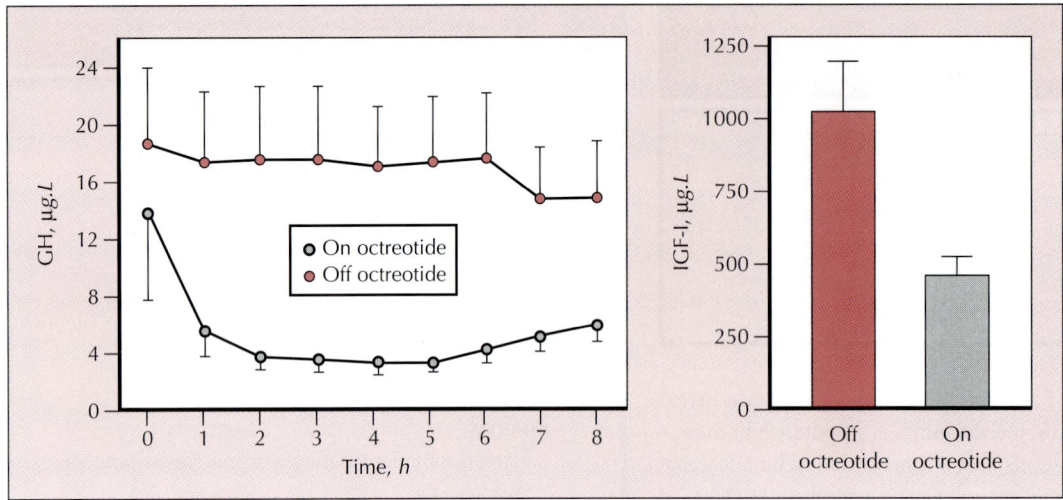

FIGURE 6 Effect of octreotide (100 μg) on growth hormone and insulin-like growth factor I- levels in 10 acromegalic patients. GH—growth hormone; IGF-I—insulin-like growth factor I. (*From* Ezzat and coworkers [7]; with permission.)

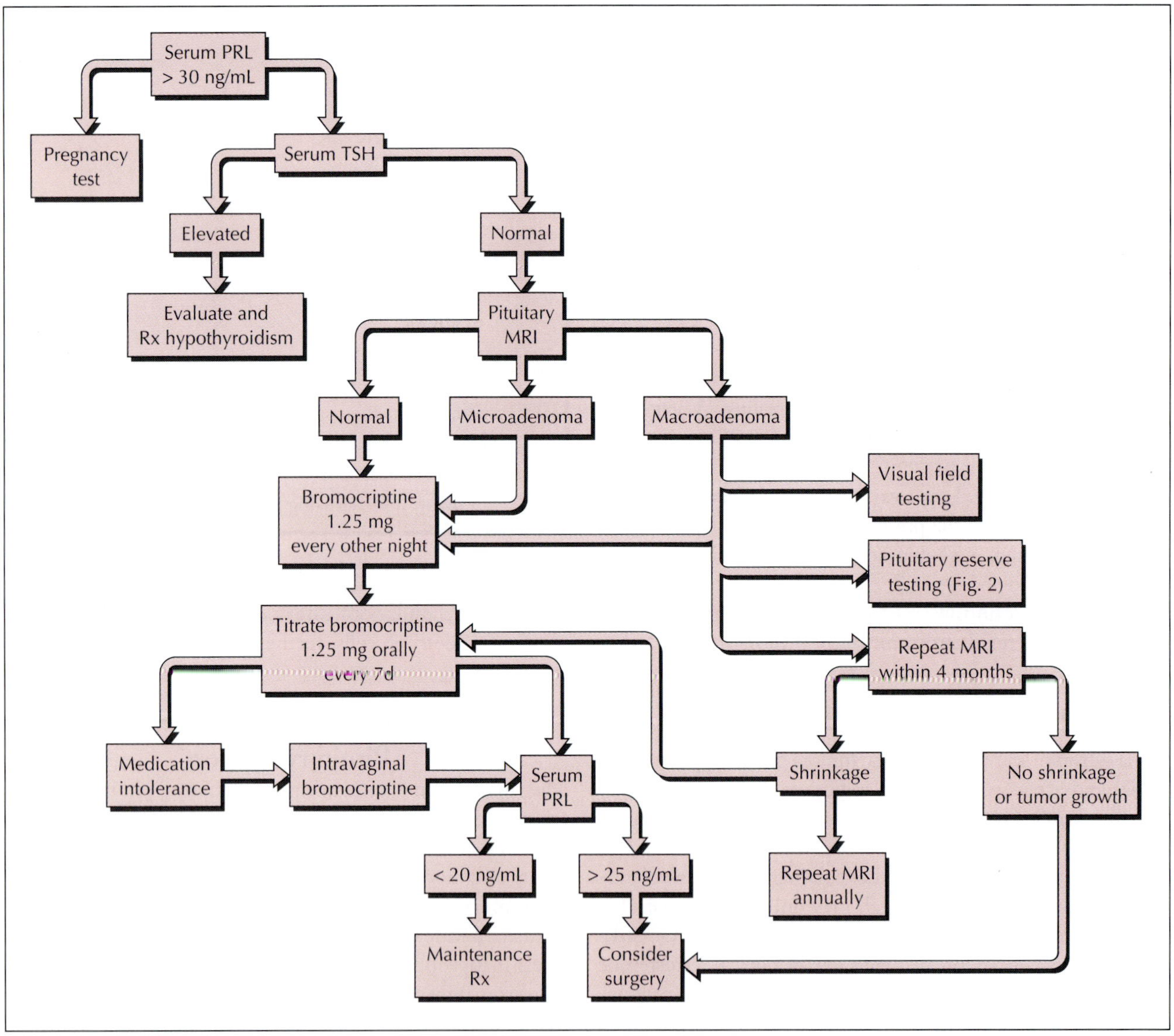

FIGURE 7 Approach to hyperprolactinemia. MRI—magnetic resonance imaging; PRL—prolactin; TSH—thyroid-stimulating hormone.

Treatment

Pituitary tumors

The aims of treatment are suppression of unrestrained hormone secretion, reduction of tumor mass, correction of visual and neurologic defects, preservation of pituitary function, and prevention of tumor progression or recurrence. Generally, treatment options include surgery, irradiation and medical therapies [11].

Acromegaly

The primary treatment is transsphenoidal surgical resection of the growth hormone-secreting adenoma [12]. In some centers, the pituitary is also irradiated, resulting in hypopituitarism in 50% of patients within 10 years [13]. Recently, a novel, long-acting somatostatin analog, octreotide, has been shown to effectively lower growth hormone and IGF-I levels when administered subcutaneously (100 µg three times daily) (Fig. 6) [14,15]. Tumors also shrink, and the soft tissue and metabolic sequelae of acromegaly are ameliorated. An important side effect of the drug is asymptomatic gallstone development.

Prolactinoma

Management outline is depicted in Figure 7 [16]. Side effects of bromocriptine are nausea and anorexia, hypotension, peripheral vasospasm, headaches, nasal stuffiness, and depression.

Other tumors

All the other pituitary tumor types, including Cushing's disease should be managed by transsphenoidal surgical resection (Fig. 8) [17].

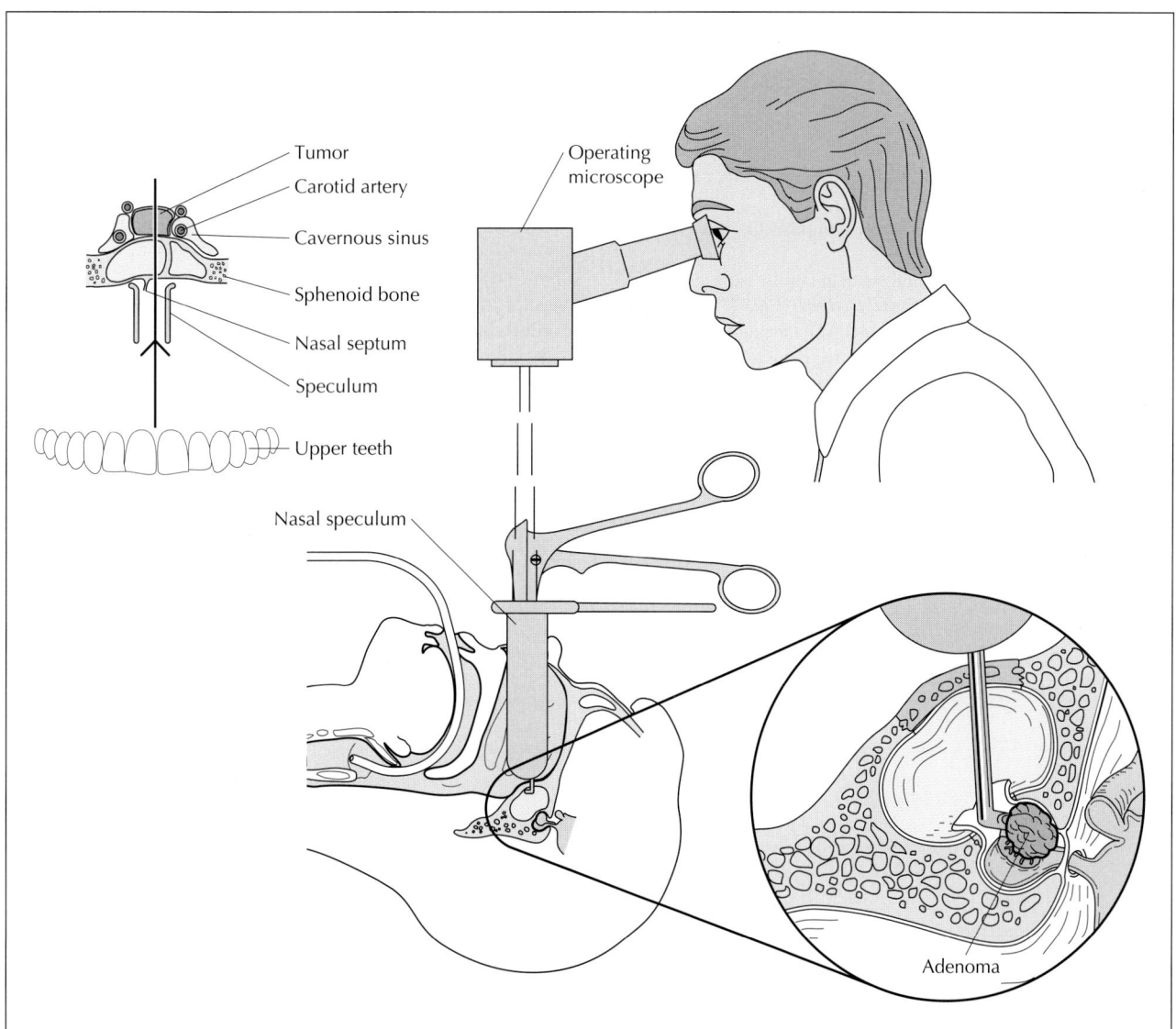

FIGURE 8 Diagram of transsphenoidal surgery for resection of pituitary adenoma.

References and Recommended Reading

Recently published papers of particular interest have been highlighted as:
- Of interest
- •• Of outstanding interest

1. Abboud CF: Anterior pituitary failure. In *The Pituitary*. Edited by Melmed S. Cambridge: Blackwell Scientific, 1995.
2. Cohen R, Bouquier D, Biot-Laporte S, *et al.*: Pituitary stimulation by combined administration of four hypothalamic releasing hormones in normal men and patients. *J Clin Endocrinol Metab* 1986, 62:892–898.
3. Asa SL, Bilbao JM, Kovacs K, *et al.*: Lymphocytic hypophysitis of pregnancy in hypopituitarism: a distinct clinicopathologic entity. *Ann Intern Med* 1981, 95:166–171.
4. • Maroldo TV, Dillon WP, Wilson CB: Advances in diagnostic techniques of pituitary tumors and prolactinomas. *Curr Opin Oncol* 1992, 4:105–115.
5. • Melmed S: Acromegaly. *N Engl J Med* 1990, 322:966–977.
6. •• Thorner ML, Perryman RL, Cronin MJ, *et al.*: Somatotroph hyperplasia: successful treatment of acromegaly by removal of a pancreatic islet tumor secreting a growth hormone-releasing factor. *J Clin Invest* 1982, 965–977.
7. •• Rajasoorya C, Holdaway M, Wrightson P, et al.: Determinants of clinical outcome and survival in acromegaly. *Clin Endocrinol* 1994, 41:95–102.
8. Cunnah D, Besser M: Management of prolactinomas. *Clin Endocrinol* 1991, 34:231–235.
9. Molitch ME: Evaluation and treatment of the patient with a pituitary incidentaloma. *J Clin Endocrinol Metab* 1995, 80:3–6.
10. Chanson P, Weintraub BD, Harris AG: Octreotide therapy for thyroid-stimulating hormone-secreting pituitary adenomas. A follow-up of 52 patients. *Ann Intern Med* 1993, 119:236–240.
11. Wilson CB: Role of surgery in the management of pituitary tumors. *Neurosurg Clin North Am* 1990, 1:139–159.
12. Melmed S, *et al.*: Consensus statement: benefits versus risks of medical therapy for acromegaly. *Am J Med* 1994, 97: 468–473.
13. Eastman RC, Gorden P, Glatstein E, Roth J: Radiation therapy of acromegaly. *Endocrinol Metab Clin North Am* 1992, 21:693–712.
14. • Lamberts SWJ, Krenning EP, Reubi J-C: The role of somatostatin and its analogs in the diagnosis and treatment of tumors. *Endocr Rev* 1991, 12:450–482.
15. •• Ezzat S, Snyder PJ, Young WF, *et al.*: Octreotide treatment of acromegaly: a randomized, multicenter study. *Ann Intern Med* 1992, 117:711–718.
16. •• Bevans JS, Webster J, Burke CW, Scanlon MF: Dopamine agonists and pituitary tumor shrinkage. *Endocr Rev* 1992, 13:220–240.
17. Trainer PJ, Grossman A: The diagnosis and differential diagnosis of Cushing's syndrome. *Clin Endocrinol* 1991, 34:317–330.
18. Ezzat S, Ren SG, Braunstein GD, Melmed S: Octreotide stimulates insulin-like growth factor binding protein-1 (IGF BP-1) lends in acromegaly. J Clin Endocrinol Metab 1991, 73:441–443.

Select Bibliography

Daneshdoost L, Gennarelli TA, Bashey HM, *et al.*: Recognition of gonadotroph adenomas in women. *N Engl J Med* 1991, 324:589–594.

Iranmanesh A, Grisso B, Veldhuis JD: Low basal and persistent pulsatile growth hormone secretion are revealed in normal and hyposomatotrophic men studied with a new ultrasensitive chemiluminescence assay. *J Clin Endocrinol Metab* 1994, 78:526–535.

Mastorakos G, Chrousos GP, Weber JS: Recombinant interleukin-6 activates the hypothalmic pituitary-adrenal axis in humans. *J Clin Endocrinol Metab* 1993, 77:1690–1694.

Mbanya J-CN, Mendelow AD, Crawford PJ, *et al.*: Rapid resolution of visual abnormalities with medical therapy alone in patients with large prolactinomas. *Brit J Neurosurg* 1993, 7:519–527.

Neely EK, Rosenfeld RG: Use and abuse of human growth hormone. *Annu Rev Med* 1994, 45:407–420.

Vance ML: Hypopituitarism. *N Engl J Med* 1994, 330(23):1651.

Thyroid Dysfunction

Jerome M. Hershman

> ### *Key Points*
> - Screening of geriatric patients for hypothyroidism is advocated.
> - The best laboratory indicator of the adequacy of therapy for hypothyroidism is the serum thyroid-stimulating hormone level, which should be in the normal range when the dose of levothyroxine is optimal.
> - A subnormal serum thyroid-stimulating hormone level indicates that the replacement dose of levothyroxine is excessive and is an indication for reducing the dose.
> - Antithyroid drugs are preferred as the definitive therapy for hyperthyroidism for patients with Graves' disease younger than 45 years of age.
> - Radioiodine therapy is recommended for older hyperthyroid patients with complicating illnesses and those with multinodular goiter or single hot nodules.

Thyroid dysfunction is common in our population. Symptoms of fatigue, weight gain, mental slowing, dry skin, and constipation should trigger the diagnostic possibility of hypothyroidism, even though these symptoms are often attributable to other causes. Nowadays, few patients present with the classic findings of myxedema; instead, the features of hypothyroidism are more subtle and often equivocal on physical examination. When physical examination reveals a goiter, the possibility of thyroid dysfunction must be considered. A family history of thyroid disease should heighten this suspicion, because autoimmune thyroid disease is familial and is the most common cause of both hypothyroidism and hyperthyroidism.

Symptoms of weight loss, fatigue, nervousness, excessive sweating, and palpitation raise the possibility of hyperthyroidism. Tremor, tachycardia, a stare, and warm, moist skin are typical findings of hyperthyroidism; in the elderly, however, depression and anorexia may be the dominant features.

Suspicion of thyroid dysfunction based on the history and physical findings should be followed by ordering specific thyroid function tests. The currently used tests are readily available and very reliable.

THYROID FUNCTION TESTS

The serum thyroxine (T_4) test measures the total amount of thyroxine in serum. The normal range is about 4.5 to 11 µg/dL serum (58 to 140 nmol/L). Serum T_4 is elevated in hyperthyroidism and low in hypothyroidism [1••,2].

The serum triiodothyronine (T_3) level is a measurement of the total amount of T_3 in serum by radioimmunoassay. The normal range is about 80 to 180 ng/dL (1.2 to 2.7 nmol/L). It is a useful test for mild hyperthyroidism, because T_3 rises earlier and more markedly than does T_4 in all common forms of hyperthyroidism. In hypothyroidism, serum T_3 is within the normal range in at least one third of patients so it is not a sensitive test for this diagnosis.

Free T_4 is measured by equilibrium dialysis, a tedious method, or newer direct immunoassay methods [2]. It is reduced in hypothyroidism and increased in hyperthy-

TABLE 1 EFFECTS OF DRUGS ON THYROID FUNCTION TESTS

Test	Drug	Effect
T_4 and FT_4	Dilantin, carbamazepine	Decrease
T_4 and FT_4	Lithium	Decrease
T_4 and FT_4	Amiodarone	Increase
T_3	Amiodarone	Decrease
T_4 and FT_4	Propranolol	Increase
T_4 and T_3	Estrogen	Increase*
T_4 and T_3	Clofibrate	Increase*
T_4 and T_3	Testosterone, high-dose	Decrease
T_4 and T_3	L-asparaginase	Decrease
T_4	Salicylate, high-dose	Decrease*
FT_4	Heparin	Increase
Thyroid-stimulating hormone	Dopamine	Decrease
Thyroid-stimulating hormone	Glucocorticoid, high-dose	Decrease

*FT_4 normal.
T_3—triiodothyronine; T_4—thyroxine; FT_4—free thyroxine.

roidism. The T_3 uptake test (T_3U) indicates the degree of saturation of the thyroid hormone–binding proteins and is used for calculation of a free T_4 index (FT_4I) ($FT_4I = T_4 \times T_3U$).

Serum thyroid-stimulating hormone is measured by sensitive methods using monoclonal antibodies. The normal range is about 0.4 to 4 mU/L (μU/mL). Serum thyroid-stimulating hormone is particularly useful in the diagnosis of primary hypothyroidism because elevated thyroid-stimulating hormone occurs early with minimal thyroid dysfunction [3]. In pituitary-hypothalamic hypothyroidism, the serum thyroid-stimulating hormone is low or sometimes normal. The normal level of thyroid-stimulating hormone in this circumstance is attributed to secretion of thyroid-stimulating hormone with reduced biologic activity. In hyperthyroidism, serum thyroid-stimulating hormone is low.

Thyrotropin-releasing hormone may be administered to test the adequacy of pituitary thyroid-stimulating hormone secretion. The peak thyroid-stimulating hormone response to thyrotropin-releasing hormone is usually proportional to the baseline thyroid-stimulating hormone level. In hyperthyroidism, the low serum thyroid-stimulating hormone does not rise after thyrotropin-releasing hormone, because the pituitary cannot overcome the negative feedback inhibition of the high circulating levels of T_4 and T_3. With the improved sensitivity of serum thyroid-stimulating hormone measurements, there is no need to measure the thyroid-stimulating hormone response to thyrotropin-releasing hormone for the evaluation of thyroid disease.

The thyroid uptake of radioiodine is mainly useful for diagnosis of the cause of hyperthyroidism and for determining the dose of ^{131}I in treating hyperthyroidism [2].

Table 1 lists the effects of various drugs on thyroid function tests.

HYPOTHYROIDISM

Hypothyroidism is the condition that results from a lack of the effects of thyroid hormone on body tissues. It is a common condition with an overall frequency in the population of approximately 0.5% to 1.0% [3]. Because the frequency of hypothyroidism in persons over age 60 is about 4%, screening of geriatric patients for hypothyroidism is advocated [4,5•].

Table 2 lists the various causes of hypothyroidism in adults. Hashimoto's lymphocytic thyroiditis is the most common cause of hypothyroidism in adults and older children. "Idiopathic atrophy" usually results from Hashimoto's thyroiditis. The antimicrosomal antibody is the most sensitive marker for the disorder, but about one fifth of patients will have positive antithyroglobulin antibody and negative antimicrosomal antibody. Table 3 lists the most frequent symptoms and signs of hypothyroidism.

DIAGNOSIS

The best diagnostic tests are measurement of serum thyroid-stimulating hormone and FT_4I [1••,2]. Figure 1 shows the scheme for diagnosis.

TABLE 2 CAUSES OF HYPOTHYROIDISM IN ADULTS

Autoimmune (Hashimoto's) thyroiditis

Thyroid ablation
Surgical
After ^{131}I therapy for hyperthyroidism
Radiation to neck for Hodgkin's disease, laryngeal cancer, other cancers

Drugs
Inorganic iodine
Amiodarone (high iodine content)
Lithium

Hypopituitarism or hypothalamic lesion

Table 3. Symptoms and Signs of Hypothyroidism

System	Clinical features
Nervous	Forgetfulness, reduced memory, mental slowing, depression, carpal tunnel syndrome, hung-up reflexes
Cardiac	Bradycardia, quiet heart sounds, pericardial effusion, dependent edema, low-voltage ECG, flat T waves
Gastrointestinal	Constipation, ascites (rare)
Renal	Reduced excretion of water load, hyponatremia (uncommon)
Pulmonary	CO_2 retention, pleural effusion (rare)
Blood	Anemia
Skin and hair	Dry cool skin, puffy sallow facies, thin lateral eyebrows and body hair, coarse scalp hair
Reproductive	Menorrhaghia from anovulatory cycles, primary or secondary amenorrhea, galactorrhea (increased serum prolactin)
Development	Retarded growth in children
Metabolism	Fatigue (most common), weight gain, hypothermia, increased serum cholesterol, or triglyceride

ECG—electrocardiogram.

In patients with a doubtful diagnosis of hypothyroidism who are taking thyroid hormone therapy, it is necessary to stop the therapy to make the diagnosis. If the patient is taking levothyroxine or desiccated thyroid, therapy must be stopped for 5 weeks; if the patient is taking triiodothyronine, therapy must be stopped for only 10 days. At the end of this period, measurement of thyroid-stimulating hormone and FT_4I will give reliable results of thyroid function.

Treatment

Levothyroxine is the preferred preparation for replacement therapy, because it is more uniform than biologic preparations, its absorption is reliable, and it is easily measured in serum. Because the circulating T_3 in T_4-treated patients comes from conversion of T_4 to T_3 in tissue, normal ranges for T_4 and T_3 can be used to monitor therapy [6]. The best laboratory indicator of the adequacy of therapy is the serum thyroid-stimulating hormone level, which should be in the normal range when the dose of thyroxine is optimal. It takes about 6 weeks for the serum thyroid-stimulating hormone level to stabilize after a change in the dose of thyroxine. The full daily replacement dose in most adults is about 100 to 150 µg of levothyroxine (1.6 µg/kg body weight) [6]. The dose in geriatric patients is 50% to 75% that of young adults [4,5•]. In hypothyroid women who become pregnant, the requirement for thyroxine increases, and it is often necessary to increase the dose of levothyroxine by 25% to 50% to maintain the serum thyroid-stimulating hormone in the normal range during the pregnancy [7].

In patients with coronary artery disease, it is preferable to initiate therapy with a small dose, such as 25 µg levothyroxine, and to increase by 25 µg at intervals of 4 to 6 weeks. If angina is exacerbated, then the dose should be reduced. Surgical treatment of the coronary artery disease may be carried out, if necessary, before optimal replacement therapy of hypothyroidism is achieved [8].

A subnormal serum thyroid-stimulating hormone indicates that the replacement dose of levothyroxine is excessive and is an indication for reducing the dose [1••]. Excessive replacement doses may cause osteoporosis, tachycardia, and other adverse cardiac effects [9].

Myxedema Coma

Myxedema coma is the end result of long-standing untreated hypothyroidism. These patients have hypothermia, bradycardia, alveolar hypoventilation, and severe obtundation or coma. Supportive therapy and treatment of underlying illness, such as infection, is essential. Specific therapy consists of giving 500 µg levothyroxine intravenously, but initial doses of 200 to 300 µg are also recommended [10,11•].

Hyperthyroidism

Hyperthyroidism is the condition that results from the effect of excessive amounts of thyroid hormones on body tissues. At one time or another, approximately 0.5% of the population has hyperthyroidism.

Table 4 lists the various causes. The most common cause of hyperthyroidism is Graves' disease. The serum IgG of patients with Graves' hyperthyroidism contains a thyroid-

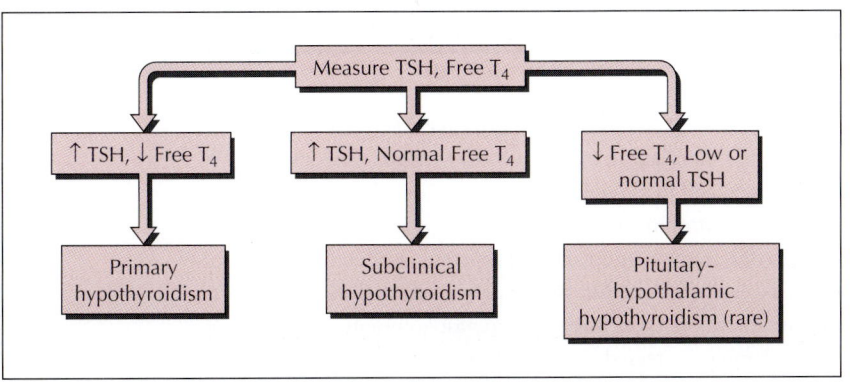

Figure 1 Diagnosis of hypothyroidism. T_4—thyroxine; TSH—thyroid-stimulating hormone.

TABLE 4 CAUSES OF HYPERTHYROIDISM
Graves' disease
Hyperfunctioning solitary thyroid adenoma ("hot" nodule)
"Toxic" multinodular goiter
Lymphocytic thyroiditis with low thyroid radioiodine uptake
Subacute (granulomatous) thyroiditis (early phase)
Ingestion of excessive amount of thyroid hormones
Thyroid-stimulating hormone-producing pituitary adenoma
Pituitary resistance to suppression of thyroid-stimulating hormone secretion by thyroid hormone because of a mutation in the T_3 receptor
Trophoblastic tumors (hydatidiform mole, choriocarcinoma) that secrete excessive amounts of chorionic gonadotropin, a weak thyroid stimulator
Follicular thyroid carcinoma with widespread metastases
Struma ovarii (ovarian teratoma with thyroid elements)

stimulating IgG. With sensitive assays, thyroid-stimulating IgG is found in the serum of over 90% of patients with active hyperthyroidism. The ophthalmopathy that occurs in about 40% of patients with Graves' hyperthyroidism probably results from antibodies directed against retro-orbital antigens such as extraocular muscle constituents.

Table 5 lists the symptoms and signs [5•].

DIAGNOSIS

Elevated serum levels of thyroid hormones are the hallmark of the diagnosis. Ordinarily, serum T_4, FT_4I, and T_3 are all elevated, and serum thyroid-stimulating hormone is suppressed [12•]. Measurement of thyroid-stimulating IgG is probably not worthwhile to diagnose Graves' disease, because the result does not alter management. With current sensitive thyroid-stimulating hormone assay, a normal or elevated serum thyroid-stimulating hormone should raise consideration of the rare forms of thyroid-stimulating hormone–induced hyperthyroidism listed in Table 4.

Although thyroid radioiodine uptake is high in most forms of hyperthyroidism, it is low in patients who are thyrotoxic because of lymphocytic thyroiditis, subacute thyroiditis, or ingestion of thyroid hormone. The thyroid scan in Graves' disease shows diffuse uptake of radioiodine. The scan is helpful if a solitary hyperfunctioning thyroid adenoma is being considered as the cause of hyperthyroidism in a patient with a palpable nodule. Figure 2 shows the plan for differential diagnosis. Patients with acute psychosis may have transient elevation of thyroid hormone levels, but these usually normalize within 1 or 2 weeks without specific therapy.

TREATMENT

Three definitive modes of treatment are available for hyperthyroidism: drugs, ^{131}I, and surgical thyroidectomy [13••,14]. Propylthiouracil and methimazole remain the principal drug therapy of hyperthyroidism and are used mainly in young and middle-aged patients. These drugs block the synthesis of thyroid hormone and may also suppress thyroid autoimmunity. Drug therapy for 1.5 to 2.0 years improves the chance of achieving a long-term remission, in contrast with treatment for only 6 months [13••]. Figure 3 illustrates a typical patient's course.

The hyperthyroidism of thyroiditis results from leakage of thyroid hormone into the circulation caused by the destructive process and does not improve with antithyroid drugs that block biosynthesis. Instead, it should be treated with β-adrenergic blocking drugs. Adrenergic blockers cause rapid improvement of many features of hyperthyroidism and are useful as adjunctive therapy while waiting for the results of definitive therapy [15].

The radiographic contrast drugs, sodium ipodate and iopanoic acid, improve severely hyperthyroid patients dramatically by blocking T_4 to T_3 conversion in peripheral tissues, thus lowering T_3 levels, and their iodine content blocks release of hormone from the thyroid. The long-term use of these drugs has been limited to a few patients, and a high proportion have escaped from control of the hyperthyroidism, a result analogous to escape from the effect of therapy with inorganic iodine.

Radioiodine is the most common therapy of Graves' hyperthyroidism; hypothyroidism is the main complication and occurs in the majority of patients, often years later. Hypothyroidism within the first 6 months after ^{131}I may be temporary. Because ^{131}I therapy may worsen preexisting

TABLE 5 SYMPTOMS AND SIGNS OF HYPERTHYROIDISM	
System	**Clinical features**
Nervous	Nervousness, emotional lability, tremor, brisk reflexes
Cardiac	Tachycardia, atrial fibrillation, congestive heart failure, flow murmurs
Gastrointestinal	Increased appetite and food intake, hyperdefecation, abnormal liver function tests
Musculoskeletal	Weakness, muscle atrophy, osteopenia
Eyes	Stare because of retraction of upper lid, proptosis, restricted ocular motility
Skin and hair	Warm-moist-velvety texture, hot sweaty palms, onycholysis
Reproductive	Oligomenorrhea, impaired fertility, gynecomastia, impotence
Metabolism	Weight loss, fatigue, increased sweating, heat intolerance

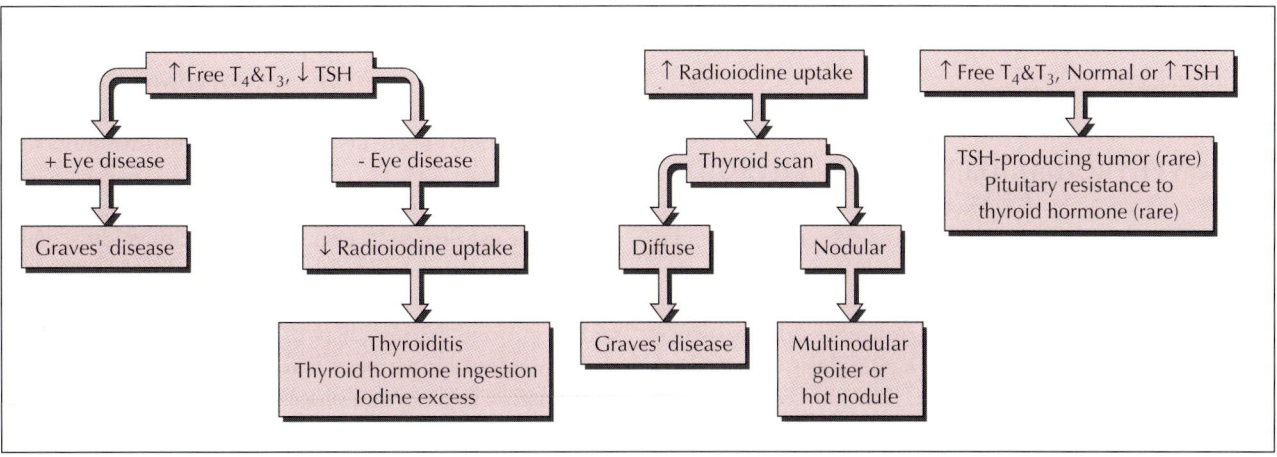

FIGURE 2 Differential diagnosis of hyperthyroidism. T₃—triiodothyronine; T₄—thyroxine; TSH—thyroid-stimulating hormone.

ophthalmopathy, patients with ophthalmopathy may benefit from a course of prednisone therapy given for a few months after the ¹³¹I [16].

Surgical thyroidectomy is usually reserved for special situations, such as obstructing goiters or allergy to antithyroid drugs or refusal to take ¹³¹I. Although some patients can be prepared for surgery with β-blockers alone to control tachycardia, common practice continues to be restoration of the euthyroid state with antithyroid drugs and stable iodine before surgery [13••,14].

CHOICE OF THERAPY

For patients less than 45 years of age, the author prefers to use antithyroid drugs as the definitive therapy. If a patient continues to require a high dose of antithyroid drug after 18 months of therapy or is noncompliant, then radioiodine therapy is recommended. For older patients with complicating illnesses and those with multinodular goiter or single hot nodules, radioiodine is recommended. However, the hyperthyroidism of these patients should be controlled with antithyroid drugs or β-adrenergic blockers before giving radioiodine.

Hyperthyroidism occurs in approximately 1 per 1000 pregnancies. It can be treated effectively with antithyroid drugs, but because they cross the placenta, the lowest possible doses should be used to control the hyperthyroidism [17]. Alternatively, surgical thyroidectomy can be performed safely during the second trimester after control of the hyperthyroidism with antithyroid drugs. Care must be exercised to avoid postoperative hypothyroidism. Radioiodine should not be given to the pregnant woman, because it crosses the placenta and could cause permanent hypothyroidism in the fetus, which has a functional thyroid by the 10th week of gestation.

THYROID STORM

Patients with thyroid storm, or severe decompensated hyperthyroidism, have tachycardia, fever, agitation or psychosis, nausea, vomiting, and diarrhea. There is usually a precipitating factor, such as infection, gastroenteritis, severe trauma, or

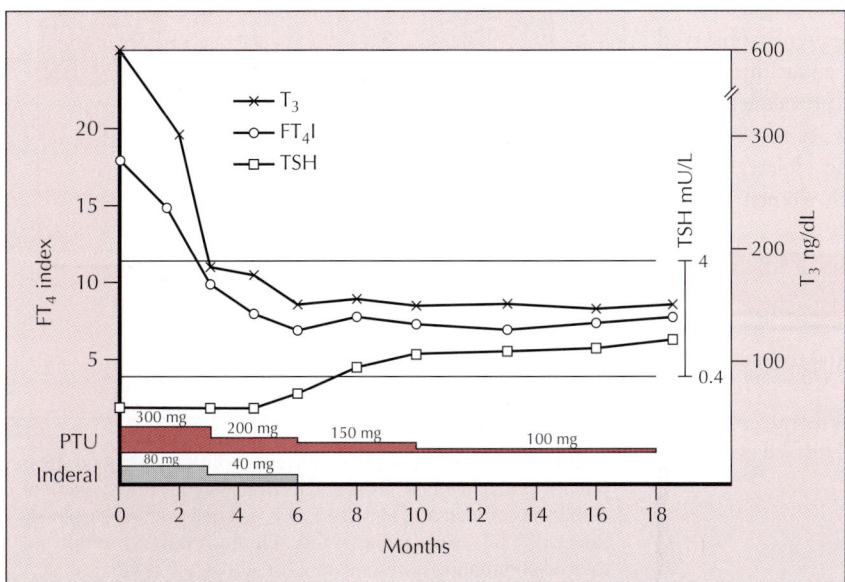

FIGURE 3 Course of therapy in a typical hyperthyroid patients treated with propylthiouracil (PTU). FT₄I—free thyroxine index; T₃—triiodothyronine; TSH—thyroid-stimulating hormone.

surgery [10,11•]. Supportive measures and treatment of the underlying causative factor are essential. Table 6 lists the specific therapy.

NONTHYROIDAL ILLNESS AND THYROID FUNCTION

Severe illnesses that do not involve the thyroid directly may cause changes in serum thyroid hormone levels [18•]. Reduction of the serum T_3 occurs commonly with many forms of metabolic stress, such as starvation, any serious illness such as pneumonia or septicemia, diabetic ketoacidosis, chronic liver disease, uremia, and major surgery. The low serum T_3 level results from impairment of 5'-monodeiodination of T_4 in peripheral tissues such as the liver, a process that usually provides 80% of the daily T_3 production. With more severe illnesses, serum T_4 concentrations also decrease, but free T_4 usually remains normal, although it may be low in some patients [18•]. Reverse T_3 is generally elevated. These patients with low T_3 and T_4 levels usually have normal serum thyroid-stimulating hormone levels, which excludes the diagnosis of primary hypothyroidism. Corticosteroids and dopamine, often used in these patients, may suppress serum thyroid-stimulating hormone levels. During recovery from the severe illness, serum T_4 and thyroid-stimulating hormone levels rise concomitantly. In this recovery phase, serum thyroid-stimulating hormone may exceed the normal range transiently. With further recovery, serum T_3 normalizes. Figure 4 diagrams the changes in thyroid function tests. Trials of therapy with T_4 or T_3 have not improved survival of the "sick euthyroid" patients [19•].

AUTOIMMUNE THYROID DISEASE

Autoimmune thyroid disease includes Hashimoto's chronic lymphocytic thyroiditis, Graves' disease, and lymphocytic thyroiditis with hyperthyroidism [20]. Several antibodies are found in the serum of these patients: antibody to thyroid microsomes (the microsomal antigen is thyroid peroxidase), antibody to thyroglobulin and antibodies to the thyroid-stimulating hormone receptor (or thyroid-stimulating IgG).

Hashimoto's thyroiditis is the most frequently observed thyroid disorder in the United States. It is about three times more common in women than in men. Its prevalence, based on antibody screening, is approximately 3% to 4% of the population, 1.4% in euthyroid asymptomatic adolescents, and about 30% to 40% of middle-aged and elderly women.

Clinically, about three fourths of the patients with Hashimoto's thyroiditis have goiter, but they are euthyroid and asymptomatic; one fourth have hypothyroidism with or without goiter, and a small proportion are hyperthyroid. Nearly one third of patients with lymphocytic thyroiditis have a nodular goiter.

Hyperthyroidism associated with low thyroid uptake of radioiodine usually results from lymphocytic thyroiditis, which is probably a variant of Hashimoto's thyroiditis [21,22]. The thyroid is not tender and is only slightly enlarged. The inflammatory process causes a leak of thyroid hormone into the circulation, but biosynthesis is reduced. Patients will usually go through a hypothyroid phase. The disease is self-limited, subsides in 1 to 3 months, and usually does not result in permanent hypothyroidism. This condition contrasts with subacute granulomatous thyroiditis, which causes very tender, irregular, firm, enlarged thyroid glands. Table 7 compares silent lymphocytic thyroiditis with hyperthyroidism and subacute granulomatous thyroiditis.

Pregnancy influences the clinical course of autoimmune thyroid disease. As pregnancy advances, the levels of thyroid autoantibodies decline. Following delivery, the titers increase, reaching a peak 3 to 4 months postpartum. This transient rebound of the autoimmune process causes postpartum thyroiditis in about 6% to 8% of postpartum women [21,22]. The most common course is transient hyperthyroidism followed by hypothyroidism and then recovery. There may be only a hypothyroid phase with spontaneous recovery in several months. In treating the hypothyroidism, one must keep in mind that it may remit, therefore therapy should be interrupted after 6 to 12 months to test for remission of the hypothyroidism [22].

TABLE 6 TREATMENT OF THYROID STORM
Propylthiouracil (600 mg) or methimazole (60 mg) stat and half this dose every 6 h
Sodium ipodate 1 g stat and 1 g daily for 14 d or 0.5 mL SSKI twice daily or 1 g sodium iodide IV infused over 8 h
Propranolol 40–80 mg every 4 to 6 h
Dexamethasone 4–8 mg daily
SSKI—saturated solution of potassium iodide.

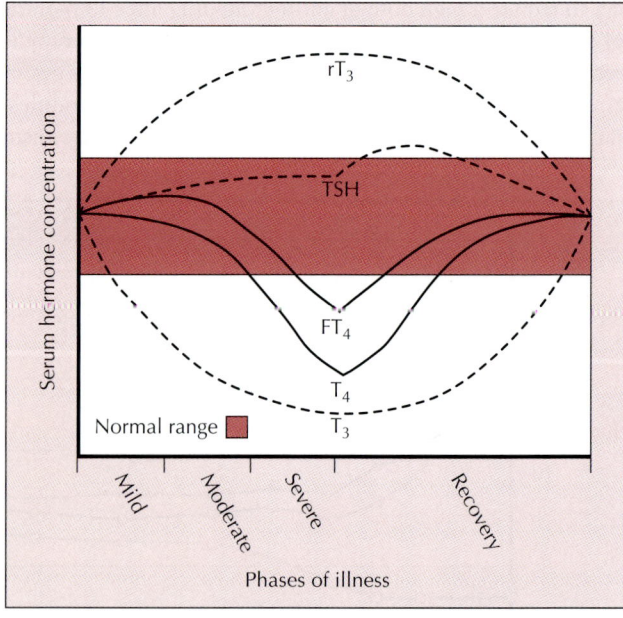

FIGURE 4 Thyroid hormone and thyroid-stimulating hormone (TSH) profiles in nonthyroidal illness and recovery. Serum T_3 is subnormal in mild illness; serum T_4 and free T_4 (FT_4) fall only with severe illness. Reverse T_3 (rT_3) rises as the T_3 falls. During recovery, serum thyroid-stimulating hormone may rise above the normal range.

Table 7. Comparison of Lymphocytic Thyroiditis with Hyperthyroidism and Subacute Granulomatous Thyroiditis

Feature	Lymphocytic	Granulomatous
Onset	Often postpartum	After viral infection
Fever	No	Yes
Thyroid gland	Symmetric, slightly enlarged or normal size, nontender	Irregular, very firm, tender
Hyperthyroid phase	1–4 mo	2–8 wk
Hypothyroid phase	Several mo	Several wk
Antithyroid antibody	Negative	Positive

References and Recommended Reading

Recently published papers of particular interest have been highlighted as:
- Of interest
- •• Of outstanding interest

1. •• Surks MI, Chopra IJ, Mariash CN, et al.: American Thyroid Association guidelines for use of laboratory in thyroid disorders. *JAMA* 1990, 2763:1529–1532.
2. Bayer MF: Effective laboratory evaluation of thyroid status. *Med Clin North Am* 1991, 75:1–26.
3. Helfand M, Crapo IM: Screening for thyroid disease. *Ann Intern Med* 1990, 112:840–849.
4. Sawin CT: Thyroid dysfunction in older persons. *Advances Intern Med* 1991, 37:223–248.
5. • Kunitake J, Pekary AE, Hershman JM: Aging and the hypothalamic-pituitary-thyroid axis. In *Problems in Geriatric Endocrinology*. Edited by Morley JE, Korenman SG. Boston: Blackwell; 1991:92–110.
6. Fish LH, Schwartz HL, Cavanaugh J, et al.: Replacement dose, metabolism, and bioavailability of levothyroxine in the treatment of hypothyroidism. *N Engl J Med* 1991, 316:764–770.
7. Mandel SJ, Larsen PR, Seely EW, Brent GA: Increased need for thyroxine during pregnancy in women with primary hypothyroidism. *N Engl J Med* 1990, 323:91–96.
8. Ladenson PW: Recognition and management of cardiovascular disease related to thyroid dysfunction. *Am J Med* 1990, 88:638–641.
9. Wartofsky L: Does replacement thyroxine therapy cause osteoporosis? *Advances Endocrinol Metab* 1993, 4:157–175.
10. Gavin LA: Thyroid crises. *Med Clin North Am* 1991, 75:179–193.
11. • Smallridge RC: Metabolic and anatomic thyroid emergencies: a review. *Crit Care Med* 1992, 20:276–291.
12. • Ross DS, Ardisson LJ, Meskell MJ: Measurement of thyrotropin in clinical and subclinical hyperthyroidism using a new chemiluminescent assay. *J Clin Endocrinol Metab* 1989, 69:684–688.
13. •• Klein I, Becker DV, Levey GS: Treatment of hyperthyroid disease. *Ann Intern Med* 1994, 121:281–288.
14. Franklyn JA: The management of hyperthyroidism. *N Engl J Med* 1994, 330:1731–1738.
15. Geffner DL, Hershman JM: β-adrenergic blockade for therapy of hyperthyroidism. *Am J Med* 1993, 93:61–68.
16. Marcocci C, Bartalena L, Bogazzi F, et al.: Relationship between Graves' ophthalmology and type of treatment of Graves' hyperthyroidism. *Thyroid* 1992, 2:171–178.
17. Burrow GN: Thyroid function and hyperfunction during gestation. *Endo Rev* 1993, 14:194–202.
18. • Wong TK, Hershman JM: Changes in thyroid function in nonthyroid illness. *Trends Endocrinol Metab* 1992, 3:8–12.
19. • Brent GA, Hershman JM: Thyroxine therapy in patients with severe nonthyroidal illnesses and low serum thyroxine concentration. *J Clin Endocrinol Metab* 1986, 63:1–8.
20. Volpe R: Autoimmune thyroiditis. In *Werner and Ingbar's The Thyroid*, edn 6. Edited by Braverman LE, Utiger RD. Philadelphia: JB Lippincott; 1991:710–727.
21. Nikolai TF: Silent thyroiditis and subacute thyroiditis. In *Werner and Ingbar's The Thyroid*, edn 6. Edited by Braverman LE, Utiger RD. Philadelphia: JB Lippincott; 1991:921–933.
22. Learoyd DL, Fung HYM, McGregor AM: Postpartum thyroid dysfunction. *Thyroid* 1992, 2:73–80.

Select Bibliography

Mandel SJ, Brent GA, Larsen PR: Levothyroxine therapy in patients with thyroid disease. *Ann Intern Med* 1993, 119:492–502.

Van Middlesworth L, ed: *The Thyroid Gland*. Chicago: Year Book; 1986.

Werner, Ingbar: *The Thyroid*, edn 6. Edited by Braverman LE, Utiger RD. Philadelphia: JB Lippincott; 1991.

Thyroid Masses

J. Francisco Fierro-Renoy
Leslie J. DeGroot

> ### Key Points
> - Diffuse thyroid enlargement (goiter) in the United States is predominantly caused by autoimmune thyroid disease.
> - Single thyroid nodules have a prevalence of approximately 2% in American women, and multinodular goiter is now much less frequent because of an abundance of iodine in our diet.
> - Multinodular goiters tend to grow slowly (despite attempts at suppression of thyroid-stimulating hormone), gradually become autonomous, and, over many years, become toxic.
> - Frontline evaluation of thyroid solitary nodules depends on fine-needle aspiration, often complemented by ultrasonography, and thyroid isotope scanning is performed much less frequently than in past years.
> - Localized, painful enlargement of the thyroid requires consideration of bleeding into a nodule, subactue thyroiditis, acute infectious thyroiditis often in a nodule or cyst, and fortunately, less frequently, rapid growth of a thyroid lymphoma or carcinoma.

Goiter, or a thyroid mass, can be defined as a diffuse or nodular enlargement of the thyroid gland. Two fundamental questions should be considered in the evaluation of a goiter. What is the metabolic status of the patient, and what is the underlying cause or nature of the goiter, including its benign or malignant character?

The evaluation of a goiter includes a detailed clinical history and physical examination and a careful examination of the thyroid gland. A family history of thyroid disease, past exposure to radiotherapy, and a history of previous thyroid disease are important considerations. Much of the subsequent diagnostic process depends on a careful examination of the thyroid. A normal gland can usually be palpated. It weighs approximately 15 to 20 g. Any enlargement should be carefully inspected to determine whether the process is diffuse or focal and whether it contains discrete nodules. The temporal pattern of the growth is important, as is evidence of compression or displacement of adjacent structures. Consistency, tenderness, and movement of the nodule when swallowing, as well as the presence of pain or regional lymph nodes may be clues to the diagnosis. A single nodule should be characterized as solid or cystic, and the presence of other nodules should be determined. It may be useful to know whether the nodule is functional. A single nodule in an otherwise normal gland requires a careful evaluation and follow-up because of the increased possibility of cancer. The presence of multiple nodules, ascertained by physical examination or other diagnostic test, is typical of multinodular goiter, a common and usually benign thyroid condition. In the United States, an autoimmune thyroid disease is the most frequent explanation for a diffuse goiter. A suggested approach to a patient with goiter is shown in Figure 1.

Goiter in Autoimmune Thyroid Disorders

Two autoimmune diseases of the thyroid, Graves' disease and Hashimoto's thyroiditis are frequent causes of diffuse goiter. In both, there is evidence of cell-mediated and humoral autoimmunity directed against thyroid antigens. The presence of antibodies against thyroid peroxidase (microsomal antigen) and thyroglobulin is a hallmark of both disorders, and thyroid stimulating antibodies are present in Graves' disease [1].

There is lymphocytic infiltration of the thyroid, with fibrosis in Hashimoto's thyroiditis and hyperplasia in Graves' disease. There is a strong hereditary component. The patients and their relatives have an increased susceptibility to other autoimmune diseases.

Graves' Disease

Clinical presentation and diagnosis

Graves' disease affects approximately 0.4% of Americans and is 10 times more frequent among women than men. It is characterized by a diffuse goiter and hyperthyroidism, often infiltrative ophthalmopathy and rarely by infiltrative dermopathy (*see* Chapter 3, Thyroid Dysfunction).

As shown in Figure 1, measurement of suppressed thyroid-stimulating hormone, and thyroid hormone levels, together with an index of hormone binding (free thyroxine index), establishes the diagnosis of hyperthyroidism. The presence of positive antithyroid antibodies is helpful and detection of thyroid-stimulating hormone receptor antibodies is useful in less clear situations, such as an isolated or unilateral exophthalmos. The demonstration of extraocular muscle swelling by ultrasound or computerized axial tomography scan suggests strongly that ophthalmopathy is a manifestation of Graves' disease.

Hashimoto's Thyroiditis

Clinical presentation and diagnosis

Hashimoto's thyroiditis, or chronic lymphocytic thyroiditis, is the most common cause of goitrous hypothyroidism in western countries. The goiter is usually moderate in size (2 to 3 times normal) painless, firm, and symmetric, with a conspicuous pyramidal lobe. Often, the surface is finely nodular, but well-defined nodules are unusual. The goiter is caused by lymphocytic infiltration and cell damage, with some compensatory hyperplasia. Hypothyroidism may be caused by thyroid cell damage or thyroid-stimulating hormone–blocking antibodies.

Although rare, sudden growth of the gland, especially if the gland is asymmetric, may suggest a malignant lymphoma. If hypothyroidism is present, the diagnosis of Hashimoto's thyroiditis is almost certain. The diagnosis is confirmed by the finding of a high titer of antimicrosomal and antithyroglobulin antibodies in serum.

Treatment

An asymptomatic patient with a small goiter due to Hashimoto's thyroiditis may not need treatment. Thyroid hormone, which can also be used to decrease the size of the goiter, should be given if there is evidence of thyroid failure, A good response is most frequently observed in patients with

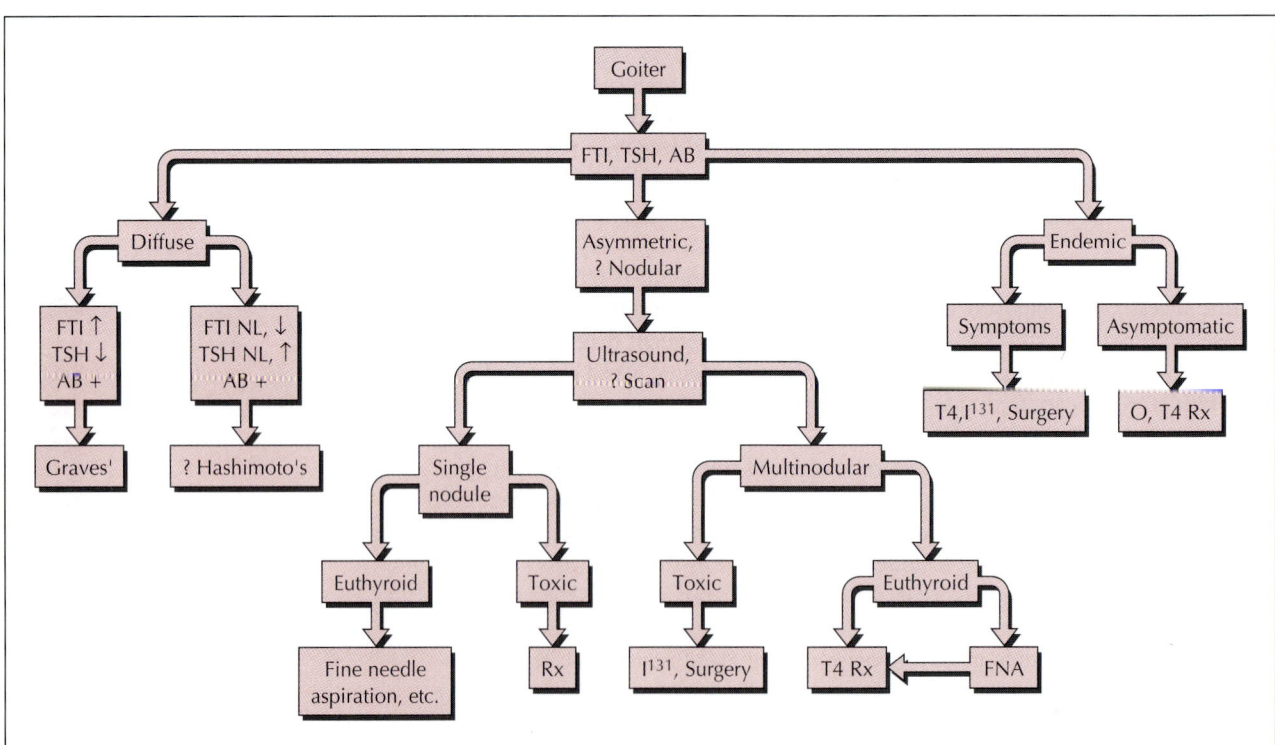

Figure 1 Suggested approach to a goiter. AB—antithyroid antibodies; FNA—fine-needle aspiration; FTI—free thyroxine index; ^{131}I—radioactive iodine; T4 Rx—levothyroxine treatment; TSH—thyroid-stimulating hormone; US—ultrasound.

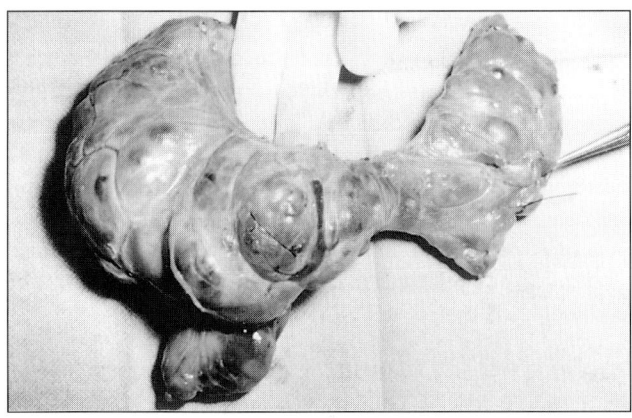

FIGURE 2 A typical, large multinodular goiter. Goiters of this size are rarely seen in the United States, but are not unusual in countries where diets are iodine deficient.

recent onset of disease. Rarely is surgery indicated. Other autoimmune diseases (*eg*, pernicious anemia, primary adrenal failure) are more frequent in these patients and should be considered during follow-up.

The relation of the silent (painless) thyroiditis syndromes, which occur postpartum and independent of pregnancy, to Hashimoto's thyroiditis, is not absolutely established, but most likely these illnesses fit within the spectrum of autoimmune thyroid disease. Both forms usually display antithyroid antibodies at low titers. Typically, a transient phase of hyperthyroidism with low radioactive iodine uptake is followed by one of transient hypothyroidism.

NONTOXIC DIFFUSE AND MULTINODULAR GOITER

Nontoxic Diffuse Goiter

Nontoxic diffuse goiter, also called colloid goiter, and multinodular goiter are two closely related common disorders of the thyroid. A long-standing colloid goiter becomes nodular as a consequence of continued stimulation of the thyroid. Factors that lead to goitrous hypothyroidism can, if less severe, give rise to a diffuse goiter. Iodine deficiency and chronic exposure to products that impair the normal function of the thyroid are possible causes, but in most patients in the United States no extrinsic goitrogenic factor can be identified. Hereditary defects in any of the steps of thyroid hormone synthesis are occasionally the cause [2], and, in a sizeable group of patients, the disorder seems to run in families. Most often, however, no intrinsic abnormality of thyroid hormone synthesis can be demonstrated, but tests to evaluate these disorders may not be sensitive enough to pick up mild defects. In the United States, a modest biosynthetic abnormality is the most likely explanation for sporadic multinodular goiter.

Clinical presentation and diagnosis

Diffuse asymptomatic colloid goiter as a cause of enlargement of the thyroid occurs occasionally in adolescent girls or during pregnancy. It occurs less often in other adults. Usually, the thyroid is 2 to 5 times normal size, symmetrically enlarged, and feels soft and spongy. This diffuse stage of the nontoxic goiter resembles the goiter of either Graves' disease or Hashimoto's thyroiditis. In Hashimoto's thyroiditis, the gland is firmer and more irregular. The finding of antithyroid antibodies is strong evidence for an autoimmune thyroid disease.

Treatment

Most patients with a colloid goiter are euthyroid, or they may have slightly elevated thyroid-stimulating hormone levels. Thyroid hormone treatment may decrease the size of the goiter or prevent it from growing. If there are significant pressure symptoms or serious cosmetic problems, surgical resection may be indicated. Thyroid hormone replacement is then needed to prevent growth of the remaining thyroid tissue.

Multinodular Goiter

It is believed that because of a number of intrinsic cellular, vascular, and connective tissue responses, nodularity becomes increasingly prominent in the initial "colloid goiter," over years giving rise to a multinodular goiter (Figs. 2 and 3). Multinodular goiter is probably the most common of all thyroid gland disorders. It is found in approximately 4% of all adults and is more common in women than men.

Clinical and anatomic features

Multinodular goiter is characterized by anatomic and functional heterogeneity and a tendency to develop functional autonomy [3,4]. Pathologic evaluation shows colloid nodules, true adenomas, and cysts. Fibrotic and sometimes calcified areas are unevenly distributed between areas of relatively normal thyroid tissue. Hypofunctional or clearly nonfunctional areas are present throughout the gland and are mixed with regions of nodular growth, exhibiting activity independent of thyroid-stimulating hormone.

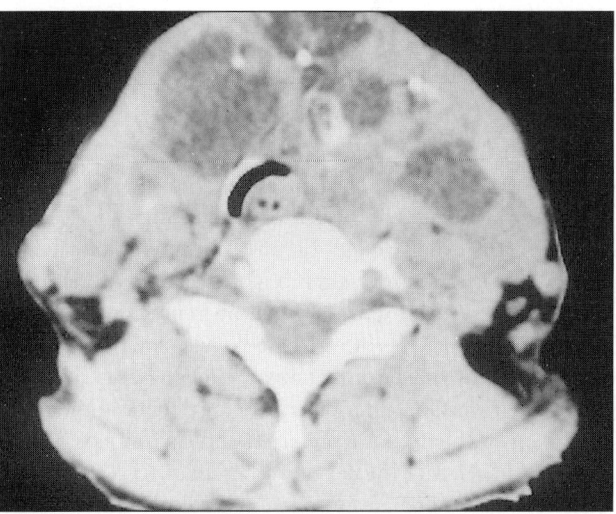

FIGURE 3 Computed tomography scan of a multinodular goiter. A bilaterally enlarged gland contains several nodules, some having less signal intensity than the rest of the gland, probably corresponding to areas of cystic and necrotic changes as well as to degenerated colloid nodules.

The amount of autonomously functioning tissue may become sufficient to suppress thyroid-stimulating hormone and eventually cause hyperthyroidism. This clinical picture is known as toxic multinodular goiter. These patients are sensitive to iodine and may develop thyrotoxicosis if exposed to an iodine load. Occasionally, a sudden increase in the size of the gland is associated with sharp pain and tenderness in one area. This event is usually caused by hemorrhage into a cyst of the nodular goiter. A clinically significant cancerous lesion in the context of a multinodular goiter occurs infrequently.

Treatment

Toxic multinodular goiter is usually treated with radioactive iodine, which reduces the size of the goiter and controls the hyperthyroidism. Sometimes, larger than usual doses of radioactive iodine are required. Alternatively, surgical subtotal thyroidectomy may be used, particularly if the gland is large. If the multinodular goiter is moderate in size and the patient has a normal thyroid-stimulating hormone level, therapy is probably not required. Thyroid hormone treatment may reduce the size of the goiter with modest results in probably less than 40% of patients. Bilateral subtotal thyroidectomy should be performed if there is sudden growth in the goiter, a hard nodule, a serious cosmetic defect, or disturbing local symptoms resulting from tracheal compression or entrapment of the goiter below the sternum. After surgery, thyroid hormone replacement helps prevent regeneration of the goiter.

GOITROUS HYPOTHYROIDISM

Iodine Deficiency

Endemic goiter (*ie*, goiter affecting 10% or more of the population) is usually caused by iodine deficiency. Although still a major public health problem in many areas of the world, it is no longer a problem in the United States. Iodine in salt, bread, other foodstuffs, and medicines is an effective prophylactic measure.

Goitrogens

Besides antithyroid drugs used in treatment of hyperthyroidism, other drugs can be goitrogenic and sometimes cause hypothyroidism. Lithium is most important among these because of its extensive use. Because lithium inhibits adenylate cyclase activity, it also inhibits the secretory function of the thyroid. Goiter with or without hypothyroidism can develop. Most patients affected are female, and patients with evidence of thyroid autoimmunity are more susceptible. The effects are reversible, and sometimes the beneficial therapeutic effects of the drug are preferred and thyroid hormone is prescribed to replace the deficit. Other drugs with goitrogenic properties are para-aminosalicylic acid, phenylbutazone, ethionamide, and topical resorcinol. These drugs rarely cause goiter with or without hypothyroidism. Naturally occurring goitrogens in certain foods, including the almond, rutabaga, white turnip, sorghum, cabbage, cauliflower, and cassava, can, if ingested in vast excess, cause goiter. At the practical level, these are not a problem.

Hereditary Defects

Genetically determined defects in hormone biosynthesis are a rare cause of goiter and hypothyroidism. Several members of a family are usually affected. All defects described so far are transmitted as autosomal recessive traits. Individuals with goiter and hypothyroidism are presumably homozygous for the defect. Initially, the goiter is diffuse, but if the hyperplastic stimulus persists, a nodular gland eventually develops. Heterozygous relatives may display a small goiter and be euthyroid [2].

Iodine Goiter

Daily requirements of iodine are about 100µg/d. Chronic exposure to more than several milligrams of iodine can block the organification of trapped iodine and can cause goiter with or without hypothyroidism in susceptible individuals. The iodine goiter is firm and diffuse. The source of excess iodine may come from the diet (*eg*, from seaweed) or drugs such as potassium iodide sometimes given to patients with chronic respiratory disorders. Patients with Hashimoto's thyroiditis or previously treated Graves' disease are known to be susceptible to this phenomenon. Patients with cystic fibrosis are also reportedly sensitive to a chronic iodine overload. Ingestion of excessive amounts of iodine by a gravid woman may cause an iodide goiter in the fetus; if the gland is large enough, it may result in asphyxia during the postnatal period.

Exposure to the antiarrhythmic drug amiodarone, which may release up to 6 mg of iodine per 200-mg tablet, can produce hypothyroidism and goiter, and occasionally thyrotoxicosis [5].

SUBACUTE THYROIDITIS

Clinical Presentation and Diagnosis

Subacute thyroiditis is an inflammatory condition of the thyroid of unknown cause. Frequently, the disorder follows a mild viral upper respiratory tract infection. In full-blown cases, the patient develops pain that is sometimes severe together with extreme tenderness of the thyroid. The pain may radiate to the jaw or ears. The overlying skin may be warm and red. The thyroid gland is enlarged, usually bilaterally and uniformly, but it may be asymmetric with predominant involvement of one lobe. A mild fever is common. Malaise, fatigue, and myalgia are common and sometimes out of proportion with the local character of the inflammatory process.

Approximately half of the patients present during the first few weeks of the illness with symptoms of thyrotoxicosis. Thyrotoxicosis is caused by an excessive release of thyroid hormone as a result of the destruction of the follicular epithelium and loss of follicular integrity induced by the inflammatory process. The radioactive iodine uptake at this time is typically low, reflecting the suppressed thyroid-stimulating hormone levels and the destructive process itself. The sedimentation rate is high, often remarkably so. Thyroglobulin levels are increased because of their release from the gland.

As the disease process subsides, a transient phase of hypothyroidism is often observed before full recovery. Ultimately, thyroid function returns to normal. Permanent hypothyroidism occurs in less than 10% of patients, usually as a consequence of a protracted course with several recurrences over many months.

Treatment

The active phase of the disease usually abates in 1 to 2 weeks, and the disease subsides within a few months. Aspirin or nonsteroidal antiinflammatory drugs are, in most instances, an effective remedy during the active inflammatory stage. Occasionally, the disease is severe enough to require narcotics and steroid therapy.

INFECTIOUS THYROIDITIS AND OTHER RARE CAUSES OF GOITER

Infectious Thyroiditis

Bacterial invasion of the gland causing an acute infectious thyroiditis is rare. It is most commonly the result of direct extension from an infected contiguous structure, an internal fistula arising from a remnant of the fourth pharyngeal pouch, an infected persistent thyroglossal duct, or metastatic seeding during bacteremia.

The dominant symptom is pain over the thyroid, which may become enlarged, hot, and tender. The patient is unable to move his or her neck freely. There are systemic signs and symptoms of infection, including fever and chills. There are usually no symptoms of hyperthyroidism or hypothyroidism, and thyroid hormone levels are normal, unless the thyroid is extensively involved. A scintiscan often shows a "cold" area corresponding to the site of abcess formation. Needle biopsy of the thyroid should be done so the infectious agent can be identified and treated with antibiotics. Surgical drainage may be required.

Systemic Diseases

Two systemic diseases, sarcoidosis and amyloidosis, can occasionally involve the thyroid gland. These diseases may present as local or diffuse growth of the thyroid. The infiltrated area appears hypofunctional on scans. Fine-needle aspiration usually makes the diagnosis.

SOLITARY THYROID NODULES

Nodularity of the thyroid gland is a nonspecific manifestation of a variety of thyroid diseases. Finding a thyroid nodule is not rare; 2% to 4% of the American population harbor clinically detectable nodular thyroids. Nodules are 4 to 6 times more common in women than in men. In most circumstances, a solitary thyroid nodule proves to be a colloid adenomatous nodule, an adenoma, a cyst, or a carcinoma; 90% to 95% are benign lesions. Table 1 lists several conditions that can present as a thyroid nodule.

Colloid Nodule

Approximately 60% of solitary nodules are colloid nodules. This nodule may be a true discrete entity or a form of follicular adenoma; both are benign growths that function and grow independently of normal regulatory mechanisms and infrequently overproduce thyroid hormones and cause hyperthyroidism. Adenomas are usually single lesions in an otherwise normal gland; colloid nodules may be solitary or form part of an inapparent multinodular gland. Colloid nodules are hypofunctional on isotope scan, but they may, especially in children, present as hyperplastic and hyperfunctional lesions.

Adenoma

Most adenomas have a follicular histology. Follicular adenomas of the thyroid are well-encapsulated lesions, with less colloid and more cellular component than colloid nodules. These lesions usually grow slowly and are typically asymptomatic. Most adenomas cannot concentrate iodine, and some have defects in the organification process, thus appearing hypofunctional and "cold" when evaluated with an isotope scan. Among follicular adenomas, the macrofollicular (*ie*, colloid) adenoma is most frequent. The microfollicular, embryonal, fetal, and Hürthle cell forms of follicular adenoma are less frequent and often cause concern. The true nature of the lesion may be difficult to determine. Occasionally, some lesions are believed to be benign and later prove to be invasive malignancies (particularly true of Hürthle cell tumors). If papillary adenomas exist, they are rare, and most observers believe that all papillary tumors should be considered as carcinomas.

Approximately 5% of solitary nodules have autonomous function. These nodules are almost always benign hyperfunctioning follicular adenomas or hyperplastic colloid nodules. The lesions tend to overproduce thyroid hormones as they increase in size. In time, they overproduce thyroid hormone and suppress thyroid-stimulating hormone levels, and the nodule becomes the only functioning tissue in the gland (hot

TABLE 1 DIFFERENTIAL DIAGNOSIS OF THYROID NODULE
Adenoma
Cyst
Carcinoma
Colloid nodule
Multinodular goiter
Hashimoto's thyroiditis
Subacute thyroiditis
Effect of prior operation or ^{131}I therapy
Thyroid hemiagenesis
Metastasis
Parathyroid cyst or adenoma
Thyroglossal duct
Nonthyroidal lesions
Inflammatory or neoplastic nodes
Cystic hygroma
Aneurysm
Bronchocele
Laryngocele
Thyroglossal duct cyst

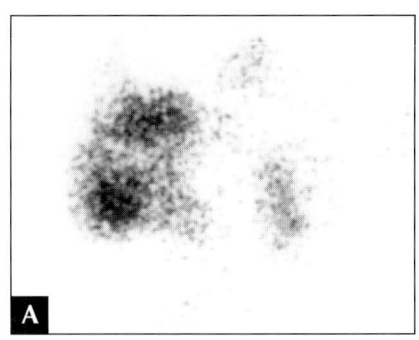 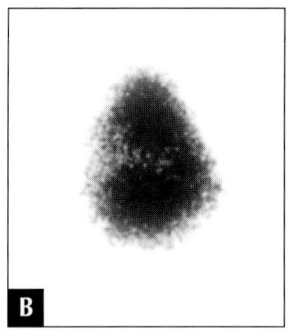

FIGURE 4 Sequential ^{131}I scan of the thyroid showing development of an autonomous-functioning thyroid nodule. **A**, A typical scan from a multinodular goiter with functioning and nonfunctioning areas. **B**, During follow-up, the functioning nodular tissue of the right lobe suppresses thyroid-stimulating hormone levels and the activity of the rest of the gland.

nodule), sometimes with elevated thyroid hormones and thyrotoxicosis [6••]. Most autonomous-functioning thyroid nodules producing excess thyroid hormones are more than 3 cm in diameter (Fig. 4). This kind of hyperfunctioning nodule is almost never malignant. Also, thyroid hormone therapy is not indicated and could be prejudicial to the patient. Fine-needle aspirates from this type of nodule may result in a hypercellular material that is interpreted as suspicious, although the cytology is usually benign. Rarely, nodules undergo spontaneous necrosis with a return of function in the formerly suppressed normal gland, leaving in place a cold area. Only 10% to 20% of functioning nodules initially found to be euthyroid become toxic.

Cyst

From 5% to 20% of all thyroid nodules are cystic [7]. Both benign and malignant lesions can present as a cyst; however, most are benign, simple cysts arising from necrotic follicular adenomas or colloid nodules. Cysts that are larger than 4 cm, cysts that are mixed solid and cystic, and cysts that recur after several aspirations have, allegedly, a greater probability of being malignant. Some thyroid cysts are necrotic papillary cancers. Thyroid ultrasound can be used to diagnose a thyroid "nodule" as a cyst (Fig. 5). Fine-needle aspiration is also simple and accurate in differentiating a cystic from a solid nodule, and it can be therapeutic [8••]. Because some cystic lesions are true malignant tumors, ultrasound helps little in discriminating benign from malignant lesions.

Carcinoma

Between 5% and 15% of solitary hypofunctioning thyroid nodules are malignant [9]. Several aspects of the medical history and the physical examination are important. Table 2 lists factors that must be considered in the evaluation of a thyroid nodule. The ratio of malignant to benign nodules is higher in young people and lower in older people. Nodules are less frequent in men, and a greater proportion are malignant. The family history is rarely helpful. Patients with the autosomal dominant disorder multiple endocrine neoplasia (MEN) type I may have thyroid adenomas, and those with MEN type II may have medullary thyroid cancer, together with hyperparathyroidism, pheochromocytomas, and mucosal neuromas. There are also familial forms of isolated medullary thyroid cancer. Patients with Gardner's and Cowden's syndromes are prone to develop thyroid tumors. Further, 6% of our patients with thyroid cancer have a history of malignant thyroid neoplasm in other family members.

Prior neck irradiation is an important consideration. Exposure to 100 to 700 rad during the first 3 to 4 years of life has been associated with a 1% to 7% incidence of thyroid cancer occurring 10 to 30 years later [10]. Radiation therapy for malignant lesions in the neck is still applied in selected patients. Because of the high incidence (30% to 40%) of carcinomas in nodules resected from irradiated glands, the finding of one or more clear-cut nodules in such a gland, or of a cold area on scan, must be considered suggestive of malignancy. In this case, multiple nodules do not indicate that the lesions are benign.

Recent onset, growth, hoarseness, nodes in the supraclavicular fossae, and local tenderness suggest malignancy. Enlarged lymph nodes should be carefully sought. Their presence suggests malignant disease, unless a good alternative diagnosis (*eg*, recent oropharyngeal sepsis or viral infection) is apparent. A history of residence in a country where diets lack iodine weighs in favor of multinodular goiter as the true diagnosis.

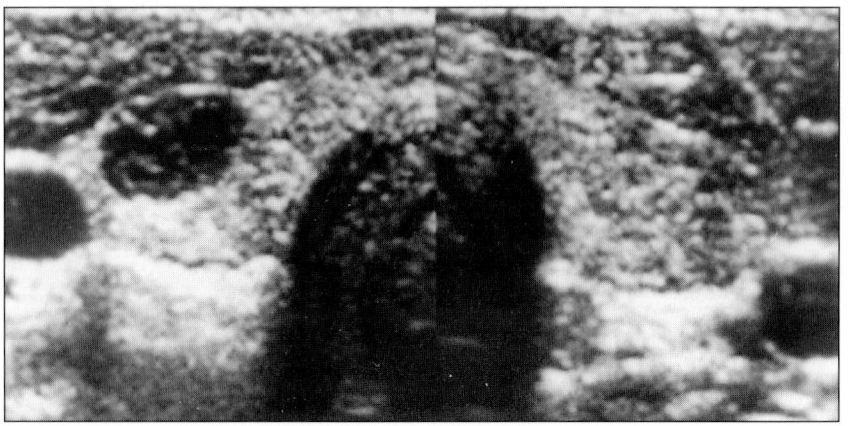

FIGURE 5 Ultrasound scan of the thyroid showing an almost purely cystic lesion of considerable size found in the left lobe of the thyroid. Note the carotid arteries at the lateral border of both thyroid lobes. The gland is slightly enlarged, and the image suggests that smaller nodules or cysts may be present on the right lobe.

Table 2 Evaluation of Solitary Thyroid Nodules

History	Physical examination
Radiation	Size
Age	Fixation
Sex	Cystic nature
Duration	Tenderness
Local symptoms	Adenopathy
Growth	Diffuse/local process
MEN syndrome	Vocal cord paralysis
Thryotoxicity	Single versus multiple nodules
Geographic residence	
Family history	

MEN—multiple endocrine neoplasia.

Fixation of the nodule to strap muscles or to the trachea is an important finding. Pain, tenderness, or sudden swelling of the nodule usually indicates hemorrhage into the nodule but can also indicate an invasive malignancy. Hoarseness may arise from pressure or from infiltration of a recurrent laryngeal nerve by a neoplasm.

The presence of a diffusely multinodular gland, ascertained on the basis of palpation or scanning, is usually interpreted as a sign of benignity. A nodule in a gland with Hashimoto's thyroiditis must be evaluated independently.

Soft tissue radiography films of the neck may show fine, stippled calcifications (psammoma bodies) through the tumor that are virtually pathognomonic of papillary cancer. Patchy or "signet ring" calcification occurs in old cysts and degenerating adenomas. Dense calcifications or calcification of lymph nodes is suggestive of medullary thyroid carcinoma.

Isotope scans are of moderate value because most malignant tumors fail to accumulate iodine to a degree equal to the normal gland (Fig. 6). However, most cold nodules are benign lesions and cysts, not cancers. Tumors smaller than 1 cm in diameter are below the discriminating power of most scanners. Some malignant tumors accumulate radioactive iodine in approximately the same concentration as the surrounding thyroid tissue. Normal tissue in front of or behind the nodule may also accumulate radioactive iodine and thus obscure a cold nodule. An iodine scintiscan has value, but it does not permit an absolute judgment concerning whether a palpable nodule is malignant or benign.

Fine-Needle Aspiration Biopsy in Management of Solitary Nodules

The regular use of fine-needle aspiration in the evaluation of thyroid nodules in the last 10 to 15 years has had an important impact on their management [8••,9–11,12••]. The procedure is safe, technically simple, and accepted by patients. Fine-needle aspiration requires the skill of an experienced endocrinologist and collaboration with a skilled cytopathologist. Used as the initial test in the evaluation of a thyroid nodule, the procedure decreases the costs needed to make a decision for management.

Fine needle aspiration appears to increase the yield of cancer among the patients who have surgery and reduces the number of patients sent for operation. If only the medical history and physical examination are used to make that decision, only 5% of patients sent to surgery have a carcinoma. Using information obtained by a scan, the yield increases to 5% to 15%. The use of fine needle aspiration biopsy increases this figure to approximately 30%.

The cytopathologic findings of a fine needle aspiration specimen are usually divided into four categories:

1. Benign cytology may suggest that the tissue obtained is normal thyroid, a colloid nodule, subacute thyroiditis, lymphocytic thyroiditis, or other benign process.
2. Suspicious cytology indicates that the cytopathologist is not able to discriminate clearly between a malignant and a benign lesion. Because 25% of patients in whom a suspicious specimen is found prove to have a malignant lesion, surgery is indicated. Also, it has been reported that a significant number of suspicious aspirates come from autonomous-functioning nodules.
3. A malignant aspirate may suggest a specific type of tumor.
4. Some samples might be considered unsatisfactory for further analysis. Cystic lesions frequently give unsatisfactory aspirates.

Results from more than 18,000 specimens demonstrated that the specimen is benign in 70% of cases, malignant in 3.5%, suspicious in 10%, and unsatisfactory in 17%. The false-negative rate is 5%. The false-positive rate is generally less of a problem, and the experience of several groups shows that approximately 1 in 100 patients have an incorrect diagnosis of cancer.

Treatment

A suggested approach to a solitary thyroid nodule as well as a flow chart used in the evaluation of a goiter is shown in Figure 7. Because of the strong association of x-ray exposure with multiple lesions and thyroid carcinoma, patients having this

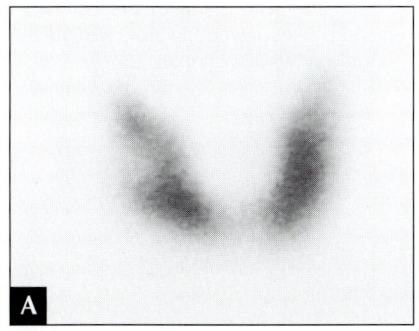
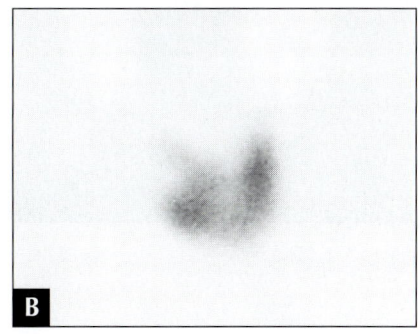

FIGURE 6 **A**, Isotope scan of the thyroid shows a cold area in the lateral part of the right lobe where a 1.5- by 2.0-cm nodule was felt. A fine needle aspirate biopsy gave a suspicious aspirate, which proved to be a papillary cancer. **B**, Functioning and nonfunctioning areas in a small multinodular goiter.

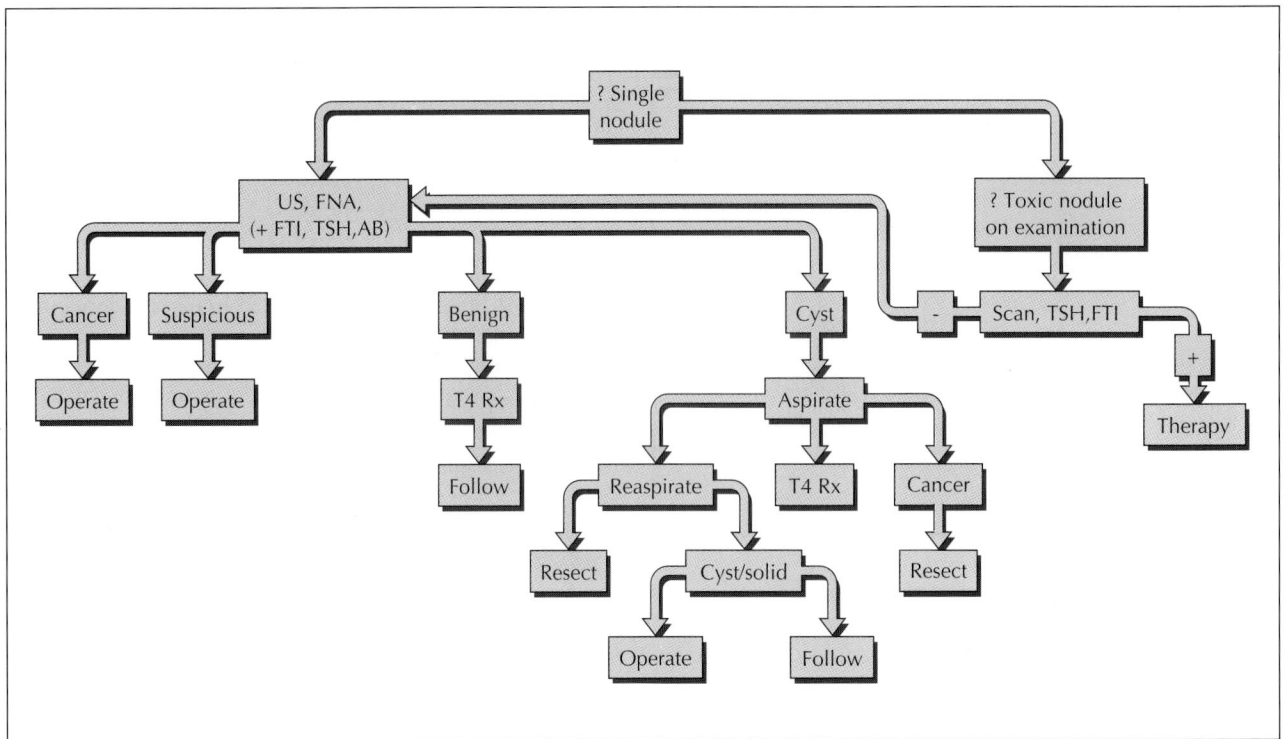

FIGURE 7 Suggested approach to a solitary thyroid nodule. AB—antithyroid antibodies; FNA—fine needle aspiration; FTI—free thyroxine index; ^{131}I—radioactive iodine; T4 Rx—levothyroxine treatment; TSH—thyroid-stimulating hormone; US—ultrasound.

history are usually examined by ultrasound or scan if the physical examination is abnormal. If there is a clearly defined single nodule, we proceed on the basis of the results of the fine-needle aspiration. If there are multiple nodules, however, because it is not possible to sample all nodules, the patient is usually referred for operation, unless there is a clear explanation for the appearance of those nodules.

Patients with a cystic lesion are treated by diagnostic and therapeutic aspiration and reaspiration of the cyst. Half of these cysts are dramatically reduced in size after multiple aspirations. In 20% to 30% of cases, recurrence may lead to its removal. The aspirated material is analyzed and may support a benign or a malignant diagnosis.

Patients with toxic nodules are treated by surgery or radioactive iodine therapy (Fig. 8). We tend to prefer surgery in younger individuals because of its speedy resolution of the problem and because it leaves normal tissue *in situ*. Radioactive iodine treatment usually requires a high dosage, such as 20 to 60 mCi of ^{131}I. There is a 10% to 20% risk of damaging normal thyroid tissue with development of hypothyroidism, and radioactive iodine often leaves behind an inactive, hard nodule that may be disconcerting during the rest of the patient's life.

Patients with a solid, nontoxic nodule are subjected to fine needle aspiration biopsy. Those with malignant or suspicious aspirates are advised to have surgical resection of the lesion. Patients with a benign cytodiagnosis are observed while treated with thyroid hormone suppressive therapy. Those with a suggestive history or physical examination and a higher risk for thyroid malignancy are recommended to have repeated aspiration biopsy within 6 to 12 months. When there is a strong clinical suspicion of malignancy, despite negative cytologic diagnosis, surgical exploration is still recommended.

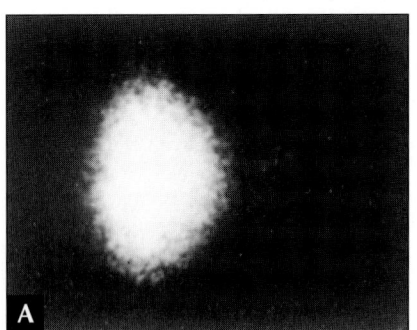
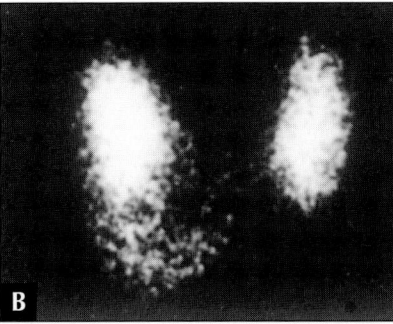

FIGURE 8 A, ^{131}I scan of the thyroid shows follow-up of 3-cm hot nodule that suppressed activity of the gland and was treated with ^{131}I. **B**, The rest of the gland has recovered function, and the nodule is hypofunctional.

References and Recommended Reading

Recently published papers of particular interest have been highlighted as:
- Of interest
- • Of outstanding interest

1. DeGroot LJ, Quintans J: The causes of autoimmune thyroid diseases. *Endocr Rev* 1989, 10:537–562.
2. Lever EG, Medeiros-Neto GA, DeGroot LJ: Inherited disorders of thyroid metabolism. *Endocr Rev* 1983, 4:213–239.
3. Studer H, Gerber H, Peter HJ: Multinodular goiter. In *Endocrinology*, edn 2. Edited by DeGroot LJ *et al*. Philadelphia: WB Saunders; 1989.
4. Aeschimann S, Kopp PA, Kimura ET, *et al.*: Morphological and functional polymorphism within clonal thyroid nodules. *J Clin Endocrinol Metab* 1993; 77:846–851.
5. Lombardi A, Martino E, Braverman LE: Amiodarone and the thyroid. *Thyroid Today* 1990, 13:2.
6. •• Hamburger JI: The autonomously functioning thyroid nodule: Goetsch' disease. *Endocr Rev* 1987, 8:439.
7. de los Santos ET, Keyhani-Rofagha S, Cunningham JJ, Mazzaferri EL: Cystic thyroid nodules: the dilemma of malignant lesions. *Arch Intern Med* 1990, 150:1422–1427.
8. •• Gharib H, Goellner JR: Fine-needle aspiration biopsy of the thyroid: an appraisal. *Ann Intern Med* 1993, 118:282–289.
9. Ridway EC: Clinical evaluation of solitary thyroid nodules. In *The Thyroid: A Fundamental and Clinical Text*, edn 6. Edited by Braverman LE, Utiger RD. Philadelphia: JB Lippincott; 1991.
10. DeGroot LJ: Clinical review 2: Diagnostic approach and management of patients exposed to irradiation to the thyroid. *J Clin Endocrinol Metab* 1989, 69:925–928.
11. DeGroot LJ, *et al.*: Thyroid neoplasia. In *The Thyroid and Its Diseases*, edn 5. Edited by DeGroot LJ, Larsen PR, Refetoff S, Stanbury JB. New York: John Wiley and sons; 1984.
12. •• Mazzaferri EL: Management of a solitary thyroid nodule. *N Engl J Med* 1993, 328:553–559.

Adrenal Cortex Glucocorticoids

Lynn Kohlmeier
David Feldman

Key Points

- Regulation of glucocorticoid synthesis is by feedback inhibition. Cortisol, for example, inhibits corticotropin-releasing hormone and corticotropin, thus modulating its own production.
- Cushing's syndrome results from an excess of glucocorticoids either endogenously overproduced or exogenously administered.
- There are two stages in the diagnosis of Cushing's syndrome: 1) hypercortisolism must be established, and 2) the source of hormone production must be determined—either pituitary adenoma, adrenal tumor, or ectopic corticotropin production.
- Cushing's disease results from a pituitary tumor oversecreting corticotropin, with subsequent adrenal stimulation and hypercortisolism.
- Addison's disease develops when the adrenal gland is unable to adequately produce glucocorticoids and mineralocorticoids.
- Autoimmune destruction of the adrenal glands and tuberculosis involving the adrenal glands are the two most common causes worldwide of Addison's disease.

BIOSYNTHESIS OF ADRENAL STEROIDS

The adrenal cortex makes up approximately 80% to 90% of the weight and volume of the whole adrenal gland, and it synthesizes more than 50 different steroids, the glucocorticoids and mineralocorticoids among them. The adrenal cortex is composed of three distinct zones, which manufacture specific steroids (Table 1). Buried within the cortex is the adrenal medulla, which is the source of catecholamine production.

The physiologic glucocorticoid, cortisol, is essential for life. Synthetic glucocorticoid derivatives, which are more potent and have longer duration of action than cortisol, are used as pharmaceutical agents in many clinical conditions. If there is an excess of glucocorticoids, either endogenously overproduced or exogenously administered, Cushing's syndrome results. On the other hand, if too little glucocorticoid and mineralocorticoid is synthesized, Addison's disease results [1••].

Aldosterone, the major mineralocorticoid, is synthesized in the zona glomerulosa. Both the zona fasciculata and the zona reticularis lack the aldosterone synthase enzymatic system necessary to synthesize aldosterone. All steroids are produced from cholesterol, either derived from circulating low-density lipoprotein or synthesized within the cortical cells from acetate by a number of well-characterized enzymes (Fig. 1). The cholesterol side chain cleavage enzyme is responsible for the rate-limiting desmolase step in which the cholesterol side chain is removed from C-21 to produce pregnenolone. Three P-450 hydroxylases, 17α-hydroxylase, 21-hydroxylase, and 11β-hydroxylase, consecutively add one hydroxyl group each to

Table 1	**Zones of the Adrenal Cortex**	
Zone	**Region**	**Steroid products**
Zona glomerulosa	Outer	Aldosterone (mineralocorticoid)
Zona fasciculata	Middle	Cortisol (glucocorticoid)
Zona reticularis	Inner	Dehydroepiandrosterone, androstenedione, testosterone (adrenal androgens)*

*The zona reticularis produces adrenal androgens, particularly dehydroepiandrosterone and androstenedione, which are converted into more potent androgens (testosterone and dihydrotestosterone) in peripheral tissues.

produce cortisol. Genetic defects in this series of enzymes cause the group of diseases known as congenital adrenal hyperplasia.

The interconversion of the active molecule cortisol to its inactive counterpart, cortisone, is demonstrated in Figure 2. By this means, the enzyme 11β-hydroxysteroid dehydrogenase regulates the intracellular concentration of active hormone and thereby plays an important role in modulating the amplitude of the response of target cells to cortisol [2].

Regulation of Cortisol Secretion

Corticotropin-releasing hormone (CRH), a 41-amino-acid peptide produced in the paraventricular nucleus of the hypothalamus, is the major stimulator of adrenocorticotropic hormone, also called corticotropin (ACTH). ACTH, a 39-amino-acid peptide, is synthesized in the pituitary gland as part of a large precursor molecule, proopiomelanocortin, and produced by posttranslational processing and cleavage of the parent proopiomelanocortin molecule. ACTH is released from the pituitary gland and is the primary regulator of cortisol production by the adrenal glands. Cortisol is secreted in a diurnal pattern, with the highest levels attained in the early morning hours and the lowest levels several hours after sleep [1••,3•]. Cortisol secretion is episodic because of the oscillatory pulses of CRH release, which causes ACTH to be secreted in an oscillatory pattern as well. Because of the diurnal rhythm and the oscillatory bursts of cortisol release, plasma cortisol measurements must be carefully interpreted relative to the time of day and individual variation between samples.

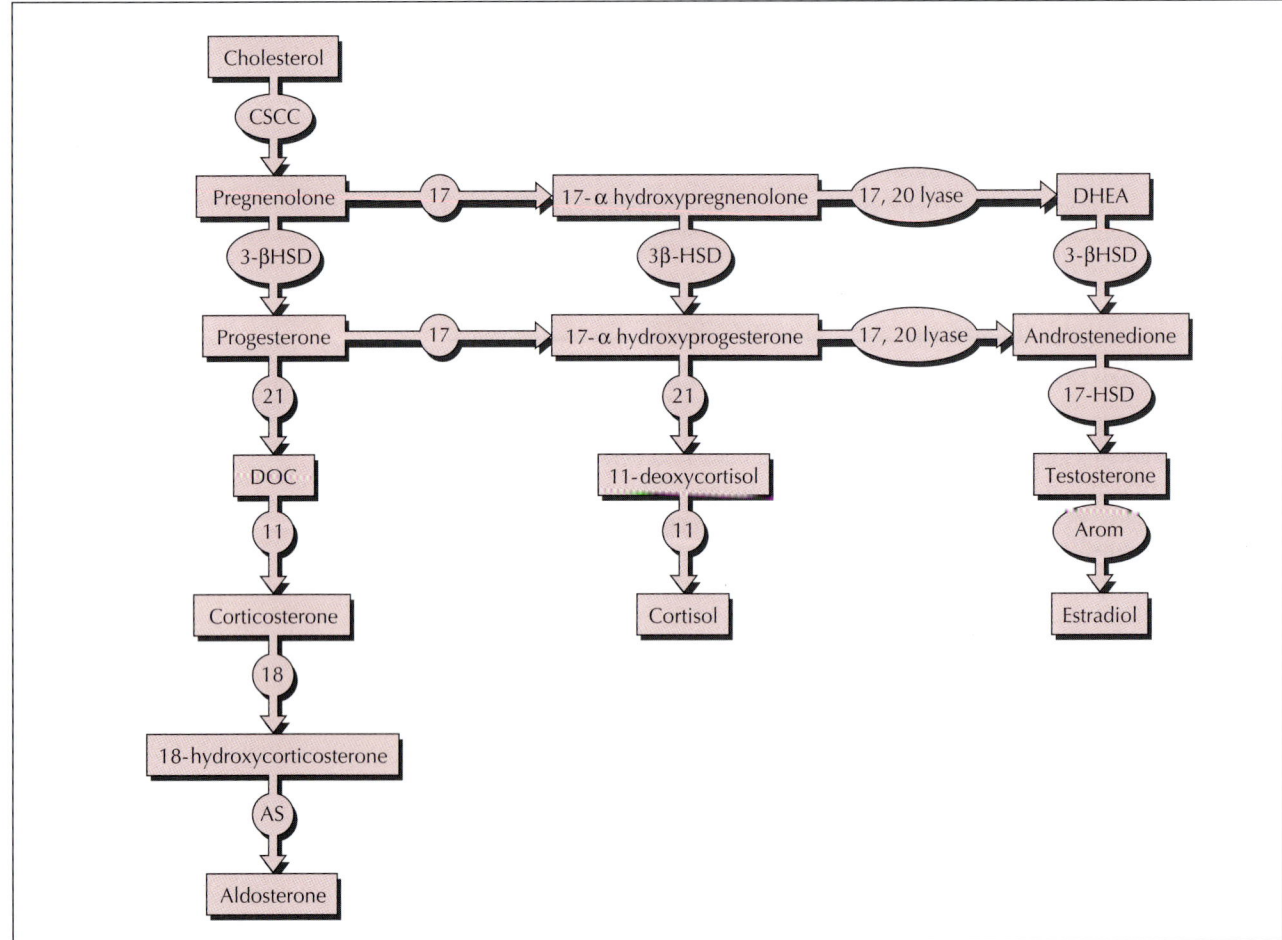

Figure 1 Pathways of steroid biosynthesis. 3β-HSD—3β-hydroxysteroid dehydrogenase; 11—11β-hydroxylase; 17—17α-hydroxylase; 17-HSD—17α-hydroxysteroid dehydrogenase; 18—18-hydroxylase; 21—21-hydroxylase; arom— aromatase; AS—aldosterone synthase; CSCC—cholesterol side chain cleavage; DHEA—dehydroepiandrosterone; DOC—11-deoxycorticosterone.

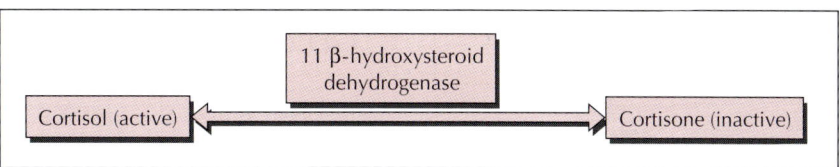

Figure 2 Conversion of cortisol to cortisone. Cortisol, the active glucocorticoid, can be converted to cortisone, an inactive analogue, by the enzyme 11β-hydroxysteroid dehydrogenase, which is present in liver and a variety of target tissues. Cortisol can bind to the glucocorticoid receptor or to the mineralocorticoid receptor, causing both actions. Cortisone does not bind well to either receptor and is therefore mostly inactive. Conversion of cortisol to cortisone therefore "protects" the mineralocorticoid receptor and reduces excessive mineralocorticoid activity.

ACTH stimulates steroidogenesis through the adenyl cyclase system (Fig. 3). The ACTH receptor is a member of the G-protein–coupled seven-transmembrane-domain receptor family, and binding results in transmembrane signals that stimulate the steroidogenic pathway at multiple sites. In addition to stimulating steroidogenesis, ACTH acts to maintain the integrity of the adrenal gland and support cellular survival. Prolonged ACTH deficiency results in cortical atrophy.

Regulation of cortisol synthesis primarily depends on feedback inhibition (Fig. 4). Cortisol inhibits CRH and ACTH release. Stresses such as illness, fever, surgery, trauma, acute cold exposure, and even motion sickness result in an increase in ACTH and cortisol. The normal feedback system is overridden in situations of stress. The rise in cortisol is immediate, and the level may remain elevated for days. Interleukins are released by activated macrophages in response to stress, and interleukin-1β is believed to directly stimulate the adrenal cortex, possibly via a prostaglandin-mediated mechanism. Interleukins may also stimulate ACTH release.

Glucocorticoid Receptors and Mechanism of Action

Cortisol, secreted by the adrenal glands, circulates bound to plasma proteins, predominantly corticosteroid-binding globulin but also albumin. The form bound to corticosteroid-binding globulin is in equilibrium with free cortisol (approximately equal to 10%), and it is the free form that is believed to have access to the intracellular compartment, where it can bind to its specific receptors and induce biologic responses (Fig. 5). The glucocorticoid receptor is a member of the steroid-thyroid-retinoid receptor superfamily, which act as hormone-dependent enhancers of gene transcription [4]. Most tissues in the body possess functional glucocorticoid receptor. By regulating the expression of specific messenger RNA transcripts, cortisol mediates a variety of biologic effects.

Glucocorticoid Effects on the Body

Cortisol mediates many effects throughout the body (Table 2) [1••,2,3•,4,5]. When cortisol is at physiologic levels, target tissues exhibit optimum function. However, when cortisol levels are higher or lower than normal, abnormalities develop.

Clinical Uses of Glucocorticoids

Cortisol is used to replace deficient endogenous glucocorticoid production; in addition, potent analogues of cortisol are used as drugs to obtain specific therapeutic benefits, espe-

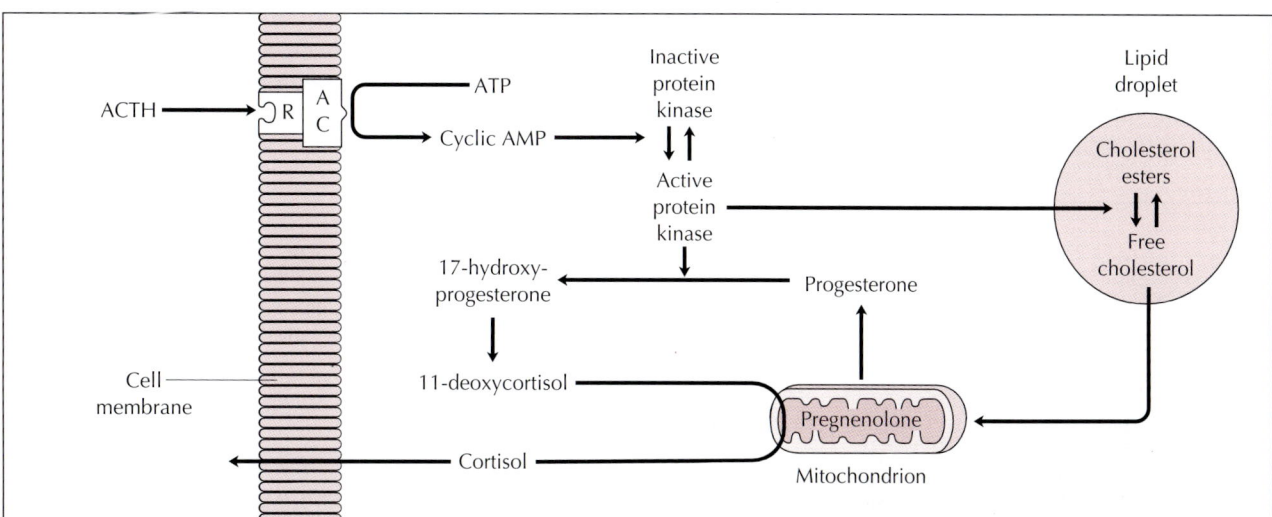

Figure 3 Pathway of corticotropin stimulation of adrenal fasiculata cells. AC—adenylate cyclase; ACTH—corticotrophin; AMP—adenosine monophosphate; ATP—adenosine triphosphate; R—receptor. (Adapted from Tyrell and Forsham [19]; with permission.)

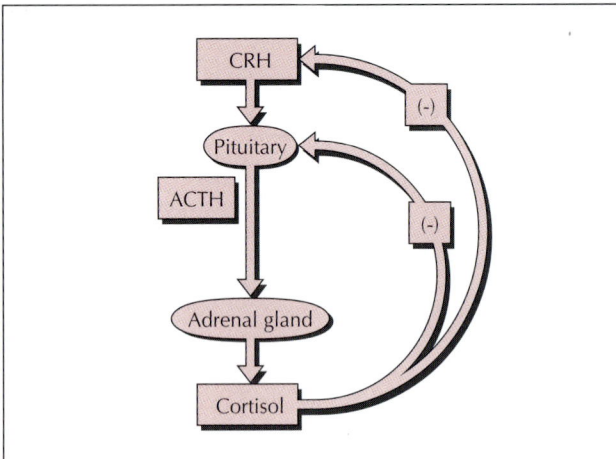

FIGURE 4 Normal hypothalamic-pituitary-adrenal axis. Corticotropin releasing hormone (CRH) is released by the hypothalamus and stimulates the pituitary to release corticotropin. Corticotropin, in turn, stimulates the adrenal gland to produce cortisol. Cortisol feeds back to inhibit CRH in the hypothalamus and corticotropin at the pituitary to regulate cortisol levels. ACTH—corticotropin.

cially to achieve antiinflammatory or immunosuppressive actions (*see* Chapter 6, Glucocorticoid Therapy and Withdrawal). The mechanism of these effects involves inhibition of proinflammatory factors such as lymphokines, prostaglandins, and histamines. Glucocorticoids are therefore of great therapeutic benefit in arthritis, asthma, bone marrow and organ transplantation, and in lymphatic malignancies. In all of these settings, pharmacologic doses of glucocorticoids can cause iatrogenic Cushing's syndrome, which is discussed in the next section.

Long-term administration (> 2 weeks) of pharmacologic levels of glucocorticoids leads to suppression of CRH and ACTH and causes adrenal atrophy. Adrenal insufficiency manifests when steroid use is discontinued. To minimize systemic absorption and side effects, glucocorticoids can be given either topically on skin or in the eye, by inhalation or nasal spray, by intraarticular injection, or as a rectal suppository. Alternate-day therapy is another strategy for diminishing the side effects of systemic pharmacologic doses while attempting to obtain adequate therapeutic benefits.

GLUCOCORTICOID EXCESS: CUSHING'S SYNDROME

Cushing's syndrome is the constellation of signs and symptoms that constitutes the clinical result of chronic hypercortisolism (Table 3) [1••,2,5]. The most common cause of Cushing's syndrome is the use of glucocorticoids to achieve pharmacologic effects. In addition, there are three major types of endogenous Cushing's syndrome and several uncommon forms (Fig. 6 and Table 4). The most common form of endogenous Cushing's syndrome is Cushing's disease, the excess production of ACTH by a pituitary adenoma causing bilateral adrenal hyperplasia and the overproduction of cortisol.

Symptoms and Signs

Whatever the cause of Cushing's syndrome, many of the features are similar. Multiple organ systems are involved, and the common features are summarized in Table 3 [1••,2,5]. The immunosuppressive effect of hypercortisolism predisposes patients with Cushing's syndrome to serious infections, particularly tuberculosis and fungal disease. Metabolic effects promote diabetes and osteoporosis.

In addition to demonstrating the glucocorticoid effects of high cortisol levels, patients often show signs of mineralocorticoid excess, such as hypokalemia and hypertension. This could result from either high levels of cortisol precursors with mineralocorticoid activity (*eg*, 11-deoxycorticosterone) or a "crossover" effect of cortisol on the mineralocorticoid receptor, for which it has a reasonably high affinity [2]. The enzyme 11β-hydroxysteroid dehydrogenase normally protects the mineralocorticoid receptor from excess cortisol by inactivating it to cortisone (Fig. 2). The high levels of cortisol in Cushing's syndrome can overwhelm this protective mechanism and result in levels of cortisol sufficient to occupy the mineralocorticoid receptor, causing hypokalemia and hypertension. Cortisol-mediated mineralocorticoid excess can similarly be seen in licorice-induced 11β-hydroxysteroid dehydrogenase blockade or in genetic defects within the 11β-hydroxysteroid dehydrogenase enzyme.

Although the clinical presentation of Cushing's syndrome can be quite convincing in itself, biochemical evaluation is critical to confirm hypercortisolism as well as to determine its etiology (Table 4).

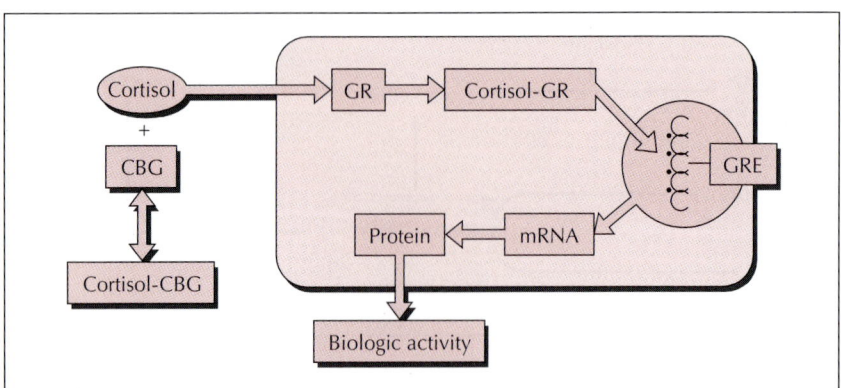

FIGURE 5 The mechanism of cortisol action. CBG—corticosteroid-binding globulin; GR—glucocorticoid receptor; GRE—glucocorticoid response element; mRNA—messenger RNA.

Table 2. Effects of glucocorticoids

Site	Effects of glucocorticoids	Possible result
Bone	↓ Osteoblast action, ↓ bone formation; ↑ osteoclast action, ↑ bone resorption	Osteoporosis
Liver	↑ Hepatic gluconeogenesis; ↓ glucose uptake in peripheral cells	Diabetes mellitus
Kidney	↑ Renal free water clearance	
Muscle and connective tissue	↓ Collagen synthesis; ↓ protein synthesis	Poor wound healing, easy bruising, thin skin, weakness, and myopathy
Gastrointestinal tract	↓ Calcium absorption	Osteoporosis
Immune system	↓ Lymphokines, prostaglandins, and histamines; thymus and lymph node involution	Antiinflammatory, immunosuppressive
Behavior	Mechanisms unclear	Depression, psychosis
Fetal and neonatal development	↑ Surfactant and fetal lung maturity; ↑ fetal hepatic and gastrointestinal enzyme systems	↑ Fetal lung maturity

Table 3. Findings in Cushing's syndrome

Findings	Frequency
Glucocorticoid effects	
Weakness	+++++
Fatigue	+++++
Thin skin	++++
Easy bruisability, ecchymoses	++
Thin extremities	++++
Truncal obesity	+++++
Round "moon" face	+++++
Supraclavicular fat pads	+++
"Buffalo hump"	++
Purple striae	++
Plethora	++++
Hirsutism	++++
Acne	++
Menstrual disorders	++++
Osteoporosis	+++
Psychiatric symptoms: depression, emotional lability, irritability, overt psychoses	+
Headache	+
Mineralocorticoid effects	
Hypertension	++
Hypokalemia	++
Edema	+

From Sheeler [5]; with permission.
+, rare (< 20%); ++, occasional (20%–50%); +++, somewhat common (50%); ++++, common; +++++, very common (> 80%).

Table 4. Etiology of endogenous Cushing's syndrome

Diagnosis	Incidence
Cushing's disease (pituitary tumor)	70%
Primary adrenal tumor (ACTH-independent)	15%
Adrenal adenoma	
Adrenal carcinoma	
Ectopic ACTH syndrome	15%
Adrenal hyperplasia syndromes	< 1%
Other etiologies	Rare
Ectopic CRH	
Food-induced	
Alcohol-induced pseudo-Cushing's syndrome	

Adapted from Sheeler [5]; with permission. ACTH—corticotropin; CRH—corticotropin releasing hormone.

Etiology

Cushing's disease—corticotropin-dependent pituitary tumor

Cushing's disease results from a pituitary tumor, either a microadenoma or a macroadenoma, oversecreting ACTH (Fig. 6). The bursts of ACTH are increased in amplitude and the diurnal rhythm is lost, leading to increased plasma ACTH levels, particularly at night. The increased ACTH levels cause bilateral adrenal hyperplasia and the overproduction of cortisol. The adenoma is usually a primary pituitary tumor, but occasionally corticotrope hyperplasia may occur, driven by excess CRH from the hypothalamus or by an ectopic CRH-producing tumor. The onset of Cushing's disease is usually between the ages of 20 and 40, and the disease is more common in women than in men [1••,3•,5]. Androgenic effects such as acne, hirsutism, and amenorrhea often occur in women because of the production of excess adrenal androgens. The elevated ACTH levels may lead to hyperpigmentation, but this is much more characteristic of ectopic ACTH syndrome or Addison's disease. In the morning, plasma cortisol and ACTH levels may overlap the normal range, but evening levels are clearly elevated. Measurement of 24-hour urine steroid excretion rates, which integrate the cortisol production of the entire day, should

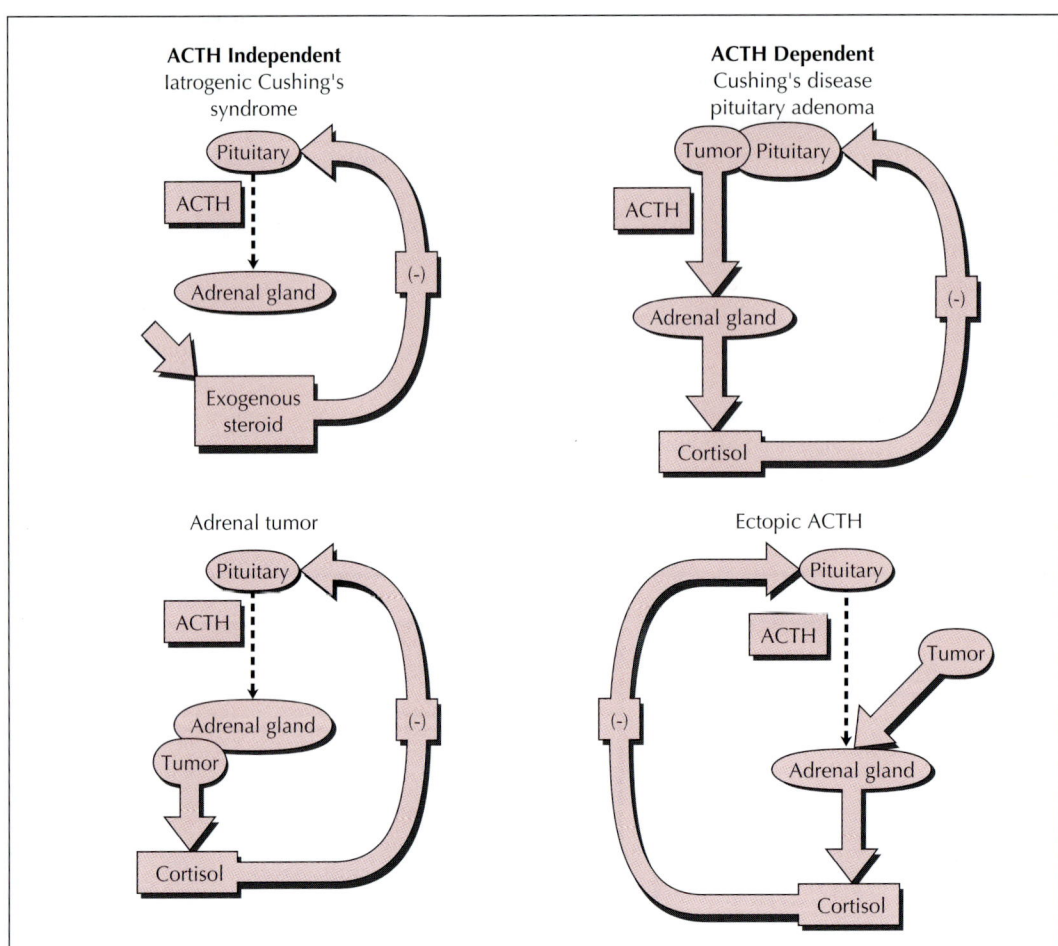

FIGURE 6 Pathogenesis of Cushing's syndrome. *Minus signs* indicate feedback inhibition; *dashed symbols* indicate suppressed levels of corticotropin (ACTH).

reflect the abnormal values. Although CRH and normal corticotropes in the pituitary are suppressed by the elevated cortisol level, the pituitary adenoma fails to be normally suppressed. However, during diagnostic dexamethasone testing, discussed later, suppression of the adenoma can be achieved at high glucocorticoid levels, indicating that the defect is actually a set-point error.

Primary adrenal tumor

Adrenal neoplasm, either adenoma or carcinoma, is a cause of ACTH-independent Cushing's syndrome (Fig. 6). The hypercortisolism causes CRH and ACTH suppression and atrophy of the contralateral adrenal gland. Onset can be gradual, and in the case of carcinoma, the adrenal tumor can grow very large and present as a palpable flank mass. Adenomas tend to be efficient producers of cortisol, whereas carcinomas are inefficient and overproduce cortisol because of the bulk of tissue involved. Carcinomas usually produce various steroid products, and urinary levels of 17-ketosteroids may be relatively greater than levels of 17-hydroxysteroids. The features of Cushing's syndrome exhibited by the patient depend on the pattern of steroid production by the cancer and may include classic Cushing's syndrome, virilization alone, predominantly mineralocorticoid excess, or no clinical endocrine abnormality. Because the steroid production is ACTH independent, high doses of dexamethasone fail to inhibit steroidogenesis. Carcinomas carry a poor prognosis: in one series, 50% to 66% of patients died within 2 years of diagnosis, and in another, only 24% survived 3 years [6•].

Ectopic corticotropin syndrome

The ectopic ACTH syndrome results from overproduction of ACTH, most commonly by nonpituitary malignant tumors (Fig. 6). The excess ACTH causes bilateral adrenal hyperplasia and hypercortisolism. Although many tumors have been reported to cause the syndrome, the most frequent is small cell lung carcinoma. Others include carcinoid tumors of bronchial, thymic, or pancreatic origin; pancreatic, prostatic, and ovarian cancers; and medullary thyroid carcinoma or pheochromocytoma. The ACTH levels can be very high, and the syndrome may therefore be associated with hyperpigmentation. Often the typical appearance of Cushing's syndrome is absent, and the clinical picture is dominated by hypertension, hypokalemia, weakness, and salt retention. This probably results from extremely high cortisol levels overwhelming the 11β-hydroxysteroid dehydrogenase enzyme, allowing cortisol to occupy mineralocorticoid receptors. On the other hand, in slow-growing tumors, the clinical presentation may be similar to that of Cushing's disease. ACTH production by the tumor is unregulated by negative feedback, and even high levels of dexamethasone fail to suppress ACTH in most cases.

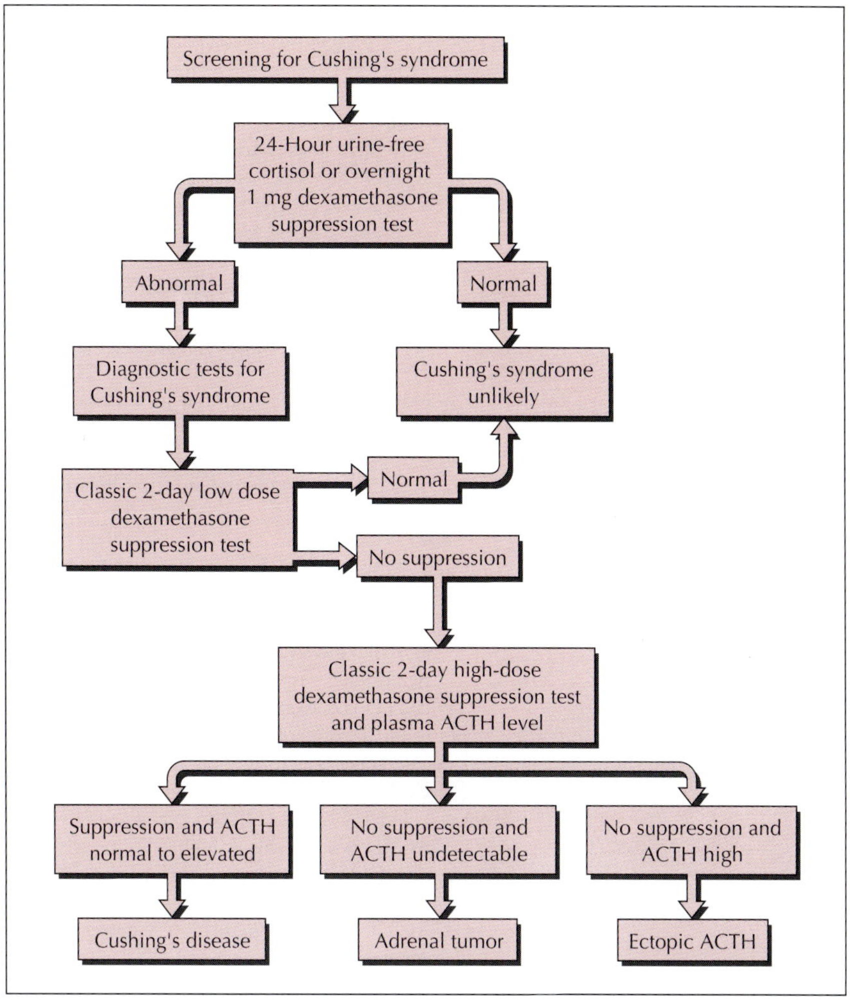

FIGURE 7 Algorithm for the evaluation of Cushing's syndrome. Suppression refers to cortisol levels. ACTH—corticotropin.

```
Screening for Cushing's syndrome
              ↓
    24-Hour urine-free
    cortisol or overnight
    1 mg dexamethasone
      suppression test
       ↓            ↓
    Abnormal      Normal
       ↓            ↓
  Diagnostic tests for   →  Cushing's syndrome
  Cushing's syndrome        unlikely
       ↓                       ↑
  Classic 2-day low dose  → Normal
  dexamethasone
  suppression test
       ↓
   No suppression
       ↓
  Classic 2-day high-dose
  dexamethasone suppression test
  and plasma ACTH level
    ↓         ↓           ↓
Suppression   No suppression   No suppression
and ACTH      and ACTH         and ACTH high
normal to     undetectable
elevated
    ↓         ↓           ↓
Cushing's    Adrenal      Ectopic ACTH
disease      tumor
```

Less common causes of Cushing's syndrome
Table 4 lists the less common causes of Cushing's syndrome.

Diagnostic Tests

Although the generalist should feel comfortable screening for Cushing's syndrome, patients should usually be referred to an endocrinologist when Cushing's syndrome is suspected by an abnormal screening result or a clinical impression. Procedures for evaluating a patient suspected of having Cushing's syndrome are depicted in Figure 7.

Screening tests

Many patients may present with some combination of hypertension, diabetes, osteoporosis, obesity, and in women, hirsutism. Although Cushing's syndrome is uncommon, the consideration of this diagnosis is not. For this reason, it is essential to have good screening tests to rule out Cushing's syndrome in the majority of cases and to identify those individuals requiring further work-up. Two tests are very useful: the overnight dexamethasone suppression test and the 24-hour urine free cortisol measurement (Table 5). The easiest test to perform is probably the overnight dexamethasone suppression test. An 8 AM plasma cortisol level suppressed to less than 5 µg/dL is normal and rules out hypercortisolism with 98% certainty. Values between 5 and 10 µg/dL are borderline, and failure to suppress below a value of 10 µg/dL is very suggestive of Cushing's syndrome [7••]. Urine free cortisol measurement performed on a 24-hour urine collection, preferably done on an outpatient basis in an otherwise healthy individual, is equally helpful as a screening test. False-positive results can occur in obese patients, depressed patients, chronically ill hospitalized patients, and patients receiving phenytoin or estrogens. Although normal values differ among laboratories, elevated free cortisol excretion is consistent with hypercortisolism.

Definitive tests

After screening tests have supported the clinical impression of Cushing's syndrome, further tests are indicated for definitive diagnosis (Fig. 7). These tests are described in detail in Table 5. Dexamethasone suppression testing remains the best means of diagnosing Cushing's syndrome. Failure to suppress cortisol normally on the low-dose test establishes the presence of Cushing's syndrome. Suppression of cortisol on the high-dose test indicates that the cause of hypercortisolism is ACTH-dependent, most likely a pituitary tumor, or Cushing's disease. Recently revised and more stringent criteria for the 2-day high-dose dexamethasone suppression test enable it to have 100% specificity and 83% sensitivity for the diagnosis of Cushing's disease. Criteria are as follows: more than 90% suppression of

Table 5 Screening and diagnostic tests for Cushing's syndrome

Use of test	Test type	Dose	Interpretation†
Screening for Cushing's syndrome	24-h urine-free cortisol		If 24-h urine-free cortisol is elevated, Cushing's syndrome is suspected
	Overnight low-dose dex suppression and AM serum cortisol	1 mg dex PO at 11 PM	If 8 AM serum cortisol is > 5 µg/dL, Cushing's syndrome is suspected
Confirm Cushing's syndrome	Classic 2-d low-dose dex suppression and 24-h urine collection	0.5 mg dex PO qid × 2 d	If 24-h urine-free cortisol after dex is > 50 µg *or* If fail low-dose dex suppression and if 24-h urine 17-hydroxycorticosteroid after dex is > 11µmol (4 mg), Cushing's syndrome is confirmed
Diagnose Cushing's disease	Classic 2-d high-dose dex suppression with baseline and day two 24-h urine collection and AM serum cortisol	2 mg dex PO qid × 2 d	If 24-h urine-free cortisol or 17-hydroxycorticosteroid is suppressed, Cushing's disease is confirmed *and*
	Overnight high-dose dex suppression and AM serum cortisol	8 mg dex PO at 11 PM	If 8 AM serum cortisol suppresses to < 10µg/dL, Cushing's disease is suspected. If 8 AM serum cortisol fails to suppress (is > 10 µg/dL), adrenal tumor or ectopic ACTH syndrome is suspected
	AM serum ACTH		If ACTH is detectable, normal, or high (> 12 pg/mL), consistent with Cushing's disease
	Inferior petrosal sinus sampling		If central:peripheral ACTH ratio is ≥ 2:1, Cushing's disease is confirmed
Diagnose ectopic ACTH syndrome vs adrenal tumor	After high-dose dex test is nonsuppressable, AM serum ACTH		If ACTH is detectable or high (> 52 pg/mL), ectopic ACTH syndrome is suspected *or* If ACTH is low (< 6 pg/mL) or undetectable, adrenal tumor is confirmed
	CRH stimulation after baseline serum cortisol and ACTH, then blood drawn at 15, 30, 60, 90, and 120 min	1 µg/kg CRH intravenously	If cortisol is unchanged or rises ≤ 20% of baseline *and* If ACTH rises ≤ 50% of baseline, ectopic ACTH syndrome or adrenal tumor is suspected
	Inferior petrosal sinus sampling		If central:peripheral ACTH ratio is ≤1.5:1, ectopic ACTH syndrome is suspected

Adapted from Kaye and Crapo [7••]; with permission.
†Normal values (all values are dependent on the specific laboratory): AM serum cortisol, 10–25 µg/dL; AM serum cortisol after 1-mg dex suppression test, < 5 µg/dL; 24-h baseline urine-free cortisol, < 50µg; 24-h baseline urine 17-hydroxycorticoids, < 10 mg; ACTH, 9–52 pg/mL (at 7–10 AM); ACTH (IRMA) after dex suppression test, 2–88 pg/mL.
ACTH—corticotropin; CRH—corticotropin releasing hormone; dex—dexamethasone; PO—orally; qid—4 times daily.

urine free cortisol or more than 64% suppression of urine 17-hydroxycorticosteroids [7••]. The overnight high-dose dexamethasone suppression test gives similar results, with 100% specificity and 89% sensitivity if the morning plasma cortisol level after 8 mg of dexamethasone is 50% or less of the baseline cortisol level [7••]. Although approximately 11% of Cushing's disease patients do not suppress with the standard high dose of dexamethasone (8 mg), they may suppress with even higher doses.

A combination of the dexamethasone suppression and the CRH stimulation tests, the dexamethasone-CRH test has recently been shown in one study to be the most accurate in distinguishing Cushing's syndrome from other non-Cushing's states in patients with mild hypercortisolism [8]. The dexamethasone-CRH test, which has 100% specificity and sensitivity, is simply the CRH stimulation test started 2 hours after completion of low-dose dexamethasone suppression. However, because CRH is not yet available for use, repeat traditional testing should be carried out, preferably when confounding conditions such as alcohol, acute illness or stress, can be minimized or eliminated.

The two common conditions that fail to suppress on the high-dose test, ectopic ACTH syndrome and primary adrenal disease, can be distinguished by the ACTH level. In ectopic ACTH syndrome, the ACTH level is elevated, whereas in primary adrenal disease, it is suppressed.

Figure 8 shows the results of the classic 2-day high-dose dexamethasone suppression test in a number of patients with

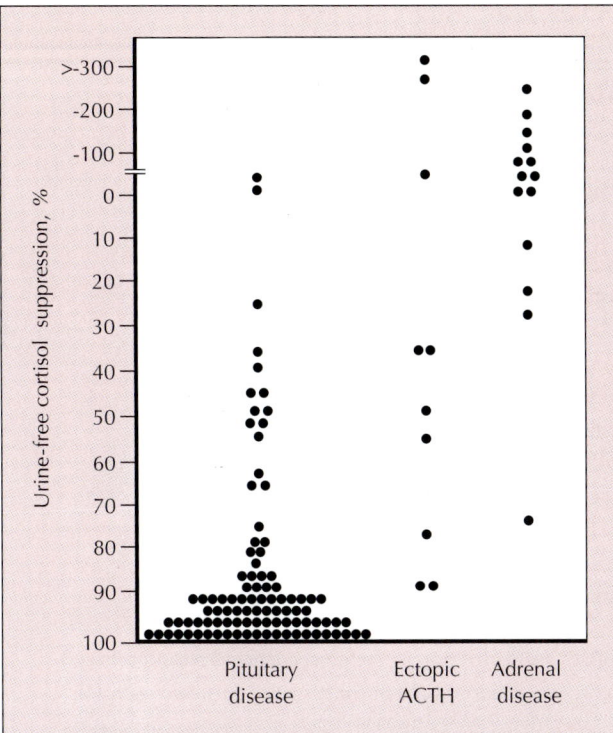

FIGURE 8 Suppression of 24-hour urine free cortisol after the high-dose dexamethasone suppression test in just over 100 patients with surgically confirmed causes of Cushing's syndrome. ACTH—corticotrophin. (*Adapted from* Flack and coworkers [9]; with permission.)

either Cushing's disease, ectopic ACTH syndrome, or adrenal disease [9]. Most cases of Cushing's disease would be identified without the need for CRH stimulation, inferior petrosal sinus sampling, or both, but these tests are now becoming available for diagnostic problems. In experienced hands, inferior petrosal sinus sampling can confirm the pituitary source of ACTH and might provide more definitive evidence indicating the need for pituitary surgery than dexamethasone testing. Together with CRH stimulation, inferior petrosal sinus sampling is considered by some investigators to be a critical adjunct to Cushing's disease evaluation [10].

Imaging

Once the type of Cushing's syndrome has been biochemically identified, localization tests are indicated (Table 6). Magnetic resonance imaging of the pituitary gland is somewhat superior to computed tomography (CT) in detecting microadenomas of the pituitary [7••]. Inferior petrosal sinus sampling may be useful if magnetic resonance imaging is not diagnostic. Abdominal CT is capable of identifying adrenal masses or atrophy in evaluating the adrenal glands for an adrenal neoplasm. Chest and abdominal CT may be useful in searching for the source of corticotropin in the ectopic corticotropin syndrome.

An incidentally discovered adrenal mass detected on abdominal CT performed for other reasons, a so-called incidentaloma, is becoming an increasingly common finding. Incidentalomas are estimated to be recognized in 0.6% to 1.3% of all abdominal CT studies performed [11]. Although the great majority of incidentalomas are nonfunctional, adrenal adenoma or carcinoma has presented in this manner. Medullary and cortical hyperfunction should be considered in this setting, and appropriate tests should be performed depending on the clinical data. It has been recommended that nonfunctional tumors larger than 3 to 6 cm be removed and that smaller ones be followed up by repeated CT and excised if they enlarge [11].

TABLE 6 IMAGING

Suspected tumor site	Test
Cushing's disease	Pituitary magnetic resonance imaging
Adrenocortical tumor	Adrenal computed tomography
Ectopic ACTH syndrome	Abdominal and chest computed tomography

ACTH—corticotropin.

Treatment of Cushing's Syndrome

The treatment of Cushing's syndrome is primarily surgical, with removal of the tumor that is causing overproduction of cortisol (Table 7).

Treatment of Cushing's disease

Primary treatment of Cushing's disease is directed at removal of the pituitary adenoma via a transphenoidal approach. In the hands of experienced neurosurgeons, microadenomas can be cured approximately 70% to 90% of the time, whereas macroadenomas are cured less than 50% of the time [1••,2,5]. Not all series of patients do this well, for reasons that are not clear [12]. Optimal results are removal of the source of hypercortisolism, restoration of a normal hypothalamic-pituitary-adrenal (HPA) axis, and restoration of normal function of other pituitary hormones. In cases in which surgery has failed, reoperation with a larger resection, radiation therapy of the pituitary gland, and bilateral adrenalectomy are options [1••,2,5,12]. New radiologic approaches, including the "gamma knife," may improve results with radiation therapy. The chance of recurrence following surgical resection is substantial in some studies, and careful follow-up is recommended. After transphenoidal surgery, thyroid and gonadal insufficiency can be found in some patients. Restoration of the normal HPA axis may take many months, and persistent adrenal insufficiency develops in some postsurgical patients, necessitating permanent steroid replacement [12].

If all attempts to treat Cushing's disease fail, bilateral adrenalectomy can be performed. Cortisol levels will obviously fall, and steroid maintenance must be instituted. In cases of Cushing's disease treated by bilateral adrenalectomy without pituitary ablation, chronic CRH stimulation may lead to enlargement of the preexisting adenoma or excessive pituitary hyperplasia. A complication known as Nelson's syndrome can result, with development of a pituitary mass that can become invasive, cause visual field impairment, elevate ACTH levels, and induce

Table 7 Treatment of Cushing's syndrome

Treatment (by tumor type)	Action or effect
Surgical	
Pituitary tumor	
Transphenoidal surgery	70%–85% cure
Adrenal tumor	
Adenoma resection	100% cure if < 3 cm
Carcinoma resection	Cure not likely; 6 mo–3 y survival only
Medical	
Pituitary tumor	
Radiotherapy (4500 cGy)	40%–60% cure
Adrenal adenoma	Inhibitors of cortisol secretion
Ketoconazole (400–1200 mg/d PO)	P-450 enzymes: ↓ 11 β-hydroxylase, ↓ CSCC
Metyrapone (2.0–4.0 g/d PO)	↓ 11 β-hydroxylase
Aminoglutethimide (500–750 mg/d PO)	↓ CSCC + ↓ aromatase
Adrenal carcinoma	
Mitotane (1.5–4.0 g/d PO; higher (as tolerated)	Mitochondrial damage with necrosis of adrenal cortex and ↓ 11 β-hydroxylase
RU486*	Antagonizes corticol action at the glucocorticoid receptor level
Spironolactone (50–300 mg/d PO)	Blocks cortisol or aldosterone at the mineralocorticoid receptor

*Not yet available in the United States.
PO—orally.
CSCC—cholesterol side-chain cleavage enzyme.

hyperpigmentation. Prior pituitary radiation can reduce the incidence of Nelson's syndrome [1••]. Because Cushing's disease is now primarily treated by transphenoidal resection, Nelson's syndrome is less commonly seen than previously.

Treatment of corticotropin-independent Cushing's syndrome

Treatment of Cushing's syndrome due to primary adrenal neoplasm is surgical and is directed at the adrenal glands (Table 7). Cure rates for surgical removal of benign adrenal tumors are very high, approaching 100% [1••,2,5]. Restoration of normal function of the contralateral, atrophic gland may take 9 to 12 months. During this period, while CRH, ACTH levels return to baseline, and the residual adrenal gland return to function, the patient requires supplementation with cortisol. Administration of ACTH does not speed the restoration of the HPA axis to normal.

Malignant tumors are rarely completely resected, and adrenal carcinoma carries a very poor prognosis [6•]. Median survival from the time of diagnosis is commonly under 15

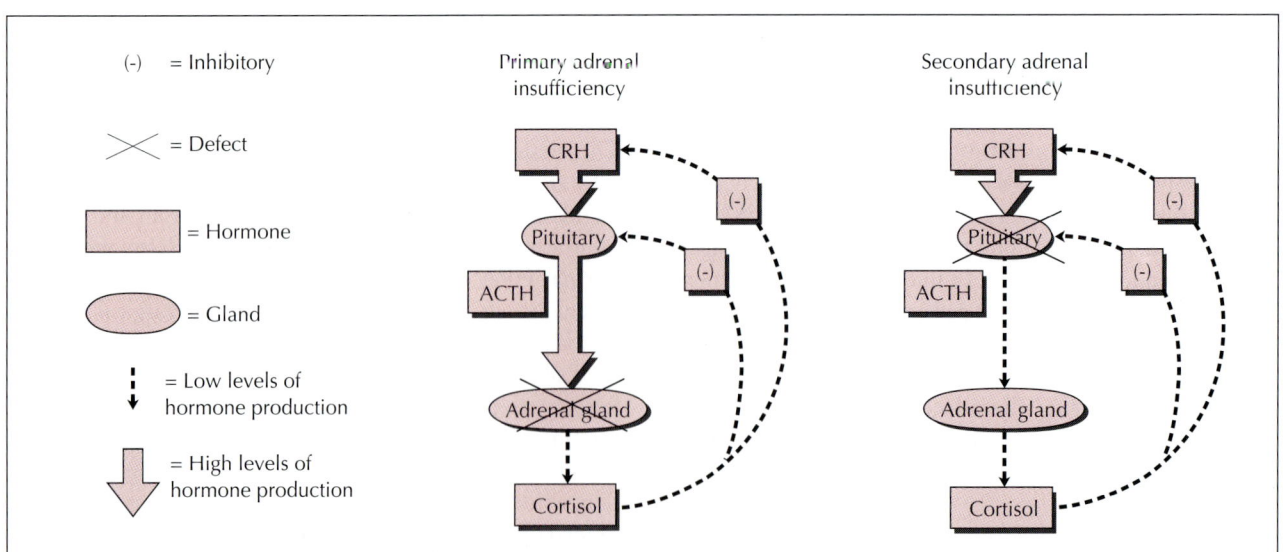

Figure 9 Primary versus secondary adrenocortical insufficiency. *Minus signs* indicate feedback inhibition; *dashed symbols* indicate suppressed levels of corticotropin (ACTH).

TABLE 8 ETIOLOGY OF PRIMARY ADRENAL INSUFFICIENCY: ADDISON'S DISEASE
Autoimmune Autoimmune polyglandular syndrome types I and II **Infection** Tuberculosis HIV infection Fungal infection **Idiopathic atrophy** **Infiltrative** Amyloidosis Sarcoidosis Hemochromatosis Adrenoleukodystrophy **Hemorrhage or infarct** Meningococcemia Disseminated intravascular coagulation Lupus (antiphospholipid antibody) Anticoagulant therapy **Neoplasm** Adrenal metastases Lymphoma **Iatrogenic** Glucocorticoid therapy Pituitary radiation therapy Surgical adrenalectomy Drugs that inhibit P-450 enzymes (ketoconazole, etomidate)

months. These bulky tumors are difficult to resect, and metastases to liver, lungs, and adjacent organs are common. Medical inhibition of cortisol synthesis with ketoconazole, aminoglutethimide, or metyrapone, for instance, is commonly used before surgery or as palliation for nonresectable cancer (Table 7). These drugs can be used individually or in combination, and they act by inhibiting various P-450 enzymes in the steroidogenic pathway. Additional benefit can be achieved by blockade of mineralocorticoid action with spironolactone. The tumor, however, is unaffected. Mitotane (ortho,paraprime-DDD) is adrenolytic, inducing necrosis of adrenal cells; although it is frequently used in adrenal carcinoma patients, it is often not effective. The drug has many side effects that limit its utility, the reduction of steroid levels is slow in onset, and there is little evidence yet that it prolongs life. However, because no other chemotherapeutic agents have been found that are effective in adrenal carcinoma and because prognosis is uniformly grim, mitotane therapy is often attempted, with transient benefits limited to the control of endocrine symptoms [13•].

Treatment of ectopic corticotropin syndrome
Treatment of ectopic ACTH syndrome is directed at the primary tumor in attempts to remove the source of ACTH and cure the patient (Table 7). However, because the tumors are frequently not resectable, medical treatment to reduce the symptoms of Cushing's syndrome is often the therapeutic goal [13•]. Bilateral adrenalectomy is an option if the patient appears likely to survive for some time and the ACTH source cannot be removed.

ADRENOCORTICAL INSUFFICIENCY

Insufficient production of cortisol may be due to primary adrenal disease or be secondary to inadequate secretion of ACTH (Fig. 9). Primary adrenal insufficiency, or Addison's disease, results from a destructive process that usually affects all zones of the adrenal cortex, leading to decreased production of cortisol, aldosterone, and adrenal androgens. Secondary adrenal insufficiency results from diminished production of ACTH and subsequent adrenal atrophy. A decreased CRH level, sometimes referred to as tertiary adrenal insufficiency, is most often a result of suppression from the pharmacologic use of glucocorticoids.

Addison's disease is most often caused by autoimmune destruction of the adrenal glands or the other conditions listed in Table 8. Pituitary tumors, or more commonly hypophysectomy for pituitary tumors, is the most frequent of a number of causes of secondary hypopituitarism (Table 9).

Symptoms and Signs

Symptoms and signs of adrenocortical insufficiency, listed in Table 10, usually do not develop until most of both adrenal

TABLE 9 ETIOLOGY OF SECONDARY ADRENOCORTICAL INSUFFICIENCY AND OTHER CAUSES
Pituitary failure Panhypopituitarism Sheehan's syndrome Pituitary apoplexy Isolated corticotropin deficiency **Familial glucocorticoid deficiency** **Cortisol resistance** **Isolated corticotropin releasing hormone**

TABLE 10 FINDINGS IN CHRONIC ADRENOCORTICAL INSUFFICIENCY	
Symptoms	Laboratory data
Weakness	Hyperkalemia
Anorexia	Hyponatremia
Nausea	Hypercalcemia
Vomiting	Hypoglycemia
Abdominal pain	Lymphocytosis
Diarrhea or constipation	Hypercalcemia
Weight loss	
Hyperpigmentation	
Hypotension	

TABLE 11 FEATURES OF ADRENAL CRISIS	
Clinical	**Laboratory**
Headache	Hyperkalemia
Shock and hypertension	Hyponatremia
Volume depletion	Eosinophilia
Weakness, lassitude	Hypoglycemia
Nausea, vomiting, anorexia	Lymphocytosis
Confusion and coma	Hypercalcemia
Fever (as high as 105° F)	

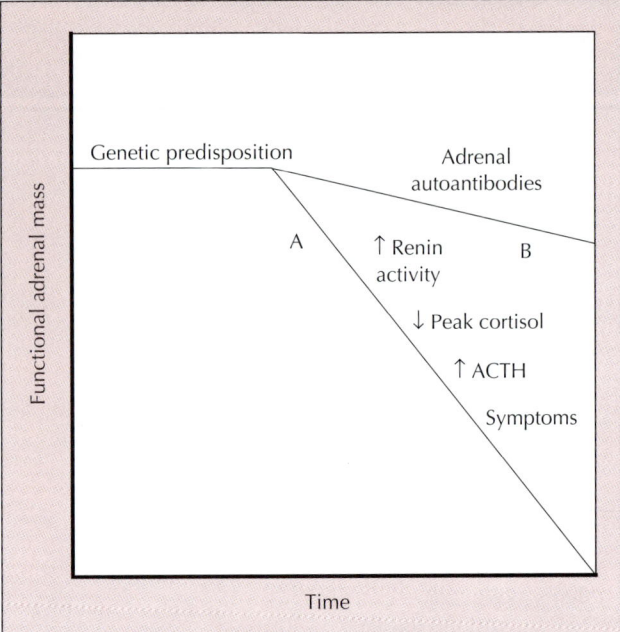

FIGURE 10 Natural history of Addison's disease. *Line A* and *line B* demonstrate courses of deterioration, *A* more progressive than *B*. ACTH—corticotropin. (Adapted from Muir and coworkers [14•]; with permission.)

glands is destroyed. In primary adrenal insufficiency, findings reflect glucocorticoid and mineralocorticoid loss, as well as deficiency of adrenal androgens in women. In secondary adrenal insufficiency, mineralocorticoid levels usually are adequate because the zona glomerulosa is not primarily regulated by ACTH but by the renin-angiotensin system, which remains intact in this setting. For this reason, secondary adrenal insufficiency often results in a pure glucocorticoid disorder, which is milder, and hypotension and adrenal crisis are less likely to develop. Hyperpigmentation of the skin and mucous membranes usually develops with long-standing ACTH elevation and is therefore seen in Addison's disease but not in secondary adrenal insufficiency, in which ACTH is diminished.

Symptoms of adrenal insufficiency usually include weight loss, fatigue, weakness, nausea, abdominal pain, and constipation or diarrhea. In this phase of the disease, a gastrointestinal problem might be suggested, particularly carcinoma. In more severely affected patients, salt craving, electrolyte disturbances, postural hypotension, hypoglycemia, hypercalcemia, and azotemia may develop. Eventually, the process may progress to vascular insufficiency, fever, and hypotension, and ultimately to shock. Signs of adrenal crisis are listed in Table 11; they are similar to but more severe than those findings in chronic glucocorticoid deficiency.

The proposed natural history of Addison's disease is schematically depicted in Figure 10 [14•]. The usual course is the gradual development of adrenal insufficiency over years. In the rapid-progression model, *eg*, when a patient with Addison's disease is subjected to substantial stress that increases the demand for steroids, acute adrenal failure or adrenal crisis can ensue. Adrenal crisis may develop in a previously undiagnosed patient or in a patient with adrenal insufficiency who does not increase his or her glucocorticoid replacement dosage in the face of severe stress (Table 12). Despite the fact that steroid therapy has been available for more than 50 years, glucocorticoid deficiency is still a potentially lethal condition.

Etiology

Primary adrenal insufficiency

Addison's disease results from primary adrenal failure (Table 8). Autoimmune Addison's disease can occur in isolation or as part of the autoimmune polyglandular syndrome. Sixty-five percent of patients with autoimmune Addison's disease have detectable levels of circulating adrenal autoantibodies [14•]. In type I autoimmune polyglandular syndrome, which is rare, Addison's disease is associated with hypoparathyroidism and candidiasis and presents most frequently in childhood. Type II autoimmune polyglandular syndrome, Addison's disease associated with autoimmune thyroid disease (Schmidt's syndrome), is more common and may also be associated with diabetes mellitus, ovarian and testicular failure, vitiligo, and pernicious anemia. The onset is usually between the ages of 20 and 50 years. It is more common in women and is associated with HLA alleles B8, DR3, and DR4.

Other causes of Addison's disease are listed in Table 9. Infection, particularly tuberculosis, was the most common cause of Addison's disease before the advent of antibiotics and improved public health measures. Worldwide, it is still responsible for approximately 30% of cases of adrenocortical insufficiency. Histoplasmosis and paracoccidioidomycosis are important causes of Addison's disease in endemic areas. HIV infection and AIDS can be associated with Addison's disease

TABLE 12 CAUSES OF ADRENAL CRISIS
Stress: trauma, surgery, infection, severe illness, or prolonged fasting in a patient with treated adrenal insufficiency
Sudden withdrawal of adrenocorticoid hormone in a patient with chronic insufficiency or with temporary insufficiency due to suppression by exogenous glucocorticoids
Removal of both adrenal glands or a functioning adrenal tumor that had suppressed the other gland
Initiation of thyroid treatment in an adrenocorticoid-deficient patient
Injury to both adrenals: hemorrhage, trauma, thrombosis, infection
Sudden pituitary destruction: necrosis, head trauma

Table 13. Diagnostic Tests for Adrenal Insufficiency

Rapid ACTH stimulation test	
250 μg IM or IV cosyntropin, synthetic ACTH (1–24)	Usually used at least 12 h after any prior steroid use
Baseline, 30 min, 60 min blood samples for cortisol (or 45 min only)	If post-ACTH cortisol is < 16–20 μg/dL or rises < 8 μg/dL from baseline level, adrenal insufficiency is confirmed
8 AM cortisol level	If 8 AM cortisol is low (< 5 μg/dL), adrenal insufficiency is suspected
ACTH level (with abnormal ACTH stimulation of cortisol)	If ACTH is elevated (> 52 pg/mL), primary adrenal insufficiency is confirmed
	If ACTH is low (< 9 pg/mL), either normal or secondary adrenal insufficiency

ACTH—corticotropin; IM—intramuscular; IV—intravenous.

and may become a more frequent cause of adrenal insufficiency in the future. Addison's disease can also be caused by the use of drugs that inhibit steroidogenic enzymes, particularly the antifungal ketoconazole and the anesthetic agent etomidate [15].

Secondary adrenal insufficiency

Corticotropin deficiency leads to adrenal gland atrophy and secondary adrenal insufficiency. ACTH deficiency is caused by multiple processes that disrupt the hypothalamic-pituitary unit and may result in complete panhypopituitarism (Table 10). Sheehan's syndrome develops after severe postpartum hemorrhagic or infectious shock and results from ischemic damage to the pituitary. Because the pituitary increases in size by 40% to 60% during pregnancy, it appears to be more susceptible to injury, although the posterior pituitary is usually spared. ACTH deficiency is rare in isolation and appears to be autoimmune [16].

The most common cause of adrenal insufficiency is inhibition of CRH following the administration of pharmacologic doses of glucocorticoids. The excess glucocorticoids suppress CRH, leading to corticotropin deficiency and adrenal atrophy.

Familial glucocorticoid deficiency

Mutations in the pathway of hormone synthesis or action can lead to adrenal insufficiency. Familial glucocorticoid deficiency is caused by unresponsiveness to corticotropin, presumably due to a defect in the corticotropin receptor [17]. Children with this condition have high corticotropin but low cortisol levels.

Glucocorticoid resistance

Glucocorticoid resistance is caused by mutations in the glucocorticoid receptor that result in hyporesponsiveness of target cells to glucocorticoids [18]. The patients are characterized by hypercortisolism without cushingoid features. Clinical manifestations result from excess mineralocorticoid or androgen action. Treatment with dexamethasone may overcome the partial resistance at the target cells and is effective in restoring the HPA axis to normal.

Diagnostic Tests

The diagnosis of adrenal insufficiency can be made using the rapid corticotropin stimulation tests (Table 13). When there is high suspicion of primary adrenal insufficiency in the face of likely adrenal crisis, blood samples for measurement of corticotropin, plasma renin activity, and aldosterone should be taken with the baseline cortisol sample, and treatment with hydrocortisone should be started immediately after the test is performed, while results are still pending.

Further testing is necessary to distinguish primary from secondary adrenal insufficiency. In primary adrenal insufficiency, corticotropin values are high, the patient is frequently pigmented and exhibits electrolyte abnormalities of aldosterone insufficiency, with hyperkalemia, elevated plasma renin activity, and decreased aldosterone. In secondary adrenal insufficiency, the corticotropin value are low and the renin-angiotensin-aldosterone system is usually intact.

Treatment of Adrenal Insufficiency

Intravenous fluids must be given in large quantities in adrenal crisis in order to gain hemodynamic control. In addition, high-dose intravenous glucocorticoids are essential (Table 14). With treatment, hyperkalemia should resolve quickly, but if electrocardiographic changes develop, calcium, insulin, and Kayexolate or cation exchange resin may be needed as well. Hypoglycemia can be corrected with intravenous glucose.

Treatment of chronic Addison's disease is less emergent, and maintenance doses of glucocorticoid and mineralocorticoid can be initiated together (Table 15). Standard recom-

Table 14. Medical Treatment of Adrenal Crisis

IV fluids
IV glucocorticoids: high dose
   Hydrocortisone, 100 mg IV immediately, then 50–100 mg q6h with gradual taper
IV glucose if hypoglycemic
Fludrocortisone, 0.05–0.2 mg PO daily to start when hydrocortisone is reduced to maintenance dose

IV—intravenous; PO—orally; q6h—every 6 h.

Table 15. Medical Treatment of Addison's Disease

Hydrocortisone, 15–30 mg PO daily
   10–20 mg AM and 5–10 mg PO daily
Fludrocortisone, 0.05–0.2 mg PO daily or every other day, adjusted according to potassium level, blood pressure, weight change, edema or a combination

PO—orally.

mended doses must be tailored to the patient to avoid iatrogenic Cushing's syndrome or inadequate replacement. Symptomatic relief, as well as blood pressure and potassium levels, can help guide therapy. Plasma renin activity also correlates well with mineralocorticoid status and can be followed to monitor the adequacy of replacement. Because hypertension may develop with mineralocorticoid therapy in Addison's patients, doses must be individually adjusted to control blood pressure and potassium levels.

Acknowledgment

The authors thank Jeff Miller and Coleman Gross for their helpful comments and critical reading of the manuscript.

References and Recommended Reading

Recently published papers of particular interest have been highlighted as:
- Of interest
- •• Of outstanding interest

1.•• Orth D, Kovacs W, Debold C: Adrenal Cortex. In *Williams Textbook of Endocrinology*, edn 8. Edited by Wilson J, Foster D. Philadelphia: WB Saunders; 1992:489–620.

2. Funder JW, Pearce PT, Myles K, *et al.*: Apparent mineralocorticoid excess, pseudohypoaldosteronism, and urinary electrolyte excretion: toward a redefinition of mineralocorticoid action. *FASEB J* 1992, 4:3234–3238.

3.• Gabrilove JL: Cushing's syndrome. *Compr Ther* 1992, 18:13–16.

4. Beato M: Gene regulation by steroid hormones. *Cell* 1989, 56:335–344.

5. Sheeler LR: Cushing's syndrome. *Urol Clin North Am* 1989, 16:447–453.

6.• Luton JP, Cerdas S, Billaud L, *et al.*: Clinical features of adrenocortical carcinoma, prognostic factors, and the effect of mitotane therapy. *N Engl J Med* 1990, 322:1195–1201.

7.•• Kaye TB, Crapo L: The Cushing's syndrome: an update on diagnostic tests. *Ann Intern Med* 1990, 112:434–444.

8. Yanovski JA, Cutler GB, Chrousos GP, *et al.*: Corticotropin-releasing hormone stimulation following low-dose dexamethasone administration. *JAMA* 1993, 269:2232–2238.

9. Flack MR, Oldfield EH, Cutler GB, *et al.*: Urine free cortisol in the high-dose dexamethasone suppression test for the differential diagnosis of the Cushing's syndrome. *Ann Intern Med* 1992, 116:211–217.

10. Oldfield EH, Doppman JL, Keiman LK, *et al.*: Petrosal sinus sampling with and without corticotropin-releasing hormone for the differential diagnosis of Cushing's syndrome. *N Engl J Med* 1991, 325:897–905.

11. Ross NS, Aron DC: Hormonal evaluation of the patient with an incidentally discovered adrenal mass. *N Engl J Med* 1990, 323:1401–1405.

12. Lindholm J: Endocrine function in patients with Cushing's disease before and after treatment. *Clin Endocrinol* 1992, 36:151–159.

13.• Miller J, Crapo L: Medical treatment of Cushing's syndrome. *Endocr Rev* 1993, 14:443–458.

14.• Muir A, Schatz DA, Maclaren NK: Autoimmune Addison's disease. *Springer Semin Immunopathol* 1993, 14:275–284.

15. Feldman D: Ketoconazole and other imidazole derivatives as inhibitors of steroidogenesis. *Endocr Rev* 1986, 7:409–420.

16. Yamamoto T, Fukuyama J, Hasegawa K, *et al.*: Isolated corticotropin deficiency in adults. *Arch Intern Med* 1992, 152:1705–1712.

17. Clark AJL, McLoughlin L, Grossman A: Familial glucocorticoid deficiency association with point mutation in the adrenocorticotropin receptor. *Lancet* 1992, 341:461–462.

18. Malchoff DM, Brufsky A, Reardon G, *et al.*: A mutation of the glucocorticoid receptor in primary cortisol resistance. *J Clin Immunol* 1993, 91:1918–1925.

19. Tyrell JB, Forsham PR: Glucocorticoids and adrenal androgens. In *Review of Medical Physiology*, edn 12. Edited by Ganong WF. Los Altos, CA: Lange Medical Publications, 1985: 277.

Select Bibliography

Liddle G: Tests of pituitary-adrenal suppressibility in the diagnosis of Cushing's syndrome. *J Clin Endocrinol Metab* 1960, 20:1539–1560.

Nugent C, Nichols T, Tyler F: Diagnosis of Cushing's syndrome-single dose dexamethasone suppression test. *Arch Intern Med* 1965, 116:172–176.

Oelkers W, Diederich S, Bahr V: Diagnosis and therapy surveillance in Addison's disease: rapid adrenocorticotropin (ACTH) test and measurement of plasma ACTH, renin activity and aldosterone. *J Clin Endocrinol Metab* 1992, 75:259–264.

Milton D, Shapiro B: Clinical review 50: clinically silent adrenal masses. *J Clin Endocrinol Metab* 1993, 77:885–888.

Miller J, Crapo L: The biochemical diagnosis of hypercortisolism. *Endocrinol* 1994, 4:7–16.

Glucocorticoid Therapy and Withdrawal

Maria Alexandra Magiakou
George P. Chrousos

> **Key Points**
> - Since 1949 glucocorticoids have been used in the therapy of a broad spectrum of nonendocrine (autoimmune, collagen, renal, gastrointestinal, respiratory, nervous, hematologic, ophthalmic) and endocrine diseases.
> - Glucocorticoids may be administered systemically or compartmentally.
> - Serious side effects are mostly associated with chronic administration of pharmacologic amounts of glucocorticoids. Acute complications occur infrequently, however.
> - To avoid complications, alternate-day administration of intermediate-acting glucocorticoids should be given, if possible.
> - Patients taking glucocorticoids should be carefully monitored for side effects. Glucocorticoids should be withdrawn gradually.

Glucocorticoids are produced by the cortices of the adrenal glands and secreted into the systemic circulation in a circadian fashion and in response to stressful stimuli. These steroid hormones play pivotal roles in the regulation of intermediary metabolism, maintenance of cardiovascular function, stimulation of behavior, and control of the immune inflammatory reaction. The major endogenous glucocorticoid in humans is cortisol, whose synthetic form has been traditionally called hydrocortisone. Cortisone, the 2-keto form of cortisol, was first used therapeutically in the management of rheumatoid arthritis by Hench and coworkers [1] in 1949. Since then, a large number of synthetic compounds with glucocorticoid activity have been developed, and glucocorticoids have been used in the therapy of a broad spectrum of nonendocrine and endocrine diseases [2•,3,4•].

Glucocorticoids may be administered systemically or compartmentally (topical, ophthalmic, inhaled, nasal, or intra-articular). Although major complications are unlikely with short-term treatment, many side effects are associated with chronic administration of pharmacologic amounts of glucocorticoids. To avoid complications, alternate-day administration of intermediate-acting glucocorticoids should be used if chronic therapy is necessary. Also, careful monitoring of patients and gradual glucocorticoid withdrawal should always be performed to avoid an adrenal crisis or reactivation of the disease under therapy [2•,4•].

SYNTHETIC GLUCOCORTICOIDS

Since the introduction of glucocorticoids in the treatment of rheumatoid arthritis in 1949, the therapeutic applications of these drugs were greatly broadened to encompass a large number of nonendocrine and endocrine diseases [1]. Intense efforts were made by science and industry to maximize the beneficial effects and to minimize the side effects of glucocorticoids. Thus, many synthetic compounds with glucocorticoid activity were manufactured and tested. The pharmacologic differences among these chemicals result from structural alterations of their basic

Table 1. Glucocorticoid Equivalencies

	Equivalent dose, *mg*	Glucocorticoid potency	Mineralocorticoid potency	Plasma half-life, *min*	Biologic half-life, *h*
Glucocorticoids					
Short-acting					
Cortisol	20.0	1.0	2	90	8–12
Cortisone	25.0	0.8	2	80–118	8–12
Intermediate-acting					
Prednisone	5.0	4.0	1	60	18–36
Prednisolone	5.0	4.0	1	115–200	18–36
Triamcinolone	4.0	5.0	0	30	18–36
Methylprednisolone	4.0	5.0	0	180	18–36
Long-acting					
Dexamethasone	0.5	25–50	0	200	36–54
Betamethasone	0.6	25–50	0	300	36–54
Mineralocorticoids					
Aldosterone	–	0.3	300	15–20	8–12
Fluorocortisone	2.0	15.0	150	200	18–36
Desoxycorticosterone acetate	–	0.0	20	70	–

From Liapi and Chrousos [2•]; with permission.

steroid nucleus and its side groups. These changes may affect the bioavailability of these compounds—including their gastrointestinal or parenteral absorption, plasma half-life, and metabolism in the liver, fat, or target tissues—and their abilities to interact with the glucocorticoid receptor and to modulate the transcription of glucocorticoid-responsive genes [5]. In addition, structural modifications diminish the natural cross-reactivity of glucocorticoids with the mineralocorticoid receptor, eliminating their undesirable salt-retaining activity. Other modifications increase glucocorticoids' water solubility for parenteral administration or decrease their water solubility to enhance topical potency [2•,6,7•,8•].

Most synthetic glucocorticoids (*eg*, methylprednisolone and dexamethasone) are minimally bound to cortisol-binding globulin and circulate mostly bound to albumin, or in the free form. The percentage of such glucocorticoids bound to plasma proteins is relatively constant, and because this binding is concentration-independent, the metabolic clearance rate of glucocorticoids remains constant regardless of dose. Table 1 shows the relative glucocorticoid and mineralocorticoid potencies of different commonly used systemic glucocorticoids and their approximate plasma and biologic effect half-lives [2•]. Glucocorticoid activity has been mostly defined in rat bioassays and may not always pertain to human responses, especially the growth-suppressing properties of synthetic glucocorticoids, which have been markedly underestimated. The biologic effect half-life of glucocorticoids divides them into short-, intermediate-, or long-acting, based on the duration of corticotropin suppression after a single dose of the compound [2•,8•].

SYSTEMIC GLUCOCORTICOID ADMINISTRATION

Therapeutic Indications

Glucocorticoids may be administered as replacement therapy in patients with primary or secondary adrenal insufficiency, as adrenal suppression therapy in congenital adrenal hyperplasia and glucocorticoid resistance, and as anti-inflammatory or immunosuppressant therapy in a broad range of mostly nonendocrine disorders affecting many different systems [4•,9•]. Thus, glucocorticoids are used in endocrine, autoimmune, collagen, renal, gastrointestinal, respiratory, nervous, hematologic, and ophthalmic diseases and are used in the suppression of the host-versus-graft or graft-versus-host reaction in cases of organ transplantation. Neoplastic disorders of the lymphoid system, such as leukemia and lymphomas, are also treated with glucocorticoids, along with the appropriate chemotherapy.

Acute administration of pharmacologic doses of glucocorticoids is necessary in a small number of nonendocrine diseases, such as malignant hyperthermia, and in patients with craniospinal trauma or brain tumors or who are undergoing major neurosurgical operations to, respectively, decrease the temperature and prevent destruction of neural tissue from the local edema and inflammatory reaction [10]. In addition, glucocorticoids have been used in the prevention of the respiratory distress syndrome in the premature neonate, when delivery is anticipated before the 34th week of gestation [11]. In this case, treatment of the pregnant woman with betamethasone, a glucocorticoid compound that readily crosses the placenta, stimulates the production of pulmonary surfactant and the maturation of the fetal lungs.

Side Effects

Side effects occur only with supraphysiologic doses of glucocorticoids and not with proper replacement, which is equivalent to 12 to 15 mg hydrocortisone/m² body surface area (Table 1) [12]. Major complications are unlikely with short-term treatment (less than 2 weeks) with high doses of glucocorticoids, although sleep disturbances and gastric irritation are common complaints, and depression, mania, or psychosis may be infrequently precipitated [13]. On the other hand, many side effects are associated with chronic daily administration of pharmacologic amounts of glucocorticoids (Table 2) [4•,6]. These side effects include the development of varying degrees of Cushing's syndrome manifestations during therapy and secondary adrenal insufficiency (adrenal suppression) after discontinuation of treatment. Growth retardation is one of the major side effects of chronic daily glucocorticoid therapy in children [9•,14].

The degree of cushingoid features and the severity and length of adrenal suppression depend on both the type and dose of the specific compound used, the duration of treatment, the idiosyncrasy, and the stress status of the patient. Most complications of glucocorticoid treatment are totally or partially reversible after discontinuation of glucocorticoid administration, with the exception of posterior subcapsular cataracts and advanced bone necrosis [15].

High doses of glucocorticoids suppress the immune defenses of the organism. Thus, individuals on glucocorticoid therapy are particularly susceptible to viral diseases against which they have not been vaccinated or naturally immunized (*eg*, varicella, which can be devastating). Also, such individuals are susceptible to contract or to sustain activation of dormant tuberculosis [16]. Individuals treated with massive doses of glucocorticoids can also develop saprophytic, fungal, or protozoan infections such as those seen in patients with severe immunodeficiency [6].

To avoid complications, alternate-day administration of intermediate-acting glucocorticoids should be used, when possible, if chronic therapy is necessary. Frequently, such a regimen can control the activity of the disease under therapy, without causing Cushing's syndrome, growth retardation, or adrenal suppression.

Nonfluorinated glucocorticoids (cortisone, cortisol, prednisone, and prednisolone) cross the placenta poorly. Fluorinated steroids, on the other hand, cross the placenta readily and should be given cautiously to women during pregnancy. Maternal–fetal plasma concentration gradients are an approximate 10:1 ratio for cortisol or prednisolone and an approximate 2.5:1.0 for betamethasone and dexamethasone. Newborns who have been exposed to high doses of synthetic fluorinated corticosteroids *in utero* should be checked for signs of adrenal insufficiency and have a Cortrosyn (Organon Inc., New Orange, NJ) stimulation test to assess for need of glucocorticoid replacement [17].

COMPARTMENTAL GLUCOCORTICOID ADMINISTRATION

Topical Glucocorticoids

Glucocorticoids are quite effective when applied topically and nontoxic to the skin in the short term. The factors that deter-

---

TABLE 2 EFFECTS OF GLUCOCORTICOIDS DURING CHRONIC THERAPY

Endocrine and metabolic
Suppression of hypothalmic-pituitary-adrenal axis (adrenal suppression)
Growth failure in children
Carbohydrate intolerance
  Hyperinsulinemia
  Insulin resistance
  Abnormal glucose tolerance test
  Diabetes mellitus
Cushingoid features
  Moon facies, facial plethora
  Generalized and truncal obesity
  Supraclavicular fat collection
  Posterior cervical fat deposition (buffalo hump)
  Glucocorticoid-induced acne
  Thin and fragile skin, violaceous striae
Impotence, menstrual disorders
Decreased thyroid-stimulating hormone and triiodothyronine
Hypokalemia, metabolic alkalosis

Gastrointestinal system
Gastric irritation, peptic ulcer
Acute pancreatitis (rare)
Fatty infiltration of liver (hepatomegaly) (rare)

Hemopoietic system
Leukocytosis
  Neutrophilia
    Increased influx from bone marrow and decreased migration from blood vessels
Monocytopenia
Lymphopenia
  Migration from blood vessels to lymphoid tissue
Eosinopenia

Immune system
Suppression of delayed hypersensitivity
  Inhibition of leukocyte and tissue macrophage migration
  Inhibition of cytokine secretion or action
Suppression of the primary antigen response

Musculoskeletal system
Osteoporosis, spontaneous fractures
Aseptic necrosis of femoral and humoral heads and other bones
Myopathy

Ophthalmic
Posterior subcapsular cataracts (more common in children)
Elevated intraocular pressure or glaucoma

Neuropsychiatric disorders
Sleep disturbances, insomnia
Euphoria, depression, mania, psychosis
Pseudotumor cerebri (benign increase of intracranial pressure)

From Laue *et al*. [6]; with permission.

Table 3 Interactions of glucocorticoids with other drugs

Drug	Side effect	Comments
Amphotericin B	Hypokalemia	Monitor potassium levels frequently
Digitalis glycosides	Digitalis toxicity	Monitor potassium levels frequently
	Hypokalemia	
Growth hormone	Ineffective	–
Potassium-depleting diuretics	Hypokalemia	Monitor potassium levels frequently
Vaccines from live attenuated viruses	Severe generalized infections	–

mine local penetration are the structure of the compound employed, the vehicle, the basic additives, occlusion versus open use, normal skin versus diseased skin, and small areas versus large areas of application. Fluorinated steroids (*eg*, dexamethasone, triamcinolone acetonide, betamethasone, and beclomethasone) penetrate the skin better than nonfluorinated steroids, such as hydrocortisone. However, fluorinated steroids also produce more local complications and may be associated with systemic absorption and side effects [2•,4•].

The complications of chronic topical skin use of glucocorticoids are mostly local (*eg*, epidermal atrophy and hypopigmentation, telangiectasia, or acne and folliculitis) or infrequently systemic, with the classic manifestations of Cushing's syndrome, retardation of growth in children, and adrenal suppression. The frequency of systemic effects by topical corticosteroids is increased in newborns and small children compared to adolescents and adults, because glucocorticoids penetrate the skin of newborns and small children more easily and in larger proportional amounts. Systemic effects may also be observed in patients with hepatic disease or idiosyncratically because of decreased drug metabolism. Although most types of dermatitis are generally responsive to topical glucocorticoids, there are rare cases in which intralesional injections should be considered (*eg*, hypertrophic scars, acne cysts, or prurigo nodularis).

Ophthalmic Glucocorticoids

Patients with autoimmune or idiopathic inflammation of the anterior segment of the eye (*eg*, iritis and uveitis) may benefit from local administration of glucocorticoids. Also, patients with postsurgical or traumatic inflammation are given topical glucocorticoids to prevent local destruction from edema. Special care should be taken to avoid treating patients with herpes simplex conjunctivitis or keratitis during the infectious stage of the disease, because major spread of the infection may be precipitated.

Inhaled Glucocorticoids

Patients with bronchial asthma may benefit from glucocorticoid inhalation therapy. The existing preparations at the recommended doses have a remarkable therapeutic effect without causing manifestations of Cushing's syndrome, growth retardation, or clinically significant adrenal suppression. Systemic effects may be observed, however, because of increased intake of such preparations or because of altered steroid metabolism.

Nasal Glucocorticoids

Aerosols containing glucocorticoids are available for the treatment of allergic rhinitis. Frequent and chronic use should be avoided to prevent local and systemic complications.

Intraarticular Glucocorticoids

The intraarticular injection of glucocorticoids may be of value in carefully selected patients if strict aseptic techniques are used and repeated, and frequent injections are avoided.

MONITORING OF PATIENTS ON GLUCOCORTICOID TREATMENT

Patients receiving chronic treatment with glucocorticoids should adhere to a high protein, calorie-restricted diet. The diet should also be rich in potassium and calcium and low in sodium. Adequate ambulation or exercise should be recommended to prevent muscular atrophy and osteopenia. Patients should concurrently take antacids or histamine$_2$ antagonists to prevent gastric irritation or peptic ulcers [18]. Growing young children should have their growth monitored every 3 months (until age 5) and older children should have their growth monitored every 6 months. All patients should have measurements of body weight, length or height, blood pressure, fasting and 2-hour postprandial blood glucose, serum electrolytes, and bone maturation or density. Because glucocorticoids decrease the organism's response to infection, care should be taken to determine whether latent infections, such as mycobacterial disease, are present before treatment begins.

Concomitant Use of Glucocorticoids with Other Drugs

Special attention is required in the concomitant use of glucocorticoids with other drugs because of potential interactions, and because some drugs may affect the metabolism of the steroids, which may lead to a decreased or increased glucocorticoid effect on their target tissues [2•,4•]. Such interactions and effects are shown in Tables 3, 4, and 5.

Glucocorticoid Withdrawal

Glucocorticoid withdrawal can present with symptoms of chronic glucocorticoid deficiency or as an acute adrenal crisis. Thus, patients may suffer from anorexia, myalgia, nausea, emesis, lethargy, headache, fever, skin desquamation, arthralgias, weight loss, and postural hypotension. In addition, they may experience exacerbation of previously present

Table 4. Effects of Glucocorticoids on Blood Levels of Other Drugs

Drug	Drug blood levels	Comments
Aspirin	Decreased	Increased metabolism or clearance
		Monitor salicylate levels
Coumarin anticoagulants	Decreased	Frequent control of prothrombin levels
Cyclophosphamide	Increased	Inhibition of hepatic metabolism
		Adjust the dosage of the drug
Cyclosporine	Increased	Inhibition of hepatic metabolism
Insulin	Decreased	Adjust the dosage of the drug
Isoniazid	Decreased	Increased metabolism and clearance
Oral hypoglycemic agents	Decreased	Adjust the dosage of the drug

autoimmune disease (*eg*, rheumatoid arthritis, atopic dermatitis, or asthma) or have new autoimmune disease (*eg*, Hashimoto's thyroiditis or Graves' disease). The occurrence of the subjective component of the steroid withdrawal syndrome does not depend on the absence of cortisol from the circulation or an impairment of the hypothalamic-pituitary-adrenal axis, because many of these symptoms may occur while on proper glucocorticoid replacement or while the patient has a normal cortisol response to Cortrosyn (Organon, Inc.). In this instance, the steroid withdrawal syndrome may be a result of difficulties in withdrawing from the high levels of glucocorticoids—a phenomenon that appears to be idiosyncratic [2•,3,4•].

Termination of chronic daily glucocorticoid therapy (longer than 2 weeks) should be gradual—both to prevent development of adrenal insufficiency and to avoid reactivation of the disease under therapy (Table 6). The likelihood of the latter depends on the activity and natural history of the disorder. When there is any chance that the underlying illness may recur, the glucocorticoids should be withdrawn slowly over a period of weeks to months with frequent reassessment of the patient's condition. Daily hydrocortisone replacement or double or triple replacement of intermediate-acting glucocorticoids given on alternate days are acceptable methods for weaning patients from glucocorticoid therapy.

Table 5. Effect of Drugs on Plasma Glucocorticoid Concentrations

Drug	Glucocorticoid blood levels	Comments
Antacids	Decreased	Possible physical adsorption to antacid
Carbamazepine	Decreased	Increased cytochrome P-450 activity
Cholestyramine	Decreased	Decreased gastrointestinal absorption of glucocorticoids
Colestipol	Decreased	Decreased gastrointestinal absorption of glucocorticoids
Cyclosporine	Increased	Inhibition of hepatic metabolism
Ephedrine	Decreased	Probably increased metabolism
Erythromycin	Increased	Impaired elimination
Mitotane	Decreased, with elevated transcortin	Total plasma cortisol unreliable
		Adjust glucocorticoid levels
Oral contraceptives	Increased	Impaired elimination, increased protein binding
Phenobarbital	Decreased	Increased cytochrome P-450 activity
		Adjust glucocorticoid dosage
Phenytoin	Decreased	Increased cytochrome P-450 activity
		Adjust glucocorticoid dosage
Rifampin	Decreased	Probably increased cytochrome P-450 activity
		Adjust glucocorticoid dosage
Troleandomycin	Increased	Partially resulting from impaired elimination

From Liapi and Chrousos [2•]; with permission.

TABLE 6 PROPOSED REGIMENS FOR TAPERING GLUCOCORTICOIDS

To prevent an adrenal crisis:
1. Switch to hydrocortisone 15 mg/m^2 body surface area/d. Perform Cortrosyn* test every 3 mo and discontinue glucocorticoids when plasma cortisol > 18 µg/dL at 30 min
2. Switch to prednisone 6 mg/m^2 body surface area on alternate days. Perform Cortrosyn* test every 3 mo and discontinue medication when plasma cortisol > 18 µg/dL at 30 min

To prevent reactivation of disease:
Decrease dose by 10% per wk until it becomes equivalent to replacement; then follow one of the above regimens

*Organon, Inc., New Orange, NJ.

ADRENAL SUPPRESSION

Recovery of the hypothalamic-pituitary-adrenal axis can take 12 months or longer [9•]. Abrupt cessation of glucocorticoid treatment or quick tapering can precipitate an acute adrenal insufficiency crisis. The main symptoms range from anorexia, fatigue, nausea, vomiting, dyspnea, fever, arthralgia, myalgia, and orthostatic hypotension to dizziness, fainting, and circulatory collapse. Hypoglycemia is occasionally observed in children and very thin adult individuals. The diagnosis is a medical emergency, and treatment should be immediate administration of fluids, electrolytes, glucose, and parenteral glucocorticoids.

To evaluate adequacy of hypothalamic-pituitary-adrenal axis recovery the rapid Cortrosyn (Organon, Inc.) test should be used. An intravenous bolus of 250 µg of corticotropin 1-24 (Cortrosyn [Organon, Inc.]) is administered and cortisol is measured after 30 or 60 minutes or both. Plasma cortisol concentration of greater than 18 or 20 µg/dL, at these times indicates adequate recovery of the hypothalamic-pituitary-adrenal axis [9•].

REFERENCES AND RECOMMENDED READING

Recently published papers of particular interest have been highlighted as:
- Of interest
- • Of outstanding interest

1. Hench PS, Kendall EC, Slocumb CH, *et al.*: The effect of a hormone of the adrenal cortex (17-hydroxy 11-dehydrocortisone), compound E and of pituitary adrenocorticotropic hormone on rheumatoid arthritis. *Proc Staff Meet Mayo Clin* 1949, 24:181–197.
2.• Liapi C, Chrousos GP: Glucocorticoids. In *Pediatric Pharmacology* edn 2. Edited by Jaffe SJ, Aranda JV. Philadelphia: WB Saunders Co; 1992:466–475.
3. Tyrell JB, Baxter JD: Glucocorticoid therapy. In *Endocrinology and Metabolism* edn 2. Edited by Felig P, Baxter JB, Broadus AE, *et al.* New York: McGraw-Hill; 1987:788–817.
4.• Magiakou MA, Chrousos GP: Corticosteroid therapy, nonendocrine disease and corticosteroid withdrawal. In *Current Therapy in Endocrinology and Metabolism* edn 5. Edited by Bardin CW. Philadelphia: Mosby-Yearbook; 1994:120–124.
5. Rousseau GG, Baxter JD, Tomkins GP: Glucocorticoid receptor: relation between steroid binding and biologic effects. *J Mol Biol* 1972, 67:99–115.
6. Laue L, Kawai S, Udelsman R, *et al.*: Glucocorticoid antagonists: pharmacological attributes of the prototype antiglucocorticoid RU 486. In *Antiinflammatory Steroid Action: Basic and Clinical Aspects*. Edited by Lichtenstein LM, Claman H, Oronsky A, *et al.* New York: Academic Press; 1989:303–329.
7.• Orth DN, Kovacs WJ, DeBold CR: The adrenal cortex. In *Williams Textbook of Endocrinology*. Edited by Wilson JD, Foster DW. Philadelphia: WB Saunders Co; 1992:489–620.
8.• Clark JH, Schrader WT, O'Malley BW: Mechanisms of action of steroid hormones. In *Williams Textbook of Endocrinology*. Edited by Wilson JD, Foster DW. Philadelphia: WB Saunders Co; 1992:35–90.
9.• Kamilaris T, Chrousos GP: Cushing's syndrome. In *Conn's Current Therapy*. Edited by Rakel R. Philadelphia: WB Saunders Co; 1991:572–578.
10. Raitt DG, Merrifield AJ: Dexamethasone in malignant hyperpyrexia [Letter]. *Br Med J* 1974, 4:656.
11. Collaborative Group on Antenatal Steroid Therapy: Effect of antenatal dexamethasone administration on the prevention of respiratory distress syndrome. *Am J Obstet Gynecol* 1981, 141:276–286.
12. Rimsza ME: Complications of corticosteroid therapy. *Am J Dis Child* 1978, 132:806–810.
13. Chrousos GA, Kattah JC, Beck RW, *et al.*: Side effects of glucocorticoid treatment. Experience of the optic neuritis treatment trial. *JAMA* 1993, 269: 16:2110–2112.
14. Morris HG: Growth and skeletal maturation in asthmatic children: effect of corticosteroid treatment. *Pediatr Res* 1975, 9:579–583.
15. Black RL, Oglesby RB, von Sallmann L, *et al.*: Posterior subcapsular cataracts induced by corticosteroids in patients with rheumatoid arthritis. *JAMA* 1960, 174:166–171.
16. Haanaes OC, Bergmann A: Tuberculosis emerging in patients treated with corticosteroids. *Eur J Respir Dis* 1983, 64:294–297.
17. Rokicki W, Bertrand J: The glucocorticoids in normal premature and small for dates newborn infants throughout the neonatal period. In *Intensive Care of the Newborn* edn 2. Edited by Stern L, Salle B, Friis-Hansen B. New York: Masson; 1981:325–342.
18. Messer J, Reitman D, Sacks HC, *et al.*: Association of adrenocorticosteroid therapy and peptic ulcer disease. *N Engl J Med* 1983, 309:21–24.

SELECT BIBLIOGRAPHY

Baxter JD, Rousseau GG: Glucocorticoid hormone action: an overview. In *Monograph in Endocrinology*. Edited by Baxter JD, Rousseau GG. Berlin and New York: Springer-Verlag; 1979: 1–24.

Boumpas DT, Chrousos GP, Wilder RL, *et al.*: NIH conference of the combined clinical staff. Glucocorticoid therapy of immune-related diseases: basic and clinical correlates. *Ann Intern Med* 1993, 119:1198–1208.

Pheochromocytoma

Vincent DeQuattro
Deping Lee

> ### Key Points
> - Pheochromocytoma, a rare but treatable cause of hypertension, can masquerade as a classical hypertensive or as an occult clinical mystery.
> - Clinical suspicion of pheochromocytoma can be confirmed by measures of urinary nometanephrine or metanephrine or plasma or urinary catecholamines.
> - Localization of the chromaffin tumor is performed with complimentary magnetic resonance imaging and octreotide or metaiodobenzylguanidine imaging or via computed tomography scan.
> - Preoperative therapy with α-blockade, usually phenoxybenzamine and often with the addition of β-blockade, should be of sufficient duration to achieve euvolemia and stable left ventricular function.
> - Operative resection requires invasive monitoring, selective anesthesia, careful dissection, and adequate supplies of α-antagonists, β-blockers, nitroprusside, colloid replacement, and autologous transfusion.

No stereotype exists for the patient with pheochromocytoma; he or she may present as an emergency room arrival with a transient ischemic attack, completed stroke, congestive heart failure, myocardial infarction, hypercalcemia, or malignant hypertension. Alternatively, the patient may present with the reverse: shock, acute respiratory distress syndrome, and lactic acidosis. The patient may present at an office visit with classic attacks of diaphoresis, headache, or feelings of impending doom, or he or she may have the symptoms and physical findings of primary hypertension. Investigators who conducted a 30-year surveillance of the population of Rochester, Minnesota found an average annual incidence of pheochromocytoma of 0.95 per 100,000 person-years [1]. In five of the 11 patients, pheochromocytoma was diagnosed at autopsy.

The tumor occurs with equal frequency in both sexes and at any age, although it is most common in the third and fourth decades. Familial tumors are less common and manifest multiplicity, especially bilateral masses, and are often associated with medullary carcinoma of the thyroid [2]. These tumors occur in patients with multiple endocrine neoplasia type II or Sipple syndrome, which is associated with medullary carcinoma of the thyroid, parathyroid adenoma, and bilateral pheochromocytoma (Table 1) [3].

Pheochromocytoma may be associated with other neuroectodermal syndromes, such as neurofibromatosis (approximately 5% of individuals with neurofibromatosis may develop pheochromocytoma), von Hippel–Lindau disease, Sturge-Weber disease, and tuberous sclerosis [4,5]. Pheochromocytoma may occur in association with other endocrine neoplasms. The cells of pheochromocytoma have similar cytochemical and ultrastructural features and a presumed common embryologic origin from the neuroectoderm, sharing amine precursor uptake and decarboxylation [6•]. Isolated tumors may arise from these tissues, or they may occur in association with other amine precursor uptake and decarboxylation cell neoplasms as part of a multiple endocrine

TABLE 1 PRESUMPTIVE DIAGNOSIS OF PHEOCHROMOCYTOMA		

Symptoms (in order of frequency)*
   Headache
   Palpitation of tachycardia
   Excessive perspiration
   Anxiety, nervousness
   Weight loss
   Tremor
   Pallor
   Chest or abdominal pains
   Nausea, vomiting
   Malaise
 Some clinical syndromes
   Hypertension (character)
     Paroxysmal (50%)
     Paradoxical response to:
       β-blockers
       Imipramine, desipramine
       Guanethidine, hydralazine
       Induction of anesthesia
	Malignant accelerated (5%–10%)
	 In pregnancy (1st, 3rd trimester)
	 Diabetes mellitus (50%)
	 Cardiomyopathy (30%)
	 In children
	 Signs (in order of frequency)
	   Hyperhidrosis
	   Paroxysmal changes in BP
	   Postural hypotension
	   Hypertension induced by
	     palpation or positioning
	   Hypertensive retinotherapy
	   Hypermetabolism
	   Neurofibromatosis
	   Cafe-au-lait spots
	   Absence of hand veins
	   Axillary freckling
	   Palpable mass (rare)
	   Acrocyanosis, shock, ARDS
		Familial (not MEN I)
		   MEN II (Sipple's syndrome)
		     Familial pheochromocytoma
		     Medullary carcinoma
		     Parathyroid adenoma
		   MEN III
		     Thickened corneal nerves
		     Ganglioneuromatosis
		     Marfanoid features
		       Mucosal neuronomas
		   von Reckinghausen's
		     neurofibramotosis
		   von Hippel–Lindau disease

*Absence of all makes diagnoses unlikely with > 90% specificity.
ARDS—adult-respiratory distress syndrome; BP— blood pressure; MEN—multiple endocrine neoplasia.

neoplasia syndrome. The screening of unselected patients with pheochromocytoma discovered 19% with von Hippel-Lindau disease and 4% with multiple endocrine neoplasia type 2 (MEN-II) [6]. When family members with von Hippel-Lindau disease or MEN-II were screened for pheochromocytoma, unsuspected pheochromocytoma was found in 46% [6].

Pheochromocytoma arising outside the chromaffin cells of the adrenal medulla are called *functional paraganglioma* [7]. These tumors occur in the posterior mediastinum; in the sympathetic chain in the neck; in the organ of Zuckerkandl, which is ventral to the aorta at the origin of the inferior mesenteric artery; in the pelvis; and in the urinary bladder [8].

ADRENAL MEDULLARY HYPERPLASIA

Whether or not this entity exists has been a topic of controversy since it was first described more than 50 years ago [9]. The normal adrenal has a weight of 6 to 6.5 g and a medullary:cortical ratio of 1:10, (thus, a medullary weight of approximately 0.6 to 0.7 g). Some investigators have reported, however, that medullary weight has approached 1.25 to 2.0 g in patients who had hypertensive crises and attacks similar to pheochromocytoma, but without chromaffin tumors [10,11].

Symptoms

The complaints of patients with pheochromocytoma may resemble those with primary hypertension (Table 1). Symptoms generally have two patterns, persistent or paroxysmal, which are related to a constant or pulsatile release of catecholamines [12]. Attacks occur from once every 2 months to 25 per day and last from 30 seconds to 1 week, with an average time of approximately 15 minutes. Paroxysmal attacks are rarely associated with malignancy [12].

Acute episodes with a constellation of symptoms may occur in patients with pheochromocytoma. Most commonly, these consist of sweating, palpitations, and anxiety with hypertension. Of course, most hypertensive patients with symptoms of pheochromocytoma do not have a chromaffin tumor but instead seem to have spontaneous adrenergic discharge without apparent reasons. Sometimes, the masquerade results from an identifiable cause, such as phenylpropanolamine ingestion or a Munchausen syndrome resulting from self-administration of vasoactive amines, like isoproterenol [13,14]. Kuchel, however, described patients who appear to have episodic dopamine surges that flood phenol sulfotransferase mechanisms that inactivate norepinephrine and epinephrine [15]. Some of our hypertensive patients have had excessive adrenergic tone and appeared to be "caricatures of pheochromocytoma," with surges of free norepinephrine and plasma concomitant with blood pressure elevation. The blood pressure rise in these patients responded to α- and β-receptor blockade [16].

Chromaffin tumors of the adrenal medulla commonly secrete only norepinephrine; less often, a mixture of norepinephrine and epinephrine; and rarely, epinephrine alone. Extra adrenal pheochromocytomas secrete only norepinephrine, which is less potent than epinephrine in causing hypermetabolism and glycogenolysis. Rarely, epinephrine-like effects are seen in patients with tumors excreting only norepinephrine. The history of attacks occurring when the patient bends to one side, wears a tight girdle, or has a full bladder may help to localize or lead to the diagnosis of the tumors.

Physical Findings

Patients with pheochromocytoma often are thin from weight loss, but some remain obese (Table 1). Sweating may be subtle or severe, with drenching night sweats and even dehydration. Facial or digital flushing may also occur, and the extremities may be pale. Vasospasm may be so severe that peripheral pulses are undetectable, and even gangrene may be present. Intense arterial constriction may result in falsely low brachial arterial pressure. The veins on the dorsum of the hands may not be seen because of intense vasoconstriction. Therefore, the clinician must determine whether central pulsations are present, and if they are strong, interarterial monitoring from the femoral region is indicated. Central nervous system findings are diverse and range from anxiety to frank psychosis and from transient ischemic attacks to completed strokes resulting from cerebral hemorrhage. The tumor is rarely palpable, and although such palpation may aid in diagnosis, it may cause a dangerous crisis. Careful quadrant-by-quadrant abdominal massage with intravenous phentolamine available may be useful in localizing the 10% to 20% of tumors in patients who harbor abdominal tumors. Patients with paroxysms related to pheochromocytoma, however, may have a completely normal physical examination during a quiescent period.

Postural hypotension is common in pheochromocytoma, perhaps because of the reduced plasma volume [17]. The hypotension or shock that occurs after removal of a pheochromocytoma results from discontinuation of the catecholamine infusion and reexpansion of the vascular compartment. This phenomenon can be minimized by the preoperative administration of oral α-blockers, such as phenoxybenzamine, and by expansion of the blood volume rapidly after removal of the pheochromocytoma with albumin or autologous blood immediately after the tumor vessels are ligated.

Acute Respiratory Distress Syndrome

We have encountered two patients with acrocyanosis and hypertension rapidly proceeding to hypotension that was associated with marked plasma volume contraction, lactic acidosis, bilateral pulmonary infiltrates, and subsequently at autopsy or surgery, a recent hemorrhage was found in the adrenal tumor. It is exceedingly important to consider the possibility of underlying chromaffin tumor in such patients.

Myocardial Sequelae

Twenty percent to 30% of patients have subjective or objective hemodynamic evidence of a catecholamine myocarditis manifested by arrhythmias, congestive heart failure, and nonspecific electrocardiographic changes of myocardiopathy [18]. This effect results partly from an increased afterload, from direct inflammatory effects of the catecholamines, and from ischemia, which produces intense arteriolar constriction [19]. Thus, α-blockade must be used for a sufficient period preoperatively for repair of this cardiac dysfunction. Echocardiography can document or detect global or segmental akinesis or hypokinesis, which usually reverts over a period of days to normal after α-blocking therapy. In one series of necropsies of patients with pheochromocytoma and sudden death, five of 10 had acute myocardial infarction. Several of the young patients had far-advanced atherosclerosis, and two of our own patients in their sixth decade required coronary revascularization. One patient with pheochromocytoma, 35 years of age, sustained an acute myocardial infarction after angiography. Thus, this complication, although relatively rare, must be considered during planning for surgical correction of these tumors. Generally, we resect the tumor and address the coronary vascular lesion after the patient recovers from the surgery. Rarely, pheochromocytoma occurs in the intraatrial groove or travels to the heart by extension inside the great veins.

Biochemical Assays

Urine

Patients should avoid stress and activities causing nonspecific elevations of catecholamines during urine collection (Table 2). We prefer to use free catecholamines for screening. We use "timed urine" or express the result as "per milligram of creatinine" (Table 2). Most specialists prefer to assess normetanephrine and metanephrine excretion rates rather than norepinephrine and epinephrine to improve both sensitivity and specificity. For patients with labile hypertension, urine should be collected during exacerbations, and this timed specimen can be compared with baseline. When the pattern of catecholamine excretion includes 20% or more as epinephrine, the tumor is usually found in the adrenals or in the organs of Zuckerkandl. Low levels of vanillylmandelic acid excretion do not exclude the diagnosis of pheochromocytoma. In our studies, the levels were normal in 10% to 15% of patients with known

Table 2 Excretion rates of catecholamines and catecholamine metabolites in normal subjects and in patients with pheochromocytoma

	Normal*, µg/h	Pheochromocytoma†, µg/h
Catecholamines (free epinephrine plus norepinephrine)	2.5±0.8	10–120
Metanephrine plus normetanephrine (free plus conjugated)	16±5	30–420
Normetanephrine (free and conjugated)	10±5	30–720
Vanillylmandelic acid	240±120	500–3500

*Mean ± standard deviation.
†Presumptive until proved otherwise.

pheochromocytoma [20]. Further, false-positive results occurring in 10% to 15% can be caused by beverages high in vanillin and food, such as bananas, coffee, nuts, and other fruits.

Plasma norepinephrine

Plasma catecholamine measurements are of value in episodic crises and before and after clonidine suppression or histamine challenge. To minimize false-positive results, blood obtained 20 to 30 minutes after supine rest avoids the effect of stress and posture on catecholamine levels. The total catecholamine value in normotensive patients ranges from 100 to 500 ng/L [21]. Patients with pheochromocytoma usually have values 10 to 15 times normal. The high predictive value of a plasma catecholamine value that is greater than 2000 ng/L is offset by the low specificity when only mild-to-moderate elevations are found (Table 3). Catecholamine values of less than 2000 ng/L in various stressful states may be considered equivocal because some patients with primary hypertension have elevations ranging from 800 to 1000 g/L. Plasma catecholamine value may be normal during normotensive or asymptomatic intervals. From our unreported experience, a fivefold or greater increase in plasma catecholamines after histamine suggests pheochromocytoma. Assay of plasma normetanephrine in pheochromocytoma is as sensitive as that of plasma norepinephrine and offers the advantage of not requiring plasma preservation [22]. We have encountered patients who have had normal plasma levels of norepinephrine and epinephrine, but elevated levels of normetanephrine that were greater than 500 ng/L [23]. Some of these patients have had metastatic pheochromocytoma. O'Connor and Bernstein [24] demonstrated elevated chromogranin A levels in the plasma of patients with pheochromocytoma. This substance may prove helpful in the diagnosis of patients with pheochromocytoma and in excluding its diagnosis in pseudopheochromocytoma.

Clonidine Suppression Test

The clonidine suppression test has practical clinical value in patients with pseudopheochromocytoma, as described previously. Because of the clinical symptoms and borderline values present in patients with pseudopheochromocytoma, the diagnosis of pheochromocytoma is entertained, and frequently the elevations of the plasma catecholamines are two SD above normal. Oral clonidine, an α_2-agonist, reduces plasma norepinephrine levels in hypertensive patients consonant with its effects in lowering central and thus peripheral sympathetic tone and blood pressure [23,25]. Bravo and coworkers [26,27] applied the method of clonidine suppression of plasma norepinephrine to a population of hypertensive patients and they found no suppression in patients with pheochromocytoma, compared with a 60% to 70% reduction of plasma norepinephrine 3 hours after an oral dose of 0.3 mg of clonidine in patients without pheochromocytoma (Fig. 1). Blood pressure was equally reduced in both groups. We do not know of any patients with pheochromocytoma in whom clonidine lowered the plasma norepinephrine level. Some of our patients have had marginally elevated plasma norepinephrine levels for many years without documentation of phcochromocytoma and have had no suppression of plasma norepinephrine level

TABLE 3 AFTER URINARY SCREENING: DIAGNOSTIC TESTS FOR PHEOCHROMOCYTOMA

Plasma
Norepinephrine and epinephrine, supine (30–60 min)
  700–1000 pg/mL (repeat, especially if urine results positive)
  1000–2000 pg/mL (use clonidine suppression test; should fall to < 50%)
  > 2000 pg/mL (usually diagnostic for pheochromocytoma)

Imaging
CT, 77% sensitivity overall
MRI
Scintigraphy:
  ^{131}I MIBG (if CT results are negative or more than one tumor suspected)
  Octreotide scan
Iodocholesterol: nonfunctional tumors in region of clips
Vena caval and regional vein sampling for catecholamine step-up
Ultrasound: pregnancy, screening, near clips
Intravenous pyelography: hypertension screening, urinary bladder
Angiography: to localize and to establish vascular connections

CT—computed tomography; MRI—magnetic resonance imaging; MIBG—metaiodobenzylguanidine.

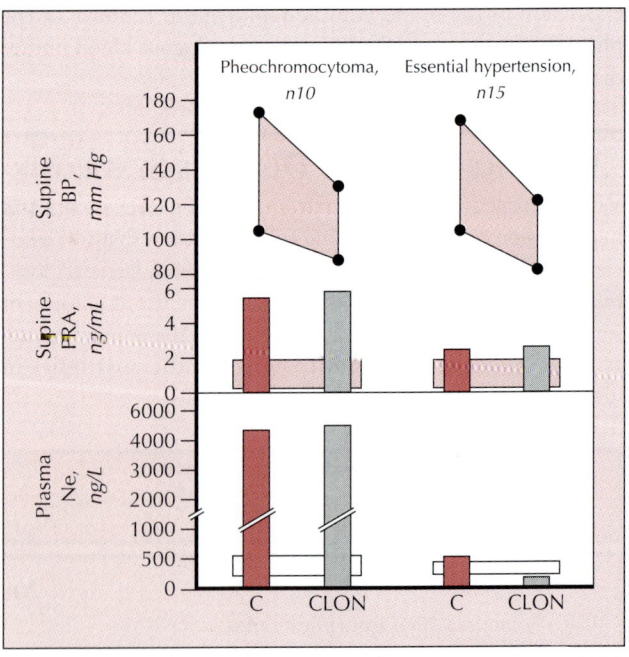

FIGURE 1 Cardiovascular and humoral responses of 10 patients with proven pheochromocytoma and 15 patients with essential hypertension who underwent the clonidine suppression test. For plasma renin activity (PRA) and plasma norepinephrine (Ne), the cross-hatched areas indicate the mean (±2 SD) of values obtained from healthy adult subjects of similar age. BP—blood pressure; C—control group; CLON—clonidine suppression test group. (From Bravo et al. [49]; with permission.)

accidents and to avert unnecessary adrenalectomy. Ninety-eight percent of pheochromocytomas are found below the diaphragm, with most sporadic cases occurring (90%) in the adrenal medulla (Fig. 2). Fifteen percent are multiple. Most of the remainder are found in the posterior mediastinum, middle ear, carotid body, and urinary bladder. Ultrasound, computed tomography, octreotide and/or metaiodobenzylguanidine (MIBG) scintigraphy, and magnetic resonance imaging have supplanted older methods of localization. They should be carried out by experienced radiologists using the most state-of-the-art equipment.

Computed Tomography, Magnetic Resonance Imaging, and Scintigraphy

Computed tomography correctly localized 89% of tumors, including single, intraadrenal, bilateral adrenal, ectopic, and malignant tumors, on initial presentation in 52 patients seen over a 7-year period at the Mayo Clinic [28]. Current state-of-the-art scanners may localize as many as 95%. The Mayo Clinic study noted a localization rate of 73% for recurrent tumors; failures were attributable to small tumor size (8 mm) and artifacts resulting from surgical clips.

Scintigraphic visualization of adrenergic tissues has been made possible by the development of an analogue of guanethidine, ^{131}I-MIBG (Fig. 3) [29]. ^{131}I-MIBG is concentrated in adrenergic neurons and chromaffin tissue by uptake into norepinephrine-containing storage sites. Discrete images after 48 hours usually represent pheochromocytomas that are rich in adrenergic storage vesicles. The method delivers 0.11 total body cGy and 17.5 cGy to the normal adrenal medullas [30]. Imaging is performed 48 and 72 hours after administration of the tracer. The method is safe, reproducible, and highly specific (Fig. 4). It provides unique functional information that may be of great value when multiple tumors are expected, as in multiple endocrine neoplasia [31]. False-negative results may occur in 4% to 10% of patients, often those with malignancy [32]. Medications known to inhibit norepinephrine uptake, such as labetalol and tricyclic antidepressants, should be discontinued 2 weeks before the study. Because ^{131}I MIBG is excreted by the bladder, imaging of this region with other methods may be necessary in some patients.

Pheochromocytomas contain a high content of somatostatin receptors. Thus, the radiologic somatostatin analog octreotide can be used to localize the primary tumor, as well as any metastases [33••]. The scintigraphy with octreotide is not specific for pheochromocytoma; other neuroendocrine (*ie*, carcinoid) and some nonendocrine (*ie*, astrocytoma) tumors, granulomas (*ie*,

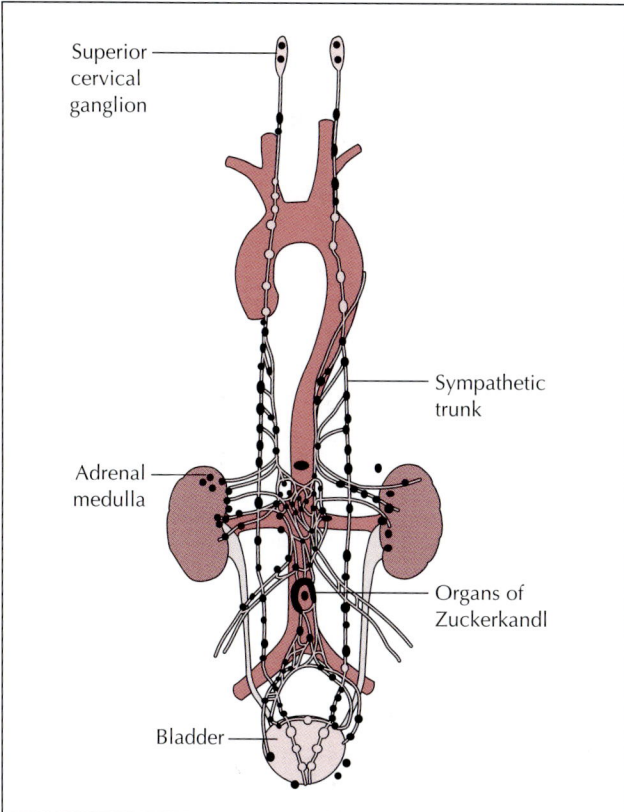

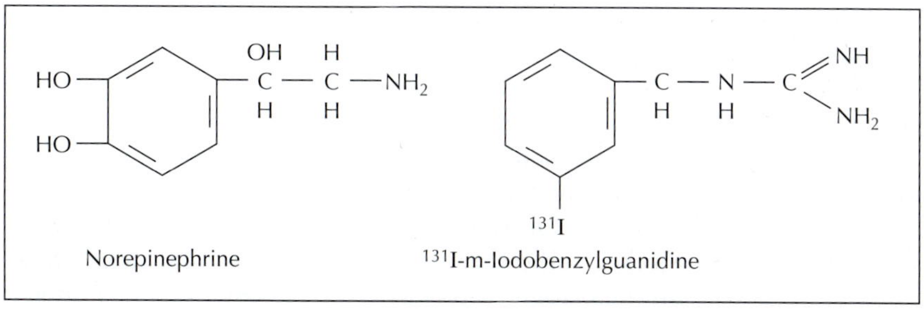

FIGURE 2 Sites of aorticosympathetic paraganglia (extramedullary chromaffin tissue) in a newborn child. Most functional paragangliomas occur below the diaphragm. (*Adapted from* Glenner and Grimbley [50]; with permission.)

after clonidine. Thus, a positive test result, that is, suppression of norepinephrine, is strongly predictive of nonpheochromocytoma, but a negative result in the presence of marginally increased catecholamines cannot be considered presumptive evidence for the presence of a chromaffin tumor.

Pharmacologic Diagnosis

The provocative tests for diagnosis of pheochromocytoma may be dangerous. These drugs have caused hypertensive crises, cardiovascular accidents, and fatalities. These tests should be carried out by experienced endocrinologists when indicated.

LOCALIZATION OF TUMORS

Localization of the tumor before surgery is required to decrease operative time and the incidence of cardiovascular

FIGURE 3 Chemical structure of metaiodobenzylguanidine.

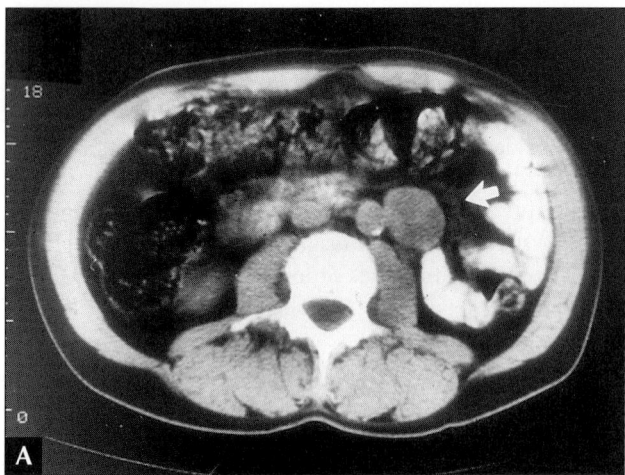 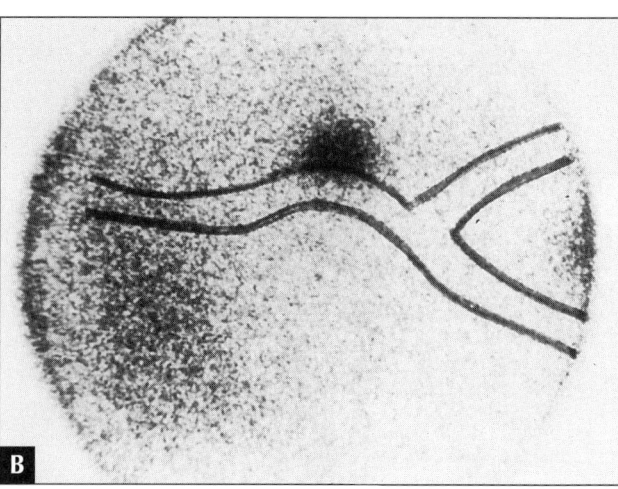

FIGURE 4 **A**, Computed tomographic scan of patient with paraganglioma. Tumor is seen at tip of arrow. **B**, Complementary role of the metaiodobenzylguanidine scan. The functional tumor is seen adjacent to the aorta. There was a plasma norepinephrine step-up increase in the left adrenal vein as well.

sarcoid), and some autoimmune processes (*ie*, Graves' disease) can be visualized using this technique. The small size of this peptide allows for rapid clearance and low background activity. In a sample of 1000 patients, 12 of the 14 patients with pheochromocytoma were somatostatin-receptor positive. Perhaps MIBG is more useful in localization of tumors in the adrenal and renal regions because of the relatively high accumulation of ligand in the kidney. A comparison study with MIBG of patients with 17 tumors yielded the following findings: 12 tumors were pheochromocytoma or paraganglioma, octreotide scans visualized 5 tumors that were not found by MIBG, MIBC localized 2 not found by octreotide scan, and both scans localized 5 tumors. The authors found that 86% of scans were positive for pheochromocytoma (compared with 88% for MIBG in the literature) and that 100% of the paragangliomas were visualized with octreotide (compared with 52% for MIBG in the literature) [33].

Computed tomography can be focused on the region likely to yield a tumor. Presently, both tests are considered complementary [34]. The presence of a mass on computed tomography does not necessarily mean a chromaffin tumor. On the other hand, some chromaffin tumors do not function or absorb MIBG [34]. If the evaluation of patients with hypertension proceeds from clinical suspicion to computed tomography without biochemical confirmation, a small number of incidental asymptomatic adrenal masses will be uncovered, most of which will not be pheochromocytoma. Autopsy data and imaging studies suggest that finding an "incidentaloma" of the adrenal gland rarely yields a functional tumor. Out of 100,000 tumors, 6500, 7000, and 35 will be pheochromocytoma, aldosteronoma, and glucocorticoid adenoma, respectively [35]. Although only 58 of 100,000 tumors will be adrenocortical carcinoma, rapid growth (or growth above 4 to 6 cm) may require excision or biopsy once pheochromocytoma is excluded [35].

Ansari and his colleagues [36] have found a sensitivity of 77% and a specificity of 92% with MIBG scanning. Their accuracy rate was 96% and 90% for MIBG and computed tomography, respectively.

Magnetic resonance imaging has demonstrated considerable promise in adrenal tissue characterization for both adrenal cortical adenoma and medullary pheochromocytoma and may be able to distinguish adrenal adenoma from adrenal medullary neoplasm on the basis of intensity difference. Patients with pheochromocytoma have demonstrated marked hyperintensity compared with normal liver on T2-weighted pulse sequences [37,38].

THERAPY

Medical Control

Advances in perioperative preparation and intraoperative patient management have had a major impact on mortality associated with pheochromocytoma surgery (Table 4). Surgical mortality was approximately 15% before 1950, and many deaths were attributable to hypovolemic shock, hypertensive hemorrhage, and anesthesia-related arrhythmias [39]. Since that time, preoperative therapy with α-blocking drugs, usually phenoxybenzamine as well as propronolol for at least 2 weeks, to allow reexpansion of blood volume, intraoperative anesthesia with improved anesthetic agents, and intraoperative or postresection volume replacement have made surgical mortality an exceptional occurrence (Table 4) [40,41]. Patients are usually prepared for surgery.

Phenoxybenzamine is a noncompetitive adrenergic blocking agent with greater selectivity for α_1 than α_2 receptors (100 to 1 compared with 3–5 to 1 for phentolamine). Therapy is initiated with one or two divided daily doses of 10 mg each. Most patients with pheochromocytoma require 20 to 40 mg per day. However, we have encountered patients who failed to respond adequately to oral phenoxybenzamine, and each has subsequently responded to intravenous phentolamine.

Prazosin hydrochloride, doxazosin mesylate, and terazosin are even more exclusive α_1-receptor blockers that have also been used with mixed success in patients with pheochromocytoma as preoperative therapy [42,43]. I do not

TABLE 4 THERAPY FOR PATIENTS WITH PHEOCHROMOCYTOMA

α-blockade
  Phentolamine: 1–5 mg IV drug of choice for surgery for rapid control of hypertension (many choose nitroprusside)
  Phenoxybenzamide: 20–80 mg/d preoperative and long-term treatment
  Specific $α_1$ blockade: prazosin, doxazosin, terazosin (less complete control that with phenoxybenzamine)
β-blockade
  Propranolol: 10–40 mg PO qid after α-blockade
α- and β-receptor blockade
  Labetalol: 300 mg/d or more
Vasodilator
  Nonspecific nitroprusside, magnesium sulfate
  Calcium channel blockade: nifedipine, diltiazem
  Converting enzyme inhibitor: captopril enalapril
Malignant or inoperable
  Methylparatyrosine (1–2 g/d)
  Vincristine, cyclophosphamide, dacarbazine (as a regimen)
  Tumoricidal ^{131}I MIBG

IV—intravenous; MIBG—metaiodobenzyguanidine; PO—by mouth; qid—four times a day.

believe that these should be relied on as the sole α-blocking agent during surgery because they only block $α_1$ receptors or they are "competitive" blockers [43]. The addition of β-receptor blockade may be indicated when tachycardia or catecholamine-induced arrhythmias are present, or when epinephrine constitutes 15% to 20% or more of total neurohormone secretion. Propranolol is added in low doses, 10 to 20 mg three to four times per day, only after α-blocking therapy has begun. Propranolol may cause paradoxical hypertension in pheochromocytoma in the absence of prior α-receptor blockade. The combined α- and β-receptor blocker labetalol has been effective in preoperative and intraoperative management [44].

Calcium channel blockade, which is useful in pheochromocytoma both preoperatively and intraoperatively, reduces smooth muscle contractility and also impairs exocytosis release of norepinephrine from storage vesicles and blocks $α_2$-receptors.

The 5-year survival of patients with benign pheochromocytoma is approximately 96%, and that small fraction of patients (< 10%) with malignant pheochromocytoma have only a 44% survival rate [45]. Therapy for these patients with malignancies and for those who cannot tolerate surgical procedures with α- and β-blocking agents is not entirely satisfactory. For these patients, alphamethyltyrosine in doses of 1 to 2 g per day can reduce tumor synthesis from active sites and can normalize blood pressure for long periods, more than 15 years in some patients [46]. However, symptoms of parkinsonism, perhaps related to reduction of basal ganglia dopamine content, have been reported [47].

Phentolamine has been the drug of choice for obtaining rapid control of hypertension during crisis, provocative testing, and surgery (Fig. 5). Doses of 1 to 5 mg are given as boluses, and side effects include nausea and tachycardia. Most recently, we have used esmolol hydrochloride (50–100 µg/kg/min) and/or sodium nitroprusside (1 µg/kg/min) infusion during induction and intraoperatively.

Chemotherapy of patients with malignant pheochromocytoma has been ineffective. However, patients treated with cyclophosphamide, vincristine, and dacarbazine have shown regression of tumor size, reduction in catecholamine excretion, and improved quality of life, at least temporarily [48].

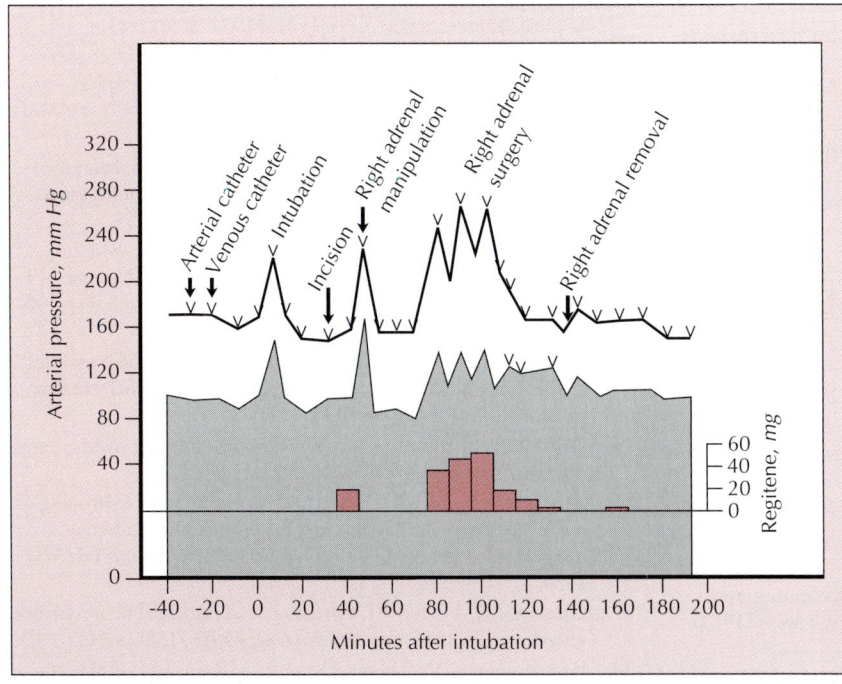

FIGURE 5 Pressor responses during operative removal of adrenal chromaffin tumor. Pressor responses were managed by bolus injections of phentolamine. Time and amount administered are given by arrows and hatched columns, respectively.

Pheochromocytoma in Pregnancy

Pregnant women with undiagnosed pheochromocytoma may die from cerebral vascular accidents, acute pulmonary edema, cardiac arrhythmias, shock, or malignancy. If pheochromocytoma is diagnosed before term, the maternal mortality is reduced to 17% or less. Few maternal deaths have been reported recently when pheochromocytoma was diagnosed before term. However, fetal mortality may remain high because of spontaneous abortion, with most deaths occurring during or, just after, labor. Increased catecholamine levels in maternal blood may cause fetal anoxia as a result of constriction of uterine arteries and also by heightened uterine contractions.

References and Recommended Reading

Recently published papers of particular interest have been highlighted as:
- Of interest
- Of outstanding interest

1. Beard C, Sheps SG, Kurland LT, *et al.*: Occurrence of pheochromocytoma in Rochester, Minnesota, 1950 through 1979. *Mayo Clin Proc* 1983, 58:802–804.
2. Moorhead EL Jr, Brenner MJ, Caldwell JR, *et al.*: Pheochromocytoma: a familial tumor. A study of 11 families. *Henry Ford Hosp Med J* 1965, 13:467–478.
3. Sipple J: The association of pheochromocytoma with carcinoma of the thyroid gland. *Am J Med* 1961, 31:163–166.
4. Glushien A, Mansuy M, Littman D: Pheochromocytoma: its relationship to the neurocutaneous syndromes. *Am J Med* 1953, 14:318–327.
5. Mulholland SG, Atuk NO, Walzak MP: Familial pheochromocytoma associated with cerebellar hemangioblastoma: a case history and review of the literature. *JAMA* 1969, 207:1709–1711.
6. • Neumann HPH, Berger DP, Sigmund G, *et al.*: Pheochromocytomas, multiple endocrine neoplasia type 2, and Von Hippel–Lindau disease. *N Engl J Med* 1993, 329(21):1531–1538.
7. Pearse AG: Common cytochemical and ultrastructural characteristics of cells producing polypeptide hormones (the APUD series) and their relevance to thyroid and ultimobranchial C cells and calcitonin. *Proc R Soc Lond [Biol]* 1968, 170:71–80.
8. Ober WB: Emil Zuckerkandl and his delightful little organ. *Pathol Annu* 1983, 18:103–119.
9. Quinan C, Berger AA: Observations on human adrenals with especial reference to the relative weight of the normal medulla. *Ann Intern Med* 1933, 6:1180–1192.
10. Visser JW, Axt R: Bilateral adrenal medullary hyperplasia: a clinicopathological entity. *J Clin Pathol* 1975, 28:298–304.
11. Carney JA, Sizemore GW, Sheps SG: Adrenal medullary disease in multiple endocrine neoplasia, type 2: pheochromocytoma and its precursors. *Am J Clin Pathol* 1976, 66:270–290.
12. Gifford R, Dvale W, Maher F, *et al.*: Clinical features, diagnosis and treatment of pheochromocytoma. A review of 76 cases. *Mayo Clin Proc* 1964, 39:281–302.
13. Hyams JS, Leichtner AM, Breiner RG, *et al.*: Pseudopheochromocytoma and cardiac arrest associated with phenylpropanolamine. *JAMA* 1985, 253:1609–1610.
14. Lurvey A, Yusin A, DeQuattro V: Pseudopheochromocytoma after self-administered isoproterenol. *J Endocrinol Metab* 1973, 36:766–769.
15. Kuchel O: Pseudopheochromocytoma. *Hypertension* 1985, 7:151–158.
16. DeQuattro V, Campese V, Miura Y, Esler M: Sympathotonia in primary hypertension and in a caricature resembling dysautonomia. *Clin Sci* 1976, 51:435–438.
17. Waldmann TA, Bradley JE: Polycythemia secondary to a pheochromocytoma with production of an erythropoiesis stimulating factor by the tumor. *Proc Soc Exp Biol Med* 1961, 108:425–427.
18. Engelman K, Sjoerdsma A: Chronic medical therapy for pheochromocytoma. *Ann Intern Med* 1964, 61:229–241.
19. Kline IK: Myocardial alterations associated with pheochromocytoma. *Am J Pathol* 1961, 38:539–551.
20. Bray GA, DeQuattro V, Fisher DA, *et al.*: Catecholamines: a symposium–teaching conference. University of California, Los Angeles and Harbor General Hospital (specialty conference). *California Med* 1972, 117:32–62.
21. DeQuattro V, Chan S: Raised plasma catecholamines in some patients with primary hypertension. *Lancet* 1972, i:806–809.
22. Kobayashi R, DeQuattro V, Kolloch R, Miano L: A radioenzymatic assay for plasma normetanephrine in man and patients with pheochromocytoma. *Life Sci* 1980, 26:567–573.
23. Foti A, Adachi M, DeQuattro V: The relationships of free to conjugated metanephrine in plasma and spinal fluid of hypertensive patients. *J Clin Endocrinol Metab* 1982, 55:81–85.
24. O'Connor DT, Bernstein KN: Radioimmunoassay of chromogranin A in plasma as a measure of exocytotic sympathoadrenal activity in normal subjects and patients with pheochromocytoma. *N Engl J Med* 1984, 311:764–770.
25. Goldstein DS, Levinson PD, Zimlichman R, *et al.*: Clonidine suppression testing in essential hypertension. *Ann Intern Med* 1985, 102:42–48.
26. Bravo EL, Tarazi RC, Fouad FM, *et al.*: Clonidine suppression test: a useful aid in the diagnosis of pheochromocytoma. *N Engl J Med* 1981, 305:623–626.
27. Bravo E: Clonidine-suppression test for diagnosis of pheochromocytoma. *N Engl J Med* 1982, 306:49–50.
28. Welch TJ, Sheedy PF, Heerden JA, *et al.*: Pheochromocytoma: value of computed tomography. *Radiology* 1983, 148:501–503.
29. Wieland DM, Wu J, Brown LE, *et al.*: Radiolabeled adrenergic neuron-blocking agents: adrenomedullary imaging with (131-I) iodobenzylguanidine. *J Nucl Med* 1980, 21:349–353.
30. Sisson JC, Frager MS, Valk TW, *et al.*: Scintigraphic localization of pheochromocytoma. *N Engl J Med* 1981, 305:12–17.
31. Valk TW, Frager MS, Gross MD, *et al.*: Spectrum of pheochromocytoma in multiple endocrine neoplasia: a scintigraphic portrayal using 131-I metaiodobenzylguanidine. *Ann Intern Med* 1981, 94:762–767.
32. Shapiro B, Copp JE, Sisson JE, *et al.*: Iodine-131 metaiodobenzylguanidine for the locating of suspected pheochromocytoma: experience in 400 cases. *J Nucl Med* 1985, 26:576–585.
33. •• Krenning EP, Kwekkeboom DJ, Bakker WH, *et al.*: Somatostatin receptor scintigraphy with [^{111}In-DPTA-D-Phe^1 and ^{123}I-Tyr^3]-octreotide: the Rotterdam experience with more than 1000 patients. *Eur J Nucl Med* 1993, 20:716–731.
34. Francis IR, Glazer GM, Shapiro B, *et al.*: Complementary roles of CT and I-MIBG scintigraphy in diagnosing pheochromocytoma. *AJR Am J Roentgenol* 1983, 141:719–725.
35. Gross MD, Shapiro B: Clinical review 50: clinically silent adrenal masses. *J Clin Endocrinol Metab* 1993, 77(4):885.
36. Ansari AN, Siegel ME, DeQuattro V, Gazarian LH: Imaging of medullary thyroid carcinoma and hyperfunctioning adrenal medulla using iodine-131 metaiodobenzylguanidine. *J Nucl Med* 1986, 27:1858–1860.
37. Glazer GM, Woolsey EJ, Borrello J, *et al.*: Adrenal tissue characterization using MR imaging. *Radiology* 1986, 158:73–79.
38. Fink IJ, Reinig JW, Dwyer AK, *et al.*: MR imaging of pheochromocytomas. *J Comput Assist Tomogr* 1985, 9:454–458.

39. Apgar V, Papper EM: Pheochromocytoma: anesthetic management during surgical treatment. *Arch Surg* 1951, 62:634–648.
40. Brunjes S, Johns V, Crane M: Pheochromocytoma: Postoperative shock and blood volume. *N Engl J Med* 1960, 262:393–396.
41. Deoreo GA Jr, Stewart BH, Tarazi RC, Gifford RW: Preoperative blood transfusion in the safe surgical management of pheochromocytoma. *J Urol* 1974, 111:715–721.
42. Wallace J, Gill DP: Prazosin in the diagnosis and treatment of pheochromocytoma. *JAMA* 1978, 240:2752–2753.
43. Nicholson JP, Vaughn ED, Pickering TG, *et al.*: Pheochromocytoma and prazosin. *Ann Intern Med* 1983, 99:477–479.
44. Rosca EA, Brown JT, Tever AF, *et al.*: Treatment of pheochromocytoma and clonidine withdrawal hypertension with labetalol. *Br J Clin Pharmacol* 1976, 3:809–815.
45. Manger WM, Gifford RW: Hypertension secondary to pheochromocytoma. *Bull N Y Acad Med* 1982, 58:139–158.
46. Sjoerdsma A, Engelman K, Spector S, Undenfriend S: Inhibition of catecholamine synthesis in man with α-methyl-tyrosine, an inhibitor of tyrosine hydroxylase. *Lancet* 1965, ii:1092–1094.
47. Gitlow SE, Pertsemlidis D, Bertani LM: Management of patients with pheochromocytoma. *Am Heart J* 1971, 83:557–567.
48. Keiser HR, Goldstein DS, Wade JL, *et al.*: Treatment of malignant pheochromocytoma with combination chemotherapy. *Hypertension* 1985, 7:18–24.
49. Bravo EL, Tarazi RC, Fouad EM, *et al.*: Blood pressure regulation in pheochromocytoma. *Hypertension* 1983, 4(suppl II):193–199.
50. Glenner G, Grimbley P: Tumors of the extra-adrenal paraganglion system. *Ann Tumor Pathol* 1974, Ser 2, fasc 9.

Select Bibliography

Aravot DJ, Banner NR, Cantor AM, *et al.* Location, localization and surgical treatment of cardiac pheochromocytoma. *Am J Cardiol* 1992, 69:283–285.

Ledger GA, Khosla S, Lindor NM, *et al.*: Genetic testing in the diagnosis and management of multiple endocrine neoplasia type II. *Ann Intern Med* 1995, 122:118–124.

Neumann HPH, Weistler OD: Clustering of features of von Hippel-Lindau syndrome: evidence for a complex genetic locus. *Lancet* 1991, 337:1052–1154.

Orchard T, Grant CS, van Heerden JA, Weaver A: Pheochromocytoma: continuing evolution of surgical therapy. *Surgery* 1993, 116 (6):1153–1159.

Schulumberger C, Gicquel C, Lumbroso J, *et al.*: Malignant pheochromocytoma: clinical, biological, histologic and therapeutic data in a series of 20 patients with distant metastases. *J Endocrinol Invest* 1992, 15:631–642.

Aldosteronism and Endocrine Blood Pressure Syndromes

Robert G. Dluhy
Gordon H. Williams

> **Key Points**
> - Primary aldosteronism (PA) is characterized by spontaneous hypokalemia on a normal sodium diet or severe diuretic-induced hypokalemia.
> - The differential diagnosis of PA includes adenoma (60%), hyperplasia (40%), and glucocorticoid-remediable aldosteronism (GRA).
> - GRA is characterized by autosomal dominant inheritance and hypertension diagnosed in the first two decades of life.
> - The mutation causing GRA has been discovered, allowing for direct genetic screening for this disorder.

Aldosterone secretion is positively regulated by the renin-angiotensin system, potassium, and, to a lesser extent, corticotropin. The primary locus of aldosterone action is in the distal tubule of the kidney, where sodium is retained and potassium and hydrogen ions are excreted into the urine. The primary functions of aldosterone include regulation of sodium and potassium homeostasis. Sodium is retained in volume-depleted states because the renin-angiotensin system has been activated (so-called secondary hyperaldosteronism). Because aldosterone is directly stimulated by potassium loading and hyperkalemia, it protects against potassium intoxication (Fig. 1). Clinical syndromes result from over- or underproduction of aldosterone because of an abnormality at the level of the adrenal gland or because of over- or underproduction of the regulating factors (usually the renin-angiotensin system). Hyperaldosteronism causes sodium retention, volume expansion, potassium wasting, hypokalemia, and alkalosis. Conversely, hypoaldosteronism is associated with sodium wasting, hypotension, acidosis, and potassium retention. This discussion focuses on states of primary aldosteronism in which the stimulus for excess aldosterone production resides within the adrenal gland (Fig. 2). States of hypoaldosteronism are also discussed because of the clinical importance of these syndromes, which are often associated with potentially life-threatening hyperkalemia.

PRIMARY ALDOSTERONISM

Primary aldosteronism occurs in approximately 1% of unselected hypertensive patients. Because of the escape phenomenon (the absence of continued sodium retention with prolonged mineralocorticoid administration), these patients seldom have edema, but most have signs and symptoms of hypokalemia, their most common distinguishing feature. Primary aldosteronism has a broad differential, including neoplasm (in approximately 60% of cases; usually adenoma, very rarely carcinoma) or bilateral hyperplasia (in 40%) [1•]. Additional mineralocorticoid excess syndromes include inherited enzyme deficiencies, ingestion of licorice, use of chewing tobacco, and an autosomal dominant form of hyperaldosteronism that

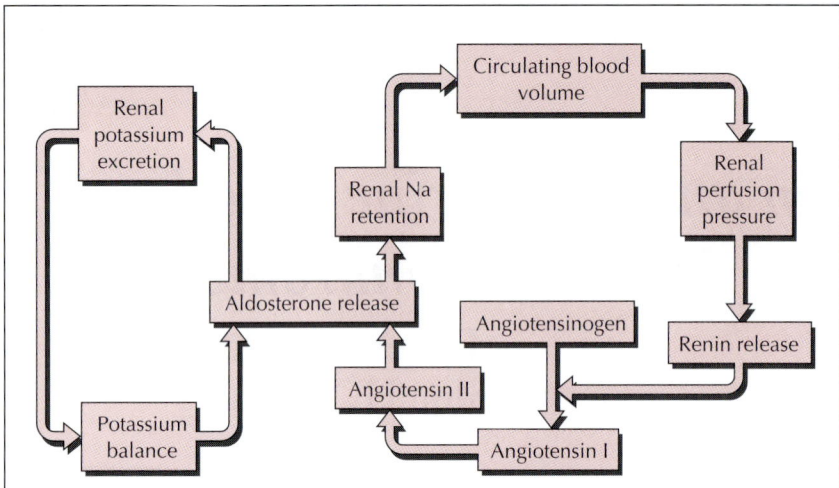

FIGURE 1 Interrelationship of volume and potassium homeostasis through actions on the renin-angiotensin system.

is corrected by the administration of glucocorticoids (so-called glucocorticoid-remediable hyperaldosteronism [GRA]) (Table 1).

Spontaneous hypokalemia, in the absence of diuretic treatment, or severe diuretic-induced hypokalemia are clues to the diagnosis of primary aldosteronism (Fig. 3). However, spontaneous hypokalemia is notably absent in such hypertensive patients if they severely restrict sodium intake or are being treated with potassium-sparing diuretics, such as spironolactone or amiloride.

Two outpatient screening tests for diagnosing primary aldosteronism have gained favor because of their ease of performance. The plasma aldosterone:plasma renin activity (PRA) ratio on a random blood sample integrates the elevated plasma aldosterone and suppressed PRA levels characteristically seen in primary aldosteronism. Although a ratio exceeding 20 to 25 points toward this diagnosis, the ratio should be interpreted with caution if the patient is hypokalemic because potassium depletion reduces plasma aldosterone and elevates PRA levels.

The second test is performed by administering 25 mg of captopril and measuring, while the patient is seated, PRA, plasma aldosterone, and cortisol levels before the test and 2 hours later. Plasma aldosterone levels should fall and PRA levels rise as angiotensin II is reduced by the converting enzyme inhibitor. Failure of PRA and plasma aldosterone levels to change suggests a diagnosis of primary aldosteronism because angiotensin II levels are profoundly suppressed in this disorder. A plasma aldosterone value of greater than 15 ng/dL and a plasma aldosterone:PRA ratio of greater than 50 after the captopril test are consistent with a diagnosis of primary aldosteronism. The next step is to perform a saline infusion [1•]. Five hundred milliliters of normal saline are infused hourly over 4 to 6 hours (Fig. 3). The normal response to volume expansion with saline is a plasma aldosterone level of less than 10 ng/dL (usually < 5 ng/dL) at the termination of the infusion. An important caveat is to restore potassium levels with oral supplementation before the infusion. Failure to suppress aldosterone secretion in association with a natriuresis can produce severe and even life-threatening hypokalemia if the patient's potassium is not repleted before the study. In addition, the patient's potassium level should always be checked at the termination of the infusion before the patient is discharged.

Because most patients with biochemical features of primary aldosteronism have an aldosterone-producing adenoma, a computed tomographic scan of the adrenals to image the

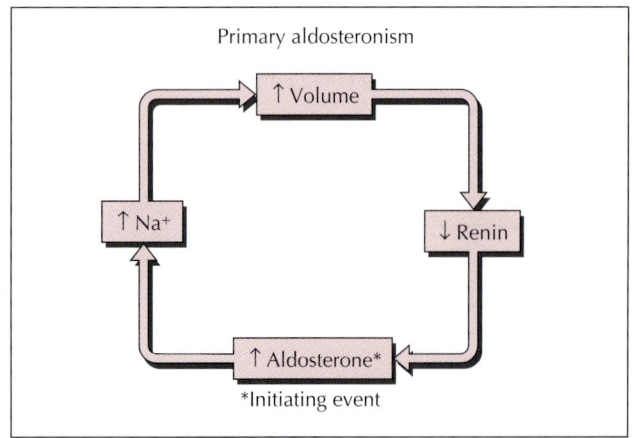

FIGURE 2 Responses of the renin-aldosterone volume control loop in primary aldosteronism.

TABLE 1 MEDICAL TREATMENT OF MINERALOCORTICOID EXCESS STATES AND HYPOALDOSTERONISM

Disorder	Drug	Dose, *mg/d*
Hyperaldosteronism (adenoma, bilateral hyperplasia, GRA†)	Spironolactone, amiloride	50–200* 5–15†
Apparent mineralocorticoid excess	Dexamethasone	0.5–1.0
Hypoaldosteronism	Fludrocortisone	0.1–1.0*

GRA—glucocorticoid-remediable hyperaldosteronism.
*Divided dosing—spironolactone, amiloride, fludrocortisone.
†An alternative treatment for GRA is glucocorticoid suppression (*eg*, prednisone, 5–10 mg/d in adults). Caution must be taken to avoid overdosing.

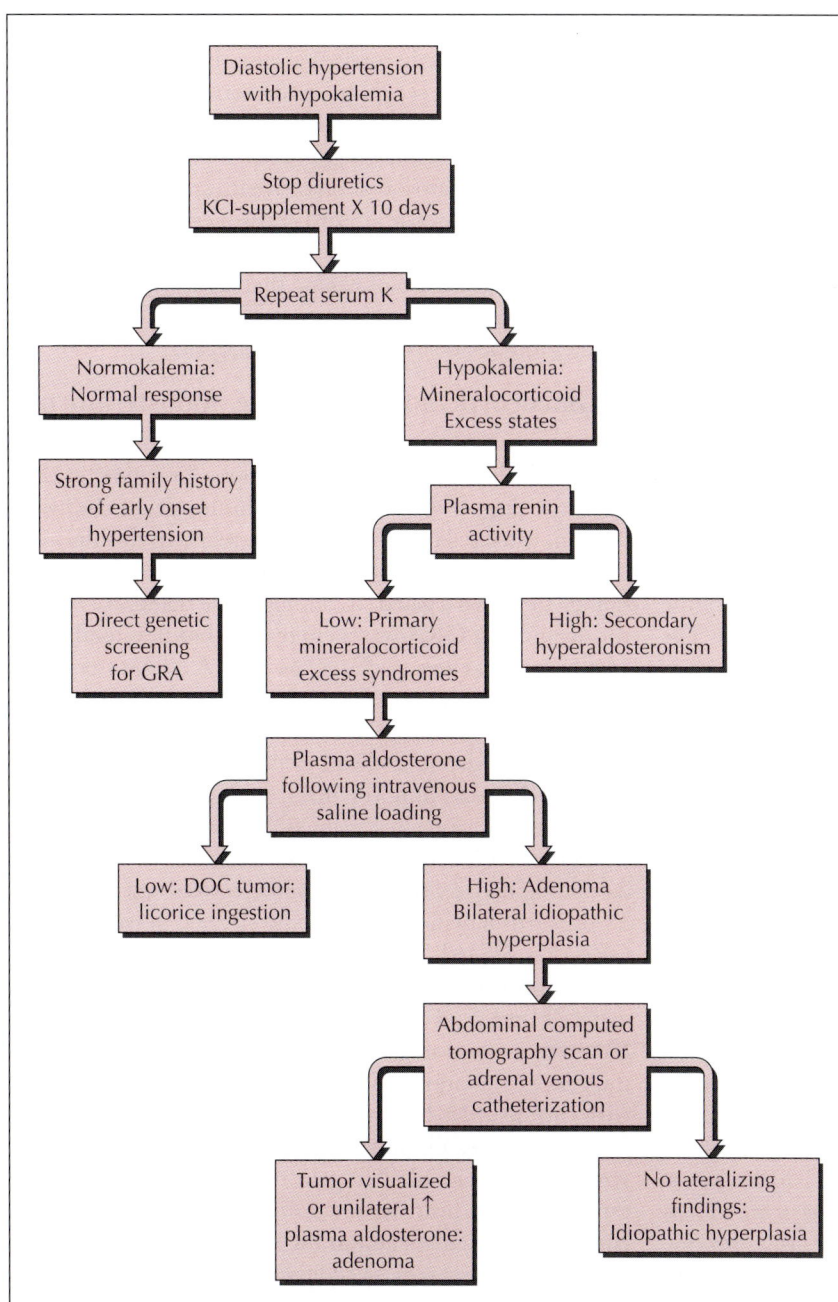

FIGURE 3 Flowchart for evaluation of a patient suspected of having primary aldosteronism. DOC—desoxycorticosterone; GRA—glucocorticoid-remediable hyperaldosteronism.

tumor should be performed next. The results of this radiologic study are diagnostic in 75% to 90% of proven cases. An additional laboratory study favoring the diagnosis of an adenoma over bilateral hyperplasia is an elevated level of the steroid 18-hydroxycorticosterone. In addition, the plasma aldosterone response to upright posture is said to distinguish these two entities; adenoma patients exhibit a fall, whereas hyperplasia patients demonstrate a postural rise. Unfortunately, in both tests, overlap often exists between these two disease states. Even the results of imaging studies may be misleading because several new entities have emerged to cloud the hormonal differences previously considered diagnostic of adenoma versus hyperplasia. For example, primary unilateral hyperplasia is characterized by hormonal responses considered diagnostic for an adenoma, but bilateral or unilateral hyperplasia findings are seen on computed tomographic scanning. Importantly, cure or significant improvement is seen in patients with unilateral adrenalectomy in patients with this disease. However, if the radiographic imaging study and hormonal findings are not clear-cut, bilateral adrenal vein catherization may be required to document unilateral versus bilateral aldosterone overproduction. Adrenal vein catheterization should be performed only in specialized centers with angiographic expertise because it is technically difficult. The finding of an adrenal nodule in a hypertensive patient does not prove its functional status, because nonfunctioning nodules are routinely found in autopsy series in up to 10% of hypertensive patients. Thus, diagnostic assessment for primary aldosteronism usually requires an experienced endocrinologist.

The treatment of patients with primary aldosteronism with a tumor is surgical removal of the tumor or long-term medical therapy if surgery is rejected or contraindicated.

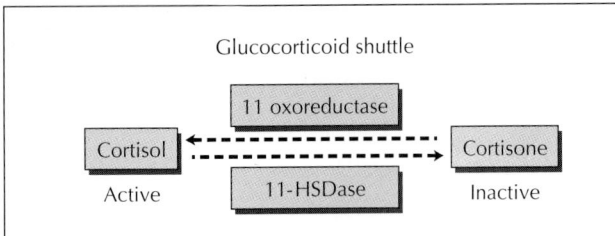

FIGURE 4 Metabolism of cortisol to cortisone in the kidney by 11β-hydroxysteroid dehydrogenase (11-HSDase).

Hypokalemia can be controlled in most patients with primary aldosteronism, regardless of etiology, with potassium-sparing diuretics. A clinically useful point is that spironolactone, an aldosterone antagonist at the mineralocorticoid receptor, also corrects the hypertension in patients with an adenoma but not in those with bilateral hyperplasia. Thus, it can be used for a therapeutic trial and provide adjunctive diagnostic as well as therapeutic information. The major problem with the long-term use of spironolactone in males is its antiandrogenic side effects, which often produce impotence and gynecomastia.

OTHER MINERALOCORTICOID SYNDROMES

Syndrome of Apparent Mineralocorticoid Excess

Ingestion of compounds in chewing tobacco or licorice, specifically glycyrrhizic acid, can produce signs and symptoms of mineralocorticoid excess. The characteristics of this syndrome, termed the *syndrome of apparent mineralocorticoid excess*, include hypertension, hypokalemia, and low renin levels, but normal or low levels of aldosterone [2]. The compound contained in chewing tobacco and licorice inhibits an enzyme in the kidney, 11 β-hydroxysteroid dehydrogenase (Fig. 4). Because the mineralocorticoid receptor *in vitro* binds cortisol with equal affinity to aldosterone, this enzyme normally inactivates cortisol by converting it to cortisone, thereby preventing mineralocorticoid effects [3•]. When the enzyme is inhibited, cortisol accumulates, binds to renal mineralocorticoid receptors, and exerts mineralocorticoid effects. A careful history establishes the diagnosis of ingestion of licorice or use of chewing tobacco. This syndrome is also inherited as an autosomal recessive disorder. An increased ratio of cortisol metabolites to cortisone metabolites in the urine is diagnostic of this disorder. Treatment consists of discontinuing the use of agents that inhibit the enzyme or low-dose dexamethasone administration in the hereditary form of this disease to suppress cortisol levels.

Glucocorticoid-Remediable Aldosteronism

Glucocorticoid-remediable aldosteronism is an autosomal dominant inherited form of hypertension. An important clinical clue to diagnosis is a strong family history of juvenile hypertension, usually dating from teenage years. In this disorder, corticotropin is the sole regulator of mineralocorticoid secretion by the adrenal gland. Accordingly, the traditional method for diagnosing GRA was a clinical trial of dexamethasone administration. Patients affected with GRA exhibit a profound decline in aldosterone secretion with the administration of exogenous glucocorticoids and secondarily experience a reduction or normalization of their blood pressure and correction of their biochemical abnormalities, such as hypokalemia and suppressed plasma renin activity. A diagnosis can be specifically established by the measurement of two abnormal steroids in a 24-hour urinary collection, 18-hydroxycortisol and tetrahydro-18-oxocortisol, which are markedly elevated in patients with GRA (Fig. 5) [4••].

Unfortunately, measurement of the steroids is technically difficult and is available in only a few research centers. However, a recent major breakthrough is the identification of the genetic mutation that causes GRA. Individuals affected with this disorder have an extra gene, a chimeric gene that fuses sequences of both the 11-hydroxylase and aldosterone syntase genes (Fig. 6). This gene duplication leads to ectopic expression of 18-hydroxylase activity in the corticotropin-regulated zona fasciculata and to the production of aldosterone from cortisol precursors. In addition, this gene mutation causes

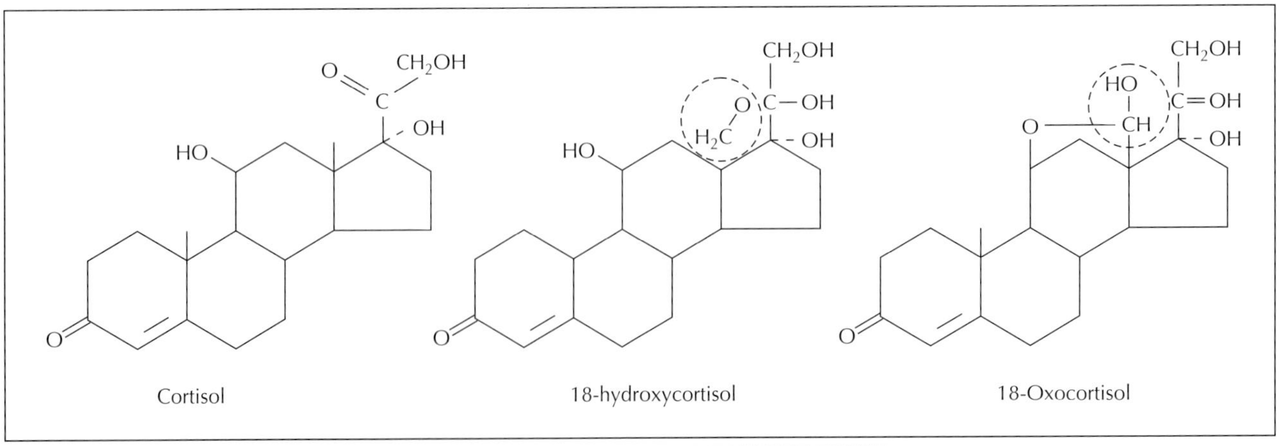

FIGURE 5 Qualitative steroid abnormality in glucocorticoid-remediable hyperaldosteronism whereby cortisol undergoes further oxidation to form C-18 oxidation products.

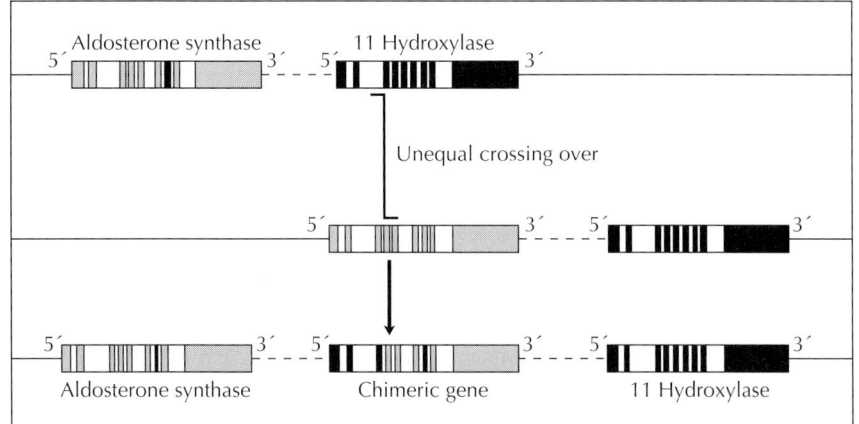

FIGURE 6 Unequal crossing over between aldosterone synthase and 11β-hydroxylase genes producing a chimeric gene.

regulation of aldosterone syntase activity by corticotropin, not by its normal regulator, angiotensin II. Because aldosterone secretion is only positively regulated by corticotropin, that is, no feedback loop exists, a mineralocorticoid excess state occurs with volume expansion and suppression of plasma renin activity; as a consequence, the adrenal glomerulosa zone that normally produces aldosterone is suppressed (Fig. 7). Cortisol is also abnormally 18-hydroxylated, producing the characteristic hybrid steroids previously described. This syndrome can be corrected by glucocorticoid administration and suppression of corticotropin secretion (Fig. 8). Confirmation of the presence of this gene duplication in 12 unrelated pedigrees with GRA establishes this genetic mutation as etiologic and diagnostic for this disorder [5••]. Moreover, this abnormal gene can readily be detected by Southern blotting, which allows direct genetic screening for this disorder with a small sample of blood. This disorder is likely to be underdiagnosed because spontaneous hypokalemia is an inconsistent finding: hypertensive patients with primary aldosteronism without demonstrable adenomata as well as hypertensive patients with suppressed levels of PRA, especially children and young adults, are candidates for this diagnosis. Moreover, for every case diagnosed, many additional cases should be discovered in extended pedigree screening because GRA is inherited as an autosomal dominant disorder.

HYPOALDOSTERONISM

Hypoaldosteronism may result from a primary defect in aldosterone production by the adrenals, or it may result from impaired stimulation by regulatory factors, usually a reduced production of renin [1]. Depending on their oral intake of sodium and potassium, such patients with hypoaldosteronism have variable clinical presentations. In uncompensated cases, volume depletion with postural hypotension and life-threatening hyperkalemia may be present. Primary adrenal hypoaldosteronism includes diseases with adrenocortical destruction (infectious or autoimmune), enzymatic defects (congenital adrenal hyperplasia), and adrenal hemorrhage. Acutely ill hospitalized patients who are anticoagulated or who have a coagulopathy may acutely develop bilateral adrenal hemorrhage and subsequent shock, hyperkalemia, or both. Hypoaldosteronism should always be considered in patients with these symptoms. AIDS has been added to the list of causes of primary adrenal insufficiency as a result of opportunistic infection with cytomegalovirus, tuberculosis, or both. The diagnosis of primary adrenal insufficiency is established by the rapid corticotropin test which indicates subnormal cortisol and aldosterone responses. Blood corticotropin levels should also be elevated to be consistent with the diagnosis of primary adrenal failure.

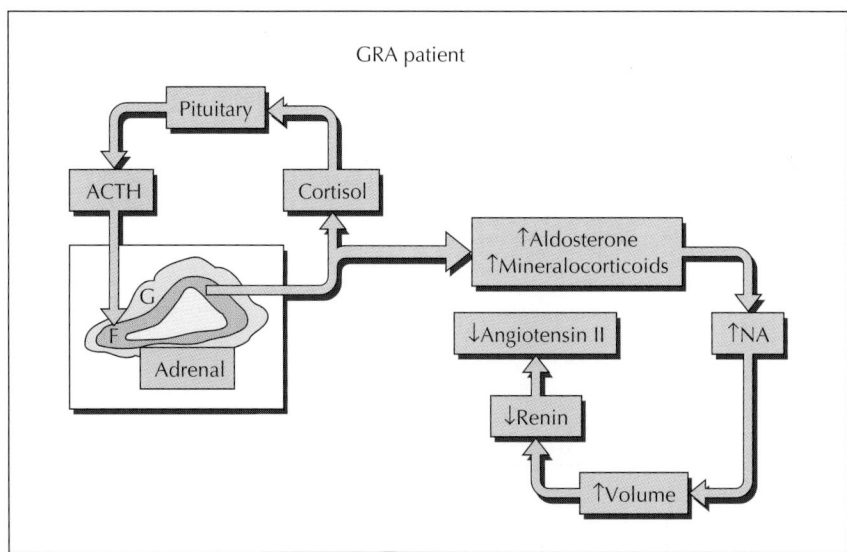

FIGURE 7 Regulation of aldosterone secretion in glucocorticoid-remediable hyperaldosteronism (GRA) solely by corticotropin. ACTH—adrenocorticotropin; F—zona fasciculata; G—zona glomerulosa; NA—sodium.

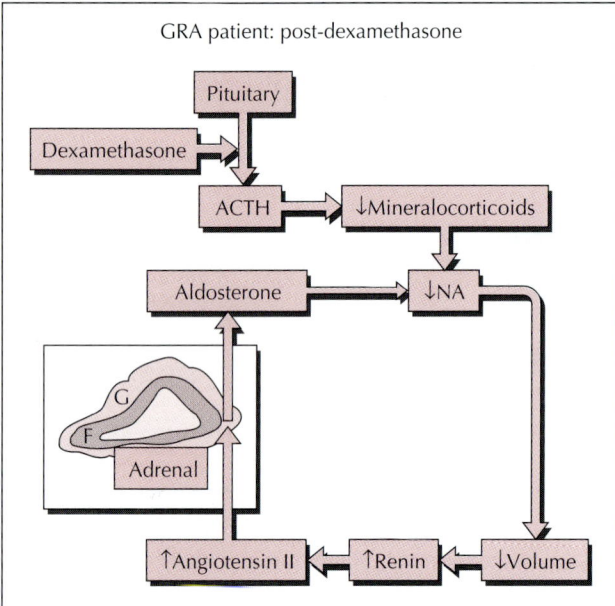

FIGURE 8 Restoration of the normal regulation of aldosterone by the renin-angiotensin system in glucocorticoid-remediable hyperaldosteronism after the administration of dexamethasone. ACTH—adrenocorticotropin; F—zona fasciculata; G—zona glomerulosa; NA—sodium.

An important clinical entity resulting from secondary failure to regulate aldosterone secretion (so-called hyporeninemic hypoaldosteronism) is typically found in patients with diabetes mellitus who exhibit hyperkalemia, metabolic acidosis and mild renal insufficiency. In such patients, the normal postural rise in renin is blunted, and the degree of hyperkalemia is typically greater than the degree of renal failure. Commonly administered medications may precipitate or exacerbate the electrolyte and hormonal findings in this disorder, including nonsteroidal anti-inflammatory drugs, which inhibit renal prostaglandin synthesis, thereby impairing renin secretion. The use of converting enzyme inhibitors to lower blood pressure in the hypertensive diabetic patient with proteinuria may also precipitate severe hyperkalemia because of the drugs' aldosterone-lowering effects. Thus, drugs that effect the renin-angiotensin-aldosterone axis should be used cautiously in diabetics, especially in older diabetic patients with mild renal insufficiency who should be presumed to be at risk for the hyporeninemic hypoaldosterone syndrome.

Why this syndrome occurs more frequently in patients with diabetes mellitus is unclear. Patients with diabetes develop autonomic dysfunction and imparied sympathetic activity that may lead to reduction in renin secretion. A role for insulin in the transmembrane movement of potassium may also be involved in such patients.

Although the hormonal assessment of renin and aldosterone levels in response to upright posture (especially in a volume-contracted state, such as a low salt diet or after diuretic administration) can confirm this diagnosis, such studies are rarely indicated. In the appropriate clinical setting, especially a diabetic patient with hyperkalemia and mild renal failure, this diagnosis should be presumed and treatment instituted. Removal of an offending drug is obviously the first step. A diet low in potassium plus the administration of furosemide may be sufficient in other patients. Some patients, however, require supraphysiologic doses of fludrocortisone (up to 1 mg/d) to correct the hyperkalemia, which suggests that renal resistance to mineralocorticoids may be an additional factor in this syndrome.

References and Recommended Reading:

Recently published papers of particular interest have been highlighted as:
- Of interest
- •• Of outstanding interest

1. • Williams GH, Dluhy RG: Disease of the adrenal cortex. In *Harrison's Principles of Internal Medicine* edn 13, Edited by Isselbacher KJ *et al*. New York: McGraw Hill; 1994 1953–1976.
2. Ulick S, Tedde R, Mantero F: Pathogenesis of the type 2 variant of the syndrome of apparent mineralocorticoid excess. *J Clin Endocrinol Metab* 1990, 70:200.
3. • Funder JW, Pearce PT, Smith R, *et al*.: Mineralocorticoid action: Target tissue specificity is enzyme, not receptor, mediated. *Science* 1988, 242:583–585.
4. •• Rich GM, Ulick S, Cook S, *et al*.: Glucocorticoid-remediable aldosteronism in a large kindred: Clinical spectrum and diagnosis using a characteristic biochemical phenotype. *Ann Intern Med* 1992, 116:813–820.
5. •• Lifton RP, Dluhy RG, Powers M, *et al*.: A chimaeric 11 β-hydroxylase/aldosterone synthase gene causes glucocorticoid-remediable aldosteronism and human hypertension. *Nature* 1992, 355:262–265.

Select Bibliography

Chu MD, Ulick S: Isolation and identification of 18-hydroxycortisol from the urine of patients with primary aldosteronism. *J Biol Chem* 1982, 257:2218–2124.

Sutherland DJ, Ruse JL, Laidlaw JC: Hypertension, increased aldosterone secretion and low plasma renin activity relieved by dexamethasone. *Can Med Assoc J* 1966, 95:1109–1119.

Abnormal Uterine Bleeding

L. Michael Kettel

> **Key Points**
> - Abnormal uterine bleeding is usually a result of either a self-limited episode of anovulation or an anatomic abnormality of the uterus.
> - The diagnosis can usually be secured with a detailed menstrual history and careful physical examination.
> - Malignancy should be excluded in women at risk. New devices are available to make endometrial biopsy less painful for the patient.
> - Isolated episodes of anovulation may resolve without treatment. A course of progestin therapy may help restore normal menstrual cyclicity.
> - Nonsteroidal antiinflammatory drugs decrease menstrual bleeding.
> - Surgical therapy is often required if anatomic defects are discovered.

Abnormal uterine bleeding commonly occurs and often presents an interesting and challenging diagnostic dilemma to the general internist. This chapter is designed to present a common sense approach to the differential diagnosis and to provide a framework on which initial treatment can be based.

The diagnosis of many disorders of the female reproductive system depends, to a great extent, on a firm understanding of the events that take place during the normal menstrual cycle (Fig. 1). Unlike the male reproductive system, the female system is a dynamic one in which day-to-day changes occur. Disorders of this system often lead to anovulation and subsequent abnormal uterine bleeding.

Vaginal bleeding separate from cyclic menstrual flow is abnormal; it can occur as either infrequent, erratic episodes of bleeding; excessive menstrual flow; intermenstrual bleeding; or prolonged episodes of bleeding. This is often referred to as dysfunctional uterine bleeding. There is no firmly established definition for dysfunctional uterine bleeding. In many instances, the degree of abnormality and the extent to which it leads to disruption of normal activities lie in an individual's perception of the problem. One woman's "hemorrhage" is another woman's "spotting" [1]. The infeasibility of quantitating vaginal bleeding hampers the clinician in accurately assessing the degree of bleeding that is occurring. The mean intermenstrual interval is 28 days (±7 days), and average menstrual blood loss is less than 60 mL (Fig. 2) [2]. Thus, if bleeding occurs more frequently than every 21 days or if blood loss exceeds 80 mL, an abnormality probably exists.

ETIOLOGY

The etiology of abnormal uterine bleeding can be divided into two broad categories—hormonal and organic. The organic disorders that can lead to abnormal bleeding include systemic diseases (*eg*, coagulopathies) and anatomic defects (*eg*, uterine fibroids or polyps). It is important that the clinician always keep in mind the possibility of malignancy and that this be excluded before a treatment regimen is initiated.

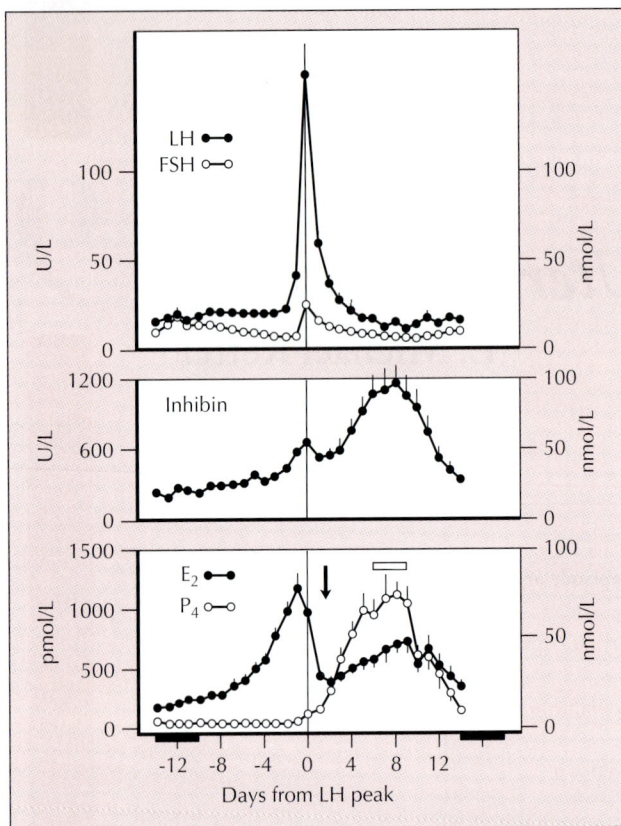

FIGURE 1 Luteinizing hormone, follicle-stimulating hormone, inhibin, estradiol, and progesterone levels in 12 women with normal cycles. The data are centered around the lutenizing hormone peak. (Values are mean ± SE.) E_2—estradiol; FSH—follicle-stimulating hormone; LH—luteinizing hormone; P_4—progesterone.

Hormonal Causes

The most common hormonal disorder leading to abnormal bleeding is anovulation. Alterations in neuroendocrine feedback mechanisms result in a failure of normal folliculogenesis and a failure of corpus luteum formation. This leads to a state

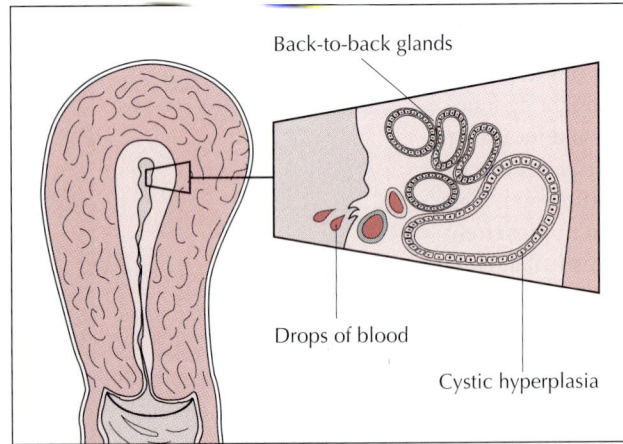

FIGURE 3 Overgrowth of endometrium following unopposed estrogen stimulation. The architecture of the endometrial glands may demonstrate cystic enlargement, back-to-back growth, and disruption of vessels.

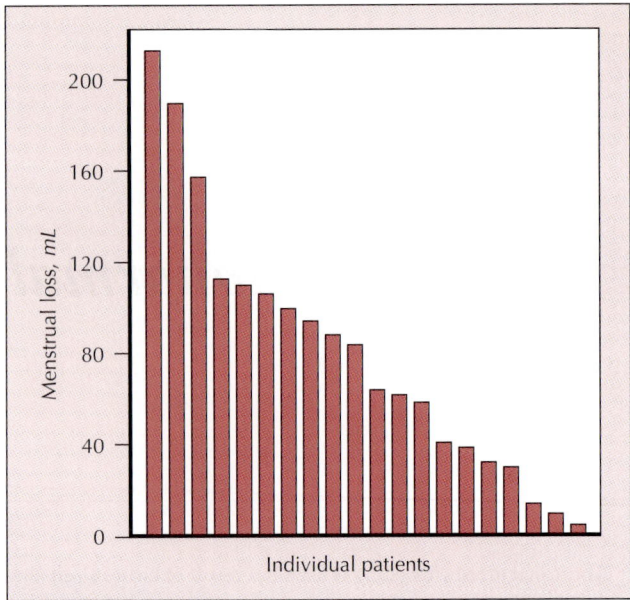

FIGURE 2 Menstrual blood loss in 20 women with normal cycles. (*Adapted from* Hallberg *et al.* [2]; with permission.)

of continuous estrogen production and, consequently, continued proliferation of the endometrium. The overgrown endometrium then sheds erratically and unpredictably as areas outgrow their blood supply (Fig. 3).

Episodes of anovulation are most common in the perimenarcheal and perimenopausal years, but they can occur at any time. Often, a woman may experience an episode of anovulation under circumstances of increased stress. Usually, these episodes are self-limited and the woman with normal cycles will revert back to her underlying menstrual cycle without treatment. Only when the abnormal bleeding episode is unusually heavy or recurrent is intervention necessary.

Organic Causes

Although systemic diseases can lead to abnormal uterine bleeding, the most frequently encountered organic causes of abnormal bleeding are anatomic defects of the uterus and endometrial cavity. The systemic diseases that should be considered include coagulopathies, cirrhosis, thyroid disease, and severe sepsis (Table 1) [3].

Uterine fibroids are the most commonly encountered pelvic tumor. Fibroids were traditionally thought to occur in approximately 30% of women, but recent reassessment of their prevalence suggests they may be found in up to 77% of uteri [4•]. They are composed of benign fibromuscular growths that can occur anywhere in the uterus. Fibroids are commonly classified into subgroups that are based on their location within the uterine wall (Fig. 4). Submucosal fibroids are located under the endometrium, intramural fibroids are within the wall of the uterus, and subserosal fibroids grow under the outer serosal surface of the uterus. Abnormal bleeding is more common with submucosal and intramural fibroids. However, regardless of their location, fibroids can distort uterine and endometrial blood flow and lead to abnormal bleeding (Fig. 5) [5]. Fibroids can grow either on pedicles off of the outer uterine wall or into the endometrial cavity.

TABLE 1 SYSTEMIC DISEASES THAT MAY RESULT IN ABNORMAL UTERINE BLEEDING
Coagulopathy von Willebrand's disease Prothrombin deficiency Leukemia Idiopathic thrombocytopenic purpura Hypersplenism **Thyroid disease** Graves' disease Hashimoto's thyroiditis **Liver disease** Cirrhosis Prothrombin deficiency

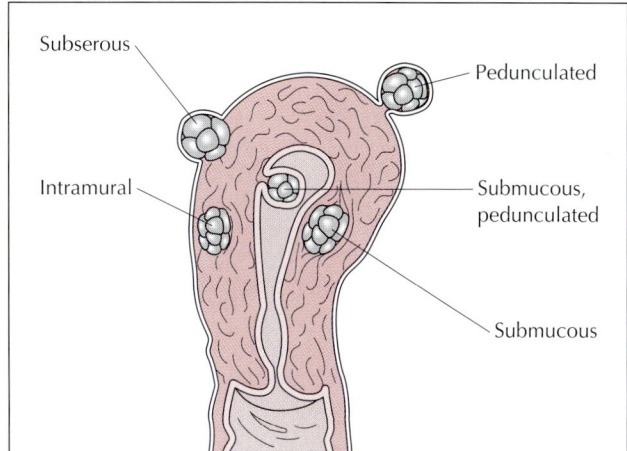

FIGURE 4 Location of fibroids within the uterus.

Fibroids may be large enough to be palpable on bimanual pelvic examination. However, ultrasonography or even magnetic resonance imaging may be necessary to secure the diagnosis (Fig. 6) [6]. In addition to causing abnormal uterine bleeding, fibroids may cause pelvic pain, urinary urgency or frequency, dyschezia, or dyspareunia.

Polyps may grow from the endocervix or endometrium and lead to abnormal uterine bleeding. Histologically, the polyp is composed of an edematous, loose fibrovascular stalk surrounded by columnar epithelium (Fig. 7). Endometrial polyps are common: they are found in as many as 10% of women when the uterus is examined at autopsy. The polyp may be broad based (sessile) or attached to the uterine wall by a pedicle (pedunculated). Usually, endometrial polyps are asymptomatic, but they may be responsible for a wide variety of bleeding abnormalities, including premenstrual and postmenstrual spotting, intermenstrual spotting, and postcoital bleeding.

Endocervical polyps are frequently seen emanating from the cervical canal. Endometrial polyps or small endocervical polyps are more difficult to diagnose. Ultrasonography is rarely able to differentiate a polyp from normal endometrial tissue. Hysterosalpingography, hysteroscopy, and dilatation and curettage are often the only reliable methods of diagnosis.

TREATMENT STRATEGIES

Diagnosis

The differential diagnosis for abnormal uterine bleeding is given in Table 2. Evaluation begins with obtaining a detailed menstrual history focusing on intermenstrual intervals, length and amount of blood flow, and changes from previous bleeding patterns. Presumptive evidence of ovulation can be gained from a history of cyclic bloating, breast tenderness, menstrual cramps, and mood changes. Anovulatory bleeding is frequently unassociated with any of these symptoms and occurs unpredictably. In women without a cyclic bleeding pattern suggestive of ovulation, hormonal screening for underlying reproductive endocrine disorders is indicated. (*See* Chapter 10, Secondary Amenorrhea.)

Whenever a woman presents with abnormal uterine bleeding, the clinician must always maintain a high index of suspi-

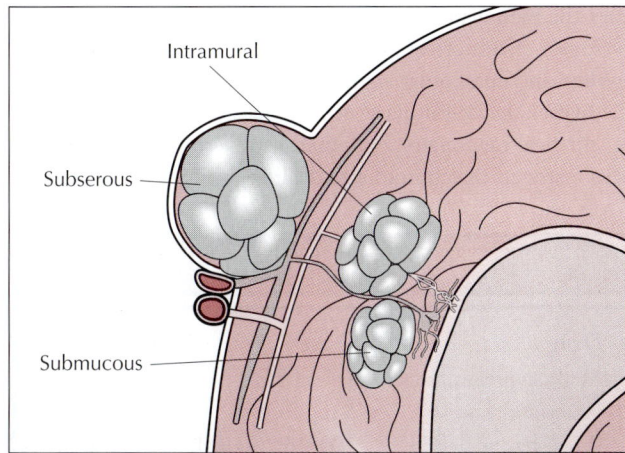

FIGURE 5 Distortion of blood flow around fibroids of various locations within the uterine wall. (*Adapted from* Buttrum and Reiter [5]; with permission.)

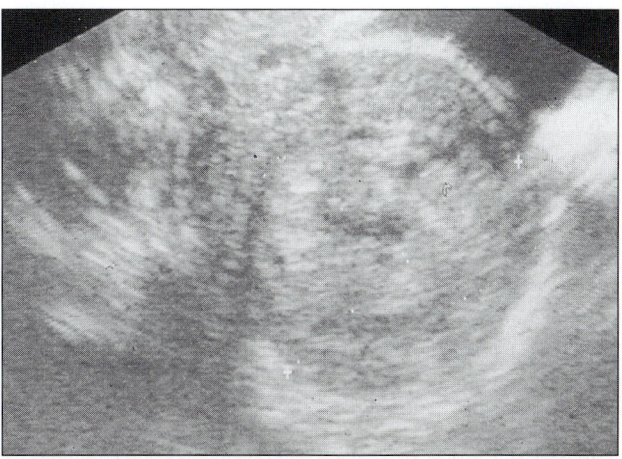

FIGURE 6 Ultrasound image of the uterus demonstrating a 4.2 × 3.7-cm intramural fibroid that was not palpable on bimanual examination.

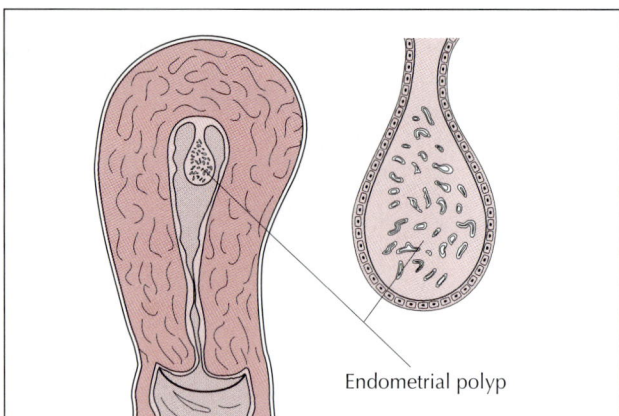

FIGURE 7 Pedunculated endometrial ployp.

TABLE 2 DIFFERENTIAL DIAGNOSIS OF ABNORMAL UTERINE BLEEDING
Malignancy
Endometrial cancer
Cervical cancer
Hormonal disorder
Anovulation
Hyperthyroidism
Hypothyroidism
Hyperprolactinemia
Polycystic ovary syndrome
Cushing's syndrome
Anatomic abnormality
Uterine fibroid
Endometrial polyp
Endocervical polyp

cion for malignancy within the reproductive tract. Often, the only sign of early endometrial cancer is abnormal bleeding [7]. These malignancies are most common in older women but have been reported in younger women who suffer from chronic anovulation [8]. Because of this possibility, the clinician must always consider performing an endometrial biopsy on any woman, regardless of age, who presents with abnormal bleeding. Endometrial biopsy was once performed with rigid stainless steel curettes, which caused a great deal of pain and often made sampling difficult. Recently developed flexible plastic suction catheters have allowed sampling of the endometrium to be regarded as a simple, almost painless procedure that can be performed easily in the office setting (Fig. 8) [9]. In the woman in whom an anatomic abnormality is suspected, pelvic ultrasonography may reveal fibroids or other structural abnormalities.

Medical Therapy

If the presumed diagnosis is anovulation, a course of progestin will transform the endometrium to a secretory pattern and lead to a synchronous withdrawal bleed. The resultant bleeding episode may be quite heavy, especially if the condition has been present for some time, and the woman should be cautioned. There are several options in selecting the progestin to be used for this treatment (Table 3). A single course of treatment may not be adequate for resolution of the abnormal bleeding and a return to cyclic bleeding. In these circumstances, anatomic abnormalities should be considered. If no etiology other than chronic anovulation can be determined, long-term menstrual cycle control with oral contraceptives can be prescribed. It is important that long-term oral contraceptives *not* be prescribed until the clinician is sure that no underlying malignancy is present and has established a diagnosis.

Nonsteroidal antiinflammatory drugs are prostaglandin synthetase inhibitors that decrease prostaglandin production within the endometrium and reduce menstrual blood loss [10]. Several studies have demonstrated a 20% to 50% decline in menstrual bleeding after treatment with nonsteroidal antiinflammatory drugs (Table 4) [11–13]. These medications are generally given to the cycling woman with heavy periods for the first 3 days of flow. Although these drugs are effective when given alone, they can be combined with oral contraceptives or progestins to enhance efficacy.

Fibroids are ovarian steroid-dependent and decrease in size after the menopause or after treatments that decrease ovarian estrogen production. Gonadotropin-releasing hormone agonist and antagonist analogues have been used to suppress the hypothalamic-pituitary-ovarian axis and create a condition of "medical menopause." Numerous investigations have now demonstrated that fibroid size declines by approximately 50%

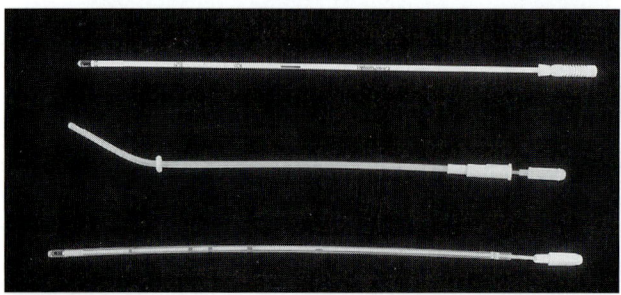

FIGURE 8 Three flexible plastic endometrial suction cannulas suitable for endometrial biopsy. (**Top**, GynoSampler, GynoPharma, Somerville, NJ. **Middle**, Uterine Explora Curette, Milex, Chicago, IL. **Bottom**, Pipelle, Unimar, Wilton, CT.)

TABLE 3 PROGESTIN THERAPY		
Drug	**Dose**	**Duration**
Medroxyprogesterone	10 mg PO	10 d
Norethindrone	5 mg PO	10 d
Progesterone in oil	100–150 mg IM	1 injection
Oral contraceptive	2 tablets bid	4 d
bid—twice daily; IM—intramuscularly; PO—orally.		

TABLE 4 NONSTEROIDAL ANTIINFLAMMATORY DRUGS THAT DECREASE MENSTRUAL BLOOD LOSS		
Drug	Dose, *mg*	Interval
Mefenamic acid	500	tid
Ibuprofen	400	tid
Meclofenamate	100	tid
Naproxen sodium	275	qid
qid—four times daily; tid—three times daily.		

after treatment with these medications (Fig. 9) [14••,15]. Unfortunately, the fibroids return to their original size within a few months after therapy has been discontinued. Long-term therapy with gonadotropin-releasing hormone analogues is not feasible because of the consequences of prolonged estrogen deprivation (*eg*, osteoporosis, hot flashes, and vaginal atrophy) [16]. Alternative hormonal therapies, such as the use of antiprogesterones, might provide acceptable long-term medical treatment [17•].

Surgical Therapy

If the diagnostic evaluation reveals an anatomic abnormality (*eg*, a fibroid or polyp), resolution of abnormal bleeding usually requires surgical resection. Endometrial or endocervical polyps are removed either by simple avulsion (curettage) or by direct resection with electrocautery through a hysteroscope.

The surgical removal of fibroids requires individualization. Many fibroids are completely asymptomatic and do not need to be removed. Only patients who experience significant problems from these anatomic abnormalities should be considered as candidates for surgical resection. Some submucosal or pedunculated fibroids may be resected with electrocautery through the hysteroscope [18]. Larger fibroids require more invasive surgery, such as abdominal myomectomy or hysterectomy [19]. The reproductive desires of the patient and the size and extent of the fibroids determine the approach and the surgical procedure to be performed.

Endometrial ablation is a surgical procedure in which the endometrial cavity is destroyed by either electrocauterization or laser vaporization [20]. The technique is performed as a relatively simple outpatient procedure using an operative hysteroscope (resectoscope). Recent prospective studies have reported very encouraging results. After 6 months, approximately 60% of women reported amenorrhea, 30% had a reduction in menstrual flow, and only 10% reported no change in bleeding pattern [2]. To date, there have been no long-term studies to verify the safety of the procedure. A very low operative complication rate has been reported, but more important will be the 5- and 10-year follow-up findings. These procedures result in partial and unpredictable obliteration of the endometrial cavity. Hypothetically, a patient could continue to cycle behind the obstruction, developing retrograde menstrual flow (and potential endometriosis) or, more importantly, a malignancy that could spread before early detection. At this point, this procedure should be considered experimental.

CONCLUSIONS

Figure 10 summarizes an appropriate management strategy for the general internist. In the woman who presents with abnormal uterine bleeding, the clinician should obtain a careful history and perform a pelvic examination. In most cases, an endometrial biopsy should be performed to rule out malignancy. If no organic disease is readily apparent, a presumptive diagnosis of anovulation is made and a course of progestin is prescribed. If cyclic bleeding does not return, pelvic ultrasonography should be performed. If no anatomic abnormality is found, long-term oral contraceptive therapy will usually result in excellent menstrual cycle control, and if necessary, oral contraceptives can be combined with a nonsteroidal antiinflammatory drug.

REFERENCES AND RECOMMENDED READING

Recently published papers of particular interest have been highlighted as:
- Of interest
- •• Of outstanding interest

1. Chimbria TH, Anderson AC, Turnbull AC: Relation between measured menstrual blood loss and patients' subjective assessment of loss, duration of bleeding, number of sanitary towels used, uterine weight and endometrial surface area. *Br J Obstet Gynecol* 1980, 87:603–610.
2. Hallberg L, Högdahl A-M, Nilsson L, *et al*.: Menstrual blood loss: a population study. Variation at different ages and attempt to define normality. *Acta Obstet Gynecol Scand* 1966, 45:320–327.

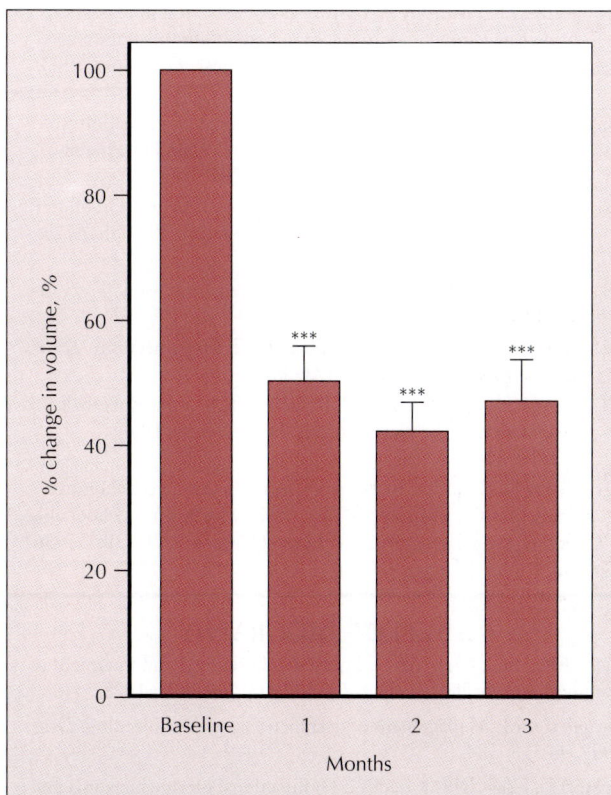

FIGURE 9 Response of uterine fibroids to 3 months of therapy with a gonadotropin-releasing hormone antagonist analogue.

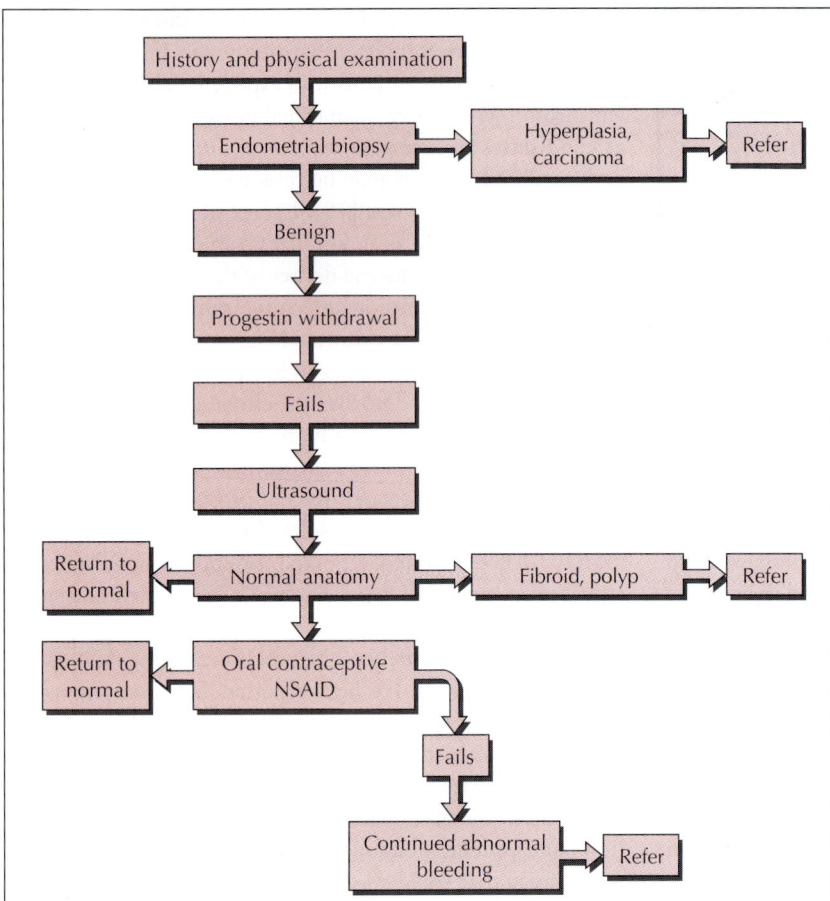

FIGURE 10 Management scheme for the general practitioner presented with a woman who complains of abnormal uterine bleeding. NSAID—nonsteroidal antiinflammatory drug.

3. Mishell DR: Abnormal Uterine Bleeding. In *Comprehensive Gynecology*, edn 2. Edited by Herbst AL, Mishell DR, Stenchever MA, *et al.* St. Louis: Mosby–Year Book; 1992:1079–1099.

4. • Cramer SF, Patel D: The frequency of uterine leiomyomas. *Am J Clin Pathol* 1990, 94:435–438.

5. Buttrum VC, Reiter R: Uterine leiomyomata: etiology, symptomatology, and management. *Fertil Steril* 1981, 36:433–445.

6. Zawin M, McCarthy S, Scoutt LM, *et al.*: High-field MRI and US evaluation of the pelvis in women with leiomyomas. *Magn Reson Imaging* 1990, 8:371–376.

7. DiSaia PJ, Creasman WT: Adenocarcinoma of the uterus. In *Clinical Gynecologic Oncology*, edn 4. Edited by DiSaia PJ, Creasman WT. St. Louis: Mosby–Year Book; 1993:157–193.

8. Dahlgren E, Friberg LG, Johansson S, *et al.* Endometrial carcinoma: ovarian dysfunction. A risk factor in young women. *Eur J Obstet Gynecol Reprod Biol* 1991, 41:143–150.

9. Stovall TG, Ling FW, Morgan PL: A prospective, randomized comparison of the Pipelle endometrial sampling device with the Novak curette. *Am J Obstet Gynecol* 1991, 165:1287–1290.

10. Vargyas JM, Campeau JD, Mishell DA: Treatment of menorrhagia with meclofenamate sodium. *Am J Obstet Gynecol* 1987, 157:944–947.

11. Dockeray CJ: The medical management of menorrhagia. In *Contemporary Obstetrics and Gynecology*. Edited by Chamberlain G. London: Butterworths; 1988:299–314.

12 Fraser IS, McCarron G, Markham R, *et al.*: Long term treatment of menorrhagia with mefenamic acid. *Obstet Gynecol* 1983, 61:109–112.

13 Hall P, Maclachlan N, Thorn N, *et al.*: Control of menorrhagia by the cyclo-oxygenase inhibitors inaproxin and mefenamic acid. *Br J Obstet Gynaecol* 1987, 94:554–558.

14. •• Friedman AJ, Hoffman DI, Comite F, *et al.*: Treatment of leiomyomata uteri with leuprolide acetate depot: A double-blind placebo-controlled, multicenter study. *Obstet Gynecol* 1992, 77:720–725.

15. Kettel LM, Murphy AA, Morales AJ, *et al.*: Rapid regression of uterine leiomyomas in response to daily administration of gonadotropin-releasing hormone antagonist. *Fertil Steril* 1993, 60:642–646.

16. Johansen JS, Riis B, Hassager C: The effect of a gonadotropin-releasing hormone agonist analog (nafarelin) on bone metabolism. *J Clin Endocrinol Metab* 1988, 67:701–706.

17. Murphy AA, Kettel LM, Morales AJ, *et al.*: Regression of uterine leiomyoma in response to the antiprogesterone RU 486. *J Clin Endocrinol Metab* 1993, 76:513–517.

18. Corson SL, Brooks PG: Resectoscopic myomectomy. *Fertil Steril* 1991, 55:1041–1044.

19. Buttrum VC, Snabes MC: Indications for myomectomy. *Semin Reprod Endocrinol* 1992, 10:378–384.

20. Townsend DE, Ricart RM, Paskowitz RA, *et al.*: Rollerball coagulation of the endometrium. *Obstet Gynecol* 1990, 76:310–314.

21. Garry R, Erian J, Grochmal SA: A multi-centre collaborative study into the treatment of menorrhagia by Nd-YAG laser ablation of the endometrium. *Br J Obstet Gynaecol* 1991, 98:357–361.

SELECT BIOGRAPHY

Bayer SR, DeCherney AH: Clinical manifestations and treatment of dysfunctional uterine bleeding. *JAMA* 1993, 269:1823–1828.

Farquhar CM: Management of dysfunctional uterine bleeding. *Drugs* 1992, 44:578–584.

Speroff L, Glass RH, Kase NG: Dysfunctional uterine bleeding. In *Clinical Gynecologic Endocrinology and Infertility*, ed 4. Edited by Speroff L, Glass RH, Kase NG. Baltimore: Williams & Wilkins; 1989:265–282.

Secondary Amenorrhea

Robert L. Rosenfield
David A. Ehrmann

10

> ### Key Points
> - Persistence of irregular menstrual cycles for 2 years beyond menarche should prompt an endocrinologic evaluation.
> - Secondary amenorrhea can occasionally result from congenital rather than acquired disturbances of the reproductive system.
> - Measurement of serum gonadotropin levels and an assessment of estrogenization are key to the diagnostic evaluation of secondary amenorrhea.
> - Hyperandrogenism must be suspected as the cause of anovulation even in the absence of hirsutism and is usually the result of functional ovarian disorders.
> - Proper management of secondary amenorrhea depends on precise diagnosis.

Menstrual cycle disturbances are among the most common disorders prompting reproductive age women to seek medical attention. Primary amenorrhea (a history of never menstruating) is a relatively uncommon disorder that indicates profound disturbances of early onset. Disorders resulting in primary amenorrhea are not covered extensively here. Secondary amenorrhea refers to the cessation of menstrual periods after menarche (the first menstrual period). The mean age of menarche is 12.7 ± 1.0 years in the United States [1•]. The normal menstrual cycle length varies with age. The median menstrual cycle lengths throughout reproductive life are depicted in Figure 1 [2]. Because of long periods of anovulation, considerable variation exists in the length of time it takes for adolescents to establish a menstrual pattern that is normal by adult standards. About half of menstrual cycles are anovulatory in the 2 years after menarche [3], and the cycles in the early postmenarcheal years tend to be several days longer than in adults. If irregular cycles persist for 2 years after menarche, an approximate 50% probability of ongoing menstrual irregularity exists. When fewer than nine menstrual periods occur per year, the term oligomenorrhea applies. Paradoxically, dysfunctional uterine bleeding has virtually the same differential diagnosis as secondary amenorrhea because both result from anovulation; the only difference is that the estrogen levels are higher in patients with dysfunctional uterine bleeding, so they bleed from a hyperplastic, uncycled endometrium.

DIFFERENTIAL DIAGNOSIS

Two general types of disorders cause amenorrhea: those that are associated with abnormalities of genital tract structure and those that result from anovulation (Table 1) [1•].

Abnormal Genital Structure

Clitoromegaly may be a clue to congenital or acquired virilization. Abnormal genital structure as a cause of secondary amenorrhea may not be obvious during pelvic examination. Endometrial atrophy may result from endometritis secondary to pelvic inflammatory disease or as a complication of radiation therapy for pelvic disease.

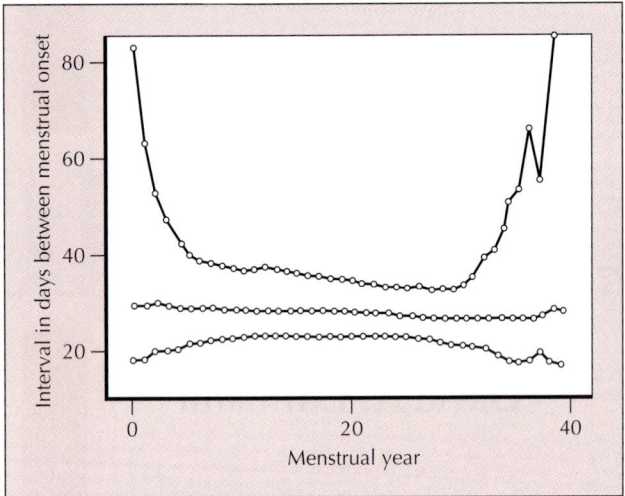

FIGURE 1 Menstrual cycle lengths throughout reproductive life from menarche to menopause. Tenth, fiftieth, and ninetieth percentials are shown. (*Adapted from* Treloar *et al.* [2]; with permission.)

TABLE 1 DIFFERENTIAL DIAGNOSIS OF SECONDARY AMENORRHEA*
I. Abnormal genital structure
A. Ambiguous genitalia
B. Endometrial atrophy
II. Anovulatory disorders
A. Hypoestrogenic
1. FSH elevated
a. Primary ovarian failure
1) Congenital
a) Anatomic, *eg*, gonadal dysgenesis
b) Functional *eg*, steroidogenic blocks, gonadotropin-resistant ovaries
2) Acquired
a) Radiotherapy or chemotherapy
b) Autoimmune oophoritis
c) Oophorectomy
2. FSH not elevated
a. Primary ovarian failure, incomplete
b. Hypogonadotropinism, acquired
1) Anorexia
2) Chronic disease
3) Structural abnormality: mass, radiotherapy
c. Virilization
B. Normoestrogenic
1. Extraovarian metabolic or endocrine disorders
a. Pregnancy
b. Hypothyroidism
c. Cushing's syndrome
d. Overnutrition or undernutrition
2. Hypothalamic anovulation
a. Psychogenic or athletic amenorrhea
b. Hyperprolactinemia
c. Idiopathic hypothalamic amenorrhea
3. Hyperandrogenism
FSH—follicle-stimulating hormone.
Adapted from Rosenfield and Barnes [1•].

Anovulatory Disorders

Anovulatory disorders can be categorized according to whether or not the patient is hypoestrogenic and whether or not gonadotropins, particularly serum follicle-stimulating hormone (FSH) levels, are elevated. Hypoestrogenism with elevated FSH levels indicates primary ovarian failure (hypergonadotropic hypogonadism), the differential diagnosis of which includes both congenital and acquired disorders. An estimated 5% of Turner syndrome patients present with secondary amenorrhea, even though they have congenitally dysgenetic ovaries.

Hypoestrogenism with normal FSH levels usually indicates secondary ovarian failure (hypogonadotropic hypogonadism) because a normal gonadotropin level is compatible with a diagnosis of gonadotropin deficiency in patients with hypoestrogenemia. However, incomplete primary ovarian failure must not be overlooked because hypergonadotropinism and frank hypoestrogenism are not found as the ovary begins to fail during premature menopause or menopause [4]. Finally, frankly virilizing disorders suppress gonadotropins, and, consequently, estrogens.

Normal estrogenization with normal FSH levels carries different diagnostic connotations: extraovarian endocrine or metabolic disorders, hypothalamic anovulation, or mild hyperandrogenic disorders. Pregnancy is always the first consideration in this setting. Iatrogenic or spontaneous glucocorticoid excess causes amenorrhea primarily by interfering with gonadotropin responsiveness to gonadotropin-releasing hormone (GnRH) [5••].

Hypothalamic anovulation occurs in patients who secrete sufficient gonadotropin tonically to estrogenize normally but lack the ability to produce a midcycle surge of luteinizing hormone. They have disturbances of cyclic or pulsatile GnRH release that interfere with the positive feedback mechanism. This phenomenon is often seen in the setting of physical, psychogenic, or athletic stress and bears some resemblance to anorexia nervosa. Such changes result from varying combinations of undernutrition and altered neurotransmission, which are caused by stress [5••].

Hyperprolactinemia disrupts the rhythmicity of the hypothalamic GnRH pulse generator. Hyperprolactinemia is quite variable in its presentation. It is in the differential diagnosis of hypothalamic amenorrhea, hypogonadotropic hypogonadism, infertility resulting from a short or inadequate luteal phase (characterized by menstrual cycles of less than 22 days), dysfunctional uterine bleeding, or a hyperandrogenic picture that clinically resembles polycystic ovary syndrome (PCOS). Half of hyperprolactinemic patients have galactorrhea.

Hyperandrogenism is a major cause of anovulation syndromes. In most cases, androgen excess arises from abnormal adrenal or ovarian function, but occasionally, it results from abnormalities in the peripheral formation of androgen. An ovarian source is more likely than an adrenal one in women with menstrual disorders [6••]. Functional abnormalities are much commoner than tumors (Table 2) [7•].

Functional adrenal hyperandrogenism
Congenital adrenal hyperplasia

Congenital adrenal hyperplasia (CAH) arises from an autosomal recessive deficiency in the activity of any one of the adrenocortical enzyme steps necessary for the biosynthesis of corticosteroid hormones. Nonclassic (late-onset) forms cause oligomenorrhea or hirsutism or both, which presents in adulthood [8] without the genital ambiguity of classic CAH. Women with this disorder may have polycystic ovaries and high serum luteinizing hormone levels. The commonest form of virilizing CAH is 21-hydroxylase deficiency; nonclassic 21-hydroxylase deficiency accounts for 2.5% of hirsute women presenting to our medical center. 3β-hydroxysteroid dehydrogenase (3β-HSD) deficiency causes ovarian hyperandrogenism to coexist with adrenal androgen excess. Although suspected in up to 20% of hirsute women because of elevated dehydroepiandrosterone sulfate (DHEAS) levels, the diagnosis can seldom be proved by ovarian function testing [9•,10]. Most patients diagnosed with nonclassic 3β-HSD deficiency have test results that we would interpret as exaggerated adrenarche.

Exaggerated adrenarche

Adrenarche is "the puberty of the adrenal gland", in which the adrenal cortex develops a zona reticularis and acquires the ability to secrete 17-ketosteroids, particularly DHEAS. Most women with adrenal hyperandrogenism do not have clear evidence of CAH. Rather, they have a pattern of steroid secretion in response to corticotropin that resembles an exaggeration of adrenarche.

Other adrenal androgenic disorders

Adrenal hyperandrogenism is sometimes associated with Cushing's syndrome. Cortisol resistance is a rare cause of hyperandrogenism: compensatory hypersecretion of corticotropin and hypercortisolemia occur without the clinical or biochemical findings of Cushing's syndrome, and hypertension with hypokalemia may accompany the syndrome. Congenitally abnormal cortisol metabolism may resemble cortisol resistance. The diagnosis of hyperprolactinemia and acromegaly must be considered.

Functional gonadal hyperandrogenism
Polycystic ovary syndrome and functional ovarian hyperandrogenism

The classic Stein-Leventhal form of PCOS is characterized by bilateral polycystic ovaries associated with amenorrhea, hirsutism, and obesity [7•,11•]. However, the signs and symptoms may vary, and not every patient has all the cardinal features (Fig. 2). Symptoms typically date from menarche, and elevation of serum luteinizing hormone or the ratio of luteinizing hormone to FSH is characteristic. However, many women with the typical clinical picture have a PCOS-like disorder of ovarian function in the absence of polycystic ovaries or gonadotropin abnormalities [6••,11•]. PCOS

TABLE 2 DIFFERENTIAL DIAGNOSIS OF HYPERANDROGENISM

I. Functional adrenal hyperandrogenism
  A. Congenital adrenal hyperplasia
  B. Exaggerated adrenarche or dysregulation
  C. Cushings's disease
  D. Growth hormone or prolactin excess
  E. Abnormal cortisol action or metabolism

II. Functional gonadal hyperandrogenism
  A. Polycystic ovary syndrome and functional ovarian hyperandrogenism
    1. Follicular maturation arrest
    2. Extraovarian virilizing disorders
    3. Ovarian steroidogenic block
    4. Dysregulation of androgen secretion
       a. LH elevation
       b. LH augmentation
    5. Insulin-resistance syndromes
  B. Hermaphroditism
  C. Chorionic gonadotropin-related

III. Peripheral androgen overproduction
  A. Obesity
  B. Other

IV. Tumoral hyperandrogenism

LH—luteinizing hormone.
From Rosenfield and Lucky [7•]; with permission.

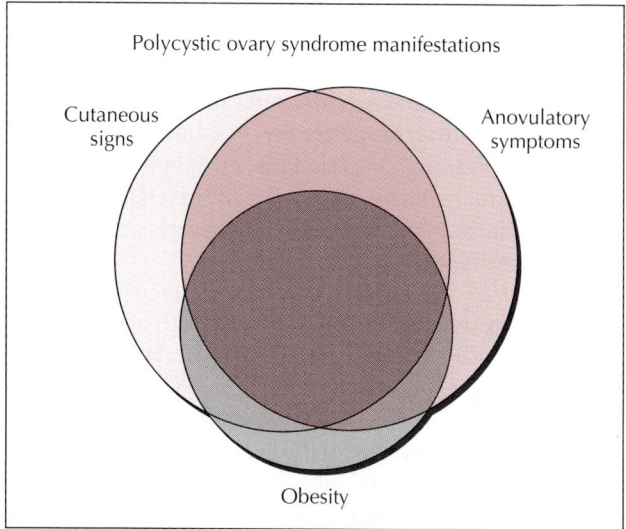

FIGURE 2 Manifestations of polycystic ovary syndrome in approximate proportion to their relative incidence and coincidence. Cutaneous symptoms include hirsutism, acne, and acanthosis nigricans. Anovulatory symptoms include amenorrhea, oligomenorrhea, dysfunctional uterine bleeding, and infertility. (Adapted from Rosenfield and Lucky [7•].)

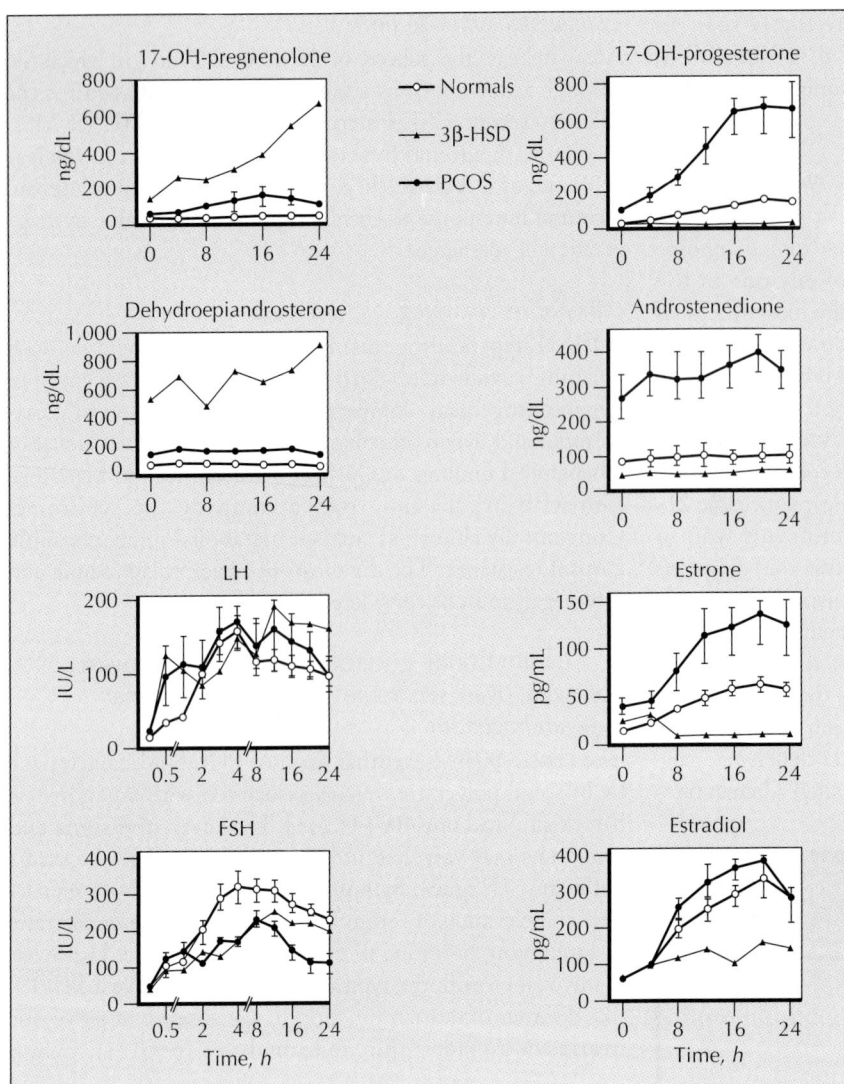

FIGURE 3 Patterns of response to gonadotropin-releasing hormone agonist (nafarelin) testing in patients with the typical ovarian hyperandrogenic type of polycystic ovary syndrome (PCOS) and a patient with late-onset 3β-hydroxysteroid dehydrogenase (3β-HSD) deficiency in comparison to normal early follicular phase females. FSH—follicle-stimulating hormone; LH—luteinizing hormone; OH—hydroxy. (*Adapted from* Rosenfield and Lucky [7•]; with permission.)

appears to be a form of functional, gonadotropin-dependent ovarian hyperandrogenism characterized by hyperresponsiveness of 17-hydroxyprogesterone to administration of a GnRH agonist (Fig. 3) [7•]. This effect appears to result from abnormal coordinate regulation (dysregulation) of ovarian androgen and estrogen synthesis rather than from a steroidogenic block.

Adrenal 17-ketosteroid hyperresponsiveness to corticotropin coexists in about half of patients with ovarian hyperandrogenism [6••]. The relationship of ovarian and adrenal hyperandrogenism is shown in Figure 4. We have hypothesized that dysregulation of androgen synthesis within the adrenal cortex explains the coexistence of exaggerated adrenarche and PCOS. Others, however, consider women with isolated exaggerated adrenarche to have an adrenal form of PCOS.

PCOS is characterized by a degree of insulin resistance that is very disproportionate to the degree of obesity [12]. Nonobese PCOS patients are as insulin resistant as obese non-PCOS patients. The association of hyperandrogenism, insulin resistance, and acanthosis nigricans, the *HAIR-AN* syndrome, is one aspect of PCOS. All syndromes of severe insulin resistance are accompanied by PCOS.

Other gonadal androgenic disorders

On rare occasions, hyperandrogenism and secondary amenorrhea can result from disorders in which rudimentary testicular tissue is present, such as true hermaphroditism, in which the testes are too rudimentary to cause aplasia of müllerian derivatives during embryogenesis. Virilization during pregnancy may result from ovarian hyperresponsiveness to chorionic gonadotropin.

Peripheral Overproduction of Androgen

Ten percent of women have idiopathic hyperandrogenemia, that is, hyperandrogenemia in which extensive testing reveals no clear adrenal or ovarian source for the androgen excess (Fig. 4). We suspect that these cases arise from increased peripheral metabolism of inactive steroid precursors to active androgens. Some of these cases can be accounted for by obesity, which can cause hyperandrogenemia and amenorrhea, thus mimicking PCOS [7•]. Other cases are unexplained and may have a genetic basis.

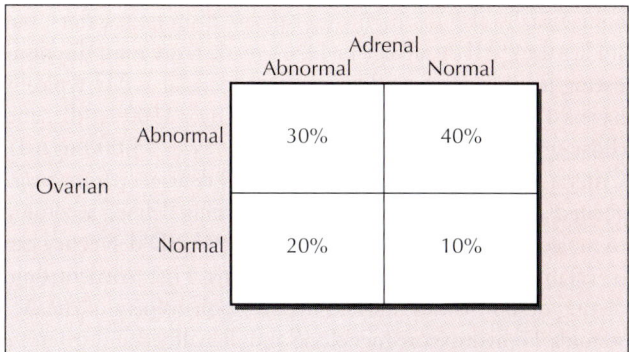

Figure 4 Relationship of adrenal and ovarian hyperandrogenism. *Data from* Ehrmann *et al.* [6••].

Tumoral Hyperandrogenism

Extreme elevation of the 17-ketosteroid DHEAS is typical of adrenal carcinoma. Ovarian virilizing tumors characteristically secrete predominantly androstenedione rather than testosterone; mild elevation of urinary 17-ketosteroid secretion characteristically results. Adrenal virilizing tumors often have some degree of gonadotropin dependency or corticotropin dependency. Arrhenoblastomas sometimes are estrogen suppressible. Ovarian lipid cell tumors are typically partly corticotropin dependent as well.

DIAGNOSTIC METHODS

The initial evaluation of amenorrhea includes a careful history and physical examination, with particular attention paid to the symptoms and signs shown in Table 3. In the absence of specific findings to focus the evaluation, the initial round of laboratory testing ordinarily should include the laboratory tests shown in Table 3.

An elevated FSH level points to hypergonadotropic hypogonadism, and, thus, primary ovarian failure (Fig. 5). A karyotype is then indicated to determine if the cause is a variant of Turner syndrome. If not, the patient should be screened for evidence of the autoimmune endocrine deficiencies (chronic lymphocytic thyroiditis, adrenal insufficiency, or hypoparathyroidism) that sometimes accompany autoimmune oophoritis.

If gonadotropins are not elevated, the assessment is further focused according to whether or not the patient is hypoestrogenic (Fig. 5). The degree of estrogenization of the sexually mature female can be estimated in several, generally imperfect ways: by measuring plasma estradiol, by obtaining a smear of the vaginal mucosa or cervical mucus, or by performing a progestin-withdrawal test. A plasma estradiol level of over 25 pg/mL normally indicates some ovarian function. However, if estradiol never rises substantially above this level, the woman is hypoestrogenic. Definitive evidence of adequate estrogenization is obtained if the Papanicolaou smear shows cornification of the vaginal mucosa or if the cervical mucus smear shows ferning. Progestin withdrawal is the simplest and lease expensive test, but it is also the least accurate; a woman who does not experience withdrawal bleeding after the administration of 100 mg of progesterone in oil intramuscularly or 10 mg of medroxyprogesterone acetate daily for 5 days probably has an ambient estradiol level of less than approximately 40 pg/mL [13].

A GnRH test or GnRH agonist test is indicated if the patient is hypoestrogenic [14•]. Hyperresponsiveness of FSH to GnRH and hyporesponse of estradiol to GnRH agonist stimulation are characteristic of incipient primary ovarian failure [4]. A normal response does not rule out gonadotropin deficiency or hypothalamic anovulation. Further evaluation for gonadotropin deficiency includes magnetic resonance imaging of the hypothalamic-pituitary area to rule out a structural lesion and an endocrine work-up for more generalized hypopituitarism. In the normally estrogenized patient with otherwise unexplained amenorrhea, hyperandrogenism, endometrial disorders, and hypothalamic amenorrhea are the major considerations [7•].

For the differential diagnosis of hyperandrogenemia, we recommend a dexamethasone androgen-suppression test (Fig. 6). The pattern of response of plasma-free testosterone, DHEAS, and cortisol segregates patients diagnostically.

Table 3 Initial assessment of the amenorrheic patient

History
Duration of symptoms
Menstrual history
Systemic, neuropsychiatric, or gynecologic symptoms

Physical examination
Weight-for-height (body mass index)
Cushingoid changes
Acanthosis nigricans
Hirsutism or acne
Visual fields and funduscopic evaluation
Sense of smell
Galactorrhea
Abdominal mass
Clitoromegaly
Pelvic mass

Blood tests
Complete blood count
Erythrocyte sedimentation rate
Chemistry panel
β–human chorionic gonadotropin
Reproductive endocrine screening tests
   Thyroid function (thyroxine, thyroid-stimulating hormone)
   Cortisol
   Prolactin
   Androgen battery (total and free testosterone, dehydroepiandrosterone sulfate)
   Estradiol
   Follicle-stimulating and luteinizing hormones

Subnormal suppressibility of free testosterone with normal adrenal suppression usually results from PCOS or functional ovarian hyperandrogenism [6••]. An elevated serum luteinizing hormone level and ultrasonographic findings may support the diagnosis of PCOS. Suppression of the plasma-free testosterone level after a therapeutic trial of estrogen-progestin is also confirmatory of functional ovarian hyperandrogenism; however, this effect does not rule out virilizing ovarian or adrenal tumors. An elevation of plasma-free testosterone (over 10 pg/mL in our laboratory) is the most common single abnormality in hyperandrogenic women. A plasma total testosterone level of over 200 ng/dL should lead the clinician to consider a virilizing tumor, and a testosterone level in the male range (over 350 ng/dL) makes a tumor the probable cause. A basal DHEAS level that is very high (over 800 µg/dL) suggests adrenal carcinoma. Ultrasound, computed tomography, or magnetic resonance imaging usually demonstrates the mass in such cases.

Normal suppression of androgens by dexamethasone indicates an adrenal source of androgens or androgen precursors. A rapid intravenous corticotropin test, using an intravenous injection of 250 µg of cosyntropin, is then indicated to rule out CAH. The 17-hydroxyprogesterone response to a rapid corticotropin test distinguishes nonclassic 21-hydroxylase deficiency CAH from normal better than baseline steroid levels (Fig. 7) [8]. The 17-hydroxyprogesterone response to a corticotropin bolus usually also distinguishes carriers from noncarriers, but studies using HLA linkage or DNA markers are most discriminating for this purpose. Those with nonclassic CAH typically have a 17-hydroxyprogesterone level of over 1500 ng/dL, and those with classic CAH have a level of over 15,000 ng/dL. Criteria for distinguishing mild 3β-HSD deficiency from exaggerated adrenarche are in the process of being defined according to molecular criteria. The diagnosis of 3β-HSD deficiency can be established only under two conditions. First, corticotropin testing demonstrates marked hyperresponsiveness of the Δ^5-steroids 17-hydroxypregnenolone and dehydroepiandrosterone both in absolute terms but relative to Δ^4-steroids (17-hydroxyprogesterone and androstenedione or cortisol) in response to corticotropin [10]. Second, GnRH agonist testing reveals evidence of 3β-HSD in the ovary [9•].

At the end of this sequence of testing, very few cases of hyperandrogenemia are left unexplained. Idiopathic hyperandrogenemia is suppressible by both dexamethasone and estrogen-progestin. Our experience with GnRH agonist testing indicates that much hyperandrogenemia that is now considered idiopathic results from ovarian hyperandrogenism [6••].

MANAGEMENT

Hypoestrogenism may be managed by its replacement or by administration of an oral contraceptive [1•]. Replacement

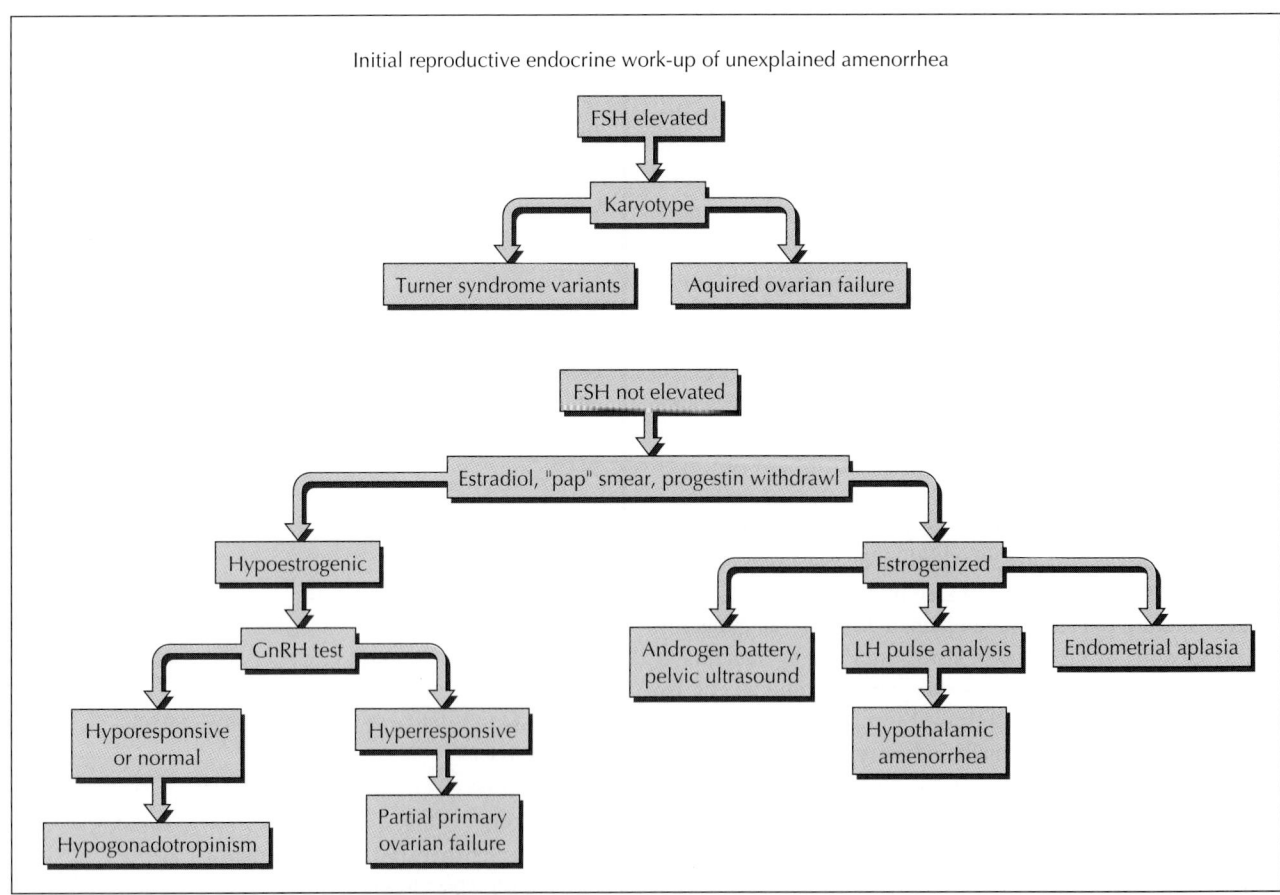

FIGURE 5 The initial reproductive endocrinologic evaluation of unexplained amenorrhea. FSH—follicle-stimulating hormone; GnRH—gonadotropin-releasing hormone; LH—luteinizing hormone.

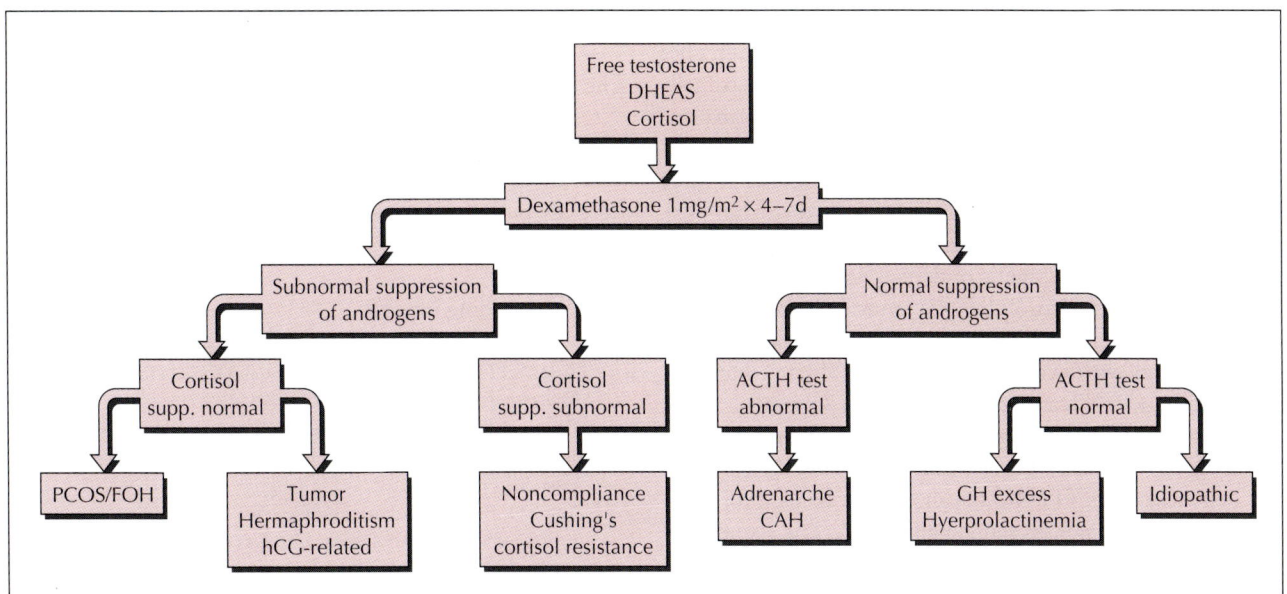

FIGURE 6 Algorithm for the differential diagnosis of hyperandrogenemia using a low-dose dexamethasone suppression test. After 4 days or more of dexamethasone administration, subnormal suppression of plasma-free testosterone suggests functional ovarian hyperandrogenism/polycystic ovary syndrome (PCOS/FOH) (if both dehydroepiandrosterone sulfate [DHEAS] and cortisol suppress normally), tumor (if only cortisol suppresses normally), or Cushing's syndrome (if cortisol does not suppress normally). Normal suppression of hyperandrogenemia is indication for corticotropin (ACTH) testing. Normal suppression of androgens is most specifically indicated by a reduction of plasma-free testosterone into the normal range for dexamethasone-suppressed women (< 8 pg/mL in our laboratory). Normal adrenal suppression is indicated by a reduction of both DHEAS and cortisol to levels below the normal range for adult controls (< 70 and < 3 μg/dL, respectively, in our laboratory). CAH—congenital adrenal hyperplasia; GH—growth hormone; hCG—human chorionic gonadotropin. (*Adapted from* Rosenfield and Lucky [7•].)

estrogen therapy customarily consists of conjugated estrogens, 0.625 mg/d, or ethinyl estradiol, 20 μg/d for 3 weeks on, 1 week off. A progestin is administered for the last 1 to 2 weeks of each course of estrogen (*eg*, medroxyprogesterone acetate, 5 to 10 mg daily). The more progestin administered, there is less risk of endometrial hyperplasia but a greater risk of premenstrual symptoms [15]. Oral contraceptive pills containing the lowest dose of estrogen that will result in normal menstrual flow are a convenient option. The lowest estrogen dosage currently available in combination contraceptive pills in the United States is 20 μg of ethinyl estradiol (*eg*, Loestrin 1/20, Parke-Davis, Morris Plains, NJ). Obese patients tend to require higher doses of estrogen. However, patients sensitive to estrogen because of such conditions as hypertension, migraine, or lymphedema are best advised to use a more physiologic form of therapy, estradiol itself in a form that bypasses the liver, such as depotestradiol, 2.5 mg given intramuscularly on a monthly basis, or ethinyl estradiol patches (Estraderm, Ciba, Woodbridge, NJ), 0.05 or 0.10 mg twice weekly. When hypoestroestrogenism results from stress or eating disorders, behavioral modification and psychological counseling are indicated rather than estrogen replacement therapy.

Hyperprolactinemia, whether idiopathic or tumoral, is usually treated with dopaminergic ergot alkaloid derivatives [16,17]. To minimize nausea, bromocriptine (Parlodel, Sandoz, East Hanover, NJ) treatment is initiated with a dose of 1.25 mg at bedtime, which is gradually increased to the usual full dosage of 2.5 mg twice or three times a day. Pergolide (Permax, Eli Lilly, Indianapolis, IN) in a dosage of

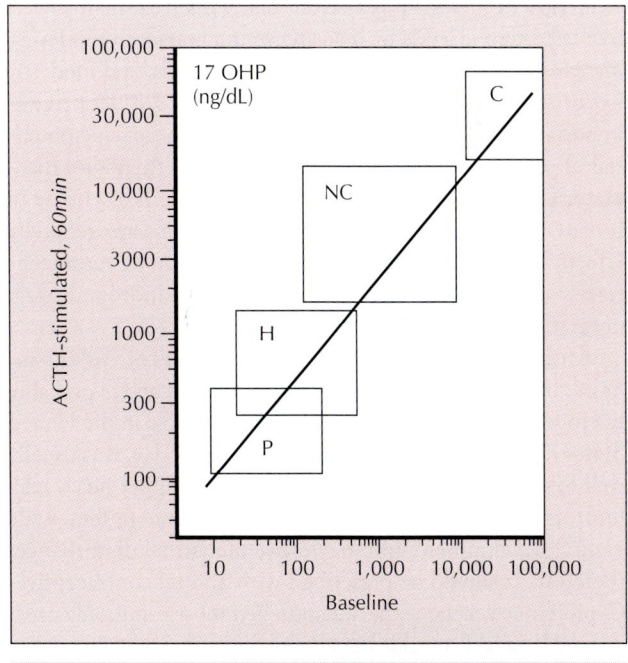

FIGURE 7 Comparison of baseline and corticotropin ACTH)–stimulated levels of 17-hydroxyprogesterone in the general population (P), heterozygotes for 21-hydroxylase deficiency (H), nonclassic variants homozygous for 21-hydroxylase deficiency (NC), and classic 21-hydroxylase–deficient patients (C). Data include males and females, regardless of phase of menstrual cycle or age. ACTH administered as 250 μg intravenous bolus. 17 OHP—17-hydroxyprogesterone (*Data from* New *et al.* [22].)

50 to 100 μg with the evening meal may be preferable to use in some patients because it often permits administration once daily. An effective dose suppresses prolactin levels maximally within a month. The reproductive cycle should be normalized within 12 weeks of administration of an effective dose.

Hyperandrogenism is treated by interrupting one or more of the steps in the pathway leading to its expression [7•]. Endocrinologic treatment of hirsutism, acne, or alopecia is indicated if standard cosmetic or dermatologic measures short of isotretinoin or minoxidil fail. The maximal effect of pharmacologic agents on hirsutism takes 9 to 12 months because of the long growth cycles of sexual hair follicles, but acne should respond to effective treatment within 2 months.

Glucocorticoids are indicated for patients whose major source of androgen is adrenal, particularly in CAH. They are occasionally beneficial in PCOS [18] but should not be used for more than 6 months if menses remain abnormal. The sequelae of glucocorticoid therapy can be minimized by use of a modest bedtime dose (about 5 to 7.5 mg of prednisone) to reduce adrenal androgen secretion selectively without causing adrenal insufficiency [7•], but classic CAH usually requires twice-a-day dosing. Significant adrenal suppression can be excluded by a rapid corticotropin (cosyntropin) test performed 2 to 3 months after initiation of therapy if plasma cortisol rises to over 8 μg/dL.

Progestin therapy is the method of choice for treatment of menstrual irregularity that is not associated with hirsutism or acne. Medroxyprogesterone, 5 to 10 mg daily for 7 to 14 days, should be given at 4-week intervals. Combination estrogen-progestin therapy arrests progression of hirsutism. Objective reduction in hirsutism is exceptional. This treatment lowers free testosterone levels by reducing serum gonadotropin levels, increasing sex-hormone binding globulin levels, and modestly lowering DHEAS levels. The choice of contraceptive is important for some patients because of the androgenic potential of some progestins. Because it contains ethynodiol diacetate, Demulen 1/35 or 1/50 has been the pill of choice in hirsute patients, although diverse preparations are generally effective in treating acne. The new generation of contraceptives contains progestins that are even less androgenic (*eg*, norgestimate or desogestrel) [19,20].

Antiandrogens are required for reversal of hirsutism. Spironolactone has been shown to be effective and is probably the most potent and safest antiandrogen available in the United States [21]. In doses of 50 to 100 mg twice a day, it is usually well tolerated; fatigue and hyperkalemia at higher doses may limit its usefulness. It is potentially teratogenic to fetal male genital development and may cause menstrual disturbance; therefore, it should be prescribed with an oral contraceptive. Cyproterone acetate is the antiandrogen most commonly used; it is only available outside the United States. It is a potent progestin, too, and in low dosage has been combined with ethinyl estradiol as an antiandrogenic contraceptive.

Weight reduction is indicated in obese hyperandrogenemic patients. This treatment is sometimes successful in reversing hyperandrogenemia and menstrual disorders.

Patients with secondary amenorrhea will probably require the expertise of an experienced reproductive endocrinologist in achieving pregnancy.

Acknowledgments

The typescript was prepared by Jean Moore.

References and Recommended Reading

Recently published papers of particular interest have been highlighted as:
- Of interest
- Of outstanding interest

1.• Rosenfield RL, Barnes RB: Menstrual disorders in adolescence. *Endocrinol Metab Clin North Am* 1993, 22:491–505.

2. Treloar AE, Boynton RE, Benn BG, Brown BW: Variation of human menstrual cycle through reproductive life. *Int J Fertil* 1967, 12:77–84.

3. Apter D, Bützow T, Laughlin G, *et al.*: Hyperandrogenism during puberty and adolescence, and its relationship to reproductive function in the adult female. In *Reproductive Medicine*. Edited by Frajese G, Steinberger E, Rodriguez-Rigau LJ. Serono Symposia Publications from Raven Press; 1993:93:265–275.

4. Winslow KL, Toner JP, Brzyski RG, *et al.*: The gonadotropin-releasing hormone agonist stimulation test — a sensitive predictor of performance in the flare-up in vitro fertilization cycle. *Fertil Steril* 1991, 56:711–717.

5.•• Chrousos GP, Gold PW: The concept of stress system disorders: Overview of behavioral and physical homeostasis. *JAMA* 1992, 267:1244–1252.

6.•• Ehrmann DA, Rosenfield RL, Barnes RB, *et al.*: Detection of functional ovarian hyperandrogenism in women with androgen excess. *N Engl J Med* 1992, 327:157–162.

7.• Rosenfield RL, Lucky AW: Acne, hirsutism, and alopecia in adolescent girls. *Endocrinol Metab Clin North Am* 1993, 22:507–532.

8. Ritzén EM: Adrenogenital syndrome. *Curr Opin Pediatr* 1992, 4:661–667.

9.• Barnes RB, Ehrmann DA, Brigell DF, Rosenfield RL: Ovarian steroidogenic responses to gonadotropin-releasing hormone testing with nafarelin in hirsute women with adrenal response to ACTH suggestive of 3β-hydroxy-delta^5-steroid dehydrogenase. *J Clin Endocrinol Metab* 1993, 76:450–455.

10. Chang YT, Zhang L, Mason JI, *et al.*: Redefining hormonal criteria for mild 3 β-hydroxysteroid dehydrogenase (3 β-HSD) deficiency (def) congenital adrenal hyperplasia (CAH) by molecular analysis of the type II 3 β-HSD gene [Abstract 563]. *Pediatr Res* 1994, 35:96A.

11.• Ehrmann DA, Barnes RB, Rosenfield RL: Polycystic ovary syndrome as a form of functional ovarian hyperandrogenism due to dysregulation of androgen secretion. *Endocrine Rev* 1995, 16:322–353.

12. Dunaif A: Insulin resistance and ovarian hyperandrogenism. *Endocrinologist* 1992, 2:248–260.

13: Rebar RW, Connolly HV: Clinical features of young women with hypergonadotropic amenorrhea. *Fertil Steril* 1990, 53:804–810.

14.• Goodpasture JC, Ghai K, Cara JF: Potential of GnRH agonists in the diagnosis of pubertal disorders in girls. *Clin Obstet Gynecol* 1993, 36:773–785.

15. Woodruff JD, Pickar JH: Incidence of endometrial hyperplasia in postmenopausal women taking conjugated estrogens (Premarin) with medroxyprogesterone acetate or conjugated estrogens alone. *Am J Obstet Gynecol* 1994, 170:1213–1223.

16. Molitch ME: Pathologic hyperprolactinemia. *Endocrinol Metab Clin North Am* 1992, 21:877–901.

17. Lamberts SWJ, Quik RFP: A comparison of the efficacy and safety of pergolide and bromocriptine in the treatment of hyperprolactinemia. *J Clin Endocrinol Metab* 1991, 72:635–641.

18. Steinberger E, Rodriguez-Rigau LJ, Petak SM, *et al.*: Glucocorticoid therapy in hyperandrogenism. *Ballieres Clin Obstet Gynaecol* 1990, 4:457–471.

19. DeCherney AH, Speroff L: Next generation of contraception: oral contraceptives in the 1990s. *Am J Obstet Gynecol* 1992, 167 (suppl):(4), part 2.

20. Burkman RT: Desogestrel: a progestin for the 1990s. *Am J Obstet Gynecol* 1993, 168 (suppl):(3), part 2.

21. Shaw JC: Spironolactone in dermatologic therapy. *J Am Acad Dermatol* 1991;24:236–243.

22. New MI, Lorenzen F, Lerner AJ: Genotyping steroid 21-hydroxylase deficiency: hormonal reference data. *J Clin Endocrinol Metab* 1983, 57:320.

Select Bibliography

Barbieri RL, Smith S, Ryan KJ: The role of hyperinsulinemia in the pathogenesis of ovarian hyperandrogenism. *Fertil Steril* 1988, 50:197–212.

Barnes RB, Rosenfield RL: Polycystic ovary syndrome: pathogenesis and treatment. *Ann Intern Med* 1989, 110:386–399.

Dunaif A, Segal KR, Futterweit W, Dobrjansky A: Profound peripheral insulin resistance, independent of obesity, in polycystic ovary syndrome. *Diabetes* 1989, 38:1165–1174.

Rittmaster RS, Givner ML: Effect of daily and alternate day low dose prednisone on serum cortisol and adrenal androgens in hirsute women. *J Clin Endocrinol Metab* 1988, 67:400–403.

Male Hypogonadism
Stephen R. Plymate

Key Points
- Hypogonadism is a prevalent condition among the male population.
- History and physical examination are the most important factors involved in making the initial diagnosis.
- Whether the hypogonadism began before or after puberty can usually be determined by history and physical examination.
- Men with secondary hypogonadism may achieve fertility with gonadotropin replacement, while those with primary hypogonadism usually have irreversible infertility.
- Long-term androgen replacement in primary or secondary hypogonadism should be accomplished with exogenous testosterone replacement.

Hypogonadism, which may be defined in the male as a failure of the testes to produce testosterone, spermatozoa, or both, is a relatively common problem. Low testosterone levels are seen in up to 20% of men with hip fractures [1]. Hypogonadism can be divided into primary and secondary etiologies: testicular failure and pituitary or hypothalamic failure, respectively. A partial list of the more common diagnoses in each of these categories is presented in Table 1. In addition, each of these categories may be subdivided into congenital and acquired causes.

Clinical recognition of hypogonadism is the crucial step in making the diagnosis. For instance, in the case of deficient sperm production resulting in infertility, the physical examination may well be normal, whereas the history is consistent with infertility if the female partner has a history of regular menses without pelvic infection or surgery, then the man has a strong likelihood of hypogonadism involving the seminiferous tubule compartment of the testes. In the case of testicular failure manifested by a deficiency in androgen secretion, the physical examination may not only provide the clues necessary for a diagnosis of hypogonadism, but it may also help determine whether the hypogonadism developed before or after puberty (Table 2).

PRIMARY HYPOGONADISM

Primary hypogonadism results from a primary testicular defect involving the Leydig cell production of testosterone, seminiferous tubule production of sperm, or both. In primary hypogonadism, the diagnosis is first suggested by a decrease in testosterone or sperm and is confirmed by a finding of elevated gonadotropin levels. In some cases in which the defect is mild, such as a decrease in sperm production in the infertile man resulting from varicocele, the basal gonadotropin levels are normal but when stimulated with gonadotropin releasing hormone, an exaggerated response is seen (Fig. 1). In addition, the progressive increase in luteinizing hormone after gonadotropin releasing hormone stimulation indicates that a defect is also present in Leydig cell function. These data confirm that a primary defect exists in these men.

TABLE 1 CLASSIFICATION OF MALE HYPOGONADISM
Primary hypogonadism
Klinefelter's syndrome
XX males
XY/XO mixed gonadal dysgenesis
Ullrich-Noonan syndrome
Myotonia dystrophica
Sertoli-cell-only syndrome
Functional prepubertal castrate
Enzymatic defects involving testosterone biosynthesis
5α-reductase deficiency
LH-gonadotropin resistant testis
Male pseudohermaphroditism involving androgen receptor defects
Mumps orchitis
Cryptorchidism
Leprosy
Testicular irradiation
Autoimmune testicular failure
Chemotherapy
Secondary hypogonadism
Hypogonadotropic hypogonadism
Isolated LH or FSH deficiency
Acquired gonadotropin deficiencies
Prolactin-secreting pituitary tumors
Severe systemic illness
Uremia
Hemochromatosis
Combined primary and secondary etiology
Aging
Hepatic cirrhosis
Sickle cell disease
FSH—follicle-stimulating hormone; LH—luteinizing hormone.

TABLE 2 MANIFESTATIONS OF TESTICULAR ANDROGEN FAILURE
Testicular failure occurring prior to onset of puberty: clinical characteristics
Testes < 2.5 cm long, volume < 5 mL
Penis < 3–5 cm long
Lack of scrotal pigmentation and rugae
Peripheral subcutaneous fat distribution over hips, face, and 0chest
Enuchoidal skeletal proportions: crown:pubis and pubis:floor ratio < 1
Arm span 6 cm > height (Normally, black men have a decreased crown:pubis and pubis:floor ratio and a longer arm span than white men)
Female escutcheon
No terminal facial hair, decreased body hair
No temporal hair recession
High-pitched voice
Decreased muscle mass
Delayed bone age
Small prostate
Crosshatching over skin lateral to the orbits
Decreased libido
Osteoporosis later in life
Postpubertal testicular failure: clinical characteristics
Normal skeletal proportions and penile length
Loss of libido
Decrease in strength and muscle mass
Normal distribution of pubic hair
Testes are soft; volume < 15 mL
Prostate is adult size, although may be smaller
No change in voice
Diminished aggressiveness
Decreased amount of axillary and pubic hair
Osteoporosis later in life

Because male infertility is common, with varicocele present in 30% to 40% of this population, the overall incidence of primary hypogonadism in men is high [2].

Klinefelter's Syndrome

The phenotypic manifestations of Klinefelter's syndrome are classic for men in whom all cells carry an XXY karyotype. However, the genetic pattern of many men with Klinefelter's syndrome is mosaic, in which only a portion of their cells have the XXY constitution and the remainder have a normal XY karyotype. In these cases, the XXY cells arise from chromosomal nondisjunction after fertilization. Before puberty, the only consistent finding in Klinefelter's syndrome is a testicular volume of less than 1.5 mL [3,4]. Regardless of age, the most characteristic finding in Klinefelter's syndrome (and most other forms of congenital primary hypogonadism) is a decreased testicular volume. This finding is thought to result from the absence of germ cells, whereas in the normal prepubertal testes and in secondary hypogonadism, primary germ cells are present. Before the age of normal puberty, gonadotropin levels are normal; however, after the age at which puberty would normally occur, gonadotropins become elevated in spite of an increase in testosterone (Fig. 2) [5•,6,7]. Also after puberty, gynecomastia occurs to varying degrees. The reason for the gynecomastia is in part the elevated estradiol levels in these men, but because a part of the gynecomastia results from stromal hyperplasia, which is not estrogen dependent as is the ductal tissue, other factors not yet identified must also be responsible. In addition to the gynecomastia and small testes, after puberty, abnormal skeletal proportions manifest by exaggerated growth of the lower extremities that results in a decreased crown:pubis and pubis:floor ratio, as is seen in other prepubertal forms of hypogonadism. In these forms, absence of androgen activity results in a delay of epiphyseal closure. However, in Klinefelter's syndrome, unlike other prepubertal eunuchoidal measurements, in which the arm span is often 6 cm greater than the height, the arm span is not greater than the height.

In Klinefelter's syndrome, muscle mass may appear normal; however, because of decreased androgen activity, strength is decreased (Fig. 3). Similar findings usually pertain to beard growth, although the amount of facial hair growth may be variable. The prostate is prepubertal in Klinefelter's syndrome but does increase in size with testosterone treatment [8]. Of further note, with age, the clinical appearance of hypogonadism tends to be more prominent, and testosterone levels decrease more than is seen with the usual aging process.

Diagnosis

Laboratory findings in Klinefelter's syndrome include testosterone levels that are low or in the lower range of normal because of the decreased testosterone production rates (Fig. 2) [5•]. In addition, the elevated sex hormone–binding globulin levels lead to a further decrease in serum free testosterone levels [6]. Luteinizing hormone and follicle-stimulating hormone levels are uniformly elevated, regardless of the serum testosterone level (Fig. 2) [5•]. In the complete form of Klinefelter's syndrome, no sperm is produced [9]. In some mosaic forms of the disease, fertility may be possible, although most of these men have spermatogenesis seen only in testicular biopsy [9]. In addition to the findings of hypogonadism in Klinefelter's syndrome, decreased intellectual development and antisocial behavior have been noted with high frequency [8]. These findings are not seen in other hypogonadal states and therefore are thought to be a manifestation of the XXY chromosome constitution. Further evidence that it is not simply the androgen deficiency that is the reason for the mental deficiency are the studies demonstrating that by the age of 7 years, boys with the XXY constitution have a significant reduction in their verbal abilities when compared with age-matched controls [10]. Other areas of psychiatric dysfunction, such as the personality traits of timidity, introspective behavior, and decreased social drive, are more common in all hypogonadal men and improve with androgen therapy [11]. Sexual drive is decreased, and no increased incidence of homosexual orientation has been described.

As we noted earlier, various mosaic forms of Klinefelter's syndrome result in different degrees of phenotypic presentation. In addition, as the number of X chromosomes increases, for example, XXXY, the manifestations become more pronounced, especially those related to intellectual dysfunction. For more complete discussion of these variants, refer to the article by Plymate and Paulsen [5•].

The treatment of Klinefelter's syndrome and other prepubertal hypogonadal problems is aimed at both the androgenic and spermatogenic functions of the testes. Because in the diseases associated with primary testicular failure gonadotropins are already elevated and therefore no significant testicular response can occur to gonadotrophin replacement, treatment

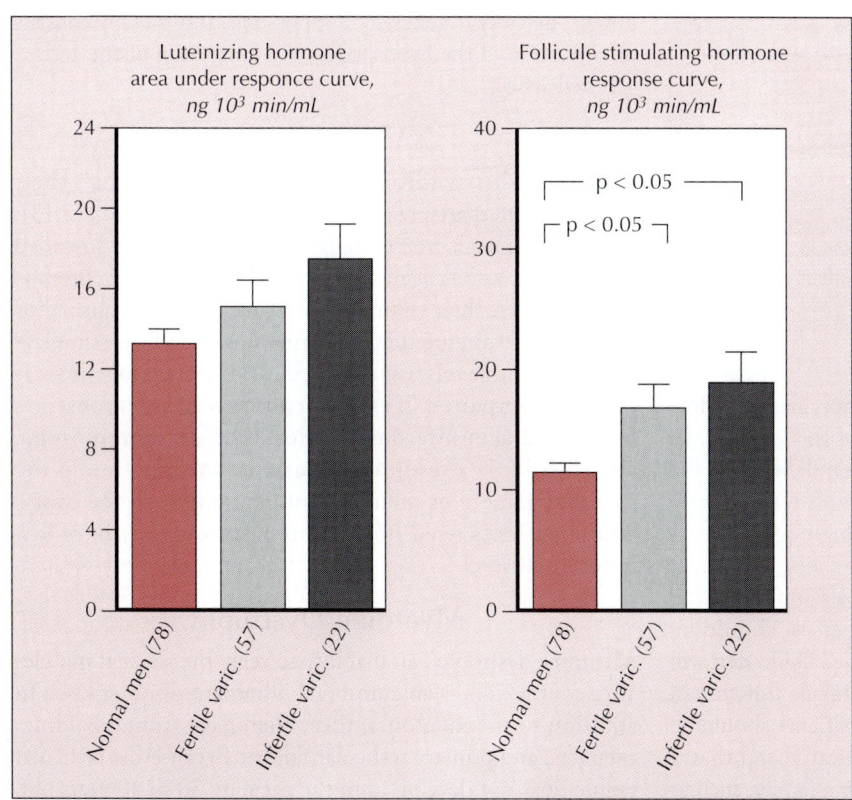

Figure 1 Exaggerated luteinizing hormone and follicle-stimulating hormone response to gonadotropin releasing hormone in fertile and infertile men with a varicocele are compared with normal men, suggesting impairment of both seminiferous tubule and Leydig cell function. (*From* Nagao *et al.* [44]; with permission.)

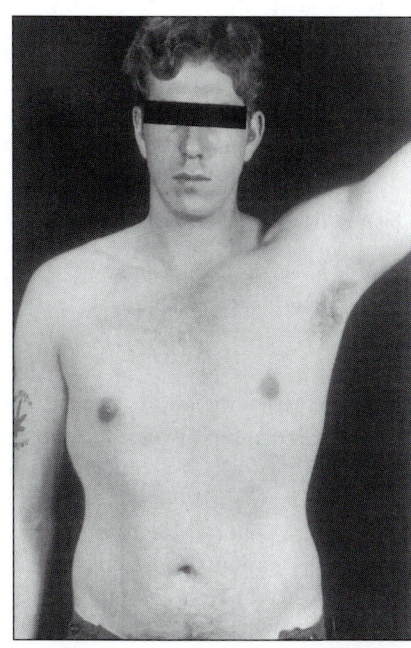

Figure 2 Patient with Klinefelter's syndrome (XXY karyotype). Note the relatively normal masculine appearance except for gynecomastia.

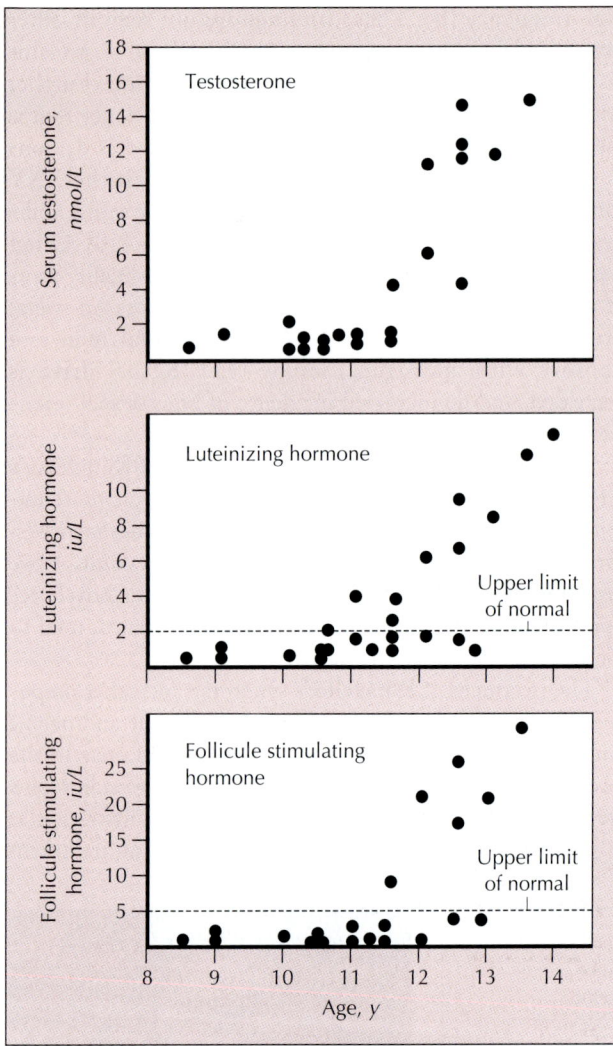

FIGURE 3 Change in serum gonadotropins and testosterone in men with Klinefelter's syndrome as they are followed through puberty. Note the lack of differentiation from normal values until after puberty has supervened. (*From* Ratcliffe [10]; with permission.)

involves replacing the missing testosterone. Specifics of androgen replacement are discussed at the end of this chapter. In general, in any form of prepubertal androgen deficiency, the man has not gone through puberty, and with testosterone replacement, puberty and all of its psychologic adjustments occurs [11]. Patients should be counseled about this effect before testosterone replacement. If they have a significant other person with whom they are living, that person should be included in the session and told of the increased libido that will be present in their partner. The semiferous tubule function of spermatogenesis cannot be corrected, and patients should be advised that they will most likely remain infertile and that if they desire children, other methods of having a family, such as adoption or donor insemination, should be considered.

XX Males

A patient with an XX chromosomal constitution may appear as a normal woman, a woman with gonadal dysgenesis, a true hermaphrodite, or a male with gonadal dysgenesis. This latter group appear to proceed through puberty, but similar to patients with Klinefelter's syndrome, after puberty have small testes, infertility, and gynecomastia. Testosterone levels are low to low-normal, and gonadotropins are normal; however, once the normal age of puberty has been reached, gonadotropins increase and remain elevated. The XX men with gonadal dysgenesis tend to be shorter than normal men, have eunuchoidal body proportions, and hypospadias. The cause of the chromosome abnormalities in most men with this syndrome is an X-to-Y translocation, with only a portion of the Y chromosome present in one of the X chromosomes. The incidence of this abnormality is 1 in 10,000 births [5•]. As with Klinefelter's syndrome, these men have irreversible infertility. Treatment involves androgen replacement and correction of the hypospadias.

XY/XO Mixed Gonadal Dysgenesis

Individuals with 45XO/46XY karyotypes may appear phenotypically male but more often are phenotypically female [12]. The gonads as usually intra-abdominal and may be either streak or dysgenetic. Depending on the timing of the arrested intrauterine development, a paramesonephric duct may be present, and a rudimentary uterus is often present. In phenotypic males, hypospadias is commonly present. Treatment of these men consists of removal of any intra-abdominal dysgenetic gonads because of the 20% chance of malignancy (dysgerminoma, gonadoblastoma, or embryonal cell carcinoma). Fertility is generally not possible, and therapy consists of correction of the hypospadias and correction of the androgen deficiency.

XYY Syndrome

Men with this syndrome are markedly taller than their normal counterparts, with a mean height of 189 cm [12,13]. In spite of their increased height, they are not the so-called super males, as has been suggested by their extra Y chromosome. Rather, their serum testosterone levels are normal or decreased, serum luteinizing hormone and follicle-stimulating hormone levels are elevated, and spermatogenesis is markedly impaired. Testicular biopsy may demonstrate hyalinized seminiferous tubules. The sex chromosome abnormality is a result of meiotic nondisjunction in the paternal gamete or meiotic nondisjunction in the ovary. These patients need no treatment unless they have low testosterone levels.

Myotonic Dystrophy

Myotonic dystrophy, an inability to relax the striated muscles after contraction, is an autosomal dominant disorder [14]. In addition to the myotonia, these men have frontal balding, cataracts, and primary testicular failure. Because the testicular failure does not develop until the men are 30 to 40 years old, the genetic disorder can be transmitted from father to son. It does not occur in women and is thought to be carried on the pseudoautosomal portion of the Y chromosome. Recent data suggest that testosterone replacement may be of some benefit to maintaining strength in these men.

Sertoli-Cell-Only (del Castillo's) Syndrome

Sertoli-cell-only syndrome is suspected in infertile men with azoospermia, small testes, and elevated follicle-stimulating hormone level. However, the diagnosis can be made only with a testicular biopsy result in which there is an absence of germ cells, thus the term *Sertoli-cell-only*. Serum testosterone levels are usually normal, although the response to human chorionic gonadotropin is decreased, and the serum luteinizing hormone levels tend to cluster in the upper range of normal [15]. The etiology of this syndrome is not known. Because serum testosterone levels are normal, no androgen replacement is necessary, and no treatment is available for the infertility.

Other Syndromes

Other syndromes associated with primary hypogonadism include the functional prepubertal castrate (vanishing testis syndrome) and enzymatic defects involving testosterone biosynthesis. The mode of inheritance and clinical and laboratory findings for the latter disorders are presented in Table 3.

5α-Reductase Deficiency

5α-Reductase deficiency is a generalized deficiency in the enzyme responsible for the reduction of the double bond in the A ring of testosterone that results in the lack of conversion of testosterone to dihydrotestosterone [16]. Dihydrotestoterone is responsible for the development of the scrotum, prostate, and testes. As a result of this defect, the men, of normal XY karyotype, appear as girls until the time of puberty because of a bifid scrotum, severe hypospadias, and a phallus that may appear as an enlarged clitoris (Fig. 4). However, at that time, the testes begin to produce a normal amount of testosterone, and the men take on a normal male appearance, hence the term *penis at 12* syndrome. At this time, because androgen receptors are normal and testosterone levels increase to normal adult levels, there is a decrease in subcutaneous fat, an increase in muscle mass, and phallic enlargement. The prostate remains rudimentary, the scrotum does not develop, and because of the severe hypospadias, a perineal urethra is present. Sperm production is either absent or markedly impaired because of decreased testicular dihydrotestosterone and abdominal testes.

The serum levels of testosterone in these individuals are either normal or slightly elevated, serum dihydrotestosterone levels are decreased significantly, and after puberty, the gonadotropin levels are mildly elevated. Diagnosis is made on the basis of the testosterone:dihydrotestosterone ratios [17]. After puberty, the ratio of testosterone:dihydrotestosterone is less than 20:1 in normal men and greater than 35:1 in men with the syndrome. Before puberty, the diagnosis is made after human chorionic gonadotropin stimulation. Normal boys maintain a ratio of 20:1 or less after stimulation, whereas this ratio increases to greater than 50:1 after stimulation in boys with 5α-reductase deficiency.

If at puberty the diagnosis has been previously unknown, a treatment decision may need to be made as to what sexual identity will make the individual most comfortable. This choice may depend on the severity of hypospadias, and, if the testes are in their usual intra-abdominal position, how the person will react to the cancer-preventing castration. In addition to the corrective surgery, if the man is to continue to be male after removal of the testes, then androgen replacement will need to be given. If the female sex is selected, after appropriate surgery, estrogen treatment is appropriate.

TABLE 3 MODE OF INHERITANCE AND CHARACTERIZATION OF ENZYME DEFECTS IN TESTOSTERONE PRODUCTION

Defects	Inheritance	Genitalia	Pubertal development	Hormone status
20,22-Desmolase	AR	Ambiguous	None	↑ LH, FSH ↓ Cortisol ↓ Mineralocorticoids ↓ Androgens
3β-ol dehydrogenase	AR	Male hypospadias	None or poor	↑ or normal LH, FSH ↓ Cortisol ↓ Androgens ↓ Mineralocorticoids
17α-hydroxylase	AR	Ambiguous	None or poor	↓ LH, ↑ FSH ↓ Androgens ↓ Cortisol ↑ Mineralocorticoids
17,20-Desmolase	AR	Male	Genitalia are prepubertal	T, LH, FSH 17-OH progesterone Normal cortisol
17-Ketosteroid reductase	AR	Female or ambiguous	Partial puberty	↓ T ↑ LH, FSH ↑ 17-OH progesterone Normal cortisol

AR—autosomal recessive; FSH—follicle-stimulating hormone; LH—luteinizing hormone; OH—hydroxycorticosteroid; T—testosterone.

Male Pseudohermaphrodism Resulting from Defects in the Androgen Receptor

Androgens enter their target cells and initiate activity by binding to the C-terminal androgen binding domain of the nuclear androgen receptor; subsequently, androgen activity is generated by transcription at the appropriate DNA binding domain of the androgen receptor. Several clinical syndromes have been described that result from defects in the androgen receptor. These defects usually result from point mutations in the hormone binding domain. These defects have been reviewed by McPhaul and coworkers [18••].

Testicular Feminization

Classically, patients with testicular feminization have no detectable binding of dihydrotestoterone to a high-affinity receptor, thereby resulting in a complete loss of androgen activity; however, the testosterone may still be converted to estrogen [19]. The chromosomal constitution of these men is XY. Because of the lack of androgen activity, they develop with the phenotypic appearance of a normal female. At puberty, because of the increase in serum estrogens from the conversion of testosterone to estradiol, these patients develop breast tissue and have female subcutaneous fat distribution [20]. Their physical examination demonstrates a normal clitoris and external genitalia, whereas on pelvic examination, a blind vaginal pouch exists. The testes may be present in the labia or may be palpated within the abdomen. Occasionally, they will be found in the canal of Nuck, when they appear as an inguinal hernia. Because these men have a normal XY karyotype, they produce antimüllerian hormone, and no müllerian structures are present. Serum levels of testosterone are normal or slightly elevated, and because of the lack of androgen feedback on the pituitary and hypothalamus, luteinizing hormone and follice-stimulating hormone levels are elevated.

In this classic form of the syndrome, the patients have been raised as female, and the syndrome is not recognized until they are evaluated for amenorrhea or a testicle is found at the time of hernia repair. Because these individuals have been raised as females, and because no treatment exists for the infertility, it is usually best to continue the female sex assignment. The testes should be removed because of the increased risk of malignancy. Because the estrogen in these women comes primarily from the peripheral conversion of testosterone to estradiol, after castration, the patient will need estrogen replacement.

Reifenstein's Syndrome

Reifenstein's syndrome, like testicular feminization, results from a defect in the androgen receptor that causes a partial rather than complete lack of sensitivity to androgens [18••]. The receptor defect appears to be heterogeneous because receptor binding studies have revealed decreased receptor numbers in some cases, whereas others show a decreased affinity or stability of the receptor [21]. Some families may have an X-linked or autosomal recessive form of the syndrome.

Phenotypically, these individuals appear as males with an XY karyotype. They have varying degrees of pseudohermaphrodism ranging from hypospadias and undescended testes to a urogenital sinus with a perineal opening to the urethra and complete lack of scrotal fusion. As adults, they have decreased

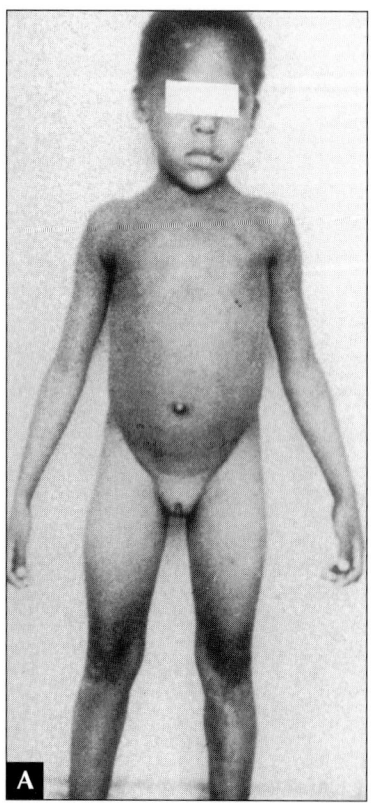
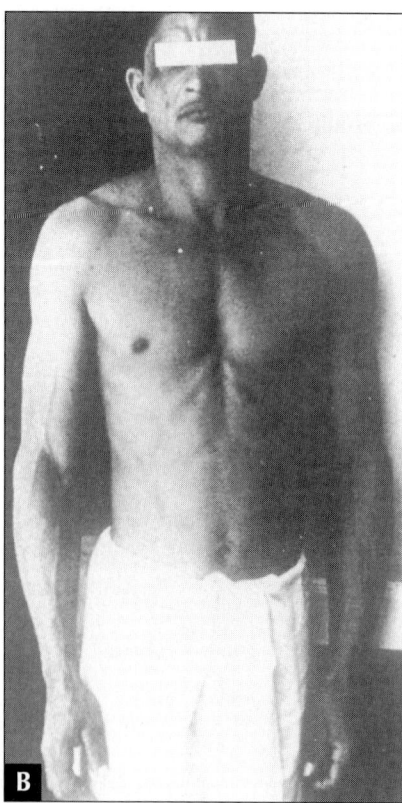

FIGURE 4 Two patients with 5α-reductase deficiencies. **A**, Before puberty, the patient presents as a phenotypic female. **B**, After puberty, a normal male body habitus develops. Note the muscular development and masculine appearance in response to endogenous testosterone. (*From* Peterson [17]; with permission.)

androgen-initiated hair growth and decreased muscle mass. Serum testosterone and gonadotropin levels are elevated. Because of the partial nature of the defect, the changes in the serum hormones are not as great as those seen in complete testicular feminization.

One of the difficulties with Reifenstein's syndrome as compared with testicular feminization is that of gender selection. Unlike their more severe counterparts, these men are not completely feminized and usually appear as males. Although they respond to very high doses of testosterone enanthate (400 mg/wk) the response is only partial. Therefore, psychologic support, as well as surgical correction of hypospadias, is important. As with testicular feminization, abdominal testes need to be removed.

Postpubertal Orchitis

After puberty, mumps are associated with clinical orchitis in 25% of cases. In addition, when a man presents with azoospermia and a history of mumps after puberty without a clinical history of orchitis, assuming he demonstrates no signs of prepubertal testicular failure, the etiology can usually be assumed to be orchitis. Of men who have a history of mumps orchitis, 60% are infertile [22]. The usual laboratory finding along with decreased spermatogenesis is a monotropic increase in follicle-stimulating hormone. However, as the time since orchitis is increased, there is an increased incidence of decreased testosterone and increased luteinizing hormone levels, suggesting involvement of the Leydig cells. No treatment is available for the infertility. If testosterone is decreased, testosterone replacement is appropriate.

Cryptorchidism

Up to 10% of men are cryptorchid at birth; however, 70% to 90% of these testes descend into the scrotum, and after puberty, the incidence of undescended testes is 0.3% to 0.4%. In addition, as we have described, undescended testes are a prominent aspect of many congenital syndromes that result in hypogonadism [23]. Cryptorchidism is associated with a 70% incidence of infertility. Treatment of cryptorchidism consists of surgically moving the undescended testicle (or testicles) into the scrotum, which decreases the 8% chance of malignancy associated with the abdominal testis, and if done early (before age 5 years), improves the chances of fertility. Unilateral cryptorchidism is also associated with infertility but to a lesser extent than bilateral disease. The treatment is the same in both cases.

Testicular Trauma

Obviously, the traumatic loss of both testes results in hypogonadism requiring testosterone replacement. In addition, a common reason for loss of a testis is testicular torsion. In addition, the torsion of a testis may have an effect (possibly immune) on the opposite testis, resulting in infertility.

Testicular Irradiation

Irradiation of the testes results from the treatment of associated diseases, such as Hodgkin's disease or prostatic carcinoma [24]. A dose as low as 15 cGy causes a significant decrease in sperm count, and by 50 cGy, azoospermia occurs. In general, the decrease in sperm production resolves until the dose reaches 400 cGy, after which the infertility is irreversible. If the dose increases to greater than 800 cGy, involvement of both the germ cells and Leydig cells occurs. Treatment of irradiation-induced Leydig cell failure is testosterone replacement, except in the case of prostate carcinoma, when it is contraindicated. If the man is of reproductive age and fertility may be desired, sperm should be obtained for this purpose before the radiation treatment.

Chemotherapy

Similar to irradiation, chemotherapy also results in seminiferous tubule failure depending on dose. Leydig cell failure may result in some cases. The appearance of gynecomastia may be an indication that Leydig cell failure has occurred. Treatment should be aimed at androgen therapy, and if appropriate, sperm should be saved before treatment.

Autoimmune Testicular Failure

Two types of autoimmune testicular failure occur. The most common of these is caused by antisperm antibodies. Most commonly, these antibodies appear after a vasovasostomy and infertility continues, despite the presence of normal sperm in the ejaculate [25]. The antisperm antibodies are IgA class in the ejaculate and IgG in the serum.

A second and much less common form of autoimmune testicular failure is caused by IgG antibodies directed at the microsomal fraction of the Leydig cell [22]. These antibodies against steroid-producing cells are more commonly produced in women with idiopathic ovarian failure; however, they are occasionally seen as a cause of primary Leydig cell failure in men. Again, treatment is aimed at replacement of testosterone.

SECONDARY HYPOGONADISM

Hypogonadotropic Hypogonadism

Hypogonadotropic hypogonadism may be caused by acquired or congenital defects. The clinical presentation depends on whether the onset of the disease has occurred before or after puberty. The distinction as to time of onset has been described in Table 2. As described earlier, secondary hypogonadotropic hypogonadism should be suspected when the end-organ products, testosterone or sperm count, are low and no increase in luteinizing hormone or follicle-stimulating hormone occurs. Because both testosterone and inhibin are involved in negative feedback on follicle-stimulating hormone, sperm counts can be markedly decreased, and follicle-stimulating hormone does not increase because of the presence of normal serum levels of testosterone, when the primary defect in the sperm production is in the testes. Therefore, as a practical matter, except for the suspicion of isolated follicle-stimulating hormone deficiency, both testosterone and sperm counts should be decreased before secondary hypogonadism is suspected. In the case of pituitary tumors, an elevation in serum prolactin with low sperm count and a normal testosterone level is also indicative of a secondary hypogonadism. A major difference in the hypogonadotropic syndromes versus those of primary gonadal failure is that spermatogenesis can often be restored in the secondary syndromes by replacement of gonadotropins or gonadotropin releasing hormone.

Classic Hypogonadotropic Hypogonadism (Kallman's Syndrome)

This syndrome is a congenital disorder manifested by isolated luteinizing hormone and follicle-stimulating hormone deficiency and hyposmia or anosmia resulting from defective development of the olfactory bulbs. Other associated findings are midline defects including cleft palate, cerebellar seizures, a short fourth metacarpal, and cardiac abnormalities [26,27].

The syndrome may result from an isolated mutation or an inherited form of the disease. The inherited forms are most often autosomal dominant, although some families demonstrate autosomal recessive or X-linked modes of inheritance. Most cases, however, result from isolated mutations.

The incidence of the syndrome is 1 in 10,000 male births. The men present as prepubertal eunuchs. Beard growth is minimal. Most patients maintain their prepubertal subcutaneous distribution of body fat. Hyposmia or anosmia is present in most of the individuals but may be missed unless specifically tested by appropriate olfactory sensing materials, such as various molar concentrations of pyridine, thiopene, and nitrobenzene [28]. The testes tend to be prepubertal, although in some patients, a modest increase in testicular size exists at the time of normal puberty. However, unlike Klinefelter's syndrome, the testes are not small in the prepubertal boys with Kallman's syndrome, because normal numbers of basal spermatogonia are present.

Serum hormones reveal low levels of testosterone, luteinizing hormone, and follicle-stimulating hormone. In some subjects, if frequent serum samples are collected over a 24-hour period for the measurement of luteinizing hormone, an occasional pulse of gonadotropin is seen. When a single bolus of gonadotropin releasing hormone is administered, the rise in luteinizing hormone and follicle-stimulating hormone is low. However, if appropriate pulses of gonadotropin releasing hormone are administered, serum luteinizing hormone and follicle-stimulating hormone levels may return to normal [29]. These studies indicate that the primary defect in these individuals is at the level of the hypothalamus rather than the pituitary.

Approximately 10% of men with hypogonadotropic hypogonadism have partial progression through puberty [29]. This can make the differential diagnosis between a physiologic delay in puberty and hypogonadotropism difficult. Currently, no reliable tests exist to differentiate these disorders in a boy up to the age of 19. However, if puberty has not begun by the age of 19 or 20 years, then hypogonadotropic hypogonadism should be considered.

Treatment of the syndrome includes androgen replacement with exogenous testosterone. When fertility is desired, the testosterone is stopped and gonadotropin replacement is undertaken. This therapy can be achieved with the combination of luteinizing hormone (human chorionic gonadotropin) and follicle-stimulating hormone or gonadotropin releasing hormone [29,30]. However, these methods are much more expensive and cumbersome for androgen replacement therapy alone, and once fertility is not needed, treatment should be converted to testosterone replacement.

Many congenital syndromes also have hypogonadotropic hypogonadism as a part of the syndrome complex. Most of these syndromes are associated with severe neurologic damage and mental retardation. These syndromes are listed in Table 4.

Isolated Deficiency of Luteinizing or Follicle-Stimulating Hormone

Isolated deficiency of luteinizing hormone has been termed the *fertile eunuch* syndrome [31]. This term was suggested because the men were androgen deficient but supposedly had enough follicle-stimulating hormone secretion to maintain

Table 4 Syndromes Associated with Congenital Gonadotropin Deficiency

Syndrome	Typical features
Lowe	Fanconi syndrome, cataracts, glaucoma, bupthalmus, hypotonia, and mental retardation
Multiple lentigines (leopard syndrome)	Generalized lentigines, sensorineural hearing loss, hypertelorism, short stature, and pulmonic stenosis
Rud	Hyposmia, congenital icthyosis, mental retardation, and epilepsy
CHARGE	Coloboma, heart disease, atresia of the choanae, and retarded growth and development
Steroid sulfatase deficiency	Hypogonadism associated with steroid sulfatase and arylsulfatase-C deficiency, congenital icthyosis, nystagmus, strabismus, decreased visual acuity, hypopigmentation of the iris, unilateral renal hypoplasia or agenesis, and hypogonadotropic hypogonadism
Martsolf	Short stature, severe mental retardation, mainly of Jewish ancestry, and X-linked or autosomal recessive inheritance
Rothmund-Thomson	Hypodontia, soft tissue contractures, short stature, anemia, and osteogenic sarcoma
Börjeson-Forssman-Lehmann	Prominent supraorbital ridges, ptosis, large ears, hypotonia, and severe mental retardation
Laurence-Moon-Biedl	Retinitis pigmentosa, polydactyly, mental retardation, and Sertoli-cell-only syndrome

fertility. Clearly, without adequate intratesticular levels of testosterone, fertility would not be possible. It is more likely that isolated luteinizing hormone deficiency with fertility occurs in men with hypogonadotropic hypogonadism with some residual follicle-stimulating hormone secretion. When treated with human chorionic gonadotropin, they become fertile but are not fertile without this treatment. Another group of men who may fit this syndrome are older men who have fathered children and maintain spermatogenesis but have lower than normal testosterone levels without an increase in luteinizing hormone. These men most likely fall on the curve of normal aging.

Isolated follicle-stimulating hormone deficiency has also been reported [32]. These men are normally androgenized but have decreased or absent sperm in their ejaculate without concomitant increases in follicle-stimulating hormone.

Acquired Forms of Gonadotropin Deficiency

Many acquired disorders may cause gonadotropin deficiency (Table 5). The deficiency may be caused either by compression and destruction of tissue, such as may occur with granulomatous diseases, or by pituitary tumors secreting other hormones that inhibit gonadotropin secretion, such as prolactin, cortisol, or corticotropin releasing hormone. As in other forms of hypogonadism, the clinical appearance of these individuals depends on whether the hypogonadism occurred before or after puberty. Patients with large, space-occupying lesions may also have other anterior pituitary hormones affected, and care must be taken to do a complete evaluation of the anterior pituitary hormone complement in these subjects, especially because deficiencies of corticotropin and thyroid-stimulating hormone may have profound effects on these individuals' well being.

Prolactin-Secreting Pituitary Adenomas

Whereas prolactin-secreting pituitary adenomas are usually detected in women as microadenomas less than 10 mm in size because of amenorrhea and galactorrhea, in men, over 80% of the tumors are macroadenomas by the time they are detected. This difference occurs either because of the lack of early signs and symptoms or the fact that in men, prolactinomas are more aggressive lesions [33]. However, little evidence exists for the latter explanation.

Because there is a decrease in testosterone and sperm production with microadenomas, it is unlikely a mass effect from the tumor is causing the hypogonadism. Rather, a direct effect of the prolactin or an increase in a neurotransmitter, such as dopamine or gamma aminobutyrate on the pituitary or hypothalamus may account for the decrease in luteinizing hormone and follicle-stimulating hormone secretory activity [34].

Diagnosis and treatment are covered more extensively in the chapter on pituitary tumors. However, although dopamine agonists such as bromocriptine decrease tumor size and prolactin levels to normal, they may not restore testosterone and sperm production to normal, and testosterone or gonadotropin replacement may be necessary to restore these functions [35].

Severe Systemic Illness

Severe stress or injury rapidly lowers serum testosterone and gonadotropin levels. Even if the serum binding protein for testosterone is decreased, free levels of serum testosterone remain low [36]. This effect appears to result from an effect on gonadotropin secretion with a decrease in immunoreactive luteinizing hormone as well as an even greater decrease in biologically active serum luteinizing hormone. Whether replacement of testosterone in these men will improve their catabolic processes associated with disease and increase survival or be detrimental to their recovery is not known.

COMBINED PRIMARY AND SECONDARY HYPOGONADISM

Aging

Whereas women have a well-demarcated loss of gonadal function with age, that is, menopause, the changes in men are far less dramatic. Initial studies designed to determine if a decrease in gonadal function occurs in men with age demonstrated a significant decline in testosterone [37••]. However, many of these initial studies were performed in men with coexisting diseases that in themselves could lower testosterone. Subsequent studies in healthy men could find no age-related decrease in testosterone. Recent studies examining frequent samples of testosterone obtained throughout the day have shown that a significant decline in testosterone occurs as healthy men age [38]. The decline in free testosterone appears

TABLE 5 ETIOLOGIES OF ACQUIRED GONADOTROPIN DEFICIENCY

Conditions that often occur before puberty
Craniopharyngioma
Eosinophilic granuloma

Conditions that usually occur after puberty
Functioning pituitary adenomas
   Prolactinoma
   Growth hormone-secreting tumor
   Corticotropin-secreting tumor
Nonfunctioning pituitary tumors
   Chromophobe adenoma
   Sarcoma
   Irradiation
Granulomatous disease: eosinophilic granuloma, sarcoidosis, tuberculosis
Tumors metastasized to the pituitary
Pituitary abscess
Pituitary apoplexy, often with the degeneration of a pituitary tumor or cyst
Postpartum pituitary hemorrhage: Sheehan's syndrome
Arteriovenous malformations
Hemochromatosis
Autoimmune pituitary hypophysitis

to be greater than the decline in total testosterone because with age, in addition to the declining testosterone-secretory capacity of the testes, an age-related increase also occurs in sex hormone–binding globulin.

Studies have shown that the reason for the decline in gonadal function with age is multifactorial and includes an increased negative feedback capacity of testosterone on luteinizing hormone secretion, decreased gonadotropin response to gonadotropin releasing hormone, and decreased testicular response to human chorionic gonadotropin [39]. Overall, associated with the decrease in testosterone with age is an increase in luteinizing hormone and follicle-stimulating hormone, suggesting that a primary testicular defect is predominant.

Treatment of the older, otherwise healthy man with testosterone has not as yet been shown to be beneficial in most cases. One exception would be the older man with osteoporosis and a decreased testosterone level. Although impotence is common in the older man, and testosterone levels are decreased in this population, treatment with testosterone does not improve their potency in most cases. In addition, the high incidence of prostate cancer in these men may put them at an additional risk for testosterone therapy.

Hepatic Cirrhosis

Both cirrhosis and ethanol intoxication affect testicular function. One pathway for ethanol's acute effect on testicular function is its higher affinity for alcohol dehydrogenase than for retinol, which prevents formation of retinoic acid. When this occurs, at a serum ethanol level of 0.10 mg/dL, testosterone production is decreased and serum luteinizing hormone level increases [40]. These findings revert to normal soon after serum ethanol levels return to normal.

Long-term ingestion of ethanol resulting in cirrhosis of the liver increases serum estradiol and sex hormone–binding globulin. The increased estradiol levels result in decreased gonadotropin levels and lower serum testosterone. In addition, elevated sex hormone-binding globulin levels decrease free testosterone levels even further.

Sickle Cell Disease

Men with sickle cell disease often appear to have characteristics of prepubertal hypogonadism [41]. They display eunuchoidal skeletal proportions and have decreased muscle mass and small testes. However, black patients have skeletal proportions that may be normal for their race (Table 2). Some men with this disease do have low serum testosterone levels and inappropriately normal serum gonadotropin levels, which suggests a secondary form of hypogonadism; however, because they also display an abnormal response to human chorionic gonadotropic, some form of primary testicular dysfunction also occurs.

Hemochromatosis

In this disease, which is manifested by iron overload, both secondary and primary elements of gonadal failure may occur that in some individuals result from specific organ iron overload and are corrected by iron removal [42].

ANDROGEN REPLACEMENT THERAPY FOR HYPOGONADISM

Androgen replacement benefits the individual in most of the diseases and syndromes that have been described. The benefits include increase in muscle mass and ability to perform physically more demanding tasks. The treatment also results in an overall increase in confidence and feeling of well-being. Finally, libido and sexual activity are increased. The individual must be made aware and counseled about the increase in libido, especially if he is an adult. If he has had prepubertal hypogonadism, the treatment takes him through puberty in a short period of time, and socially he is interacting with a peer group that is not experiencing similar feelings. In addition, his sexual partner also needs to be counseled about the changes that can be expected. This becomes especially important if the couple has been together for a period of time and are comfortably settled into their relationship. In addition to the behavioral changes, physical changes, such as increased beard growth and transient pubertal acne, also occur. Finally, contraindications to androgen therapy need to be considered, including prostate cancer and hypertrophy, sleep apnea, and inappropriate sexual activity in those with such conditions as hypogonadism and mental retardation.

The methods available for androgen replacement are relatively limited at the present time. In the United States, the only available replacements are the intramuscular injection of testosterone esters, such as testosterone enanthate or cypionate scrotal testosterone patches. Esters are given in a dose of 200 to 300 mg intramuscularly every 3 weeks. With this injection schedule, the subject has markedly elevated serum levels of testosterone during the first few days after injection, and the serum levels are well below normal in hypogonadal men. Regardless of these alterations in serum levels of testosterone, this schedule of injections has well maintained normal androgenization in hypogonadal men with no significant side effects. If serum levels in the normal range are desired, injections of 75 to 100 mg weekly are needed. However, most patients prefer the less frequent injection schedule, and no evidence exists that the more frequent schedule offers any significant clinical benefit.

Several newer methods of androgen replacement are in the developmental stage, including transdermal testosterone patches, sublingual tablets, and implants of testosterone pellets [43•]. The transdermal patches have been applied to the scrotum as well as to the back and legs. Patches that need to be applied to the scrotum produce levels of dihydrotestosterone in the serum that are slightly above normal because of the increased level of 5α-reductase in scrotal skin as opposed to nonsexual skin. However, no adverse effects are seen with this mild elevation of dihydrotestosterone. The sublingual tablets contain testosterone bound to cyclodextrins for solubility. The testosterone is absorbed through the buccal mucosa, and the cyclodextrins are eliminated through the gastrointestinal tract. These tablets taken three to four times a day produce spikes of testosterone levels that give a normal total daily dose. Finally, the subcutaneous inserts are effective but require a qualified health professional for insertion.

References and Recommended Reading

Recently published papers of particular interest have been highlighted as:
- Of interest
- •• Of outstanding interest

1. Stanley HL, Schmitt BP, Poses PM, Deiss WP: Does hypogonadism contribute to the occurrence of minimal trauma hip fracture in the older man? *J Am Geriatr Soc* 1991, 39:766–771.
2. Mosher WD: Infertility trends among U.S. couples: 1965–1976. *Family* 1982, 14:22–27.
3. Laron Z, Hochman H: Small testes in prepubertal boys with Klinefelter syndrome. *J Clin Endocrinol Metab* 1971, 32:671–677g.
4. Ratcliffe SG: The sexual development of boys with the chromosome constitution of 47 XXY (Klinefelter's syndrome). *Endocrinol Metab Clin North Am* 1982, 11:703–716.
5. • Plymate SR, Paulsen CA: Klinefelter's syndrome. In *The Genetic Basis of Common Diseases*. Edited by King RA, Rotter JI, Motulsky A. Oxford University Press; 1992:876–894.
6. Plymate SR, Leonard JM, Paulsen CA, *et al.*: Sex hormone-binding globulin changes with androgen replacement. *J Clin Endocrinol Metab* 1983, 57-645–648.
7. Ratcliffe SG, Bancroft J, Axworthy D, McCloren W: Klinefelter's syndrome in adolescence. *Arch Dis Child* 1982, 57:6–12.
8. Swanson DW, Stipes AN: Psychiatric aspects of Klinefelter's syndrome. *Am J Psychiatry* 1969, 126:814–822.
9. Nistal M, Paniagua R, Abaurrea MA, Santamaria L: Hyperplasia and the immature appearance of Sertoli cells in primary testicular disorders. *Hum Pathol* 1982, 13:3–12.
10. Ratcliffe SG: Klinefelter's syndrome in children: a longitudinal study of 47, XXY boys identified by population screening in Klinefelter's syndrome. In *Klinefelter's Syndrome*. Edited by Bandmann HJ, Breit R, Perwein E. New York: Springer-Verlag; 1984:38–47.
11. Becker KL: Clinical and therapeutic experiences with Klinefelter's syndrome. *Fertil Steril* 1972, 23:568–578.
12. Davidoff F, Federman DD: Mixed gonadal dysgenesis. *Pediatrics* 1973, 52:725–738.
13. Phillip J, Lundsteen C, Owen D: The frequency of chromosome aberrations in tall men with special reference to 47,XYY and 47,XXY. *Am J Hum Genet* 1976, 28:404–416.
14. Welle S, Josefowicz R, Forbes G, Griggs RC: Effect of testosterone on metabolic rate and body composition in normal men and men with muscular dystrophy. *J Clin Endocrinol Metab* 1992, 74:332–335.
15. de Kretser DM, Burger HG, Fortune D, *et al.*: Hormonal, histological and chromosomal studies in adult males with testicular disorder. *J Clin Endocrinol Metab* 1972, 35:392–399.
16. Imperato-McGinley JL, Guerrero L, Gautier T, Petersen RC: Steroid 5α-reductase deficiency in man: an inherited form of male pseudohermaphroditism. *Science* 1974, 186:1213–1215.
17. Peterson RE, Imperato-McGinley J, Gauiter T, Sturla E: Male pseudohermaphroditism due to steroid 5α-reductase deficiency. *Am J Med* 1977, 62:170–182.
18. •• McPhaul MJ, Marcelli M, Zoppi S, *et al.*: Genetic basis of endocrine disease: the spectrum of mutations in the androgen receptor gene that causes androgen resistance. *J Clin Endocrinol Metab* 1993, Jan 76:17–23.
19. Kovacs WJ, Griffin JE, Weaver DD, *et al.*: A mutation that causes lability of the androgen receptor under conditions that normally promote transformation to the DNA-binding state. *J Clin Invest* 1984, 73:1095–1103.
20. MacDonald PC, Madden JD, Brenner PF, *et al.*: Origin of estrogen in normal men and in women with testicular feminization. *J Clin Endocrinol Metab* 1979, 49:905–912.
21. Gyorki S, Warne GL, Khalid BAK, Funder JW: Defective nuclear accumulation of androgen receptors in disorders of sexual differentiation. *J Clin Invest* 1983, 72:819.
22. Charney CW: The spermatogenic potential for the undescended testis before and after treatment. *J Urol* 1960, 83:697–703.
23. Rajfer J, Walsh PC: Testicular descent: normal and abnormal. *Urol Clin North Am* 1978, 5:223–230.
24. Clifton DK, Bremner WJ: The effect of testicular x-irradiation on spermatogenesis in man. *J Androl* 1983, 4:387–392.
25. Haas GGJ, Cines DB, Schreiber AD: Immunologic infertility: Identification on patients with antisperm antibody. *N Engl J Med* 1980, 303:722–730.
26. Santen RJ, Paulsen CA: Hypogonatropic eunuchoidism: part 1. Clinical study of the mode of inheritance. *J Clin Endocrinol Metab* 1973, 36:47–53.
27. Schwankhaus JD, Currie J, Jaffe MJ, *et al.*: Neurological findings in men with isolated hypogonadotropic hypogonadism. *Neurology* 1989, 39:223–228.
28. Henkin RF, Barter FC: Olfactory thresholds in normal men and in patients with adrenocortical insufficiency. *J Clin Invest* 1966, 45:1631–1637.
29. Hoffman AR, Crowley WF Jr: Induction of puberty in men by long-term pulsatile administration of low-dose gonadotropin-releasing hormone. *N Engl J Med* 1982, 307:1237–1241.
30. Sherins RJ: Clinical aspects of treatment of male infertility with gonadotropins: testicular response of some men given HCG with and without pergonal. In *Male Infertility and Sterility*. Edited by Mancini RE, Mortini L. New York: New York Academic Press; 1974:545.
31. McCullagh EP, Beck JC, Jones HW: A syndrome of eunuchoidism with spermatogenesis, normal urinary FSH and low or normal ICSH (fertile "eunuchs"). *J Clin Endocrinol Metab* 1953, 13:489–494.
32. Mozaffarian GA, Higley M, Paulsen CA: Clinical studies in an adult male patient with "isolated follicle stimulating hormone (FSH) deficiency." *J Androl* 1983, 4:393–399.
33. Rodman EF, Goodman R: Prolactinomas in males. In *Prolactinomas—Contemporary Issues in Endocrinology and Metabolism*, vol 2. Edited by Olefsky JM, Robbins RI. New York: Churchill Livingston; 1986:115–127.
34. Fuchs E, Mansky T, Stock KW, *et al.*: Involvement of catecholamines and glutamate in gabaergic mechanisms regulatory to luteinizing hormone and prolactin. *Neuroendocrinology* 1984, 38:484–493.
35. Murray FT, Cameron DF, Ketchum C: Return of gonadal function in men with prolactin-secreting pituitary tumors. *J Clin Endocrinol Metab* 1984, 59:79–84.
36. Plymate SR, Vaughan GM, Mason AD Jr, Pruitt BA Jr: Central hypogonadism in burned men. *Horm Res* 1987, 27:152–158.
37. •• Vermeulen A: Androgens in the aging male. *J Clin Endocrinol Metab* 1991, 73:221–226.
38. Bremner WJ, Vitiello MV, Prinz PN: Loss of circadian rhythmicity in blood testosterone levels with aging in normal men. *J Clin Endocrinol Metab* 1983, 56:1278–1285.
39. Tenover JS, Matsumoto AM, Plymate SR, Bremner WJ: The effects of aging in normal men on bioavailable testosterone and luteinizing hormone secretion: response to clomiphene citrate. *J Clin Endocrinol Metab* 1987, 65:1118–1126.
40. Galvao-Teles A, Monteiro E, Gavaler JS, Van Thiel DH: Gonadal consequences of alcohol abuse: lessons from the liver. *Hepatology* 1986, 6:135–142.
41. Landefeld CS, Schambelan M, Kaplan SL, Embury SH: Clomiphene-responsive hypogonadism in sickle cell anemia. *Ann Intern Med* 1983, 99:480–485.
42. Duranteau L, Chanson P, Blumberg-Tick P, Thomas G: Non-responsiveness of serum gonadotropins and testosterone to pulsatile GnRH in hemochromatosis suggesting a pituitary defect. *Acta Endocrinol (Copenh)* 1993, 128:351–354.

43.• Bhasin S: Androgen treatment of hypogonadal men. Clinical review 34. *J Clin Endocrinol Metab* 1992, 74:1221–1225.

44. Nagao RR, Plymate SR, Berger RE, *et al.* Comparison of gonadal function between fertile and infertile men with varicoceles. *Fertil Steril* 1986, 46:930–933.

45. Peterson RE, Impertato-McGinley J, Gautier I, Sturla E: Male pseudohermaphroditism due to steroid 5α-reductase deficiency. *Am J Med* 1977; 62:170.

SELECT BIBLIOGRAPHY

de Kretser DM, Burger HG, Fortune D: Hormonal, histological, and chromosomal studies in adult males with testicular disorders. *J Clin Endocrinol Metab* 1972, 35:392–380.

Plymate SR, Paulsen CA: *Male Hypogonadism in Principles and Practice of Endocrinology and Metabolism.* Edited by Becker KL. Philadelphia: Lippincott 1990:948–970.

Male Reproductive Problems

Shalender Bhasin

> ### Key Points
> - Male infertility is a common medical problem; the cause of infertility is not determinable in most infertile men.
> - Treatable causes of infertility are present in only a small number of infertile men, but most of the diagnostic work-up is directed at identifying these few potentially correctable causes.
> - Impotence is often a multifactorial organic problem; most men presenting with impotence have diabetes, hypertension, or arteriosclerotic disease. Optimization of therapy of coexisting medical problems, exclusion of treatable factors, counseling of the couple, and usage of vacuum devices and intracavernosal injections of prostaglandin E_2 are the cornerstones of the medical management of impotence.
> - Vasectomy and condom usage remain the only available male contraceptives. Hormonal methods, such as androgens and gonadotropin-releasing hormone (Gn-RH) antagonists, have not been shown to effectively inhibit spermatogenesis, but many practical problems remain to be resolved before these agents can be advocated for general use as contraceptives.
> - Vasectomy is a highly effective and safe, but essentially irreversible method of contraception. Microsurgical reversal of vasectomy is possible but does not always restore fertility.

Infertility, impotence, and contraception are common reproductive problems that significantly affect a couple's relationship, reproductive health, and overall quality of life. The practicing internist is often ill prepared to manage these medical problems and is content to refer the patient to a urologist, even though the role of surgery is limited in the treatment of these patients. This chapter presents an algorithmic approach to the management of men with infertility and impotence and an update on the currently available male contraceptive methods, including vasectomy, from a physician's perspective.

MALE INFERTILITY

Infertility, defined as the inability of a couple to achieve pregnancy despite unprotected intercourse for a period of at least 12 months, affects about 15% of couples. In about 33% of these couples, the primary problem resides in the man, in 33% in the woman, and in an additional 33% in both the man and the woman [1–5].

Pathogenesis

Common causes of infertility are listed in Table 1. Several large surveys of infertile men have been published in recent years [4]. Although differences exist in the frequency of various etiologic factors in surveys from different centers, based in part on the patient referral patterns, the nature and extent of investigation, and geography, salient features stand out.

Table 1. Major etiologic diagnoses in infertile men

Diagnosis	Incidence, %
Idiopathic infertility	60–80
Primary testicular failure	8–10
(Chromosomal disorders including Klinefelter's syndrome, undescended testes, irradiation, orchitis, drugs)	
Genital tract obstruction	5
(Congenital absence of vas, vasectomy, epididymal obstruction)	
Coital disorders	1
Hypogonadotropic hypogonadism	<1
(Pituitary adenomas, panhypopituitarism, idiopathic hypogonadotropic hypogonadism, hyperprolactinemia)	
Varicocele*	15–35
Others	5
(Sperm autoimmunity, drugs, toxins, systemic illness)	

Adapted from Baker *et al.* [4]; with permission.
*Although the prevalence of varicocele in infertile men is higher than in general population, it is not known whether the presence of varicocele causes or contributes to infertility.

- Male infertility is a heterogeneous group of disorders. A specific cause of infertility is not determinable in most men.
- Fifteen percent to 20% of infertile men are azoospermic. An additional 10% are severely oligozoospermic (sperm density less than 1 million/mL). The prognosis for fertility in these men is very poor.
- Correctable or treatable causes, such as gonadotropin deficiency and obstruction, are present only in a small number of men.
- Most infertile men have idiopathic oligospermia or male factor infertility.
- Although varicoceles are present in 10% to 35% of infertile men, their role, if any, in the pathogenesis of male infertility remains controversial.

Diagnosis

History

The man and the woman should be evaluated simultaneously. The history should focus on duration of infertility, previous evidence of fertility in the man or the woman, contraceptive use, sexual function, frequency and timing of intercourse in relation to the menstrual cycle, pubertal development, shaving frequency, hair loss, and hair distribution. A history of scrotal trauma, genitourinary infection, scrotal surgery or inguinal surgery may be pertinent. Details of other medical problems and medications should be obtained.

Physical examination

The physical examination should focus on body proportions (height-to-span and upper segment to lower segment ratios);

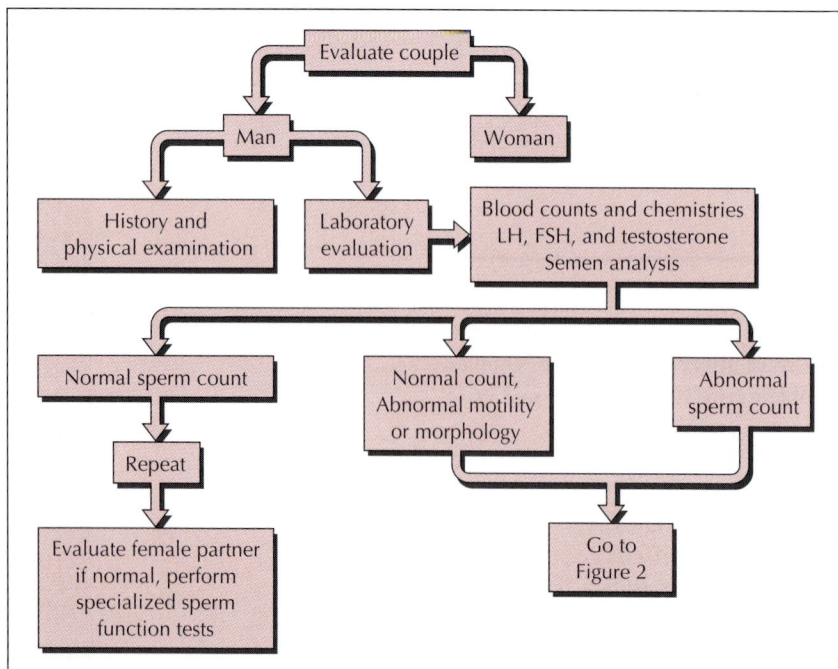

FIGURE 1 Initial evaluation of an infertile couple. Both partners should be evaluated simultaneously. Further work-up of an infertile man with abnormal sperm count, motility, or morphology is outlined in Figure 2. LH—luteinizing hormone; FSH—follicle stimulating hormone.

voice (high pitched or not); hair distribution, including the escutcheon, muscle mass, and body habitus, and the absence or presence of gynecomastia. Cryptorchidism, varicocele, and nodularity of the vas deferens should be recorded. prostate size should be recorded on rectal examination. Testis size can be accurately measured with a Prader orchidometer.

Laboratory evaluation

An outline of the laboratory evaluation is provided in Figures 1 through 4. Initial evaluation should begin with a complete blood count, serum chemistries, and urinalysis. Three or more semen samples obtained by masturbation after a 48-hour abstinence should be assessed for volume, sperm count, sperm motility, and sperm morphology. According to World Health Organization criteria [3,6], a normal semen specimen should have a volume of more than 2 mL, a concentration of more than 20 million/mL, or a total sperm count of greater than 40 million/ejaculate. More than 50% of the sperm should show forward motility, and more than 30% of the cells should have normal morphology.

The significance of leukocytes in semen is not clear. The presence of leukocytes does not always indicate male accessory gland infection. Measurements of luteinizing hormone, follicle-stimulating hormone (FSH), and testosterone can help diagnose hypogonadism and ascertain whether hypogonadism is hypogonadotropic or hypergonadotropic. High luteinizing hormone and FSH (hypergonadotropic) levels suggest primary testicular failure, and a karyotype can be obtained to exclude Klinefelter's syndrome (47 XXY) or its variants. However, karyotyping is expensive, and it rarely alters treatment of the patient.

Elevated testosterone and luteinizing hormone levels in a patient who appears hypogonadal suggest androgen insensitivity. Analysis of skin fibroblasts in research laboratories can help confirm androgen receptor defect or 5 α-reductase deficiency. An isolated increase in serum FSH levels with normal luteinizing hormone and testosterone levels suggests failure of the germ cell compartment.

If the patient has hypogonadotropic hypogonadism, a history of eating disorders, excessive exercise, and systemic illness should be ascertained. Serum prolactin level should be measured to exclude hyperprolactinemia. Magnetic resonance imaging may be performed to exclude the presence of a pituitary or hypothalamic tumor. Detailed preoperative evaluation of pituitary function, apart from checking free thyroxine and thyroid-stimulating hormone levels in patients with pituitary tumors, is not indicated because most of these patients receive glucocorticoid replacement in the perioperative period anyway and must be evaluated postoperatively. In older men

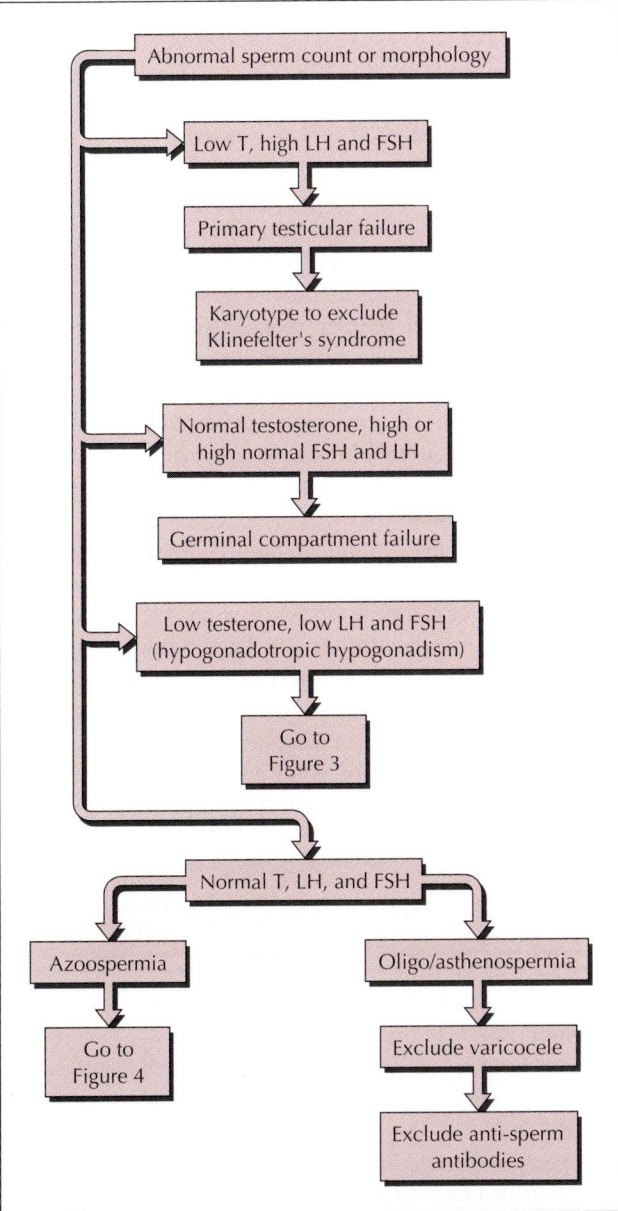

FIGURE 2 Evaluation of an infertile male with abnormal sperm count, motility, or morphology. Algorithms for further evaluation of men with hypogonadotropic hypogonadism and those with normal luteinizing hormone (LH), follicle-stimulating hormone (FSH), and testosterone (T) levels and azoospermia are depicted in Figures 3 and 4, respectively.

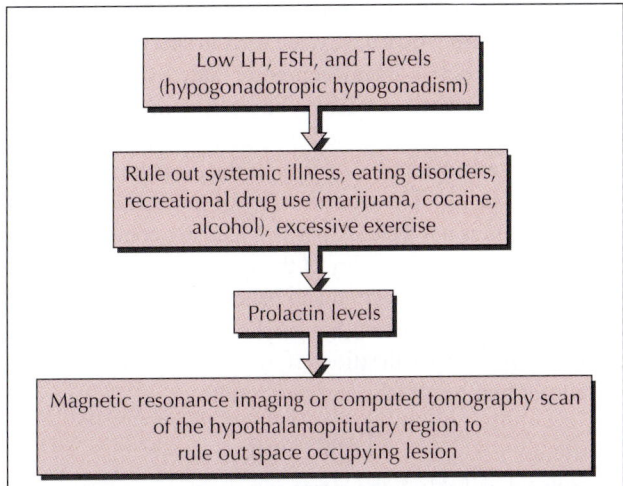

FIGURE 3 An algorithm for further evaluation of infertile men with hypogonadotropic hypogonadism (low luteinizing hormone (LH), follicle-stimulating hormone (FSH), and testosterone (T) levels).

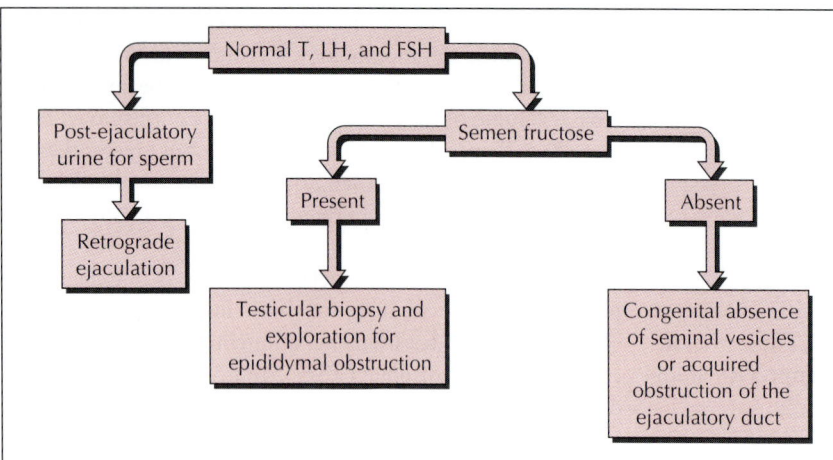

FIGURE 4 An algorithm for further evaluation of infertile men with normal luteinizing hormone (LH), follicle-stimulating hormone (FSH), and testosterone (T) levels and azoospermia.

with mild hypogonadotropic hypogonadism, the search for additional causes of hypogonadotropism is often unrewarding, and the cost effectiveness of a detailed pituitary evaluation, including magnetic resonance imaging, remains to be established. However, older men with severe hypogonadism should have serum prolactin, free thyroxine, and thyroid-stimulating hormone levels checked, and magnetic resonance imaging performed.

Men with azoospermia and normal luteinizing hormone, FSH, and testosterone concentrations may have an obstructive lesion, such as congenital absence of vas or epididymis or an acquired obstruction. In such patients, postejaculatory urine should be examined to exclude retrograde ejaculation, and seminal plasma fructose should be measured. Very low fructose concentrations suggest the absence of seminal vesicles or obstruction. In such patients, exploration and testicular biopsy are indicated to rule out a correctable obstructive lesion or germ cell failure.

In men who have normal hormone levels and low or normal sperm count, specialized sperm function tests are indicated. Various sperm function tests, including the cervical mucus penetration test, acrosome reaction, zona-free hamster egg penetration test, human zona pellucida binding test, and specialized sperm biochemistry, are used in specialized andrology laboratories [6]. Many computer-aided sperm analysis systems are currently available. These systems offer no real advantage over manual methods for sperm morphology classification and are susceptible to error in the estimation of sperm concentrations [6]. The clinical utility of measuring the acrosome reaction is not clear. A positive hamster oocyte penetration is indicative of the ability of the sperm to undergo capacitation and acrosome reaction and penetrate and fuse with the hamster egg. This reaction has good concordance with fertilization in *in vitro* fertilization efforts. Unfortunately, it has a significant number of false-negative results.

Treatment

As outlined in Table 2, the internist can play an important role in the treatment of infertile men by initiating a rational diagnostic evaluation and referring those who require more specialized care. If a specific cause of infertility can be identified, it should be treated first. Patients with hypogonadotropic hypogonadism can be treated with human chorionic gonadotropin, which has luteinizing hormone–like activity with or without human menopausal gonadotropin, which has FSH-like activity. Treatment is initially started with approximately 1500 U of human chorionic gonadotropin three times a week. If after 4 to 6 months the patient has not responded, human chorionic gonadotropin should be added at a dose of 37.5 to 75.0 U subcutaneously three times a week. Men with a prepubertal onset of gonadotropin deficiency often require both luteinizing hormone and FSH replacement, whereas in those with postpubertal onset, luteinizing hormone alone can reinitiate spermatogenesis. A successful response to gonadotropin therapy may take 6 to 15 months and patients should be forewarned about the long duration of therapy.

Some treatments continue to draw controversy (Table 3). Conditions associated with untreatable infertility are azoospermia and severe or complete teratozoospermia [1]. In the case of varicocele, confounding factors and flaws in study design have prevented a consensus on whether varicocelectomy improves fertility in infertile men with varicoceles. However, physicians often feel compelled to recommend varicocelectomy

Microsurgical techniques for correction of obstructive lesions have markedly improved. Although the success rates

---

TABLE 2 THE ROLE OF THE INTERNIST IN THE TREATMENT OF THE INFERTILE MALE

Perform initial evaluation and rule out a systemic disorder.
Identify and treat gonadotropin deficiency.
Identify primary testicular failure and Klinefelter's syndrome.
Separate coital disorders from true infertility.
Refer those with idiopathic male factor infertility for more specialized sperm function assessment and consideration of assisted reproductive technologies.
Recognize that the assisted reproductive technology is expensive, and its benefits remain unproved and quite limited in idiopathic oligospermia (male factor infertility).
Recognize conditions that are untreatable, *eg*, azoospermia, total teratozoospermia, and convey that information empathetically to the patient.

Table 3. Questionable Treatments in Male Factor Infertility*

Clomiphene and other antiestrogens
Varicocelectomy
Luteinizing and follicle-stimulating hormones
Testosterone rebound
Antibiotics
Vitamins and minerals
Low-dose glucocorticoid administration
Artificial insemination husband

*The role of in vitro fertilization in the treatment of male factor infertility remains controversial: no data demonstrate that in vitro fertilization or other assisted reproductive technologies alter the natural history of male factor infertility.
Adapted from Burger and Baker [1]; with permission.

for restoration of patency are high (70% to 90%), the pregnancy rates remain considerably lower (40% to 50%).

Assisted Reproductive Technologies

Assisted reproductive technology, including such techniques as *in vitro* fertilization of the wife's egg with the husband's sperm, transfer of the male gamete (gamete intrafallopian transfer) or zygote (zygote intrafallopian transfer), or tubal embryo transfer, are now in wide use. However, in men with male factor infertility, it is still not clear if assisted reproductive technology has altered the natural history of the disease. Although the fertilization rates have increased steadily with improvement in technology, the overall pregnancy rates have stayed around 15% per cycle. With the ability to micromanipulate the gamete and perform subzonal injections of sperm, some groups are reporting considerably higher success rates. These early results from small series of patients need further confirmation. Adoption and artificial insemination by donor sperm are always reasonable options and should be discussed with the couple.

IMPOTENCE

"Impotence is the inability to achieve an erection that is sufficiently rigid to allow vaginal penetration in at least half the attempts" [7]. Impotence is an extremely common problem that affects 50% diabetic men and 10% to 15% of the general population. The incidence of impotence increases rapidly after age 50 and approaches 50% at age 90. Contrary to previous belief, more than 80% of men with impotence have an organic etiology; psychological factors often exacerbate an underlying organic disorder [7].

Pathophysiology

The etiology of impotence is often multifactorial, particularly in the elderly diabetic. Vascular, neurogenic, and hormonal factors often coexist and play a synergistic role. Performance anxiety, relationship conflict, avoidance, and guilt and depression associated with sexual dysfunction create a self-perpetuating cycle.

Common diseases associated with impotence are diabetes mellitus; hypertension, peripheral vascular disease; hypogonadism; prostate, renal transplant, or other extensive pelvic surgery; depression; spinal cord injury; chronic debilitating illness; and drug therapy for hypertension and depression [7]. Over 90% of older men presenting with sexual dysfunction after a period of normal sexual life have hypertension, diabetes, or atherosclerotic disease [7]. Sexual dysfunction in diabetics usually results from a combination of factors, including impaired vascular supply, venous leak, autonomic neuropathy, and decreased tactile sensation, and usually fails to improve even after achievement of optimum glycemic control [7]. Hypogonadism is not a common cause of impotence; however, because it is so easily treatable, it must always be excluded.

Diagnosis

Because relationship conflicts often accompany sexual dysfunction in men, the couple should be initially evaluated together, and their motivation in undergoing the diagnostic and therapeutic interventions should be gauged. The major objectives of the diagnostic evaluation are shown in Table 4.

Underlying disorder

Detect and evaluate the underlying medical problem, such as diabetes, hypertension, peripheral vascular disease, pelvic surgery, uremia, neurologic disease, and drug use or side effects.

Hypogonadism

Exclude hypogonadism. Look for clinical evidence of underVirilization, and obtain serum testosterone luteinizing hormone and FSH levels on pooled samples. The diagnosis of hypogonadism in older men is not always easy. Korenman [7] recommends using serum bioavailable testosterone levels of 70 ng/dL as the cut-off level in elderly men. Gonadotropins are rarely elevated above the upper limit of normal in older men with low bioavailable testosterone levels.

Diabetes

In diabetics, ascertain the duration of diabetes, the quality of glycemic control, and the presence or absence of autonomic neuropathy, peripheral vascular disease, or renal dysfunction.

Penile vascular flow

Evaluate the penile vascular flow. Numerous diagnostic tests have been described for assessment of penile vasculature. Of these, determination of the penile brachial blood pressure index (PBPI) and response to an intracavernosal injection of prostaglandin E (10 µg) are the easiest to perform and are also the most useful. More complicated procedures, such as duplex scanning, penile arteriography, cavernosometry, and cavernosography should be performed only by an experienced specialist. The criteria for the interpretation of PBPI are outlined in Table 5. A good erectile response to intracavernosal injection of prostaglandin E rules out severe vascular insufficiency only; many men with definite vascular impotence by PBPI or duplex scanning have good responses to intracavernosal vasodilator injection. A poor erectile response to intracavernosal injection suggests arterial insufficiency or venous leak.

Treatment

General measures

The physician should discuss risks and benefits of all the diagnostic procedures and treatment modalities with the couple. The treatment of associated medical disorders should be optimized. Testosterone replacement should be instituted in hypogonadal men, as discussed in Chapter 11. In diabetic men, every effort should be made to improve glycemic control, although improved glycemic control may not improve sexual function. Hypertension should be medically controlled, and if possible, the therapeutic regimen should be modified to remove antihypertensive agents that impair sexual function. This strategy may not always be possible, because almost all antihypertensive agents, including the converting enzyme inhibitors, have been associated with sexual dysfunction. In men with vascular lesions, surgical correction of occlusive lesions or venous leak should be considered.

Specific treatment modalities

Vacuum devices
Intracavernosal injection of vasoactive agents
Penile prostheses
Pentoxifylline
Miscellaneous, unproven agents, such as yohimbine, nitroglycerin, and minoxidil.

Vacuum devices

Various suction devices are commercially available. The most commonly used systems consist of a plastic cylinder, a vacuum pump, and an elastic constriction band. The plastic cylinder fits over the penis and is connected to a vacuum pump. The vacuum within the cylinder draws blood into the penis, producing an erection. An elastic band slipped around the base of the penis from the proximal end of the cylinder traps the blood in the penis. After removal of the cylinder, the erection-like state is maintained for sufficient length of time to permit intercourse. The constriction band should not be left in place for more than 30 minutes.

These devices are safe, reasonably effective, and relatively inexpensive. With a cooperative and understanding partner, precoital activity associated with the application of the device can become part of satisfactory foreplay. Caution should be used by those on anticoagulant therapy.

Intracavernosal injections of vasoactive compounds

Pharmacologic agents that lead to arteriolar and cavernosal smooth muscle relaxation increase blood flow into the penis, thus facilitating erection [8]. The commonly used agents include prostaglandin E_1, papaverine hydrochloride, and phentolamine. Although all of these agents are effective, prostaglandin E_1 is reported to have a lower incidence of prolonged erection and priapism and fewer systemic side effects, presumably because it is metabolized locally within the penis. Many physicians use a mixture of two or all three of these agents.

Relative contraindications include a significant venous leak, significant cardiovascular disease, sickle cell disease, poor vision, and lack of ready access to medical care in the event of complications, such as priapism. The dose of the agent must be initially established for each patient. In general, men whose impotence has a neurogenic cause appear to display greater sensitivity and require a lower dose.

Intracavernosal injections can cause rare but serious side effects, including hematoma, cavernositis, fibrosis, and penile angulation. Persistent erection and priapism are serious complications that need immediate attention. The use of 60 mg of pseudoephedrine when the erection persists for an hour usually results in detumescence. Persistent erection can be treated by intracavernosal injection of an α-adrenergic agent or by withdrawal of 50 mL of corporal blood. Orthostatic hypotension can occur if significant amount of the drug leaks into the systemic circulation [8].

Penile implants

Two types of penile implants are available: malleable and self-inflatable devices [9]. Implantation of a penile prosthesis should always be considered the last therapeutic option in the treatment of impotence. The inflatable devices are aesthetically more attractive because they can simulate tumescent and detumescent states, but they have a greater incidence of

TABLE 4 DIAGNOSTIC EVALUATION OF THE IMPOTENT MALE

History

Evaluate marital relationship

Evaluate depression

Rule out or detect other medical disorders: diabetes mellitus, hypertension, claudication, chest pain, pelvic surgery, other systemic diseases, uremia, stroke

Evaluate drug use: α- and β-adrenergic blocking agents, antidepressants, methyldopa, reserpine, diuretics, cimetidine, antipsychotics, tranquilizers, sympatholytic agents, calcium channel blockers, cocaine, antihistamines, alcohol, nicotine

Obtain surgical history: previous prostate, pelvic, pituitary, or penile surgery

Physical examination

Undervirilization

Peyronie's plaque or fibrous tissue

Autonomic neuropathy (postural hypotension)

Bulbocavernosus reflex, rectal tone

Peripheral vascular disease

Laboratory tests

Fasting blood sugar and Hb A_1C

Total and bioavailable testosterone luteinizing hormone

Prolactin

Thyroxine, triiodothyronine resin uptake, and thyroid-stimulating hormone

Penile brachial blood pressure index

Diagnostic intracavernosal vasodilator injection*

Others: duplex scanning, penile arteriography, and cavernosography*

*These tests should be performed only by those with considerable experiences with their use. Invasive tests are rarely indicated.

mechanical failure. Use of penile implants is undergoing a rapid decline because of the availability of less invasive procedures and concerns about long-term implantation of silicone. Other methods, such as the administration of yohimbine, nitroglycerin, or minoxidil, are unproved.

Male Contraception

The ideal male contraceptive that is easily available, immediately effective, completely reliable, free of adverse effects, rapidly and assuredly reversible, and does not interfere with the spontaneous and pleasurable aspects of sexual intercourse is not yet available [10]. The only two methods that can truly be considered male directed are condom and vasectomy.

Condom

Condoms are the oldest and most effective of the easily reversible forms of male contraceptive. Condoms not only serve as barrier contraceptives but also provide protection from sexually transmitted diseases. Their use has increased in recent years because of the fear of AIDS and other sexually transmitted diseases.

In the British Family Planning Study, a use-pregnancy rate of 4.0/100 woman-years was reported. Failure rates appear to be related to improper condom use. Proper application of the condom onto the penis, to allow a reservoir space for the ejaculate, and care on withdrawal of the penis from the vaginal vault, to minimize spillage, may influence failure rates. The combined use of condom and spermicidal agents not only reduces the failure rates but also lowers the risk of sexually transmitted diseases substantially [11] and is highly desirable.

Hormonal Methods

Observations that men who have congenital deficiency of luteinizing hormone and FSH and those who have undergone surgical hypophysectomy are predictably azoospermic led to the hypothesis that pharmacologic inhibition of luteinizing hormone and FSH might lead to suppression of spermatogenesis.

Pharmacologic inhibitors of luteinizing hormone and FSH secretion that have been explored for suppression of spermatogenesis include testosterone esters, gonadotropin-releasing hormone (Gn-RH) agonists and antagonists, and progestational agents alone and in combination. Clinical trials with suppressive doses of testosterone enanthate in China have shown extremely high azoospermia rates (> 90%) in men treated with 200 mg/w testosterone enanthate alone [12]. Recent studies in predominantly white populations have also demonstrated azoospermia rates approaching 80% in those taking testosterone enanthate alone.

Hormonally induced azoospermia

A recent multicenter study has clearly demonstrated that men who are rendered azoospermic by testosterone enanthate treatment are infertile [12]. Thus, hormonally induced azoospermia confers very effective reversible contraception that has failure rates comparable to, or even better than oral contraceptives.

The issue of whether men who become significantly oligospermic (< 3 million/mL) during testosterone enanthate treatment are also infertile is now being examined in a multicenter clinical trial. Thus, in some ethnic groups, testosterone administration alone might be revealed as an inexpensive and effective contraceptive method. However, many issues related to the safety of long-term testosterone treatment remain to be resolved.

Gonadotropin-releasing hormone analogues

Recent studies have shown that inhibition of luteinizing hormone and FSH by combined Gn-RH antagonist and testosterone treatment leads to azoospermia in most men [13]. However, the currently available Gn-RH antagonist analogues cause significant local skin reactions at the injection site. Similarly, Gn-RH antagonists, like other inhibitors of luteinizing hormone secretion, are associated with a decrease in serum testosterone levels and therefore require concomitant androgen replacement. Because of the long time required to achieve suppression of spermatogenesis, both the onset of and recovery from the contraceptive action of hormonal methods is slow.

Immunologic approaches

Immunization against Gn-RH is being explored as a potential male contraceptive method. Active or passive immunization against FSH has not been consistently effective in suppressing spermatogenesis. Great interest exists in targeting sperm surface antigens as a female contraceptive; however, concern exists that their use in men may lead to autoimmune orchitis.

Vasectomy

Vasectomy is the surgical ligation of the vas deferens. The operation results in permanent sterilization, although there is increasing interest in easily reversible mechanical devices to interrupt the vas [14]. A "no-scalpel" technique has been in use in China and India and has recently been introduced in this country. The procedure should be performed by a specialist, but key points are shown in Table 6.

TABLE 5 PENILE BRACHIAL BLOOD PRESSURE INDEX

Procedure
Brachial and penile blood pressure measurements are taken on either side in supine position before and after leg exercise. The ratio of the penile to brachial systolic blood pressure is calculated on both sides under each condition.

Interpretation
An abnormal response is defined as any penile to brachial systolic blood pressure ratio of ≤ 0.65 or a decrease in penile brachial blood pressure index (PBPI) of ≥ 0.15 after exercise.

Caveat
The PBPI is a relatively specific but not very sensitive marker of vascular insufficiency. The PBPI and the response to intracavernosal injection of vasodilators may diverge in about 20% of men with vascular problems—a venous leak should be suspected in these individuals.

TABLE 6 KEY POINTS ABOUT VASECTOMY FOR THE INTERNIST
Have the patient's spouse be present at counseling.
Stress that vasectomy is an irreversible procedure
After vasectomy, recommend continued use of alternate methods of contraception until the subject becomes azoospermic. Perform semen analysis after 12 ejaculates or after about 3 months.
Stress that vasectomy is a highly effective and safe procedure and that concerns about atherosclerosis and prostate and testicular cancer have not been substantiated.
Indicate that antisperm antibodies are present in a large percent of vasectomized men. Indicate that reversal is achievable by microsurgery, but that restoration of fertility occurs in fewer than 50%.

Adapted from Goldacre *et al*. [16] and Silber [17]; with permission.

Sperm Antibodies

After vasectomy, sperm can no longer be ejaculated and are absorbed by the body, resulting in production of antibodies against the sperm antigens. Sperm-agglutinating and sperm-immobilizing antibodies are detectable in 60% and 40%, respectively, of men who have undergone vasectomy [15]. These antigen-antibody complexes may result in the formation of postvasectomy sperm granuloma and epididymitis. In addition, these antibodies may interfere with subsequent fertility after vasectomy reversal.

Complications

Scrotal discomfort, edema, or hematoma can occur as a result of the procedure. Epididymitis, epididymal ruptures, and sperm granuloma are reported in fewer than 5% of patients. Spontaneous recanalization occurs extremely rarely, and no evidence of an adverse systemic effect of vasectomy has been demonstrated [16].

Reversal

Microsurgical techniques to reverse vasectomy have been considerably refined [17]. Although the restoration of patency is achieved in over 85% to 90% of vasectomized men, fertility is restored in only 50% of men. The success of the vasectomy reversal partly depends on the development of sperm antibodies, the occurrence of sperm granuloma, and the presence of sperm in the vas fluid at the time of vasovasostomy.

Acceptability

Vasectomy remains the most common mode of contraception in men in many countries. In the United States, 500,000 vasectomies are performed each year. It is particularly attractive for men who do not desire, or no longer desire, to conceive.

Achievement of azoospermia after vasectomy takes variable amounts of time. Patients should be advised to have semen analysis performed after 8 to 10 ejaculates or after about 3 to 4 months. Only after two consecutive semen samples have been free of sperm should the patient be pronounced sterile.

REFERENCES AND RECOMMENDED READING

Recently published papers of particular interest have been highlighted as:
- Of interest
- • Of outstanding interest

1. Burger HG, Baker HWG: The treatment of infertility. *Annu Rev Med* 1987, 38:29–40.
2. Swerdloff RS, Boyers SP: Evaluation of the male partner in an infertile couple: an algorithmic approach. *JAMA* 1982, 247:2418–2422.
3. World Health Organization: *Laboratory Manual for the Examination of Human Semen and Semen-Cervical Mucus Interaction.* Cambridge: Cambridge University Press; 1987:1–67.
4. Baker HWG, Burger HG, deKretser DM, Hudson B: Relative incidence of etiological disorders in male infertility. In *Male Reproductive Dysfunction: Diagnosis and Management of Hypogonadism, Infertility and Impotence.* Edited by Santen RJ, Swerdloff RS. New York: Marcel Dekker; 1986:341–372.
5. Paulson RJ: Human in vitro fertilization and related reproductive techniques. In *Infertility, Contraception, and Reproductive Endocrinology,* edn 3. Edited by Mishell D, Davajan V, Lobo R. Boston: Blackwell Scientific; 1991:807–823.
6. Wang C: Diagnostic value of sperm function tests and routine semen analyses in fertile and infertile men. *J Androl* 1988, 9:384–389.
7. Korenman SG: Sexual dysfunction. In *Williams Textbook of Endocrinology,* edn 8. Edited by Wilson JD, Foster DW. 1992:1033–1048.
8. Kursh ED, Bodner DR, Resnick MI, *et al.*: Injection therapy for impotence. *Urol Clin North Am* 1988, 15:625–629.
9. Krane RJ: Penile prosthesis. *Urol Clin North Am* 1988, 15:103–109.
10. Bhasin S, Swerdloff RS: Toward development of a male contraceptive. In *Male Reproductive Dysfunction.* Edited by Swerdloff RS, Santen RJ. New York: Marcell Dekker; 1988:579–601.
11. Kestelman P, Trussel J: Efficacy of the simultaneous use of condoms and spermicides. *Fam Plann Perspect* 1991, 23:226–232.
12. World Health Organization Task Force on Methods for the Regulation of Male Fertility: Contraceptive efficacy of testosterone-induced azoospermia in normal men. *Lancet* 1990, 336:955–999.
13. Tom L, Bhasin S, Salameh W, *et al.*: Induction of azoospermia in normal men with combined GnRH antagonist and testosterone enanthate. *J Clin Endocrinol Metab* 1992, 75:476–483.
14. Rajfer J, Bennett CJ: Vasectomy. *Urol Clin North Am* 1988, 15:631–634.
15. Sotolongo JR: Immunologic effects of vasectomy. *J Urol* 1982, 127:1063–1066.
16. Goldacre MJ, Holford TR, Vessey MP: Cardiovascular disease and vasectomy: findings from 2 epidemiological studies. *N Engl J Med* 1983, 308:805–808.
17. Silber SJ: Reversal of vasectomy in the treatment of male infertility. *J Androl* 1980, 1:261–268.

SELECT BIBLIOGRAPHY

Bhasin S, De Kretser DM, Baker HWG: Natural history and pathophysiology of male infertility. *J Clin Endo Metab* 1994, 79:1525–1530.

Fahrner EM: Sexual dysfunction in male alcohol addicts: prevalence and treatment. *Arch Sex Behav* 1987, 16:247–257.

Kaiser FE, Korenman SG: Impotence in diabetic men. *Am J Med* 1988, 85:147–152.

Melman A: Iatrogenic causes of erectile dysfunction. *Urol Clin North Am* 1988, 15:33–39.

Wein AJ, VanArsdale KN: Drug-induced male sexual dysfunction. *Urol Clin North Am* 1988, 15:13–31.

Disorders of Serum Calcium Concentration

13

Robert Marcus

> **Key Points**
> - Most patients who are discovered by routine laboratory testing to have hypercalcemia will prove to have primary hyperparathyroidism.
> - Contemporary assays for intact parathyroid hormone provide accurate diagnosis in approximately 90% of cases.
> - Many patients with asymptomatic hyperparathyroidism can be monitored long-term without specific intervention.
> - For symptomatic patients with hyperparathyroidism, surgery remains the treatment of choice.
> - Accuracy of noninvasive parathyroid localization procedures is not sufficiently great to relieve the surgeon of the necessity for careful and systematic examination of all parathyroid glands.

In human plasma, calcium normally circulates within a narrow concentration range of 8.5 to 10.5 mg/dL (2.1 to 2.6 mmol/L). Maintenance of this concentration requires the coordinated activity of the kidneys, the intestine, and the skeleton. Primary hormonal regulation of this system is carried out by parathyroid hormone (PTH), the 84–amino acid secretory product of the parathyroid glands. The physiologic role of PTH is to support the serum calcium concentration. When plasma-ionized calcium activity falls, PTH secretion increases and results in more efficient renal calcium reabsorption. When reductions in ionized calcium are sustained, PTH stimulates renal production of 1,25 dihydroxyvitamin D (calcitriol), the active metabolite of vitamin D, which promotes intestinal calcium absorption. When decreases in ionized calcium activity are severe or prolonged, hypersecretion of PTH leads to activation of bone remodeling and support of extracellular fluid calcium at the expense of the skeleton. This chapter discusses a small group of clinical disorders of the calcium–parathyroid axis. Primary hyperparathyroidism (HPT) is the most common cause of hypercalcemia in the general population. In contrast, hypoparathyroidism and pseudohypoparathyroidism are uncommon to rare, but pose complexities for clinical management and provide insight into the basic features of PTH action.

HYPERCALCEMIA AND HYPOCALCEMIA

Under standard conditions of hydration and fasting, total serum calcium concentrations in adults approximate 9.6 ± 0.3 mg/dL. Hypercalcemia and hypocalcemia are defined as any value that is 2 standard deviations from the normal mean. By this criterion, 9.0 to 10.2 mg/dL denotes the normal range. Commercial and hospital laboratories often quote 8.5 to 10.4 mg/dL as the normal range to accommodate samples that are not collected under standard conditions. Few laboratories still report normal ranges beyond 10.5 mg/dL, and these cannot be relied on for accurate diag-

Table 1	**Correction of the Calcium Values with Abnormal Plasma Albumin Levels***		
	Patient 1		**Patient 2**
Total serum calcium value	8.0 mg/dL		10.0 mg/dL
Plasma albumin value	2.5 g/dL		2.5 g/dL
Corrected level	[(4.0–2.5) × 0.8] + 8.0 = 9.2 mg/dL (normal value)		(4.0–2.5) × 0.8) + 10.0 = 11.2 mg/dL (hypercalcemic)

*Formula: Add or subtract 0.8 mg/dL calcium for every 1 g/dL deviation of albumin from its nominal level of 4 g/dL.

nosis. Many patients with mild calcium abnormalities found on a single specimen prove to be eucalcemic. For patients with calcium levels between 10.5 and 10.8 mg/dL, this figure may be as high as 63%. Thus, hypercalcemia must be confirmed before a patient is subjected to additional evaluation.

Approximately 50% of circulating calcium is bound to plasma proteins, primarily albumin, so the plasma-ionized calcium level is about 5 mg/dL (1.25 mmol/L or 2.5 mEq per liter). Measured properly, ionized calcium provides great diagnostic sensitivity. The accuracy of this measurement depends on fastidious and timely specimen handling, which is not likely when specimens are not obtained under anaerobic conditions and are analyzed under the conditions of most commercial laboratories, using thawed serum days after collection. Therefore, unless there is rapid access to a high-quality ionized calcium analysis, adjustment of total calcium for the serum protein concentration is a satisfactory compromise. In malnutrition or liver disease, abnormal levels of plasma albumin may change the apparent serum calcium concentration. When this occurs, it is essential to correct the calcium value (Table 1). Correction formulas are approximations, and when there is ambiguity concerning the presence of hypercalcemia, proper determination of ionized calcium is indicated.

Causes

Hypercalcemic disorders vary in prevalence depending on the setting in which patients come to attention. Recognized during the course of in-hospital medical evaluations, elevated blood calcium is most often a manifestation of clinically obvious systemic malignancy [1,2]. When discovered during routine health surveillance, most cases prove to be caused by primary HPT [3,4]. A differential diagnosis for hypercalcemia is presented in Table 2.

Hypocalcemia is frequently encountered in patients with malnutrition, intestinal malabsorption, or chronic renal failure. In the absence of these systemic illnesses, hypoparathyroidism and pseudohypoparathyroidism must be considered.

Primary Hyperparathyroidism

Hyperfunction of one or more parathyroid glands accounts for the clinical and laboratory findings of hypercalcemia or primary HPT. When PTH secretion is increased as a compensatory response to hypocalcemia (so-called secondary HPT), blood calcium levels are low to normal. In about 80% of patients with primary HPT, hypersecretion of PTH comes from a single adenoma. In the remainder of cases, multiple gland hyperplasia is generally found, although parathyroid carcinoma occurs, accounting for less than 1% of cases.

The specific cause of HPT is not known in most cases. Previous exposure of the head and neck area to ionizing radiation is clearly a predisposing factor. It is not known whether the biological or clinical behavior of the parathyroid adenoma differs in patients whose disorder is radiation-related. Evidence suggests that some adenomas are associated with a rearrangement of the PTH gene on chromosome 11 to a site on the same chromosome where a gene (cyclin) that is involved in control of cellular proliferation is located [5]. Lithium carbonate treatment promotes secretion of

Table 2	**Differential Diagnosis of Hypercalcemia**

Primary hyperparathyroidism
   Sporadic
      Adenoma 80%
      Hyperplasia 18%
      Carcinoma 1%–2%
      Lithium-related
   Familial
      Multiple endocrine adenomatosis Types I and IIa
      Familial hyperparathyroidism

Familial benign (hypocalciuric) hypercalcemia

Malignancy-associated hypercalcemia
   Humoral hypercalcemia of malignancy
   Multiple myeloma
   Bony metastasis

Vitamin D–mediated hypercalcemia
   Hypervitaminosis D
   Granulomatous disease (sarcoidosis, tuberculosis)

Hypervitaminosis A

Thiazide diuretics

Thyrotoxicosis

Immobilization (during growth years)

Milk-alkali syndrome

Table 3. Clinical Manifestations of Hyperparathyroidism

Characteristic features
Kidney stones
Bone fractures
Constipation
Abnormal cognitive function
Depression
Hypertension

Uncommon features
Peptic ulcer
Pancreatitis
Pseudogout

PTH and growth of parathyroid tissue [6], and several dozen cases of HPT have been described in the setting of long-term lithium therapy.

The most plausible model for HPT is that a single cell undergoes a change in its sensitivity, or set-point, for inhibition by calcium. The cell then misreads the ambient calcium environment and secretes PTH as though the ionized calcium activity were lower than normal and undergoes cell proliferation. This response continues until a new equilibrium is established. Such a model is compatible with clinical experience that serum calcium and PTH concentrations generally remain stable for many years after the diagnosis is recognized.

Clinical Features

The diverse clinical manifestations of HPT are listed in Table 3. When HPT was first described, skeletal involvement was a hallmark of disease. In the mid-1960s, introduction of multichannel autoanalyzers permitted routine determination of serum calcium concentrations, resulting in a huge increase in case-finding of HPT, usually in postmenopausal women with few, if any, characteristic symptoms [7]. Although patients with severe bone disease are still occasionally encountered, and about 15% of patients with HPT relate a history of nephrolithiasis, most patients have few, if any, symptoms of their disorder. In recent years, the issue of greatest interest to students of this disease is not diagnosis or treatment for symptomatic patients, but appropriate management for asymptomatic patients.

Biochemical Features

The characteristic biochemical changes in HPT, hypercalcemia, hypercalciuria, and hypophosphatemia, are caused by the actions of PTH. Hypercalcemia reflects the composite effect of increased renal tubular calcium reabsorption, increased bone turnover, and increased gastrointestinal calcium absorption. Although renal calcium reabsorption is more efficient than normal in patients with HPT, hypercalciuria is observed because hypercalcemia increases the filtered load of calcium through the glomerulus. Hypophosphatemia reflects the renal action of PTH to decrease renal phosphorus reabsorption.

Diagnosis

The availability of specific and unequivocal tests for circulating parathyroid hormone has simplified the diagnostic assessment of hypercalcemia. Moreover, accurate tests are available for some of the entities that should be distinguished from HPT (*see* Table 2).

Measurement of Circulating Parathyroid Hormone

The newest advance in assay methodology is the immunoradiometric assay (IRMA) for the intact PTH molecule, which should be selected as the assay of choice [8]. IRMA for intact PTH constitutes a standard for diagnosis. Normal ranges for circulating intact PTH_{IRMA} are generally 10 to 65 pg/mL. Circulating hormone fragments do not interfere with these assays, and the results provide true representations of circulating intact PTH. The simultaneous presence of hypercalcemia and an elevated PTH_{IRMA} provides solid evidence for primary HPT with a diagnostic accuracy of greater than 90%.

Although more than 90% of patients with HPT have elevated PTH_{IRMA} values, occasional patients with intermittent PTH hypersecretion may require more than one blood sample to document an elevated concentration. Furthermore, because intact PTH concentrations rise significantly with age [9], it may be necessary to use age-specific normal ranges for younger patients whose PTH_{IRMA} values are near the published normal upper limits.

An occasional patient has no other apparent cause of hypercalcemia and has PTH concentrations consistently within the normal range on multiple occasions when multiple laboratory assays, including IRMA are used. In our experience with four such patients, two underwent surgical removal of single parathyroid adenomas with resolution of hypercalcemia and two declined surgery.

Surgical Treatment

Surgical removal of the abnormal parathyroid gland is the standard treatment against which all other approaches must be compared. An experienced parathyroid surgeon can anticipate cure of HPT in about 90% of single operations. Key to a successful operation is a systematic and careful dissection with identification of all parathyroid glands. Failure to adhere to such an approach is the most common reason for an unsuccessful operation.

In recent years, several techniques have been developed for preoperative localization of parathyroid adenoma. These include fine-parts ultrasound, technetium–thallium scanning, and magnetic resonance imaging. The sensitivity and specificity of any of these methods do not generally exceed 60% [10], thus reinforcing the need for a careful surgical exploration and direct visualization of all four parathyroid glands. Localization studies are reserved for patients who have persistent hypercalcemia after an operation or for patients who have undergone thyroid or other neck surgery and in whom anatomic landmarks may be distorted or uncertain. Under such circumstances, other localization procedures, such as venous catheterization with measurement of PTH, can be helpful.

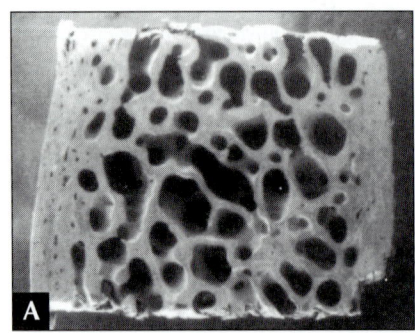 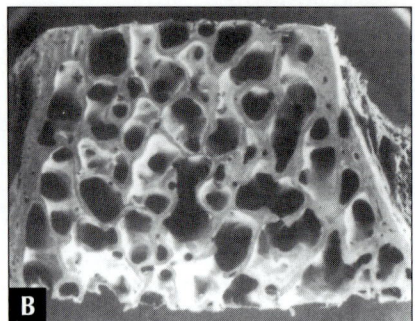

FIGURE 1 Scanning electron micrographs of iliac crest biopsies of a patient with primary hyperparathyroidism (**A**) and a control subject (**B**). The hyperparathyroid bone shows marked cortical thinning, but trabecular mass and connectivity are well preserved. (*From* Bilezikian and coworkers [20•]; with permission.)

Nonsurgical Treatments

Several pharmacologic approaches to managing patients with HPT have been explored. These include attempts to lower PTH secretion as well as to blunt hormone responsiveness. No useful pharmacologic means to lower PTH secretion has yet been established. Oral therapy with inorganic phosphorus provides short-term reduction of serum and urinary calcium concentrations, and may be useful in managing a patient until surgery. Calcitonin and parenteral bisphosphonates may help to control serum calcium levels for short periods, but do not provide effective long-term treatment. For postmenopausal women, treatment with estrogen may control blood and urinary calcium long-term, although hypersecretion of PTH persists [11]. These treatments and other non-operative approaches should be carried out by an endocrinologist experienced in the management of parathyroid disease.

Asymptomatic Patients

Long-term studies of patients with HPT who have been conservatively followed suggest that many asymptomatic patients require only periodic surveillance [12,13]. The degree of hypercalcemia appears to remain stable over at least a decade, and few patients experience important reductions in glomerular filtration rates over time. A critical issue regarding these patients is the degree to which sustained hypersecretion of PTH places the skeleton in jeopardy. Although there are devastating skeletal consequences of severe HPT, most individuals with mild or asymptomatic HPT have little skeletal involvement. Modest deficits in bone mineral content in the cortical skeleton (*eg*, longbones) are characteristically observed, but axial (*eg*, vertebral) bone mass appears to be relatively spared, with excellent maintenance of trabecular connectivity [14,15] (Fig. 1). Recent epidemiologic studies indicate that patients with HPT may not experience an increased risk for fracture. A National Institutes of Health Consensus Conference on Mild Hyperparathyroidism concluded that many patients with asymptomatic disease can be safely followed without active intervention, but recommended that physicians assess cortical bone mineral density to identify patients who might be at increased risk for fracture [16•]. Compliance is an important drawback to long-term observation as a treatment strategy; about 30% of patients are lost to follow-up by 10 years.

Hyperparathyroidism does not undergo spontaneous remission; therefore, affected patients are expected to remain affected indefinitely. Results of observational follow-up for about 10 years are reassuring for most patients, but there is no basis for such reassurance over 20 or 30 years. I, therefore, recommend surgery to all patients younger than age 50 years. For older women with asymptomatic HPT, hypercalcemia and hypercalciuria may be controlled with replacement estrogen. For older men and women who are poor surgical candidates or whose symptoms of HPT are minimal, I embark on long-term surveillance. The steps necessary for this approach are outlined in Table 4. The physician who undertakes such an observational approach must develop clear guidelines for referring patients to surgery. Such a list of criteria is provided in Table 5.

HYPOPARATHYROIDISM AND PSEUDOHYPOPARATHYROIDISM

Hypoparathyroidism

Hypoparathyroidism is an unusual disorder that may be iatrogenic, metabolic, or idiopathic. Most commonly, parathyroid hormone deficiency is a consequence of neck surgery, particularly when an attempt is made to perform a complete thyroidectomy, when the surgeon is inexperienced, or when a previously operated patient undergoes another neck explo-

---

TABLE 4 LONG-TERM OBSERVATION OF ASYMPTOMATIC HYPERCALCEMIC PATIENTS

Physician periodically monitors

Serum and urinary calcium; serum alkaline phosphatase activity

Creatinine clearance

Blood pressure

Cortical bone density (hip or forearm)

Patients should

Maintain a reasonable calcium intake, about 1000 mg/d (total intake)

Maintain adequate hydration (> 2 L/d), particularly during warm months

Avoid extended bed rest or immobilization

Avoid thiazide diuretics

TABLE 5 CRITERIA FOR REFERRING PATIENTS FOR SURGERY
Increase of serum calcium concentration to > 12 mg/dL on multiple occasions
Decrease in endogenous creatinine clearance > 20% from baseline
Decrease in bone mineral density > 3% per year
Presence of nephrolithiasis
Development of symptoms that might be related to hyperparathyroidism
Poor compliance with surveillance procedures

TABLE 6 CLINICAL FEATURES OF HYPOPARATHYROIDISM AND PSEUDOHYPOPARATHYROIDISM
Hypoparathyroidism
Neuromuscular irritability
Paresthesias
Muscle cramps
Chvostek's sign
Facial spasm
Trousseau sign
Pseudohypoparathyroidism
Phenotypic abnormalities
Short stature
Round face
Foreshortening of metacarpal and metatarsal bones
Mild mental retardation

ration. In surgical hypoparathyroidism, postoperative hypocalcemia develops within a few hours and is associated with a rise in the serum concentration of inorganic phosphorus. This latter feature distinguishes hypoparathyroidism from the "hungry bone syndrome," which is seen in patients with parathyroid bone disease and which reflects the uptake of calcium by bone as the parathyroid stimulus for hyper-remodeling is removed.

Idiopathic hypoparathyroidism is a rare disorder. It begins early in life and is sometimes associated with autoimmune multiple endocrine gland failure. It is frequently associated with mucocutaneous candidiasis, vitiligo, and alopecia, and may be complicated by primary adrenal or gonadal failure and pernicious anemia. For technical reasons, early radioimmunoassays showed low-normal values for circulating PTH in hypoparathyroidism. PTH_{IRMA} assays, however, clearly identify hypoparathyroid patients by showing no detectable PTH.

Pseudohypoparathyroidism

Pseudohypoparathyroidism is a rare condition that mimics true hypoparathyroidism insofar as levels of calcium and phosphorus are concerned. However, patients with hypoparathyroidism have undetectable serum levels of PTH and show robust responses to exogenously administered PTH, whereas patients with pseudohypoparathyroidism have high-normal to elevated circulating levels of PTH and have severely blunted responses to exogenous PTH [17]. The clinical features of hypoparathyroidism and pseudohypoparathyroidism are listed in Table 6.

Recent application of molecular techniques has shown that patients with classical pseudohypoparathyroidism and hereditary osteodystrophy may have discrete mutations in the guanine nucleotide binding protein that is necessary for activation of the adenylate cyclase complex by PTH [18,19•]. Careful evaluation of patients with classical pseudohypoparathyroidism frequently elicits evidence for subtle abnormalities in the response to other peptide hormones, such as glucagon or thyrotropin-releasing hormone. Relatives of patients with pseudohypoparathyroidism occasionally display the characteristic phenotypic abnormalities, but maintain normal calcium homeostasis. These patients are said to have pseudo-pseudohypoparathyroidism. Occasionally patients with pseudohypoparathyroidism enter spontaneous remission, at which time they may be difficult to distinguish from those with pseudo-pseudohypoparathyroidism. Patients with hypoparathyroidism or pseudohypoparathyroidism may be overlooked for many years before their serum calcium level is evaluated.

Treatment of Hypocalcemia

Treatment of the hypocalcemia improves cognitive function. In the acute postoperative state, laryngospasm may be a life-threatening complication of hypocalcemia. Patients should be frequently monitored during the first 24 hours, with frequent assessment of the Chvostek and Trousseau tests and periodic monitoring of the serum calcium concentration. Such monitoring is of particular importance for patients who have undergone radical neck dissections, complete thyroidectomies, and repeat parathyroid explorations. Urgent treatment of hypocalcemia is accomplished by intravenous infusion of 10 to 15 mg/kg of calcium as calcium gluconate over several hours in isotonic saline or dextrose and water. The usual ampule of 10% calcium gluconate contains only about 100 mg of calcium, so to achieve 15 mg/kg for a 70-kg man requires 1050 mg of calcium, or about 10.5 ampules. In an emergency, that is, with laryngospasm, 1 or 2 ampules of calcium gluconate can be rapidly administered by vein. It is best not to give calcium chloride in this manner, because it is highly sclerotic to peripheral veins.

For long-term management of hypocalcemic patients, vitamin D and oral calcium are the mainstay of treatment. Early in the course of therapy, until blood calcium levels reach a reasonable equilibrium, 1,25 dihydroxyvitamin D (calcitriol) can be given orally. This agent is the most potent form of vitamin D and has a rapid onset. Its half-life is also brief, so that most patients require 0.25 to 0.5 µg as twice-daily therapy. Calcitriol is expensive and is, therefore, not ideal for long-term treatment. After calcium levels are corrected, I customarily switch to ordinary vitamin D, which can be given in doses ranging from 50,000 to 150,000 U/d. Vitamin D therapy is effective only if sufficient dietary calcium is available (*see* Brust, Nutritional Disorders of the Nervous System, Neurology). I, therefore, issue patients an oral calcium supplement, generally calcium carbonate, because it consists of 40% calcium and the number of pills can be minimized.

Patients with hypoparathyroidism should not have serum calcium levels raised much beyond 9 mg/dL. In the absence of PTH, there is a higher urinary calcium excretion at any given calcium level. Thus, maintaining a hypoparathyroid patient at a serum calcium level of 10 mg/dL may be associated with unacceptably high urinary calcium excretion and kidney stone risk. I, therefore, try to maintain serum calcium levels between 8 and 9 mg/dL. It is occasionally difficult to achieve this level of calcemia because of high serum concentrations of inorganic phosphorus. In such patients, phosphorus-binding antacids such as aluminum hydroxide given with each meal may assist therapy.

REFERENCES AND RECOMMENDED READING

Recently published papers of particular interest have been highlighted as:
- Of interest

1. Fisken RA, Heath DA, Bold AM: Hypercalcemia—a hospital survey. *Q J Med* 1980, 49;405.
2. Fisken RA, Heath DA, Somers S, Bold AM: Hypercalcemia in hospital patients. Clinical and diagnostic aspects. *Lancet* 1981, 1:202.
3. Christensson T, Hellstrom K, Wengle B, *et al.*: Prevalence of hypercalcemia in a health screening in Stockholm. *Acta Med Scand* 1976, 200:131.
4. Christensson T, Hellstrom K, Wengle B: Clinical and laboratory findings in subjects with hypercalcemia. *Acta Med Scand* 1976, 200:355.
5. Arnold A, Kim HG, Gaz RD, *et al.*: Molecular cloning and chromosomal mapping of DNA rearranged with the parathyroid hormone gene in a parathyroid adenoma. *J Clin Invest* 1989, 83:2034–2040.
6. Spiegel AM, Rudorfer MV, Marx SJ, Linnoila M: The effect of short-term lithium administration on suppressibility of parathyroid hormone secretion by calcium in vivo. *J Clin Endocrinol Metab* 1984, 59:354–359.
7. Heath H III, Hodgson SF, Kennedy M: Primary hyperparathyroidism: incidence, morbidity and potential economic impact in a community. *N Engl J Med* 1980, 302:189–193.
8. Nussbaum SR, Zahradnik RJ, Lavigne JR: Highly sensitive two-site immunoradiometric assay of parathyrin, and its clinical utility in evaluating patients with hypercalcemia. *Clin Chem* 1988, 33:1364–1367.
9. Young G, Marcus R, Minkoff JR, *et al.*: Age-related rise in parathyroid hormone in man: the use of intact and midmolecule antisera to distinguish hormone secretion from retention. *J Bone Miner Res* 1987, 2:367.
10. Doppman JL, Miller DL: Localization of parathyroid tumors in patients with asymptomatic hyperparathyroidism and no previous surgery. *J Bone Miner Res* 1991, 6(suppl 2):S153–S158.
11. Marcus R, Madvig P, Crim M, *et al.*: Conjugated estrogens in the treatment of post-menopausal women with hyperparathyroidism. *Ann Intern Med* 1984, 100:633–640.
12. Mitlak BH, Daly M, Potts JT Jr, *et al.*: Asymptomatic primary hyperparathyroidism. *J Bone Miner Res* 1991, 6(suppl 2):S103–S110.
13. Heath DA, Heath EM: Conservative management of primary hyperparathyroidism. *J Bone Miner Res* 1991, 6(suppl 2):S117–S120.
14. Silverberg SJ, Shane E, De La Cruz L, *et al.*: Skeletal disease in primary hyperparathyroidism. *J Bone Miner Res* 1989, 4:283–291.
15. Parisien M, Silverberg SJ, Shane E, *et al.*: Bone disease in primary hyperparathyroidism. *Endocrinol Metab Clin North Am* 1990, 19:19–34.
16.• Potts JT Jr, ed.: Proceedings of the NIH Consensus Development Conference on diagnosis and management of asymptomatic primary hyperparathyroidism. *J Bone Miner Res* 1991, 6(suppl 2):S1–S166.
17. Chase LR, Melson GL, Aurbach GD: Pseudohypoparathyroidism: defective excretion of 3′,5′-AMP in response to parathyroid hormone. *J Clin Invest* 1969, 48:1832–1844.
18. Levine MA, Jap TS, Mauseth RS, *et al.*: Activity of the stimulatory guanine nucleotide-binding protein is reduced in erythrocytes from patients with pseudohypoparathyroidism and pseudo-hypoparathryroidism: biochemical, endocrine, and genetic analysis of Albright's hereditary osteodystrophy in six kindreds. *J Clin Endocrinol Metab* 1986, 62:497–502.
19.• Miric A, Vechio JD, Levine MA: Heterozygous mutations in the gene encoding the alpha subunit of the stimulatory G protein of adenylyl cyclase in Albright hereditary osteodystrophy. *J Clin Endocrinol Metab* 1993, 76:1560–1568.
20.• Bilezikian JP, Silverberg SH, Shane E, *et al.*: Characterization and evaluation of asymptomatic hyperparathyroidism. *J Bone Miner Res* 1991, 6(suppl 2):S85–S89.

SELECT BIBLIOGRAPHY

Arnold A: Molecular basis of primary hyperparathyroidism. In *The Parathyroids: Basic & Clinical Concepts*. Edited by Bilezikian JP, Marcus R, Levine MA. New York: Raven Press; 1994:107–422.

Bilezikian JP: Guidelines for the medical or surgical management of primary hyperparathyroidism. To operate or not to operate. In *The Parathyroids: Basic & Clinical Concepts*. Edited by Bilezikian JP, Marcus R, Levine MA. New York: Raven Press; 1994:567–574.

Kleerekoper M: Clinical course of primary hyperparathyroidism. In *The Parathyroids: Basic & Clinical Concepts*. Edited by Bilezikian JP, Marcus R, Levine MA. New York: Raven Press; 1994:471–484.

Levine MA, Schwindinger WF, Downs RW Jr, Moses AM: Pseudohypoparathyroidism: clinical, biochemical, and molecular features. In *The Parathyroids: Basic & Clinical Concepts*. Edited by Bilezikian JP, Marcus R, Levine MA. New York: Raven Press; 1994:781–800.

Stock J, Marcus R: Medical management of primary hyperparathyroidism. In *The Parathyroids: Basic & Clinical Concepts*. Edited by Bilezikian JP, Marcus R, Levine MA. New York: Raven Press; 1994:519–530.

Diabetes Mellitus and Hypoglycemia

Martin J. Abrahamson
Jeffrey S. Flier

Key Points

- Diabetes mellitus should be regarded as a heterogeneous group of disorders with the common feature of hyperglycemia.
- Type 1 (insulin-dependent diabetes mellitus [IDDM]) is an autoimmune disorder characterized by autoantibodies to the beta cell and insulitis.
- The management of IDDM should ideally be aimed at achieving blood glucose concentrations as close to normal as possible because good glucose control may delay or prevent development of the chronic microvascular complications of the disease.
- Noninsulin-dependent diabetes (NIDDM) represents a heterogeneous group of disorders with different pathophysiologic mechanisms. Insulin resistance and impaired insulin secretion occur in the majority of patients.
- Diet and exercise form the mainstay of therapy for most patients with NIDDM, particularly when associated with obesity.
- The cause of fasting (postabsorptive) hypoglycemia, based on the history, clinical examination, and relevant biochemical investigations, must be sought in every case.

HYPERGLYCEMIC SYNDROMES: DIABETES MELLITUS

Diabetes mellitus is a disorder of metabolism of carbohydrate, fat, and protein associated with an absolute or relative deficiency of insulin and varying degrees of insulin resistance. It results from the interaction between genetic factors and environmental influences. Diabetes mellitus should be regarded as a syndrome because the disease is a heterogeneous group of disorders—with the common feature of hyperglycemia. This chapter outlines the classification of the syndrome, reviews current diagnostic criteria, discusses the clinical presentation of diabetes, and provides a simple approach to the principles of management.

Classification

The present classification of diabetes (Table 1), which is derived from the National Diabetes Data Group (NDDG) of the National Institutes of Health, includes three general groups [1]:

1. *Diabetes mellitus*: characterized by fasting hyperglycemia or plasma glucose concentrations above defined limits following a standard glucose tolerance test (GTT). Diabetes mellitus is divided into four different types that appear to differ in etiology and pathogenesis—type 1 or insulin-dependent diabetes (IDDM); type 2 or noninsulin-dependent diabetes (NIDDM); malnutrition-related diabetes; and diabetes associated with conditions that predispose to the development of insulin resistance and hyperglycemia.
2. *Impaired glucose tolerance (IGT)*: describes plasma glucose concentrations outside the normal range following a GTT, but not high enough to be labeled diabetic.

3. *Gestational diabetes*: refers to glucose intolerance discovered or developing during pregnancy. This class also includes patients statistically thought to be at risk for the development of diabetes—those who have had a previous abnormality of glucose tolerance and those with a potential abnormality of glucose tolerance.

Diagnosis

The clinical diagnosis of diabetes is often suggested by the presence of classic symptoms and can be confirmed by measuring a fasting or random plasma glucose concentration rather than by performing provocative tests. A fasting plasma glucose concentration of 140 mg/dL or higher or a random plasma glucose concentration of 200 mg/dL or more on more than one occasion confirms the diagnosis of diabetes. The finding of a random plasma glucose concentration of between 140 and 200 mg/dL does not exclude diabetes. Indeed, in the presence of a random plasma glucose concentration of between 140 and 200 mg/dL, and a fasting plasma glucose concentration of less than 140 mg/dL, but a high index of suspicion, further investigation with an oral glucose tolerance test (oGTT) may be indicated.

The high-risk situations in which an oGTT may be indicated include the following:

Borderline blood glucose values, as measured in previous testing, or overt hyperglycemia during stress
Pregnancy
Obesity or strongly positive family history of NIDDM
Development of microvascular complications of diabetes—in particular, retinopathy or neuropathy

The oGTT is the only form of glucose tolerance testing recommended for the diagnosis of diabetes and is the only test for IGT. The use of glycosuria as a diagnostic criterion for diabetes is obsolete, and the measurement of glycated proteins such as glycosylated hemoglobin may be helpful in assessing the duration and extent of hyperglycemia, but has not been validated for diagnostic purposes. The NDDG report recommended standardized methods for performing the oGTT as well as diagnostic criteria for confirming diabetes in nonpregnant adults. These methods are summarized in Tables 2 and 3.

Diagnosis in pregnancy

Plasma glucose levels obtained during the oGTT that are lower than those proposed for a diagnosis of diabetes in nonpregnant adults may impart an increased risk to the newborn of pregnant women. Thus, diagnostic criteria during pregnancy are set lower than those given for the nonpregnant state, as summarized in Table 3. In the United States, it is currently recommended that all pregnant women receive a 50-g glucose load followed by measurement of blood glucose 1 hour

---

TABLE 1   CLASSIFICATION OF DIABETES MELLITUS AND OTHER CATEGORIES OF GLUCOSE INTOLERANCE

Clinical classes
Diabetes mellitus
  Insulin-dependent diabetes mellitus (IDDM)
  Noninsulin-dependent diabetes mellitus (NIDDM)
    Obese
    Nonobese
    Maturity-onset diabetes in the young (MODY)
  Malnutrition-related diabetes mellitus
  Other types of diabetes associated with specific conditions or syndromes
    Diabetes due to pancreatic disease
      Chronic pancreatitis
      Hemochromatosis
    Diabetes due to other endocrine disease
      Cushing's syndrome
      Acromegaly
      Pheochromocytoma
      Glucagonoma
      Thyrotoxicosis
    Diabetes due to drugs and toxins
      Glucocorticoids
      Diuretics
      Phenytoin
      Pentamidine
    Diabetes due to abnormalities of insulin or the insulin receptor
      Leprechaunism
      Type A syndrome of insulin resistance
      Rabson-Mendenhall syndrome
    Diabetes associated with genetic syndromes
      Lipodystrophic syndromes
      Type 1 glycogen storage disease
      Cystic fibrosis
Impaired glucose tolerance (IGT)
Gestational diabetes mellitus

Statistical risk classes
Previous abnormality of glucose tolerance
Potential abnormality of glucose tolerance

TABLE 2   PROCEDURE FOR THE ORAL GLUCOSE TOLERANCE TEST

1. Patients should be on a diet containing at least 150 g of carbohydrate per day for at least 3 days prior to the test.
2. The test should be administered in the morning after an overnight fast of 10–16 hours, during which time only water can be taken.
3. Smoking and strenuous activity should be avoided during the test.
4. A fasting blood sample is taken before giving the glucose load.
5. The subject then drinks 75 g of glucose (or a 75-g glucose equivalent containing starch hydrolysate) in 250–300 mL of water. In children, 1.75 g/kg body weight of glucose is given, up to a maximum of 75 g. The glucose load should be consumed over 5 minutes.
6. Further blood samples are collected at 30, 60, 90, and 120 minutes after the glucose has been consumed for a measurement of whole blood or plasma glucose.
7. Glucose should be measured by formal laboratory procedure. The less accurate glucose-oxidase test strips should not be used.

TABLE 3 NATIONAL DIABETES GROUP CRITERIA FOR INTERPRETATION OF THE ORAL GLUCOSE TOLERANCE TEST WITH THE USE OF VENOUS PLASMA OR SERUM*

Fasting (F) or hours after glucose load	Normal glucose tolerance	Impaired glucose tolerance†	Diabetes†	Gestational diabetes‡ (100 g glucose)
F	≤115 (6.4)	≤140 (7.8)	≥140 (7.8) or	≥105
0.5	≤200 (11.1)			
1	≤200 (11.1)	≤200 (11.1)	≥200 (11.1)	≥190
1.5	≤200 (11.1)		and	
2	≤140 (7.8)	140–199	≥200 (11.1)	≥165
3		(7.8–11.1)		≥145

*Values are given in mg/dL; values in parentheses are in mM; a 75-g carbohydrate load was used.
†In nonpregnant adults. In children, a fasting glucose concentration of >140 mg/dL in addition to the 1- and 2-h elevations in glucose are required for the diagnosis.
‡If any two or more of the four values meet the criteria described; based on the criteria of O'Sullivan and Mahan.

later between the 24th and 28th week of gestation. Patients who have a positive screening test then undergo a 100-g oGTT, which is interpreted according to O'Sullivan and Mahan's criteria (Table 3)[2].

Diagnosis in children

Most children will present with classic symptoms of diabetes and severe hyperglycemia. In unusual situations in which a GTT is required for diagnosis, the dose of glucose administered is 1.75 g/kg body weight, up to a maximum of 75 g. The diagnostic criteria are the same as for nonpregnant adults, except that a fasting glucose concentration of more than 140 mg/dL is also required.

Insulin-Dependent Diabetes Mellitus

Pathogenesis and epidemiology

Insulin-dependent diabetes mellitus (IDDM) is an autoimmune disorder characterized by the development of autoantibodies to β-cell antigens or to insulin itself, as well as cellular infiltration (insulitis) and β-cell destruction, eventually causing insulinopenia, and ultimately ketoacidosis [3,4••]. Genetic factors are important, and expression of certain histocompatibility antigens (HLAs) is associated with the disorder. IDDM accounts for approximately 10% of all diabetes in the western world.

Most studies of the incidence and prevalence of IDDM have been conducted in children, adolescents, and young adults. These studies show two major characteristics: First, the incidence of the disease rises from birth to 12 years, reaching a peak between 11 and 13 years, and then falls progressively. Second, there is a seasonal variation in incidence of the disease in older children and adolescents, with the lowest rates occurring in the spring and summer. Although an infectious cause could be speculated on the basis of these data, it is unlikely because it is now known that the disease has a protracted preclinical period and that biochemical and immunologic abnormalities typically exist for months or years before clinical onset of the disease. IDDM may occur at any age, but the risk of developing it after the age of 20 years appears to be one half the risk up to this age, and the risk then remains constant for the remainder of life. Genetic susceptibility plays an important role in the development of the disease. On the other hand, there is evidence that environmental factors play a critical role in the development of the disease. This evidence includes the fact that there is enormous geographic variation in incidence. There is also ethnic variation in the incidence of IDDM, which may be accounted for by differences in genetic susceptibility to the disease [5].

Clinical presentation

The common clinical features with which patients with IDDM present are summarized in Table 4. IDDM usually presents in an acute manner, with classic symptoms of polyuria, polydipsia, loss of weight, lethargy, blurring of vision, and recurrent infections. Unfortunately, many patients still present with varying degrees of severity of ketoacidosis, ranging from mild to severe ketoacidotic coma. Immunologic and biochemical abnormalities may precede clinical onset of

TABLE 4 COMMON PRESENTING SYMPTOMS OF DIABETES MELLITUS

Symptoms common to IDDM and NIDDM
Thirst
Polyuria
Weight loss
Fatigue
Blurred vision
Candidiasis
Recurrent furunculosis

Symptoms present in patients with ketoacidosis
Nausea
Vomiting
Abdominal pain
Drowsiness, stupor, or coma

IDDM—insulin-dependent diabetes mellitus;
NIDDM—noninsulin-dependent diabetes mellitus.

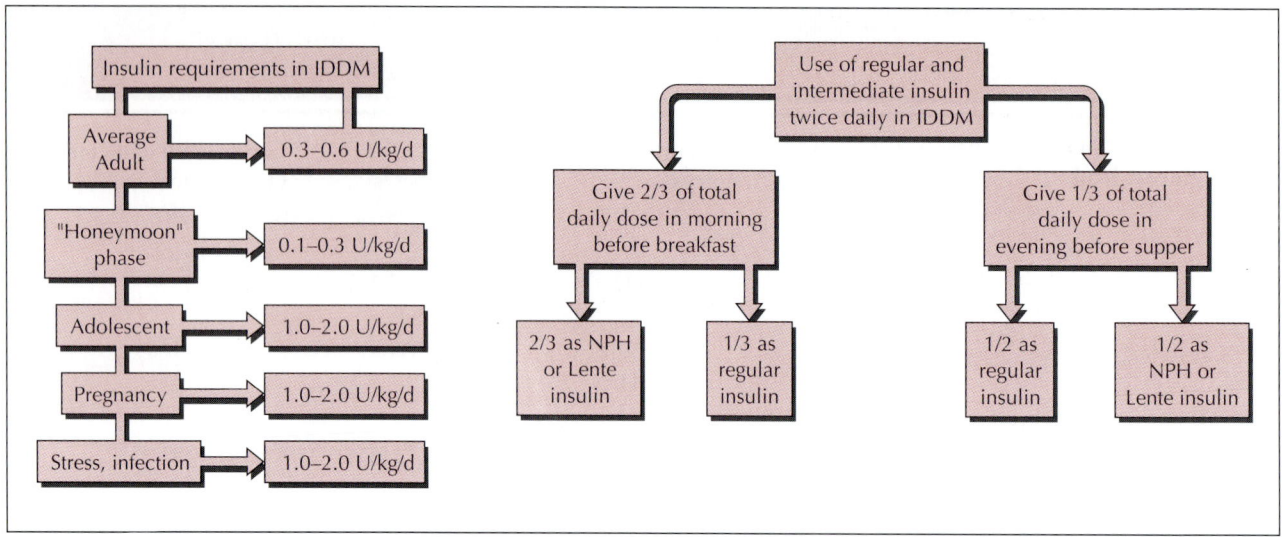

Figure 1 Insulin requirements in IDDM. Occasionally, the evening dose of intermediate insulin is given at bedtime instead of before supper. Regular insulin is always given before meals, usually half an hour before ingestion of the meal. When mixing insulin, always draw up the regular insulin first. IDDM—insulin-dependent diabetes mellitus.

the disease for months or years, and are being used clinically to predict the development of IDDM in individuals with positive family histories of the disorder.

Treatment

Treatment is initiated only when individuals become hyperglycemic. These individuals are insulinopenic and require insulin, which is administered (usually) two or more times daily, using combinations of short- and intermediate-acting insulin preparations. An algorithm outlining the average daily insulin requirements and relative proportions of regular and intermediate insulin used to treat patients with IDDM is shown in Figure 1. Combinations of ultralong-acting and regular insulin can also be used in the treatment of IDDM. All patients should also receive nutritional counseling. They should also be offered instruction in current methods of monitoring blood glucose concentrations at home, through the use of blood glucose reflectance meters, and be encouraged to maintain blood glucose concentrations as close to normal as possible. This will reduce the risk for long-term complications from the disease [6••].

Soon after the onset of IDDM, many patients achieve excellent glycemic control when using low doses of insulin. This so-called "honeymoon phase" is characterized by partial recovery of beta-cell function, and usually lasts for 2 to 3 months. During this time some patients may be able to stop taking insulin completely, but this is only temporary and is eventually followed by absolute insulinopenia, which is associated with a significant increase in insulin requirements.

Noninsulin-Dependent Diabetes Mellitus

Pathogenesis and epidemiology

Noninsulin-dependent diabetes mellitus (NIDDM) is the most prevalent form of diabetes encountered in the western world, accounting for more than 90% of all cases of diabetes. It may remain undetected for years and, even in countries where health care is of a high standard, there is typically one undiagnosed case of NIDDM for every one that is known. NIDDM is not a single disease. It represents a heterogeneous group of disorders with different pathophysiologic mechanisms contributing to hyperglycemia. These mechanisms range from uncommon but well-defined genetic abnormalities, *eg*, mutations in insulin or its receptor, to as-yet-unexplained insulin resistance and impaired insulin secretion in the majority of patients—often, but not always, associated with obesity [7].

Variations in the prevalence of NIDDM are seen among populations. In the United States the prevalence of NIDDM in persons aged 18 years or more is approximately 7.0% [8]. The prevalence increases with age and is higher in nonwhites than in whites, and higher in females than in males. The prevalence in some population groups exceeds that of the general population. The highest prevalence and incidence of NIDDM in the world is seen in the Pima Indians of Arizona where the age-adjusted prevalence rate is ten times greater than that in the general US population [9]. Variations in the prevalence of NIDDM are also seen in other parts of the world, with considerable differences in prevalence noted in populations of different ethnic origin living in similar environments.

Expatriate communities often develop NIDDM with a different frequency compared with that seen in their country of origin. For example, Indian communities in many parts of the world have much higher prevalences of NIDDM than in most regions of India itself [10]. This higher prevalence may be related to a certain amount of inbreeding within the population group itself, and suggests that genetic factors play an important role in the development of diabetes in these populations. The strongest evidence for a genetic predisposition to NIDDM comes from twin studies—concordance rates for monozygotic twins range from 55% to 100% [11]. Although the pattern of inheritance for most forms of NIDDM has yet to be elucidated, inheritance of one form of NIDDM is known. This form is maturity-onset diabetes of the young (MODY), which is inherited as an autosomal dominant condition [12••].

Although there is strong evidence to support a genetic predisposition to NIDDM, environmental factors also influence development of the disorder. The prevalence of NIDDM in migrant population groups is different from that observed in their country of origin. Changes in lifestyle, different eating patterns, and the development of obesity increase the risk of developing NIDDM in the individual who is genetically predisposed to development of the disorder.

Clinical presentation

The classic symptoms of NIDDM are those of hyperglycemia (Table 4). However, the onset of the disease is usually more insidious than in IDDM, and marked weight loss is often not a feature. Approximately 50% of patients with NIDDM present with classic symptoms. The rest of the cases are discovered indirectly—*eg*, during routine screening (during insurance or general medical check-ups), during hospitalization for unrelated illnesses, or during intercurrent infections (usually, urinary tract or genital). A few patients (approximately 2%) present with established microvascular complications of diabetes. Patients rarely present with hyperosmolar coma. Ketoacidosis is infrequent, but may occur under certain precipitating conditions.

Treatment

Diet and exercise are mainstays of therapy for most patients with NIDDM, particularly when associated with obesity. After an adequate trial of this treatment, oral hypoglycemic agents are usually prescribed if blood glucose concentrations remain elevated. Currently two groups of drugs are available for the treatment of NIDDM in the United States: sulphonylureas and biguanides. Sulphonylureas were the only group of drugs available until recently. A list of these drugs, as well as their relative potencies, duration of action, and dosage used, is provided in Table 5. Sulphonylureas act by stimulating endogenous insulin secretion and reducing basal hepatic glucose production. They have the potential to cause prolonged and severe hypoglycemia, and should be used with caution, especially in the elderly. They should be commenced at the lowest possible dose, increasing the dose gradually until the desired target glucose ranges are met. The biguanide metformin (glucophage) was recently approved by the FDA for use in the treatment of NIDDM. Metformin acts by increasing insulin sensitivity and does not stimulate endogenous insulin secretion. It also decreases hepatic glucose production and reduces intestinal glucose absorption. Side effects include anorexia, diarrhea, and flatulence, and are reduced by taking the drug with meals. Metformin is commenced at a dose of 500 mg twice daily with meals and can be increased to a maximum of 2.5 g daily in divided doses. The drug is contraindicated in patients with renal or hepatic dysfunction; when used in these situations it is more likely to cause lactic acidosis. Metformin can be used in combination with sulphonylureas. When used in this way, further reduction in fasting and postprandial glucose concentrations have been observed [13]. Failure to respond to these drugs, despite adherence to appropriate diet and exercise regimens, provides an indication for the institution of insulin therapy. Temporary use of insulin is also indicated for patients under certain circumstances, *eg*, during pregnancy, and during times of stress when glucose tolerance deteriorates [14].

Other Conditions

Malnutrition-related diabetes occurs in certain parts of the world including India, parts of Africa, and the West Indies. It is found in young people and is associated with protein–calorie malnutrition and emaciation, and, in some patients, pancreatic calculi. These individuals are severely hyperglycemic and require insulin but do not have an increased propensity to develop ketosis.

Impaired glucose tolerance describes biochemical indices between normal glucose concentrations and those diagnostic of diabetes documented during a standard glucose tolerance test. This impairment may represent a stage in the natural development of IDDM or, more commonly, NIDDM. Indeed, 10% to 25% of patients with IGT will develop diabetes within 5 years, many will return to normal glucose tolerance, and some will continue to have IGT. Individuals with continuing IGT do not develop significant microvascular

TABLE 5 SULPHONYLUREAS USED IN THE TREATMENT OF NONINSULIN-DEPENDENT DIABETES MELLITUS*

Compound	Potency ratio, mg	Duration of action, h	Dosage range (mg), frequency	Metabolites	Excretion
Tolbutamide	1	6–12	500–2000, usually divided	Inactive	Urine
Acetohexamide	2.5	12–24	125–1000, single/divided	Active and inactive	Urine
Chlorpropamide	5	up to 60	100–500, single	Less active	Urine
Tolazamide	5	14–24	100–1000, usually single	Active and inactive	Urine
Glipizide†	100–200	12–24	2.5–40, single/divided	Inactive	Urine
Glyburide†	100–200	12–24	1.25–20, single/divided	Active	Urine and bile

*All sulphonylureas can potentially cause hypoglycemia. Therapy with them should be commenced at the lowest possible dose and the dose increased thereafter to achieve target-range glucose concentrations.
†Glipizide and glyburide are "second-generation" sulphonylureas—usually given twice daily, particularly when doses of more than 10 or 5 mg, respectively, per day are required.

disease but have an increased prevalence of coronary artery and peripheral vascular disease associated with premature death when compared with age-matched normoglycemic individuals. These patients also show an increased prevalence of hypertension, hyperlipidemia, and obesity.

Gestational diabetes describes glucose intolerance developing or discovered during pregnancy. The diagnostic criteria differ from those for the nonpregnant adult. Gestational diabetes occurs in about 3% of all pregnancies and is associated with increased perinatal morbidity and mortality. Although most women with gestational diabetes mellitus have normal glucose tolerance postpartum, up to 60% will develop NIDDM within 15 years after parturition. It is therefore important to reclassify these patients as patients with impaired glucose tolerance, diabetes, or a *previous abnormality of glucose tolerance* after the termination of pregnancy.

Persons with normal glucose tolerance who have had a previous abnormality of glucose tolerance or who have a close genetic relationship with individuals with diabetes are statistically at risk for the development of diabetes in the future. They are regarded as having a *potential* abnormality of glucose tolerance [15].

Although this classification of diabetes can be applied to the majority of patients, there are situations in which it is difficult to assign an individual to one particular class with certainty. Fortunately, an incorrect designation is not critical because therapy remains the same.

HYPOGLYCEMIC SYNDROMES

Maintenance of the plasma glucose concentration within the normal range is essential for health. Hypoglycemia is dangerous because glucose is the primary energy substrate of the brain, and its absence leads to deranged function and, if untreated, permanent damage or death. The brain is vulnerable to hypoglycemia because it cannot use circulating free fatty acids as an energy substrate, unlike other parts of the body.

Diagnosis

Hypoglycemia is defined as a venous plasma glucose concentration of less than 45 mg/dL (2.2 mmol/L). It is diagnosed by a classic triad of symptoms known as the "Whipple" triad—symptoms consistent with hypoglycemia, confirmation of a low plasma glucose concentration, and relief of symptoms when plasma glucose concentrations are raised to normal levels.

The symptoms of hypoglycemia fall into two main groups—those caused by the central nervous system manifestations of hypoglycemia (*neuroglycopenia*), and those caused by the release of counterregulatory hormones in response to hypoglycemia, mainly epinephrine (*adrenergic symptoms and signs*). The neuroglycopenic manifestations range from subtle impairment of mental function to confusion, convulsions, coma, and death. The adrenergic manifestations include a nonspecific sense of arousal, anxiety, or impending doom, and are coupled with tremulousness, palpitations, and diaphoresis [16].

Classification

There are two categories of hypoglycemia: *postabsorptive* (fasting), and *postprandial* (reactive). Fasting hypoglycemia implies the presence of serious disease, and requires diagnostic explanation and therapy. Postprandial hypoglycemia may occur during the latter portion of any postabsorptive state and usually does not imply a serious underlying disorder. Thus, the distinction between postprandial and fasting hypoglycemia is fundamental.

Fasting (Postabsorptive) Hypoglycemia

The causes of fasting hypoglycemia are listed in Table 5. A diagnosis of the cause is made from the history, physical examination, and biochemical investigations, which are ideally performed when the patient is hypoglycemic before emergency treatment is administered. Drugs are the commonest cause of hypoglycemia. For insulin-dependent diabetics, hypoglycemia is a fact of life. In any year 10% of diabetics receiving conventional and 25% of those receiving intensive therapy with multiple injections of insulin will experience at least one episode of severe hypoglycemia. Four percent of deaths of patients with IDDM are attributable to hypoglycemia. Patients with IDDM often have deficient counterregulatory responses to hypoglycemia and, after many years of disease, may lose the (adrenergic) warning symptoms of hypoglycemia. They are thus at increased risk for developing severe neuroglycopenia. Risks for the development of hypoglycemia in IDDM include excessive insulin administration combined with exercise, alcohol consumption, and relatively little food ingestion.

Hypoglycemia is sometimes seen in patients with critical organ failure. In hepatic failure, the inability to maintain endogenous glucose production (via gluconeogenesis and glycogenolysis) in the fasting state leads to hypoglycemia. The mechanisms of hypoglycemia in cardiac and renal failure are not completely understood. These mechanisms include inanition, hepatic congestion, failure of gluconeogenesis, and hepatic hypoxia in cardiac failure. Abnormal glucose counterregulatory mechanisms may be a dominant feature in the hypoglycemia associated with renal failure.

Endogenous (non–drug-induced) hyperinsulinism and hormonal deficiencies (mainly, cortisol) account for the major causes of hypoglycemia in the absence of the conditions already mentioned. Endogenous hyperinsulinism may be caused by either an insulin-secreting pancreatic tumor (insulinoma) or by a variety of autoimmune mechanisms leading to reduced metabolic clearance of insulin. Insulinomas are rare pancreatic tumors with a frequency of occurrence estimated to be one in a million. They are usually small (1–1.5 cm in diameter), may be multifocal, and are benign in 85% to 90% of cases. Insulinomas invariably come to attention because of symptoms of hypoglycemia rather than secondary to a mass effect of the tumor.

The diagnosis of insulinoma is suggested by finding inappropriate hyperinsulinism in the presence of hypoglycemia in a single sample. Thus, blood sampling at the time of fasting hypoglycemia is critical in making the diagnosis. If the diagnosis is suspected from the history, the patient may be required to undergo a fast, during which glucose and insulin concentrations are determined once hypoglycemia is confirmed. Up to 98% of patients with insulinomas will become hypoglycemic within 72 hours of fasting. Attempted localization of these tumors(s) preoperatively is usually undertaken by using a computed tomographic scan, magnetic resonance imaging scan, or angiography, but success is achieved in only about 50% of cases. Occasionally, pancreatic venous sampling via the percutaneous route may be used to localize these small tumors preoperatively [17•]. Insulin antibodies or the presence of antibodies to the insulin receptor are rare causes of hypoglycemia, and often occur in association with other autoimmune diseases. They should be considered when all other causes of hypoglycemia have been excluded.

Except in patients with IDDM, glucoregulatory abnormalities causing hypoglycemia are uncommon. Cortisol deficiency is a recognized cause of hypoglycemia in nondiabetic patients. Isolated growth hormone deficiency rarely, if ever, causes hypoglycemia in adults but may cause hypoglycemia in infants and children. Epinephrine and glucagon deficiencies do not cause hypoglycemia in adults with normal insulin secretion.

Treatment

The initial treatment of severe fasting hypoglycemia producing confusion, coma, or both, is the intravenous administration of a bolus of 25% or 50% glucose followed by a constant infusion of glucose until the patient is able to eat a meal. Frequent measurement of the glucose concentration is required to ensure that the patient is receiving an adequate infusion of glucose. Surgery is the treatment of choice for insulinoma. In situations in which tumors cannot be localized and/or removed, or surgery has failed, medical treatment is indicated. Drugs used in these circumstances include diazoxide or octreotide, an analogue of somatostatin [18]. Therapy for other causes of hypoglycemia, apart from hormone replacement therapy in hypopituitarism or adrenal insufficiency, is dietary. In most cases, avoidance of fasting is all that is required.

Postprandial Hypoglycemia

The causes of postprandial hypoglycemia are listed in Table 6. Postprandial (reactive) hypoglycemia classically occurs after meals, usually within 4 hours after the ingestion of food. It is commonly seen in patients who have undergone gastric surgery that results in the rapid movement of food into the small intestine, and is thought to be the result of marked hyperinsulinemia that follows the rapid absorption of ingested nutrients, or the increased secretion of insulinotropic hormones that may be associated with rapid bowel transit of food. Symptoms of hypoglycemia classically occur within 1.5 to 3 hours after a meal. Idiopathic reactive hypoglycemia is often erroneously diagnosed by physicians and patients. In one series, less than 15% of patients thought to have this condition actually had blood glucose levels lower than the 10th percentile of asymptomatic subjects after an oral glucose load, and less than one third of these patents had symptoms of hypoglycemia after their regular meals [19]. The pathogenesis of this condition is incompletely understood—there is no evidence that insulin secretion is increased. Increased sensitivity to insulin has been postulated, as has deficient glucagon secretion. Treatment is empirical and comprises the ingestion of frequent small meals containing small amounts of complex carbohydrate rich in protein and the complete elimination of simple sugars. Congenital deficiencies of enzymes of carbohydrate metabolism are rare causes of postprandial hypoglycemia in infancy and childhood, but discussion of them is beyond the scope of this chapter.

TABLE 6 CLASSIFICATION AND CAUSES OF HYPOGLYCEMIA

Postabsorptive (fasting) hypoglycemia
Drugs
    Insulin, sulphonylureas, alcohol
    Pentamidine, quinine
    Salicylates, sulfonamides (rare)
Organ failure
    Hepatic disease
    Cardiac disease
    Renal disease
    Sepsis
    Inanition
Hormonal deficiencies
    Cortisol deficiency
    Growth hormone deficiency (in children only)
    Glucagon and epinephrine
Non–β-cell tumors
    Tumors secreting insulin-like growth factors (mainly, insulin-like growth factor type 2)
Endogenous hyperinsulinism
    Pancreatic β-cell disorders
        Insulinoma
        Nesidioblastosis
    β-cell secretagogues (*eg*, sulphonylureas)
    Autoimmune hypoglycemia
        Insulin antibodies
        Insulin receptor antibodies
Hypoglycemia of infancy and childhood
    Neonatal hypoglycemia
    Glycogen storage diseases
    Ketotic hypoglycemia of childhood

Postprandial (reactive) hypoglycemia
Congenital deficiencies of enzymes of carbohydrate metabolism
    Galactosemia
    Hereditary fructose intolerance
Alimentary hypoglycemia
Usually following bowel resection
Idiopathic (functional) reactive hypoglycemia

References and Recommended Reading

Recently published papers of particular interest have been highlighted as:
- Of interest
- •• Of outstanding interest

1. National Diabetes Data Group: Classification and diagnosis of diabetes mellitus and other categories of glucose intolerance. *Diabetes* 1979, 28:1039–1057.

2. O'Sullivan JB, Mahan CM: Criteria for the oral glucose tolerance test in pregnancy. *Diabetes* 1964, 13:278–285.

3. Eisenbarth GE: Type 1 diabetes mellitus: a chronic autoimmune disease. *N Engl J Med* 1986, 314:1360–1368.

4. •• Atkinson MA, Maclaren NK: Mechanisms of disease: the pathogenesis of insulin-dependent diabetes mellitus. *N Engl J Med* 1994, 331:1428–1436.

5. Krolewski AS, Warram JH, Rand LI, Kahn CR: Epidemiologic approach to the etiology of type 1 diabetes mellitus and its complications. *N Engl J Med* 1987, 317:1390–1398.

6. •• The Diabetes Control and Complications Trial Research Group: The effect of intensive treatment of diabetes on the development and progression of long-term complications in insulin-dependent diabetes mellitus. *N Engl J Med* 1993, 329:977–986.

7. DeFronzo R: The triumvirate: Beta-cell, muscle and liver—a collusion responsible for NIDDM. *Diabetes* 1988, 37:667–687.

8. Harris MI, Hadden WC, Knowler WC, Bennett PH: Prevalence of diabetes and impaired glucose tolerance and plasma glucose levels in U.S. population aged 20-74 yr. *Diabetes* 1987, 36:523–534.

9. Knowler WC, Pettitt DJ, Saad MF, Bennett PH: Diabetes mellitus in the Pima Indians: incidence, risk factors and pathogenesis. *Diabet Metab Rev* 1990, 6:1–27.

10. Omar MAK, Seedat MA, Dyer RB, *et al.*: The prevalence of diabetes mellitus in a large group of South African Indians. *S Afr Med J* 1985, 67:924–926.

11. Barnett AH, Eff C, Leslie RD, Pyke DA: Diabetes in identical twins: a study of 200 pairs. *Diabetologia* 1981, 20:87–93.

12. •• Froguel P, Zouali H, Vionnet N, *et al.*: Familial hyperglycemia due to mutations in glucokinase—definition of a subtype of diabetes mellitus. *N Engl J Med* 1993, 328:697–702.

13. Bailey CJ: Biguanides and NIDDM. *Diabetes Care* 1992, 15:755–784.

14. Lebovitz HE: *Physicians' Guide to Non-insulin-dependent (Type II) Diabetes Mellitus: Diagnosis and Treatment*, edn 2. Alexandria, VA: American Diabetes Association; 1988.

15. Diabetes Mellitus: Report of WHO study group. *Tech Rep Ser* 1985, 727:1–113.

16. Service FJ: Hypoglycemias. *J Clin Endocrinol Metab* 1993, 76:269–272.

17. • Service FJ, McMahon MM, O'Brien PC, Ballard DJ: Functioning insulinoma—incidence, recurrence, and long-term survival: a 60 year study. *Mayo Clin Proc* 1991, 66:711–719.

18. Glaser B, Rosler A, Halperin Y: Chronic treatment of a benign insulinoma using the long-acting somatostatin analogue SMS 201-995. *Isr J Med Sci* 1990, 26:16–19.

19. Palardy J, Havrankova J, Lepage R, *et al.*: Blood glucose measurements during symptomatic episodes in patients with suspected postprandial hypoglycemia. *N Engl J Med* 1989, 321:1421–1425.

Select Bibliography

Moller DE, Flier JS: Insulin resistance—mechanisms, syndromes and mutations. *N Engl J Med* 1991, 325:938–948.

O'Rahilly S, Wainscoat JS, Turner RC: Type 2 (non-insulin dependent) diabetes mellitus: new genetics for old nightmares. *Diabetologia* 1988, 31:407–414.

Summary and Recommendations of the 3rd International Workshop-Conference on Gestational Diabetes Mellitus. *Diabetes* 1991, 40(suppl 2):197–201.

Warram JH, Rich SS, Krolewski AS: Epidemiology and genetics of diabetes mellitus. In *Joslin's Diabetes Mellitus*, edn 13. Edited by Kahn CR, Weir GC. Malvern, PA: Lea & Febiger; 1994:201–215.

Management of Hyperglycemic Emergencies and Other Hyperglycemic States

15

Jane E-B. Reusch
Karl E. Sussman

Key Points
- Diabetic ketoacidosis still remains a relatively common complication of insulin-dependent diabetes mellitus.
- Mortality rate resulting from diabetic ketoacidosis increases in elderly patients, reaching 15% to 28% in patients over age 65 years.
- The two most urgent interventions required in the treatment of diabetic ketoacidosis are rehydration and insulin administration.
- Hyperosmolar, hyperglycemic nonketotic coma, a profound state of dehydration associated with a relative or absolute insulin deficiency, may be difficult to diagnose and causes significant mortality in the diabetic patient population.
- In diabetic patients undergoing surgery, it is important to establish adequate metabolic control and to optimize cardiovascular status before undertaking surgery.
- The transient occurrence of diabetes in the face of glucocorticoid therapy suggests compromised insulin reserve and indicates that these persons are at increased risk for the development of diabetes in the future.

Two of the major acute metabolic complications of diabetes are diabetic ketoacidosis and hyperosmolar hyperglycemic nonketotic coma (HHNK). The differential diagnosis between HHNK and diabetic ketoacidosis is often difficult, as these two conditions are two ends of a continuous spectrum. Table 1 outlines the major differences between the two syndromes. Often, there is considerable overlap between the disorders. As both are emergencies, priorities in initiating therapies are fluid resuscitation and potassium and insulin administration to reverse the process.

Management of diabetic patients who are being treated surgically or with glucocorticoids or chemotherapy is important. Because of the increased incidence of cardiovascular disease and poor wound healing in this population, it is important that these patients have a thorough preoperative evaluation as well as well-targeted perioperative and postoperative care. Also, many of the drugs used in clinical practice have an ability to alter insulin sensitivity and may lead to difficulty in the treatment of patients with known diabetes or may induce diabetes in non-diabetic individuals. Glucocorticoids often induce diabetes and chemotherapy often complicates diabetes management secondary to decreased appetite and high catabolic state.

DIABETIC KETOACIDOSIS

Diabetic ketoacidosis seen in patients with insulin-dependent diabetes mellitus (IDDM) and rarely in patients with noninsulin-dependent diabetes mellitus (NIDDM) is frequently encountered in general clinical practice [1,2]. Diabetic ketoacidosis is a common complication of IDDM with approximately 45,000 cases annually and an overall mortality rate of 5% to 9% (or at least 2500 deaths per year). The mortality rate resulting from diabetic ketoacidosis increases in elderly patients reaching between 15% to 28% in patients over age 65 [3,4]. Diabetic ketoacidosis

Differential diagnosis of DKA versus HHNK	DKA	HHNK
Population at risk	IDDM <40 years	NIDDM >40 y
Symptoms	12%–20% new onset	50% no prior diagnosis
Laboratory studies	<2 d polyuria, polydipsia, nausea, vomiting	>5 d polyuria, polydipsia, decreased mental status
Glucose	<800	>800
Sodium	Normal or ↓	Normal or ↑
Potassium	↑, normal, ↓	↑, normal, ↓
Bicarbonate	<15	Normal
Ketones	Positive	Negative/trace
pH	<7.3	Normal
Osmolarity	<350	>350
Prognosis (in most cases HH)	5%–10% mortality	30%–50% mortality

Table 1. Hyperosmolar nonketotic coma/hyperosmolar dehydration syndrome. DKA—diabetic ketoacidosis; HH—hyperosmolar hyperglycemic; HHNK—hyperosmolar hyperglycemic nonketotic coma. IDDM—insulin-dependent diabetes mellitus; non-insulin-dependent diabetes mellitus.

accounts for 8% to 10% of all diabetes-related deaths annually. Death may result from diabetic ketoacidosis alone or the underlying condition that precipitated the ketoacidosis.

Diagnosis and Differential Diagnosis

Diabetes ketoacidosis is the result of insulin deficiency, or relative insulin deficiency, when systemic counter-regulatory hormones—especially glucagon—are elevated [5,6••]. The disease has two primary aspects. The first is hyperglycemia and dehydration occurring secondary to insulin deficiency. The insulin deficiency leads to increased blood sugars from decreased peripheral fat and muscle glucose utilization and increased hepatic glucose production. The resultant hyperglycemia leads to an osmotic diuresis with loss of free water and electrolytes. The second essential event leading to diabetic ketoacidosis is the increased production of ketone bodies by the liver [7]. Normally, free fatty acids (FFAs) presented to the liver are oxidized. With insulin deficiency and glucagon excess, FFA metabolism shifts so that ketone bodies (β-hydroxybuterate and acetoacetate) are produced. These weak acids deplete the body's bicarbonate stores and acidosis ensues. Thus, the triad associated with ketoacidosis includes hyperglycemia, dehydration, and acidemia.

The differential diagnosis for diabetic ketoacidosis is outlined in Table 2 [8•,9]. The blood glucose level and rapidity of onset are the major clinical aids to distinguish between diabetic ketoacidosis and hypoglycemia. Alcoholic ketoacidosis and other anion gap acidosis can usually be distinguished by history or toxicology screen. Hypoglycemia may present with a mild ketonemia but without the associated acidosis. Brainstem hemorrhage and cerebrovascular accidents may be difficult to distinguish and are also known precipitants of diabetic ketoacidosis. Viral syndromes can both mimic diabetic ketoacidosis, with dehydration, nausea, vomiting, and lethargy, and cause diabetic ketoacidosis if managed inappropriately with regard to insulin therapy. The signs and symptoms of diabetic ketoacidosis are detailed in Table 3 and the diagnostic criteria in Table 4.

In various series, the most common precipitating factor leading to the onset of diabetic ketoacidosis was the omission of insulin either by the patient or by the doctor or clinic staff. The next most common were new diagnoses of diabetes and infection, followed by myocardial infarction and cerebrovascular accident (stroke). Beyond these, it is often difficult to determine the etiology of the diabetic ketoacidosis, except to note that patients with erratic control tend to drift into diabetic ketoacidosis more commonly than do well-controlled patients. Because infection figures so prominently among the precipitating factors, it is important to evaluate the patient for infection.

Therapy

There is no exact formula for rehydration except that the usual free water deficit is 3 to 5 L in adults. Rehydration is usually undertaken with normal saline especially if the patient is orthostatic. If the patient has hypernatremia, half-normal saline may be used. Lactated ringers are usually avoided because severe diabetic ketoacidosis with hypovolemia can have concomitant lactic acidosis.

Insulin administration, both to reverse the ketone body production and to lower blood sugar, is the other urgent intervention. Much controversy has surrounded the optimal insulin schedule (*ie*, low-dose vs high-dose therapy) [10]. Both treat-

Table 2. Differential diagnosis of diabetic ketoacidosis

Diabetic ketoacidosis
Alcoholic ketoacidosis
Anion gap acidosis (methanol, ethylene glycol [anti-freeze], salicylate ingestion, uremia, lactic acidosis)
Viral syndrome
Hypoglycemia
Cerebrovascular accident/brainstem hemorrhage

Table 3 Symptoms and signs of diabetic ketoacidosis	
Symptoms	**Signs**
Polyuria, polydipsia	Tachycardia
Nausea and vomiting	Hypothermia
Anorexia	Dehydration
Fatigue	Kussmaul respirations
Weakness	Acetone breath
Abdominal pain	"Acute abdomen"
Dyspnea	Hypotonia/hyporeflexia
	Altered mental status
	Focal neurologic signs

Table 4 Diagnostic criteria for diabetic ketoacidosis

Hyperglycemia (300–800 mg/dL)
Acidemia pH 6.8–7.3
Bicarbonate depletion <15
Positive ketones
Incidental increased liver function tests, elevated leukocyte (with or without infection) count, increased amylase, hypertriglyceridemia
Electrolyte abnormalities
Free water deficit

ments are equally efficacious. We recommend a low-dose continuous intravenous insulin infusion of 5 to 7 units per hour (or 0.1 U/kg/h) with a goal of lowering the blood sugar about 10% over the first 2 hours. If the glucose decreases more rapidly, the insulin infusion should be cut by half; if the decline in glucose is inadequate, the infusion should be doubled. Occasionally, patients will require an extremely high insulin infusion (50 to 60 U/h of insulin); this insulin resistance suggests an underlying disorder such as infection.

At presentation, the patient's electrolytes (Na^+, K^+, Mg^{2+}, PO_4) may be high or low as measured by the laboratory. Those results can be misleading because of a combination of volume depletion, acidosis, and insulin deficiency. The osmotic diuresis will have caused a significant total body depletion of these electrolytes, and their repletion is essential to successfully managing these patients. Sodium will be replenished with intravenous fluids as mentioned earlier. The measured serum sodium may be falsely lowered by hyperglycemia or hypertriglyceridemia.

Of the electrolytes depleted, potassium needs to be monitored with the most care. Initially, the serum potassium level is often elevated whereas the body's potassium stores are severely depleted. If the patient is urinating, it is advisable to administer potassium early even if serum levels are in the high normal range. Fluid and insulin administration will lower serum potassium by dilution, by reequilibration with hydrogen ions as the acidemia resolves, and also by cellular transport of potassium and phosphate into the cells with glucose. An electrocardiogram can be used to monitor potassium [11]. Tall, symmetric, peaked T waves indicate hyperkalemia, whereas flattened T waves with U waves indicate hypokalemia. Commonly, patients need 120 to 160 mEq of potassium in the first 24 hours of therapy. Potassium replacement is continued orally for 5 to 7 days to replete total body stores.

The use of bicarbonate for managing diabetic ketoacidosis is controversial [12,13]. If the pH is less than 7.10 or cardiovascular compromise is impending, or both, bicarbonate is often added to intravenous fluids (one to two ampules, 44 to 88 mEq) or in hypotonic fluid (one third to one half normal saline). Bicarbonate should not be given by intravenous push and may precipitate a dramatic decline in potassium. Thus, even more careful monitoring and replacement of potassium is required for patients receiving bicarbonate. There are no data that bicarbonate therapy alters the clinical outcome regardless of the level of acidemia; hence, bicarbonate therapy is not routine [12].

Therapy for diabetic ketoacidosis can lead to profound hypophosphatemia associated with muscle weakness, respiratory failure, hemolytic anemia, hemorrhage, rhabdomyolysis, and neurologic dysfunction. Despite this phenomenon, intercurrent phosphate administration has no effect on recovery rates or mortality from diabetic ketoacidosis in studies done over the last 50 years [14,15]. Because the low phosphate levels are disconcerting to most practitioners, most groups recommend repleting potassium losses with potassium phosphate solutions, unless there is renal failure, and monitoring patients for hyperphosphatemia and hypocalcemia (do not exceed 90 mM PO_4 in 24 hours) [14]. Once the patient's blood glucose has normalized and the ketonemia cleared, usually within 24 to 48 hours, the patient should be switched over to subcutaneous insulin and oral food and fluids. Other options for therapy include infection work-up with treatment and cardiac evaluation for older patients.

A flow sheet of the usual course of monitoring patients is shown in Table 5. Flow sheets are essential in the successful management of diabetic ketoacidosis.

It has become commonplace for well-educated patients with mild diabetic ketoacidosis to be treated as outpatients. That regimen requires frequent subcutaneous injections of regular insulin, monitoring of blood glucose levels, and oral hydration with potassium-containing solutions.

Complications

Most of the complications of diabetic ketoacidosis therapy (hypoglycemia, fluid overload, hypokalemia, hypophosphatemia) can and should be anticipated and therapy modified accordingly. Hyperchloremic metabolic acidosis is a frequently anticipated consequence of treatment and should resolve spontaneously over 5 to 7 days. Hypoxia is frequently observed but seldom is of clinical significance. Cerebral edema is poorly understood and happens most frequently in young persons [16,17]. Treatment of this condition with mannitol, dexamethasone, and mechanical ventilation is not well studied [17]. A change in mental status during therapy should prompt an

Table 5. Diabetic ketoacidosis—A guide to management

Time (clock)										
Hours since admission	0	1/2	1	2	3	4	5	6	7	8
Vital signs										
Blood pressure	x	x	x	x	x	x	x	x	x	x
Temperature	x			x		x				x
Pulse	x	x	x	x	x	x	x	x	x	x
EKG	x									x
Fluid therapy										
Type of fluid (NS, D, 1/2 NS, etc.)										
Amount of fluid, L										
Urine output										
Insulin therapy										
Infusion rate, U/h										
Injection										
Units/route (IV, IM, SQ)										
Laboratory data										
Glucose	x	x.	x	x	x	x	x	x	x	x
Potassium	x		x	x		x		x		x
Bicarbonate	x		x	x		x				x
Sodium chloride	x/x			x/x		x/x				x/x
pH (blood gases)	x									x
Calcium/phosphate	x/x									x/x
BUN/Creatine	x/x					x/x				x/x
Anion gap (calculate)	x					x				x
Mental status	x		x			x				x
Oral intake										

BUN—blood urea nitrogen; D—dextrose; EKG—electrocardiogram; IM—intramuscular; IV—intravenous; NS—normal saline; SQ—subcutaneous.

examination of eye grounds and evaluation for increased central nervous system pressure. The incidence of clotting abnormalities is increased during recovery, especially if patients have been bedridden or comatose. The use of subcutaneous heparin is recommended for such patients.

Prevention

The largest percentage of cases of diabetic ketoacidosis are secondary to the omission of insulin by the patient or by care providers [8•]. It is especially common for patients to omit insulin when they have mild gastrointestinal distress because they are consuming fewer calories. At times, mild gastrointestinal distress may be a sign of impending diabetic ketoacidosis and it is evident that more, not less, insulin is required then. Education on sick-day rules should be part of all patients' education and frequent monitoring with ketone checks for sugars greater than 300 mg/dL should be routine.

HYPEROSMOLAR HYPERGLYCEMIC NONKETOTIC COMA

Hyperosmolar hyperglycemic nonketotic coma is a profound state of dehydration associated with a relative or absolute insulin deficiency [18,19••,20,21•]. The dehydration results from decreased effective insulin action leading to increased hepatic glucose production and decreased peripheral glucose utilization, leading, as in diabetic ketoacidosis, to an osmotic diuresis with loss of free water and electrolytes. This disorder has no significant ketone body formation or acidosis, which is associated with gastrointestinal distress. The polyuria and polydipsia are well tolerated, although loss of fluids and electrolytes is profound, and patients often do not seek medical attention until near cardiovascular collapse or in coma. As discussed earlier, diagnosis is difficult (Table 1).

Precipitating Factors

The most common initiating factor for the development of HHNK is undiagnosed NIDDM and lack of recognition of the early symptoms. A group of conditions and medications associated with decompensation and development of HHNK including infections, pancreatitis or pancreatic carcinoma, acromegaly, Cushing's syndrome, thyrotoxicosis, burns, drugs (diuretics, dilantin, glucocorticoids, propranolol, diazoxide), hypothermia, and heat stroke. Most of the conditions either lead to a severe decline in insulin secretion or induce an insulin-resistant state.

Treatment

The treatment of HHNK largely parallels that of diabetic ketoacidosis. Rigorous fluid repletion is essential to successful treatment. When this condition was first treated with insulin, there were a few instances of cardiovascular collapse secondary to rapid shift of glucose intracellularly. Because these patients are elderly and often have a compromised cardiovascular status, central venous pressure monitoring is recommended. Following the same treatment algorithm as is used for diabetic ketoacidosis is beneficial. The complications are similar to diabetic ketoacidosis. Patients will not need bicarbonate or pH monitoring and normalization of blood glucose and serum sodium are the main therapeutic endpoints. The risk of hypokalemia and hypophosphatemia is similar to that for diabetic ketoacidosis, so their levels should be monitored, with replacement as needed. Renal function dictates the clearance of potassium and phosphate, as such renal status must be assessed before administering these electrolytes to elderly patients.

Management of Patients After Hyperosmolar Hyperglycemic Nonketotic Coma

Many patients with HHNK have new-onset NIDDM and still have a good amount of endogenous insulin production. For this reason, once the patient is stable for a month or so (usually on insulin), it is reasonable to assess the best medical management as for any patient with diabetes. An episode of HHNK does not necessitate chronic life-long insulin therapy.

Preventing HHNK is mainly a matter of education. Repeated episodes of HHNK are seldom seen except in debilitated patients *ie*, s/p cerebrovascular accident (stroke), renal insufficiency, occult or recurrent infections) with poor thirst mechanisms or a functional inability to access appropriate fluids.

SURGICAL MANAGEMENT

Preoperative Surgical Evaluation

The key points for preoperative evaluation are listed in Table 6 [22]. The two most important aspects of preoperative evaluation are to establish adequate metabolic control and to optimize cardiovascular status. For elective surgery, the evaluation should be completed a few days before the scheduled operation so that changes in management can be made. Poor metabolic control will be exacerbated by the physiologic stress of the surgery and hyperglycemia will impair wound healing.

Any electrocardiogram abnormalities should be assumed to represent silent ischemia or silent infarction and the operation should be postponed until after complete cardiovascular evaluation. Evidence of peripheral vascular disease is often associated with increased cardiac risk, and patients should be treated expectantly. Autonomic neuropathy with orthostatic changes may predict anesthesia-induced hypotension, and the hydration status of the patient should be carefully assessed.

Surgical Management

Many different strategies can be used to treat patients during surgery and most are effective as long as hyperglycemia and hypoglycemia can be avoided. All surgery should be done early in the day.

A general schema for management is given in Table 7 [23]. The insulin infusion should be adjusted as noted in Table 8. During cardiovascular bypass surgery, patients can be extremely insulin resistant, requiring as many as 50 units of insulin an hour. Blood glucose should be monitored hourly in operations longer than 2 hours and postoperatively every 2 hours until stable, then every 4 hours. The optimal glycemic range is 125 to 200 mg/d as this range minimizes risk of hypoglycemia.

Postoperative Management

Many patients with diabetes have complicated postoperative courses, with 15% to 25% having complications. These include wound infections, genitourinary tract infections, cardiovascular complications, and delayed wound healing. Optimal metabolic control and careful fluid management can minimize these complications, but careful postoperative management with early recognition of problems is the key to successful outcomes.

TABLE 6 PREOPERATIVE SURGICAL EVALUATION

History
Angina, claudication, prior cardiovascular events, family history—coronary diagnosis, duration and control of diabetes

Physical
Blood pressure (with orthostatics), eye examination, neurologic examination (peripheral and autonomic), cardiovascular examination (S_4, S_3, peripheral pulses, bruits)

Laboratory
Fasting blood glucose, HgbA$_1$C, electrolytes plus creatinine, electrocardiogram, urine screen (ketones/protein)

S_3—third heart sound: S_4—fourth heart sound.

TABLE 7 SURGICAL MANAGEMENT

Minor surgery
NIDDM: Hold oral agents until after procedure and resume with the resumption of oral intake.
IDDM: One half of usual morning dose (NPH or Lente), remainder with resumption of oral regular as needed. (If blood sugar is >200 mg/d on insulin, infusion may be considered.)

Major surgery
NIDDM: If well controlled by diet or oral medication, manage as above with measured blood sugars every 4 h and insulin/glucose infusion for blood sugar >200.
NIDDM on insulin and IDDM: Insulin/glucose infusion.
Insulin infusion 1–3 U/h
10% dextrose in 0.45% normal saline at 100 mg/h (20 mEq/KCl)
Check glucose and adjust insulin drip every 1–2 h

Diabetic Management of Patients on Glucocorticoids or Chemotherapy

Glucocorticoids

Patients are placed on a regimen of glucocorticoids for many chronic diseases and occasionally for acute medical interventions. Glucocorticoids interfere with peripheral glucose utilization and enhance hepatic glucose production. That places an increased burden on the pancreas and will exacerbate diabetes. It may also unmask early diabetes in a diabetes-prone individual. These patients can occasionally be managed with diet, but more often need insulin or an oral agent. For patients requiring medications, the dosage will usually vary directly with the glucocorticoid dosage. As the steroid dose is being tapered, it is not uncommon that the diabetic state may suddenly resolve and hypoglycemic therapy may no longer be required. The occurrence of diabetes in the face of glucocorticoids suggests a deficient insulin reserve and these persons will be prone to the development of diabetes in the future.

Chemotherapy

Insulin-dependent diabetes mellitus

Patients receiving chemotherapy with cancer generally tend to have poor nutrition and weight loss. For patients with IDDM, that usually means a decrease in insulin requirements, especially regular insulin, and frequent monitoring will be needed to avoid hypoglycemia. Patients will need to remain adequately insulinized to avoid diabetic ketoacidosis, especially on severe sick days at the time of highest chemotherapy toxicity. Perhaps the most difficult aspect is to have the patients maintain adequate oral intake to avoid recurrent hypoglycemia. The acute and chronic renal failure that often results from tumor lysis syndromes will also radically diminish insulin requirements. Overall, patients with IDDM given chemotherapy will usually require lower insulin dosage and frequent glucose monitoring.

Noninsulin-dependent diabetes mellitus

For patients with NIDDM treated by diet regulation or oral agents, the weight loss and anorexia associated with cancer and chemotherapy will often improve their blood sugars. Patients taking oral agents, especially long-acting agents such as chlorpropamide, are at risk for hypoglycemia. This complication needs to be anticipated and medication dosage decreased. Patients taking oral agents frequently do not do home glucose monitoring and will need to be instructed in this technique.

Patients with NIDDM on an insulin regimen may also see a decline in insulin requirements. Some will be able to discontinue their insulin and others will need to be treated similarly to patients with IDDM. Once again, frequent home glucose monitoring will be useful to titrate the patient to the appropriate insulin dose.

Infection

Patients receiving chemotherapy are prone to infections. Infections will frequently elevate counter-regulatory hormones, blood sugar will increase, and insulin requirements may increase. Because hyperglycemia can impair leukocyte function (as can chemotherapy), it is best to optimize blood glucose levels during the treatment of the infection. As the infection resolves, the insulin requirements will return to baseline.

After chemotherapy

Once the chemotherapy is completed, the patients' diabetes treatment will depend on their weight and calorie consumption. For most IDDM patients, the regimen will be similar to that before therapy. For patients with NIDDM, body weight and activity levels will be key determinants. If patients with NIDDM have been taken off of diabetic medications during chemotherapy, they should be observed for the need to resume therapy.

References and Recommended Reading

Recently published papers of particular interest have been highlighted as:
- Of interest
- •• Of outstanding interest

1. Hospitalizations for diabetic ketoacidosis–Washington State, 1987–1989. *MMWR Morb Mortal Wkly Rep* 1992, 41:837–839.
2. Wetterhall SF, Olson DR, DeStefano F, *et al.*: Trends in diabetes and diabetic complications, 1908–1987. *Diabet Care* 1992, 15:960–967.
3. Basu A, Close CF, Jenkins D, *et al.*: Persisting mortality in diabetic ketoacidosis. *Diabet Med* 1993, 10:282–284.
4. Malone ML, Gennis V, Goodwin JS: Characteristics of diabetic ketoacidosis in older versus younger adults. *J Am Geriatr Soc* 1992, 40:1100–1104.
5. Barrett EJ, DeFronzo RA: Diabetic ketoacidosis: diagnosis and treatment. *Hosp Pract (Off Ed)* 1984, 19:89–95, 99–104.
6.•• Kreisberg RA: Diabetic ketoacidosis. In *Diabetes Mellitus: Theory and Practice*. Edited by Rifkin H, Porte D. New York: Elsevier; 1990:591–603.
7. McGarry JD, Foster DW: Regulation of hepatic fatty acid oxidation and ketone body production. *Annu Rev Biochem* 1980, 49:395–420.
8.• Cefalu WT: Diabetic ketoacidosis. *Crit Care Clin* 1991, 7:89–108.
9. Fleckman AM: Diabetic ketoacidosis. *Endocrinol Metab Clin North Am* 1993, 22:181–207.
10. Alberti KG: Low-dose insulin in the treatment of diabetic ketoacidosis. *Arch Intern Med* 1977, 137:1367–1376.

Table 8. Insulin infusion rates

Blood sugar, *mg/dL*	Infusion rate, *U/h*
<100	0–1
101–200	1–2
201–300	2–3
301–400	3–4
>400	4–8 or more

Adapted from Kolterman [23]; with permission.

11. Soler NG, Bennett MA, Fitzgerald MG, Malins JM: Electrocardiogram as a guide to potassium replacement in diabetic ketoacidosis. *Diabetes* 1974, 23:610–615.

12. Gamba G, Oseguera J, Castrejon M, Gomez-Perez FJ: Bicarbonate therapy in severe diabetic ketoacidosis. A double-blind, randomized, placebo-controlled trial. *Rev Invest Clin* 1991, 43:234–238.

13. Beech JS, Iles RA, Cohen RD: Bicarbonate in the treatment of metabolic acidosis: effects on hepatic intracellular pH, gluconeogenesis, and lactate disposal in rats. *Metabolism* 1993, 42:341–346.

14. Zipf WB, Bacon GE, Spencer ML, *et al.*: Hypocalcemia, hypomagnesemia, and transient hypoparathyroidism during therapy with potassium phosphate in diabetic ketoacidosis. *Diabetes Care* 1979, 2:265–268.

15. Sinclair AJ, Bouloux PM, Sanders PG, Gale EA: Persistent normal anion gap acidosis in the recovery phase of diabetic ketoacidosis. *Br J Clin Pract* 1991, 45:59–60.

16. Fein IA, Rachow EC, Sprung CL, Grodman R: Relation of colloid osmotic pressure to arterial hypoxemia and cerebral edema during crystalloid volume loading of patients with diabetic ketoacidosis. *Ann Intern Med* 1982, 96:570–575.

17. Kalis NN, van der Merwe PL, Schoeman JF, Smith RM: Cerebral oedema with coning in diabetic ketoacidosis. Report of 2 survivors. *S Afr Med J* 1991, 79:727–731.

18. Wachtel TJ: The diabetic hyperosmolar state. *Clin Geriatr Med* 1990, 6:797–806.

19.•• Matz R: Hyperosmolar nonacidotic diabetes (HNAD). In *Diabetes Mellitus: Theory and Practice*. Edited by Rifkin H, Porte D. New York: Elsevier; 1990:604–616.

20. Wachtel TJ, Tetu-Mouradjian LM, Goldman DL, *et al.*: Hyperosmolarity and acidosis in diabetes mellitus: a three-year experience in Rhode Island. *J Gen Intern Med* 1991, 6:495–502.

21.• Siperstein MD: Diabetic ketoacidosis and hyperosmolar coma. *Endocrinol Metab Clin North Am* 1992, 21:415–432.

22. Alberti KGMM: Diabetes and surgery. In *Diabetes Mellitus: Theory and Practice*. Edited by Rifkin H, Porte D. New York: Elsevier; 1990:626–633.

23. Kolterman OG: Surgery and the care of the diabetic patient. In *Clinical Guide to Diabetes Mellitus*. Edited by Sussman KE, Draznin B, James WE. New York: Alan R. Liss; 1987:175–181.

Select Bibliography

Raskin P, ed: *Medical Management of Non-Insulin Dependent (Type II) Diabetes*. Alexandria, VA: American Diabetes Association; 1994.

Rifkin H, Porte D, eds: *Diabetes Mellitus: Theory and Practice*. New York: Elsevier Publishers; 1990.

Santiago JV, ed: *Medical Management of Insulin-Dependent (Type I) Diabetes*. Alexandria, VA: American Diabetes Association; 1994.

Complications of Diabetes

Fredric B. Kraemer

> ### Key Points
> - Microvascular complications are related to the duration of diabetes and the degree of glucose control, whereas macrovascular complications are related to known cardiovascular risk factors and diabetes itself.
> - Diagnosis of complications depends on close surveillance and is based on careful patient history, physical examination, and laboratory studies.
> - Near normal glycemic control to prevent complications is the goal of therapy and is also recommended to delay the progression of complications when they occur.
> - Control of hypertension with angiotensin-converting enzyme inhibitors is important.
> - Patient education and reduction of cardiovascular risk factors should be emphasized.
> - Drug therapy should be tailored for the patient's complications and symptoms.

A summary of recommendations for the generalist to follow for the early recognition, prevention, or retardation of complications in patients with diabetes is provided in Table 1. Patients with diabetes mellitus, whether insulin-dependent (type I) or non-insulin-dependent (type II), are prone to develop a number of complications that have historically been classified as affecting primarily either small blood vessels (causing microvascular complications) or large blood vessels (causing macrovascular complications) (Table 2). It is less certain whether the metabolic perturbations of diabetes itself are responsible for the development of the complications or whether diabetes simply exaggerates other factors that are then responsible for the complications, but patients with diabetes manifest a markedly increased incidence or an accelerated progression of complications.

Over the past decade, studies in humans, animal models, and experimental systems have tended to support a link between the development of diabetic complications and the degree of glucose control [1,2•,3]. Several epidemiologic studies have shown a strong relationship between the degree of glucose control and the development or extent of retinopathy, neuropathy, and nephropathy. A few trials of intensive insulin therapy in type I diabetics, who had evidence of microvascular complications, have generally, though not always, demonstrated a stabilization or improvement in complications. Intensive insulin therapy has usually resulted in an improvement in measurements of nerve conduction velocity, but this therapy frequently has not translated into any perceptible changes in symptoms. The effects of intensive insulin therapy on nephropathy in these trials have been quite variable, with some reversibility or stabilization demonstrated in early stages but not in later ones.

Most importantly, the results of the Diabetes Control and Complications Trial have recently been reported and demonstrate a significant effect of improved glycemic control [4••]. Intensive insulin therapy was associated with 50% to 70% reduction in the development of microvascular complications (retinopathy,

TABLE 1 SECONDARY PREVENTION FOR PATIENTS WITH DIABETES MELLITUS
Medical history
Symptoms suggestive of development of any diabetic complications
Development of any other medical conditions that could affect complications
Assessment of symptoms related to glucose control and results of glucose monitoring
Physical examination
Comprehensive physical exam at least annually
Complete eye exam annually
Assessment of blood pressure at each visit
Examination of the feet at each visit
Examination of areas previously noted to be abnormal or areas of abnormalities suggested by the history
Laboratory evaluation
Glycosylated hemoglobin at least twice per year
Fasting lipids (triglycerides, cholesterol, high-density lipoprotein cholesterol) annually
Routine urinalysis annually
24-hour urinary protein excretion annually, including glomerular filtration rate if proteinuria detected
Indications for referrals to specialists
Patients with recurrent diabetic ketoacidosis or decompensation of glucose control should be referred to a diabetes specialist
Patients with diabetes who desire pregnancy should be referred to an obstetrician and a medical specialist in diabetes before pregnancy begins and should be followed by these specialists during pregnancy
Patients with evidence of diabetic retinopathy or visual disturbances should be referred to an ophthalmologist
Patients with evidence of clinical nephropathy should be referred to a specialist in diabetic renal disease
Patients with evidence of foot problems should be referred to a podiatrist, orthopedic surgeon, or vascular surgeon as indicated
Patients with manifestations of autonomic neuropathy should be referred to an appropriate specialist
Adapted from ADA Position Statement [9]; with permission.

TABLE 2 COMPLICATIONS IN PATIENTS WITH DIABETES	
Microvascular	**Macrovascular**
Retinopathy	Peripheral vascular disease
Nephropathy	Foot ulcers
Neuropathy	Amputations
	Myocardial infarction
	Cerebrovascular accidents

TABLE 3 FACTORS RELATED TO THE PATHOGENESIS OF DIABETIC COMPLICATIONS
Hyperglycemia
Duration, magnitude
Leading to:
1. Abnormalities in blood flow and vascular permeability
2. Cell damage
Hypertension
Hyperlipidemia
Genetic factors
HLA phenotype
Variations in enzymes in the polyol pathway
Variations in enzymes regulating heparan sulfates
HLA—human antigen leukocyte

TABLE 4 ALTERATIONS INDUCED BY HYPERGLYCEMIA
↑ **Sorbitol (polyol) pathway**
→ Altered redox state
↑ **Diacylglycerol and ↑protein kinase C activity**
↓ **Myoinositol and ↓ Na/K–ATPase activity**
↑ **Glycation (nonenzymatic modification of proteins)**
Reversible
Irreversible → advanced glycation end products

neuropathy, nephropathy) in patients without previous evidence of complications and a similar reduction in the progression of these complications in patients who had preexisting complications. Therefore, the Diabetes Control and Complications Trial has conclusively demonstrated in a study of sufficient statistical power that optimizing glucose control can prevent the development and slow the progression of diabetic complications.

A vast amount of data has been generated concerning potential mechanisms responsible for the development of micro- and macrovascular complications in diabetes (Table 3). Most of the data suggest that hyperglycemia is the central factor in the pathogenesis of microvascular complications; however, hyperglycemia is clearly not the only factor involved, because not all patients with diabetes develop microvascular complications. Thus, a number of genetic factors have also been suggested as modulating the response to hyperglycemia and the subsequent development of complications. It has been proposed that the effects of hyperglycemia are mediated by glucose through changes in several different pathways (Table 4) [5•]. It seems likely that each mechanism might play a variable role in the development or propagation of a particular complication.

Retinopathy

Natural History

Ophthalmologic classifications of diabetic retinopathy, based on stereoscopic fundus photography or fluorescein angiography, are not suitable for most internists. For nonophthalmologists, diabetic retinopathy is most easily divided into a first stage of background retinopathy and a later progressive stage of proliferative retinopathy.

The prevalence of diabetic retinopathy appears to vary with the duration of diabetes and, to a lesser extent, with the type of diabetes, as shown by several large epidemiologic studies [6•]. The onset of diabetic retinopathy is heralded by capillary microaneurysms, which appear as small red dots with smooth edges (punctate hemorrhages tend to have irregular borders). The increase in vascular permeability gives rise to retinal hemorrhages or hard exudates. When these are found within one disk diameter of the center of the macula, the patient is at risk for developing macular edema, which is a threat to visual acuity and warrants a referral to an ophthalmologist. Likewise patients with a large number of retinal hemorrhages or hard exudates, even if these lesions do not involve the macula, as well as patients with evidence of cotton-wool spots (soft exudates) should also be referred to an ophthalmologist, because they probably have intraretinal microvascular abnormalities.

Proliferative retinopathy is heralded by the formation of new blood vessels. With the proliferation of new blood vessels and formation of fibrous tissue, there is contraction of the vitreous and a tendency to pull the retina forward (detachment), causing preretinal or vitreous hemorrhages that will be associated with visual symptoms ranging from a few floating specks to loss of all vision but light perception. A massive hemorrhage will usually occur within a few days or weeks of the initial event. Thus, patients with vitreous hemorrhages require prompt attention from an ophthalmologist.

Screening

The ability to detect retinopathy is dependent on the skill of the observer and on the methods utilized. Stereoscopic fundus photography is the gold standard and is similar in sensitivity to fluorescein angiography. However, dilated ophthalmoscopy is more cost-effective and easily available, even though up to 20% of individuals with retinopathy can be missed. Guidelines for screening for diabetic retinopathy have been developed by several groups, including the American Diabetes Association, the American Academy of Ophthalmology, and the American College of Physicians (Table 5). In general, their recommendations are similar and utilize dilated ophthalmoscopy as the procedure of choice.

Risk Factors for Retinopathy

The major risk for the development of diabetic retinopathy relates to the duration of diabetes and the degree of hyperglycemia. The prevalence of retinopathy increases the longer the disease has been present and occurs earlier in individuals who have been poorly controlled. Of the other risk factors suggested to be associated with an increased risk of retinopathy, few have been consistently found to be statistically significant. No differences in the prevalence of nonproliferative or proliferative retinopathy are observed among men versus women. Some studies have suggested a higher frequency of retinopathy among Mexican-Americans and blacks, but this has not been a consistent finding. A genetic predisposition has been suggested by an association of retinopathy with several different human leukocyte antigens. Hypertension, both systolic and diastolic, alcohol consumption, and cigarette smoking have been associated, but not uniformly, with the development and progression of retinopathy. Proteinuria, either microalbuminuria or macroalbuminuria, is associated with an increased prevalence of nonproliferative and proliferative retinopathy, as is pregnancy.

Therapy

The mainstay of medical therapy for diabetic retinopathy is prevention through the achievement of near normal glycemic control. The achievement of near normoglycemia is also recommended when retinopathy is already present. The only caveat is that caution should be exercised in establishing near normoglycemia in individuals with retinopathy who have had long-standing poor glucose control (requiring a fall in $HgbA_{1c}$

TABLE 5 SCREENING GUIDELINES FOR DIABETIC RETINOPATHY

1. Patients with type I diabetes should be screened annually starting 5 years after the onset of diabetes; however, screening is generally not required prior to the onset of puberty.
2. Patients with type II diabetes should be screened when the diagnosis of diabetes is made. If dilated ophthalmoscopy is utilized, screening should be repeated annually. If stereoscopic fundus photography is performed and shows no evidence of retinopathy, screening need not be repeated for 4 years. As an exception, patients who have persistent hyperglycemia (≥ 280 mg/dL) or proteinuria should be screened annually even if the initial screening is normal. After the 4 years following an initial normal screening, subsequent screening should be performed annually.
3. Women with preexisting diabetes who become pregnant should have a comprehensive eye exam during the first trimester of pregnancy and should be followed closely throughout the pregnancy. These recommendations do not apply to women with gestational diabetes, because they are not at risk for developing retinopathy.
4. Finally, individuals with macular edema, moderately to advanced nonproliferative retinopathy, and any evidence of proliferative retinopathy should be referred to an ophthalmologist experienced in the management of diabetic retinopathy.

Adapted from ADA Position Statement [22] and Screening Guidelines for Diabetic Retinopathy [23]; with permission.

>3%), because an acceleration of retinopathy is often observed within the first 6 to 12 months after initiation of intensive therapy. Although no trials have established similar efficacy of glucose control on retinopathy in type II diabetics, it seems reasonable to take a similar approach with these patients.

Antiplatelet agents have been investigated for efficacy in retinopathy, with a small beneficial effect noted in some studies but not in others. It should be noted that antiplatelet agents could be used without increasing the risks of vitreous hemorrhage and can be used safely for other indications, such as prevention of atherosclerotic complications (*see* below), even in patients with advanced retinopathy.

The major therapeutic modality for treating diabetic retinopathy is retinal photocoagulation. Photocoagulation reduces new vessel formation and macular edema, leading to an improvement in vision and preservation of sight. It is important to advise patients undergoing panretinal photocoagulation that there is a loss of peripheral vision resulting from the therapy, but that the treatment reduces the rate of blindness by over 50%. Finally, the early use of pars plana vitrectomy in patients with severe vitreous hemorrhage or retinal detachment has been shown to preserve visual acuity.

Nephropathy

Natural History

The natural history of renal disease has been established for patients with type I diabetes but is relatively unclear for patients with type II diabetes [7,8]. Before the development of clinical nephropathy resulting from diabetes, there are effects on renal function (Fig. 1). Abnormalities observed at the time of diagnosis are reversed by institution of insulin therapy and achievement of optimal glycemic control. Renal function is then typically stable for a number of years. During this time, no clinical signs are apparent; however, morphologic lesions of the glomeruli develop. In approximately 30% to 50% of patients, there will be progression after 7 to 15 years to incipient nephropathy, where urinary albumin excretion rates are continuously elevated between 30 and 300 mg/24 h (microalbuminuria). Glomerular filtration rates are usually normal or still elevated during this stage, and a rise in blood pressure is frequently observed.

Microalbuminuria is highly predictive for the occurrence of clinical nephropathy over the ensuing 5 to 15 years. Clinical diabetic nephropathy, manifest by urinary protein excretion of more than 300 mg/24 h, occurs in approximately 40% of patients with type I diabetes after 40 years of follow-up. At this stage glomerular filtration rates are normal or reduced and elevations in blood pressure are seen. If hypertension is left untreated, rates of glomerular filtration will decline, on the average, at 1 mL/min/mo. At this rate, end-stage renal disease, manifest by uremia and the need for dialysis or transplantation, develops in a mean of 7 years, with 75% of patients developing end-stage renal disease by 10 years.

As many as 13% to 41% of patients with type II diabetes have microalbuminuria at the time of diagnosis, and up to 5% already manifest clinical nephropathy. Microalbuminuria in patients with type II diabetes also predicts the development of clinical proteinuria; however, a steady decline in glomerular filtration rate has been difficult to document. In fact, microalbuminuria is a stronger predictor of cardiovascular mortality than renal disease in these patients. Although there appear to be variations among different ethnic groups, the progression to end-stage renal disease in patients with type II diabetes seems to be similar to that seen in patients with type I diabetes.

Predisposing Factors

Hyperglycemia and, in particular, poor glucose control are strong predictors of the development of clinical diabetic nephropathy. In addition, age and the duration of diabetes are

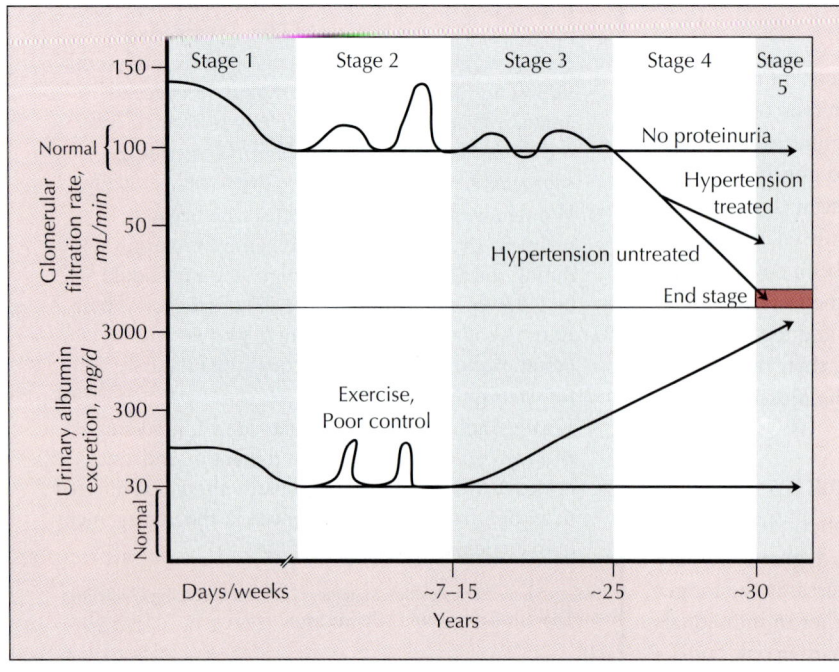

Figure 1 Course of diabetic nephropathy. (*Adapted from* Mogensen and coworkers [24]; with permission.)

strongly associated, with little evidence for nephropathy developing before puberty or after 30 years of disease if it has not already done so. However, it is clear that other factors are also involved because less than 40% of all patients with diabetes, whether type I or II, develop clinical diabetic nephropathy. Genetic predisposition is suggested by the clustering of nephropathy within families and by a strong family history of hypertension or cardiovascular disease in patients who develop nephropathy. Race also seems to confer a susceptibility, because the incidence of clinical nephropathy is two- to sixfold higher in blacks, Mexican-Americans, and American Indians than in whites. Whether this results from an increased frequency of hypertension, less access to medical care, or greater poverty is not clear. Cigarette smoking and hyperlipidemia could possibly play roles in the development of nephropathy, but this association has not been conclusively established. Body weight and gender have no impact on the development of nephropathy.

Screening

Recommendations for surveillance and screening for diabetic nephropathy have been published by the American Diabetes Association and the Canadian Diabetes Advisory Board [9,10]. These groups suggest that a urinalysis and serum creatinine be performed initially and annually thereafter. In adults, a 24-hour urine for protein excretion (detecting microalbuminuria if possible) and creatinine clearance should be obtained. After 5 years of diabetes in children and in all adults, yearly determinations of urinary protein (and particularly microalbumin) excretion and glomerular filtration rate should be made. Attention to the control of risk factors should routinely be given. If clinical nephropathy develops, the patient should be referred to a specialist in diabetic renal disease.

Therapy

The goal of therapy is primary prevention through the achievement of near normoglycemia. Several trials have shown improved glucose control can decrease the incidence of microalbuminuria as well as the progression of microalbuminuria to overt nephropathy in type I diabetes. It seems reasonable to infer that patients with type II diabetes would similarly benefit from improved glucose control and that end-stage renal disease would thus be delayed or prevented. Unfortunately, once overt clinical nephropathy has developed, the achievement of near normoglycemia does not influence the progression of renal disease.

Aggressive management of hypertension is very useful in preserving renal function at all stages of renal involvement. Reducing elevated blood pressure results in a decrease in proteinuria and an improvement in glomerular filtration rate [11••]. Low-dose angiotensin-converting enzyme inhibitors have been shown to be effective in reducing proteinuria and maintaining glomerular filtration rate in normotensive type I and type II diabetics with microalbuminuria without affecting blood pressure. In addition, angiotensin-converting enzyme inhibitors are associated with a significant reduction in risk of death, dialysis, and transplantation in patients with clinical diabetic nephropathy [12]. Thus, they should be the antihypertensive agents of choice for treating hypertension in diabetic patients, whether type I or type II. In addition, low-dose angiotensin-converting enzyme inhibitors should be considered in normotensive patients with evidence of microalbuminuria. Given the results of recent clinical studies, it seems reasonable to try to reduce blood pressure to at least 130/80 in patients with diabetes and albuminuria.

Decreasing dietary protein to approximately 0.6 g/kg body weight/d has been shown to reduce proteinuria and slow the rate of decline of the glomerular filtration rate in some patients with overt nephropathy as well as decrease proteinuria in some patients with microalbuminuria. No longer-term studies have yet documented that decreasing dietary protein is effective in preventing the development of clinical nephropathy. Thus, although some protein restriction (0.8 g/kg body weight/d) or more severe protein restriction if the patient has symptoms of uremia might be indicated, the routine use of low-protein diets is not currently advised.

When patients develop overt nephropathy and progress to end-stage renal disease, they should be under the care of a specialist in diabetic renal disease. If no contraindications exist, renal transplantation is currently the therapy of choice. Many centers now perform pancreas transplantation at the time of renal transplantation in patients with type I diabetes with very favorable results. If transplantation is not an option, a decision must be made between hemodialysis and continuous ambulatory peritoneal dialysis.

NEUROPATHY

Clinical Syndromes

The term *diabetic neuropathy* refers to a number of different clinical syndromes that develop in patients with diabetes [13–15]. Estimates of the prevalence of neuropathy in patients with diabetes range up to 90%, with most studies suggesting approximately 50% of patients will have clinical evidence of neuropathy after 15 to 20 years. Development of neuropathy is related to the degree of hyperglycemia and the duration of disease, although acute hyperglycemia can cause reversible abnormalities on nerve conduction studies.

A classification used for diabetic neuropathy is shown in Table 6. The most common form of neuropathy observed in diabetics is a diffuse, distal, symmetric sensorimotor neuropathy that affects the lower extremities first and can later affect the upper extremities. The pathogenesis of diffuse neuropathies appears to relate to metabolic derangements. The sensory component usually predominates, with the insidious onset of diminished sensation, proprioception, or temperature discrimination in a stocking-glove distribution. Ankle jerks are generally absent early, whereas muscle weakness and atrophy are usually late manifestations. Occasionally, patients may complain of lancinating, burning, or aching pain, pins and needles, numbness, or coldness. These symptoms are usually worse at night and exacerbated by contact with clothing or other objects. Diffuse neuropathy affecting the autonomic system has a wide variety of manifestations that are

| **Table 6** | **Classification of diabetic neuropathy** |

Subclinical

Clinical
  Diffuse neuropathy
    Distal symmetrical sensorimotor
    Autonomic
  Focal neuropathy
    Mononeuropathy
    Cranial mononeuropathies
    Mononeuropathy multiplex
    Femoral neuropathy (amyotrophy)
    Radiculopathy

important to identify because treatment can often improve the quality of the patient's life.

Focal neuropathies occur primarily on a vascular or traumatic basis. Focal neuropathies affect single or multiple peripheral or cranial nerves, with symptoms and signs dependent on the distribution of the nerve or nerves involved. The presentation is usually acute and may be painful in half the cases. It is important to exclude internal carotid artery aneurysms or a space-occupying lesion as the underlying cause. Symptoms generally resolve in 2 to 6 months. Femoral neuropathy is a proximal motor neuropathy with weakness and wasting of the quadriceps (girdle area). It is characteristically associated with severe wasting; however, there is generally complete recovery after several months to years. Radiculopathy usually presents as unilateral pain in the distribution of a thoracoabdominal nerve root. It can be confused with herpes zoster if vesicles are not seen. Diabetic radiculopathies will generally resolve within 6 months.

Therapy

Maintenance of near normal glucose control is the recommended therapy for the prevention of diabetic neuropathy. In addition, it will often improve symptoms of painful neuropathy, although rapid insulinization is occasionally associated with a transient worsening of symptoms.

Figure 2 displays a scheme for treating patients with painful diabetic neuropathy. Simple physical measures and mild analgesics should be tried first. If the patient has burning pain, capsaicin cream can be applied. Side effects include burning, rash, and inhalation reactions. If the patient does not respond to capsaicin or has gnawing, deep-seated pain, tricyclic antidepressants (preferably without fluphenazine, which increases the sedative effects) have been shown to be effective in more than 50% of patients. The major side effects are anticholinergic symptoms and drowsiness. Other interventions include carbamazepine (whose use is curtailed by the risk of unacceptable adverse side effects, predominantly leukopenia) and mexiletine, whose side effects include gastrointestinal upset, dizziness, and the potential for worsening arrhythmias. Interventions that are occasionally effective, but that have not been rigorously studied, include clonidine, clonazepam, baclofen, and pentoxifylline.

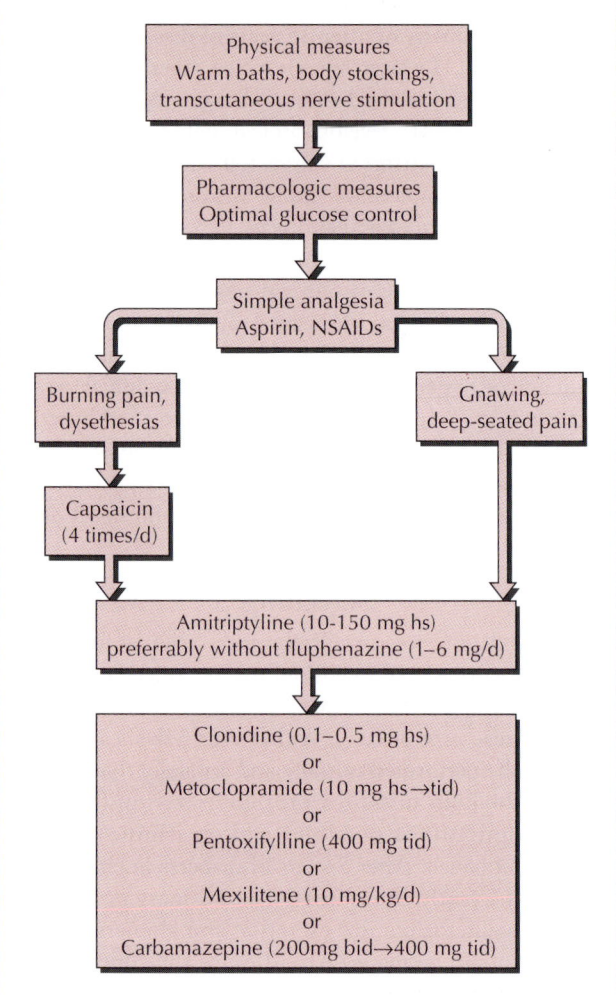

Figure 2 Treatment strategy for painful diabetic neuropathy. bid—twice daily; NSAIDs—nonsteroidal antiinflammatory drugs; tid—three times daily. (*Adapted from* Vinik and coworkers [15]; with permission.)

Treatment of symptoms of autonomic neuropathy is often very difficult and may require referral to a specialist (Table 7). Patients with orthostatic hypotension should be evaluated for volume depletion, anemia, hypothyroidism, and adrenal insufficiency before therapy is initiated. Therapeutic measures consist of use of body stockings, volume expansion with increased salt intake or fludrocortisone, phenylephrine, or clonidine. Gastrointestinal symptoms can be improved with metoclopramide, cisapride, or erythromycin, but it is important to exclude intrinsic gastrointestinal pathology with endoscopy or an upper gastrointestinal series before initiating therapy. Diabetic diarrhea can be extremely frustrating to treat. Once laxative abuse, excess alcohol intake, pancreatic insufficiency, and infectious or inflammatory processes have been excluded, diphenoxylate, loperamide, or codeine can be tried. Bile acid sequestrants or clonidine are sometimes helpful, as is a short (2-week) course of a broad-spectrum antibiotic such as tetracycline. Urinary incontinence can sometimes be treated successfully with bethanechol or may require recurrent self-catheterization. Erectile impotence is very common.

It is important to exclude psychogenic causes, gonadal deficiency, and vascular insufficiency (buttock claudication). Therapy can involve counseling, avoidance of medications associated with impotence (β-blockers, etc.), vacuum suction devices, intracavernous injections of vasoactive drugs (papaverine, phentolamine), and penile implants. Referral to a specialist should be made for these latter interventions. Retrograde ejaculation can often be improved with brompheniramine.

PERIPHERAL VASCULAR DISEASE—FOOT ULCERS

Pathogenesis

The occurrence of foot ulcers and other foot problems in diabetics is a major cause of morbidity and expense, because diabetics account for approximately 50% of all nontraumatic amputations performed in the United States. It is estimated that at least half of these procedures could be prevented with proper intervention and education. A combination of different factors leads to foot ulcers (Table 8). The typical patient developing a foot ulcer is one with neuropathy and loss of distal sensation in the feet who has unknowingly suffered trauma to the foot from a foreign object in the shoe, improperly fitting shoes, walking barefoot, or placing the foot in scalding water. If this trauma is left unattended, infection and ischemia threaten the foot [16].

Therapy

When a patient develops a foot ulcer, it is necessary to introduce proper care promptly. This care should be done in consultation with a specialist (podiatrist, orthopedic surgeon, vascular surgeon). The etiology of the ulcer, its size and the depth of involvement, the presence of purulent drainage, necrosis, and evidence of edema or cellulitis should be evaluated. Systemic infection should be excluded and a vascular exam performed. Radiologic examination to evaluate the presence of gas or a foreign body and to determine the presence of a Charcot joint is useful. Osteomyelitis can be difficult to assess with standard bone radiographs; often, radionuclide triple-phase bone scans or leukocyte scans are required.

Because diabetic foot ulcers are commonly polymicrobial in origin, broad-spectrum antibiotics are required. Débridement of the ulcer with removal of all nonviable tissue is essential for healing and provides a diagnostic means for bacterial culture. Wound care should consist of continued débridement as required. Foot soaks and applications of topical agents have not been rigorously studied and thus are not recommended. If there is evidence of ischemia of the foot (distal necrosis, absent pulses, or diminished arterial pressures by Doppler examination), vascular reconstruction should be considered. Improved glucose control should be an important priority because hyperglycemia can decrease the patient's ability to fight infection. Finally, treatment of a diabetic foot ulcer should include properly fitting footwear and patient education for prevention of recurrent ulcers.

Prevention

Because neuropathic changes are not reversible, peripheral vascular disease (PVD) tends to be progressive, and many of the structural deformities of the foot will persist, primary and secondary prevention are critical for foot care in the diabetic

TABLE 7 SYMPTOMS AND SIGNS OBSERVED IN DIABETIC AUTONOMIC NEUROPATHY

System	Symptoms or signs
Cardiovascular	Dizziness due to postural hypotension
	Resting tachycardia
Gastrointestinal	Dysphagia due to esophageal dysmotility
	Early satiety, nausea, vomiting due to gastroparesis diabeticorum
	Constipation
	Diarrhea
	Fecal incontinence
Genitourinary	Overflow incontinence due to atonic bladder
	Postmicturition dribbling
	Impotence
	Retrograde ejaculation
	Dyspareunia due to decreased vaginal lubrication
Thermoregulatory	Diminished or excessive sweating
	Gustatory sweating
	Dependent edema (neuropathic)
Metabolic	Hypoglycemia unawareness
Pupillary	Miosis
	Diminished dilation
	Argyll-Robertson-like pupil

TABLE 8 FACTORS CONTRIBUTING TO THE DEVELOPMENT OF FOOT ULCERS

Neuropathy
Distal, symmetrical, sensorimotor—loss of pain or temperature sensation, loss of proprioception with abnormal gait
Autonomic—abnormal sweating

Structural factors
Hammerhead deformity of the toes
Bunions
Calluses
Poorly trimmed toenails
Improperly fitted shoes
Neuroosteoarthropathy (Charcot joint)

Vascular
Large vessels (proximal—aortoiliac, femoral)
Small vessels (distal—below the knee)
Cigarette smoking

patient. Prevention is undertaken through surveillance by the health care provider and through patient education (Table 9) [10,17]. This recommended approach has been shown to be effective in improving patient outcome [18].

Atherosclerosis

Macrovascular disease, manifest by coronary artery disease (CAD), PVD, and cerebrovascular disease, constitutes the leading cause of mortality among patients with diabetes [19,20]. Patients with type II diabetes have a two- to fourfold increased risk for CAD, and the protective effect of female gender in premenopausal women is lost when diabetes is present. Similarly, PVD is about four- to sixfold higher among type II diabetics than nondiabetic subjects, and cerebrovascular disease is about two- to fourfold higher among diabetics. Type I diabetics have about an 11-fold higher risk of CAD than nondiabetics, and there is a cumulative mortality from CAD of approximately 35% among type I diabetics by 55 years of age.

Cardiovascular Risk Factors

The prevalence of many of the risk factors predisposing to atherosclerosis and cardiovascular disease is increased in patients with diabetes; however, factors such as aging, male gender, and genetic predisposition are similar to diabetics and nondiabetics. Among the known cardiovascular risk factors, several are potentially reversible; they include cigarette smoking, hypertension, obesity, hyperglycemia, hyperinsulinemia, hypercholesterolemia, hypertriglyceridemia, and low high-density lipoprotein cholesterol. A strong relationship between the duration of diabetes and the development of CAD is seen in type I diabetics. Albuminuria is a powerful predictor of cardiovascular mortality in both type I and type II diabetics. How these risk factors combine to influence the atherosclerotic process and how diabetes causes an acceleration of this process are not fully understood, but lipid and lipoprotein abnormalities, alterations in thrombotic and antithrombotic factors, growth factors or cytokines, insulin resistance and hyperinsulinemia, and glycation or oxidation of proteins and lipids could all contribute to the pathogenesis of atherogenesis [21].

Lipoprotein Abnormalities

There are a number of quantitative and qualitative abnormalities in lipid and lipoproteins in patients with diabetes. These abnormalities differ in type I and type II diabetics. Most patients with type I diabetes have normal concentrations of plasma lipids and lipoproteins, although qualitative defects can be discerned using investigational measurements. The prevalence of hyperlipidemia is relatively similar in type I diabetics and age-matched nondiabetics with the exception that hypertriglyceridemia is a little more common among women with type I diabetes. In fact, hypercholesterolemia tends to be less frequent among men and women with type I diabetes than among nondiabetic subjects. In contrast to type I diabetes, dyslipidemia (including elevated lipids or low high-density lipoprotein cholesterol) is very common among patients with type II diabetes. The prevalence of hyperlipidemia is generally two- to threefold that seen among nondiabetics, with approximately 60% or more of type II diabetics having evidence of dyslipidemia.

Therapy

Therapy of atherosclerosis should be directed at improving known vascular disease and reducing overall cardiovascular

TABLE 9 GUIDELINES FOR DIABETIC FOOT CARE PREVENTION

Examination
A qualified health care professional should examine the legs and feet at every visit
A comprehensive exam of the vascular, musculoskeletal, and neurologic systems should be performed at least annually. If significant evidence of ischemia, deformities of the foot, or abnormalities in the gait or wear patterns of the shoes are found, the patient should be referred to a specialist for consultation

Patient education
Low-risk patients without evidence of abnormalities on exam
  Provide instruction in:
    Foot hygiene
    Proper footwear
    Avoidance of trauma
    Smoking cessation
    Notify physician if blister, sore, or cracks in skin appear.
High-risk patients with evidence of vascular, musculoskeletal, or neurologic abnormalities on exam
  Instruct patient in all of above and to:
    Inspect inside of shoes for foreign objects before putting on shoes.
    Inspect feet daily for blisters, cuts, cracks, redness, infection.
    Wash feet daily and dry carefully
    Avoid exposure of feet to hot water, heating pads, hot water bottles.
    Do not cut corns or calluses or use chemical removal agents. These procedures to be performed by qualified health care provider.
    Avoid using adhesive tape on feet.
    Clip nails in contour with toes; do not cut deeply down sides.
    If patient is visually impaired, this task should be performed by family member or qualified health care provider.
    Notify physician if blister, sore, or cracks in skin appear.
Instruction on proper footwear
  Shoes should fit properly at purchase.
  Break in new shoes slowly.
  Wear shoes that breathe.
  Avoid high heels and pointed-toe shoes; also sandals and thongs.
  Do not walk barefoot anywhere.
  Always wear socks or stockings with shoes. Avoid tight elastic bands on socks or rolling hose.

risk. Thus, attempts should be made to modify reversible risk factors—such as cigarette smoking, hypertension, and obesity—through patient education, reinforcement, and medications. It is recommended that optimal glucose control remain a goal of therapy in view of its beneficial effects on the development and progression of microvascular complications and the improvements seen in dyslipidemias. Treatment of dyslipidemia in patients with diabetes is vitally important for reducing cardiovascular risk.

The treatment of dyslipidemia in diabetes requires a stepwise approach, starting with effective dietary therapy, weight reduction if the patient is obese, and a decrease in the intake of dietary saturated fat. Patients should be referred to a nutritionist for dietary evaluation and instruction. Optimal glucose control should be attained through a combination of diet, exercise, oral hypoglycemic agents, or insulin therapy. If hyperlipidemia persists, pharmacologic therapy with hypolipidemic agents should be instituted; patients should be monitored for the effectiveness of the lipid-lowering agent and for specific toxicities associated with these agents. Consideration should be given to referring to a specialist patients with significant hyperlipidemia that has not responded to dietary therapy and improved glucose control. Unless contraindications to its use exist, aspirin is recommended for secondary prevention of cardiovascular and cerebrovascular disease in diabetics based on its proven effectiveness in trials involving nondiabetics.

References and Recommended Reading

Recently published papers of particular interest have been highlighted as:
- Of interest
- •• Of outstanding interest

1. Hanssen KF, Bangstad H-J, Brinchmann-Hansen O, Dahl-Jorgensen K: Blood glucose control and diabetic microvascular complications: long-term effects of near-normoglycemia. *Diabetic Med* 1992, 9:687–705.
2. • Strowig A, Raskin P: Glycemic control and diabetic complications. *Diabetes Care* 1992, 15:1126–1140.
3. Nathan DM: Long-term complications of diabetes mellitus. *N Engl J Med* 1993, 328:1676–1685.
4. •• The Diabetes Control and Complications Research Group: The effect of intensive treatment of diabetes on the development and progression of long-term complications in insulin-dependent diabetes mellitus. *N Engl J Med* 1993, 329:977–986.
5. • Ruderman NB, Williamson JR, Brownlee M: Glucose and diabetic vascular disease. *FASEB J* 1992, 6:2905–2914.
6. • Davis M: Diabetic retinopathy. *Diabetes Care* 1992, 15:1844–1874.
7. Selby JV, Fitzsimmons SC, Newman JM, *et al.*: The natural history and epidemiology of diabetic nephropathy—implications for prevention and control. *JAMA* 1990, 263:1954–1960.
8. Viberti GC, Yip-Messent J, Morocutti A: Diabetic nephropathy: future avenue. *Diabetes Care* 1992, 15:1216–1225.
9. ADA Position Statement: Standards of medical care for patients with diabetes mellitus. *Diabetes Care* 1995, 18(suppl 1):8–15.
10. Expert Committee of the Canadian Diabetes Advisory Board: Clinical practice guidelines for treatment of diabetes mellitus. *Can Med Assoc J* 1992, 147:697–712.
11. •• Kisaske BL, Kalil RSN, Ma JZ, *et al.*: Effect of antihypertensive therapy on the kidney in patients with diabetes: A meta-regression analysis. *Ann Intern Med* 1993, 118:129–138.
12. Lewis EJ, Hunsicker LG, Bain RP, Rohde RD: The effect of angiotensin-converting enzyme inhibition on diabetic nephropathy. *N Engl J Med* 1993, 329:1456–1462.
13. Harati Y: Diabetic peripheral neuropathies. *Ann Intern Med* 1987, 107:546–559.
14. Greene DA, Sima AAF, Pfeifer MA, Albers JW: Diabetic neuropathy. *Annu Rev Med* 1990, 41:303–317.
15. Vinik AI, Holland MT, Le Beau JM, *et al.*: Diabetic neuropathies. *Diabetes Care* 1992, 15:1926–1975.
16. Grunfeld C: Diabetic foot ulcers: Etiology, treatment, and prevention. *Adv Intern Med* 1992, 37:103–132.
17. ADA Position Statement: Foot care in patients with diabetes mellitus. *Diabetes Care* 1993, 16(suppl 2):19–20.
18. Litzelman DK, Slemenda CW, Langefeld CD, *et al.*: Reduction of lower extremity clinical abnormalities in patients with non-insulin-dependent diabetes mellitus: a randomized, controlled trial. *Ann Intern Med* 1993, 119:36–41.
19. Merrin PK, Feher MD, Elkeles RS: Diabetic macrovascular disease and serum lipids: is there a connection? *Diabetic Med* 1992, 9:9–14.
20. Donahue RP, Orchard TJ: Diabetes mellitus and macrovascular complications: an epidemiological perspective. *Diabetes Care* 1992, 15:1141–1155.
21. Bierman EL: Atherogenesis in patients. *Arterioscler Thromb* 1992, 12:647–656.
22. ADA Position Statement: Screening for diabetic retinopathy. *Diabetes Care* 1995, 18(suppl 1):21–23.
23. Screening guidelines for diabetic retinopathy. *Ann Intern Med* 1992, 116:683–685.
24. Mogensen CE, Christensen CK, Vittinghus E: The stages in diabetic renal disease with emphasis on the stage of incipient diabetic nephropathy. *Diabetes* 1983, 32(suppl 2):64–78.

Select Bibliography

Alberti KGMM, DeFronzo RA, Keen H, Zimmet P, eds: *International Textbook of Diabetes Mellitus*. Chicester: John Wiley & Sons; 1992.

Kahn CR, Weir GC, eds: *Joslin's Diabetes Mellitus*. Philadelphia: Lea & Febiger; 1994.

Pirart J: Diabetes mellitus and its complications: a prospective study of 4400 patients observed between 1947 and 1973. *Diabetes Care* 1978, 1:168–188, 252–263.

Report 7. A modification of the Airlie House classification of diabetic retinopathy. *Invest Ophthalmol Vis Sci* 1981, 21:210–226.

Breast Disease   17
David Heber

> ### *Key Points*
> - Approximately 50% of all women will experience some form of benign breast disease; this condition can include fibrosis, cysts, duct ectasia, and breast ductal cell atypical hyperplasia.
> - A fibroadenoma can be observed in patients younger than 25 years of age without removal once the diagnosis has been determined with certainty; in women older than 25 years, the slight risk of cancer dictates removal of the lesion.
> - Known risk factors for breast cancer include pregnancy after 30 years of age, nulliparity, proliferative benign breast disease, and history of breast cancer in mother or sister; however, most patients with breast cancer do not have known risk factors for the disease.
> - It is logical to recommend both a low-fat diet and maintenance of desirable body weight in women with breast cancer or an increased risk of breast cancer.
> - Nonpalpable lesions seen on mammography should result in referral for stereotactic needle biopsy or fine-needle aspiration of the breast mass; however, these diagnostic methods are not to be viewed as alternatives to open surgical biopsy and frozen section of suspicious lesions.

One of every nine women in the United States will develop breast cancer at some time during her life. Despite advances in screening and various treatment modalities, the overall mortality from breast cancer has not changed in the past 20 years. Both animal studies and studies of populations migrating to Western industrialized nations from countries with lower fat intake suggest that diet may be an important factor in the etiology and development of breast cancer [1]. Studies conducted among women living in the United States, where the variability in dietary intake is much less than in international studies, suggest that genetic predisposition may have a major effect [2]. In fact, the etiology of breast cancer is related both to genetic and to environmental and dietary factors. Widespread screening will probably lead to the earlier diagnosis of breast cancer, but only prevention has the potential to decrease the incidence of breast cancer. Developments in the areas of molecular biology and genetics may someday make it possible to provide more specific counseling about diet and lifestyle to individuals who are at increased risk for developing breast cancer. Approximately half of all women will have some form of benign breast disease, and these women will seek consultations for problems of nodularity, pain, and breast discharge, including galactorrhea [3]. In addition to providing a brief consideration of breast cancer, this chapter outlines the common forms of benign breast disease that the generalist may encounter.

BREAST CANCER

Most patients with breast cancer do not have known risk factors for the disease (Table 1). Cases of familial breast cancer represent a special subset, accounting for 5% to 10% of all breast cancer cases [4]. These forms of cancer represent inheritance

TABLE 1 RECOGNIZED RISK FACTORS FOR BREAST CANCER
Pregnancy after age 30 y Nulliparity Proliferative benign breast disease History of breast cancer in mother or sister

via the germline and have in common early onset (before 50 years of age) and an association with other forms of cancer, including ovarian cancer. Such women are the targets of increased attention in high-risk breast clinics and may be participating in research trials of antiestrogens and other agents for risk reduction. The most common form of breast cancer, which is sporadic, is the result of multiple somatic genetic changes at the level of the breast ductal cell. Changes have been described in the expression of both protooncogenes and tumor suppressor genes that regulate cell growth (Table 2) [5]. Because the known risk factors do not provide an adequate assessment of risk in most women who develop breast cancer, preventive strategies at this stage must be applied to all women to reduce the incidence of breast cancer significantly.

HORMONAL FACTORS

Breast cancer is frequently dependent on estrogen stimulation for growth, both *in vivo* and in experimental model systems. For the purposes of this chapter, premenopausal breast cancer in women younger than 40 years of age should be regarded as a separate disease in which high-fat diets and obesity are not related to incidence as they are for postmenopausal women. In postmenopausal women, the amount of estrogen produced from adrenal androgens and the percentage of bioavailable estradiol circulating (as opposed to that bound to serum proteins) are higher in obese than in lean women [6]. Obesity has repeatedly been associated with more advanced breast cancer at the time of diagnosis, higher rates of recurrence, and shorter survival times, even after tumor size and the stage of disease at diagnosis have been controlled [7–12]. A meta-analysis of epidemiologic studies relating body weight, body mass index, or relative body weight to breast cancer incidence demonstrated a significant positive relationship in 9 of 11 studies [13]. This association has been explained in the past as resulting from delayed diagnosis in obese women rather than from enhanced tumor promotion caused by increased estrogen production. However, Verreault and coworkers [14] found that the apparent effects of obesity on the invasiveness of breast cancers at the time of diagnosis were very different in patients with estrogen receptor–positive tumors than in those with estrogen receptor–negative tumors. Among patients with estrogen receptor–positive tumors, the incidence of involved nodes at diagnosis was 65.6% in obese patients (body mass index > 27 kg/m^2), compared with 32.9% in lean patients (body mass index < 21 kg/m^2). This highly significant difference was noted even after adjustment for age and tumor size. However, no such associations were seen among patients with estrogen receptor–negative tumors. If the effects of obesity on breast tumor nodal invasion, and therefore on prognosis, simply resulted from delayed diagnosis, then similar associations should have been seen for both the receptor-positive and the receptor-negative patients. The fact that such an effect of obesity was observed only in the receptor-positive patients strongly suggests that a hormonal mechanism accounts for the effects of obesity on breast tumor promotion. Potential hormonal mechanisms are summarized in Table 3.

DIETARY FACTORS

Adult weight gain increases the risk of postmenopausal breast cancer and is a predictor of breast cancer risk independent of body weight [15–17]. These findings suggest that positive energy balance may have a promotional effect independent of weight status. Such an effect could be mediated by estrogens in the opposite direction of the hormonal changes noted with short-term negative energy balance in postmenopausal women (discussed later). Several studies have demonstrated that patients with breast cancer are more likely to have abdominal obesity [17–19]. The relative risks of breast cancer are increased significantly for any given level of obesity by consid-

TABLE 2 GENETIC ALTERATIONS IN SPORADIC BREAST CANCER
Tumor suppressor genes p53 on 17p13.3 (lost in 60% of tumors) RB-1 on 13q14 **Protooncogenes** Protein kinases: src, yes, fgk, abl, erb B GTP binding proteins: H-ras, K-ras Growth factors: sis Nuclear proteins: myc, myb, fos, ski Hormone receptors: HER-2/neu, erb A

TABLE 3 HORMONAL AND NUTRITIONAL MECHANISMS PROMOTING BREAST CANCER IN POSTMENOPAUSAL WOMEN
Increased conversion of androstenedione to estrone in obese versus lean postmenopausal women Increased adrenal production of androstenedione in obese versus lean women Increased non–protein-bound estradiol in obese versus lean postmenopausal women with breast cancer Increased nodal invasion in obese versus lean postmenopausal women with estrogen receptor–positive tumors Increased estrogen receptor number in breast cancers in obese versus lean postmenopausal women

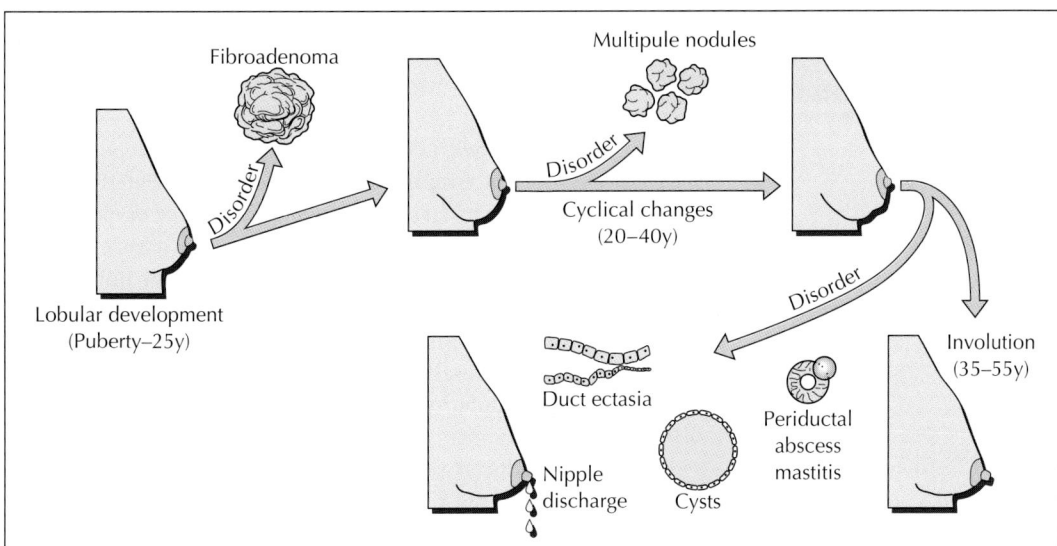

FIGURE 1
Breast disorders of development and involution.

ering fat distribution. Calculations based on the increased risk associated with abdominal obesity indicate that obese women who lose more than 4.5 kg of body weight decrease abdominal obesity and thereby decrease their relative increased risk of breast cancer by 45% [20].

Because added fat increases the caloric density as well as the palatability of processed foods, increased caloric intake is likely to result from free access to high-fat foods. A carefully designed study by Lissner and coworkers [21] demonstrated that when normal subjects were given a high-fat diet (45% to 50% of calories from fat) ad libitum, they consumed 600 more calories per day than subjects given a low-fat diet (15% to 20% of calories from fat) ad libitum. Therefore, in humans a high-fat and a high-calorie diet are necessarily associated and lead to obesity. It is logical to recommend both a lower-fat diet and the achievement of a desirable body weight in women with breast cancer or an increased risk of breast cancer.

BENIGN BREAST DISEASE

Fibrocystic Disease

In the past, there was a tendency to consider all benign breast disease as one disorder called fibrocystic breast disease. This condition has also been called a "nondisease" to differentiate it from cancer. In fact, this condition can include fibrosis, cysts, duct ectasia, and breast ductal cell atypical hyperplasia. It has been estimated that up to 50% of all women develop breast nodular disease at some time in their lives, and most of the clinical presentations of benign breast disease occur during the reproductive years of a woman's life (Fig. 1).

Abnormalities

Most of the benign abnormalities presenting in the breast are minor aberrations of normal development (Fig. 1) [22]. These presentations include fibroadenoma at younger ages; pain and nodularity in the mid-30s; and cysts, duct ectasia, and epithelial hyperplasia toward menopause. These periods in which different abnormalities appear to coincide with different periods in the development of the breast tissue. From menarcheal to approximately 25 years of age, lobular development is occurring. Then, between 20 and 40 years of age, the cyclic changes occurring with normal menstrual function take place. Between 35 and 55 years of age, involution of the breast ducts is occurring. Patchy changes in breast histology occur after pregnancy. During pregnancy, there is maximal stimulation of the growth and development of lobular tissue. After pregnancy, regression is patchy, with some areas regressing rapidly and others remaining hyperplastic for months to years. Therefore, the fibroadenomas and other abnormalities of ductal function can be regarded as aberrations rather than benign tumors [22]. The implication for management is that not all of these lesions require surgical removal.

RISK OF BREAST CANCER

The risk factors related to specifics of a woman's reproductive history as well as to a family history of breast cancer are associated with a magnitude of cancer risk that is less than twice that of comparable women from the general population and appropriately are not considered premalignant lesions (Table 4). The largest prospective study performed of the risk of breast cancer associated with breast lesions was conducted by Dupont and Page, who studied cancer incidence and its relationship to various pathologic features, including the proliferative status of the epithelium [23]. They defined three groups: 1) nonproliferative lesions, 2) proliferative lesions without atypia, and 3) atypical hyperplasia. In this study of more than 10,000 women, 70% were in the first group and had no increased risk of breast cancer. Approximately 25% of women were in the second group and had a 1.5- to twofold increased risk of breast cancer. About 4% of women had atypical hyperplasia, with a fourfold increased risk of breast cancer. Women who had both atypical hyperplasia and a family history of breast cancer had an eightfold increased risk of breast cancer. The actual increase in risk is distributed over a number of years, so that the absolute risk in this highest-risk group is 8% to 10% in 10 to 15 years. This risk is comparable to that of

Table 4 Breast cancer risk and pathology of benign breast disease
Not at increased risk
Adenosis
Apocrine metaplasia
Cysts (macrocysts, microcysts, or both)
Mild hyperplasia
Duct ectasia
Fibroadenoma
Mastitis
Squamous metaplasia
At slightly increased risk (1.5- to 2-fold)
Hyperplasia (moderate or florid)
Papilloma
Sclerosing adenosis (well developed)
At moderately increased risk (4- to 5-fold)
Atypical ductal hyperplasia
Atypical lobular hyperplasia

developing breast cancer in a contralateral breast after conservative treatment of invasive breast cancer. This famous study was done in the era before the widespread use of screening mammography. In a more recent study of biopsies done on mammographically suspicious lesions, the incidence of atypical hyperplasia increased from 4% to 10% of the study population [24].

When to Refer

Serious lesions can occur even in the breast with multiple nodules, and women should always be referred to comprehensive consultative services when any doubt exists as to the nature of the breast lesion. This step should certainly be taken before any hormonal treatment is instituted. Unfortunately, the mammographic appearance of dense breasts that are thought to correlate with increased amounts of proliferative tissue correlates poorly with the histologic pathology of masses that undergo biopsy [25].

A fibroadenoma can be safely observed in anyone younger than 25 years of age without removal once the diagnosis has been determined with certainty. In women older than 25 years of age, the slight risk of cancer dictates removal of the lesion. In a balanced discussion with younger patients, the decision can be made to remove the fibroadenoma simply to reassure the patient rather than because of the risk of leaving the lesion in place.

In the case of multiple areas of nodularity, the condition loses significance as a precancerous lesion, and the treatment is related to the impact on the patient. With cyclic mastalgia, a hormonal or dietary approach may be taken. In several studies, a low-fat, high-fiber diet with weight loss reduced symptoms of cystic mastalgia. Accepted hormonal manipulations include the use of bromocriptine and danazol.

In women who develop large cysts (so-called macrocysts), there is little concern about cancer, and simple aspiration adequately treats most such lesions in the breast with multiple nodules.

In women with duct ectasia, treatment is dependent on the severity of symptoms, which are usually related to breast nipple discharge. In simple discharge of milky or clear breast ductal fluid, women should be reassured. This condition commonly occurs for more than 1 year after nursing has been completed, and the discharge can be maintained by inadvertent nipple stimulation. Women should be made aware of the causal connection between nipple discharge and breast manipulation. If bloody discharge is observed, then referral for biopsy is necessary to rule out epithelial hyperplasia or intraductal cancer.

Periductal mastitis with abscess formation can also occur. This condition is usually treated simply with antibiotics and local surgical drainage.

In the modern mammographic era, nonpalpable lesions seen on mammography should result in referral for stereotactic needle biopsy or fine-needle aspiration of the breast mass. Although these biopsies do not supply adequate amounts of tissue for the examination of duct architecture, they do provide fragments and cells that can be used to diagnose cancerous changes based on the histopathology and cytopathology. These diagnostic methods require highly experienced units to be reliable alternatives to open surgical biopsy and frozen section of suspicious lesions.

The generalist should have adequate familiarity with breast lesions to know when to refer to experts. Only under unusual circumstances should any lesion be followed without proper diagnostic measures being used.

References and Recommended Reading

Recently published papers of particular interest have been highlighted as:
- Of interest
- Of outstanding interest

1. Willett WC: *Nutritional Epidemiology*. New York: Oxford University Press; 1990.
2. Council on Scientific Affairs, American Medical Association: Diet and cancer: where do matters stand?. *Arch Intern Med* 1993, 153:50–56.
3. Love SM, Gelman RS, Silen W: Fibrocystic "disease" of the breast: a non-disease? *N Engl J Med* 1982, 307:1010–1014.
4. Anderson DE: Genetic study of breast cancer: identification of a high risk group. *Cancer* 1974, 34:1090–1097.
5. King MC: Breast cancer genes: how many, where and who are they? *Nature Genet* 1990, 2:125–129.
6. MacDonald PC, Edman CD, Hemsell DL, *et al.*: Effect of obesity on conversion of plasma androstenedione to estrone in postmenopausal women with and without endometrial cancer. *Am J Obstet Gynecol* 1978, 130:448–455.
7. Kalish L: Relationship of body size with breast cancer. *J Clin Oncol* 1984, 2:287–293.
8. Abe R, Kumagai N, Kimura M: Biological characteristics of breast cancer in obesity. *Tohoku J Exp Med* 1976, 120:351–359.
9. Donegan WL, Hartz AJ, Rimm AA: The association of body weight with recurrent cancer of the breast. *Cancer* 1978, 41:1590–1594.

10. Howson CP, Kinne D, Wynder EL: Body weight, serum cholesterol and stage of primary breast cancer. *Cancer* 1986, 58:2372–2381.

11. De Waard F: Epidemiology of breast cancer: a review. *Eur J Clin Oncol* 1983, 19:1671–1676.

12. Lew EA, Garfinkel L: Variations in mortality by weight among 750,000 men and women. *J Chronic Dis* 1979, 32:563–576.

13. Albanes D: Total calories, body weight, and tumor incidence in mice. *Cancer Res* 1987, 47:1987–1991.

14. Verreault R, Brisson J, Deschenes L, Naud F: Body weight and prognostic indicators in breast cancer. *Am J Epidemiol* 1989, 129:260–268.

15. Le Marchand L, Kolonel LN, Earle ME, *et al.*: Body size at different periods of life and breast cancer risk. *Am J Epidemiol* 1988, 128:137–152.

16. Ballard-Barbash R, Schatzkin A, Carter C, *et al.*: Body fat distribution and breast cancer risk in the Framingham study. *J Natl Cancer Inst* 1990, 82:286–290.

17. Folsom AR, Kaye SA, Prineas RJ, *et al.*: Increased incidence of carcinoma of the breast in association with abdominal adiposity in postmenopausal women. *Am J Epidemiol* 1990, 131:794–803.

18. Schapira DV, Kumar NB, Lyman GH, Cox CE: Abdominal obesity and breast cancer risk. *Ann Intern Med* 1990, 114:182–186.

19. Ota DM, Jones LA, Jackson GI, *et al.*: Obesity, non-protein bound estradiol levels, and distribution of estradiol in sera of breast cancer patients. *Cancer* 1986, 57:558–562.

20. Schapira DV, Kumar NB, Lyman GH: Estimate of breast cancer risk reduction with weight loss. *Cancer* 1991, 67:2622–2625.

21. Lissner L, Levitsky DA, Strupp BJ, *et al.*: Dietary fat and the regulation of energy intake in human subjects. *Am J Clin Nutr* 1987, 46:886–892.

22. Hughes LE, Mansel RE, Webster DJT: Aberrations of normal development and involution (ANDI): a new perspective.

23. Dupont WD, Page DL: Risk factors for breast cancer in women with proliferative breast disease. *N Engl J Med* 1985, 312:146–151.

24. Rubin E, Alexander RW, Visscher DW, *et al.*: Proliferative disease and atypia in biopsies performed for mammographically detected nonpalpable lesions. *Cancer* 1988, 61:2077–2082.

25. Arthur JE, Ellis IO, Flowers C, *et al.*: The relationship to "high risk" mammographic patterns to histologic risk factors for development of cancer in the human breast. *Br J Radiol* 1990, 63:845–855.

Nutrition and Lipids
David Heber

> **Key Points**
> - Humans are adapted to starvation and poorly adapted to overnutrition.
> - Familial hyperlipidemias are less common than obesity-associated dyslipidemia.
> - Hypertriglyceridemia with low levels of high-density lipoprotein are obesity-related.
> - The majority of cholesterol is synthesized, not taken in from the diet.
> - Weight loss and exercise can improve lipid profiles and reduce risk.
> - Preventive strategies are critical to reducing heart disease risk.

LIPIDS

Humans are adapted to starvation and have developed methods to store fat efficiently as the primary store of energy in the body [1]. Lipids and lipoproteins play an essential role in transporting fat-derived metabolites between organs for absorption, metabolism, and distribution [2]. However, overnutrition and underactivity can lead to metabolic overload, in which susceptible individuals are no longer able to regulate their circulating lipid levels within a normal range. Susceptibility to dietary-induced elevations in blood lipids, including cholesterol, is extremely common, and the interaction of genetic predisposition and a high-fat, high-calorie diet coupled with underactivity can lead to heart disease, hypertension, hypertriglyceridemia, and diabetes in a significant proportion of the US population. Regular exercise, healthy nutrition, and achievement of desirable body weights can prevent or reduce the incidence of common chronic diseases, such as heart disease associated with elevations of blood lipid levels [3••].

Male gender is a risk factor for coronary artery disease, and the susceptibility to overnutrition effects on lipids and lipoproteins may be mediated more easily by diet in men compared with women based on the metabolic effects of differences in body fat distribution. Women with upper body obesity (the distribution usually seen in men) are more likely to develop atherosclerosis and diabetes than women with lower body obesity [4]. In societies with low rates of heart disease, sex differences in levels of high-density lipoprotein (HDL) cholesterol, and mortality from coronary artery disease are reduced greatly. An analysis of the various dietary factors important in hypercholesterolemia leads to the conclusion that the primary approach to this disorder should include calorie and fat restriction, as well as increased physical activity, to attempt to reduce body weight to a desirable level. The loss of small amounts of upper body fat in men and postmenopausal women can reduce cholesterol levels significantly. Only after this goal has been attained should attention be given to avoiding high-cholesterol foods and switching from saturated to polyunsaturated fats. Increased fiber from fruits, vegetables, and certain grains such as oat bran and psyllium also can be used to lower cholesterol via diet.

CORONARY ARTERY DISEASE RISK

High serum cholesterol is a major risk factor for coronary artery disease. The National Cholesterol Education Program used the data obtained from the Multiple Risk Factor Intervention Trial (MRFIT) study [5] to establish a risk profile for coronary heart disease versus serum cholesterol level (Fig. 1). Although there is a continuous risk as cholesterol levels rise, the number of affected individuals decreases markedly at higher levels of cholesterol where genetic hyperlipidemias predominate. In fact, lesser degrees of hypercholesterolemia (about 240 mg/dL) more commonly increase cardiovascular risk than the less common greater elevations of serum cholesterol (> 300 mg/dL).

GENETIC FACTORS

Hypercholesterolemia is a laboratory finding that can result from a number of causes, least commonly from purely genetic hyperlipidemias. Hypercholesterolemia is a phenotype that is most commonly polygenically inherited, and its expression is environmentally influenced. Although genetic hyperlipidemias (especially type II hypercholesterolemia) are emphasized in medical education, these disorders account for less than 5% of all incident cases of hypercholesterolemia [6]. The frequency of the gene for type II hypercholesterolemia in the US population is one in 500 in the heterozygous state and one in 1 million in the homozygous state. Most investigators agree that the association between high cholesterol levels and increased incidence of heart disease is multifactorial, with important cellular mediators and intermediates involved, but the concentration of low-density lipoprotein (LDL) containing apolipoprotein B-100 (apoB-100) is the major determinant of cholesterol levels.

TRIGLYCERIDE LEVELS

Other associated lipid abnormalities, including hypertriglyceridemia, especially in the presence of lowered HDL cholesterol levels, have been recognized as influencing the risk of cardiovascular disease as well. There is a reciprocal relationship between elevated triglyceride levels and lowered HDL levels, and the elevations in triglyceride levels contribute to total cholesterol elevations according to the following equation [7]:

Total cholesterol = LDL cholesterol + HDL cholesterol + triglycerides/5

This estimation recognizes that very low-density lipoproteins (VLDL), which are 80% triglyceride and 20% cholesterol, contribute significantly to hypercholesterolemia. The primary apoB-100–containing particle synthesized and secreted by the liver is VLDL, and this is an important source of circulating LDL. The production of VLDL in the liver is stimulated by insulin and is commonly elevated in "syndrome X" or the "deadly quartet" (hypertension, hypertriglyceridemia, hyperglycemia, and hyperinsulinemia) [8].

HOMEOSTATIC MECHANISMS

The majority of circulating cholesterol is synthesized endogenously in the liver and is not derived from dietary cholesterol. In fact, as discussed below, the level of cholesterol in the diet is only the third most important nutritional factor influencing cholesterol levels (after total calories and saturated fat intake). There are a number of homeostatic mechanisms in humans, including changes in absorption of cholesterol from the gastrointestinal tract, that make serum cholesterol levels relatively resistant to changes in serum cholesterol in the range between 200 to 800 mg of dietary cholesterol per day. The primary dietary sources of cholesterol, which are eggs and organ meats, also provide significant fat and calories in most foods in which they are included.

SECONDARY FACTORS

The level of cholesterol in the circulation results from the balance between production of this particle and its removal from the circulation (Fig. 2). There are a number of factors, including estrogen and thyroid hormone, that affect the levels of LDL receptor activity and cholesterol removal

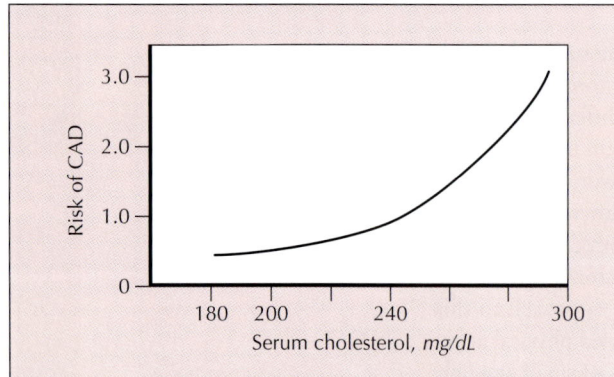

FIGURE 1 Relative risk of coronary artery disease versus serum cholesterol levels (mg/dL) in men from the Multiple Risk Factor Intervention Trial study. CAD—coronary artery disease. (*From* Kissebah and coworkers [4]; with permission.)

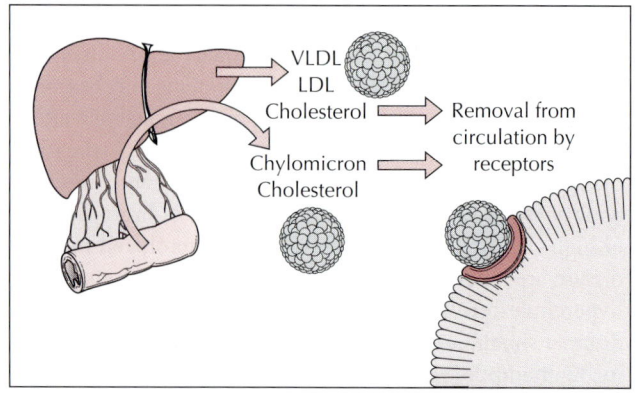

FIGURE 2 The level of serum cholesterol depends on both the rate of hepatic production and export to the circulation and the rate of receptor-mediated removal from the circulation. LDL—low-density lipoprotein; VLDL—very low density lipoprotein.

TABLE 1 SECONDARY CAUSES OF LIPID ELEVATIONS

Primarily increased LDL cholesterol levels
Hypothyroidism
Diabetes mellitus*
Nephrotic syndrome
Obstructive liver disease
Progestins
Anabolic steroids

Primarily increased triglycerides
Obesity*
Diabetes mellitus*
Lack of exercise*
Excess alcohol intake
Renal insufficiency
Estrogens
β blockade

Low levels of HDL
Hypertriglyceridemia*
Obesity*
Diabetes mellitus*
Cigarette smoking
Lack of exercise*
β blockade
Progestins
Anabolic steroids

*Indicates areas in which nutrition plays an important role.
HDL—high-density lipoprotein; LDL—low-density lipoprotein.

TABLE 2 NUTRITIONAL FACTORS AND ABNORMAL LIPIDS

Total fat and calories
Polyunsaturated, monounsaturated, and saturated fats
Dietary cholesterol
Soluble fiber

---

ered either for medical treatment or for a primary nutritional approach, in the case of obesity, diabetes mellitus, or a lack of exercise (Table 1).

NUTRITION AND LIFESTYLE

The nutritional factors that promote hypercholesterolemia and the practical steps the general internist can take to lower cholesterol levels through implementation of strategies for nutrition and lifestyle changes are shown in Table 2. It is generally agreed that diet is the cornerstone of treatment of hypercholesterolemia, but the implementation of dietary strategies is unfamiliar and difficult for the general internist. As a result drug approaches, which are more costly, usually are selected as the treatment modality. The official recommendations of the National Cholesterol Education Program can be implemented by physicians and office staff using educational materials provided by the American Heart Association Step 1 Diet (Fig. 3). If this approach fails, patients should be referred to a dietitian for the Step 2 Diet, which restricts total fat and more severely restricts cholesterol (Fig. 4). It generally is recommended that dietary approaches be used for up to 6 months before any drug therapy is instituted. This chapter provides some basic nutrition information for the general internist to communicate accurately to the patient.

from the circulation. Before considering institution of a dietary approach to cholesterol regulation, these secondary causes of elevated hypercholesterolemia should be consid-

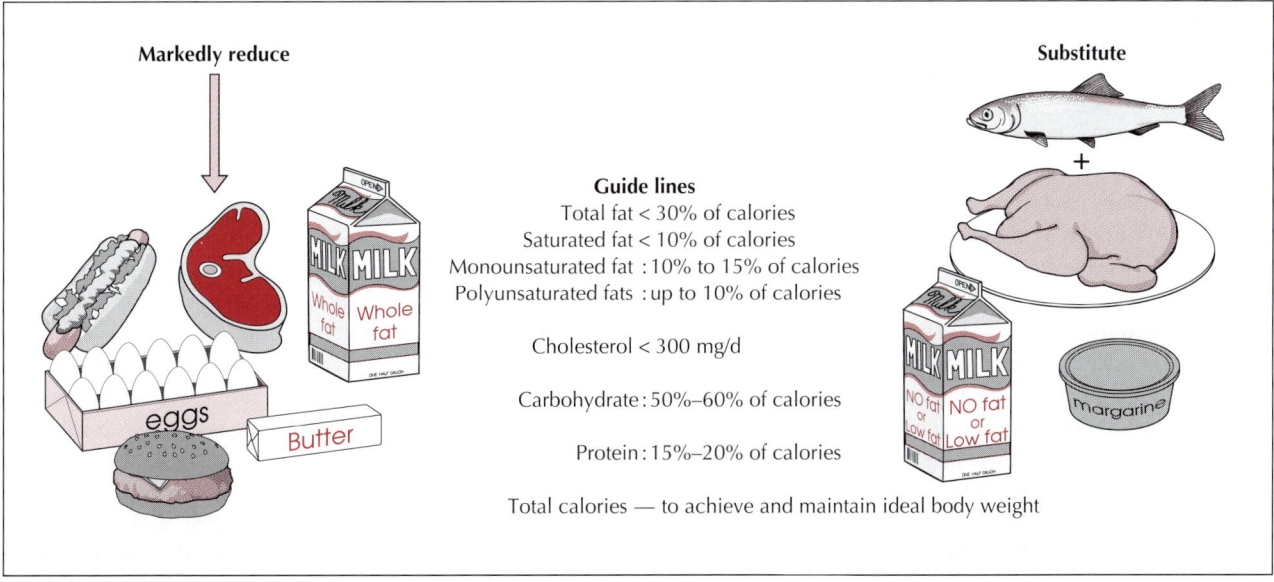

Guide lines
Total fat < 30% of calories
Saturated fat < 10% of calories
Monounsaturated fat : 10% to 15% of calories
Polyunsaturated fats : up to 10% of calories

Cholesterol < 300 mg/d

Carbohydrate : 50%–60% of calories

Protein : 15%–20% of calories

Total calories — to achieve and maintain ideal body weight

FIGURE 3 American Heart Association Step 1 Diet.

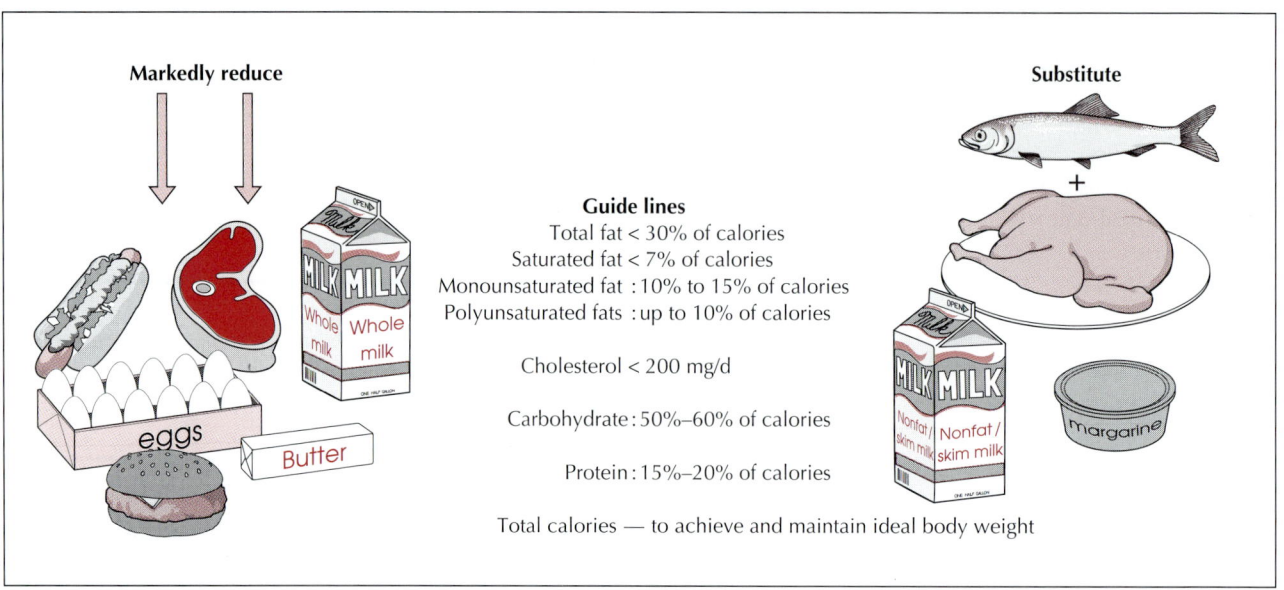

FIGURE 4 American Heart Association Step 2 Diet.

Low-Fat Diets

Low-fat diets at 30% of total calories without caloric restriction will not lower cholesterol levels in many patients in whom the primary disorder is obesity. Massive obesity is associated less commonly with hypercholesterolemia than mild obesity, especially in an upper body or abdominal distribution, which commonly is found in men and postmenopausal women. Elevations of lipids also can be found in premenopausal women with inherited upper body obesity and syndrome X. Obesity is extremely common in women over the age of 45 in the United States, with estimates of up to a 50% prevalence [9]. In fact, excess body fat is detected frequently by patients because one of three American women is on a diet at any given time. These women do not appear obviously overweight to the untrained eye because much of the excess fat is abdominally distributed, and a girdle can hide up to 23 kg of excess fat.

It is very common to find that in obese or diabetic women, a low-fat diet fails to lead to lowering of serum cholesterol levels. In some women, weight gain can even follow the institution of a low-fat diet without regard for caloric restriction. On average, there is maintenance of body weight with little change in serum cholesterol. Particular problem foods that cannot be consumed in unlimited amounts are low-fat cheeses and yogurts. Moreover, low-fat salad dressings used in large amounts, large portions of low-fat meats, such as chicken, or even increased intake of beans in salads can all lead to weight gain through excess caloric intake of ostensibly healthy foods. Therefore, calories do count, and the use of portion-controlled foods, including low-fat, low-cholesterol frozen foods and liquid meal replacements, can be effective strategies for limiting caloric intake to achieve weight loss.

Dietary Sources of Fat

Fats and oils provide the most concentrated source of calories of any foodstuff. Over 95% of the weight of most fats and oils is comprised of triglycerides. Excess calories, regardless of source, also are stored as triglycerides. They provide essential fatty acids (linoleic and linolenic acids), which are precursors for prostaglandins, require prolonged digestion, and contribute to satiety; they also carry fat-soluble vitamins and concentrate the tastes of food to make them more palatable.

The principal dietary sources of fat are meats, dairy products, poultry, fish, nuts, vegetable oils, and fats used in processed foods. Vegetables and fruits contain only small amounts of fat, so that vegetable oils are only sources of fat due to processing of vegetables. The most commonly used oils and fats for salad and cooking oils, shortenings, and margarines in the United States include soybean, corn, cottonseed, palm, peanut, olive, canola (low-erucic acid rapeseed oil), safflower, sunflower, coconut, and palm kernel oils and tallow and lard. These fat sources contain varying compositions of fatty acids that have particular physiologic properties. However, none of these fats have beneficial effects on serum cholesterol levels when consumed in excess quantities. Keeping calories constant, the substitution of polyunsaturated fats for saturated fats can lead to some lowering of cholesterol [10]. However, the marketing of extra virgin olive, corn, canola, and other oils for their cholesterol-lowering effects misrepresents the fact that hidden fats added to the diet raise cholesterol levels by contributing to obesity. Fish oils, which are enriched in the ω-3 fatty acids, can play a role in lowering triglycerides, but the primary effect of eating fish is an overall lowering of fat and calorie intake [11]. In fact, when fish oil capsules are administered to diabetics with hypertriglyceridemia, their glucose levels increase secondary to increased calorie intake.

The body can make saturated and monounsaturated fatty acids by modifying other fatty acids or by *de novo* synthesis from carbohydrate and protein. However, the polyunsaturated fatty acids linoleic acid and linolenic acid are essential fatty acids and must be supplied in the diet. The minimum intake of linoleic acid is said to be 3% of total calories. Because linoleic acid makes up about 60% of corn oil fatty acids, most diets should contain over 5% of total calories as fat. Needless to say, the problem of fatty acid deficiency is not widespread in the free-living population in this country. The average American eats between 35% and 40% of total calories as fat. High-fat diets eaten *ad lib* account for as much as 600 excess kcal/d compared with low-fat *ad lib* diets [12].

In starvation and overfeeding, the body regulates the metabolism of carbohydrates and protein closely but allows the stores of fat to expand easily in overfeeding and to contract with underfeeding. Because fat yields 9 kcal/g and requires little water for storage, it is a very efficient store of calories. In the nonobese 70-kg mythical man, 13.5 kg of fat will carry 130,000 to 160,000 kcal, whereas 13.5 kg of muscle will carry over 54,000 kcal. Using the fat stores and sparing protein stores is essential to surviving starvation. Because many populations have been exposed to epidemics of starvation and abuse, the tendency to retain fat stores is relatively common and is inherited polygenically, with a strong environmental influence.

The emphasis on obesity and fat content in the diet is purposeful because obesity is the most common nutritional disorder in the United States and clearly accounts most frequently for the lipid abnormalities encountered in general internal medicine practice. Failure to correct body weight toward desirable levels is inevitably associated with a failure of diet to lower cholesterol levels.

Exercise

Sedentary lifestyle leads to muscle atrophy, with increased body fat and increased metabolic efficiency promoting obesity. Increased physical activity, including supervised weight-lifting, can lead to increased muscle mass and improved removal and oxidation of circulation triglycerides through lipoprotein lipase found in skeletal muscle [13]. Muscle activity also leads to increased glucose use leading to a lowering of circulating insulin levels. In turn, lowered insulin levels lead to decreased synthesis of VLDL-carrying triglycerides and cholesterol (Fig. 5). Increased emphasis on counteracting muscle atrophy in the aging US population has led to the use of these strategies in many physical therapy facilities where patients can be referred when muscle atrophy is present.

Dietary Fiber

Beyond a consideration of total calories and fat, types of fat, and dietary cholesterol content, patients also may have questions regarding the role of fiber in lowering cholesterol levels. The type of fiber that lowers cholesterol levels is soluble fiber, including oat bran, and the soluble fibers, such as pectin and guar, found in fruits and vegetables. These fibers are different from insoluble fibers, such as wheat bran commonly found in whole-wheat cereals and grains [14]. These insoluble fibers have no effect on cholesterol but do aid digestion.

Micronutrient Antioxidants

A high-fat, low-fiber diet is also a diet usually low in fruits and vegetables, which are important sources of micronutrients. These micronutrients include antioxidants such as vitamin E and beta carotene, which can affect lipid oxidation. Atherosclerosis is clearly a multifactorial cellular process, and recent work has shown that an oxidized lipid is more avidly taken up by macrophages (Fig. 6) [15]. This oxidation can be prevented in the laboratory by adding antioxidants, and in humans an increased intake of vitamin E has been associated with a reduced incidence of coronary artery disease. The levels at which the beneficial effects of vitamin E are seen in these studies are greater than those usually obtained from the diet, where many of the rich sources of vitamin E are also high in fat (*eg*, nuts, grains, and vegetable oil) [16•]. Although the Recommended Dietary Allowance is 15 IU/d to prevent nutritional deficiency, the beneficial antioxidant effects usually are demonstrated at doses more than 10 times higher. It is not feasible to obtain this antioxidant from the diet in these amounts, and some cardiologists are recommending that patients with established coronary artery disease take vitamin E supplement pills at doses of 200 to 800 IU/d [17]. Beta carotene can be obtained from carrots or carrot juice and other yellow, orange, and green vegetables and also can prevent lipid oxidation. The Physicians Health Study demonstrated a lowering of the expected rate of heart disease deaths in 333

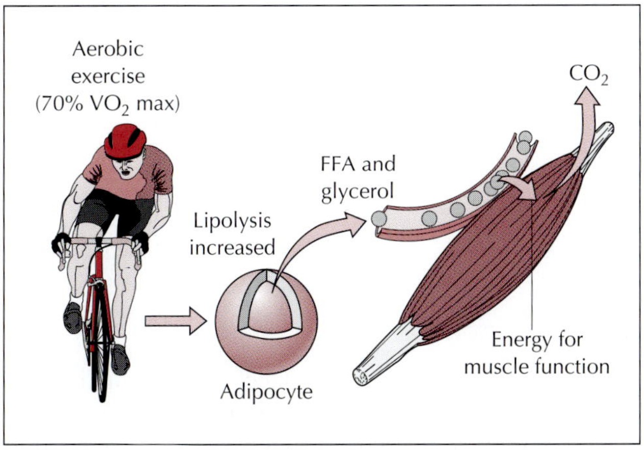

FIGURE 5 Exercise increases lipid removal from the circulation by lipoprotein oxidation in muscle.

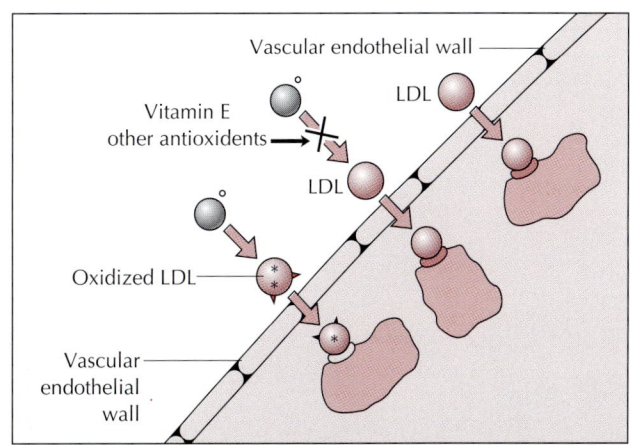

FIGURE 6 Dietary antioxidants inhibit the oxidation of lipoprotein cholesterol, reducing its rate of uptake macrophage for entry into the endothelial wall.

physicians with established heart disease at the time of entry into the study [18]. There are other trace minerals and vitamins with antioxidant effects, including folic acid and selenium, but these can be obtained in adequate amounts in most multivitamin and multimineral supplement preparations to provide beneficial effects based on our current understanding. All of these emerging data, together with the observation that only about 10% of Americans eat the recommended amounts of fruits and vegetables, have led to the wider use of vitamin supplements, especially vitamin E, among heart disease patients in an attempt to prevent lipid oxidation and progression of their disease.

REFERENCES AND RECOMMENDED READING

Recently published papers of particular interest have been highlighted as:
- Of interest
- •• Of outstanding interest

1. Felig P, Wahren J: Fuel homeostasis during exercise. *N Engl J Med* 1975, 293:1078–1084.
2. Frederickson DS, Levy RI, Lees RS: Fat transport in lipoproteins—an integrated approach to mechanisms and disorders. *N Engl J Med* 1967, 276:34, 94, 148, 214, 273.
3.•• Pi-Sunyer FX: Health implications of obesity. *Am J Clin Nutr* 1991, 53:1595S–1603S.
4. Kissebah AH, Alfarsi S, Adams PW: Integrated regulation of very low density lipoprotein triglyceride and apolipoprotein B kinetics in man: normolipidemic subjects, familial hypertriglyceridemia, and familial combined hyperlipidemia. *Metabolism* 1981, 30:856–868.
5. Kannel WB, Neaton JD, Wentworth, *et al.*: Overall and CHD mortality rates in relation to major risk factors in 325,348 men screened for MRFIT. *Am Heart J* 1986, 112:825–836.
6. Schaefer EJ, Levy RI: Pathogenesis and management of lipoprotein disorders. *N Engl J Med* 1985, 312:1300–1310.
7. Friedewald WT, Levy RI, Frederickson DS: Estimation of low density lipoprotein cholesterol in plasma without use of the preparative ultracentrifuge. *Clin Chem* 1972, 18:499–502.
8. Kaplan NM: The deadly quartet: Upper body obesity, glucose intolerance, hypertriglyceridemia, and hypertension. *Arch Intern Med* 1989, 149:1514–1520.
9. Bray GA: Obesity in America: an overview. In *Obesity in American*. Edited by Bray GA. Washington DC: Public Health Service; 1979:1–19. [NIH Publ 79-359]
10. National Cholesterol Education Program Expert Panel: Report on detection, evaluation, and treatment of high blood cholesterol in adults. *Arch Intern Med* 1988, 148:36–69.
11. Connor WE, Connor SL: Nutrition management of hyperlipidemia. *Curr Concepts Nutr* 1979, 8:179–216.
12. Lissner L, Levitsky DA, Strupp BJ, *et al.*: Dietary fat and the regulation of energy intake in human subjects. *Am J Clin Nutr* 1987, 46:886.
13. Horton ES: Metabolic fuels, utilization, and exercise. *Am J Clin Nutr* 1989, 49:931–932.
14. Asp N-G, Furda I, Schweizer TF, Prosky L: Dietary fiber definition and analysis. *Am J Clin Nutr* 1988, 48:688–690.
15. Steinberg D, Pathasarathy S, Carew TE, *et al.*: Beyond cholesterol: modification of low density lipoprotein that increase its atherogenicity. *N Engl J Med* 1989, 320:915–924.
16.• Rimm EB, Stampfer MJ, Ascherio A, *et al.*: Vitamin E consumption and the risk of coronary heart disease in men. *N Engl J Med* 1993, 328:1450–1456.
17. Bendich A, Machlin LJ: Safety of oral intake of vitamin E. *Am J Clin Nutr* 1988, 48:612–619.
18. Gaziano JM, Manson JE, Ridker M, *et al.*: Beta carotene therapy for chronic stable angina [Abstract]. *Circulation* 1990, 82(suppl III):201.

SELECT BIBLIOGRAPHY

Brown ML: *Present Knowledge in Nutrition*. Washington DC: International Life Sciences Institute Nutrition Foundation Inc; 1990.

Frankle RT, Yang M-U: *Obesity and Weight Control*. Rockville, MD: Aspen Publishers; 1988.

Endocrine Manifestations of Cancer

Andrée C. de Bustros
Stephen B. Baylin

> ### Key Points
> - Hormone secretion by nonendocrine tumors is not completely understood. There is often an association between tumor type and individual hormone production.
> - It is important to recognize and manage the endocrine manifestations of cancer because they can cause significant morbidity and mortality.
> - Tumor-related hypercalcemia is quite common. The role of parathyroid hormone–related peptide in this entity is being elucidated, and the newer bisque, such as pamidronate, are useful therapeutic agents.
> - Hyponatremia in cancer patients often results from the syndrome of inappropriate antidiuresis. Management is mainly by fluid restriction.
> - Cushing's syndrome, hypoglycemia, acromegaly, and osteomalacia are rare manifestations of cancer. Evaluation of these entities often requires specialized tests, and management can be challenging.

Nonendocrine tumors occasionally produce hormones that are often biologically inactive, or their serum levels are too low to cause symptoms. Rarely, they result in hormonal syndromes that have significant morbidity and mortality. Criteria for the diagnosis of a tumor-related hormonal syndrome are as follows:

Evidence of hormonal activity in conjunction with a tumor
Absence of primary endocrine gland dysfunction
Elevated serum or urine levels of hormone
Demonstration of hormone gradient across the tumor
Normalization or improvement of the hormonal syndrome by treatment of the underlying tumor
In vitro hormone production by tumor cells

The relationship between histologic tumor type and individual hormone is outlined in Table 1, and an example of hormone production by a neuroendocrine tumor is shown in Figure 1.

COMMON CLINICAL SYNDROMES

Tumor-Related Hypercalcemia

In patients with solid tumors and no evidence of bone metastases, hypercalcemia is thought to result from parathyroid hormone–related peptide (PTH-RP) [1,2]. PTH-RP is primarily secreted by squamous tumors (lung, skin, head and neck, cervix, or vulva), renal cell carcinomas, and less frequently, by other tumors, such as bladder, breast and ovarian carcinomas, lymphomas, pancreatic islet cell tumors, and pheochromocytomas. Like parathyroid hormone, PTH-RP causes hypercalcemia and hypophosphatemia by increasing bone resorption and renal phosphate clearance.

TABLE 1 RELATIONSHIP BETWEEN TUMOR CELL TYPE AND HORMONE PRODUCED	
Tumor cell type	**Hormone**
Neuroendocrine	Corticotropin
	Arginine vasopressin
	Corticotropin-releasing factor
	Growth hormone-releasing hormone
	Somatostatin
	Calcitonin
Squamous	Parathyroid hormone-related peptide
Large cell	Human chorionic gonadotropin
Mesenchymal	Insulin-like growth factor II
	Phosphaturic factor

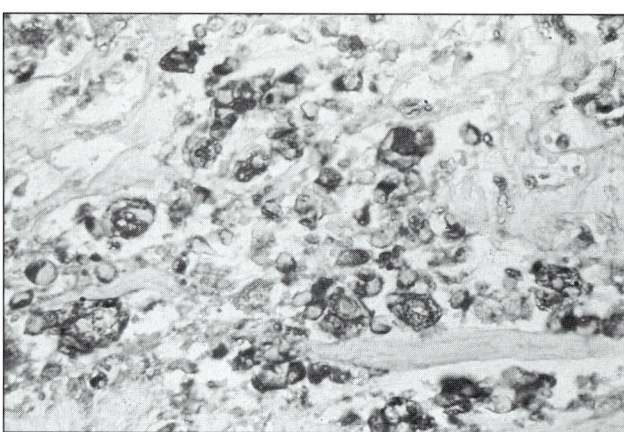

FIGURE 1 Positive immunostaining for corticotropin in small cell lung carcinoma (see Color Plate).

Other mediators of hypercalcemia are locally produced osteolytic factors, in conjunction with skeletal metastases from tumors, such as those occurring in breast cancer, or with bone marrow involvement by hematologic malignancies, such as multiple myeloma. Some lymphomas can cause hypercalcemia by overproducing 1,25-dihydroxyvitamin D.

Diagnosis

In a patient with suspected tumor-related hypercalcemia, potentially reversible causes of hypercalcemia, such as primary hyperparathyroidism and vitamin D intoxication, must be excluded (Table 2). When hypercalcemia results from PTH-RP production, parathyroid hormone and 1,25-dihydroxyvitamin D levels are suppressed.

Treatment

Treatment of hypercalcemia should be directed at reducing symptoms rather than at reducing serum calcium level [3•]. However, a calcium level of more than 15 mg/dL should be treated irrespective of symptoms because of the high risk of arrhythmias and heart blocks.

For mild hypercalcemia, hydration with normal saline in addition to a loop diuretic, such as furosemide, may be sufficient. Furosemide enhances the renal excretion of calcium and prevents fluid overload. For moderate hypercalcemia, a bisphosphonate, such as pamidronate, should be administered (Table 3) [4,5]. Normocalcemia is usually achieved within 2 to 6 days of a single intravenous dose of pamidronate, and the effect lasts for 2 to 3 weeks. For severe life-threatening hypercalcemia, calcitonin, because of its rapid onset of action, may be added to the pamidronate regimen. Gallium nitrate or plicamycin may be used if pamidronate is unavailable or ineffective. Unfortunately, these two drugs have significant toxicities.

The hypercalcemia of hematologic malignancies and breast cancer may respond to steroid therapy, and the somatostatin analogue octreotide may be useful when hypercalcemia is associated with PTH-RP production by pancreatic islet tumors.

When to refer

Hypercalcemic patients who present diagnostic difficulties should be referred to an endocrinologist for an efficient and cost-effective evaluation; however, the generalist usually performs initial management of mild-to-moderate hypercalcemia with hydration and diuretics. For moderate-to-severe hypercalcemia requiring pamidronate, gallium nitrate, or

TABLE 2 DIAGNOSTIC APPROACH TO TUMOR-RELATED HYPERCALCEMIA
Skeletal radiographs or bone scan
Rule out primary hyperparathyroidism (intact PTH level)
Rule out vitamin D-induced hypercalcemia resulting from excessive intake (25-hydroxyvitamin D level) or endogenous production by granulomatous diseases such as sarcoidosis or lymphoma (1,25-dihydroxyvitamin D level, chest radiograph)
PTH-RP if necessary (A PTH-RP assay is now commercially available, and there seems to be a good correlation between high PTH-RP levels and presence of hypercalcemia.)
PTH—parathyroid hormone; PTH-RP—parathyroid hormone-related peptide.

TABLE 3 TREATMENT OF HYPERCALCEMIA OF MALIGNANCY	
Pamidronate	30–90 mg by 24-h intravenous infusion. Repeat after 1 wk if necessary
Plicamycin	25 µg/kg, intravenously, over 4–6 h Repeat after 48 h if necessary
Gallium nitrate	200 mg/m^3, intravenously, over 24 h/d for 5 d
Salmon calcitonin	200–400 U, subcutaneously, every 6–8 h

TABLE 4 DIAGNOSIS OF THE SYNDROME OF INAPPROPRIATE ANTIDIURESIS
Hyponatremia (serum Na less than 135 mEq/L)
Low serum osmolarity (less than 275 mOsm/L)
Elevated urine osmolarity (more than 100 mOsm/L)
Urinary sodium loss (urinary Na more than 40 mEq/L)
Serum arginine vasopressin levels should not be used for diagnosis, but they may be helpful in assessing severity of the disorder. Some patients with SIAD have elevated serum atrial natriuretic factor levels. Atrial natriuretic factor may play a role in the high urinary sodium excretion seen in SIAD.
SIAD—syndrome of inappropriate antidiuresis.

TABLE 5 DRUGS CAUSING SYNDROME OF INAPPROPRIATE ANTIDIURESIS
Cyclophosphamide
Tricyclic antidepressants
Phenothiazines
Carbamazepine
Chlorpropamide
Clofibrate
Colchicine

plicamycin, the patient should be referred to an endocrinologist or an oncologist who is experienced in administering these drugs.

Syndrome of Inappropriate Antidiuresis

The syndrome of inappropriate antidiuresis (SIAD) should be considered in patients with signs and symptoms outlined in Table 4 [6•]. By far, the most common tumor associated with SIAD is small-cell lung carcinoma (SCLC). An estimated 10% of patients with SCLC have SIAD. Occasionally, hyponatremia is the first clue to the presence of SCLC. Other tumors associated with SIAD are mesotheliomas, thymomas, lymphomas, leukemias, and pancreatic, prostatic, and uterine carcinomas. Some of these tumors have been clearly shown to produce the antidiuretic hormone arginine vasopressin. However, in most patients, circulating arginine vasopressin levels are in the normal range, although they are inappropriately high for the serum osmolarity.

Before hyponatremia is attributed to tumor arginine vasopressin production, sodium depletion induced by diuretic use, salt-losing nephropathy, or mineralocorticoid deficiency all must be ruled out. Endocrine disorders associated with impaired free water clearance, such as hypocortisolism or hypothyroidism, should also be considered. Finally, certain drugs are known to cause SIAD (Table 5).

Diagnosis

The criteria listed in Table 4 are usually sufficient for the diagnosis of SIAD. However, not all patients with this syndrome fulfill these criteria. For example, concomitant SIAD and dehydration may result in low urinary sodium. A careful trial of normal saline hydration (500 to 1000 mL administered over 12 hours) may be helpful: correction of hyponatremia favors dehydration, whereas further dilution and worsening of hyponatremia suggest SIAD.

Treatment

Treatment of SIAD consists of fluid restriction, to about 750 to 500 mL/d. Administering ice chips helps to insure compliance. Usually, biochemical and clinical improvement take several days to occur. For severe chronic hyponatremia associated with mental obtundation, a careful infusion of hypertonic saline is required, with the aim of increasing serum sodium level to about 120 mEq/L by no more than 12 mEq/L over 24 hours. Acute symptomatic hyponatremia can be treated more aggressively.

Demeclocycline, 150 mg four times a day, may be used to treat SIAD on a long-term basis. This agent induces a nephrogenic diabetes insipidus–like state and improves free water clearance. If no response is observed after 3 to 4 days, the dose can be doubled. Renal function should be carefully monitored in patients taking demeclocycline. Oral urea (30 g/d) has been used for faster relief of symptoms.

When to refer

The patient should be referred to an endocrinologist when the etiology of hyponatremia is not clear, and particularly when hypoadrenalism is suspected. Treatment of patients with severe hyponatremia and mental changes may result in life-threatening complications and is preferably done in consultation with an endocrinologist or nephrologist [7•]. Also, long-term treatment of chronic SIAD should be performed in conjunction with an endocrinologist who is familiar with the treatment of such patients.

Ectopic Cushing's Syndrome

Fifteen percent of all cases of Cushing's syndrome result from the ectopic production of corticotropin. Rarely, tumors may secrete corticotropin-releasing factor, and some tumors secrete both corticotropin and corticotropin-releasing factor. Tumors with neuroendocrine differentiation account for most cases of ectopic Cushing's syndrome, particularly SCLC, carcinoid, pancreatic islet cell tumors, medullary thyroid carcinomas, and pheochromocytomas. Other tumors include thymomas and prostate, stomach, colon, and ovarian carcinomas.

The clinical manifestations of ectopic Cushing's syndrome depend on the underlying tumor. For example, patients with rapidly progressive SCLC present with hyperpigmentation, muscle weakness, hypertension, and hypokalemic alkalosis. By contrast, patients with slow-growing carcinoid tumors develop the full phenotypic features of Cushing's syndrome, including central obesity, facial plethora, and striae (Fig. 2).

Diagnosis

A diagnostic approach to ectopic Cushing's syndrome is as follows [8•,9]. The 24-hour urinary free cortisol is usually

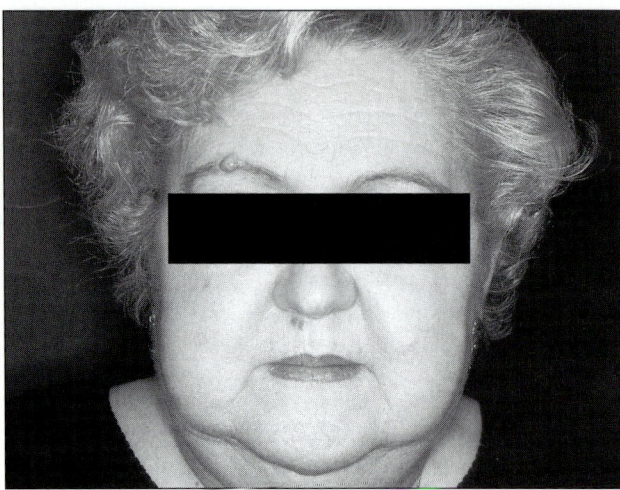

FIGURE 2 Patient demonstrating some of the typical signs of Cushing's syndrome (moon facies, supraclavicular and cervical fat pads).

elevated in patients with Cushing's syndrome, and cortisol production in these patients is not suppressible by low-dose dexamethasone administration. Some increase in cortisol production may occur in patients who are under stress, are depressed, or are alcohol abusers.

Once the diagnosis of Cushing's syndrome has been established, the major challenge is to distinguish ectopic from pituitary Cushing's syndrome. Circulating corticotropin levels tend to be higher in ectopic Cushing's syndrome, and patients with this syndrome usually fail to respond to corticotropin-releasing factor and to suppress cortisol production in response to high-dose dexamethasone. However, occasionally, patients with bronchial carcinoids have a response to both tests that is indistinguishable from that of patients with pituitary Cushing's.

To complicate matters further, bronchial carcinoids can be very small and may escape detection by chest radiography or computed tomography. In addition, these tumors may be metabolically inactive, and therefore, 5-hydroxyindoleacetic acid levels may be normal. Often, elaborate studies, such as inferior petrosal sinus catheterization, may be necessary to establish the source of corticotropin production.

Treatment

In the case of benign corticotropin-producing tumors, such as carcinoids or pheochromocytomas, tumor resection may result in complete cure of Cushing's syndrome. Unfortunately, in patients with malignant tumors, such as SCLC, tumor eradication is not feasible, and medical management with adrenal inhibitors is necessary. The antifungal agent ketoconazole (given orally 400 to 1000 mg/d) is very effective and has fewer side effects than metyrapone or aminoglutethimide. Most patients' conditions can be maintained on ketoconazole for long periods of time. Liver function should be monitored, and the drug should be discontinued if hepatotoxicity develops. In rare instances, palliative bilateral adrenalectomy is indicated for occult, slow-growing corticotropin-producing tumors [10].

When to refer

Generalists are urged to obtain help from endocrinologists as soon as the diagnosis of Cushing's syndrome is entertained because of the many pitfalls in diagnostic tests (as discussed earlier). The evaluation for Cushing's syndrome should be systematic. A common mistake is to obtain pituitary and adrenal imaging studies before or even at the exclusion of a biochemical evaluation. Such short-cuts result in both false positive and false negative results: first, incidental benign masses are often found on adrenal and pituitary scans; second, up to half of all corticotropin-producing pituitary adenomas are too small to be visualized by current imaging techniques. With regard to treatment, generalists are advised to refer their patients to endocrinologists who are familiar with the management of this rare disorder.

TABLE 6 DIAGNOSTIC APPROACH TO ECTOPIC CUSHING'S SYNDROME

Establish diagnosis
Elevated 24-h urinary-free cortisol (more than 300 µg)
Nonsuppression on low-dose dexamethasone
  (0.5 mg every 6 h for 2 d)*

Establish etiology
Elevated plasm corticotropin
Nonsuppression on high-dose dexamethasone
  (2 mg every 6 h for 2 d)†
No response to corticotropin-releasing factor stimulation

Localization
Chest and abdominal computed tomographic scan
Inferior petrosal sinus sampling

*Urinary 17-hydroxycorticosteroids should decrease to below 2.5 mg/g of creatinine on the 2nd day of dexamethasone administration.
†The diagnostic performance of the high-dose dexamethasone test is improved by requiring suppression of 17-hydroxycorticosteroids to less than 50% of baseline and suppression of free cortisol to less than 90% of baseline [9].

TABLE 7 DIAGNOSTIC EVALUATION OF PATIENTS WITH CANCER AND HYPOGLYCEMIA

Consider pseudohypoglycemia resulting from high leukocyte count
Rule out hepatic and renal disease
Consider sepsis
Rule out hypopituitarism and hypoadrenalism. Obtain thyroid function tests and perform short corticotropin stimulation test*
Insulin levels if indicated

*Serum cortisol should be greater than 18 mg/dL 30–60 min after intravenous injection of 250 µg of cosyntropin

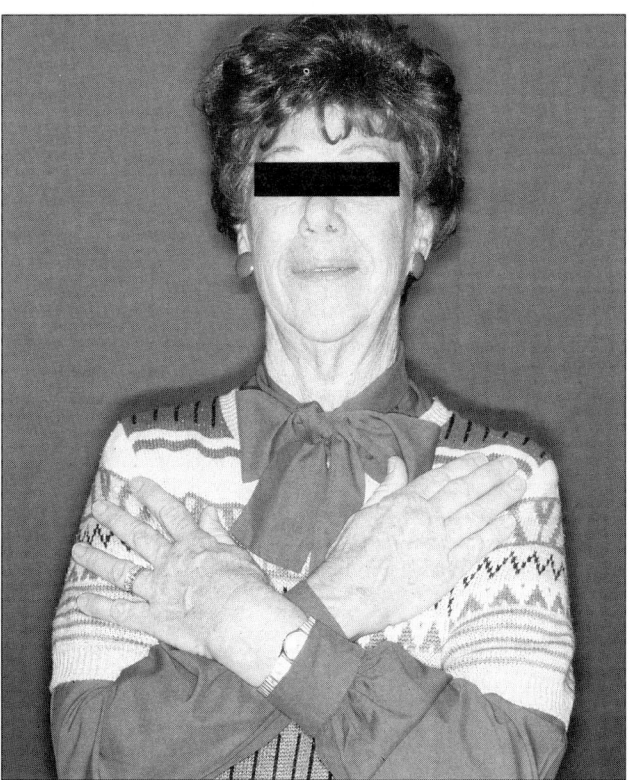

FIGURE 3 Patient with subtle signs of acromegaly: mild coarsening of facial features, thickened skin folds, and enlarged hands.

Tumor-Related Hypoglycemia

Nonislet tumor-related hypoglycemia is thought to be caused by insulin-like growth factor II [11•]. Insulin-like growth factor II may induce hypoglycemia by suppressing hepatic glucose output, increasing glucose consumption by the tumor, and impairing growth hormone release. Insulin itself or insulin-like growth factor I (or somatomedin C) has not been associated with tumor hypoglycemia. Tumors that cause hypoglycemia are mesenchymal tumors (fibromas, sarcomas), hepatomas, adrenal carcinomas, and rarely, colon and renal cell carcinomas. The mesenchymal tumors are often very large and are located in either the mediastinum or the retroperitoneum.

Diagnosis

Patients with cancer and hypoglycemia are often very sick and tend to have neuroglycopenic symptoms, such as confusion and lethargy, as opposed to adrenergic symptoms. Before hypoglycemia is attributed to hormonal activity of the tumor, other etiologies of hypoglycemia should be ruled out (Table 7). Marked leukocytosis may result in spurious hypoglycemia. Extensive liver infiltration by tumor, passive liver congestion, chronic renal failure, and sepsis may all cause hypoglycemia because of interference with carbohydrate metabolism. In addition, hypopituitarism or hypoadrenalism should be ruled out based on results obtained from thyroid function and short corticotropin tests. Serum cortisol level should be higher than 18 mg/dL 30 to 60 minutes after intravenous injection of 250 μg of cosyntropin. An insulin level should be obtained when the tumor cell type is unclear. Circulating levels of insulin-like growth factor II are not always elevated, and therefore, the diagnosis of insulin-like growth factor II–related hypoglycemia is by exclusion of other etiologies of hypoglycemia.

Treatment

Tumor eradication is rarely possible in this setting, and tumor recurrences are common. Palliative treatment consists of infusion of a 10% glucose solution. Diazoxide, 50 mg orally twice a day, may be helpful. Addition of a thiazide diuretic may decrease the fluid retention seen with this drug and may improve its efficacy as well. Steroids and glucagon are of transient benefit.

When to refer

Patients with severe and persistent hypoglycemia should be referred to an endocrinologist for efficient evaluation and treatment. The endocrinologist will help rule out life-threatening but treatable causes of hypoglycemia, such as hypoadrenalism or hypopituitarism, which may result from tumor metastases.

UNCOMMON SYNDROMES
Acromegaly

Fewer than 1% of all cases of acromegaly are ectopic, and almost all result from the secretion of growth hormone–releasing hormone by nonpituitary tumors [12]. Growth hormone–releasing hormone–producing tumors are of neuroendocrine origin (carcinoids, islet cell tumors, hypothalamic and pituitary gangliocytomas, and pheochromocytomas). Bronchial carcinoids represent most of the tumors associated with growth hormone–releasing hormone production and acromegaly.

Patients with acromegaly may present with nonspecific findings, such as arthritis, excessive sweating, hypertension, glucose intolerance, or carpal tunnel syndrome, and only subtle evidence of bone and soft tissue hypertrophy (Fig. 3). Diagnosis is established from elevated serum growth hormone levels that fail to suppress after glucose ingestion. A nonpituitary source is suggested by elevated serum levels of growth hormone–releasing hormone. Treatment of ectopic acromegaly is primarily surgical resection of the underlying tumor. The long-acting somatostatin analogue octreotide is very effective when acromegaly occurs in conjunction with a nonresectable tumor.

When to refer

The role of the generalist is essential in the recognition of acromegaly, because early treatment substantially reduces morbidity and mortality. Once the diagnosis is suggested by clinical evidence, patients should be referred to endocrinologists for diagnosis and treatment. Acromegaly is rare, and most generalists are not experienced in its management.

Tumor-Related Osteomalacia

Tumor-related osteomalacia should be suspected in patients with musculoskeletal pain and muscle weakness who have hypophosphatemia in the absence of intestinal malabsorption or renal tubular acidosis [13,14]. Tumors causing this disorder are generally benign mesenchymal tumors, such as hemangiomas, giant cell tumors, and fibromas. Malignant neoplasms have been implicated as well (SCLCs and prostate and breast carcinomas).

Serum levels of phosphorus and 1,25-dihydroxyvitamin D are low in these patients, but calcium levels are usually normal. Skeletal films may show decreased bone density or pseudofractures. Treatment consists of large doses of 1,25-dihydroxyvitamin D and phosphate supplements, but only tumor eradication results in regression of all signs and symptoms.

When to refer

Patients with severe hypophosphatemia of unclear etiology should be referred to an endocrinologist for metabolic evaluation and optimal treatment with vitamin D and phosphorus.

Human Chorionic Gonadotropin Production by Tumors

The most common human chorionic gonadotropin–producing tumors are testicular tumors in men and trophoblastic uterine tumors in women. Rarely, human chorionic gonadotropin secretion occurs from extragonadal choriocarcinomas, large-cell lung tumors, pancreatic carcinomas, and hepatomas.

In men, human chorionic gonadotropin–producing tumors may result in gynecomastia and impotence. In both men and women with very high levels of human chorionic gonadotropin, hyperthyroidism may occur [15]. Sometimes, prolonged use of antithyroid drugs is necessary in these patients.

Hypertension

Renin-secreting tumors should be suspected in patients with hypertension, hypokalemia, high renin and aldosterone levels, and no evidence of renal artery stenosis [16]. These tumors are often renal, but they may also occur in the ovaries, pancreas, lungs, adrenals, and testes. Tumor removal may decrease renin and aldosterone levels. If cure is not achieved, angiotensin-converting enzyme inhibitors are indicated for the management of hypertension.

Conclusions

Only the most common and best-defined tumor-related endocrine syndromes have been outlined in this short review. A high index of suspicion is necessary to diagnose hormonal syndromes in cancer patients with unexplained symptoms or metabolic abnormalities. Treatment of hormonal excess often decreases morbidity and mortality in patients with malignancies.

Increasingly, the role of hormones as local autocrine and paracrine factors in tumor cells is being appreciated. New therapeutic approaches for cancer may involve blocking hormonal action, either by using antibodies or antisense messenger RNA to decrease hormone levels or interfere with hormone function.

References and Recommended Reading

Recently published papers of particular interest have been highlighted as:
- Of interest
- •• Of outstanding interest

1. Budayr A, Nissenson R, Klein R *et al.*: Increased serum levels of parathyroid hormone-like protein in malignancy-associated hypercalcemia. *Ann Intern Med* 1989, 111:807–812.
2. Burtis W, Brady T, Orloff J, *et al.*: Immunochemical characterization of circulating parathyroid hormone-related protein in patients with humoral hypercalcemia of cancer. *N Engl J Med* 1990, 322:1106–1112.
3. • Bilezikian J: Management of acute hypercalcemia. *N Engl J Med* 1992, 326:1196–1203.
4. Fitton A, McTavish D: Pamidronate—a review of its pharmacological properties and therapeutic efficacy in resorptive bone disease. *Drugs* 1991, 4:289–318.
5. Grill V, Murray R, Ho P, *et al*: Circulating PTH and PTHrP levels before and after treatment of tumor-induced hypercalcemia with pamidronate disodium (APD). *J Clin Endocrinol Metab* 1992, 74:1468–1470.
6. • Kovacs L, Robertson GL: Syndrome of inappropriate antidiuresis. *Endocrinol Metab Clin North Am* 1992, 21:859–875.
7. • Sterns R: The treatment of hyponatremia: first, do no harm. *Am J Med* 1990, 88:557–560.
8. • Kaye T, Crapo L: The Cushing Syndrome: an update on diagnostic tests. *Ann Intern Med* 1990, 112:434–444.
9. Flack M, Oldfield E, Cutler G, *et al.*: Urine free cortisol in the high-dose dexamethasone suppression test for the differential diagnosis of the Cushing syndrome. *Ann Intern Med* 1992, 116:211–217.
10. Goellner J, Salomao D, Ebersold J, *et al.*: Surgical strategy in the management of non-small cell ectopic adrenocorticotropic hormone syndrome. *Surgery* 1992, 112:994–1001.
11. • LeRoith D, Clemmons D, Nissley P, Rechler MM: Insulin-like growth factors in health and disease. *Ann Intern Med* 1992, 116:854–862.
12. Melmed S: Extrapituitary acromegaly. *Endocrinol Metab Clin North Am* 1991, 20:507–518.
13. Hewison M, Karmali R, O'Riordan JLH: Tumour-induced osteomalacia. *Clin Endocrinol (Oxf)* 1992, 37:379–382.
14. Nuovo M, Dorfman H, Sun C, Chalew S: Tumor induced osteomalacia and rickets. *Am J Surg Pathol* 1989, 13:588–599.
15. Giralt SA, Dexeus F, Amato R, *et al.*: Hyperthyroidism in men with germ cell tumors and high levels of β-human chorionic gonadotropin. *Cancer* 1992, 69:1286–1290.
16. Anderson P, Macaulay L, Do Y, *et al.*: Extrarenal renin-secreting tumors: Insights into hypertension and ovarian renin production. *Medicine* 1989, 68:257–268.

Select Bibliography

Daughaday W, Deuel T: Tumor secretion of growth factors. *Endocrinol Metab Clin* 1991, 20:539–552.

de Bustros A, Baylin S: Ectopic hormone production by tumors. In *Diagn Endocrinol* Edited by Moore WT, Eastman RC. Toronto, Philadelphia: BC Decker, Inc; 1990:283–299.

Mundy G: Ectopic production of calciotropic peptides. *Endocrinol Metab Clin North Am* 1991, 20:473–487.

Moses A, Scheinman S: Ectopic secretion of neurohypophyseal peptides in patients with malignancy. *Endocrinol Metab Clin North Am* 1991, 20:489–506.

Schteingart D: Ectopic secretion of peptides of the proopiomelanocortin family. *Endocrinol Metab Clin North Am* 1991, 20:453–471.

Aging: Prostatic Disease, Benign Prostatic Hyperplasia, and Carcinoma

20

Jack Geller

Key Points

- Dihydrotestosterone plays a major role in the pathogenesis benign prostatic hyperplasia because prostates of men with 5α-reductase deficiency and decreased dihydrotestosterone are atrophic.

- Medical treatment of benign prostatic hyperplasia with finasteride, a 5α-reductase inhibitor, has been shown in studies of continuous therapies for up to 5 years to produce a sustained arrest of benign prostatic hyperplasia— *ie*, the prostate shrinks by 20%, maximum urinary flow rates increase, and clinical symptom scores or prostatism improve.

- If primary care physicians treat patients with benign prostatic hyperplasia with finasteride, they must do a few simple tests to rule out other causes of prostatism in the differential diagnosis, select patients for treatment who have moderate stage disease by symptom score and have shown some progression, and monitor serum prostate-specific antigen and digital rectal examination on a yearly basis while the patient is taking the drug.

- Though not yet proven to save lives, prostate-specific antigen screening of men with 10 years or more of expected life enables diagnosis of prostate cancer in 3.6% of healthy men over age 50 years; 70% of the cancers are localized and potentially curable when diagnosed with prostate-specific antigen testing compared with less than 50% before the prostate-specific antigen era.

- For advanced stage D2 prostate cancer (widely metastatic), total androgen blockade with medical or surgical castration and flutamide, an antiandrogen, significantly increases time to progression of disease (3 months) and median time to survival (7-month increase).

- Alternative therapies to total androgen blockade are or will soon be available for stage D2 prostate cancer patients whose quality of life is threatened by potential side effects of total androgen blockade.

BENIGN PROSTATIC HYPERPLASIA

Benign prostatic hyperplasia (BPH) commonly affects two thirds of men over 55 years of age. A large number of patients with varying degrees of symptomatic BPH are living with their symptoms.

Pathogenesis of Benign Prostatic Hyperplasia

In recent years, both epidemiologic and experimental data have strongly supported that BPH is an endocrinopathy related to dihydrotestosterone (DHT) and aging. Epidemiologic data include 1) males castrated before age 40 are protected from BPH, implicating an essential role of the testes; and 2) males with congenital 5 α-reductase deficiency with elevated testosterone, but very low levels of DHT in the prostate, have small vestigial prostates implicating DHT in BPH (Fig. 1) [1,2]. Patients with testicular feminization who lack an androgen receptor have no identifiable prostate. Prostate weight increases steadily after age 50 in autopsy studies (Fig. 2) [3].

The 5 α-reductase enzyme, which converts testosterone to DHT, is higher in BPH prostates than in normal prostates (age less than 40). Prostate enzymes that metabolize prostatic DHT are lower in BPH prostate than normal prostates [4]. Finally, experimental data in which DHT levels are lowered with a variety of drugs or surgical techniques uniformly demonstrate prostate gland size reduction (Table 1) [5–8].

Symptoms of Benign Prostatic Hyperplasia

The symptoms of BPH, referred to as prostatism, include both irritative and obstructive symptoms (Table 2). Outlet obstruction of the bladder causing prostatism primarily results from mechanical enlargement of the prostate that narrows the prostatic urethra. In addition, activation of α_1-adrenergic receptors that are concentrated in the bladder neck and in the prostate smooth muscle, contribute to prostatism by constriction of the bladder outlet and increasing the intraurethral pressure. The mechanical factor would appear to be more important than the α_1-adrenergic tone, since BPH has been successfully treated for the past 90 years with TURP, which removes the mechanically obstructing peri-urethral adenoma.

Differential Diagnosis of Benign Prostatic Hyperplasia

The therapy for BPH is highly specific and must be initiated only after eliminating other conditions to be considered in the differential diagnosis. These other conditions include chronic prostatitis, chronic and acute urinary tract infections, prostate cancer, bladder cancer, neurogenic bladder, and urethral stricture. Checking a urine for erythrocytes, leukocytes, and cell cytology will help to diagnose infection and bladder cancer; comparison of leukocytes and bacteria in urethral and bladder urine with post-prostatic massage urine will aid recognition of prostatitis; a serum prostate-specific antigen (PSA) and digital rectal exam will tend to rule out prostate cancer, and a post-void, catheterized or ultrasound residual urine will help to diagnose neurogenic bladder or advanced decompensated BPH if present. Although the digital rectal examination provides only an approximation of prostate size, the examination is very useful in suspecting carcinoma if hard areas, nodules, or asymmetry are present. Patients with PSA levels above normal should be referred to a urologist for transrectal ultrasound and biopsy if indicated.

Medical Treatment of Benign Prostatic Hyperplasia

Once the diagnosis of BPH has been established by appropriate history, physical examination, and tests, the question of therapy is raised. Until recently, transurethral prostatectomy was the only acceptable therapy for BPH. However, as mentioned, the epidemiologic and experimental data pointing to the significant role of DHT in the pathogenesis of the disease make a 5 α-

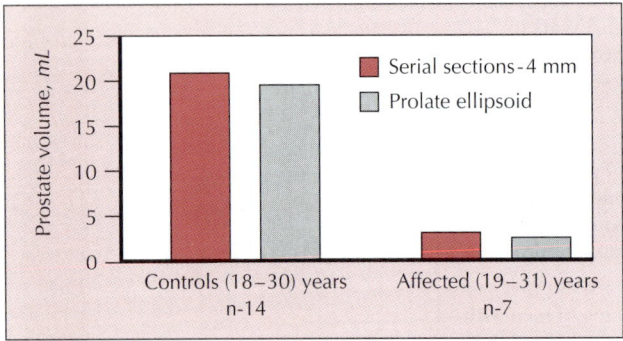

FIGURE 1 Comparison of prostate volumes in young and old control male subjects. The *darker bar* represents prostate volume calculated by the slice method, and the *lighter bar* represents calculations by the prolate ellipsoid method.

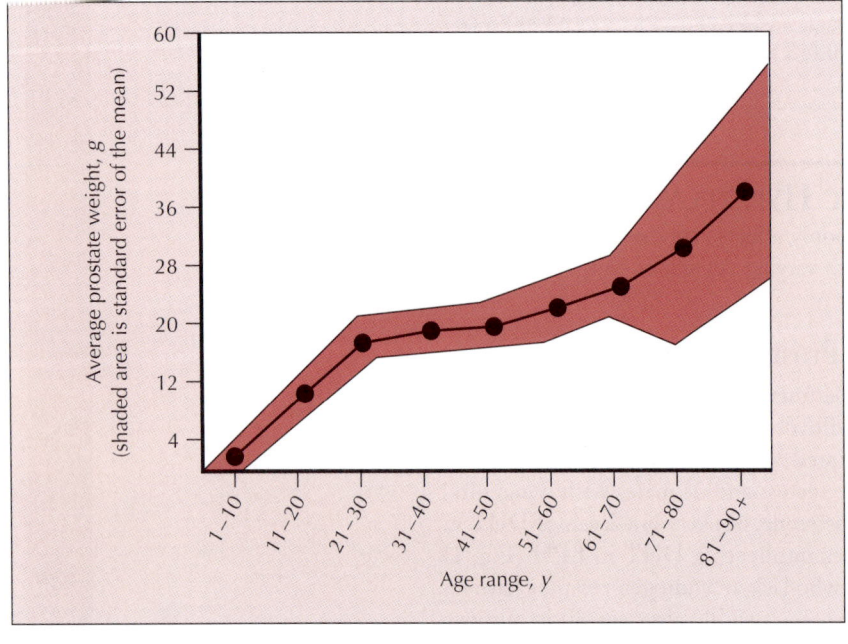

FIGURE 2 Mean prostate weight in grams for each decade is shown. Prostates were obtained at autopsy. Note progressive increase in weight following age 40.

Table 1. Effect of Androgen Withdrawal on Prostate Size

Androgen blockers	Mean decrease in prostate volume, % (Type of measurement)	Average time for maximal decrease in size, *mo*	Large double-blind studies of clinical effects
Surgical castration	30 (TRUS)	3–6	No
Progestational anti-androgens (cyproterone acetate)	30 (TRUS)	3–6	No
Flutamide	40 (TRUS)	3–6	No
Gonadotropin-releasing hormone agonists	25 (TRUS)	3–6	No
5 α-reductase inhibitors (finasteride)	20 (MRI)	3–6	Yes

From Geller [23]; with permission.
MRI—magnetic resonance imaging; TRUS—transrectal ultrasound.

reductase inhibitor, which blocks the formation of DHT and decreases prostate size, a logical choice for treatment. Such a drug, finasteride, has recently been approved by the Food and Drug Administration for use in BPH.

Finasteride reduces plasma dihydrotestosterone concentration by approximately 70% whereas plasma testosterone values remain within the normal range [8]. The drug has no other apparent effects. Five mg a day of finasteride significantly reduced prostate size by approximately 20%, significantly increased maximal urinary flow rates, and significantly reduced clinical symptoms of BPH in treated patients compared with controls (Figs. 3 and 4) [8]. The drug had minimal side effects, which was important in elevating it to the status of an effective medical treatment for BPH.

Monitoring During Finasteride Therapy

Initial therapy should be given for at least 6 months to all patients because it takes that long for a significant decrease in prostate size. Improvement in obstructive and irritative symptoms of BPH lag behind size reduction by several months or more. If therapy is effective in improving symptoms, treatment should be continued indefinitely, because the gland will regrow if therapy is discontinued.

Patients should be seen at 3-month intervals for reevaluation of symptoms during the 1st year of finasteride therapy. Digital rectal examination and plasma PSA (blood for test should be drawn before digital rectal examination) should be done every 6 months for the 1st year.

If the baseline PSA decreases by the expected 30% to 50% after 1 year, PSA testing and digital rectal examination should be conducted annually [8]. An increase of PSA to above upper normal test limits at any time or of greater than 1 ng/mL within 1 year, but still within the normal range, should initiate a referral for transrectal ultrasound to rule out prostate cancer.

In a double-blind study, prostate cancer was discovered as frequently in patients on finasteride as those on placebo [8]. However, the agent may delay the increase of PSA associated with an early prostate cancer. Because PSA is a good tumor marker for prostate cancer and predicts tumor mass, a small, undiagnosable early prostate cancer present at initiation of finasteride therapy would not become inoperable if the instructions outlined in the previous section of monitoring PSA are followed.

Side Effects During Finasteride Therapy

Statistically significant differences between the placebo and 5.0-mg finasteride-treated groups occurred in the following parameters: 1) decreased libido occurred in 4.7% of the finasteride

Table 2. Obstructive and Irritative Symptoms of Benign Prostatic Hyperplasia

Obstructive	Irritative
Hesitancy	Frequency
Straining	Urgency
Weak stream	Nocturia
Terminal dribbling	Urge incontinence
Prolonged micturition	Small voided volume
Retention	
Overflow incontinence	

From Walsh [24]; with permission.

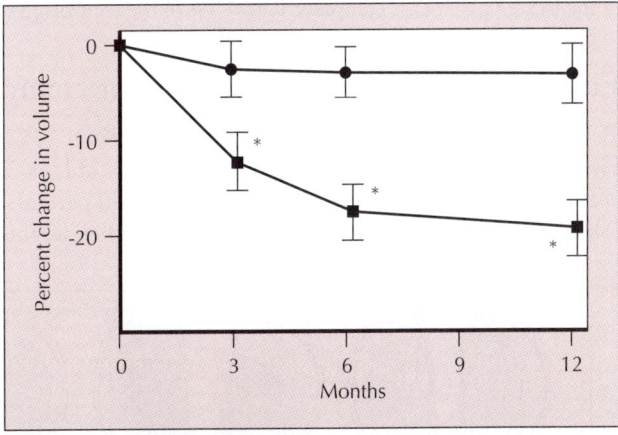

Figure 3 The changes in prostate volume at three monthly intervals, measured with magnetic resonance imaging, in placebo patients (*circles*) compared with finasteride-treated patients (*squares*) in a large double-blind randomized placebo-controlled study. *$P < 0.05$.

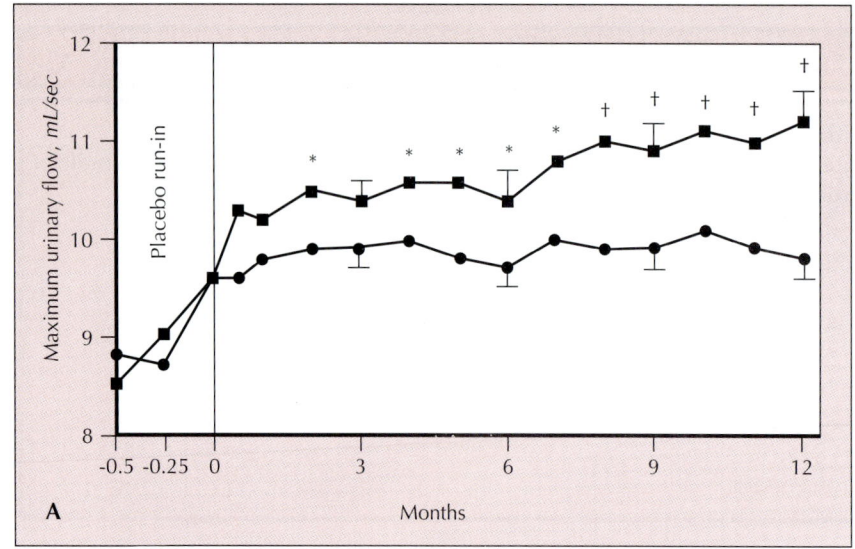

FIGURE 4 **A**, Maximum urinary flow rate changes in placebo-treated patients (*circles*) and finasteride-treated patients (*squares*) in a large, double-blind randomized placebo-controlled study are shown. Notice the statistically significant increase in the drug-treated group. **B**, Changes in the symptom score measured with modified Boyarsky scale in placebo-treated patients (*circles*) and finasteride-treated patients in a large (*squares*) double-blind, randomized placebo-controlled study are shown. *$P < .05$; †$P < .01$.

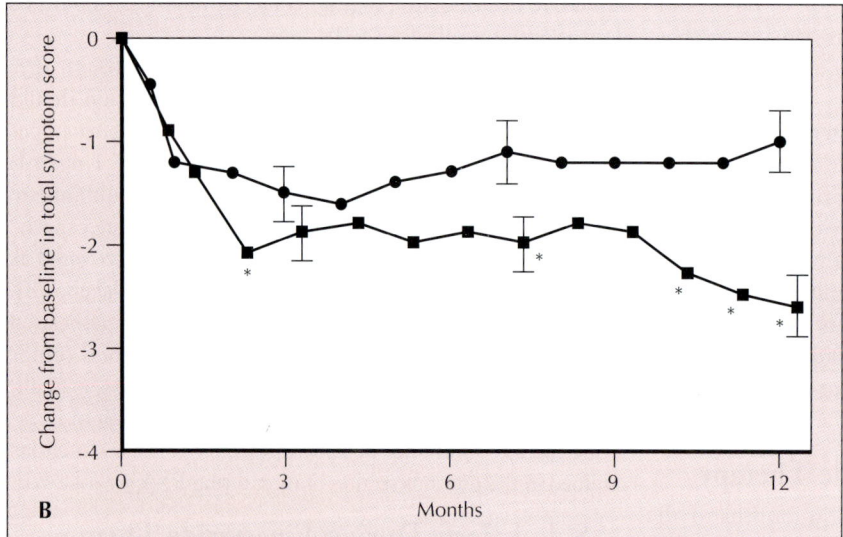

patients compared with 1.3% of the placebo group; 2) decreased ejaculate was reported in 4.4% of the finasteride group compared with 1.7% of the placebo group; 3) impotence was noted in 3.4% of the treated patients as compared with 1.7% of the controls [8].

Finasteride Versus Transurethral Prostatectomy for Benign Prostatic Hyperplasia

Finasteride sustains a reduction in prostate size for at least 5 years in unpublished studies of approximately 50 patients followed by us in open extension to date. Nevertheless, the symptomatic improvement in prostatism was only half as much in patients on finasteride compared to transurethral prostatectomy 1 year following surgery [8]. The mean improvement of flow rates in patients on finasteride was considerably less than that reported following transurethral prostatectomy.

At advanced stages of prostatism, symptoms are usually sufficiently severe to affect quality of life, mandating aggressive therapy. This stage characterizes most patients undergoing surgery who have gone through "watchful waiting" for years before transurethral prostatectomy. Therefore, with advanced BPH, surgery is clearly preferable in most cases (Fig. 5).

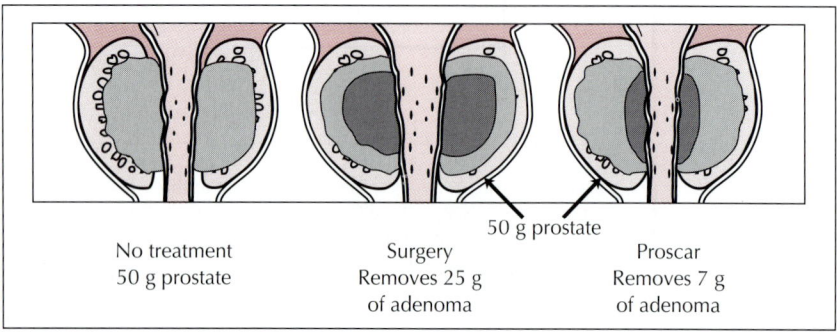

FIGURE 5 An example of the comparison of surgery versus finasteride in the treatment of advanced benign prostatic hypertrophy is shown. Notice the three- to fourfold greater removal of tissue with surgery as compared to medical therapy.

Table 3 International prostate symptom score

	Not at all	Less than 1 time in 5	Less than half the time	About half the time	More than half the time	Almost always
Incomplete emptying Over the past month, how often have you had a sensation of not emptying your bladder completely after you finished urinating?	0	1	2	3	4	5
Frequency Over the past month, how often have you had to urinate again less than 2 hours after you finished urinating?	0	1	2	3	4	5
Intermittency Over the past month, how often have you found you stopped and started again several times when you urinated?	0	1	2	3	4	5
Urgency Over the past month, how often have you found it difficult to postpone urination?	0	1	2	3	4	5
Weak stream Over the past month, how often have you had a weak urinary stream?	0	1	2	3	4	5
Straining Over the past month, how often have you had to push or strain to begin urination?	0	1	2	3	4	5
	None	1 time	2 times	3 Times	4 times	≥ 5 times
Nocturia Over the past month, how many times did you most typically get up to urinate from the time you went to bed at night until the time you got up in the morning?	0	1	2	3	4	5
Total international prostate symptom score =	Your score					
	Delighted	Pleased	Mostly satisfied	Mixed—about equally satisfied and dissatisfied	Mostly dissatisfied	Unhappy
Quality of life resulting from urinary symptoms If you were to spend the rest of your life with your urinary condition just the way it is now, how would you feel about that?	0	1	2	3	4	5

From Berry et al. [25]; with permission.

If, on the other hand, internists initiate drug therapy at a moderate stage of disease where symptoms are annoying or the patient wants to avoid surgery, finasteride will arrest and improve the disease. Because only 40% of patients with symptomatic BPH progress to advanced disease, treatment with finasteride carries the risk of being unnecessary. However, transurethral prostatectomy for patients with moderate BPH would not be acceptable to most individuals and would be subject to a much higher recurrence rate, because the patients would undergo surgery at an earlier age and stage of disease.

Staging of Benign Prostatic Hypertrophy

Three factors must be evaluated to stage BPH into mild, moderate, or severe disease. First is the symptom score. Table 3 shows the standardized scoring system for bladder outlet obstruction recently published by the American Urology Association (AUA). Scores of less than nine indicate mild disease, nine to 18 indicate moderate disease, and above 18 indicate severe disease. Uroflow rates are also helpful, and maximal flow rates less than 10 mL/s indicate severe disease, with values above 10 mL/s indicating moderate to mild disease. In addi-

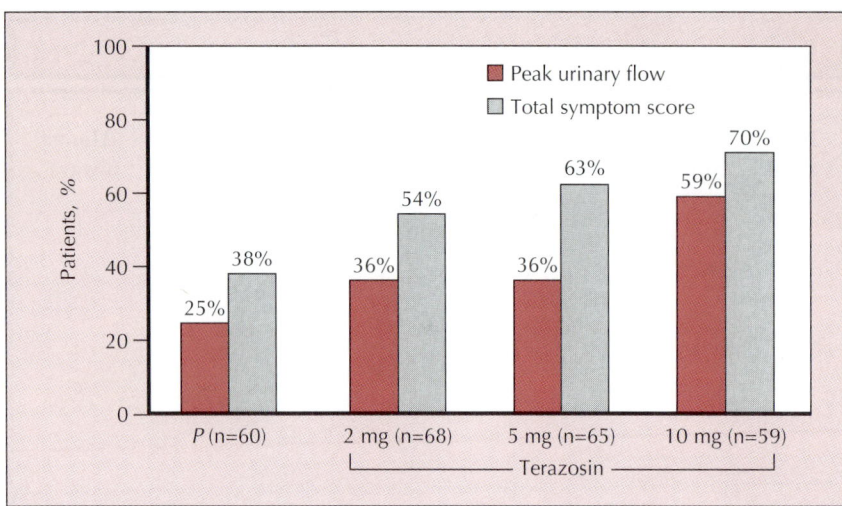

FIGURE 6 The effects of varying doses of terazosin is shown for its effect on peak urinary flow and total symptom score in patients with benign prostatic hypertrophy.

tion, residual urine should be estimated with either straight catheterization or the use of a bladder ultrasound. Values over 200 mL indicate significant longstanding outlet obstruction and early bladder failure and point to advanced disease.

Use of α Blockers as Medical Treatment for Benign Prostatic Hypertrophy

$α_1$-adrenergic blockers, terazosin and doxazosin, have recently been approved by the FDA for medical treatment of BPH. Although these drugs improve clinical symptoms of prostatism (Figure 6), they don't control prostatic growth, and therefore may not provide long-term medical treatment for BPH. Increasing prostate volume over time would appear to have overriding importance in the natural history of disease progression in at least 25% of patients with mild or early BPH who go on to advanced disease and in the past have required a TURP. The TURP is successful by virtue of removing a large part of the periurethral adenoma. Finasteride is a medical therapy that decreases prostate size, and that for at least five years prevents any subsequent growth. This is not the case at all with α blockers, and there is a major concern as to their long-term effectiveness in patients whose prostates continue to grow. Therefore, finasteride is our choice as a long-term therapy for medical management of BPH. However, α blockers may be used as initial therapy together with finasteride to provide quick symptomatic relief of BPH or may be added to finasteride after 6 months in patients desiring a better clinical response.

PROSTATIC CARCINOMA

Prostatic carcinoma is the most prevalent cancer in men. More than 130,000 cases are currently diagnosed per year. As a cause of cancer death, prostatic cancer ranks second to lung cancer.

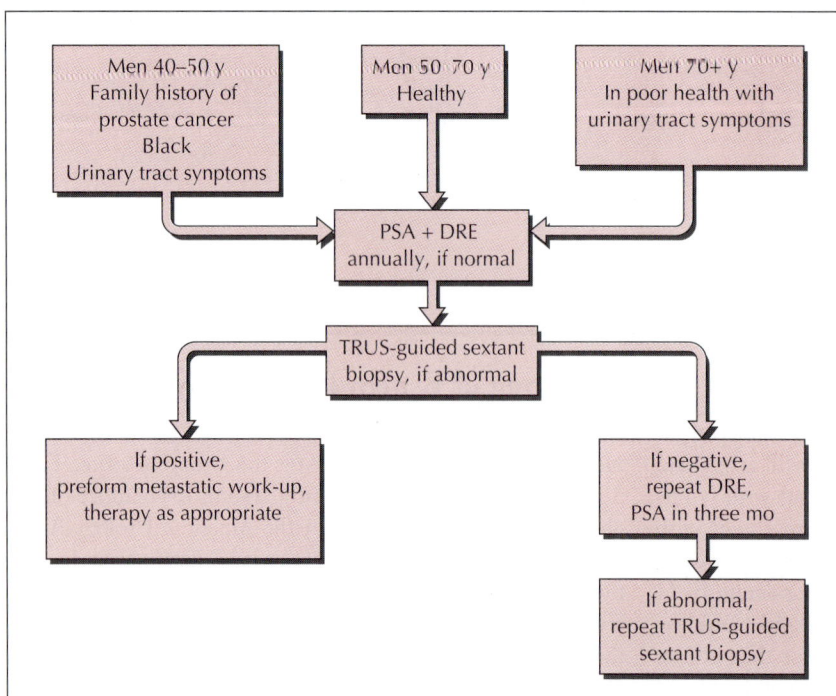

FIGURE 7 Algorithm for prostate cancer screening. DRE—digital rectal examination; PSA—prostate-specific antigen; TRUS—transrectal ultrasound.

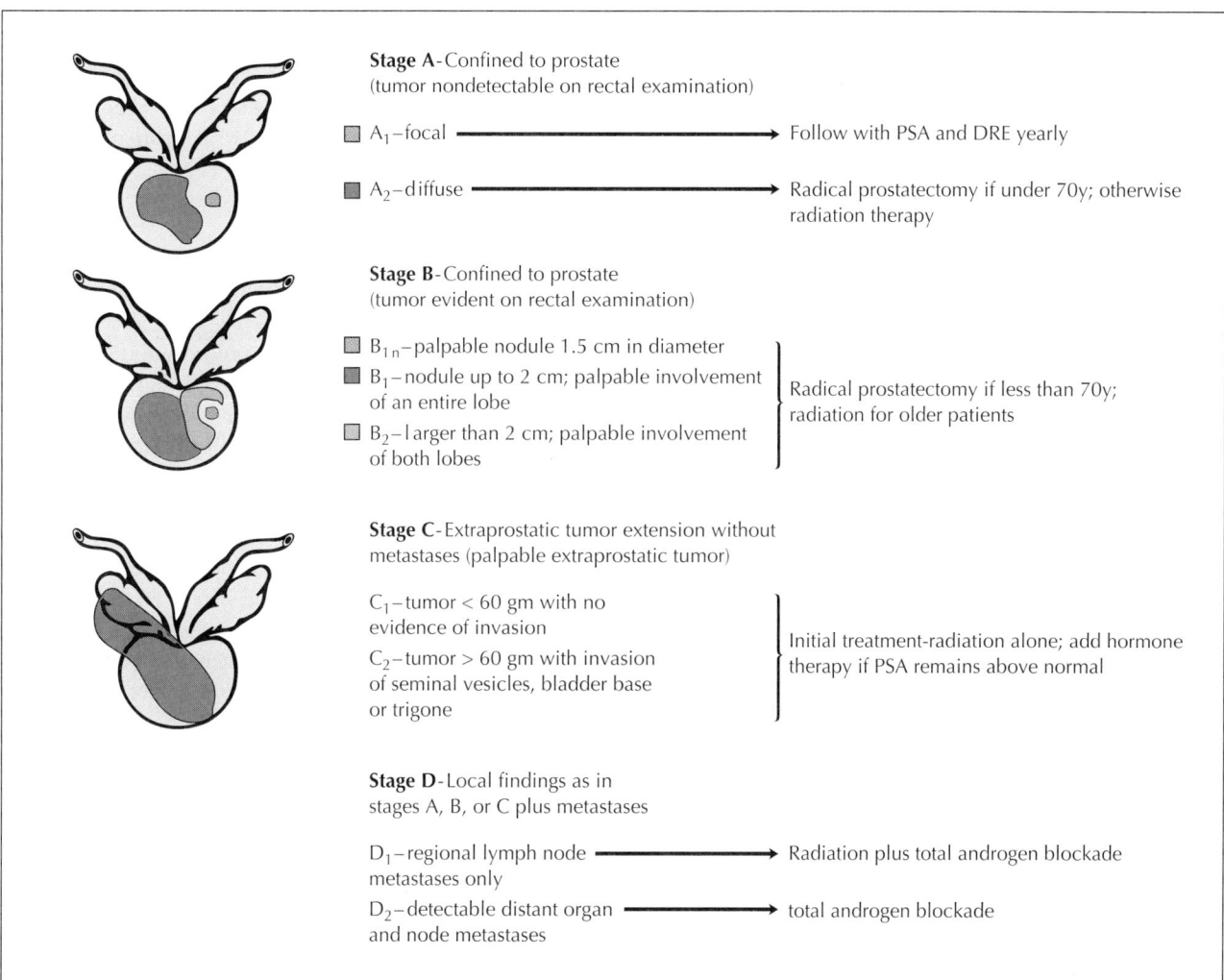

FIGURE 8 Staging and treatment of prostate cancer.

The diagnosis of prostatic cancer has been considerably augmented by the availability of new screening techniques, particularly the PSA. This test has been shown by Catalona and coworkers [10], as well as others, to have the highest sensitivity (79%) and specificity (59%) as an individual test for prostate cancer. When combined with digital rectal examination, the sensitivity and specificity climbs even higher [10]. Catalona and coworkers [10] have shown that in men with PSA levels between 4.0 and 10.0 ng/mL (upper limits of normal = 4.0 ng/mL), the detection of prostate cancer was approximately 22% in a group of asymptomatic men. At levels above 10 ng/mL, the incidence of prostate cancer in a group of asymptomatic men above age 50 was 67%.

Diagnosis of Prostate Cancer

The current policy, endorsed by the American Cancer Society and AUA for diagnostic screening for prostate cancer, is to do a PSA test and a digital rectal examination yearly in men older than 50 years of age (Fig. 7). A controlled clinical trial to evaluate the effectiveness of screening with PSA and DRE has been started by the National Cancer Institute, but it will take 15 years to complete. Meanwhile, Catalona and coworkers [10] have demonstrated that screening with serial PSA alone resulted in the discovery of prostate cancer in approximately 3.6% of over 10,000 asymptomatic men who were screened and over age 50 years. The very encouraging aspect of this study was that 70% of the patients discovered with prostate cancer using serial PSA assays had disease confined to the prostate. This finding represents a highly significant improvement in the detection of potentially curable early disease compared with a comparison group in whom only 43% of tumors confined to the gland were detected using DRE. Concerns that tumors detected by PSA may be small and insignificant have been answered by two studies in which nonpalpable prostate cancer detected by PSA screening was compared with cancers detected by DRE. All patients in these studies had radical prostatectomies so that their tumor volume and grade could be compared, and they were very similar regarding these parameters [13,14].

Staging of Prostate Cancer

Before the development of the PSA test, the majority of prostate cancers were discovered in advanced stages. Prostate cancer staging in the United States is shown in Figure 8.

Since the development of the PSA test, more patients with earlier stage prostate disease are being discovered. An algorithm for staging following the diagnosis of prostate cancer is shown in Figure 9.

Treatment of Prostate Cancer

There are major differences in opinion regarding the effectiveness of various treatments for early prostate cancer. Johansson and coworkers [13] and Chodak and coworkers [14] have published data showing a 91% and 87% 10-year survival rate respectively in patients with early prostate cancer treated with deferred therapy. Many patients in these studies were older than age 75 years, and there were four to five times as many patients who died before the 10-year period as those who survived.

In a meta-analysis of 10-year survival rate of early prostate cancer, Adolfsson and coworkers [15] showed that the best results were achieved using radical prostatectomy (93% 10-year survival rate) compared with an 83% 10-year survival rate for deferred therapy. All of these studies indicated a high metastatic rate for the 10-year survivors who were treated with deferred therapy [13–15]. Therefore it seems likely that radical prostatectomy for patients with a 10-year life expectancy will cure more patients and leave fewer with metastatic disease at 10 years than any other therapy. It is likely that screening for prostate cancer will focus on patients with a 10-year life expectancy. Because most patients with less than a 10-year life expectancy will die of other causes before the relatively slow growing prostate cancer becomes a major clinical problem, the role of screening and even therapy for such patients is uncertain. A test to determine the clinical aggressiveness of the tumor is needed to choose appropriate therapy for patients with early prostate cancer.

One scheme of therapy for clinically localized disease is shown in Figure 8. Figure 8 also contains recommendations for treatment in metastatic cancer for which there is much less of a consensus. In stage C, for instance, radiation therapy alone or radiation therapy plus hormonal therapy is usually used. In stage D_1 with positive lymph nodes, orchiectomy of medical castration is usually associated with a median 5-year survival of 50%. Recent studies have indicated that radiation therapy plus castration (medical or surgical) or radical prostatectomy plus orchiectomy provides a longer time to progression and survival than hormonal therapy alone [16].

Over the past 5 years, the major debate in treating prostate cancer has been in stage D_1 disease, specifically regarding the question of the benefits of total androgen blockade (*ie*, blocking both adrenal and testicular androgens) versus blocking testicular androgens alone. Geller and coworkers [17] showed that following castration, residual DHT levels in the prostate averaged 25% of that found in untreated prostates. This residual DHT is important in regulating epithelial cell growth and

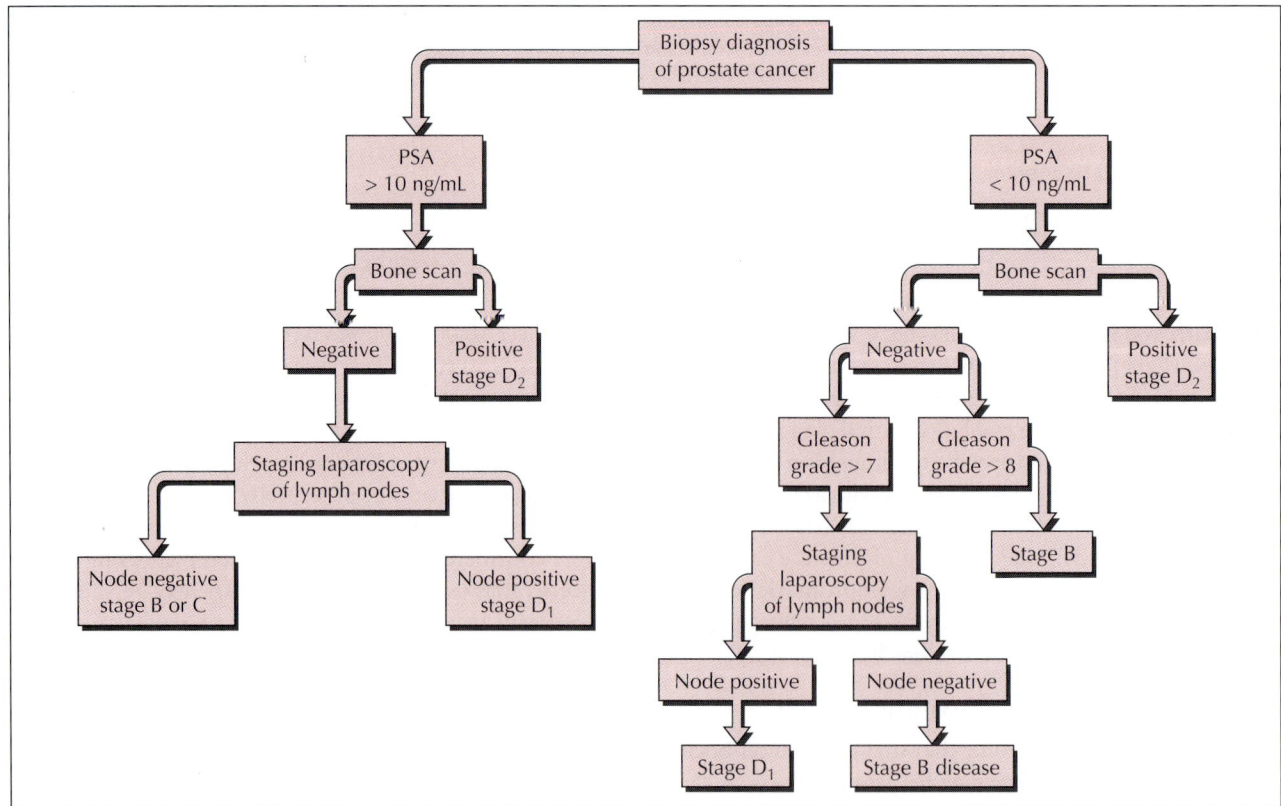

FIGURE 9 Staging algorithm. PSA—prostate specific antigen.

TABLE 4 EFFECT OF COMBINED ANDROGEN BLOCKADE COMPARED WITH CASTRATION (MEDICAL OR SURGICAL) ALONE ON MEDIAN SURVIVAL IN STAGE D_2 PROSTATE CANCER TRIALS

Trial	Treatment arms	Patients, n	Median time to progression Mo	P value	Median time to survival Mo	P value
SWOG, NCI Crawford et al. [18]	Leuprolide and placebo	300	13.9	0.039	28.3	0.035
	Leuprolide and flutamide	303	16.5		35.6	
EORTC 30853 Keuppens et al. [19]	Orchiectomy	155	11.5	0.002	36.0	0.04
	Zoladex and flutamide	162	18.0		52.0	
Canadian Beland et al. [20]	Orchiectomy and placebo	96	11.7	0.152	18.3	0.04
	Orchiectomy and nilutamide	98	12.4		24.3	
DAPROCA [21]	Orchiectomy	129	16.3	0.09	27.6	0.11
	Zoladex and flutamide	119	16.6		22.8	

DAPROCA—Danish Prostate Cancer Study; EORTC—European Organization on Research Treatment of Cancer; NCI—National Cancer Institute; SWOG—Southwestern Oncology Group.

PSA; it is also important clinically because further reduction of DHT levels has provided second clinical remissions in about one third of patients with stage D_2 prostate cancer who were previously castrated [12].

Three of four international trials have provided evidence that there is a benefit regarding both time to progression and median time to survival in patients treated with total androgen blockade as opposed to medical or surgical castration. A summary of these four trials is shown in Table 4 [18–21].

Issues Relating to the Use of Total Androgen Blockade in Stage D_2 Prostate Cancer

One of the strong points that favors blocking all androgens is the heterogeneity of prostate cancer. According to the Southwestern Oncology Group data, administration of total androgen blockade at the start of therapy was more effective than sequential blockade (Table 4). Recent analysis of subsets of patients in the largest of the double-blind, randomized studies of the effect of total androgen blockade indicates that patients with minimal D_2 disease have very dramatic benefits averaging 30 months compared to the group as a whole regarding median time to progression and survival (Fig. 10). Total androgen blockade may not be useful in patients who have poor performance status along with extensive metastatic disease.

Alternative Therapies to Reduce Cost of Total Androgen Blockade

Total androgen blockade using a gonadotropin-releasing hormone agonist plus flutamide costs $600 to $700 a month. Of course, the orchiectomy is much cheaper and much more cost-effective, but less popular with patients. An alternative to medical castration with gonadotropin-releasing hormone agonists is the use of megestrol acetate, 120 mg/d, in combination with low-dose estrogen such as 0.1 mg diethylstilbestrol or 0.5 to 1.0 mg of estradiol, which has minimal estrogenic side effects. This therapy has been shown to provide a medical castration along with at least a 50% reduction in circulating adrenal androgens and an antiandrogenic effect at the cell level (Fig. 11) [22]. The cost of such therapy excluding flutamide costs would be about $80 per month, as compared to the levprolide acetate (luteinizing hormone-releasing hormone agonist) cost of $300 to $400 a month.

Downstaging of Clinical Stage C Prostate Cancer, with Total Androgen Blockade

Recent studies have shown that prostate tumor size can be significantly reduced by 3 or more months of therapy with total androgen blockade using lupron and flutamide. Such therapy may reduce or eliminate tumor cells at the margin of the prostate and allow for radical prostatectomy with cure. In addition, 10% of patients who have had malignant biopsy specimens do not show any residual tumor microscopically following removal of the prostate after 3 months of downstaging with total androgen blockade. The long-term results and effectiveness of this technique are currently under study. Patients with PSAs less than 38 ng/mL and tumor Gleason grading of less than 7 are candidates for such downstaging treatment.

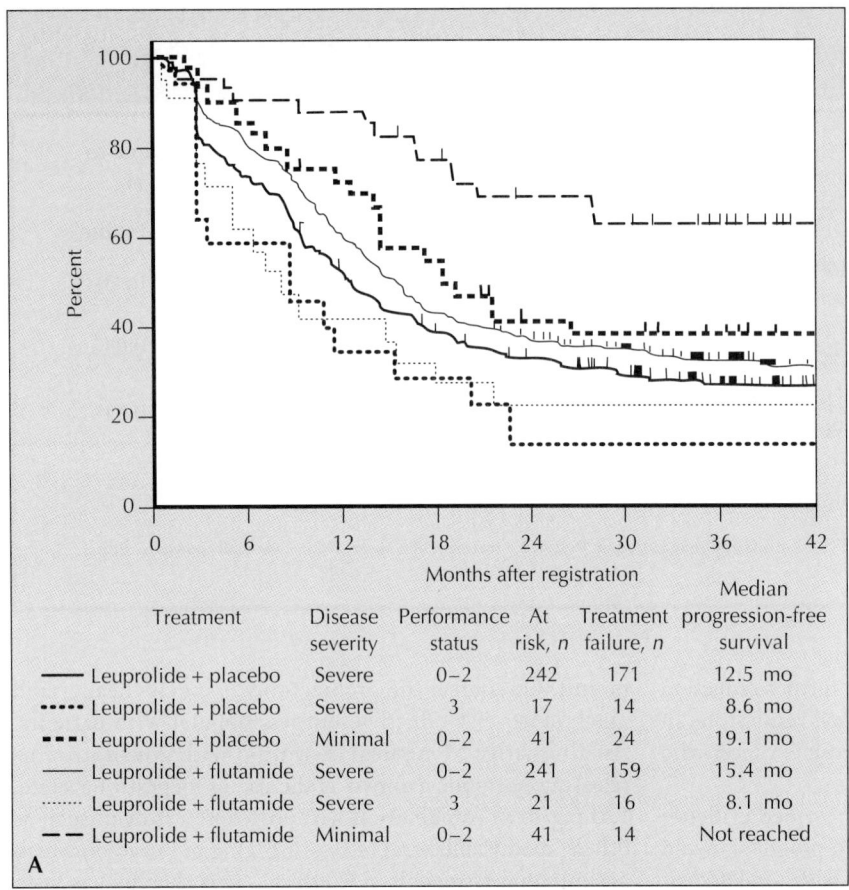

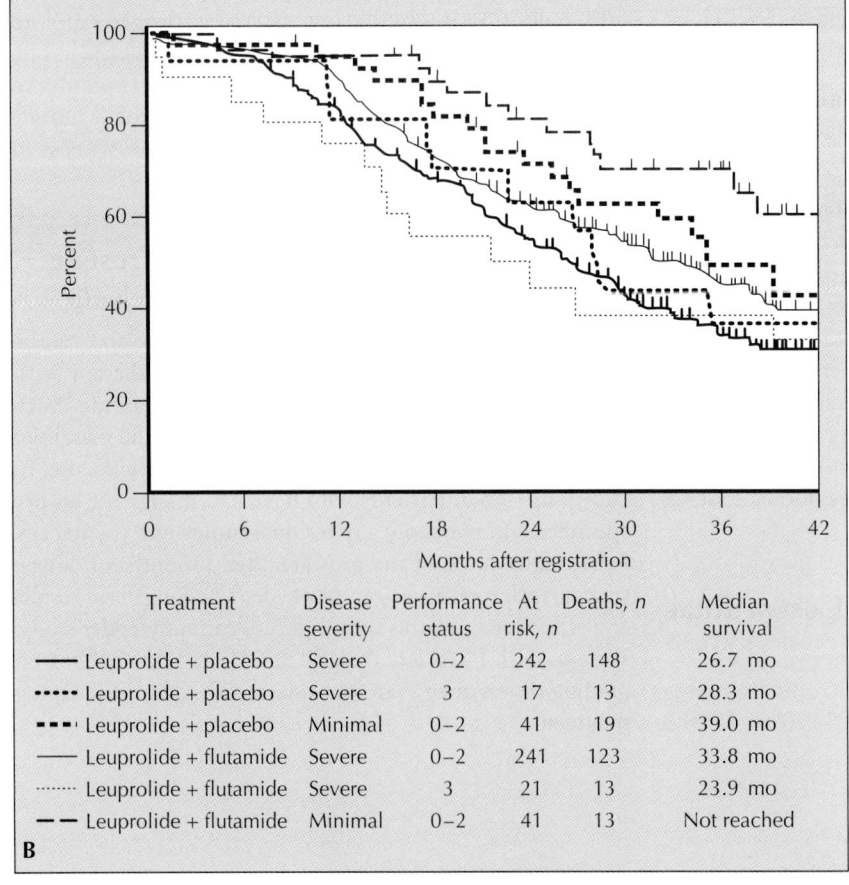

FIGURE 10 A, This is a Kaplan-Meier curve showing median progression-free survival for patients treated with either leuprolide plus placebo or leuprolide plus flutamide. The patients are broken down into subsets according to the disease severity and performance status. Notice the markedly greater benefits of leuprolide plus flutamide versus leuprolide alone in the patients with minimal disease severity and good performance status. B, Median time to survival for patients treated with either leuprolide plus placebo or leuprolide plus flutamide. The entire group is broken down into subsets according to severity of disease and performance status. Note the very large benefits of leuprolide plus flutamide compared to leuprolide alone in patients who had good performance status and minimal disease severity.

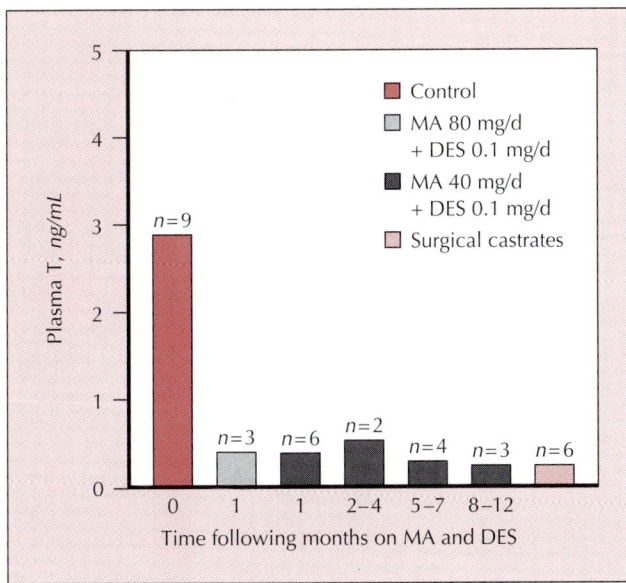

FIGURE 11 Demonstration of the effect of the administration of megestrol acetate (MA) combined with diethylstilbestrol (DES) on plasma T.

REFERENCES AND RECOMMENDED READING

Recently published papers of particular interest have been highlighted as:
- Of interest
- •• Of outstanding interest

1. Moore RA: Benign hypertrophy and carcinoma of the prostate: occurrence and experimental production in animals. *Surgery* 1944, 16:152–167.
2. Imperato-McGinley J, Gautier T, Zirinsky K, *et al.*: Steroid 5 α-reductase deficiency in man: an inherited form of male pseudohermaphroditism. *Science* 1974, 186:1213–1215.
3. Berry SJ, Coffey DS, Walsh PC, *et al.*: The development of human benign prostatic hyperplasia with age. *J Urol* 1984, 132:474–479.
4. Isaacs J, Brendler C, Walsh P: Changes in the metabolism of dihydrotestosterone in the hyperplastic human prostate. *J Clin Endocrinol Metab* 1983, 56:139.
5. Schroeder FH, Westerhof M, Bosch RJ, *et al.*: Benign prostatic hyperplasias treated by castration or the LHRH analogue buserelin: a report on 6 cases. *Eur Urol* 1986, 12(5):318–321.
6. Ekman P, Johansson B, Ohlsen H, *et al.*: Drug therapy in benign prostatic hyperplasia. *Scand J Urol Nephrol* 1981, 60(suppl):72–80.
7. Peters CA, Walsh PC: The effect of nafarelin acetate, a luteinizing-hormone-releasing agonist, on benign prostatic hyperplasia. *N Engl J Med* 1987, 317:599.
8. Gormley JG, Stoner E, Bruskewitz RC, *et al.*: The effect of finasteride in men with benign prostatic hyperplasia. *N Engl J Med* 1992, 327:1185–1191.
9. Lepor H, Auerbach S, Puras-Baez A: A randomized placebo-controlled multicenter study of the efficacy and safety of terazosin in the treatment of benign prostatic hyperplasia. *J Urol* 1992, 148:1467–1474.
10. Catalona WJ, Smith DS, Ratliff TL, *et al.*: Measurement of prostate-specific antigen in serum as a screening test for prostate cancer. *N Engl J Med* 1991, 324:1156–1161.
11. Stormont TJ, Farrow GM, Myers RP, *et al.*: Clinical stage B_0 in T1c cancer: nonpalpable disease identified by elevated serum prostate-specific antigen concentration. *Urol* 1993, 41:3–8.
12. Walsh PC: Using prostate-specific antigen to diagnose prostate cancer: sailing in uncharted waters. *Ann Int Med* 1993, 119:948–949.
13. Johansson JE, Adami HO, Andersson SO, *et al.*: High 10-year survival rate in patients with early, untreated prostatic cancer. *JAMA* 1992, 267:2191–2196.
14. Chodak GW, Thisted RA, Gerber GS, *et al.*: Results of conservative management of clinically localized prostate cancer. *N Engl J Med* 1994, 330:242–248.
15. Adolfsson J, Steineck G, Whitmore WF: Recent results of management of palpable clinically localized prostate cancer. *Cancer* 1993, 72:310–322.
16. Cheng CWS, Bergstrálh EJ, Zincke H: Stage D_1 prostate cancer: a randomized comparison of conservative treatment options versus radical prostatectomy. *Cancer* 1993, 71(suppl 3):996–1004.
17. Geller J, Albert J, Loza D: Steroid levels in cancer of the prostate—markers of tumor differentiation and adequacy of anti-androgen therapy. *J Steroid Biochem Mol Biol* 1979 11:631–636.
18. Crawford ED, Eisenberger MA, McLeod DG, *et al.*: A controlled trial of leuprolide with and without flutamide in prostatic carcinoma. *N Engl J Med* 1989, 321:419–424.
19. Keuppens F, Denis L, Smith P, *et al.*: Zoladex and flutamide versus bilateral orchiectomy—a randomized phase III EORTC 30853 study. *Cancer* 1990, 66:1045–1057.
20. Béland G, Elhilali M, Fradet Y, *et al.*: A controlled trial of castration with and without nilutamide in metastatic prostatic carcinoma. *Cancer* 1990, 66:1074–1079.
21. Iversen P, Christensen MG, Friis E, *et al.*: A phase III trial of zoladex and flutamide versus orchiectomy in the treatment of patients with advanced carcinoma of the prostate. *Cancer* 1990, 66:1058–1066.
22. Geller J, Albert J, Yen SSC, *et al.*: Medical castration of males with megestrol acetate and small doses of diethylstilbestrol. *J Clin Endocrinol Metab* 1981, 52:3,576–580.
23. Geller J: Therapeutic controversies: clinical treatment of benign prostatic hyperplasia. *J Clin Endocrinol Metab* 1995; 80(3):745–747.
24. Walsh PC: Benign prostatic hyperplasia. *Campbell's Urology*, 6th edn. Edited by Walsh, Redick, Philadelphia: WB Saunders; 1994:1018.
25. Berry, Fowler, O'Leary, *et al.*: The American Urological Association Symptom Index for Benign Prostatic Hyperplasia. *J Urol* 1992, 148:1549–1557.

Special Presentation of Endocrine Disease in the Elderly

Itamar B. Abrass
Robert S. Schwartz

> **Key Points**
> - In older adults, diagnosis of diabetes mellitus should be made on the basis of fasting-glucose abnormality, not by post-glucose load abnormality.
> - Acceptable glucose control must be carefully individualized to avoid hypoglycemia.
> - Diet and exercise regimens are the cornerstones of diabetic treatment.
> - Despite the marked hyperglycemia of the hyperosmolar nonketotic state, initial therapy must first be directed to fluid resuscitation.
> - Any older patient who presents with new medical complaints and who has not had thyroid function tests in the past year should be screened for hypothyroidism.
> - Unexplained congestive heart failure or tachyarrhythmia, recent onset psychiatric disorder, or profound myopathy should raise suspicion of hyperthyroidism.

GLUCOSE INTOLERANCE AND DIABETES MELLITUS

Aging Effects on Glucose Tolerance

Glucose tolerance worsens with age. While fasting plasma glucose levels increase only 1 to 2 mg/dL (0.05–0.10 mmol/L) for each decade after 30 years of age, the 2-hour postprandial glucose level rises by 10 to 20 mg/dL (0.5–1.0 mmol/L). This more prominent post-load abnormality has led to a conundrum in the diagnosis of diabetes in the elderly [1••]. According to World Health Organization or National Diabetes Data Group criteria, it is possible to make the diagnosis of diabetes mellitus without the presence of fasting hyperglycemia; however, we consider this diagnosis not to be clinically relevant in older adults and reserve the diagnosis of diabetes mellitus for those who have two separate fasting plasma glucose levels that are greater than or equal to 140 mg/dL (7.8 mmol/L). This definition obviates the need for oral glucose tolerance tests under almost all clinical circumstances. This conservative approach to diagnosing diabetes also reduces the likelihood of inappropriate labeling with its potentially profound social and economic consequences. We consider those who have a fasting plasma glucose level less than 140 mg/dL but an elevated postprandial glucose level (>200 mg/dL) to have impaired glucose tolerance, a condition that may or may not progress to true diabetes mellitus.

Epidemiology

Data from the National Health and Nutrition Examination Survey II find diabetes mellitus to be the fifth most prevalent chronic condition in persons 65 years of age or older in the United States [2]. Diabetes mellitus occurs in 18% to 20% of the population older than 65 years, and half of these cases (9% to 10%) are undiagnosed. In addition to the 20% of the elderly population with frank diabetes, another 20% to 25% fit criteria for impaired glucose tolerance. The clinical importance of this state of abnormal glucose tolerance is emphasized by the twofold greater incidence of macrovascular complications in this group, despite there being no significant increase in microvascular or neuropathic disorders.

Clinical Presentation and Management

Almost all primary diabetes in the elderly is non–insulin-dependent diabetes mellitus (NIDDM). Some of the more common signs and symptoms that might initially lead to the diagnosis of diabetes mellitus are as follows:

- Classic triad of polyuria, polydipsia, and polyphasia occurs less frequently than in young
- Systemic symptoms such as weight loss, fatigue, or weakness
- Cataracts or sudden change in visual acuity
- Recurrent or slowly healing bacterial or fungal infections of the skin, genitalia, or urinary or respiratory tract
- Neurologic findings including peripheral neuropathy, isolated cranial nerve palsies, autonomic neuropathy (*eg*, diarrhea, orthostatic hypotension, atonic bladder with incontinence)
- Microangiopathy involving the kidney (*eg*, proteinuria, reduced glomerular function, uremia) or eyes (*eg*, maculopathy with hemorrhages and exudates)
- Cardiovascular (silent ischemia or infarction), cerebrovascular, or peripheral vascular disease
- Changed mental status (*eg*, delirium, dementia, depression, coma)
- Impotence

Physicians should consider the diagnosis of diabetes when older patients complain of diffuse symptoms that are often ascribed to "aging."

The overall approach to the management of diabetes mellitus and its cardinal finding of hyperglycemia has been debated for many years. Recent findings from the Diabetes Control and Complications Trial have demonstrated the effectiveness of tight glucose control in mitigating the progression of microvascular complications of diabetes in a highly select group of young insulin-dependent (Type I) diabetic patients. The application of these findings to NIDDM (Type II) is being debated. Most authorities agree that glucose levels should be controlled tightly while avoiding hypoglycemia. Because physiologic heterogeneity of the elderly ranges from healthy and active to frail, the physician's approach to what constitutes acceptable glucose control must be carefully individualized.

The major risk of tight glucose control in any diabetic population is hypoglycemia. Even with the highly select population of the Diabetes Control and Complications Trial, the incidence of severe hypoglycemic episodes was 2.5-fold greater in the tight glucose control group. Many of these episodes were at night and unrecognized. Furthermore, tight glucose control may blunt the usual warning symptoms of hypoglycemia, even in patients who are awake. The symptoms related to hypoglycemia may be partially masked by or misdiagnosed as other chronic illnesses common in the elderly such as cerebrovascular accidents, dementia, delirium, depression, sleep abnormalities, and myocardial ischemia. The following are factors that may predispose the older patient with NIDDM to frequent or severe hypoglycemia:

- Poor or erratic nutritional intake
- Changes in cognitive status that impair the perception or response to hypoglycemia
- Forgetfulness leading to noncompliance with medications or meals
- Dependence or isolation that limits receipt of early treatment for a hypoglycemic episode
- Impaired renal or hepatic metabolism or impaired clearance of drugs
- Reduced early morning growth hormone secretion

Drugs that can potentiate hypoglycemia include coumarin, cimetidine, salicylates, phenylbutazone, monoamine oxidase inhibitors, β-blockers, alcohol, sulfonamides, angiotensin converting enzyme inhibitors [3•].

The goal for many otherwise healthy elderly patients is the same as for younger patients, that is, near-normal fasting plasma glucose levels without hypoglycemia. This strategy must include a thorough evaluation to exclude occult hypoglycemic episodes that can be quickly followed by a secondary hyperglycemia (Somogyi effect). In elderly patients whose care is complicated by chronic medical illnesses, frailty, isolation, dependence, abnormal mental status, or a short life expectancy, the therapeutic goal must be realistic and should be aimed at reducing the symptoms of polyuria, fatigue, and weight loss rather than attaining euglycemia. In most cases, a fasting plasma glucose level of less than 200 mg is attainable with few hypoglycemic episodes. As in younger diabetic patients, careful attention to and aggressive treatment of other cardiovascular risk factors (*eg*, hypertension and smoking) are clearly indicated in older diabetic patients.

Diet and Exercise

Diet and exercise regimens are the cornerstones of diabetic treatment. However, stable weight reduction is seldom accomplished. The high level of recidivism leads us to recommend a simple, noncalorically restricted, low-fat (≤ 30% of calories), high-carbohydrate (> 50% of calories) diet, in combination with endurance exercise for older diabetics. A low-fat diet and endurance exercise each can reduce insulin resistance and both are associated with mild spontaneous weight loss. Endurance exercise also appears helpful in maintaining any lost weight. The exercise prescribed for the elderly diabetic patient need not be intense (50% to 70% of maximal heart rate; maximal heart rate = 200 − age) and even moderate leisure time activity has been associated with a reduced risk of developing diabetes mellitus [4].

Drug Therapy

If significant hyperglycemia persists after a concerted attempt at diet and exercise, a trial of an oral hypoglycemic agent is indicated. Because of their once-a-day dosing, lack of an antidiuretic effect, and lesser displacement from plasma-binding proteins by other drugs, the second generation sulfonylureas are generally preferred. Of these, glyburide is excreted as an active metabolite by both the kidney and liver, and glipizide is metabolized to an inactive form before excretion by the kidney. Of the two, glipizide has been associated with fewer episodes of hypoglycemia, an important concern in the elderly. The drug chlorpropamide should not be used in the elderly because of long half-life, antidiuretic effect, and association with severe and prolonged hypoglycemia. Oral agents should be started at the low end of the dosing range and cautiously increased, while adverse effects (hypoglycemia) and efficacy (glycosylated hemoglobin or fructosamine levels) are monitored. Because of the frequency of problems, such as poor vision, arthritis, and memory deficits, and the added potential for hypoglycemia, insulin therapy may be problematic in many older diabetic patients. Overall, regimens for insulin treatment in the elderly are similar to those in the young and should include the use of home glucose monitoring. Devices to aid in accurate insulin dose withdrawal and the use of premixed insulins or predrawn syringes may be necessary in the elderly diabetic patient who requires insulin therapy.

Hyperosmolar Nonketotic State

Hyperosmolar nonketotic state is seen primarily in the elderly, with about one third to one half of cases occurring in patients without a previous diagnosis of NIDDM. Typically, the onset is insidious, and long delays in the diagnosis may account for the near 50% mortality in this disorder. Days to weeks of increasing hyperglycemia, glycosuria, and osmotic diuresis lead to marked free water (10 to 12 L) and sodium deficits, hyperglycemia (glucose > 600 mg/dL), hyperosmolarity (osmolarity > 320 mosm/L where osm = [2 Na + K] + glucose/18 + blood urea nitrogen [BUN]/2.8), and a spectrum of neurologic abnormalities including confusion, seizures, focal neurologic deficits, and coma. Although overlap with ketoacidosis has been described, in most cases, the available insulin in hyperosmolar nonketotic state patients appears to suppress ketosis and, thus, acidosis. In many cases, the development of hyperosmolar nonketotic state is associated with an inciting illness (usually an acute infection), procedure, or drug (Table 1).

Despite the marked hyperglycemia associated with hyperosmolar nonketotic state, initial therapy must first be directed toward fluid resuscitation. Volume replacement should begin with aggressive use of normal saline to increase blood pressure and blood flow. Once volume is repleted, the remaining water deficit is corrected at a 2-mEq/L/h rate of decrease in the serum sodium concentration. Approximately half of the calculated fluid deficit should be corrected over the first 12 hours and the rest within 36 hours.

Insulin therapy is less important but should begin with an intravenous bolus of 20 U of regular insulin, followed by a continuous infusion of 5 to 20 U/h if necessary. Plasma glucose, BUN, and electrolytes should be monitored hourly and glucose added to the intravenous solutions once a plasma glucose concentration of approximately 250 mg/dL is reached. Fluid status should be carefully monitored, and treatment in an intensive care unit is usually necessary in these critically ill elderly patients. An often overlooked part of therapy is the identification and treatment of the initial inciting event or illness.

DYSLIPIDEMIA

Prospective population studies have clarified the important relation between coronary heart disease (CHD) endpoints and total cholesterol (positive), low-density lipoprotein (LDL) cholesterol (positive), and high-density lipoprotein (HDL) cholesterol (negative). Furthermore, recent large clinical studies have demonstrated that exercise, diet, and drug treatment can mitigate against these CHD endpoints in both primary and secondary prevention trials. However, most of these data pertain to middle-aged individuals. The question of screening and treatment of dyslipidemias in patients older than 65 years of age is disputed [5•,6,7•]. This controversy stems from several observations listed in Table 2.

Due to the efforts of the National Cholesterol Education Program, many elderly individuals have been found to have total cholesterol levels greater than 240 mg/dL or LDL cholesterol levels greater than 160 mg/dL (or greater than 130 mg/dL with additional risk factors), thus requiring additional therapeutic decisions.

Diet and exercise regimens are the initial recommended modes of therapy. If LDL cholesterol remains elevated and the LDL to HDL ratio is greater than 3.0, drug treatment should be considered. Because the likelihood of benefit is greater in a secondary prevention situation, the most serious consideration for drug therapy should arise in patients with

TABLE 1 FACTORS ASSOCIATED WITH DEVELOPMENT OF HYPEROSMOLAR NONKETOTIC STATE

Demographic factors
Older age
Female sex
Nursing home residence or dependency

Inciting illnesses and procedures
Infection
Myocardial infarction
Cerebrovascular accident or subdural hematoma
Pancreatitis
Gastrointestinal bleeding
Pulmonary embolism
Burns
Renal failure
Peritoneal- or hemodialysis
Hyperalimentation
Surgery

Medication
Glucocorticoids
Diuretics (thiazide)
β-Blockers
Phenytoin
Diazoxide

Comorbid conditions
Known non–insulin-dependent diabetes mellitus
Abnormal mental status
Heart failure
Renal disease

Table 2 Controversy about screening and treatment of dyslipidemias in elderly patients	
In favor	**Against**
Because of the exponential increase in coronary heart disease with age, aggregate risk is great	Total and low-density lipoprotein cholesterol are less powerful risk factors with age
Efficacy of drug treatment is not different than in younger patients	Increased number of other diseases and drugs enhances the risk for adverse side effects
	Despite improvement in coronary heart disease endpoints with drug treatment, mortality is not decreased

known CHD. Drug therapy should be undertaken only in subjects whose life expectancy makes benefit likely.

Each drug type used for treatment of dyslipidemia has significant potential side effects in elderly patients, which may primarily determine their usage. A nonabsorbable bile acid binding resin may be preferred in subjects with significant renal or hepatic dysfunction. However, these drugs can worsen constipation, a common and important problem in elderly patients. Fibric acids should be avoided in patients with gallbladder disease, and nicotinic acid may worsen both gout and diabetes mellitus. Lovastatin, a hepatic hydroxymethyl glutaryl coenzyme A reductase inhibitor, was found to be effective and associated with low side effects in elderly patients in one recent study. The 40-mg/d dosage showed no benefit over the 20-mg/d dosage. The role of probucol, a drug that appears to inhibit the oxidation of LDL, thus reducing its atherogenicity, is unclear in elderly patients. Possibly the most effective therapy for dyslipidemia in women is estrogen replacement. Estrogen has been shown to reduce CHD endpoints by up to 50% in large prospective population studies. Estrogen replacement therapy seems to have beneficial effects on LDL and HDL cholesterol even when given with progestational agents. It is not clear whether estrogens can be as effective in reducing the risk of CHD when therapy is started in old age.

The presence of dyslipidemia should always signal the clinician to review and attempt to modify the status of other potential risk factors for CHD such as smoking and hypertension.

Thyroid Disease

Thyroid function tests are generally normal in elderly patients [8•]. Thyroxine levels are normal, but some studies have reported low triiodothyronine levels in healthy older people, possibly reflecting underlying undiagnosed nonthyroidal disease or the decreased secretory rate of thyroid hormone. Thyroid-stimulating hormone level is normal, but thyroid-stimulating hormone response to thyrotropin-releasing hormone is decreased in males and normal in females. The metabolic clearance rate of thyroid hormone is decreased. With an intact feedback loop, thyroid hormone secretory rate is diminished, and thyroxine is maintained in the normal range.

Hypothyroidism

Hypothyroidism is a disease of aging with peak incidence in the fifth to seventh decades. Goiter occurs rarely; when present, it suggests iodide-induced goiter and hypothyroidism. Laboratory evaluation should include TSH determination, because thyroxine may be depressed by nonthyroidal illness.

The diagnosis of hypothyroidism can be overlooked, especially in elderly patients. Symptoms of fatigue, memory loss, or decreased hearing should not just be ascribed to aging. Several studies suggest that general screening of the elderly population is not cost-effective. However, any older patient who presents with new symptoms and who has not had thyroid function tests in the past year should be screened with a free-thyroxine and thyroid-stimulating hormone test [9].

Treatment should be initiated with low-dose levothyroxine (0.025 to 0.05 mg/d). Heart rate (to avoid resting tachycardia), symptoms of angina, and thyroid-stimulating hormone levels should be monitored. When possible thyroid-stimulating hormone levels should be returned to the high normal range. Doses are increased at 1- to 3-week intervals. Because of the decreased metabolic clearance rate, maintenance doses in elderly patients are lower [10•].

Myxedema Coma

Most patients with myxedema coma are older than 60 years of age. This syndrome is induced by sedative hypnotics in approximately 50% of patients. Thus, patients with hypothyroidism should not receive sedative hypnotics. The presence of a neck scar may assist in the diagnosis, because the patient may have previously had thyroid surgery for hyperthyroidism. Hypothermia occurs in about 60% of patients. Delayed relaxation of the deep tendon reflexes is a helpful diagnostic sign. Respiratory failure is common, and apnea is the usual cause of death.

Therapy includes levothyroxine (500 μmg intravenously) and glucocorticoids (200 to 300 mg/d of hydrocortisone). Glucocorticoids are given to treat potential associated adrenal insufficiency until that diagnosis is excluded. The most important therapy, however, is respiratory care in an intensive care unit. Endotracheal intubation and elective tracheotomy should be considered if respiratory failure ensues.

Hyperthyroidism

Approximately 20% of patients with hyperthyroidism are elderly. About 75% present with classic symptoms. Ophthalmopathy occurs infrequently, and about one third of patients present without a goiter. Toxic multinodular goiter occurs more frequently in elderly than in younger patients.

Hyperthyroidism can be disguised by other illness, especially congestive heart failure, stroke, or infection. There should be a low threshold for recognition of this disorder. Unexplained congestive heart failure or tachyarrhythmia, recent onset psychiatric disorder, or profound myopathy should raise suspicion of hyperthyroidism. After cancer is ruled out, the triad of weight loss, anorexia, and constipation should suggest evaluation for hyperthyroidism.

In the absence of nonthyroidal disease, ultrasensitive thyroid-stimulating hormone assays can confirm the clinical diagnosis of hyperthyroidism. In the presence of acute illness, concomitant determination of thyroid-stimulating hormone and free-thyroxine may be more appropriate [11].

The mainstay of treatment is radioactive iodine, although most patients should first be treated with an antithyroidal agent. Surgery is reserved for cosmetic reasons, or rarely, when obstructive symptoms occur. With severe disease, antithyroidals to block hormone synthesis, iodides to block hormone release, and β-blockers to block peripheral manifestations are given. If antithyroidals or β-blockers cannot be given, then radiographic agents used for gallbladder imaging (Sodium ipodate, 3 g every 3 days or 500 mg/d) can be used to block peripheral conversion of thyroxine to triiodothyronine.

Hyperparathyroidism

Approximately one third of patients with hyperparathyroidism are older than 60 years of age. Diagnosis is frequently made by calcium measurements on multichannel screening chemistries in patients with few or no symptoms. Symptoms are similar in older and younger adults, but may be overlooked. Bone demineralization, fatigue, weakness, impaired cognition, recent-memory loss, depression, hypertension, constipation, anorexia, and joint complaints may be ascribed to aging when they indicate parathyroid disease.

Older patients may have impaired renal function and, therefore, accumulate C-terminal fragments of parathyroid hormone. Therefore, the combination of N- and C-terminal assays, or assays for intact parathyroid hormone, may be better discriminators of hyperparathyroidism in elderly patients. Table 3 contrasts basic patterns of common laboratory tests in hyperparathyroidism with those of other metabolic bone diseases common in elderly patients.

There is no effective chronic medical therapy for primary hyperparathyroidism. β-blockers, estrogen therapy in postmenopausal women, phosphate supplementation, diphosphonate therapy, and calcium restriction may lower calcium levels, but other aspects of the disease may progress. Surgery is the primary mode of therapy. In patients with mild elevation of calcium and no symptoms, the surgical risks must be carefully weighed.

Fluid and Electrolyte Disorders

Under normal circumstances, there is no change in sodium or potassium levels, hydrogen ion concentration, or fluid volume with age. However, adaptive mechanisms are impaired, and acute illness is often complicated by derangements in fluid and electrolyte balance.

The response to sodium restriction is blunted. Older individuals can reach fluid and electrolyte balance with sodium restriction, but the response is sluggish and the sodium deficit before balance is reached is greater than in younger individuals. Several factors contribute to this salt-losing tendency in elderly patients: 1) nephron loss increases osmotic load per nephron; 2) renin, both in the basal and stimulated state, decreases; consequently, 3) aldosterone levels decrease. Patient confusion and inadequate fluid volume repletion during illness and hospitalization may aggravate the deficit.

Regardless of preexisting myocardial disease, older adults are at increased risk for fluid volume expansion. They are less able to excrete an acute salt load, requiring a longer time to reestablish fluid and electrolyte balance. These changes relate to a decrease in glomerular filtration rate and decreased baroreceptor reflex sensitivity.

Older individuals are at increased risk for developing hyperkalemia. With a reduced glomerular filtration rate and decreased aldosterone levels, renal potassium excretion is altered. Insulin and catecholamines modulate potassium transport into cells. With decreased insulin and β-adrenergic responsiveness, these adaptive mechanisms are diminished with age.

Dehydration (*ie*, water depletion) is a particular problem in older adults when fluid intake is limited and insensible loss is increased. Water conservation and urine-concentrating ability are impaired with aging. Thirst mechanisms are also impaired, compromising the adaptive response to dehydration. Combined with the salt-losing tendency, hypertonic volume depletion is a common presentation.

Possibly the most serious and least recognized fluid and electrolyte problem in older adults is water intoxication (*ie*, hyponatremia). Patients may present with depression, confusion, lethargy, anorexia, weakness, stupor, or seizures. Again, changes in physiologic parameters contribute to this disorder. Basal vasopressin levels are unaltered in normal aging. However, infusion of hypertonic saline leads to a greater increase in plasma vasopressin levels than in younger individuals. Conversely, infusion of alcohol leads to a lesser suppres-

TABLE 3 LABORATORY FINDINGS IN METABOLIC BONE DISEASE

Disease	Ca	P	Alk	PTH
Hyperparathyroidism	High	Low/normal	High/normal	High
Osteomalacia	Low/normal	Low	High/normal	High
Hyperthyroidism	High	High	High/normal	Low
Osteoporosis	Normal	Normal	Normal	Normal/high
Paget's disease	Normal/high	Normal/high	High	Normal

Alk—alkaline phosphate; Ca—calcium; P—phosphorus; PTH—parathyroid hormone.

sion of vasopressin in older individuals. These data suggest increased osmoreceptor sensitivity in older adults with a higher "set-point" for vasopressin secretion. Thus, certain drugs, pulmonary and central nervous system disorders, and stress are more likely to precipitate the inappropriate antidiuretic syndrome in older patients.

In all these disorders, therapy is similar for older adults to that for younger individuals. However, patients may be monitored closely for adverse effects. For example, volume depletion should be treated with volume expanders, such as normal saline. The anticipation of fluid volume overload should not lead to use of inappropriate solutions, such as half-normal saline; instead, smaller volume boluses should be given and the patient should be monitored more closely.

Trophic Hormone Supplementation in the Elderly

The importance of estrogen replacement therapy in reducing the risk of osteoporosis and cardiovascular disease, as well as its effectiveness in the treatment of symptoms of vasomotor instability, vaginal and introital atrophy, and the psychologic symptoms of menopause are discussed in detail elsewhere (*see* Chapter 22, Menopause and the Postmenopausal State). Recently, interest has been kindled in the effects of supplementation of other trophic hormones known to decline with aging.

Normal aging in men is associated with declines in total and bioavailable testosterone, although, in most men, not into the hypogonadal range. Because of the concomitant reductions in strength and muscle mass and in increases in central adiposity, recent studies have evaluated the effect of testosterone supplementation on these parameters in older men [12,13]. These studies suggest improvements in the body composition with greater lean mass and less fat (especially central fat), improvement in lipid profiles, and possibly reductions in blood pressure and fasting plasma glucose levels. Potential side effects are concerning; one study found an increase in prostate specific antigen that remained elevated even after discontinuation of the testosterone supplementation.

The activity of the growth hormone–insulin-like growth factor I axis also declines with age in both men and women. A recent study suggested that growth hormone supplementation was associated with improvements in body composition (increased lean and reduced fat mass), as well as increased skin thickness [14]. Other studies, which will more carefully evaluate effects on bone mass, strength, and fat distribution, are pending. In preliminary studies, administration of growth hormone has been associated with a significant incidence of new carpal tunnel symptoms, arthralgias, fluid retention, and deterioration in glucose tolerance. Whether this adverse effects profile can be reduced by changes in dose or by inclusion of exercise in the study protocols awaits further results.

References and Recommended Reading

Recently published papers of particular interest have been highlighted as:
- Of interest
- •• Of outstanding interest

1. •• Kahn SE, Schwartz RS, Porte D Jr, Abrass IB: The glucose intolerance of aging: implications for intervention. *Hosp Pract* 1991, 26:29–38.
2. Harris MI: Epidemiology of diabetes mellitus among the elderly in the United States. *Clin Geriatr Med* 1990, 6:703–719.
3. • Pandit MK, Burke J, Gustafson AB, *et al.*: Drug-induced disorders of glucose tolerance. *Ann Intern Med* 1993, 118:529–539.
4. Helmrich SP, Ragland DR, Leung RW, Paffenbarger RS: Physical activity and reduced occurrence of non–insulin-dependent diabetes mellitus. *N Engl J Med* 1991, 325:147–152.
5. • Denke MA, Grundy SM: Hypercholesterolemia in elderly persons: resolving the treatment dilemma. *Ann Intern Med* 1990, 1112:780–792.
6. Kronmal RA, Cain KC, Zhan Y, Omenn GS: Total serum cholesterol levels and mortality risks as a function of age. *Arch Intern Med,I>* 1993, 653:1065–1073.
7. • Hazzard WR: Dyslipoproteinemia in the elderly. Should it be treated? *Clin Geriatr Med* 1992, 8:89–102.
8. • Hershman JM, Pekary AE, Bergh, *et al.*: Serum thyrotropin and thyroid hormone levels in elderly and middle-aged euthyroid persons. *J Am Geriatr Soc* 1993, 41:823–828.
9. Sawin CT, Castelli WP, Hershman JM: The aging thyroid: thyroid deficiency in the Framingham Study. *Arch Intern Med* 1985, 145:1386–1388.
10. • Mandel SJ, Brent GA, Larson PR: Levothyroxine therapy in patients with thyroid disease. *Ann Intern Med* 1993, 119:492–502.
11. Sawin CT, Geller A, Kaplan MM, *et al.*: Low serum thyrotropin (thyroid-stimulating hormone) in older persons without hyperthyroidism. *Arch Intern Med* 1991, 151:165–168.
12. Tenover JS: Effects of testosterone supplementation in the aging male. *J Clin Endocrinol Metab* 1992, 75:1092–1098.
13. Marin P, Holmang S, Gustafsson C, *et al.*: Androgen treatment of abdominally obese men. *Obesity Res* 1993, 1:245–251.
14. Rudman D, Feller AG, Nagrai HS, *et al.*: Effects of human growth hormone in men over 60 years old. *N Engl J Med* 1990, 323:1–6.

Select Bibliography

Abrass IB: Endocrine disease. In *Essentials of Clinical Geriatrics*, edn 3. Edited by Kane RL, Ouslander JG, Abrass IB: New York: McGraw-Hill; 1993:280–294.

Goldberg AD, Coon PJ: Diabetes mellitus and glucose metabolism in the elderly. In *Principles of Geriatric Medicine and Gerontology*, edn 3. Edited by Hazzard WR, Bierman EL, Blass JP, *et al.*. New York: McGraw-Hill; 1993:825–842.

Gregerman RI, Katz MS: Thyroid diseases. In *Principles of Geriatric Medicine and Gerontology*, edn 3. Edited by Hazzard, WR, Bierman EL, Blass JP, *et al.*. New York: McGraw-Hill; 1993:807–823.

Hazzard WR: Dylipoproteinemia. In *Principles of Geriatric Medicine and Gerontology*, edn 3. Edited by Hazzard WR, Bierman EL, Blass JP, *et al.*. New York: McGraw-Hill; 1993:855–866.

Lyles KW: Hyperparathyroidism. In *Principles of Geriatric Medicine and Gerontology*, edn 3. Edited by Hazard WR, Bierman EL, Blass JP, *et al.* New York: McGraw-Hill; 1993:923–928.

Menopause and the Postmenopausal State

Valery T. Miller

22

Key Points
- Menopause is a natural state that comes to all women, but many women will develop a deficiency state because of it.
- Oral contraceptives in the perimenopause will prevent unintended pregnancies, irregular, anovulation bleeding, and hot flashes.
- Hormone replacement therapy is the management choice for postmenopausal hot flashes, urogenital atrophy, and prevention of osteoporosis.
- Women who receive hormone replacement therapy are more likely to undergo cholecystectomy but are not more likely to experience thromboembolism.
- The risk of heart disease, which kills more women than all cancers combined, appears to be reduced by hormone replacement therapy.

Menopause is a natural state but it is characterized by a decline in endogenous estrogen and, consequently in most women, estrogen deprivation develops. This deprivation is a condition now recognized as unhealthy and leading to pathologic conditions. The lack of estrogen may go unrecognized for many years until incontinence develops, as with urogenital atrophy, or until a hip is fractured. On the other hand, early symptoms may be quite serious, interfering with everyday activities. The diminished levels of estrogen promote atherosclerotic and osteoporotic processes that are significant causes of increased morbidity and mortality in women. The demonstrated ability of estrogen replacement to prevent the consequences of estrogen deprivation has led to renewed interest in its use over the last decade. Every physician should be aware of the significance of the menopausal state and of the benefits of hormone replacement.

THE BEGINNING OF MENOPAUSE

Recognition of the impending menopause begins with the identification of the start of menopause or the perimenopause. The perimenopause extends over a 4- to 6-year period with variable levels of gonadotropins and ovarian hormones, often causing irregular and anovulatory menses [1•]. Although many women will present at the appropriate age (average age is 51.4 years) with cessation of menses and signs of estrogen deficiency such as vaginal dryness and hot flashes, others will not. Some women will continue to have regular periods, ovulate, and still have hot flashes. Indeed, it has been estimated that 30% of women ages 50 to 54 theoretically remain fertile. When in doubt concerning a patient's menopausal status (*eg*, in the woman who has had a hysterectomy), the most expedient way to assess the menopause is to measure the follicle-stimulating hormone level. Although not an absolute predictor, a follicle-stimulating hormone level greater than 40 mIU/mL in an age-appropriate woman indicates the menopausal state. It is usually not necessary to measure luteinizing hormone levels but until both the luteinizing hormone levels and follicle-

TABLE 1 TESTS OF HORMONAL AND MENOPAUSAL STATUS

Ovulation	Perimenopause	Menopause
Basal body temp >98°F, 3 consecutive days, 1 wk before menses	FSH–variable 5–30 mIU/mL* LH–normal* 5–20 mIU/mL	FSH >40 mIU/mL LH >25 mIU/mL
Blood progesterone >3 ng/mL, 1 wk before menses	Anovulation Irregular bleeding	Estradiol <25 pg/mL No menses × 6 mo Age >55 y

*With ovulation, mid-cycle peak can be three times normal.

stimulating hormone are elevated, menopause can not be assured. Table 1 depicts tests used to determine ovulation and perimenopausal and menopausal status.

Endometrial Risk in the Perimenopause

As perimenopausal women gradually become anovulatory, the absence of opposing progesterone places them at increasing risk for over-stimulation of the endometrium by endogenous estrogen and for endometrial hyperplasia and cancer. Characteristics of women at increased risk for endometrial cancer include obesity, dysfunctional uterine bleeding, anovulation, hirsutism, high alcohol intake, hepatic disease, diabetes, and family history. In a patient who has a lengthy perimenopause with irregular bleeding, consideration should be given to monitoring the endometrium by biopsy or to treatment with either a progestogen, like medroxyprogesterone acetate, 5 to 10 mg 12 days of the month, or a low-dose oral contraceptive.

It is not uncommon for the perimenopausal woman to complain of periodic vasomotor symptoms severe enough to prompt her physician to consider hormone-replacement therapy (HRT). Although there is no controversy over initiation of HRT in the age-appropriate woman who has not bled for many months, there is disagreement over whether it is safe to prescribe HRT to a woman who still produces endogenous estrogen, however inconsistently. Most clinicians believe that it is inappropriate to treat such a woman with HRT because not only will the patient be receiving more estrogen than she needs (endogenous plus exogenous), but HRT does not prevent conception. The doses of estrogen currently used in HRT do not inhibit gonadotropin sufficiently to prevent pregnancy. Thus there are two considerations that speak against HRT at this time: irregular bleeding may be worsened and no HRT regimen provides contraception.

Contraception in Perimenopause

Women are at continued risk of pregnancy in their perimenopausal years and advice concerning this and about appropriate contraceptive methods should be a part of patient education. By age 54, 43% of women have experienced natural menopause and another 28% are surgically menopausal. Theoretically 30% of women 50 to 54 years of age remain fertile. Although it is true that fecundity is age related, in 1989 in the United States, 1,599 births were to women aged 45 to 49. Most pregnancies in this age group are unintended and abortion rates in women older than 40 years of age are second only to the rate in women younger than 20. The problem worsened when the intrauterine device was removed from use; unintended pregnancies increased from 24% (1979–1982) to 53% (1984–1988). Table 2 lists the risks of pregnancy to older women and the contraceptive methods appropriate for them.

For perimenopausal women who are otherwise healthy and do not smoke, low-dose oral contraceptives have been approved by the Food and Drug Administration and offer advantages that other methods do not, such as improved cycle regularity, decreased menstrual flow, prevention of endometrial pathology because of anovulation, relief from vasomotor symptoms, enhanced bone density, and a decreased risk of ovarian cancer [2].

MENOPAUSE

All women have in common the drastic decline in ovarian estrogen and progesterone production. Heavy women (> 200 pounds) can convert circulating adrenal androstenedione to estradiol in their fat cells, and thus, may have enough hormone in their blood to cause endometrial pathology. Nevertheless, these women may still experience severe vasomotor symptoms.

Estrogen deprivation is reflected in a variety of body systems, and the expression of this lack of hormone varies greatly from woman to woman. Problems associated with low levels of estradiol can be divided into early, middle, and late depending on when they more commonly appear through the menopausal years (Table 3). It is not understood why some women experience severe vasomotor symptoms and others do

TABLE 2 RISKS OF PREGNANCY TO OLDER WOMEN AND CONTRACEPTION

Risks	Methods of contraception
Chromosomal abnormalities	Condom
Age 35 1:192	Diaphragm, cap, sponge
Age 40 1:66	Spermicide
Age 45 1:21	Intrauterine device
Increased mortality rates	Periodic abstinence
Unacceptability of abortion	Oral contraceptive
	Tubule ligation

TABLE 3 POSTMENOPAUSAL SIGNS AND SYMPTOMS OF ESTROGEN DEFICIENCY	
Early postmenopausal	**Middle postmenopausal**
Vaginal dryness	Vaginal dryness
Dyspareunia	Urogenital atrophy
Hot flashes	Incontinence
Night sweats	Abacterial cystitis
Insomnia	Urethral caruncle
Irritability	**Late postmenopausal**
Mood swings	Atherosclerosis
Anxiety	Osteoporosis
No menses	Bone fractures

TABLE 4 RISK FACTORS FOR HEART DISEASE IN WOMEN
1. Smoking—voids the advantage of higher HDL-C level
2. Diabetes—voids the gender advantage
3. HDL-C <40 mg/dL
4. Triglyceride >200 mg/dL—more readily identifiable as independent risk factor in women than in men
5. LDL-C—in absence of other risk factors, less risk than for men
6. Hypertension
7. Estrogen deficiency
8. Six or more pregnancies*
*From Ness et al [4]; with permission.

not. An unfortunate myth still exists that the woman who proceeds through early menopause without significant symptomatology is better adjusted emotionally. Certainly the mentally healthy woman can better handle sleep disturbance caused by night sweats and embarrassing daytime flushes, but vasomotor symptoms can be so severe as to seriously disrupt an otherwise healthy woman's life.

Cardiovascular Disease in Menopause

Cardiovascular disease is the major cause of death in women—surpassing all cancer deaths combined. In general, women appear to be protected from atherosclerosis as a group compared with men. The high incidence of heart disease recognized in men at 55 years of age is seen in women at 65 years of age. Menopause is not the cause of heart disease in women, but contributes to a woman's prior burden of risks such as cigarette smoking or hypertension. Careful observation of a group of women progressing through menopause—matched with premenopausal women of similar age, weight, and habits—demonstrates that, in addition to the adverse lipid changes associated with aging, women do experience modest atherogenic changes in their lipid and lipoprotein levels with the decline in estrogen levels [3••]. The risk factors commonly associated with heart disease in men also increase risk in women, but with some important differences (Table 4).

Osteoporosis

Osteoporosis in women, like atherosclerosis, is accentuated by menopause. Between age 40 and the menopause, bone is lost at a rate of approximately 0.5% per year, but accelerates postmenopausally to 1.0% to 1.5% per year of total bone mass, which may continue for the next 10 to 15 years. Far more important, however, is the loss specifically of trabecular bone (comprising much of the spine and the hip), which may be as much as 5%, resulting in a 50% reduction in trabecular bone mass in the postmenopausal years.

Urogenital Atrophy

Significant disability in older women is seen resulting from urogenital atrophy. The vagina, urethra, and parts of the bladder originate from similar embryologic tissue and are estrogen dependent. Consequently, not only vaginal problems occur postmenopausally, but atrophy of other pelvic tissues contribute to dysuria, frequency, urgency, and incontinence in older women. Urethral closure pressure is significantly reduced in elderly women and is thought to be associated with the decline in submucosal vascular supply, tissue turgor, and muscle bulk of the urethra resulting from estrogen deprivation. Mucosal changes also disrupt vaginal flora, alter tissue resistance, and give rise to urethritis and urethral and meatal stenosis with obstructive sequelae.

ESTROGEN REPLACEMENT

Efficacy

Lack of knowledge about the benefits of estrogen and fear of cancer are the main reasons why many women do not take estrogen postmenopausally. Each woman should be evaluated for the possible risks to her from estrogen replacement and for the prevention of problems or diseases that estrogen will offer her [5•,6••]. Physicians owe it to their patients to discuss with each woman her individual risks and benefits so that she can assist in the decision-making process.

No treatment has been found to compare with the efficacy of HRT for the relief of vasomotor symptoms. Similarly urogenital atrophy and urinary incontinence, a much underreported problem to which it contributes, can be prevented and often even corrected by estrogen. Simultaneous administration of oral and vaginal estrogen may be required initially to restore healthy tissue quickly.

Estrogen is the acknowledged treatment of choice for the prevention of osteoporosis and hip fractures, surpassing combinations of exercise and calcium [7]. Decreased bone loss resulting from HRT has been translated into a 50% to 60% reduction in fractures of the arm and hip.

Most importantly, cardiovascular disease, the leading cause of death in older women, has been reported by numerous observational studies to be reduced 40% to 50% by estrogen therapy [8•,9••]. As much as half of the reduction in cardiovascular risk, attributed to estrogen replacement, may be due to changes in lipid and lipoprotein levels. (Table 5) [10].

Table 5. Beneficial effects of conjugated equine estrogen, 0.625 mg/dL, replacement on lipids and lipoproteins in normal women

	Percent change
Total cholesterol	-5.0
Total triglyceride	+19.4
LDL-C	-14.6
HDL-C	+11.5
HDL2-C	+19.2
HDL3-C	+5.9
Apoprotein B	-9.4
Apoprotein A-I	+12.7
Apoprotein A-II	+9.6

From Muesing and coworkers [10]; with permission.

Risks

Despite the fact that the risk–benefit ratio of estrogen has been demonstrated to be so much in favor of HRT, women often fail to continue their prescriptions or do not fill them. This largely results from fear of cancer. Only two cancers are related to HRT: breast and endometrial cancer. Breast cancer continues to be an issue because there are no prospective trials and, unlike endometrial cancer, the more than 50 observational studies are in disagreement [11,12].

There is no controversy, however, about the association between endometrial cancer and estrogen use. The evidence is clear that unopposed estrogen use leads to hyperplasia, atypia, and cancer. Endometrial cancers are well-differentiated and less aggressive; they are usually identified early and cure rates approach 100%. Women who have had stage I endometrial cancer are being prescribed HRT after hysterectomy [13]. Progestogen use to prevent endometrial cancer is discussed in the next section.

Although thrombophlebitis has been reported with HRT in uncontrolled studies, this association has not been observed in controlled trials. Caution should be exercised in administering HRT to women who are at risk for thrombosis or embolism.

Stone formation in the gallbladder is enhanced with hormone replacement. Women who use HRT are two times more likely to have a cholecystectomy than nonusers [14]. There are contraindications to prescribing HRT (Table 6) [15••].

Prescribing

Conjugated equine estrogen, 0.625 mg/dL or its equivalents, is the dose of estrogen required by most women to prevent bone loss and has become the most common dose prescribed (Table 7) [16•]. Table 8 shows the various progestogens and doses used in combination regimens [16•]. Transdermal estrogen does not alter lipids as does oral estrogen, because it does not reach the liver in high enough concentrations. Thus, this form of estrogen administration is superior for preventing hypertriglyceridemia (see below) and may be useful in women who are at risk for thrombosis.

Progestogens are prescribed in combination with estrogen to women who have uteri because the progestogens inhibit the estrogen-induced endometrial DNA synthesis, thus preventing cancer. Progestogens were initially administered cyclically, 10 to 15 days of the month to mimic the normal premenopausal hormone cycle. Cycle A in Figure 1 depicts that HRT regimen. Cycles B and C depict preferable regimens. Cycle B may be preferable because it is easier to remember to start the progestogen at the first of each month and because vasomotor symptoms return in some women when estrogen is discontinued even for a few days. The bleeding associated with cyclic administration of the progestogen (85%) is a common complaint among women and cycle C was devised to answer this problem. A lower dose of progestogen is administered daily with the estrogen in the continuous combined regimen and, although irregular spotting may be experienced for the initial 6 months, most women will ultimately have no bleeding.

A recent controlled clinical trial of 3 years revealed that 33% of women who were assigned estrogen, unopposed by a progestin developed adenomatous hyperplasia or atypia [17••]. While these severe endometrial changes resulted in no deaths, they did result in the need for lengthy progestational therapy, extensive monitoring and hysterectomy in some women. The extent of these pathological findings is surprising and should alert physicians to be particularly careful to advise their patients that the need to take their progestin is very real.

Table 6. Contraindications and relative contraindications to hormone replacement therapy

Contraindications	Relative contraindications
Unexplained vaginal bleeding	Seizure disorders
Active liver disease	Hypertension
Chronic impaired liver function	Uterine leiomyomas
Recent vascular thrombosis	Familial hypertriglyceridemia
Carcinoma of the breast	Migraine headaches
Carcinoma of endometrium	Thrombophebitis
	Endometriosis
	Gallbladder disease

From Lindsay and coworkers [15••]; with permission.

Table 7. Equivalent estrogen doses used in unopposed and combination regimens*

Generic name	Equivalent Doses
Conjugated equine estrogen	0.625 mg, daily
Micronized estradiol	1.0 mg, daily
Estropipate†	0.75 mg, daily
Transdermal estradiol	0.05 mg, patch every 3 d

*Higher doses of estrogen may be required for symptom relief in younger women, in women initially after surgery, or for a limited time in women for whom the lower dose does not relieve symptoms.
†Formerly piperazine estrone sulfate.

TABLE 8 PROGESTOGENS AND DOSES USED IN CYCLIC COMBINED REGIMENS

Conjugated equine estrogen or equivalent	0.625 mg, daily, equivalent
Progestogens used in cyclic regimens:	
Medroxyprogesterone acetate	5 mg, 10 mg, 10–15 d/mo
Norethindrone	1 mg, 2.5 mg, 10–15 d/mo
Micronized progesterone*	200 mg, 300 mg, 10–14 d/mo
Progestogens used in continuous combination regimens:	
Medroxyprogesterone acetate	2.5 mg, daily
Norethindrone acetate	5 mg, daily

*Not approved for HRT

Women who have had hysterectomies should not be prescribed combination therapy. Progestogens have not been shown to protect the breast as previously reported. Furthermore, progestogens cause side affects (bloating, weight gain, irritability, and depression) and, although it appears progestogens do not reduce many of the beneficial effects of estrogen, their long-term and full effects are unknown at this time [17].

SYMPTOMS NOT ATTRIBUTABLE TO ESTROGEN DEPRIVATION

Not all problems in the postmenopausal period of women's life are related to estrogen deficiency. Clearly not all emotional problems should be attributed to the lack of estrogen, but when vasomotor instability is concurrent or when sleep is disturbed, serious attention to estrogen replacement should be given. Side effects of estrogens include bloating, headache, and breast tenderness. Not all hot flashes are related to estrogen deficiency. When an adequate blood level of estradiol is attained, rather than increasing the dose, other medical and psychologic causes should be explored (Table 9). Serum estradiol levels between 50 to 100 pg/mL are adequate and prove intestinal absorption.

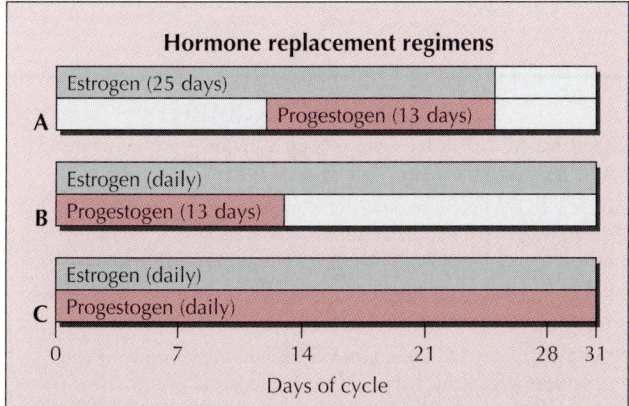

FIGURE 1 Three estrogen and progestogen combination regimens are shown. A, The standard cyclic regimen. B, Does not interrupt estrogen and starts the progestogen at the beginning of the month. C, Estrogen and progestogen are administered continuously through the month. The progestogen is prescribed at a lower dose.

DYSLIPOPROTEINEMIA

Cholesterol and lipoprotein abnormalities should be corrected in postmenopausal women because, as in men, they are significant risk factors for heart disease. As indicated above, oral estrogen influences lipids and lipoproteins beneficially. Indeed, estrogen has been recommended as an intermediary treatment between diet and lipid-lowering drugs in women who have high cholesterol by the recently published guidelines from the Adult Treatment Panel II [18]. Women who have heart disease or who are at high risk for heart disease should be prescribed HRT.

Estrogen can also cause lipid problems, notably in women who exhibit high triglyceride levels. Estrogen is known to increase triglyceride levels to some extent in all women, but this increase may become a significant clinical problem in women who have even modest baseline triglyceride levels of 250 to 400 mg/dL, as seen in type III, IV, or V hyperlipoproteinemia. In these women, triglyceride levels may exceed 1000 mg/dL with estrogen therapy and place the patient at risk for pancreatitis. Patients should not be at risk if physicians routinely identify cholesterol abnormalities in their patients as is recommended. The answer to this treatment dilemma is to prescribe the transdermal estrogen patch. Estrogen delivered through the skin does not affect the liver, and therefore, does not alter lipids as does oral estrogen. If the patient has a uterus, she must take an oral progestogen as well as apply the patch.

FOLLOW-UP

Postmenopausal women with or without HRT require the recommended annual follow-up monitoring tests of younger

TABLE 9 CAUSES OF VASOMOTOR INSTABILITY AND CONDITIONS COMMONLY CONFUSED WITH MENOPAUSE

Side effects of antidepressants	Pheochromocytoma
Carcenoid tumor	Panic attacks
Alcohol consumption	Depression

women plus closer monitoring of diseases associated with the older women's age group. Postmenopausal women need breast and pelvic examinations and Papanicolaou's tests. Their age dictates an annual mammography. They need monitoring of cardiovascular risk factors: blood pressure, cholesterol profile, body mass index, and blood sugar. Women at risk for heart disease should have annual electrocardiograms because silent heart attacks also occur in women. Because of the frequency of unsuspected hypothyroidism in this population, thyroid-stimulating hormone is recommended every 3 years. Bone mass measurements have been recommended in women to help decide whether or not to prescribe HRT. Some women will require endometrial biopsy, dilettation and curettage, or transvaginal ultrasound to investigate heavy or lengthy bleeding.

Any physician who does pelvic and breast examinations can prescribe HRT. Proficiency with endometrial sampling by the pipelle can easily be mastered but referral to the gynecologist for the few patients who require investigation of their bleeding is also an acceptable alternative (Table 10).

TABLE 10 INDICATIONS FOR ENDOMETRIAL BIOPSY

1. Any postmenopausal bleeding not associated with HRT
2. Any prolonged (10–14 days) or heavy bleeding associated with any HRT regimen
3. At initiation of HRT: Usually not, if there has been no bleeding for greater than 6 months
4. With unopposed estrogen regimen: annually and with any prolonged or heavy bleeding
5. With cyclical combined HRT: only with unusual, irregular, prolonged or heavy bleeding—most women on this regimen never require a biopsy
6. With continuous combined: Possibly at start to reassure when spotting occurs longer than 4–6 months

HRT—hormone replacement therapy.

References and Recommended Reading

Recently published papers of particular interest have been highlighted as:
- Of interest
- •• Of outstanding interest

1.• Sherwin BM, West JH, Korenman SG: The menopause transition: analysis of LH, FSH, estradiol, and progesterone concentrations during menstrual cycles of older women. *J Clin Endocrinol Metab* 1976, 42:629–636.

2. Mishell DR Jr: Oral contraception for women in their 40s. *J Reprod Med* 1990, 35(s):447–481.

3.•• Kuller LH, Gutai JP, Meilahn E, *et al.*: Relationship of endogenous sex steroid hormones to lipid apoproteins in postmenopausal women. *Arteriosclerosis* 1990, 10:1058–1066.

4. Ness RB, Harris T, Cobb J, *et al.*: Number of pregnancies and the subsequent risk of cardiovascular disease. *N Engl J Med* 1993, 328:1528–1533.

5.• Grady D, Rubin SM, Petitti DB, *et al.*: Hormone therapy to prevent disease and prolong life in postmenopausal women. *Ann Intern Med* 1992, 117:1016–1041.

6.•• Clinical Guideline: Guidelines for counseling postmenopausal women about preventive hormone therapy. *Ann Intern Med* 1992, 117:1038–1041.

7. Aloia JF, Vaswani A, Yeh JK, *et al.*: Calcium supplementation with and without hormone replacement therapy to prevent postmenopausal bone loss. *Ann Intern Med* 1994, 120:97–103.

8.• Bush TL, Barrett-Connor E, Cowan LD, *et al.*: Cardiovascular mortality and noncontraceptive use of estrogen in women: Results from the Lipid Research Clinics Program Follow-Up Study. *Circulation* 1987, 75:1102–1109.

9.•• Stampfer MJ, Colditz GA: Estrogen replacement therapy and coronary heart disease: A quantitative assessment of the epidemiologic evidence. *Preventive Med* 1991, 20:47–63.

10. Muesing RS, Miller VT, La Rosa JC, *et al.*: Effects of unopposed conjugated equine estrogen on lipoprotein composition and apolipoprotein-E distribution. *J Clin Endocrinol Metab* 1992, 75:1250–1254.

11. Steinberg KK, Thacker SB, Smith SJ, *et al.*: A meta-analysis of the effect of estrogen replacement therapy on the risk of breast cancer. *JAMA* 1991, 265:1985–1990.

12. Dupont WD, Page DL: Menopause estrogen replacement therapy and breast cancer. *Arch Intern Med* 1991, 151:67–70.

13. Creaseman WT, Henderson D, Hinshaw W, *et al.*: Estrogen replacement therapy in the patient treated for endometrial cancer. *Obstet Gynecol* 1986, 67:326–329.

14. Grodstein F, Colditz GA, Stampfer MJ: Postmenopausal hormone use and cholecystectomy in a large prospective study. *Obstet Gynecol* 1994; 83:5–11.

15.•• ACOG Technical Bulletin: Hormone replacement therapy. 1992; Number 166.

16.• Lindsay R, Hart DM, Clark DM: The minimum effective dose of estrogen for prevention for postmenopausal bone loss. *Obstet Gynecol* 1984, 63:759–763.

17.•• Effects of estrogen/progestin regimens on heart disease risk factors in postmenopausal women. The Postmenopausal Extrogen/Progestin Interventions (PEPI) Trial. *JAMA* 1995; 273:199–208.

18. Summary of the second panel report of the National Cholesterol Education Program (NCEP) Expert Panel on detection, evaluation, and treatment of high blood cholesterol in adults (Adult Treatment Panel II). *JAMA* 1993, 269:3015–3023.

Select Bibliography

Creaseman WT: Estrogen replacement therapy: is previously treated cancer a contraindication? *Obstet Gynecol* 1991, 77:308–312.

Miller VT: Dyslipoproteinemia in women: special considerations. In *Endocrinology and Metabolism Clinics of North America*, Edited by LaRosa JC. Philadelphia: WB Saunders Co.: 1990:381–398.

NIH Consensus Development Conference Summary: Osteoporosis. *JAMA* 1984, 252:799–802.

Saleh AA, Dorey LG, Dombrowski MD, *et al.*: Thrombosis and hormone replacement therapy in postmenopausal women. *Am J Obstet Gynecol* 1993, 169:1554–1557.

Wenger NK, Speroff L, Packard B: Cardiovascular health and disease in women. *N Engl J Med* 1993, 329:247–256

Volume Index

Note: section numbers appear in boldface; page numbers followed by *f* indicate figures, and numbers followed by *t* indicate tables.

A

Abbreviated Injury Scale, **II:27**.4*t*, 27.5, 27.5*t*
Abdomen
    guarding, **I:3**.10
    palpation, **I:3**.9–3.10
    physical examination, **I:3**.8*t*, 3.8–3.10, 3.9*t*
    rebound tenderness, **I:3**.10
Abdominal aortic aneurysm(s), **II:28**.1–28.2
    clinical presentation, **II:28**.1, 28.2*f*
    diagnosis, **II:28**.2
    imaging, **II:28**.2, 28.2*f*
    pathophysiology, **II:28**.1, 28.2*t*
    and popliteal artery aneurysm, **II:29**.6
    prognosis for, **II:28**.2
    treatment, **II:28**.2
Abdominal distention, etiology, maneuvers to differentiate, **I:3**.9*t*
Abdominal pain, **I:3**.8–3.10
    evaluation
        by location, **I:3**.9*t*
        maneuvers for, **I:3**.9*t*
    physical examination with, **I:3**.8*t*, 3.8–3.10, 3.9*t*
Abnormal uterine bleeding, **IV:9**.1–9.6, 10.1
    with anatomic defects, **IV:9**.2–9.3
    definition, **IV:9**.1
    diagnosis, **IV:9**.3–9.4, 9.4*t*
    differential diagnosis, **IV:9**.3–9.4, 9.4*t*
    etiology, **IV:9**.1–9.3
    hormonal causes, **IV:9**.2, 9.2*f*
    with malignancy, **IV:9**.3–9.4, 9.4*t*
    management strategy for, **IV:9**.6*f*
    medical therapy for, **IV:9**.4*t*, 9.4–9.5
    organic causes, **IV:9**.1–9.3
    surgical therapy for, **IV:9**.5
    with systemic disease, **IV:9**.2–9.3, 9.3*t*
Accidents, as cause of death, **III:2**.2*t*
Accuracy, of screening test, **I:2**.2
Acetazolamide, for central sleep apnea, **III:9**.7
Acetohexamide, for non-insulin-dependent diabetes mellitus (NIDDM), **IV:14**.5, 14.5*t*
Acidemia, in diabetic ketoacidosis, **IV:15**.2
Acquired immunodeficiency syndrome. *See also* Human immunodeficiency virus infection
    cardiac involvement in, **II:19**.6, 19.6*t*
    pericarditis in, **II:21**.1
Acromegaly, **IV:2**.7, 2.7*f*
    clinical features, **IV:2**.8, 2.8*t*
    diagnosis, **IV:2**.8, 2.8*f*
    extrapituitary causes, **IV:2**.7–2.8
    treatment, **IV:2**.10*f*, 2.11
    tumor-related, **IV:19**.5, 19.5*f*
Acromioclavicular separation, **I:3**.6
Acute respiratory distress syndrome, pheochromocytoma and, **IV:7**.3
Addison's disease, **IV:5**.11
    etiology, **IV:5**.11, 5.11*t*, 5.12–5.13
    in HIV-infected (AIDS) patient, **IV:5**.12–5.13
    natural history, **IV:5**.12, 5.12*f*
    treatment, **IV:5**.13*t*, 5.13–5.14
Adenoma(s)
    adrenal
        aldosterone-producing, **IV:8**.2–8.3
        treatment, **IV:5**.10, 5.10*t*
    parathyroid, **IV:13**.2–13.3
    pituitary. *See* Pituitary adenoma(s)
    thyroid, **IV:4**.5–4.6
Adiposity, mesenteric, diagnosis, maneuvers for, **I:3**.9*f*
Adrenal adenoma(s)
    aldosterone-producing, **IV:8**.2–8.3
    treatment, **IV:5**.10, 5.10*t*
Adrenal androgenic disorder(s), **IV:10**.3
Adrenal atrophy, **IV:5**.3, 5.4
Adrenal cortex
    glucocorticoids, **IV:5**.1–5.14
    zones, **IV:5**.1, 5.2*t*
Adrenal crisis
    causes, **IV:5**.12, 5.12*t*
    features, **IV:5**.12, 5.12*t*
    with glucocorticoid withdrawal, **IV:6**.6
    treatment, **IV:5**.13*t*, 5.13–5.14
Adrenal gland
    carcinoma, treatment, **IV:5**.10*t*, 5.10–5.11
    weight, **IV:7**.2
Adrenal hyperplasia, vs. adenoma, **IV:8**.3
Adrenal medulla
    hyperplasia, **IV:7**.2–7.3
    weight, **IV:7**.2
Adrenal steroids, biosynthesis, **IV:5**.1–5.2
Adrenal tumor(s)
    primary, Cushing's syndrome with, **IV:5**.6, 5.6*f*
    treatment, **IV:5**.10, 5.10*t*
    virilizing, **IV:10**.5
Adrenal vein catheterization, **IV:8**.3
Adrenarche, exaggerated, **IV:10**.3
β-Adrenergic agonists, for COPD, **III:2**.7
    efficacy, **III:2**.8*f*
$β_2$-Adrenergic agonists, for acute severe asthma, **III:10**.4
α-Adrenergic blockers
    for benign prostatic hyperplasia, **IV:20**.6, 20.6*f*
    dosage and administration, **IV:7**.7*t*
    for elderly, advantages and disadvantages, **II:32**.5*t*
    indications for, **IV:7**.3, 7.6–7.7
    for pheochromocytoma, **IV:7**.6–7.7, 7.7*t*
β-Adrenergic blockers
    for angina, **II:9**.5
    for congestive cardiomyopathy, **II:17**.9
    for congestive heart failure, **II:17**.9
    effects on myocardial oxygen supply and demand, **II:9**.3*f*
    for elderly, advantages and disadvantages, **II:32**.5*t*, 32.8
    for hyperthyroidism, **IV:3**.4
    for hypertrophic cardiomyopathy, **II:16**.3–16.4
    indications for, **II:3**.6, 13.8–13.9, **IV:7**.7
    mechanism of action, **II:9**.5
    for MI, **II:11**.4
        for secondary prevention, **II:11**.7*t*
    with mitral stenosis, **II:12**.4
    for pheochromocytoma, **IV:7**.7, 7.7*t*
    precautions with, **II:9**.5
Adrenocortical insufficiency, **IV:5**.11–5.14
    diagnostic tests for, **IV:5**.13, 5.13*t*
    primary, **IV:8**.5–8.6. *See also* Addison's disease
        diagnosis, **IV:5**.13
        etiology, **IV:5**.11, 5.11*t*, 5.12–5.13
        vs. secondary, **IV:5**.10*f*, 5.13
    secondary, **IV:5**.10*f*, 5.11
        diagnosis, **IV:5**.13
        etiology, **IV:5**.11, 5.11*t*, 5.13
    signs and symptoms, **IV:5**.11*t*, 5.11–12
    treatment, **IV:5**.13*t*, 5.13–5.14
Adrenocorticotropic hormone (corticotropin), **IV:2**.2*f*
    actions, **IV:5**.2–5.3, 5.3*f*
    deficiency, **IV:2**.5
        causes, **IV:5**.13
    ectopic. *See* Ectopic corticotropin syndrome
    hypersecretion, test for, **IV:2**.2
    reserve, test for, **IV:2**.1–2.2
    secretion, by pituitary tumor, **IV:5**.5–5.6
    in steroidogenesis, **IV:5**.2–5.3, 5.3*f*
    stimulants, **IV:5**.2
    synthesis, **IV:5**.2
    tumors producing, ectopic Cushing's syndrome due to, **IV:19**.3–19.4
Adson maneuver, in occlusive arterial disease, **II:29**.4*f*
Adult respiratory distress syndrome, **III:10**.2–10.3
    acute respiratory failure with, **III:10**.1
    clinical presentation, **III:10**.2, 10.2*t*
    diagnosis, criteria for, **III:10**.2*t*
    mechanical ventilation for, **III:7**.7
    radiographic findings in, **III:10**.2, 10.2*f*
    with toxic fume inhalation, **III:7**.6
    treatment, **III:10**.2–10.3
Adventitious sounds, in physical diagnosis, **I:3**.4, 3.4*t*
AFASAK study. *See* Danish Atrial Fibrillation, Aspirin, Anticoagulation study
Afterload, **II:3**.2, 3.2*t*
Age
    cardiovascular disease risk and, **II:7**.1, 7.2*f*, 7.3*f*, 8.2
    congestive cardiomyopathy and, **II:17**.1, 17.3*t*
Agency for Health Care Policy and Research, **I:7**.4
Aging. *See also* Elderly
    cardiovascular changes with, **II:32**.1–32.10
    cardiovascular disease and, **II:32**.2, 32.4*t*
    glucose tolerance and, **IV:21**.1
    prostatic changes and disorders in, **IV:20**.1–20.11
AHCPR. *See* Agency for Health Care Policy and Research
AIDS. *See* Acquired immunodeficiency syndrome
Airflow obstruction
    causes, **III:2**.2, 2.2*f*
    in occupational asthma, **III:7**.2
Airway obstruction, in interstitial lung disease, **III:6**.5
Albendazole, for echinococcosis, **II:19**.8
Albuterol, for acute severe asthma, **III:10**.4
Alcohol consumption, congestive cardiomyopathy and, **II:17**.1, 17.3*t*
Alcoholism
    male hypogonadism with, **IV:11**.10
    screening recommendations for, **I:2**.7*t*

Aldosterone
   actions, IV:8.1
   pharmacology, IV:6.2t
   secretion, IV:8.1
      in glucocorticoid-remediable aldosteronism, IV:8.5, 8.5f
   synthesis, IV:5.1, 5.2t
Aldosteronism
   glucocorticoid-remediable, IV:8.1–8.2, 8.4f, 8.4–8.5, 8.5f
   primary, IV:8.1–8.4
      diagnosis, IV:8.2, 8.3f
      diagnostic tests for, IV:8.2
      differential diagnosis, IV:8.1–8.2
      treatment, IV:8.3–8.4
Alkaline phosphatase, serum, findings in interstitial lung disease, III:6.5t
Allen test, II:29.2–29.3, 29.3f
Allied health professionals, I:6.6
Alphamethyltyrosine, for pheochromocytoma, IV:7.7
Alveolar gas equation, III:9.2
Alveolar hemorrhage syndrome, III:6.8
Amenorrhea
   in anorexia nervosa, IV:1.6, 1.7
   primary, IV:10.1
   with prolactinoma, IV:2.8
   secondary, IV:2.5, 10.1–10.9
      with abnormal genital structure, IV:10.1, 10.2t
      and achievement or pregnancy, IV:10.8
      with anovulation, IV:10.1, 10.2t, 10.2–10.4
      causes, IV:10.1–10.5
      definition, IV:10.1
      diagnosis, IV:10.5–10.6
      differential diagnosis, IV:10.1–10.5
      endocrinologic evaluation, IV:10.6f
      management, IV:10.6–10.8
      physical findings with, IV:10.5, 10.5t
      signs and symptoms with, IV:10.5, 10.5t
American Heart Association
   Step 1 Diet, IV:18.3, 18.3f
   Step 2 Diet, IV:18.3, 18.4f
Amiloride, for diabetes insipidus, IV:1.4t
Amine precursor uptake and decarboxylation, pheochromocytoma and, IV:7.1
Aminoglutethimide, for adrenal tumor, IV:5.10t, 5.11
Aminoglycosides
   for nosocomial pneumonia, III:4.7t
   plus clindamycin, for nosocomial pneumonia, III:4.7t
Aminophylline, for acute severe asthma, III:10.4
Amiodarone
   goitrogenic properties, IV:4.4
   for hypertrophic cardiomyopathy, II:16.4
Amoxicillin, for acute bronchitis, III:4.2
Amphotericin B, drug interactions, with glucocorticoids, IV:6.4t
Amrinone, for congestive heart failure, II:17.8t, 17.9
Amylase, pleural fluid, III:8.2
Amyloidosis
   cardiac involvement in, II:31.2t, 31.7–31.8, 31.7t
      treatment, II:31.8
   prognosis for, II:31.8
   restrictive cardiomyopathy with, II:18.4f, 18.4–18.6, 18.5f
   thyroid involvement in, IV:4.5
   treatment, II:18.5–18.6, 31.8
Androgen(s)
   peripheral overproduction, in females, IV:10.4, 10.5f

replacement
   behavioral effects, IV:11.10
   contraindications to, IV:11.10
   dosage and administration, IV:11.10
   in male hypogonadism, IV:11.10
   in prepubertal testicular failure, IV:11.3–11.4
   psychosexual effects, IV:11.10
   withdrawal, effects on prostate size, IV:20.3t
Androgen receptor defects, male pseudohermaphroditism with, IV:11.6
Anemia
   physiologic, of pregnancy, II:33.1
   screening recommendations for, I:2.7t
Aneurysm(s)
   aortic. See Abdominal aortic aneurysm(s); Aortic aneurysm(s)
   mycotic, II:20.3
   peripheral arterial, II:29.6–29.7
      complications, II:29.6, 29.6t
      diagnosis, II:29.6
      differential diagnosis, II:29.6
      distribution, II:29.6
      referrals for, II:29.6–29.7
      sex distribution, II:29.6
   sinus of Valsalva, repair, II:23.6
Angina equivalent, II:1.3, 9.1–9.2
Angina pectoris, II:1.1–1.3. See also Chest pain
   with aortic stenosis, II:14.2
   atypical, II:1.2–1.3, 1.4, 9.1–9.2
   characteristics, II:1.3f, 1.3–1.4
   classic, II:9.1
   duration, II:1.3
   emergency evaluation, II:1.7
   epidemiology, II:1.7
   in hypertrophic cardiomyopathy, II:16.2
   inciting factors, II:1.3–1.4
   management, II:9.4–9.6
   mixed, II:9.2
   noninvasive evaluation, II:1.7–1.8
   patterns of relief, II:1.4
   postinfarction, II:11.4t
   prognosis for, II:9.3–9.4
   at rest, II:1.4
   risk stratification with, II:9.3–9.4, 9.6t
   second-wind, II:1.4
   threshold for, II:9.2, 9.2f
   unstable, II:1.2, 1.4, 10.1–10.6
      alternative terminology for, II:10.1
      cardiology consultation and, II:10.5
      coronary arteriography and intervention with, II:10.5, 10.5f
      creatine kinase with, II:10.4, 10.4t
      diagnosis, II:10.1–10.2
      diagnostic testing with, II:10.2–10.4
      ECG findings with, II:10.2–10.4, 10.3f
      emergency treatment, II:10.5
      history-taking with, II:10.2
      hospitalization for, II:10.5
      initial assessment for, II:10.2
      laboratory testing with, II:10.2
      pathophysiology, II:10.1
      physical examination with, II:10.2
      treatment, II:10.4f, 10.4–10.5
   variant, II:1.4, 9.2
   walk-through, II:1.4
Angiocardiography, with pulmonary arteriovenous fistula, II:22.11, 22.11f
Angiography. See also Aortography; Coronary arteriography; Radionuclide angiography
   of aortic dissection, II:28.4–28.5, 28.5f
   of cardiac tumors, II:26.6
   in heart failure, II:2.6, 2.6f

pulmonary, III:1.4, 1.4f
   complications, II:25.5–25.6
   for pulmonary embolism, II:25.5–25.6, 25.6f
   in pulmonary hypertension, II:24.3
   in restrictive cardiomyopathy, II:18.3
Angioplasty, for MI treatment, II:11.7
Angiosarcoma, cardiac, clinical manifestations, II:26.3t
Angiotensin-converting enzyme, in interstitial lung disease, III:6.5t
Angiotensin converting enzyme inhibitors
   for congestive heart failure, II:17.8–17.9
   contraindications to, in pregnancy, II:33.4
   for elderly, advantages and disadvantages, II:32.5t, 32.8
   indications for, II:23.5
   for mitral regurgitation, II:12.6
   precautions with, II:18.3, 18.5
   for restrictive cardiomyopathy, II:18.3
   teratogenicity, II:33.4
Ankylosing spondylitis, I:3.4
   aortitis in, II:28.6
   cardiac involvement in, II:31.2t, 31.6–31.7
Anorexia nervosa, IV:1.6–1.7
   clinical features, IV:1.6t, 1.6–1.7
   hormonal features, IV:1.7, 1.7t
   management, IV:1.7
   referrals for, IV:1.7–1.8
Anovulation, IV:10.1
   abnormal uterine bleeding with, IV:9.2, 9.2f
   amenorrhea with, IV:10.1, 10.2t, 10.2–10.4
   hypothalamic, IV:10.2
   medical therapy for, IV:9.4t, 9.4–9.5
Antacids, drug interactions, with glucocorticoids, IV:6.5t
Anterior cruciate ligament, tear, I:3.4
Anterior glenohumeral dislocation, I:3.6
Anthracycline toxicity, congestive cardiomyopathy and, II:17.2
Antiandrogens, for hirsutism, IV:10.8
Antianginal drugs, II:9.4–9.6
Antiarrhythmic therapy
   for congestive cardiomyopathy, II:17.9, 17.9f
   for hypertrophic cardiomyopathy, II:16.3–16.4
   indications for, II:3.6
   proarrhythmic, II:5.2, 6.2
Antibiotic(s)
   for acute bronchitis, III:4.2
   for acute rheumatic fever, II:31.3, 31.3t
   for Chagas' disease, II:19.8
   with COPD, III:2.7–2.9
      efficacy, III:2.9t
   for inhalation injury, III:7.7
   for Lyme disease, II:31.3, 31.4t
   for nosocomial pneumonia, III:4.7, 4.7t, 10.8
   prophylactic
      after rheumatic fever, II:31.3, 31.3t
      after surgical repair for congenital heart disease, II:23.4, 23.6, 23.7
      with heart murmurs, I:3.2
      for infectious endocarditis, II:12.3, 12.3t, 12.6, 14.5, 20.7, 20.7t
      auscultatory findings and, II:20.3–20.5
   for septic shock, III:10.6
Antibiotic prophylaxis, with heart murmur, I:3.6–3.7
Anticholinergics, for COPD, efficacy, III:2.8f
Anticoagulation
   for chronic thromboembolic pulmonary hypertension, III:5.4
   for deep venous thrombosis, II:25.2, 25.3t, 29.7, 29.8f
   with mitral stenosis, II:12.4
   pericarditis and, II:21.3–21.4

in pregnancy, II:33.4
for primary pulmonary hypertension, III:5.4
in stroke prevention, II:30.4–30.5, 30.4t
Antidiuretic hormone. *See also* Syndrome of inappropriate antidiuretic hormone secretion
actions, IV:1.1–1.2
deficiency, IV:1.2t
regulation, IV:1.1–1.2
releaser/enhancer, for diabetes insipidus, IV:1.4, 1.4t
renal response to, IV:1.2
resistance, IV:1.2t
Antimyosin antibody imaging, in viral myocarditis, II:19.4
Antineutrophil cytoplasmic antibody, findings in interstitial lung disease, III:6.5t
Antioxidants, effects on serum lipids, IV:18.5f, 18.5–18.6
Antistreplase
dosage and administration, II:11.5t
for MI, II:11.5–11.6
pharmacology, II:11.5t
stroke risk with, II:11.6
Antithrombotic therapy
for deep venous thrombosis, II:25.3t
for pulmonary embolism, II:25.3t, 25.7, 25.7t
Antithymocyte globulin, for viral myocarditis, II:19.5
Antithyroid drug(s), for hyperthyroidism, IV:3.4, 3.5
Antitumor agents, toxicity, congestive cardiomyopathy and, II:17.2
Anxiety, trait, mitral valve prolapse and, II:13.6, 13.6t, 13.7t
Aorta
diseases, II:28.1–28.7, 28.2t
thromboembolic disease, II:28.6
Aortic aneurysm(s), arteriosclerotic, II:28.1–28.3. *See also* Abdominal aortic aneurysm(s); Thoracic aortic aneurysm(s)
Aortic arch
right-sided, II:22.2
ulcerated plaques in, stroke risk with, II:30.4
Aortic arteritis, II:28.5–28.6. *See also* Giant cell arteritis; Takayasu's arteritis
Aortic coarctation. *See* Coarctation of the aorta
Aortic dissection
causes, II:28.3
clinical presentation, II:28.4
DeBakey classification, II:28.3, 28.3t, 28.4f
diagnosis, II:28.4f, 28.4–28.5
iatrogenic causes, II:28.3
imaging, II:28.4f, 28.4–28.5
location, II:28.3
pain with, II:1.3, 28.4
pathophysiology, II:28.3
physical findings with, II:1.5
predisposing factors, II:28.3, 28.3t
prognosis for, II:28.5
treatment, II:28.5
Aortic embolism
atheromatous, II:28.6
cholesterol emboli syndrome and, II:28.6
clinical features, II:28.6
diagnosis, II:28.6
pathophysiology, II:28.6
predisposing factors for, II:28.6, 28.6t
prognosis for, II:28.6
treatment, II:28.6
Aortic root dissection, Marfan syndrome and, II:33.4–33.5
Aortic valve
acommissural, II:22.7

bicuspid, II:14.1, 14.2f, 22.1–22.2, 22.7
in adult, II:22.2
with aortic coarctation, II:22.8–22.9
intracardiac repair for, sequelae and residua after, II:23.2, 23.3t
disease, manifestations, II:14.1
flow gradient, calculation, II:14.3–14.4
insufficiency, diagnosis, II:3.5t
lesions, differential diagnosis, maneuvers for, I:3.7, 3.7t
normal anatomy, II:14.2f
regurgitation, II:14.1, 14.6–14.9
age and, II:32.8
auscultatory findings with, II:14.7–14.8, 20.5, 20.5t
chronic vs. acute, II:14.6–14.7, 14.7t
ECG findings with, II:14.8
echocardiography, II:14.8, 14.8f
etiology, II:14.6–14.7, 14.7t
evaluation, II:14.7–14.8
and infectious endocarditis, II:20.5
management, II:14.8–14.9, 14.9f
manifestations, II:20.5, 20.5t
pathogenesis, II:14.6–14.7
postoperative, with intracardiac repair for congenital heart disease, II:23.3–23.4
in pregnancy, II:33.4
referrals for, II:14.9
rheumatic, II:14.6
surgical management, II:14.9
replacement
age and, II:32.8, 32.9f
for aortic regurgitation, II:14.9
for aortic stenosis, II:14.5–14.6, 14.6f
rheumatic, II:14.1, 14.2f, 14.6
sclerosis, I:3.7
differential diagnosis, maneuvers for, I:3.7, 3.8t
sclerosis, differential diagnosis, I:3.2, 3.3t
stenosis, I:3.6–3.7, II:14.1–14.6. *See also* Idiopathic hypertrophic subaortic stenosis
in adult, II:22.2
vs. aortic sclerosis, I:3.7, 3.8t
auscultatory features, II:14.2–14.3, 16.2f
with bicuspid aortic valve, II:22.1
congenital
anatomy, II:22.7
complications, II:22.8
diagnosis, II:22.7, 22.8f
ECG findings with, II:22.7, 22.8f
intracardiac repair for, sequelae and residua after, II:23.3–23.4
pathophysiology, II:22.7
physical findings with, II:22.7
treatment, II:22.8
diagnosis, II:3.5t
differential diagnosis, I:3.2, 3.2t, 3.3t, II:14.2–14.3, 14.2t
ECG findings with, II:14.3, 14.3f
echocardiography with, II:14.3–14.4, 14.4f
epidemiology, II:14.1
etiology, II:14.1–14.2, 14.2f
evaluation, II:14.2–14.4
exercise testing and, II:14.3
management, II:14.4–14.5, 14.5f
natural history, II:14.4, 14.4f, 32.8, 32.8f
pathophysiology, II:14.1–14.2
pharmacologic therapy with, II:14.5
physical findings with, II:1.5
in pregnancy, II:33.3–33.4
referrals for, II:14.5–14.6
rheumatic, II:14.1, 14.2f
senile calcific, II:14.1, 14.2f
subvalvular, II:22.7

supravalvular, II:22.7
valve replacement for, II:14.5–14.6, 14.6f
unicuspid, II:22.7
Aortitis, II:28.5–28.6
Aortography
of abdominal aortic aneurysm, II:28.2f
of aortic dissection, II:28.5, 28.5f
of thoracic aortic aneurysm, II:28.2f
Aortopulmonary shunts, II:23.5, 23.6
Apical pulmonary tumor, diagnosis, III:3.4
Arcus cornealis, II:1.5, 9.2
ARF. *See* Rheumatic fever, acute
Arginine vasopressin
plasma, and plasma osmolality, IV:1.3, 1.3f
urinary, and plasma osmolality, IV:1.3, 1.3f
Arrhenoblastoma, IV:10.5
Arrhythmia(s). *See also specific arrhythmia*
with acute MI, II:11.3
atrial, with atrial septal defect, II:22.3
of Chagas' disease, II:19.7–19.8
in elderly
diagnosis, II:32.8
prevalence, II:32.8
treatment, II:32.8
evaluation, II:6.5–6.6, 6.6f
in patients with palpitations, II:4.5, 4.6t, 4.7f
non-life-threatening. *See also* Palpitations
characteristics, II:4.3–4.4, 4.5t
patient evaluation with, II:4.3–4.5
postoperative, with intracardiac repair for congenital heart disease, II:23.2, 23.2t
symptomatic manifestations, II:4.1
in viral myocarditis, II:19.5
Arterial blood gases, III:1.2
measurement, in diagnosis of respiratory failure, III:10.1
regulation, III:9.1
Arterial compression syndrome(s), II:29.3, 29.5
Arterial disease. *See* Peripheral arterial disease
Arterial switch procedure, II:23.5
Arteriography, cardiac, II:1.8
Arteriosclerosis. *See also* Aortic aneurysm(s), arteriosclerotic
prognosis for, II:29.5
Arteriosclerosis obliterans, prognosis for, II:29.5
Arteritis. *See also* Aortic arteritis; Giant cell arteritis; Takayasu's arteritis
occlusive arterial disease and, II:29.3
prognosis for, II:29.5
in rheumatoid arthritis, II:31.5
temporal. *See* Giant cell arteritis
Arteritis obliterans, in polymyositis and dermatomyositis, II:31.6
Arthritis
of inflammatory bowel disease, cardiac involvement in, II:31.6–31.7
psoriatic
aortitis in, II:28.6
cardiac involvement in, II:31.6–31.7
reactive, cardiac involvement in, II:31.6–31.7
Asbestos inhalation, effects, III:7.3
Asbestosis, III:7.3
clinical features, III:6.1–6.2
diagnosis, III:7.4, 7.5t
differential diagnosis, III:7.5t
exposure settings for, III:7.4t
treatment, III:7.5
Ascites
in constrictive pericarditis, II:21.6
diagnosis, maneuvers for, I:3.9t
Aspartate aminotransferase, II:11.2
Aspergillosis, allergic bronchopulmonary, differential diagnosis, III:6.9t
Asphyxiants, inhalation, III:7.6–7.7

3

Aspirin, drug interactions, with glucocorticoids, IV:6.5*t*
Aspirin therapy
  for flushing, with niacin, II:8.8
  for MI, II:11.4, 11.6
    for secondary prevention, II:11.7*t*
  in stroke prevention, II:30.4–30.5
  for unstable angina, II:10.4, 10.5
Assisted reproductive technologies, IV:12.5
Asthma
  acute respiratory failure with, III:10.1
  acute severe, III:10.3–10.4
    clinical presentation, III:10.3–10.4
    prognosis in, III:10.4
    treatment, III:10.4
  clinical course, III:2.4, 2.4*f*
    long-term, III:2.4, 2.4*f*
  definition, III:2.1
  differential diagnosis, III:2.4*t*, 2.4–2.5
  exacerbations, causes, III:10.3–10.4
  exercise-induced, diagnosis, III:1.3
  and hypoventilation, III:9.2
  mortality with, III:2.1
  occupational. *See* Occupational asthma
  physical diagnosis, I:3.3, 3.4*t*
  physical findings with, I:3.11*t*
  severity, classification, by blood gases, III:10.3*t*
Asthmatic bronchitis, III:2.4
Atelectasis
  lobar, and bronchogenic carcinoma, III:3.4, 3.4*f*
  segmental, and bronchogenic carcinoma, III:3.4, 3.4*f*
Atherosclerosis
  accelerated, II:8.1
  coronary, prevalence, age and, II:32.3, 32.4
  in diabetes mellitus, IV:16.8–16.9
  initiating event, II:8.1
  occlusive arterial disease due to, II:29.2
  pathogenesis, II:8.1
  risk factors for, II:8.2, 8.2*f*, 8.2*t*
Atherosclerotic cardiovascular disease, II:7.1–7.10. *See also* Cardiovascular disease
  risk factors for, II:7.1–7.10
Atrial arrhythmias, with atrial septal defect, II:22.3
Atrial fibrillation, II:6.2, 6.3*f*
  with acute MI, II:11.3
  with mitral regurgitation, II:12.4, 12.5, 12.6
  with mitral stenosis, II:12.2
    management, II:12.4
  nonvalvular, stroke risk with, II:30.2
Atrial flutter, with acute MI, II:11.3
Atrial myxoma. *See* Myxoma(s)
Atrial natriuretic factor, in congestive cardiomyopathy, II:17.2
Atrial natriuretic hormone
  renal response to, IV:1.2
  secretion, IV:1.2
Atrial septal defect, II:22.2–22.3. *See also* Eisenmenger's syndrome
  in adult, II:22.2
  anatomy, II:22.2
  atrial arrhythmias with, II:22.3
  complications, II:22.2–22.3
  congestive heart failure with, II:22.3
  Doppler echocardiography with, II:22.2, 22.3*f*
  ECG findings with, II:22.3*t*
  intracardiac repair for, II:23.4–23.5
  ostium primum, II:22.2
    intracardiac repair for, sequelae and residua after, II:23.2, 23.3*t*
  ostium secundum, II:22.2
    intracardiac repair for, II:23.4
      sequelae and residua after, II:23.2, 23.3*t*
  pathophysiology, II:22.2
  physical findings with, II:22.3*t*
  pulmonary hypertension with, II:22.2–22.3
  radiographic findings with, II:22.3*f*, 22.3*t*
  sinus venosus, II:22.2
  treatment, II:22.3
  types, II:22.2
Atrial tachycardia
  with acute MI, II:11.3
  in pregnancy, II:33.3
Atrioventricular valve
  incompetence, auscultatory findings, II:20.5
  regurgitation, postoperative, with intracardiac repair for congenital heart disease, II:23.2, 23.2*t*
Atropine, for MI, II:11.6*t*
At-work challenge, in diagnosis of occupational asthma, III:7.2
Auscultation. *See also* Heart murmur(s); Heart sound(s)
  with aortic regurgitation, II:14.7–14.8, 20.5, 20.5*t*
  with bicuspid aortic valve, II:22.1–22.2
  of chest pain patient, II:1.5
  in congestive cardiomyopathy, II:17.2–17.3
  in constrictive pericarditis, II:21.6
  with Ebstein's anomaly, II:15.2
  in hypertrophic cardiomyopathy, II:16.2*f*, 16.2–16.3, 20.4, 20.4*f*
  in infectious endocarditis, II:20.3–20.5
  with mitral regurgitation, II:16.2*f*, 20.5, 20.6*t*
  with mitral stenosis, II:15.3, 15.3*t*
  with mitral valve prolapse, II:13.1–13.4, 13.2*f*, 13.6*t*, 20.4, 20.4*f*, 20.5
  with myxoma, II:26.2
  of patent ductus arteriosus, II:22.6
  in physical diagnosis, I:3.2–3.3, 3.4*t*
  with syncope, II:5.3
  of systolic murmurs
    loudest at apex, I:3.3
    loudest at base, I:3.2
  technique, II:20.4*f*, 20.4–20.5
  with tricuspid regurgitation, II:15.4
  with tricuspid stenosis, II:15.3, 15.3*t*
Austin-Flint murmur, with aortic regurgitation, II:14.8
Autoimmune disease, thyroid, IV:3.6, 4.1–4.3
Autoimmune polyglandular syndrome, IV:5.12
Autonomic nervous system, testing, and syncope, II:5.4
Azathioprine
  for collagen vascular disorders, III:6.8
  for viral myocarditis, II:19.5
Azithromycin
  for acute bronchitis, III:4.2
  for community-acquired pneumonia, III:4.5*t*
Azlocillin, for nosocomial pneumonia, III:4.7*t*
Azoospermia, hormonally induced, for contraception, IV:12.7
Aztreonam, for nosocomial pneumonia, III:4.7*t*

B

BAATAF. *See* Boston Area Anticoagulation Trial for Atrial Fibrillation
Back. *See also* Low back
  acute musculoskeletal or ligamentous strain, I:3.3
  pain in, I:3.3–3.4
  physical examination, I:3.3*t*
  sciatica in, I:3.3, 3.4*t*
  stiffness in, I:3.3–3.4

Bacteremia, vs. infectious endocarditis, II:20.6*t*, 20.7
Bacterial myocarditis, II:19.3*t*, 19.7
Bacterial pericarditis, II:21.1, 21.2, 21.3
  management, II:21.3
Bacteriuria, asymptomatic, screening recommendations for, I:2.7*t*
Balloon valvuloplasty
  for congenital heart disease, sequelae and residua, II:23.3
  indications for, II:3.7
  mitral
    age and, II:32.8
    evaluation of candidates for, II:12.2–12.3
  pulmonic, indications for, II:15.5, 15.5*t*
  tricuspid, indications for, II:15.3
Barotrauma, definition, III:10.7
Bayes' theorem, I:4.4–4.5
  nomogram for, I:4.5, 4.5*f*
Bed rest, pulmonary embolism and, II:25.1, 25.2*t*
Behçet's syndrome, aortitis in, II:28.6
Benign prostatic hyperplasia, IV:20.1–20.6
  differential diagnosis, IV:20.2
  epidemiology, IV:20.1
  finasteride therapy for, IV:20.3–20.5
  medical therapy, α-adrenergic blockers for, IV:20.6, 20.6*f*
  medical treatment, IV:20.2–20.3
  pathogenesis, IV:20.1–20.2
  signs and symptoms, IV:20.2, 20.3*t*
  staging, IV:20.5*t*, 20.5–20.6
Benznidazole, for Chagas' disease, II:19.8
Berylliosis
  differential diagnosis, III:7.5*t*
  exposure settings for, III:7.4*t*
Beta lactam/beta lactamase inhibitor combination
  for acute bronchitis, III:4.2
  for community-acquired pneumonia, III:4.5*t*
  for nosocomial pneumonia, III:4.7*t*
Betamethasone, pharmacology, IV:6.2*t*
Bias, in screening recommendations, I:2.4, 2.5*f*
Bicipital tendinitis, I:3.6
Biguanides, for non-insulin-dependent diabetes mellitus (NIDDM), IV:14.5
Bile-acid sequestrants, in lipid-lowering therapy, II:8.7, 8.8*t*
Bleeding, abnormal uterine. *See* Abnormal uterine bleeding
Bleomycin
  adverse effects, III:8.9
  as sclerosing agent, for malignant pleural effusions, III:8.9
Blood culture, in infectious endocarditis, II:20.1, 20.6–20.7
Blood pressure
  ankle and brachial, in occlusive arterial disease, II:29.3, 29.4*t*
  cardiovascular disease and, II:7.2*f*, 7.2–7.4, 7.3*f*, 7.3*t*
  J-shaped curve for, II:7.2
  with mitral valve prolapse, II:13.6
  normal, determinants, II:3.1–3.2
  systolic
    age-related changes in, II:32.1, 32.2*f*
    in occlusive arterial disease, II:29.3, 29.4*t*
Blood volume
  determinants, II:3.1–3.2
  in pregnancy, II:33.1
Body fat, IV:18.1
  distribution, cardiovascular disease and, II:7.7, 8.2
Body fluid tests, findings in interstitial lung disease, III:6.5*t*
Body water. *See* Water balance

Body weight. *See also* Obesity
    cardiovascular disease and, II:7.7
Bone(s), in primary hyperparathyroidism, IV:13.4, 13.4f
Borborygmi, I:3.8
Börjeson-Forssman-Lehmann syndrome, IV:11.8t
Boston Area Anticoagulation Trial for Atrial Fibrillation, II:30.4
Bouchard's nodes, I:3.2
Boutonnière deformity, I:3.2
Bowel sounds, auscultation, I:3.8
Boxer's fracture, I:3.2
Bradycardia, II:1.5
Breast cancer
    cardiac metastases, II:26.2
    dietary (nutritional) factors in, IV:17.2t, 17.2–17.3
    epidemiology, IV:17.1
    etiology, IV:17.1
    familial, IV:17.1–17.2
    genetic alterations in, IV:17.2, 17.2t
    hormonal factors in, IV:17.2, 17.2t
    and malignant pleural effusions, III:8.7t
    metastasis to pleura, III:8.3
    mortality with, IV:17.1
    pathogenesis, IV:17.1
    risk factors for, IV:17.1, 17.2t, 17.3–17.4, 17.4t
    screening recommendations for, I:2.6t
Breast disease
    benign, IV:17.1, 17.3
        abnormalities as, IV:17.3
        breast cancer risk and, IV:17.3–17.4, 17.4t
        of development and involution, IV:17.3, 17.3f
    fibrocystic, IV:17.3
    malignant. *See* Breast cancer
    referral guidelines, IV:17.4
Breast duct ectasia, IV:17.3, 17.4
Breathing, control, III:9.1, 9.2f
    controller in, III:9.1
    disorders, III:9.1–9.8
    effectors in, III:9.1
    sensors in, III:9.1
Breathing patterns, disordered, III:9.5
Breath sounds, I:3.10
    evaluation, I:3.3t, 3.3–3.4, 3.4t
Bromocriptine, for hyperprolactinemia, IV:10.7
Bronchial diseases, occupational, development, III:7.3f
Bronchitis
    acute, III:4.1–4.2
        clinical features, III:4.2
        diagnosis, III:4.2
        prevention, III:4.2
        therapy for, III:4.2
    asthmatic, III:2.4
    chronic
        acute exacerbation, differential diagnosis, III:4.2
        in COLD, III:1.2t
        definition, III:2.1
        physical findings with, I:3.11t
        simple, III:2.2
    physical diagnosis, I:3.3, 3.4t
    physical findings with, I:3.11t
Bronchocentric granulomatosis, III:6.8
Bronchodilators
    response to, in COLD, III:1.2t
    therapy, for COPD, III:2.7–2.9
    use with spirometry, III:1.1
Bronchogenic carcinoma, III:3.1–3.6
    adenocarcinoma, III:3.2
        clinical features, III:3.2t
    classification, III:3.2
    clinical manifestations, III:3.2–3.3
    diagnostic tests for, III:3.5
    etiology, III:3.1–3.2
    incidence, III:3.1
    large cell, III:3.2
        clinical features, III:3.2t
    mortality with, III:3.1
    non-small cell, management, III:3.6
    paraneoplastic syndromes, III:3.3, 3.3t
    radiologic manifestations, III:3.3f, 3.3–3.4, 3.4f
    risk factors in, III:3.1–3.2
    role of generalist in, III:3.7
    small cell, III:3.2
        clinical features, III:3.2t
        management, III:3.6
    squamous cell, III:3.2
        clinical features, III:3.2t
    staging, III:3.5, 3.5t
    therapy for, III:3.5–3.6
Bronchogenic cyst, clinical manifestations, II:26.3t
Bronchography, III:1.4
Bronchoscopy
    diagnostic, II:1.5–1.6
        of bronchogenic carcinoma, III:3.5
        indications for, III:1.5t
        specimens obtained by, III:1.5t
    therapeutic, with inhalation injury, III:7.7
Brucellosis, differential diagnosis, III:6.9t
Bruit(s)
    carotid, II:9.2
    femoral, II:9.2
Bucindolol, for congestive heart failure, II:17.9
Buerger's disease
    clinical features, II:29.3, 29.5t
    occlusive arterial disease due to, II:29.2
Bulimia nervosa, IV:1.7–1.8
    clinical features, IV:1.7, 1.8t
    management, IV:1.7
    referrals for, IV:1.8
Bullae, on chest x-ray or CT, in COLD, III:1.2t
Bullous lesion, differential diagnosis, III:8.3
Bumetanide, for right ventricular failure, III:5.5
Bundle branch block, left, in viral myocarditis, II:19.2–19.3
Bursitis
    infrapatellar, I:3.4
    prepatellar, I:3.4
    semimembranous, I:3.4
    subacromial, I:3.6
Butorphanol, for SIADH, IV:1.6t

C

Calcitonin, salmon, for hypercalcemia of malignancy, IV:19.2t
Calcium, serum
    adjustment for plasma albumin values, IV:13.2, 13.2t
    disorders, IV:13.1–13.6. *See also* Hypercalcemia; Hypocalcemia
    findings in interstitial lung disease, III:6.5t
    normal values, IV:13.1
    regulation, IV:13.1
Calcium channel blockers
    for angina, II:9.5
    for congestive cardiomyopathy, II:17.9
    effects on myocardial oxygen supply and demand, II:9.3f
    for elderly, advantages and disadvantages, II:32.5t, 32.8
    for hypertrophic cardiomyopathy, II:16.3–16.4
    indications for, II:3.6, IV:7.7
    mechanism of action, II:9.5
    with mitral stenosis, II:12.4
    for pheochromocytoma, IV:7.7, 7.7t
    for pulmonary hypertension, II:24.3f, 24.5–24.6, III:5.4–5.5
    for restrictive cardiomyopathy, II:18.3
    side effects, III:5.5
Calcium–parathyroid axis, IV:13.1
Canadian Atrial Fibrillation Study, II:30.4
Cancer. *See also* Tumor(s)
    adrenal gland, treatment, IV:5.10t, 5.10–5.11
    breast. *See* Breast cancer
    cervical, screening recommendations for, I:2.6t
    colorectal, screening recommendations for, I:2.6t
    endocrine manifestations, IV:19.1–19.6
    gastric, and malignant pleural effusions, III:8.7t
    gonadal, screening recommendations for, I:2.6t
    lung. *See* Bronchogenic carcinoma; Lung cancer
    lymphangitic carcinoma, III:6.1
        interstitial, differential diagnosis, III:6.3t
    oral, screening recommendations for, I:2.6t
    ovarian, and malignant pleural effusions, III:8.7t
    pancreatic
        screening recommendations for, I:2.6t
        SIADH with, IV:1.4, 1.5t
    prostatic. *See* Prostate cancer
    skin, screening recommendations for, I:2.6t
    in solitary thyroid nodules, IV:4.6–4.7, 4.7t
    thyroid, IV:4.6–4.7, 4.7t
        medullary, IV:7.1
Captopril
    for MI, II:11.4–11.5
        for secondary prevention, II:11.7t
    in viral myocarditis, II:19.5
Captopril test, for aldosteronism, IV:8.2
Carbamazepine, drug interactions, with glucocorticoids, IV:6.5t
Carbon dioxide, arterial partial pressure, III:1.2
    elevation, in hypoventilation, III:9.3
Carbon monoxide poisoning, III:7.6–7.7
    management, III:7.9f
    treatment, III:7.7
Carcinoid heart disease, II:18.6
Carcinoma. *See* Cancer; *specific carcinoma*
Cardiac arrest, II:6.1–6.7. *See also* Sudden (cardiac) death
    causes, II:6.1, 6.2t
    electrophysiologic abnormalities with, II:6.2, 6.4
    iatrogenic causes, II:6.2
    prevention, II:6.5–6.6, 6.6f
    risk stratification, II:6.6, 6.6f
    survival rates, II:6.1
    survivors
        approach to, II:6.2–6.5
        evaluation, II:6.2–6.4
        referral, II:6.7
        treatment, II:6.4–6.5, 6.5f
Cardiac Arrhythmias Suppression Trial, II:11.3
Cardiac catheterization, II:1.8
    with cardiac tamponade, II:21.5
    with cardiac tumors, II:26.6
    in congestive cardiomyopathy, II:17.5
    in constrictive pericarditis, II:21.6
    in heart failure, II:2.6, 2.6f
    with hypertrophic cardiomyopathy, II:16.3
    indications for, II:4.6t
    with mitral regurgitation, II:12.5
    with mitral stenosis, II:12.3
    in pulmonary hypertension, II:24.3
Cardiac enzyme(s). *See also* Creatine kinase
    in pericarditis, II:21.3

Cardiac index
  calculation, II:3.7t
  normal value, II:3.7t
Cardiac murmurs. *See* Heart murmur(s)
Cardiac output, II:3.1, 3.2
  age-related changes in, II:32.1, 32.2f
  in pregnancy, II:33.1–33.2, 33.2f
Cardiac performance, determinants, II:3.2, 3.2t
Cardiac rupture, postinfarction, II:11.4t
Cardiac tamponade, II:21.4–21.5
  clinical features, II:21.4
  diagnosis, II:3.5t
  hemodynamic parameters for, II:3.6t
  low-pressure, II:21.5
  management, II:21.5
  pathogenesis, II:21.4
  physical findings in, II:21.4, 21.4t
Cardiac trauma. *See* Trauma, cardiac
Cardiac tumors, II:26.1–26.7. *See also specific tumor*
  angiography, II:26.6
  benign
    prognosis for, II:26.6, 26.6t
    treatment, II:26.6, 26.6t
  computed tomography with, II:26.5
  diagnosis, techniques for, II:26.4–26.6
  diagnostic work-up, II:26.4, 26.4t
  echocardiography with, II:26.4, 26.4f, 26.5f
  magnetic resonance imaging with, II:26.5–26.6
  malignant, II:26.2, 26.3t
    prognosis for, II:26.6, 26.6t
    treatment, II:26.6, 26.6t
  metastatic, II:26.2–26.4
    clinical manifestations, II:26.3–26.4, 26.3t
    prognosis for, II:26.6, 26.6t
    treatment, II:26.6, 26.6t
  primary, II:26.1–26.2
    benign, II:26.1–26.2, 26.2t
    clinical manifestations, II:26.1
    incidence, II:26.1, 26.2f
  radiologic findings with, II:26.4, 26.4t
  secondary, II:26.2–26.4
  transesophageal echocardiography with, II:26.4–26.5
Cardiogenic shock, II:3.1–3.8, 11.4t
  causes, II:3.3, 3.3t
    differential diagnosis, II:3.3
  clinical manifestations, II:3.2
  complicating MI, incidence, II:3.3
  diagnostic benchmarks in, II:3.4t–3.5t
  diagnostic evaluation, II:3.3
  hemodynamic monitoring in, II:3.3, 3.6t, 3.7t
  hemodynamic parameters in, II:3.6t
  initial stabilization in, II:3.2, 3.2t
  intraarterial monitoring in, II:3.3
  laboratory findings in, II:3.2
  management, II:3.3–3.7
  mechanical intervention for, II:3.6–3.7
  pathology, II:3.3, 3.3f
  pharmacologic therapy, II:3.3–3.6
  surgical intervention in, II:3.7
Cardiomegaly, with amyloid heart disease, II:31.7–31.8
Cardiomyopathy, II:6.6
  of Chagas' disease, II:19.7–19.8
  congestive. *See* Congestive cardiomyopathy
  dilated. *See also* Congestive cardiomyopathy
    diagnosis, II:3.4t
    genetics, II:2.2
    infectious myocarditis and, II:19.1
    sudden cardiac death due to, II:6.2
  hypertrophic. *See* Hypertrophic cardiomyopathy
  peripartum, II:33.4
  restrictive. *See* Restrictive cardiomyopathy

Cardiopulmonary support, percutaneous, II:3.6
Cardiovascular disease
  aging and, II:32.2, 32.4t
  blood lipids and, II:7.4–7.6
  blood pressure and, II:7.2f, 7.2–7.4, 7.3f, 7.3t
  body weight and, II:7.7
  cigarette smoking and, II:7.6, 7.7f
  diabetes mellitus and, II:7.6–7.7
  glucose tolerance and, II:7.6–7.7
  hypertension and, II:7.2f, 7.2–7.4, 7.3f, 7.3t
  incidence, age and, II:7.1, 7.2f
  left ventricular hypertrophy and, II:7.7
  in menopause, IV:22.3
  physical activity and, II:7.7
  prevention, II:7.8
  risk factors for, II:7.1–7.8
Cardiovascular risk, age and, II:32.5, 32.6f, 32.7f
Cardiovascular risk profiles, II:7.8, 7.8f, 7.9t
Cardiovascular system, age-related changes in, II:32.1–32.2, 32.2f, 32.2t, 32.4t
Cardioversion, indications for, II:3.6, 11.3
Carditis
  in acute rheumatic fever, II:31.1
  in systemic lupus erythematosus, II:31.4
Carotid sinus massage, indications for, II:5.4
Carotid vessels, auscultation, in patient with syncope, II:5.3
Carpal tunnel syndrome, I:3.3
Carvallo sign, II:15.4, 20.5
Case finding, definition, I:2.2
Catecholamines
  excretion, with pheochromocytoma, IV:7.2, 7.3t
  metabolites, with pheochromocytoma, IV:7.2, 7.3t
  myocarditis caused by, IV:7.3
  plasma, with pheochromocytoma, IV:7.4, 7.4t
  urinary, with pheochromocytoma, IV:7.3t, 7.3–7.4
Catheter aspiration, for primary spontaneous pneumothorax, III:8.3
Caval to pulmonary arterial connections, for congenital heart disease, II:23.2t, 23.6f, 23.7
Cefoperazone, for nosocomial pneumonia, III:4.7t
Ceftazidime, for nosocomial pneumonia, III:4.7t
Central autonomic insufficiency, IV:1.2
Central nervous system disorders, SIADH with, IV:1.4, 1.5t
Cephalosporin
  second-generation
    for community-acquired pneumonia, III:4.5t
    for nosocomial pneumonia, III:4.7t
  third-generation
    for community-acquired pneumonia, III:4.5t
    for nosocomial pneumonia, III:4.7t
Cerebellar degeneration, and bronchogenic carcinoma, III:3.3t
Cerebrovascular complications. *See also* Stroke
  of cardiac disorders, II:30.1–30.6
  of cardiac therapy, II:30.5
Cerebrovascular disease, II:7.1
  as cause of death, III:2.2t
  screening recommendations for, I:2.6t
Cervical cancer, screening recommendations for, I:2.6t
Chagas' disease, II:19.7–19.8
  clinical course, II:19.7
  ECG findings in, II:19.7–19.8
  etiology, II:19.7
  treatment, II:19.8
Chagoma, II:19.7
CHARGE syndrome, IV:11.8t
CHD. *See* Coronary heart disease
Chemoreceptors, III:9.1

Chemotherapy
  for bronchogenic carcinoma, III:3.6
  in diabetic patient, IV:15.6
  effects on testicular function, IV:11.7
Chest pain. *See also* Angina pectoris
  of aortic dissection, II:28.4
  in carcinomatous pleurisy, III:8.6
  causes, II:1.1, 1.2t
  ECG findings with, II:1.5–1.6, 1.6f
  echocardiographic findings in, II:1.6–1.7
  emergency evaluation, II:1.7
  esophageal, II:1.1
    patterns of relief, II:1.4
  evaluation, II:1.1–1.9
  laboratory findings with, II:1.7
  with mitral stenosis, II:12.2
  mitral valve prolapse and, II:13.6, 13.6t, 13.7t
  musculoskeletal, II:1.4, 1.7
  of myocardial infarction, II:11.1
  with myocardial ischemia, II:1.1–1.3
  noninvasive evaluation, II:1.7–1.8
  nonischemic, II:1.4
  with non-Q wave MI, II:10.2
  in pericarditis, II:21.2
  physical examination with, II:1.4–1.5
  with pleurisy, III:8.2
  in pregnancy, II:33.2
  in primary spontaneous pneumothorax, III:8.2
  radiographic findings with, II:1.6
  in secondary spontaneous pneumothorax, III:8.3
  with unstable angina, II:10.1–10.2
Chest radiography
  in chest pain patient, II:1.6
  in congestive cardiomyopathy, II:17.3, 17.4f
  in heart failure, II:2.3, 2.3f
  with hypertrophic cardiomyopathy, II:16.3
  with mitral regurgitation, II:12.5
  with mitral stenosis, II:12.3
  with pericardial effusion, II:21.4–21.5, 21.4t, 21.5f
  in pericarditis, II:21.3
  in pulmonary hypertension, II:24.2, 24.2f
Cheyne-Stokes respirations, III:9.4f, 9.5
Child(ren)
  diabetes in, diagnosis, IV:14.3
  hypoglycemia in, IV:14.7, 14.7t
Childress' test, I:3.4
Chlamydia infection, screening recommendations for, I:2.7t
Chlamydia pneumoniae, III:4.3, 4.3t, 4.4t
Chloroquine, for sarcoidosis, III:6.5
Chlorpropamide
  contraindications to, in elderly, IV:21.3
  for diabetes insipidus, IV:1.4t
  for non-insulin-dependent diabetes mellitus (NIDDM), IV:14.5, 14.5t
Chlorthalidone, for diabetes insipidus, IV:1.4t
Cholesterol, serum. *See also* Hypercholesterolemia
  antioxidants and, IV:18.5f, 18.5–18.6
  beneficial effects of estrogen replacement therapy on, IV:22.4t
  and cardiovascular disease, IV:18.2
  cardiovascular disease and, II:7.4f, 7.4–7.6
  and coronary artery disease risk, IV:18.2, 18.2f
  dietary fiber and, IV:18.5
  in elderly, IV:21.3–21.4
  exercise and, IV:18.5
  homeostatic mechanisms, IV:18.2, 18.2f
  measurement, II:8.2–8.4
  and risk of coronary death, II:8.2, 8.2f
Cholesterol emboli syndrome, II:28.6
Cholesterol/HDL ratio, coronary heart disease risk and, II:7.5, 7.6f

Cholesterol Lowering and Atherosclerosis Study, II:8.6
Cholestyramine
  drug interactions, with glucocorticoids, IV:6.5*t*
  lipid-lowering therapy, II:8.8*t*
Chromaffin tumor(s), IV:7.2, 7.3
Chronic indurated cellulitis, II:29.8, 29.8*f*, 29.9*f*
Chronic obstructive pulmonary disease, III:2.1–2.10
  acute respiratory failure with, III:10.1
  airflow obstruction in, III:2.2
  bronchodilator therapy for, III:2.7–2.9
    algorithm for approach to, III:2.8*f*
  clinical course, III:2.4, 2.4*f*
    long-term, III:2.4, 2.4*f*
  costs, III:2.1
  definition, III:2.1
  diagnosis, III:2.2–2.5
  diagnostic findings in, III:1.1, 1.2*t*
  differential diagnosis, III:2.4*t*, 2.4–2.5
  etiology, III:2.2
  hypoventilation in, III:9.2
  infectious diseases with, prevention, III:2.6–2.7
  lung volumes in, III:1.3*t*
  management, III:2.5–2.9
  mortality with, III:2.1, 2.2*t*
  oxygen therapy for, III:2.9
    and survival rates, III:2.9, 2.9*f*
  physical diagnosis, I:3.3, 3.4*t*
  pulmonary hypertension in, II:24.6
  rehabilitation in, III:2.9
Chronic venous insufficiency, II:29.7–29.8
Churg-Strauss disease, III:6.8
Churg-Strauss syndrome, cardiac involvement in, II:31.6
Cigarette smoking, cardiovascular disease and, II:7.6, 7.7*f*, 8.2, 8.2*t*
Ciprofloxacin
  for community-acquired pneumonia, III:4.5*t*
  for nosocomial pneumonia, III:4.7*t*
  plus clindamycin, for nosocomial pneumonia, III:4.7*t*
Circulatory assist devices, indications for, II:3.7
Cirrhosis
  cardiac, in constrictive pericarditis, II:21.6
  hepatic, male hypogonadism with, IV:11.10
  with portal-pulmonary hypertension, differential diagnosis, III:5.3
Clarithromycin
  for acute bronchitis, III:4.2
  for community-acquired pneumonia, III:4.5*t*
CLAS. *See* Cholesterol Lowering and Atherosclerosis Study
Clavicular fracture, I:3.6
Click-like sounds, II:20.5, 20.5*t*
Clicks, systolic, and antibiotic prophylaxis, II:20.5
Clinical guidelines, I:7.4–7.5
Clitoromegaly, IV:10.1
Clofibrate
  for diabetes insipidus, IV:1.4*t*
  lipid-lowering therapy, clinical intervention trial, II:8.6
Clonidine suppression test, with pheochromocytoma, IV:7.4*f*, 7.4–7.5, 7.4*t*
Clubbing
  of fingers, III:6.2, 6.2*f*
  of nails, I:3.4, 3.10–3.11
  of toes, with patent ductus arteriosus, II:22.6, 22.6*f*
Coarctation of the aorta, II:22.8–22.9
  in adult, II:22.2
  anatomy, II:22.8–22.9
  complications, II:22.9
  diagnosis, II:22.9
  pathophysiology, II:22.9
  physical findings with, II:22.9
  repair, II:23.6
    sequelae and residua after, II:23.3*t*
  treatment, II:22.9
Coccidioidomycosis, differential diagnosis, III:6.9*t*
COLD (chronic obstructive lung disease). *See* Chronic obstructive pulmonary disease
Colestipol
  drug interactions, with glucocorticoids, IV:6.5*t*
  lipid-lowering therapy, II:8.8*t*
Collagen vascular disorders, III:6.1, 6.7*f*, 6.7–6.8
  characteristics, III:6.7
  pulmonary hypertension in, II:24.6
  treatment, III:6.8
Colorectal cancer, screening recommendations for, I:2.6*t*
Coma
  hyperosmolar hyperglycemic nonketotic. *See* Hyperosmolar hyperglycemic nonketotic coma
  myxedemic, IV:3.3
  in elderly, IV:21.4
Complete blood count, in interstitial lung disease, III:6.5*t*
Compression fracture, vertebral, I:3.3
Computed tomography
  of aortic dissection, II:28.4–28.5
  with cardiac tumors, II:26.5
  chest
    in diagnosis of bronchogenic carcinoma, III:3.4, 3.4*f*
    in diagnosis of pneumoconiosis, III:7.4
  in Cushing's syndrome, IV:5.9, 5.9*t*
  of pheochromocytoma, IV:7.5–7.6, 7.5–7.6, 7.6*f*
  pulmonary, III:1.4*f*, 1.5
  in restrictive cardiomyopathy, II:18.3
Condom(s), IV:12.7
Conduction abnormalities
  with acute MI, II:11.3
  in rheumatoid arthritis, II:31.5
  in scleroderma, II:31.5
  in systemic lupus erythematosus, II:31.5
Conduits, intracardiac, II:23.2, 23.2*t*
Congenital adrenal hyperplasia, IV:5.2, 10.3, 10.3*t*
  diagnosis, IV:10.6
  management, IV:10.8
Congenital heart disease, II:22.1–22.12
  in adults
    common presentations, II:22.1, 22.2*t*
    general considerations, II:23.1–23.3
    intracardiac repair for, surgical procedures, II:23.4–23.7
    postoperative residua and sequelae, II:23.1–23.7
    recognition, II:22.2–22.12
  caval to pulmonary arterial connections for, II:23.2*t*, 23.6*f*, 23.7
  cyanotic, II:22.9–22.12
  intracardiac repair for
    prosthetic materials in, II:23.2–23.3, 23.2*t*
    residua, II:23.1, 23.2*t*, 23.3*t*
      anatomic, II:23.2
    sequelae, II:23.1, 23.2*t*, 23.3*t*
      anatomic, II:23.2
      electrophysiologic, II:23.2
      surgical procedures, II:23.4–23.7
  magnetic resonance imaging in, II:23.3
  minor lesions, II:22.1–22.2
  in pregnant woman, II:33.4
  pulmonary hypertension with, II:24.6
  sudden cardiac death due to, II:6.2
    transesophageal echocardiography in, II:23.2–23.3
Congestive cardiomyopathy, II:17.1–17.10. *See also* Cardiomyopathy, dilated
  auscultatory findings with, II:17.2–17.3
  chest radiography in, II:17.3, 17.4*f*
  clinical course, II:17.6–17.7
  clinical features, II:17.2–17.7
  with diastolic failure, treatment, II:17.9
  differential diagnosis, II:17.6, 17.7*t*
  ECG findings in, II:17.3–17.4, 17.4*f*, 17.5*f*
  echocardiography in, II:17.4–17.5, 17.5*f*, 17.6*f*, 17.6*t*
  electrophysiology in, II:17.4
  etiology, II:17.1, 17.3*t*
  functional abnormalities in, II:17.2, 17.3*f*, 17.3*t*, 17.4*f*
  functional status in, assessment, II:17.5–17.6, 17.7*t*
  hemodynamic parameters in, II:17.5, 17.6*t*
  laboratory findings in, II:17.3–17.5
  pathophysiology, II:17.1, 17.2*f*
  physical findings with, II:17.2–17.3
  prognosis for, II:17.7, 17.8*t*
  referrals for, II:17.9
  signs and symptoms, II:17.2–17.3
  with systolic failure, II:17.2, 17.3*t*
    treatment, II:17.7–17.9
  treatment, II:17.7–17.9
Congestive heart failure. *See also* Congestive cardiomyopathy
  with amyloid heart disease, II:31.7–31.8
  with atrial septal defect, II:22.3
  incidence, age and, II:7.1, 7.2*f*
  in polymyositis and dermatomyositis, II:31.6
  with viral myocarditis, treatment, II:19.5
Connective-tissue disorders. *See also* Ehlers-Danlos syndrome; Marfan syndrome
  cardiac involvement in, II:31.7
  differential diagnosis, III:5.2
  occlusive arterial disease and, II:29.3
Consolidation, physical diagnosis, I:3.3–3.4, 3.4*t*
Constrictive pericarditis, II:21.5–21.7
  auscultatory findings with, II:21.6
  clinical features, II:21.6
  differential diagnosis, II:21.6
  ECG findings with, II:21.6
  echocardiography in, II:21.6
  etiology, II:21.6, 21.6*t*
  laboratory findings with, II:21.6, 21.7*t*
  management, II:21.7
  pathophysiology, II:21.6
  referrals for, II:21.7
  vs. restrictive cardiomyopathy, II:21.6, 21.7*f*
Consultant(s)
  contacting, I:5.2
  information to be provided to, I:5.2–5.3, 5.3*t*
  selection, I:5.2
Consultation, I:5.1, I:5.1, I:5.3, I:5.3
  awkward issues in, I:5.3–5.4, I:5.3–5.4
  communicating conclusions and recommendations in, I:5.3, 5.4*f*
  effective, rules for, I:5.3, I:5.3, I:5.3*t*, I:5.3*t*
  information for consulting physician in, I:5.2–5.3, 5.3*t*
  reasons for, I:5.1, I:5.1–5.2, I:5.2*t*, I:5.2*t*
  results, communication, I:5.3, 5.4*f*
  steps in, I:5.2*t*, 5.2–5.3
  timing, I:5.2
Consumer Price Index (CPI), I:6.2, 7.3
  medical, I:6.2, 6.3*f*, 7.3
Continuous positive airway pressure
  nasal, for central sleep apnea, III:9.7
  for obstructive sleep apnea, III:9.6

7

Contraception
  male, IV:12.7
  in perimenopause, IV:22.2, 22.2t
Contractility, II:3.2, 3.2t
Contusion, myocardial. See Myocardial contusion
COPD. See Chronic obstructive pulmonary disease
Coronary angioplasty
  advantages and disadvantages, II:9.6
  in elderly, results, II:32.4, 32.5t
  indications for, II:3.7, 9.6
Coronary arteriography, II:1.8
Coronary artery(ies)
  obstruction, II:1.5
  in polymyositis and dermatomyositis, II:31.6
  rupture, posttraumatic, II:27.8–27.9
  in systemic lupus erythematosus, II:31.4
Coronary artery bypass grafting
  cerebrovascular complications, II:30.5
  in elderly, results, II:32.4, 32.5t
  indications for, II:6.4–6.5, 9.6
Coronary artery disease, II:6.6. See also Coronary heart disease
  accelerated, in heart transplant recipient, II:34.8, 34.8f
  asymptomatic, screening recommendations for, I:2.6t
  and blood pressure, age and, II:32.5, 32.6f
  in diabetes mellitus, IV:16.8–16.9
  diagnosis, II:1.7–1.8, 9.2–9.3
  differential diagnosis, II:17.6
  ECG findings with, II:1.5
  in elderly, IV:21.3–21.4
  epidemiology, II:1.4, 1.4f, 1.7
  heart sounds with, II:1.5
  and hypothyroidism, management, IV:3.3
  likelihood, estimation, II:1.4, 1.4f, 1.5f
    nomogram for, II:9.4f, 9.5f
  lipid-lowering therapy and, II:8.6–8.7, 8.7f
  noninvasive tests for, II:1.7–1.8
  physical findings in, II:1.5
  posttest risk, II:9.3, 9.5t
  pretest risk, II:9.2–9.3
  prevalence, by age and sex, II:1.4, 1.4f
  prognosis in, II:9.3–9.4
  revascularization in, II:9.6
  risk factors for, II:9.2–9.3, IV:18.1, 18.2, 18.2f
  risk stratification in, II:9.3–9.4, 9.6t
  serum lipids in, II:8.3
  sudden cardiac death due to, II:6.1–6.2, 6.2f
  treatment, II:9.4–9.6
Coronary Artery Surgery Study, II:32.4
Coronary artery trauma, II:27.7–27.9
  acute myocardial infarction and, II:27.8
  case material on, II:27.7–27.8
  consequences, II:27.8f, 27.9, 27.9f
  mechanism of injury, II:27.8
  treatment, II:27.8–27.9
Coronary Drug Project, II:8.6
Coronary heart disease, II:7.1. See also Coronary artery disease
  blood lipids and, II:7.4f, 7.4–7.6
  familial risk for, II:7.8
  incidence, age and, II:7.1, 7.2f
  prevention, II:7.8
  risk for, assessment, II:7.8, 7.8f, 7.9t
Corrigan's pulse, II:14.7
Corticosteroids
  for acute bronchitis, III:4.2
  for COPD, III:2.7
  for hypersensitivity pneumonitis, III:6.7
  for idiopathic pulmonary fibrosis, III:6.10
  for inhalation injury, III:7.7
  intravenous, for acute severe asthma, III:10.4
  for lupus pleuritis and postcardiac injury syndrome, III:8.2
  for pulmonary infiltration with eosinophilia, III:6.8
  for sarcoidosis, III:6.5
  for viral myocarditis, II:19.5
Corticotropin-releasing factor, response to, IV:2.2
Corticotropin-releasing hormone, IV:2.2f, 5.2
  stimulation test, IV:5.8, 5.8t
Corticotropin test, rapid intravenous, IV:10.6
Cortisol, IV:5.1, 5.2t, 6.1
  clinical applications, IV:5.3–5.4
  conversion to cortisone, IV:5.2, 5.3f, 8.4, 8.4f
  24-h urine free, IV:5.7, 5.8t
  mechanism of action, IV:5.3, 5.4f
  pharmacology, IV:6.2t
  receptors, IV:5.3
  resistance, hyperandrogenism in, IV:10.3
  secretion, regulation, IV:5.2–5.3
  synthesis, feedback inhibition, IV:5.3, 5.4f
Cortisone, IV:6.1
  pharmacology, IV:6.2t
Cortrosyn stimulation test, IV:2.2, 6.6
  for neonate, IV:6.3
Cost containment. See Health care cost(s), containment
Costoclavicular maneuver, in occlusive arterial disease, II:29.4f
Cosyntropin test, IV:10.6
Cough
  in carcinomatous pleurisy, III:8.6
  productive, in COLD, III:1.2t
Coumarin anticoagulants, drug interactions, with glucocorticoids, IV:6.5t
Country of origin, and interstitial lung disease, III:6.2
Coxsackievirus, myocarditis due to, II:19.6
Crackles, I:3.4, 3.10, 3.11t
Creatine kinase
  elevations, causes, II:11.2
  MB isoenzymes, II:1.7, 11.2
    in blunt myocardial injury, II:27.6–27.7
  MM isoenzymes, II:11.2
  with non-Q-wave MI, II:10.4, 10.4t
  with Q-wave MI, II:11.2
  with unstable angina, II:10.4, 10.4t
CREST syndrome, I:3.2, II:31.5
Critical care, III:10.1–10.8
Crohn's disease, cardiac involvement in, II:31.6–31.7
Cryptogenic fibrosing alveolitis. See Idiopathic pulmonary fibrosis
Cryptorchidism, IV:11.7
CT. See Computed tomography
Cushing's disease, IV:5.4, 5.5t, 5.5–5.6
  treatment, IV:5.9–5.10, 5.10t
Cushing's syndrome, IV:5.1, 5.4–5.11
  adrenal hyperandrogenism in, IV:10.3
  with adrenal tumors, IV:5.6, 5.6f
  and bronchogenic carcinoma, III:3.3t
  corticotropin-independent, treatment, IV:5.10t, 5.10–5.11
  definitive tests for, IV:5.7–5.9
  diagnostic tests for, IV:5.7f, 5.7–5.9
  ectopic, IV:19.3–19.4
    clinical features, IV:19.3–19.4, 19.4f
    diagnosis, IV:19.3–19.4, 19.4t
    referral guidelines, IV:19.4
    treatment, IV:19.4
  with ectopic corticotropin syndrome, IV:5.6, 5.6f
  endogenous, IV:5.4, 5.5t
  etiology, IV:5.4, 5.5–5.7
  findings in, IV:5.5t
  imaging in, IV:5.9, 5.9t
  with pituitary tumors, IV:5.5–5.6
  screening tests for, IV:5.7, 5.8t
  signs and symptoms, IV:5.4, 5.5t
  treatment, IV:5.9–5.11, 5.10t
CVD. See Atherosclerotic cardiovascular disease; Cardiovascular disease
Cyanosis, differential, II:22.6, 22.6f
Cyanotic lesions, congenital, II:22.9–22.12
Cyclophosphamide
  for collagen vascular disorders, III:6.8
  drug interactions, with glucocorticoids, IV:6.5t
Cyclosporine. See also Immunosuppressive therapy
  drug interactions, with glucocorticoids, IV:6.5t
  drug interactions with, II:34.6, 34.7t
  for viral myocarditis, II:19.5
Cyproterone acetate, for hirsutism, IV:10.8
Cyst(s), thyroid, IV:4.6, 4.6f
Cytomegalovirus infection, in heart transplant recipient, II:34.7
Cytotoxic agents
  for idiopathic pulmonary fibrosis, III:6.10
  for restrictive cardiomyopathy, II:18.3

D

Dallas criteria, for myocarditis, II:19.4, 19.4t
Danish Atrial Fibrillation, Aspirin, Anticoagulation study, II:30.4
Death, causes of, leading, III:2.2t
DeBakey classification, of aortic dissection, II:28.3, 28.3t, 28.4f
Decisions of conscience, I:8.2
Deep venous thrombosis, II:25.1–25.2, 29.7
  diagnosis, II:25.1–25.2, 29.7
  differential diagnosis, II:29.7
  prevention, II:25.2, 25.3t
  pulmonary embolism and, II:25.1
  recurrence, II:29.7, 29.8t
  treatment, II:25.2, 25.3t, 29.7, 29.8f
Defensive medicine, I:7.4
  costs, I:6.3
Degenerative joint disease, in knee, I:3.5
Dehydration
  in diabetic ketoacidosis, IV:15.2
  in elderly, IV:21.5
  in hyperosmolar hyperglycemic nonketotic coma, IV:15.4–15.5
Dehydroepiandrosterone sulfate, elevation, in females, IV:10.3, 10.5
3β-ol Dehydrogenase, deficiency, IV:11.5t
del Castillo's syndrome, IV:11.5
Demeclocycline, for SIADH, IV:1.6t
Dementia, screening recommendations for, I:2.7t
Depression, screening recommendations for, I:2.7t
de Quervain's disease, I:3.2
Dermatomyositis
  cardiac involvement in, II:31.2t, 31.6
  diagnosis, II:31.6
Dermoid cysts, clinical manifestations, II:26.3t
17,20-Desmolase deficiency, IV:11.5t
20,22-Desmolase deficiency, IV:11.5t
Desmopressin acetate, for diabetes insipidus, IV:1.3–1.4, 1.4t
Desoxycorticosterone acetate, pharmacology, IV:6.2t
Dexamethasone, pharmacology, IV:6.2t
Dexamethasone androgen-suppression test, IV:10.5–10.6, 10.7f
Dexamethasone-CRH test, IV:5.8, 5.8t
Dexamethasone suppression test, IV:2.2, 5.7–5.9, 5.8t, 5.9f

Dextrocardia, II:22.2
Diabetes Control and Complications Trial (DCCT), IV:16.1–16.2
Diabetes insipidus, IV:1.2–1.4
  causes, IV:1.2*t*
  central, IV:1.2, 1.2*t*, 1.3
  diagnosis, IV:1.2–1.3
  nephrogenic, IV:1.2
  treatment, IV:1.3–1.4, 1.4*t*
Diabetes mellitus, IV:14.1–14.6
  atherosclerosis in, IV:16.8–16.9
  cardiovascular disease and, II:7.6–7.7, 8.2
  cardiovascular risk factors in, IV:16.8
  chemotherapy and, IV:15.6
  classification, IV:14.1–14.2, 14.2*t*
  complications, IV:16.1–16.9, 16.2*t*. *See also* Diabetic nephropathy; Diabetic neuropathy; Diabetic retinopathy
    glucose control and, IV:16.1
    macrovascular, IV:16.1, 16.2*t*
    microvascular, IV:16.1, 16.2*t*
    pathogenesis, IV:16.2, 16.2*t*
  congestive cardiomyopathy and, II:17.2
  coronary artery disease in, IV:16.8–16.9
  diabetes insipidus with, IV:1.2
  diagnosis, IV:14.2*t*, 14.2–14.3, 14.3*t*
    in children, IV:14.3
    in pregnancy, IV:14.2–14.3, 14.3*t*
  in elderly, IV:21.1–21.3
  foot care in, IV:16.7–16.8, 16.8*t*
  foot ulcers in, IV:16.7–16.8
  glucocorticoid therapy and, IV:15.6
  and hyporeninemic hypoaldosteronism, IV:8.6
  impotence in, IV:12.5
  insulin-dependent (IDDM), IV:14.1–14.2, 14.2*t*, 14.3–14.4
    chemotherapy and, IV:15.6
    clinical features, IV:14.3*t*, 14.3–14.4
    diabetic ketoacidosis in, IV:15.1–15.4
    epidemiology, IV:14.3
    insulin requirements in, IV:14.4, 14.4*f*
    pathogenesis, IV:14.3
    treatment, IV:14.4
  lipoprotein abnormalities in, IV:16.8–16.9
  malnutrition-related, IV:14.5
  non-insulin-dependent (NIDDM), IV:14.1–14.2, 14.2*t*
    chemotherapy and, IV:15.6
    clinical features, IV:14.3*t*, 14.5
    diabetic ketoacidosis in, IV:15.1
    epidemiology, IV:14.4–14.5
    pathogenesis, IV:14.4–14.5
    treatment, IV:14.5, 14.5*t*
  occlusive arterial disease in, prognosis for, II:29.5
  peripheral vascular disease in, IV:16.7–16.8
  postoperative management in, IV:15.5
  in pregnancy. *See* Gestational diabetes
  preoperative surgical evaluation in, IV:15.5, 15.5*t*
  screening recommendations for, I:2.6*t*
  secondary prevention in, IV:16.1, 16.2*t*
  surgical management, IV:15.5, 15.5*t*, 15.6*t*
Diabetic ketoacidosis, IV:15.1–15.4
  complications, IV:15.3–15.4
  diagnosis, IV:15.2
  diagnostic criteria for, IV:15.2, 15.3*t*
  differential diagnosis, IV:15.2, 15.2*t*
  epidemiology, IV:15.1–15.2
  vs. hyperosmolar hyperglycemic nonketotic coma, IV:15.2*t*
  monitoring patients with, IV:15.3, 15.4*t*
  mortality with, IV:15.1–15.2
  precipitating factors, IV:15.2
  prevention, IV:15.4
  signs and symptoms, IV:15.2, 15.3*t*
  treatment, IV:15.2–15.3, 15.4*t*
Diabetic nephropathy, IV:16.4–16.5
  natural history, IV:16.4, 16.4*f*
  predisposing factors, IV:16.4–16.5
  screening for, IV:16.5
  treatment, IV:16.5
Diabetic neuropathy, IV:16.5–16.7
  autonomic, signs and symptoms, IV:16.6, 16.7*t*
  classification, IV:16.5–16.6, 16.6*t*
  clinical syndromes, IV:16.5–16.6
  treatment, IV:16.6*f*, 16.6–16.7
Diabetic retinopathy, IV:16.3–16.4
  natural history, IV:16.3
  risk factors for, IV:16.3
  screening for, IV:16.3, 16.3*t*
  treatment, IV:16.3–16.4
Diagnosis. *See also* Physical diagnosis
  hypothetico-deductive process, I:4.1
  pattern recognition in, I:4.1
  process, I:4.1
  strategies for, I:4.1
Diagnosis-related groups, I:6.4, 7.4
Diagnostic evaluation, II:4.5, 4.6*t*
Diagnostic tests, I:4.1–4.6
  for adrenocortical insufficiency, IV:5.13, 5.13*t*
  for Cushing's syndrome, IV:5.7*f*, 5.7–5.9
  interpretation, I:4.3–4.6
  likelihood ratios and, I:4.4*f*, 4.4–4.5, 4.5*t*
  for pheochromocytoma, IV:7.4, 7.4*t*
  post-test probability of disease and, I:4.5
  predictive value, I:4.3*f*, 4.3–4.4
  pretest probability of disease and, I:4.4, 4.5
  for primary aldosteronism, IV:8.2
  selection, I:4.2*t*, 4.2–4.3
  sensitivity, I:4.3*f*, 4.3–4.4
  specificity, I:4.3–4.4
  and treatment threshold, I:4.6
Diazepam, for MI, II:11.4
Diet, breast cancer and, IV:17.2*t*, 17.2–17.3
Dietary therapy
  for diabetes in elderly, IV:21.2
  for hypercholesterolemia, IV:18.3*f*, 18.3–18.6, 18.4*f*
  for hyperlipidemia, II:8.4–8.5
    practical aspects, II:8.5, 8.5*t*
  low-fat, IV:18.4
Differential cyanosis, II:22.6, 22.6*f*
Diffusing capacity, III:1.2
  alterations in, III:1.3*t*
  in asthma vs. COPD, III:2.4–2.5
  and degree of emphysema, III:2.4–2.5, 2.5*f*
  reduced, in COLD, III:1.2*t*
Digitalis glycosides
  for congestive heart failure, II:17.8
  drug interactions, with glucocorticoids, IV:6.4*t*
Digital rectal examination, in diagnosis of prostate cancer, IV:20.6*f*, 20.7
Digoxin
  for atrial fibrillation, with mitral regurgitation, II:12.6
  indications for, II:13.8–13.9
  with mitral stenosis, II:12.4
Dihydrotestosterone, in benign prostatic hyperplasia, IV:20.1–20.2, 20.2*f*
Diltiazem. *See also* Calcium channel blockers
  for angina, II:9.5
  dosage and administration, II:10.5
  indications for, II:10.5
Diphtherial myocarditis, II:19.7
Dipyridamole, perfusion imaging with, II:1.8
Dipyridamole-thallium imaging, in coronary artery disease, II:9.3

Disease interest groups, historical perspective on, I:7.2
Disk(s), intervertebral, herniation, I:3.3
Disopyramide, for hypertrophic cardiomyopathy, II:16.4
Diuretic therapy
  for congestive cardiomyopathy, II:17.9
  for congestive heart failure, II:17.8
  for elderly, advantages and disadvantages, II:32.5*t*, 32.6–32.8
  with mitral regurgitation, II:12.5–12.6
  with mitral stenosis, II:12.3–12.4
  potassium-depleting, drug interactions, with glucocorticoids, IV:6.4*t*
  for restrictive cardiomyopathy, II:18.3
  for right ventricular failure, III:5.5
Dizziness
  with myxoma, II:26.1
  in pregnancy, II:33.2
Dobutamine
  for congestive heart failure, II:17.8*t*, 17.9
  indications for, II:3.6
  for MI, II:11.6*t*
  for septic shock, III:10.6
Dopamine, IV:2.2*f*
  for cardiogenic shock, II:3.3–3.6
  for congestive heart failure, II:17.8*t*, 17.9
  for MI, II:11.6*t*
  prolactin secretion and, IV:2.3–2.4
  for septic shock, III:10.6
Doppler echocardiography. *See* Echocardiography, Doppler
Dowager's hump, I:3.3
Doxazosin
  for benign prostatic hyperplasia, IV:20.6, 20.6*f*
  indications for, IV:7.6–7.7
Doxazosin mesylate, for pheochromocytoma, IV:7.6–7.7, 7.7*t*
Doxorubicin, toxicity, congestive cardiomyopathy and, II:17.2
Doxycycline
  for malignant pleural effusions, III:8.9
  for secondary spontaneous pneumothorax, III:8.3
DRGs. *See* Diagnosis-related groups
Drug(s). *See also specific drug*
  abuse, screening recommendations for, I:2.7*t*
  associated with palpitations, II:4.5*t*
  effects, on thyroid function tests, IV:3.2*t*
  goitrogenic, IV:4.4
  hypoglycemia caused by, IV:14.6, 14.7*t*
  SIADH caused by, IV:1.4, 1.5*t*
  syncope and, II:5.2, 5.3
  syndrome of inappropriate antidiuresis caused by, IV:19.3, 19.3*t*
  toxicity, congestive cardiomyopathy and, II:17.1–17.2, 17.3*t*
Drug therapy, economics, I:6.6
Dry cough, in interstitial lung disease, III:6.1
Duck waddle test, I:3.4
Dupuytren's disease, I:3.2
Duroziez's sign, II:14.7
Duty of care, I:10.2
  breach, I:10.2–10.3
DVT. *See* Deep venous thrombosis
Dysfunctional uterine bleeding. *See* Abnormal uterine bleeding
Dyslipidemias, II:7.4–7.6. *See also* Hyperlipidemia
  in elderly, IV:21.3–21.4, 21.4*t*
Dyslipoproteinemia, postmenopausal, IV:22.5
Dyspnea
  in congestive cardiomyopathy, II:17.2
  exertional

Dyspnea (*continued*)
    in carcinomatous pleurisy, III:8.6
    with mitral stenosis, II:12.2
    in pregnancy, II:33.2
    in hypertrophic cardiomyopathy, II:16.2
    in interstitial lung disease, III:6.1
    mitral valve prolapse and, II:13.6, 13.6*t*, 13.7*t*
    with myxoma, II:26.1
    in pleurisy, III:8.2
    in pneumoconiosis, III:7.4
    in pregnancy, II:33.2, 33.3
    in primary spontaneous pneumothorax, III:8.2
    with pulmonary embolism, II:25.2
    in secondary spontaneous pneumothorax, III:8.3

E

Earlobe creases, II:1.5
Eating disorder(s), IV:1.1, 1.6–1.8. *See also* Anorexia nervosa; Bulimia nervosa
Eaton-Lambert syndrome, and bronchogenic carcinoma, III:3.3*t*
Ebstein's anomaly, II:14.9–14.10
    clinical features, II:14.9–14.10
    ECG findings with, II:14.10
    intracardiac repair for, sequelae and residua after, II:23.4
    management, II:14.10
    pathophysiology, II:14.9
Ebstein's disease, II:22.11–22.12
    in adult, II:22.2
    anatomy, II:22.11–22.12
    complications, II:22.12
    diagnosis, II:22.12
    echocardiography in, II:22.12, 22.12*f*
    pathophysiology, II:22.12
    physical findings with, II:22.12
Echinococcosis, myocarditis in, II:19.8
Echocardiography. *See also* Stress echocardiography; Transesophageal echocardiography
    of aortic dissection, II:28.4–28.5
    of aortic regurgitation, II:14.8, 14.8*f*
    with aortic stenosis, II:14.3–14.4, 14.4*f*
    for cardiac arrest survivor, II:6.4
    of cardiac sources for emboli, II:30.4
    with cardiac tumors, II:26.4, 26.4*f*, 26.5*f*
    in chest pain patient, II:1.6–1.7
    in congestive cardiomyopathy, II:17.4–17.5, 17.5*f*, 17.6*f*, 17.6*t*
    in constrictive pericarditis, II:21.6
    Doppler
        with atrial septal defect, II:22.2, 22.3*f*
        with interventricular septal defect, II:22.4, 22.5*f*
        left ventricular diastolic filling patterns on, aging and, II:32.2, 32.3*f*, 32.4*f*
        in restrictive cardiomyopathy, II:18.2
    in Ebstein's disease, II:22.12, 22.12*f*
    in evaluation for pericardiocentesis, II:21.7
    in heart failure, II:2.5, 2.5*f*
    in hypertrophic cardiomyopathy, II:16.3, 16.3*f*
    indications for, II:4.6*t*
    in infectious endocarditis, II:20.1, 20.6, 20.6*t*
    of mitral regurgitation, II:12.5, 12.5*f*
        with mitral valve prolapse, II:13.4, 13.5*f*
    with mitral stenosis, II:12.2, 12.3*f*
    of mitral valve prolapse, II:13.3*f*, 13.3–13.4, 13.4*f*, 20.3
    of myocardial contusion, II:27.7
    with myocardial infarction, II:11.2–11.3
    of patent ductus arteriosus, II:22.6, 22.6*f*
    of pericardial effusions, II:21.4–21.5

    in pulmonary hypertension, II:24.3
    in restrictive cardiomyopathy, II:18.2
    and syncope, II:5.4
    in viral myocarditis, II:19.3*f*, 19.3–19.4
Echovirus, myocarditis due to, II:19.6
Ectopic corticotropin syndrome, IV:5.6, 5.6*f*
    diagnosis, IV:5.8–5.9
    treatment, IV:5.10*t*, 5.11
Edema
    in constrictive pericarditis, II:21.6
    pharmacologic therapy for. *See* Diuretic therapy
Edinburgh Declaration of the World Council on Medical Education, I:9.3, 9.4*t*
Effusive-constrictive pericarditis, II:21.6
Ehlers-Danlos syndrome
    cardiac involvement in, II:31.2*t*, 31.7
    mitral valve prolapse with, II:13.1, 31.7
Eisenmenger's syndrome, II:22.4, 22.9–22.10, 22.10*f*, III:5.3
Ejection fraction, age-related changes in, II:32.1, 32.2*f*
Elderly. *See also* Aging
    acute myocardial infarction in, II:32.4–32.5, 32.6*t*
    arrhythmias in, II:32.8
    cardiovascular disease in, II:32.2, 32.4*t*
    chronic ischemic heart disease in, II:32.3–32.4, 32.5*f*, 32.5*t*
    coronary artery disease in, IV:21.3–21.4
    dehydration in, IV:21.5
    diabetes mellitus in, IV:21.1–21.3
        clinical features, IV:21.2
        dietary therapy for, IV:21.2
        drug therapy for, IV:21.2–21.3
        epidemiology, IV:21.1–21.2
        exercise therapy for, IV:21.2
        management, IV:21.2
    dyslipidemia in, IV:21.3–21.4, 21.4*t*
    endocrine disease in, IV:21.1–21.6
    fluid and electrolyte disorders in, IV:21.5–21.6
    hyperkalemia in, IV:21.5
    hyperosmolar nonketotic state in, IV:21.3, 21.3*t*
    hypertension in, II:32.5–32.8, 32.6*f*, 32.7*f*
    hyperthyroidism in, IV:21.4–21.5
        laboratory findings in, IV:21.5*t*
    hypothyroidism in, IV:21.4
        management, IV:3.3
    insulin therapy in, IV:21.3
    metabolic bone disease in, laboratory findings in, IV:21.5, 21.5*t*
    myxedema coma in, IV:21.4
    osteomalacia in, laboratory findings in, IV:21.5*t*
    osteoporosis in, laboratory findings in, IV:21.5*t*
    Paget's disease in, laboratory findings in, IV:21.5*t*
    salt-losing tendency in, IV:21.5
    serum cholesterol in, IV:21.3–21.4
    thyroid disease in, IV:21.4–21.6
    trophic hormone supplementation in, IV:21.6
    valvular heart disease in, II:32.8, 32.8*f*, 32.9*f*
    vasopressin secretion in, IV:21.5–21.6
    water intoxication in, IV:21.5–21.6
Electrocardiography. *See also* Signal-averaged electrocardiograms
    abnormalities on
        mitral valve prolapse and, II:13.6, 13.6*t*, 13.7*t*
        in scleroderma, II:31.5
    ambulatory, in patient with syncope, II:5.3–5.4
    with aortic regurgitation, II:14.8
    with aortic stenosis, II:14.3, 14.3*f*, 22.7, 22.8*f*
    in Chagas' disease, II:19.7–19.8
    in chest pain patient, II:1.5–1.6, 1.6*f*

    in congestive cardiomyopathy, II:17.3–17.4, 17.4*f*, 17.5*f*
    in constrictive pericarditis, II:21.6
    with Ebstein's anomaly, II:14.10
    event recording, II:2.5
        indications for, II:4.6*t*
    in heart failure, II:2.4*f*, 2.4–2.5
    in hypertrophic cardiomyopathy, II:16.3
    indications for, II:4.6*t*, 9.2
    in ischemia/infarction, II:1.5–1.6, 1.6*f*, II:10.2–10.4, 10.3*f*, 11.2, 11.2*f*, 11.3*t*
    with mitral stenosis, II:12.3
    with myocardial contusion, II:27.2
    with myocardial infarction, II:1.5–1.6, 1.6*f*, 10.2–10.4, 10.3*f*, 11.2, 11.2*f*, 11.3*t*
    with non-Q wave MI, II:10.2–10.4, 10.3*f*
    with palpitations, II:4.2, 4.2*f*, 4.4
    with pericardial effusion, II:21.4
    in pericarditis, II:1.6, 21.2, 21.2*f*
    pseudoinfarct findings, II:31.8
    with pulmonary embolism, II:1.6, 25.2–25.4, 25.4*t*
    with pulmonic stenosis, II:15.4, 15.5*f*
    in restrictive cardiomyopathy, II:18.2
    transtelephonic, in patient with syncope, II:5.3–5.4
    with tricuspid regurgitation, II:15.4
    with tricuspid stenosis, II:15.3, 15.3*f*
    24-hour monitoring, II:1.8
    with unstable angina, II:10.2–10.4, 10.3*f*
    in viral myocarditis, II:19.2–19.3
Electrophysiologic testing
    for cardiac arrest survivor, II:6.2, 6.4
    in congestive cardiomyopathy, II:17.4
    in heart failure, II:2.4–2.5
    in hypertrophic cardiomyopathy, II:16.3
    indications for, II:4.6*t*
Embolism/emboli. *See also* Thromboembolism
    aortic. *See* Aortic embolism
    cerebral. *See* Stroke, cardioembolic
    cholesterol. *See* Cholesterol emboli syndrome
    in infectious endocarditis, II:20.2–20.3
    with mitral stenosis, II:12.2
    paradoxical, stroke risk with, II:30.3–30.4
    pulmonary. *See* Pulmonary embolism
    systemic, with myxoma, II:26.1
Emphysema
    airflow obstruction in, III:2.2
    in COLD, III:1.2*t*
    definition, III:2.1
    physical diagnosis, I:3.4*t*
    physical findings with, I:3.11*t*
Employee Retirement Income Security Act, underfunding, I:7.4
End-diastolic volume, age-related changes in, II:32.1, 32.2*f*
End-inspiratory rales, III:6.1–6.2
Endocardial masses, noninfectious, II:20.6*t*, 20.7
Endocarditis
    culture-negative, II:20.6, 20.6*t*
    infective/infectious, II:20.1–20.8
        antibiotic prophylaxis for, II:12.3, 12.3*t*, 12.6, 14.5, 20.3–20.5, 20.7, 20.7*t*
        with aortic stenosis, II:14.5
        auscultatory findings in, II:20.3–20.5
        vs. bacteremia, II:20.7
        with bicuspid aortic valve, II:22.1
        blood culture in, II:20.1, 20.6–20.7
        clinical features, II:20.1–20.3
        complications, II:20.7, 20.7*t*
        diagnosis, II:20.5
        diagnostic criteria, II:20.1, 20.2*t*
        echocardiography in, II:20.1, 20.6, 20.6*t*
        etiologic agents, II:20.1

with mitral stenosis, II:12.2
with mitral valve prolapse, II:13.7–13.8, 13.8*t*
predisposing conditions for, II:20.1
prevention, II:20.3–20.5
after surgical repair for congenital heart disease, II:23.4, 23.6, 23.7
referrals for, II:20.7
severity, determination, II:20.5
signs and symptoms, II:20.1–20.3
tricuspid regurgitation caused by, II:15.4
with ventricular septal defect, II:22.5
Libman-Sacks, in systemic lupus erythematosus, II:31.4
mitral regurgitation with, II:12.4, 12.6
nonbacterial
thrombotic, stroke risk with, II:30.3
verrucous, in systemic lupus erythematosus, II:31.4
noninfectious, II:20.6*t*, 20.7
Endocardium, in rheumatoid arthritis, II:31.5
Endocrine disease, in elderly, IV:21.1–21.6
Endometrial ablation, IV:9.5
Endometrial biopsy
indications for, IV:9.4
in postmenopausal patient, IV:22.6*t*
suction cannulas for, IV:9.4, 9.4*f*
Endometrium, in perimenopause, IV:22.2
Endomyocardial biopsy
in infectious myocarditis, II:19.2
in myocarditis, II:19.4–19.5, 19.6
in restrictive cardiomyopathy, II:18.3
technique, II:19.4
Endomyocardial fibrosis, restrictive cardiomyopathy with, II:18.3
Endothelium, vascular, injury, atherosclerosis and, II:8.1
Endotracheal intubation, III:7.7
complications, III:10.7
End-systolic volume, age-related changes in, II:32.1, 32.2*f*
Enzyme-linked immunosorbent assay, in diagnosis of occupational asthma, III:7.3
Eosinophilia
pulmonary infiltration with, III:6.8
causes, III:6.9*t*
differential diagnosis, III:6.9*t*
drug-induced, differential diagnosis, III:6.9*t*
tropical, differential diagnosis, III:6.9*t*
Eosinophilic myocardial disease, restrictive cardiomyopathy with, II:18.3–18.4, 18.4*f*
Eosinophilic pneumonia, III:6.10*f*
chronic, differential diagnosis, III:6.9*t*
Ephedrine, drug interactions, with glucocorticoids, IV:6.5*t*
Epidural disease, I:3.4
Epinephrine
plasma, with pheochromocytoma, IV:7.2, 7.3*t*, 7.4, 7.4*t*
urinary, with pheochromocytoma, IV:7.3*t*, 7.3–7.4
EPOs. *See* Exclusive provider organizations
ERISA. *See* Employee Retirement Income Security Act
Erythema chronicum migrans, II:19.7
Erythema nodosum, III:6.2, 6.2*f*
Erythromycin
for acute bronchitis, III:4.2
for community-acquired pneumonia, III:4.5*t*
drug interactions, with glucocorticoids, IV:6.5*t*
Escape phenomenon, IV:8.1
Esmolol hydrochloride, intraoperative, with pheochromocytoma surgery, IV:7.7
Esophageal manometry, II:1.8

Esophageal pain, patterns of relief, II:1.4
Esophageal rupture
differential diagnosis, III:8.2
spontaneous, clinical features, III:8.4*t*
Essential hypertension. *See* Hypertension
Estradiol, plasma, measurement, IV:10.5
Estrogen(s)
and breast cancer, IV:17.2
deprivation
menopausal, IV:22.1
in menopause, IV:22.2–22.3, 22.3*t*
lipid-lowering therapy and, II:8.6, 8.7
Estrogenization
assessment, IV:10.5
normal, with normal FSH, and amenorrhea, IV:10.2, 10.2*t*
Estrogen replacement therapy, IV:21.6. *See also* Hormone replacement therapy
for dyslipidemia, in elderly females, IV:21.4
for hypoestrogenism, IV:10.6–10.7
postmenopausal, IV:22.3–22.5
beneficial effects, IV:22.3, 22.4*t*
contraindications to, IV:22.4, 22.4*t*
dosage and administration, IV:22.4*t*, 22.4–22.5, 22.5*f*, 22.5*t*
efficacy, IV:22.3
prescribing, IV:22.4*t*, 22.4–22.5, 22.5*f*, 22.5*t*
risks with, IV:22.4
Ethacrynic acid, for congestive heart failure, II:17.8
Ethical decisions, I:8.2
collaborative process for reasoned analysis in, I:8.4
Ethical norms, I:8.3
for medicine, I:8.3*t*, 8.3–8.4
Ethics, I:8.1–8.4
definition, I:8.1
grounding in human need, I:8.1–8.2, 8.2*t*
values and, I:8.2
ETT. *See* Exercise treadmill test
European Atrial Fibrillation Trial, II:30.5
Event monitor, II:2.5
indications for, II:4.6*t*
Exclusive provider organizations, I:6.4
Exercise
effects on serum lipids, IV:18.5, 18.5*f*
therapy, for diabetes in elderly, IV:21.2
Exercise echocardiography. *See* Stress echocardiography
Exercise perfusion scintigraphy, II:1.8. *See also* Myocardial perfusion imaging
Exercise radionuclide ventriculography, in coronary artery disease, II:9.3
Exercise (stress) testing
age and, II:32.4
aortic stenosis and, II:14.3
in asthma vs. COPD, III:2.5
cardiopulmonary, III:1.3
contraindications to, III:1.3*t*
indications for, III:1.3*t*
in coronary artery disease, II:9.2
in heart failure, II:2.5
indications for, II:4.6*t*
with mitral stenosis, II:12.3
Exercise tolerance, in pulmonary hypertension, II:24.2
Exercise treadmill test, II:1.7–1.8
Expert testimony, I:10.2–10.3, 10.3*t*
Expiratory film, in diagnosis of primary spontaneous pneumothorax, III:8.3, 8.6*f*
Exposure history, in diagnosis of pneumoconiosis, III:7.4
Extrinsic allergic alveolitis, III:6.1. *See also* Hypersensitivity pneumonitis
interstitial, differential diagnosis, III:6.3*t*

F

Fabry's disease, II:18.6
Facet disease, I:3.3–3.4
Familial Atherosclerosis Treatment Study, II:8.6, 8.7*f*
Farmer's lung, III:6.5
Fat, dietary
breast cancer and, IV:17.2*t*, 17.2–17.3
sources, IV:18.4–18.5
Fatigue
in congestive cardiomyopathy, II:17.2
in hypertrophic cardiomyopathy, II:16.2
FATS. *See* Familial Atherosclerosis Treatment Study
FDA. *See* Food and Drug Administration
Felon, I:3.2
Femoral artery, aneurysm, II:29.6
Fertile eunuch, IV:11.8–11.9
Fever
in infectious endocarditis, II:20.1–20.3
with noninfectious endocarditis or endocardial masses, II:20.6*t*, 20.7
Fiber, dietary, effects on serum lipids, IV:18.5
Fibric-acid derivatives, in lipid-lowering therapy, II:8.7–8.8, 8.8*t*
Fibrinogen, plasma, cardiovascular disease and, II:7.7
Fibroadenoma, of breast, IV:17.3, 17.4
Fibrocystic breast disease, IV:17.3
Fibroma, cardiac
clinical manifestations, II:26.3*t*
treatment, II:26.6
Fibrosis
endomyocardial, restrictive cardiomyopathy with, II:18.3
pulmonary. *See also* Idiopathic pulmonary fibrosis
caused by inorganic dust exposure, III:7.3
Finasteride therapy, for benign prostatic hyperplasia, IV:20.3, 20.3*f*, 20.4*f*
monitoring during, IV:20.3
side effects, IV:20.3–20.4
vs. transurethral prostatectomy, IV:20.4*f*, 20.4–20.5
Fine-needle aspiration biopsy, of solitary thyroid nodules, IV:4.7
Finger(s)
clubbing, III:6.2, 6.2*f*
locked, I:3.2
pain, stiffness, or dysfunction, I:3.2–3.3
trigger, I:3.2
Finklestein's sign, I:3.2
Flow volume loop
with emphysema, III:2.2, 2.3*f*
normal, III:2.3*f*
Fluid and electrolyte disorders, in elderly, IV:21.5–21.6
Fluid resuscitation, for septic shock, III:10.6
Fluorocortisone, pharmacology, IV:6.2*t*
Flushing, with niacin therapy, II:8.8
Fluvastatin, lipid-lowering therapy, II:8.8, 8.8*t*
Follicle-stimulating hormone, IV:2.2*f*
actions, IV:2.2–2.3
deficiency, in males, IV:11.8–11.9
immunization against, for male contraception, IV:12.7
inhibition, for male contraception, IV:12.7
response to GnRH, with varicocele, IV:11.1, 11.3*f*
response to gonadotropin-releasing hormone, IV:2.3
serum, in Klinefelter's syndrome, IV:11.3, 11.4*f*
Fontaine classification, of peripheral arterial disease, II:29.2, 29.2*t*

Fontan shunt, **II**:23.2*t*, 23.6*f*, 23.7
Food and Drug Administration, **I**:7.4
Foot ulcer(s), in diabetes mellitus, **IV**:16.7–16.8
Foramen ovale, patent, stroke risk with, **II**:30.3
Forced expiratory flow, in occupational asthma, **III**:7.2
Forced expiratory flow rate, during midportion of FVC, **III**:1.1
Forced expiratory volume, in 1 second, **III**:1.1, 1.2*f*
   in COPD, **III**:2.2, 2.3*f*
   ratio to forced vital capacity, **III**:1.1
   in COLD, **III**:1.2*t*
Forced vital capacity, **III**:1.1, 1.2*f*
Fractures and dislocations. *See also* Compression fracture
   anterior glenohumeral, **I**:3.6
   clavicular, **I**:3.6
Free thyroxine
   measurement, **IV**:3.1–3.2
   and nonthyroidal illness, **IV**:3.6, 3.6*f*
Free thyroxine index, **IV**:3.2
Friction rub(s)
   pericardial, **II**:1.5, 21.2
   in pericarditis, **II**:21.2
   pleural, **II**:1.5
Functional paraganglioma, **IV**:7.2
Functional residual capacity
   measurement, **III**:1.1–1.2
   in normal and disease states, **III**:1.3*t*
Fungal myocarditis, **II**:19.3*t*
Furosemide
   for congestive heart failure, **II**:17.8
   for right ventricular failure, **III**:5.5
   for SIADH, **IV**:1.6, 1.6*t*

G

Galactorrhea, with prolactinoma, **IV**:2.8
Gallium nitrate, for hypercalcemia of malignancy, **IV**:19.2*t*
Ganglion, **I**:3.2
Ganglion cyst, **I**:3.2
Gastric cancer, and malignant pleural effusions, **III**:8.7*t*
Gastrointestinal bleeding, with aortic stenosis, **II**:14.2
Gastrointestinal hemorrhage, diagnosis, **III**:10.7
Gemfibrozil, lipid lowering therapy, **II**:8.7–8.8, 8.8*t*
   clinical intervention trial, **II**:8.6
General anesthesia, SIADH caused by, **IV**:1.4, 1.5*t*
Genital(s), female, abnormal structure, **IV**:10.1, 10.2*t*
Gestational diabetes, **IV**:14.2, 14.2*t*, 14.6
   diagnosis, **IV**:14.2–14.3, 14.3*t*
Giant cell arteritis, **II**:28.5–28.6
   occlusive arterial disease and, **II**:29.2, 29.3
Giant cell myocarditis, **II**:19.6
Gigantism, **IV**:2.7
Glaucoma, screening recommendations for, **I**:2.7*t*
Glenn shunt, **II**:23.2*t*, 23.7
Glipizide
   for diabetes in elderly, **IV**:21.2–21.3
   for non-insulin-dependent diabetes mellitus (NIDDM), **IV**:14.5, 14.5*t*
Glucocorticoid(s)
   actions, **IV**:6.1
   adrenal cortex, **IV**:5.1–5.14
   clinical applications, **IV**:5.3–5.4
   deficiency, **IV**:5.1
      familial, **IV**:5.13
   drug interactions, **IV**:6.4, 6.4*t*, 6.5*t*
   effects on body, **IV**:5.3, 5.5*t*
   excess, **IV**:5.1, 5.4–5.11
   inhalation therapy, **IV**:6.4
   inhibition, **IV**:5.13
   intraarticular, **IV**:6.4
   mechanism of action, **IV**:5.3
   nasal, **IV**:6.4
   ophthalmic, **IV**:6.4
   plasma protein binding, **IV**:6.2
   receptors, **IV**:5.3
   resistance, **IV**:5.13
   for restrictive cardiomyopathy, **II**:18.3
   secretion, **IV**:6.1
   synthesis, **IV**:6.1
   synthetic, **IV**:6.1–6.2
   therapy with, **IV**:6.1–6.6
      adrenal suppression due to, **IV**:6.6
      compartmental administration, **IV**:6.3–6.4
      concomitant use of other drugs with, **IV**:6.4, 6.4*t*
      for congenital adrenal hyperplasia, **IV**:10.8
      in diabetic patient, **IV**:15.6
      dosage and administration, **IV**:6.1, 6.3
      indications for, **IV**:6.2–6.3
      monitoring of patient on, **IV**:6.4–6.6
      in pregnancy, **IV**:6.3
      side effects, **IV**:6.3, 6.3*t*
      systemic administration, **IV**:6.2–6.3
      tapering, **IV**:6.5, 6.6*t*
      termination, **IV**:6.5
   topical, **IV**:6.3–6.4
      complications with, **IV**:6.4
   withdrawal, **IV**:6.4–6.5
Glucocorticoid-remediable aldosteronism, **IV**:8.1–8.2, 8.4*f*, 8.4–8.5, 8.5*f*
   aldosterone secretion in, **IV**:8.5, 8.5*f*
   treatment, **IV**:8.5, 8.6*f*
Glucophage. *See* Metformin
Glucose tolerance
   abnormalities. *See also* Diabetes mellitus
      potential, **IV**:14.6
   age-related changes in, **IV**:21.1
   cardiovascular disease and, **II**:7.6–7.7
   impaired. *See* Impaired glucose tolerance
Glucose tolerance test, oral, **IV**:14.2*t*, 14.2–14.3, 14.3*t*
Glyburide
   for diabetes in elderly, **IV**:21.2–21.3
   for non-insulin-dependent diabetes mellitus (NIDDM), **IV**:14.5, 14.5*t*
Glycemic control, in prevention of diabetic complications, **IV**:16.1–16.2
Goiter
   approach to, **IV**:4.1, 4.2*f*
   in autoimmune thyroid disorders, **IV**:4.2–4.3
   colloid. *See* Goiter, nontoxic diffuse
   evaluation, **IV**:4.1, 4.8*f*
   in Graves' disease, **IV**:4.2
   in Hashimoto's thyroiditis, **IV**:4.2
   hereditary defects causing, **IV**:4.4
   in infectious thyroiditis, **IV**:4.5
   iodine, **IV**:4.4
   with lymphocytic thyroiditis, **IV**:3.6, 3.7*t*
   multinodular, **IV**:4.1, 4.3*f*, 4.3–4.4
      anatomic features, **IV**:4.3–4.4
      clinical features, **IV**:4.3–4.4
      treatment, **IV**:4.4
   nontoxic diffuse, **IV**:4.3
      clinical features, **IV**:4.3
      diagnosis, **IV**:4.3
      treatment, **IV**:4.3
   in systemic disease, **IV**:4.5
   toxic multinodular, **IV**:4.4
      treatment, **IV**:4.4
   treatment, **IV**:4.2–4.3
Goitrogens, **IV**:4.4
Gonadal cancer, screening recommendations for, **I**:2.6*t*
Gonadal dysgenesis, **IV**:11.4
Gonadotropin(s), **IV**:2.3
   deficiency, **IV**:2.3, 2.5
      acquired, in males, **IV**:11.9, 11.9*t*
   secretion, by pituitary tumors, **IV**:2.6*t*, 2.9
Gonadotropin-releasing hormone, **IV**:2.2*f*
   actions, **IV**:2.2
   agonist, test, **IV**:10.5
   analogues
      for male contraception, **IV**:12.7
      for uterine fibroids, **IV**:9.4–9.5, 9.5*f*
   FSH response to, **IV**:2.3
   immunization against, for male contraception, **IV**:12.7
   LH response to, **IV**:2.3
   response to, with varicocele, **IV**:11.1, 11.3*f*
   test, **IV**:10.5
Gonorrhea, screening recommendations for, **I**:2.7*t*
Goodpasture's syndrome, **III**:6.8
Graham Steell murmur, **II**:12.2, 33.2
Granulomatous vasculitis, chronic, differential diagnosis, **III**:5.2
Graves' disease, **IV**:3.3–3.4, 3.4*t*
   clinical features, **IV**:4.2
   diagnosis, **IV**:4.2
Ground glass haziness, **III**:6.4
Growth hormone, **IV**:2.2*f*
   actions, **IV**:2.3
   deficiency, **IV**:2.5
   drug interactions, with glucocorticoids, **IV**:6.4*t*
   hypersecretion, testing for, **IV**:2.3
   recombinant, **IV**:2.5
   replacement, **IV**:2.5, 2.6*t*
   reserve, testing for, **IV**:2.3
   secretion, **IV**:2.3
      by pituitary tumor, **IV**:2.6*t*, 2.6–2.8
   supplementation, in older men, **IV**:21.6
Growth hormone-releasing hormone
   actions, **IV**:2.3
   tumors producing, **IV**:19.5
Growth hormone-somatomedin axis, in anorexia nervosa, **IV**:1.7, 1.7*t*
Gynecomastia, and bronchogenic carcinoma, **III**:3.3*t*

H

Haemophilus influenzae
   in acute bronchitis, **III**:4.2
   in pneumonia, **III**:4.3, 4.3*t*, 4.4*t*
Haemophilus parainfluenzae, in acute bronchitis, **III**:4.2
HAIR-AN syndrome, **IV**:10.4
Hamartoma, cardiac, treatment, **II**:26.6
Hand(s)
   nerves in, screening examination, **I**:3.3*t*
   occlusive arterial disease from repetitive trauma, **II**:29.5, 29.5*f*
      clinical features, **II**:29.3, 29.5*t*
   pain, stiffness, or dysfunction, **I**:3.2*t*, 3.2–3.3
   physical examination, **I**:3.2, 3.2*t*
Hashimoto's lymphocytic thyroiditis, **IV**:3.2, 3.6
   clinical features, **IV**:4.2
   diagnosis, **IV**:4.2
HCM. *See* Hypertrophic cardiomyopathy
Head-up tilt testing. *See* Tilt-table testing
Health care
   access to, **I**:6.6–6.7
   and cost, **I**:7.2
   and quality, **I**:7.2

quality
    and cost, I:7.2
    threats to, I:7.4
rationing, I:6.4
Health care cost(s), I:6.1–6.3, 6.2f
    and changes in intensity of health care, I:6.3
    changes in volume and, I:6.2
    containment, I:6.3–6.4, 7.3–7.4
        possibilities for, I:7.5
        price controls and, I:6.4
        utilization review and, I:6.4
    defensive medicine and, I:6.3
    factors affecting, I:6.1–6.3, 7.2, 7.3
    health care system's responses to, I:6.4–6.6
    increased access to health care and, I:6.3, 7.3
    population changes and, I:6.2–6.3
    price inflation in, I:6.2, 6.3f, 7.3
    and technology, I:6.3
Health insurance
    availability, I:6.4
    cost containment and, I:6.3–6.4
    costs, public policy and, I:7.4
    data on, I:6.6
    expenditures, I:6.2
    historical perspective on, I:7.2
    and increased access to health care, I:6.3
    lack, I:6.6, 7.4
    models, I:6.4–6.5
Health maintenance organizations, I:6.4, 6.4f, 7.4
Health policy, I:6.1, 6.2, 7.1–7.5
    historical perspective on, I:7.1–7.2
Hearing loss, screening recommendations for, I:2.7t
Heart
    age-related changes in, II:32.1–32.2, 32.2f, 32.2t
    anatomy, age-related changes in, II:32.1–32.2, 32.2t
    left. See Heart failure, left-sided; Left heart; Left ventricular
    physiology, age-related changes in, II:32.1–32.2, 32.2f, 32.2t
    in pregnancy, II:33.1–33.5
    right. See Heart failure, right-sided; Right ventricle
    trauma to. See Trauma, cardiac
Heart disease
    amyloid, II:31.7–31.8, 31.7t
    carcinoid, II:18.6
    as cause of death, III:2.2t
    ischemic. See also Myocardial ischemia
        chronic, II:9.1–9.7
    in pregnancy, II:33.1
    risk factors for, in females, IV:22.3, 22.3t
    sudden cardiac death due to, II:6.1–6.2
    valvular. See specific valve; Valvular heart disease
Heart failure, II:2.1–2.10. See also Congestive cardiomyopathy; Congestive heart failure; Constrictive pericarditis
    angiography in, II:2.6, 2.6f
    blood/serum studies in, II:2.3
    in cardiac amyloidosis, II:31.8
    cardiac catheterization in, II:2.6, 2.6f
    causes, II:2.2
        clues for, II:2.2–2.3
    chronic moderate to severe (New York Heart Association functional class III or IV), management, II:2.8
    chronic stable mild (New York Heart Association functional class I or II), management, II:2.8
    clinical evaluation, II:2.7–2.8
    decompensation, management, II:2.8–2.9
    diastolic
        mechanisms, II:17.2, 17.3f, 17.4f
        treatment, II:17.9
    ECG findings in, II:2.4f, 2.4–2.5
    echocardiography in, II:2.5, 2.5f
    electrophysiologic testing in, II:2.4–2.5
    exercise testing in, II:2.5
    extent or severity, indicators, II:2.2
    follow-up evaluation, II:2.7–2.9
    in HIV-infected (AIDS) patient, II:19.6
    hypertensive, II:2.2
    hypotensive, II:2.2
    initial evaluation, II:2.1–2.7
    laboratory findings in, II:2.3, 2.8–2.9
    left-sided, II:11.4t
        with aortic regurgitation, II:14.7
        with aortic stenosis, II:14.2
        signs and symptoms, II:2.2
    management, II:2.7
    medical history-taking with, II:2.1–2.2
    myocardial biopsy in, II:2.7
    myocardial perfusion imaging in, II:2.7
    neurohumoral mechanisms, II:17.2, 17.3f
    pathophysiology, II:2.2
    pharmacohemodynamic evaluation, II:2.7
    physical diagnosis, I:3.3, 3.4t
    physical findings in, II:2.2–2.3
    physical findings with, I:3.11t
    prevalence, II:2.1
    prognosis for, II:2.2, 34.3, 34.4t
    pulmonary function testing in, II:2.7
    radiographic findings in, II:2.3, 2.3f
    right, signs and symptoms, II:2.2
    right-sided, II:11.4t
    signs and symptoms, II:2.1–2.2
    systemic diseases associated with, II:2.2–2.3
    systolic, in congestive cardiomyopathy, II:17.2, 17.3t
    treatment, II:17.7–17.9
    with ventricular septal defect, II:22.4
Heart murmur(s), I:3.6–3.8, II:1.5. See also specific murmur
    in acute rheumatic fever, II:31.1
    antibiotic prophylaxis with, I:3.6–3.7
    with aortic regurgitation, II:14.7–14.8
    with aortic stenosis, II:14.2–14.3, 22.7
    associated manifestations, I:3.2, 3.2t
    with bicuspid aortic valve, II:22.1–22.2
    coincident with first heart sound, II:20.2f, 20.3
    coincident with second heart sound, II:20.3, 20.3f
    continuous, differential diagnosis, II:22.6, 22.6t
    diagnosis, bedside maneuvers in, I:3.2, 3.2t, 3.3t
    diagnostic features, I:3.2, 3.2t, 3.7t
    diastolic, II:20.4
    differential diagnosis, I:3.2, 3.2t
    flow, II:20.2f, 20.3
        endocarditis prevention and, II:20.3
    Graham Steell, II:12.2, 33.2
    high-frequency, II:20.5
    holosystolic, II:20.3f, 20.3–20.4
    in hypertrophic cardiomyopathy, II:16.2f, 16.2–16.3
    in infectious endocarditis, II:20.1–20.2, 20.2f, 20.3f, 20.3–20.5
    intensity, I:3.2, 3.2t
    during isovolumetric contraction, II:20.3–20.4
    during isovolumetric relaxation, II:20.3–20.4
    lesions with, differential diagnosis, I:3.6, 3.7t
    location, I:3.2, 3.2t
    low-frequency, II:20.5
    with mitral regurgitation, II:12.4
    with mitral stenosis, II:12.2
    with mitral valve prolapse, II:13.1–13.4, 13.3f
    pansystolic, II:20.3f, 20.3–20.4
    physical findings with, I:3.2–3.3
    in pregnancy, II:33.2
    radiation, I:3.2, 3.2t
    referral for, II:5.5
    regurgitant, II:20.2f, 20.3, 20.3f
        endocarditis prevention and, II:20.3–20.5
        identification, II:20.3–20.5
        in infectious endocarditis, II:20.5
    systolic
        loudest at apex, I:3.3, 3.7t, 3.7–3.8
        loudest at base, I:3.2, 3.6–3.7, 3.7t
    timing, I:3.2, 3.2t
Heart rate, age-related changes in, II:32.1, 32.2f
Heart sound(s). See also Auscultation
    with aortic stenosis, II:14.2–14.3
    with coronary artery disease, II:1.5
    fourth, II:20.5
    with mitral stenosis, II:12.2
    in physical diagnosis, I:3.2, 3.3t, 3.4t
    second, with aortic valve lesions, I:3.2, 3.3t
    third, II:20.5
Heart transplantation, II:3.7, 34.1–34.9
    allograft
        physiology, II:34.5–34.6
        rejection, II:34.6, 34.6f, 34.7t
    for amyloidosis, II:18.5–18.6
    candidate for, evaluation, II:2.9
    complications, II:34.8, 34.8t
    contraindications to, II:17.8t, 34.4, 34.5t
    current results, II:34.1
    donor heart, physiology, II:34.5–34.6
    indications for, II:34.3f, 34.3–34.4, 34.3t
    infections after, II:34.6–34.7, 34.8f
    maintenance immunosuppression, II:34.6, 34.7f, 34.7t
    management, II:34.4–34.8
    in myocarditis, II:19.6
    number performed per year, II:34.1, 34.2f
    recipient
        accelerated coronary artery disease in, II:34.8, 34.8f
        hypertension in, II:34.8
        malignancy in, II:34.8
        pretransplant medical evaluation, II:34.4, 34.5t
        selection, II:34.3–34.4
        status criteria, II:34.4, 34.5t
    role of generalist in, II:34.8
    survival after, II:34.1, 34.2f
    waiting list for, II:34.3, 34.3f
    waiting time for, II:34.4
Heart valve(s). See also specific valve
    disease. See Valvular heart disease
    prosthetic, II:23.2, 23.2t
        pregnancy and, II:33.4
        stroke risk with, II:30.3
    replacement, for congenital heart disease, sequelae and residua, II:23.4
Heberden's nodes, I:3.2
Heerfordt's syndrome, III:6.5
Helminthic myocarditis, II:19.3t, 19.8
Helsinki Heart Trial, II:8.6
Hemangioma, cardiac
    clinical manifestations, II:26.3t
    treatment, II:26.6
Hematocrit, cardiovascular disease and, II:7.7
Hematologic disease, screening recommendations for, I:2.7t
Hemochromatosis, II:18.6–18.7
    male hypogonadism in, IV:11.10
Hemoglobinopathy, screening recommendations for, I:2.7t

Hemoptysis
  with mitral stenosis, II:12.2
  in pregnancy, II:33.3
Hemopump, indications for, II:3.7
Heparin therapy
  for deep venous thrombosis, II:25.2
  for MI, II:11.4, 11.6
    for secondary prevention, II:11.7t
  in pregnancy, II:33.4
  for pulmonary thromboembolism, III:5.6
Hepatitis B, screening recommendations for, I:2.7t
Hermaphroditism, true, IV:10.4
Herpes simplex, genital, screening recommendations for, I:2.7t
HHNK. See Hyperosmolar hyperglycemic nonketotic coma
High-density lipoprotein(s)
  coronary heart disease risk and, II:7.4–7.5, 7.5f, 8.4
  low levels
    cardiovascular disease risk with, II:8.2, 8.3
    management, II:8.3, 8.9
  serum, measurement, II:8.3–8.4
Hilar adenopathy, in interstitial lung disease, III:6.4t
Hilar enlargement, unilateral, and bronchogenic carcinoma, III:3.4, 3.4f
Hirsutism, management, IV:10.8
Hirudin therapy, for MI, II:11.6
Hirulog therapy, for MI, II:11.6
Histiocytosis X, III:6.8
  differential diagnosis, III:6.9t
  interstitial, differential diagnosis, III:6.3t
Histoplasmosis, differential diagnosis, III:6.9t
History-taking, in interstitial lung disease, III:6.3t
HMOs. See Health maintenance organizations
Hoarseness, with mitral stenosis, II:12.2
Holter monitoring, II:1.8
  in heart failure, II:2.5
Honeycombing
  with eosinophilic pneumonia, III:6.10f
  in interstitial lung disease, III:6.4, 6.4f
Hormone replacement therapy. See also Estrogen replacement therapy
  in perimenopause, IV:22.2
Hospital(s)
  bed availability in, I:6.6
  numbers of, in US, I:6.6
    historical perspective on, I:7.2
  use, trends in, I:6.6, 6.6f
Human chorionic gonadotropin production, by tumors, IV:19.6
Human immunodeficiency virus infection
  myocarditis due to, II:19.6
  screening recommendations for, I:2.7t
Humanitas, I:9.1–9.2
Humanities
  domain, I:9.1–9.2
  in medicine, I:9.1–9.6
  and sciences
    bidirectional relationship between, I:9.2–9.3
    dichotomy between, I:9.2
    metaphorical split between, I:9.3
Hümle cell tumors, IV:4.5
Hydralazine, for congestive heart failure, II:17.8
Hydrochlorothiazide, for diabetes insipidus, IV:1.4t
Hydrocortisone, IV:6.1
18-Hydroxycortisol, urinary, IV:8.4, 8.4f
11β-Hydroxylase, IV:5.1–5.2
17α-Hydroxylase, IV:5.1–5.2
  deficiency, IV:11.5t
21-Hydroxylase, IV:5.1–5.2
  deficiency, IV:10.3
    diagnosis, IV:10.6, 10.7f

Hydroxymethylglutaryl-CoA reductase inhibitors, in lipid-lowering therapy, II:8.8, 8.8t, 8.9
11β-Hydroxysteroid dehydrogenase, IV:5.2, 5.3f, 5.4, 8.4, 8.4f
3β-Hydroxysteroid dehydrogenase deficiency, IV:10.3
Hyperabduction maneuver, in occlusive arterial disease, II:29.4f
Hyperaldosteronism, IV:8.1
  treatment, IV:8.2t
Hyperandrogenemia
  differential diagnosis, IV:10.5–10.6, 10.7f
  idiopathic, in females, IV:10.4, 10.5f
Hyperandrogenism
  differential diagnosis, IV:10.5–10.6, 10.7f
  in females, IV:10.2–10.3
    adrenal and ovarian, relationship, IV:10.3–10.4, 10.5f
    differential diagnosis, IV:10.3t
    functional adrenal, IV:10.3, 10.3t
    functional gonadal, IV:10.3–10.4
    functional ovarian, IV:10.3–10.4
    management, IV:10.8
    tumoral, IV:10.5
Hypercalcemia, IV:13.1–13.2
  and bronchogenic carcinoma, III:3.3t
  causes, IV:13.2
  differential diagnosis, IV:13.2t
  tumor-related (hypercalcemia of malignancy), IV:19.1–19.5
    diagnosis, IV:19.2, 19.2t
    pathogenesis, IV:19.1–19.2
    referral guidelines, IV:19.2–19.3
    treatment, IV:19.2, 19.2t
Hypercapnia, differential diagnosis, III:5.2
Hypercholesterolemia, IV:18.1. See also Hyperlipidemia
  and cardiovascular disease, IV:18.2
  causes, II:8.2, 8.3, 8.3t
  dietary therapy for, IV:18.3f, 18.3–18.6, 18.4f
  familial, II:8.3
  genetic factors in, IV:18.2
  and nutrition, IV:18.3–18.6
  obesity and, IV:18.4
  screening recommendations for, I:2.6t
  secondary causes, IV:18.2–18.3, 18.3f
Hypercortisolism. See Cushing's disease; Cushing's syndrome
Hypereosinophilic syndrome, restrictive cardiomyopathy with, II:18.3–18.4, 18.4f
Hyperglycemia. See also Diabetes mellitus
  and diabetic complications, IV:16.2, 16.2t
  in diabetic ketoacidosis, IV:15.2
  management, IV:15.1–15.7
Hyperglycemic emergencies, IV:15.1–15.7
Hypergonadotropic hypogonadism, IV:10.2, 10.5
Hyperinflation, in occupational asthma, III:7.2
Hyperinsulinism, endogenous, IV:14.6, 14.7t
Hyperkalemia
  with aldosteronism, IV:8.1
  in elderly, IV:21.5
Hyperlipidemia, II:8.1–8.10
  causes, II:8.2, 8.3t
  coronary heart disease risk and, II:7.4–7.6
  dietary therapy for, II:8.4–8.5
    practical aspects, II:8.5, 8.5t
  drug treatment for, II:8.5–8.9
    clinical intervention trials, II:8.5–8.7
  familial combined, II:8.3
  management, II:7.6, 8.1–8.10
  treatment, nonpharmacologic modification trials, II:8.4–8.5

Hyperosmolar hyperglycemic nonketotic coma, IV:15.1, 15.4–15.5
  vs. diabetic ketoacidosis, IV:15.2t
  management of patients after, IV:15.5
  precipitating factors, IV:15.4
  treatment, IV:15.4–15.5
Hyperosmolar nonketotic state, in elderly, IV:21.3, 21.3t
Hyperparathyroidism
  in elderly, IV:21.5, 21.5t
  primary, IV:13.1, 13.2–13.4
    in asymptomatic patients, IV:13.4
      conservative management, IV:13.4
    biochemical features, IV:13.3
    bone changes in, IV:13.4, 13.4f
    clinical features, IV:13.3, 13.3t
    diagnosis, IV:13.3
    long-term follow-up, IV:13.4, 13.4t
    nonsurgical treatment, IV:13.4
    surgical treatment, IV:13.3
    surgical treatment, referral for, IV:13.4, 13.5t
  secondary, IV:13.2
Hyperprolactinemia, IV:10.2
  diagnosis, IV:2.9, 2.9t
  management, IV:2.10f, 2.11
  treatment, IV:10.7–10.8
Hyperreactive airway disease, in COLD, III:1.2t
Hyperresponsive airway disease, diagnosis, III:1.2
Hypersensitivity pneumonitis, III:6.5–6.7
  acute, symptoms, III:6.7
  clinical features, III:6.1
  diagnosis, III:6.7
  vs. sarcoidosis, III:6.7t
Hypertension. See also Glucocorticoid-remediable aldosteronism
  age and, II:32.5–32.8
  with aortic stenosis, II:14.2
  cardiovascular disease and, II:7.2f, 7.2–7.4, 7.3f, 7.3t, 8.2, 8.2t
  congestive cardiomyopathy and, II:17.1, 17.3t
  in elderly
    diagnosis, II:32.6
    treated, and cardiovascular risk, II:32.6, 32.7f
    treatment, II:32.6–32.8
  in heart transplant recipient, II:34.8
  prevalence, age and, II:32.5–32.6
  screening recommendations for, I:2.6t
  tumor-related, IV:19.6
Hyperthyroidism
  causes, IV:3.3–3.4, 3.4t
  clinical features, IV:3.1
  definition, IV:3.3
  diagnosis, IV:3.4
  differential diagnosis, IV:3.4, 3.5f
  in elderly, IV:21.4–21.5
    laboratory findings in, IV:21.5t
  goitrous, IV:4.2
  laboratory findings in, IV:3.1–3.2
  with lymphocytic thyroiditis, IV:3.6, 3.7t
  postpartum, IV:3.6, 4.3
  in pregnancy, management, IV:3.5
  signs and symptoms, IV:3.4, 3.4t
  treatment, IV:3.4–3.5, 3.5f
    choice of therapy, IV:3.5
Hypertriglyceridemia. See also Hyperlipidemia
  causes, II:8.2, 8.3, 8.3t
Hypertrophic cardiomyopathy, II:16.1–16.5, 22.7
  auscultatory features, II:16.2f, 16.2–16.3
  cardiac catheterization with, II:16.3
  chest radiography with, II:16.3
  classification, II:16.2f
  clinical course, II:16.3
  clinical features, II:16.2–16.3
  diagnosis, II:3.5t, 16.3, 16.3f

differential diagnosis, II:14.2t, 17.6, 17.7t
ECG findings with, II:16.3
echocardiography, II:16.3, 16.3f
electrophysiology in, II:16.3
etiology, II:16.1
familial, II:16.1
medical therapy for, II:16.3–16.4
morphologic features, II:16.1
nonobstructive, II:16.1, 16.2
obstructive, II:16.1–16.2, 16.2f
auscultatory findings in, II:20.4, 20.4f
in pregnant woman, II:33.5
pathophysiology, II:16.1–16.2, 16.2f
prevalence, II:16.1
prognosis for, II:16.3
subaortic pressure gradients in, II:16.1–16.2, 16.2f
sudden death and, II:6.2, 16.1
surgical therapy for, II:16.4
treatment, II:16.3–16.4
Hypoaldosteronism, IV:8.1, 8.5–8.6
treatment, IV:8.2t
Hypocalcemia, IV:13.1–13.2
causes, IV:13.2
in hypoparathyroidism, IV:13.4–13.5
hypoventilation with, III:9.2
in pseudohypoparathyroidism, IV:13.5
treatment, IV:13.5–13.6
Hypoestrogenism
with elevated FSH, IV:10.2, 10.2t
evaluation of patient with, IV:10.5
management, IV:10.6–10.7
with normal FSH, IV:10.2, 10.2t
Hypoglycemia, IV:14.6–14.7
classification, IV:14.6
definition, IV:14.6
diagnosis, IV:14.6
drug-induced, IV:14.6, 14.7t
fasting (postabsorptive), IV:14.6t, 14.6–14.7
treatment, IV:14.7
in infants and children, IV:14.7, 14.7t
in organ failure, IV:14.6, 14.7t
postprandial (reactive), IV:14.7, 14.7t
tumor-related, IV:19.4t, 19.5
Hypogonadism, IV:2.5
in males, IV:11.1–11.12
secondary, IV:11.7–11.9
Hypogonadotropic hypogonadism, IV:10.2
in males, IV:11.7–11.8, 12.3–12.4. *See also* Male hypogonadism
classic, IV:11.8, 11.8t
in systemic illness, IV:11.9
Hypokalemia, with aldosteronism, IV:8.1–8.2
management, IV:8.4
Hypomagnesemia, hypoventilation with, III:9.2
Hyponatremia, in SIADH, IV:1.4–1.5
management, IV:1.5–1.6, 1.6t
Hypoparathyroidism, IV:13.1, 13.4–13.5, 13.5t
Hypoperfusion
in cardiogenic shock, II:3.2
definition, II:3.2
detection, II:3.2
Hypophosphatemia
hypoventilation with, III:9.2
tumor-related, IV:19.5–19.6
Hypopituitarism, IV:2.1, 2.5
acquired, causes, IV:2.3t
congenital, causes, IV:2.3t
treatment, IV:2.5, 2.6t
Hyporeninemic hypoaldosteronism, IV:8.6
Hypospadias, IV:11.4, 11.5
Hypotension
in cardiogenic shock, II:3.2
definition, II:3.2

and shock, II:3.1–3.8. *See also* Cardiogenic shock
Hypothalamic disorder(s), diabetes insipidus in, IV:1.2
Hypothalamic failure, idiopathic, IV:1.2
Hypothalamic hormones, IV:2.1
Hypothalamic-pituitary-adrenal axis, IV:2.1–2.2, 5.3, 5.4f
in anorexia nervosa, IV:1.7, 1.7t
recovery, IV:6.6
Hypothalamic-pituitary axis, IV:2.1, 2.2f
Hypothalamic-pituitary-gonadal axis, IV:2.2–2.3
in anorexia nervosa, IV:1.7, 1.7t
Hypothalamic-pituitary growth hormone system, IV:2.3
Hypothalamic-pituitary prolactin system, IV:2.3–2.4
Hypothalamic-pituitary-thyroid axis, IV:2.1
in anorexia nervosa, IV:1.7, 1.7t
Hypothyroidism
after radioiodine therapy for hyperthyroidism, IV:3.4–3.5
causes, IV:3.2, 3.2t
clinical features, IV:3.1
definition, IV:3.2
diagnosis, IV:3.2–3.3, 3.4f
in elderly, IV:3.4
goitrous, IV:4.2, 4.4
laboratory findings in, IV:3.1–3.2
with lymphocytic thyroiditis, IV:3.6, 3.7t
postpartum, IV:3.6, 4.3
and respiratory drive, III:9.2
signs and symptoms, IV:3.3t
treatment, IV:3.3
Hypoventilation, III:9.2–9.3
carbon dioxide tension in, III:9.2f
causes, III:9.3t
clinical features, III:9.3, 9.3t
diagnosis, III:9.3
idiopathic alveolar, III:9.2
oxygen tension in, III:9.2f
treatment, III:9.3, 9.4f
Hypovolemia, hemodynamic parameters in, II:3.6t
Hypoxemia
differential diagnosis, III:5.2
exercise-induced, diagnosis, III:1.3
in pregnancy, II:33.3

I

Ideational environment, I:9.2
Idiopathic hypertrophic subaortic stenosis, I:3.6–3.7
differential diagnosis, I:3.2, 3.2t
maneuvers for, I:3.7, 3.7t
and syncope, II:5.4
Idiopathic pulmonary fibrosis, III:6.10
clinical features, III:6.1–6.2
diagnosis, III:6.10
interstitial, differential diagnosis, III:6.3t
Idiopathic pulmonary hemosiderosis, III:6.8
IHSS. *See* Idiopathic hypertrophic subaortic stenosis
Ileus, I:3.8
Iliac artery aneurysm, II:29.6
Imaging techniques, for lungs, III:1.3–1.5
Imipenem, for nosocomial pneumonia, III:4.7t
Imipenem/cilastatin
for community-acquired pneumonia, III:4.5t
for nosocomial pneumonia, III:4.7t
Immunoradiometric assay, of parathyroid hormone, IV:13.3
Immunosuppressive therapy

for heart transplant recipient, II:34.6, 34.7t
complications, II:34.6–34.8
and infections, II:34.6–34.7
for pneumoconiosis, III:7.5
for sarcoidosis, III:6.5
side effects, II:34.6, 34.7t
toxicity, II:34.6, 34.7t
in viral myocarditis, II:19.5
Impaired glucose tolerance, IV:14.1, 14.2t, 14.5–14.6
in elderly, IV:21.1–21.3
Impedance plethysmography, in deep venous thrombosis, II:25.1–25.2
Implantable cardioverter defibrillator, indications for, II:6.4–6.5, 17.9
Impotence, IV:12.5–12.7
definition, IV:12.5
diagnosis, IV:12.5, 12.6t
diseases associated with, IV:12.5
pathophysiology, IV:12.5
prevalence, IV:12.5
treatment, IV:12.6–12.7
intracavernosal injections of vasoactive compounds for, IV:12.6
penile implants for, IV:12.6–12.7
vacuum devices for, IV:12.6
Incidentaloma, IV:5.9
Indomethacin, for diabetes insipidus, IV:1.4t
Infection(s). *See also* Endocarditis; Myocarditis
after heart transplantation, II:34.6–34.7, 34.8f
cytomegalovirus, in heart transplant recipient, II:34.7
in diabetic patient, chemotherapy and, IV:15.6
streptococcal, and acute rheumatic fever, II:31.1–31.3
viral
congestive cardiomyopathy and, II:17.1–17.2, 17.3t
myocarditis due to, II:19.1–19.4
Infectious disease, screening recommendations for, I:2.7t
Infectious thyroiditis, IV:4.5
Inferior petrosal sinus sampling, IV:5.8t, 5.9
Inferior vena cava interruption, III:5.7
Infertility
definition, IV:12.1
history-taking with, IV:12.2
initial evaluation of couple, IV:12.2f
male, IV:11.4, 12.1–12.5
diagnosis, IV:12.2–12.4
etiology, IV:12.1–12.2, 12.2t
laboratory findings in, IV:12.2f, 12.3f, 12.3–12.4, 12.4t
pathogenesis, IV:12.1–12.2, 12.2t
treatment, IV:12.4t, 12.4–12.5, 12.5t
with varicocele, IV:11.1–11.2
physical findings with, IV:12.2–12.3
prevalence, IV:12.1
Inflammatory bowel disease, cardiac involvement in, II:31.6–31.7
Influenza
as cause of death, III:2.2t
myocarditis due to, II:19.6
vaccination for, III:2.6
Infrapatellar bursitis, I:3.4
Inhalants, toxic, classification, III:7.5t
Inhalation
of asphyxiants, III:7.6–7.7
of irritant-corrosive gases, III:7.6
of toxic fumes
causes, III:7.6
clinical manifestations and course, III:7.6–7.7
effects, III:7.6t

15

Inhalation challenge tests, III:1.2
Inhalation injury, III:7.5–7.7
    treatment, III:7.7
Injury Severity Score, and cardiac complications, in blunt chest-wall injury, II:27.4t, 27.5t, 27.5–27.6, 27.6t
Inorganic dusts
    fibrosis caused by, III:7.3
    in pneumoconiosis, III:7.3
Inotropic support. *See also specific agent(s)*
    in cardiogenic shock, II:3.3–3.6
Insulin
    deficiency
        in diabetic ketoacidosis, IV:15.2
        in hyperosmolar hyperglycemic nonketotic coma, IV:15.4–15.5
    drug interactions, with glucocorticoids, IV:6.5t
    resistance, in polycystic ovary syndrome, IV:10.4
Insulin hypoglycemia, IV:2.2
Insulin-like growth factor binding protein, IV:2.3
Insulin-like growth factor-I
    in acromegaly, IV:2.7, 2.8, 2.8f
    actions, IV:2.3
    production, IV:2.3
Insulinoma, IV:14.6–14.7
    treatment, IV:14.7
Insulin therapy
    in elderly, IV:21.3
    for insulin-dependent diabetes mellitus (IDDM), IV:14.4, 14.4f
    perioperative
        in diabetes mellitus, IV:15.5, 15.5t
        infusion rate, IV:15.6t
    in prevention of diabetic complications, IV:16.1–16.2
Interatrial septal defect. *See* Atrial septal defect
Interferon therapy, for viral myocarditis, II:19.6
Interleukin(s), and cortisol synthesis, IV:5.3
Intermediate coronary syndromes, II:10.1
Intermittent claudication, II:29.2, 29.2t
Interpreters, using, in interviewing, I:1.4, 1.4t
Interstitial lung disease, diagnosis, histologic, III:6.4
Interventricular septal defect, II:22.4–22.5. *See also* Eisenmenger's syndrome
    in adult, II:22.2
        prevalence, II:22.4
    complications, II:22.4–22.5, 22.5t
    diagnosis, II:22.4
    Doppler echocardiography with, II:22.4, 22.5f
    intracardiac repair for, II:23.5f, 23.5–23.6, 23.6f
    large
        pathophysiology, II:22.4
        physical findings with, II:22.4
    moderate-sized
        pathophysiology, II:22.4
        physical findings with, II:22.4
    pathophysiology, II:22.4
    physical findings with, I:3.3
    postinfarction, II:11.4t
    small
        pathophysiology, II:22.4
        physical findings with, II:22.4
    treatment, II:22.5
Interview, medical, I:1.1–1.6
    barriers to communication in, I:1.3
    chief complaint in, I:1.3
    collecting information in, I:1.1–1.2, 1.2t
    communicating information in, I:1.2, 1.3t
    developing therapeutic relationship in, I:1.2, 1.2t
    of difficult patient, I:1.5, 1.5t
    eliciting patient's belief system in, I:1.4, 1.4t
    environment for, I:1.2
    functions, I:1.1–1.2, 1.2t, 1.3t
    greeting the patient for, I:1.3
    interpreters for, I:1.4, 1.4t
    introduction phase, I:1.3
    narrative thread in, I:1.3–1.4
    negotiated priority in, I:1.3
    patient education in, I:1.4
    preparing for, I:1.3
    problem list in, I:1.3
    sexual history-taking in, I:1.4, 1.4t
    skills, improving, I:1.5–1.6
    skills for, I:1.1–1.2, 1.2t, 1.3t
    structural elements, I:1.2–1.4
    terminating, I:1.4
    in unusual or difficult situations, I:1.4–1.5
Intra-aortic balloon counterpulsation
    indications for, II:3.6–3.7
    for MI, II:11.4
    with mitral regurgitation, II:12.6
Intracerebral hemorrhage, with thrombolytic therapy, II:30.5
Intravenous immunoglobulin, for viral myocarditis, II:19.5–19.6
Iodine
    deficiency, IV:4.4
    radioactive. *See* Iodine-131
    requirements, IV:4.4
Iodine-131
    for hyperthyroidism, IV:3.4–3.5
    for thyroid nodule, IV:4.8
Iodine goiter, IV:4.4
Iopanoic acid, for hyperthyroidism, IV:3.4
Ipratropium bromide
    for acute severe asthma, III:10.4
    for COPD, III:2.7
        efficacy, III:2.8f
        effects, III:2.7
Irritant-corrosive gases, inhalation, III:7.6
Irritant gases, III:7.6t
Ischemic heart disease
    with amyloidosis, II:31.8
    chronic
        aging and, II:32.3–32.4
        diagnosis, age and, II:32.3–32.4
        prevalence, age and, II:32.3
        treatment, age and, II:32.4, 32.5t
    in pregnancy, II:33.4
    stroke risk with, II:30.2
Ischemic rest pain, II:29.2
Ischemic ulceration, II:29.2, 29.2f, 29.2t
Isoniazid, drug interactions, with glucocorticoids, IV:6.5t

J

Janeway lesions, II:20.2
Jones criteria, for acute rheumatic fever, II:31.1, 31.3t

K

Kallmann's syndrome, IV:11.8
Kawasaki syndrome, cardiac involvement in, II:31.6
Kerley's B lines, II:17.3
Ketoconazole, for adrenal tumor, IV:5.10t, 5.11
17-Ketosteroid reductase, deficiency, IV:11.5t
Kidney disease. *See* Renal failure; Uremia
Klinefelter's syndrome, IV:11.2–11.3, 11.3f, 11.4f
    laboratory findings in, IV:11.3, 11.4f
    phenotypic features, IV:11.3, 11.3f
    treatment, IV:11.3–11.4
Knee
    degenerative joint disease in, I:3.5
    examination, I:3.4–3.5, 3.5t
    pain or dysfunction, I:3.4–3.5, 3.5t
Kussmaul's sign, II:18.1, 21.6
Kveim-Stilzbach test, findings in interstitial lung disease, III:6.5t
Kyphoscoliosis, lung volumes in, III:1.3t
Kyphosis, thoracic, I:3.3

L

Labetalol, for pheochromocytoma, IV:7.7, 7.7t
Laboratory testing
    for cardiac arrest survivor, II:6.4
    in heart failure, II:2.3, 2.8–2.9
    with syncope, II:5.3–5.4, 5.4t
Lachman's sign, I:3.4
Lactate dehydrogenase, with MI, II:11.2
Lactic dehydrogenase, serum, findings in interstitial lung disease, III:6.5t
Lancisi's sign, I:3.3, 3.8
Langerhans' cell granuloma. *See* Histiocytosis X
Laser therapy
    for secondary spontaneous pneumothorax, III:8.3
    with thoracoscopy, for primary spontaneous pneumothorax, III:8.3
Lateral collateral ligament, tear, I:3.5
Lateral meniscus tear, I:3.4–3.5
Laurence-Moon-Biedl syndrome, IV:11.8t
Lead poisoning, screening recommendations for, I:2.7t
Left heart
    dilated, II:17.2f
    normal, II:17.2f
Left-to-right shunts, predominant, with normal or moderately increased pulmonary vascular resistance, II:22.2–22.7
Left ventricular diastolic dysfunction, pulmonary hypertension with, II:24.6
Left ventricular function, assessment, after surgery for congenital heart disease, II:23.6
Left ventricular hypertrophy, I:3.6–3.7
    with aortic stenosis, II:22.7
    cardiovascular disease and, II:7.7
    in elderly, and cardiovascular risk, II:32.5–32.6, 32.7f
    with hypertrophic cardiomyopathy, II:16.1, 16.2f
Left ventricular remodeling, postinfarction, II:11.4t
Left ventricular thrombus, postinfarction, II:11.4t
Left ventricular wall thickness, age-related changes in, II:32.1, 32.2f
Legionella species, in pneumonia, III:4.3, 4.3t, 4.4t
Legionella pneumophila, in pneumonia, III:4.3
Leopard syndrome, IV:11.8t
Leukemia, cardiac metastases, II:26.2–26.3
Leuprolide
    and flutamide, for prostate cancer, IV:20.8–20.9, 20.9t, 20.10f
    for prostate cancer, IV:20.8–20.9, 20.9t, 20.10f
Levothyroxine, for hypothyroidism, IV:3.3
Libman-Sacks endocarditis, in systemic lupus erythematosus, II:31.4
Licorice, and syndrome of apparent mineralocorticoid excess, IV:8.4
Lidocaine
    indications for, II:11.3
    for MI, II:11.6t
Lifestyle, cardiovascular disease risk and, II:8.2
Lightheadedness, with aortic stenosis, II:14.2
Likelihood ratios, I:4.4f, 4.4–4.5, 4.5t

Lipid(s), **IV**:18.1. *See also* Dyslipidemia
   beneficial effects of estrogen replacement therapy on, **IV**:22.4*t*
   blood/serum. *See also* Hyperlipidemia
      cardiovascular disease and, **II**:7.4*f*, 7.4–7.6, 7.5*f*, 7.6*f*
      measurement, **II**:8.2–8.4
         laboratory variation in, **II**:8.3–8.4, 8.4*t*
   elevation, secondary causes, **IV**:18.2–18.3, 18.3*f*
Lipid-lowering therapy
   clinical intervention trials, **II**:8.5–8.7
      effects on coronary artery disease, **II**:8.6–8.7, 8.7*f*
   combination therapy, **II**:8.8–8.9, 8.8*t*
   drug selection, **II**:8.7–8.9, 8.8*t*
Lipid Research Clinics Primary Prevention Trial, **II**:8.5–8.6
Lipodermatosclerosis, **II**:29.8, 29.8*f*
Lipoma, cardiac, clinical manifestations, **II**:26.3*t*
Lipomatous hypertrophy, cardiac, clinical manifestations, **II**:26.3*t*
Lipoprotein(s), **IV**:18.1
   beneficial effects of estrogen replacement therapy on, **IV**:22.4*t*
   serum, measurement, **II**:8.2–8.4
   triglyceride-rich, visual inspection, **II**:8.3, 8.4*f*
Lipoprotein abnormalities, in diabetes mellitus, **IV**:16.8–16.9
Lithium, goitrogenic properties, **IV**:4.4
Lithium carbonate, for SIADH, **IV**:1.6*t*
Liver, physical assessment, **I**:3.8–3.9
Locked finger, **I**:3.2
Loffler's syndrome, differential diagnosis, **III**:6.9*t*
Long-QT syndrome, **III**:6.2
Long-term care, **I**:6.6
Loop diuretics, for congestive heart failure, **II**:17.8
Los Angeles Veterans Administration Study, **II**:8.5
Lovastatin
   for dyslipidemia, in elderly, **IV**:21.4
   lipid-lowering therapy, **II**:8.8, 8.8*t*
Low back pain, **I**:3.3–3.4
Low back stiffness, **I**:3.3–3.4
Low-density lipoprotein(s)
   in atherosclerosis, **II**:8.1–8.2, 8.2*t*
   coronary heart disease risk and, **II**:7.4, 7.5*f*, 8.3–8.4
   serum
      decision cutoffs with, **II**:8.3, 8.3*t*
      measurement, **II**:8.3–8.4
Lower extremity
   neurological examination, **I**:3.3, 3.4*t*
   weakness, **I**:3.4, 3.4*t*
Lowe's syndrome, **IV**:11.8
Lung(s). *See also* Pulmonary
   abscess
      computed tomography scans, **III**:1.4*f*
      radiography, **III**:1.4*f*
      SIADH with, **IV**:1.4, 1.5*t*
   biopsies, in interstitial lung disease, **III**:6.4
   imaging techniques for, **III**:1.3–1.5
   in interstitial lung disease
      diffuse involvement, **III**:6.4*t*
      upper lobe involvement, **III**:6.4*t*
   neoplasms, **III**:3.1–3.7
   occupational and environmental exposure effects on, **III**:7.2*t*
   thermal injury to, **III**:7.7
      management, **III**:7.8*f*
      treatment, **III**:7.7, 7.8*f*
   transplantation
      for idiopathic pulmonary fibrosis, **III**:6.10
      for pneumoconiosis, **III**:7.5
      for pulmonary hypertension, **III**:5.5–5.6
   tumors
      benign, **III**:3.6–3.7
      malignant, **III**:3.7. *See also* Lung cancer
      metastatic, **III**:3.7
Lung cancer. *See also* Bronchogenic carcinoma
   cardiac metastases, **II**:26.2
   and malignant pleural effusions, **III**:8.7*t*
   metastasis to pleura, **III**:8.3
   screening recommendations for, **I**:2.6*t*
   SIADH with, **IV**:1.4, 1.5*t*
Lung compliance, decreased, **III**:6.4, 6.5*f*
Lung disease
   drug-induced, **III**:6.8
      interstitial, differential diagnosis, **III**:6.3*t*
   drugs and agents causing, **III**:6.8*t*
   hypersensitivity, **III**:6.1
   infectious, **III**:4.1–4.8
   interstitial, **III**:6.1–6.10
      causes, classification, **III**:6.2*f*
      chest roentgenographic changes in, **III**:6.2–6.4, 6.4*t*
      clinical features, **III**:6.1–6.4
      differential diagnosis, **III**:6.3*t*
      disease activity in, **III**:6.4
      history in, **III**:6.2
      inflammation in, evaluation, **III**:6.4
      laboratory and immunologic tests in, **III**:6.4, 6.5*t*
      lung function tests in, **III**:6.4
      lung volumes in, **III**:1.3*t*
      rheumatoid, differential diagnosis, **III**:6.3*t*
   occupational and environmental, **III**:7.1–7.10
   parenchymal, differential diagnosis, **III**:5.3–5.4
   restrictive
      differential diagnosis, **III**:1.2
      indicators, **III**:1.1–1.2
   rheumatoid, **III**:6.7*f*
Lung volumes
   in interstitial lung disease, **III**:6.5
   in normal and disease states, **III**:1.3*t*
   tests, **III**:1.1–1.2
Lupus pleurisy, clinical features, **III**:8.4*t*
Luteinizing hormone, **IV**:2.2*f*
   actions, **IV**:2.2
   deficiency, in males, **IV**:11.8–11.9
   inhibition, for male contraception, **IV**:12.7
   response to GnRH, with varicocele, **IV**:11.1, 11.3*f*
   response to gonadotropin-releasing hormone, **IV**:2.3
   serum, in Klinefelter's syndrome, **IV**:11.3, 11.4*f*
Lyme disease, **II**:19.7
   antibiotic therapy for, **II**:31.3, 31.4*t*
   cardiac involvement in, **II**:31.2*t*, 31.3
   myocarditis in, **II**:19.7
Lymphangioma, cardiac, clinical manifestations, **II**:26.3*t*
Lymphangitic carcinoma, **III**:6.1
   interstitial, differential diagnosis, **III**:6.3*t*
Lymphocyte transformation, findings in interstitial lung disease, **III**:6.5*t*
Lymphocytic thyroiditis, **IV**:3.6, 3.7*t*
Lymphoma(s)
   cardiac metastases, **II**:26.2
   and malignant pleural effusions, **III**:8.7*t*
Lymphomatoid granulomatosis, **III**:6.8
Lymphosarcoma
   cardiac, treatment, **II**:26.6
   SIADH with, **IV**:1.4, 1.5*t*
Lysine vasopressin, for diabetes insipidus, **IV**:1.4*t*

M

Machado-Guerreiro test, **II**:19.7

Macrolides
   for community-acquired pneumonia, **III**:4.5*t*
   plus rifampin, for community-acquired pneumonia, **III**:4.5*t*
Magnetic resonance imaging
   of aortic dissection, **II**:28.4–28.5
   with cardiac tumors, **II**:26.5–26.6
   in central diabetes insipidus, **IV**:1.3
   in congenital heart disease, **II**:23.3
   in deep venous thrombosis, **II**:25.1–25.2
   in diagnosis of bronchogenic carcinoma, **III**:3.4
   of pheochromocytoma, **IV**:7.5–7.6
   of pituitary, in Cushing's syndrome, **IV**:5.9, 5.9*t*
   of pituitary adenoma, **IV**:2.6, 2.6*f*
   in restrictive cardiomyopathy, **II**:18.3
Malathion inhalation, effects, **III**:7.5–7.6
Male hypogonadism, **IV**:11.1–11.12. *See also* Hypogonadotropic hypogonadism, in males
   in aging, **IV**:11.9–11.10
   in alcoholism, **IV**:11.10
   androgen replacement therapy for, **IV**:11.10
   combined primary and secondary, **IV**:11.9–11.10
   definition, **IV**:11.1
   diagnosis, **IV**:12.3, 12.5
   etiology, **IV**:11.1, 11.2*t*
   in hemochromatosis, **IV**:11.10
   with hepatic cirrhosis, **IV**:11.10
   in hypothalamic failure, **IV**:11.1, 11.2*t*
   laboratory findings in, **IV**:12.3–12.4
   prevalence, **IV**:11.1
   primary, **IV**:11.1–11.7, 11.2*t*
      diagnosis, **IV**:11.1, 11.3*f*
   secondary, **IV**:11.1, 11.2*t*
   in sickle cell disease, **IV**:11.10
   in systemic illness, **IV**:11.9
   in testicular failure, **IV**:11.1, 11.2*t*
Male pseudohermaphroditism, with androgen receptor defects, **IV**:11.6
Malignancy. *See also* Cancer
   as cause of death, **III**:2.2*t*
   SIADH with, **IV**:1.4, 1.5*t*
Malpractice, **I**:10.1–10.5
   definition, **I**:10.1
   medical. *See also* Negligence, medical
      and breach of duty of care, **I**:10.2–10.3
      and damages, **I**:10.4
      defenses against, **I**:10.4
      definition, **I**:10.1
      and proximate cause, **I**:10.3–10.4
Malpractice insurance, costs, **I**:7.4
Malpractice litigation, **I**:7.4
   defendant in, **I**:10.4, 10.4*t*
   defenses in, **I**:10.4
   potential claims as part, **I**:10.1, 10.2*t*
   and statute of limitations, **I**:10.4
Mammography, lesions seen on, referral guidelines for, **IV**:17.4
Managed care, **I**:6.4
Marfan syndrome
   cardiac involvement in, **II**:31.2*t*, 31.7
   mitral regurgitation with, **II**:12.4
   mitral valve prolapse with, **II**:13.1, 31.7
   in pregnant woman, **II**:33.4–33.5
Martsolf syndrome, **IV**:11.8
Mastalgia, cyclic, **IV**:17.3, 17.4
Mastitis, **IV**:17.4
McMurray's test, **I**:3.4, 3.5
Mean arterial pressure
   calculation, **II**:3.7*t*
   normal value, **II**:3.7*t*
Mebendazole, for trichinosis, **II**:19.8

Mechanical ventilation, III:10.6–10.7
　for adult respiratory distress syndrome, III:7.7
　assist-control, III:10.6
　for hypoventilation, III:9.3
　mechanism, III:10.6
　pressure-cycled, III:10.6
　synchronized intermittent mandatory, III:10.6
　volume-cycled, III:10.6
　weaning from, III:10.6–10.7
Medial collateral ligament, tear, I:3.5
Medial meniscus tear, I:3.4
Median nerve
　dysfunction, I:3.3
　screening examination, I:3.3t
Mediastinoscopy, in diagnosis of bronchogenic carcinoma, III:3.5
Medicaid
　coverage provided by, I:7.3
　expenditures, I:6.2
　historical perspective on, I:7.3
　and increased access to health care, I:6.3
　underfunding, I:7.4
Medical economics, I:6.1–6.7
Medical education, I:9.3
Medical history-taking, with heart failure, II:2.1–2.2
Medical interview. *See* Interview, medical
Medicare
　coverage provided by, I:7.3
　expenditures, I:6.2
　funding of graduate medical education, I:7.3
　historical perspective on, I:7.3
　and increased access to health care, I:6.3
　price controls and, I:6.4
　underfunding, I:7.4
MEDICS questionnaire, II:8.5, 8.6t
Medroxyprogesterone
　for anovulation, IV:9.4, 9.4t
　for menstrual irregularity, IV:10.8
Megestrol acetate, plus diethylstilbestrol or estradiol, for prostate cancer, IV:20.9, 20.11f
Melanoma, cardiac metastases, II:26.2
Menarche, age at, IV:10.1
Menopause, IV:22.1–22.6
　beginning, IV:22.1–22.2
　cardiovascular disease in, IV:22.3
　symptoms, not attributable to estrogen deprivation, IV:22.5
　tests for, IV:22.2t
　vasomotor symptoms in, IV:22.2–22.3
Menstrual blood loss, IV:9.1, 9.2f
　NSAIDs that decrease, IV:9.4, 9.5t
Menstrual cycle, IV:9.1, 9.2f
　length, IV:10.1, 10.2f
Mental disorder(s), screening recommendations for, I:2.7t
Mesothelioma
　cardiac, II:26.2
　pericardial, clinical manifestations, II:26.3t
Metabolic bone disease, in elderly, laboratory findings in, IV:21.5, 21.5t
[131I]Metaiodobenzylguanidine
　structure, IV:7.5, 7.5f
[131I]Metaiodobenzylguanidine scan
　of adrenal tissue, IV:7.5–7.6, 7.6f
　of pheochromocytoma, IV:7.5–7.6, 7.6f
Metanephrine, urinary, with pheochromocytoma, IV:7.3t, 7.3–7.4
Metaproterenol, for acute severe asthma, III:10.4
Metazoal myocarditis, II:19.3t, 19.8
Metformin, for non-insulin-dependent diabetes mellitus (NIDDM), IV:14.5
Methacholine challenge test, III:1.2

　in asthma vs. COPD, III:2.5
　contraindications to, III:1.2
　positive, in COLD, III:1.2t
Methimazole, for hyperthyroidism, IV:3.4
Methotrexate, for collagen vascular disorders, III:6.8
Methylprednisolone
　for acute severe asthma, III:10.4
　pharmacology, IV:6.2t
Methylxanthine, side effects, III:10.4
Metolazone
　for congestive heart failure, II:17.8
　for right ventricular failure, III:5.5
Metoprolol
　for congestive heart failure, II:17.9
　for MI, II:11.4
Metyrapone, for adrenal tumor, IV:5.10t, 5.11
Metyrapone test, IV:2.2
Mezlocillin, for nosocomial pneumonia, III:4.7t
MIBG. *See* [131I]Metaiodobenzylguanidine
Micronutrients, effects on serum lipids, IV:18.5–18.6
Miliary tuberculosis, interstitial, differential diagnosis, III:6.3
Milrinone. *See* Amrinone
Mineralocorticoid(s)
　deficiency, IV:5.1
　excess, IV:8.1–8.2. *See also* Syndrome of apparent mineralocorticoid excess
　　treatment, IV:8.2t
　pharmacology, IV:6.2t
Minocycline
　intrapleural, for primary spontaneous pneumothorax, III:8.3
　as sclerosing agent, for malignant pleural effusions, III:8.9
　for secondary spontaneous pneumothorax, III:8.3
Mitotane
　for adrenal tumor, IV:5.10t, 5.11
　drug interactions, with glucocorticoids, IV:6.5t
Mitral facies, II:12.2
Mitral valve
　insufficiency, acute, diagnosis, II:3.4t
　leaflet, systolic anterior motion, in hypertrophic cardiomyopathy, II:16.1–16.2, 16.2f
　prolapse, I:3.7t, 3.7–3.8, II:13.1–13.9
　　artifactual, II:13.4, 13.5f
　　auscultatory features, II:13.1–13.4, 13.2f, 13.6t, 20.4, 20.4f, 20.5
　　clinical features, II:13.5–13.6, 13.6t
　　complications, II:13.6–13.8, 13.7t
　　in connective-tissue disorders, II:13.1, 31.7
　　diagnosis, II:13.1–13.4
　　echocardiography with, II:13.3f, 13.3–13.4, 13.4f
　　echo-only, II:20.3
　　extracardiac features, II:13.5–13.6, 13.6t
　　management, II:13.8–13.9, 13.8t
　　maneuvers affecting, II:13.2f, 13.2–13.3, 13.3f
　　overdiagnosis, by echocardiography, II:20.3
　　pathophysiology, II:13.1, 13.2f
　　physical findings with, I:3.3, II:1.5
　　in pregnancy, II:33.4
　　prevalence, II:13.1
　　primary, II:13.1
　　secondary, II:13.1
　　sex distribution, II:13.1
　　stroke risk with, II:30.3
　regurgitation, II:12.4–12.6
　　auscultatory features, II:16.2f, 20.5, 20.6t
　　clinical features, II:12.5
　　differential diagnosis, II:14.2t

　　echocardiography with, II:12.5, 12.5f, 13.4, 13.5f
　　etiology, II:12.4, 12.4t
　　laboratory findings with, II:12.5
　　management, II:12.5–12.6
　　with mitral valve prolapse, II:13.6–13.7, 13.7f
　　pathophysiology, II:12.4
　　physical findings with, I:3.3
　　postoperative, with intracardiac repair for congenital heart disease, II:23.2, 23.2t
　　in pregnancy, II:33.4
　　referrals for, II:12.6
　　with rheumatic fever, II:12.4
　regurgitation (insufficiency), I:3.7t, 3.7–3.8
　replacement, age and, II:32.8
　rheumatic, stroke risk with, II:30.2–30.3
　stenosis, II:12.1–12.4
　　age and, II:32.8
　　auscultatory features, II:15.3, 15.3t
　　clinical features, II:12.2
　　diagnosis, II:3.5t
　　ECG findings with, II:12.3
　　echocardiography with, II:12.2, 12.3f
　　etiology, II:12.1–12.2, 12.2t
　　laboratory findings with, II:12.2–12.3
　　management, II:12.3–12.4, 12.4t
　　pathophysiology, II:12.1–12.2
　　postoperative, with intracardiac repair for congenital heart disease, II:23.2, 23.2t
　　pulmonary hypertension with, II:24.6
　　referral for, II:12.4
　　in reproductive-age women, II:33.2–33.3
　　rheumatic fever and, II:12.1–12.2, 12.2t
　　scoring system for, II:12.2–12.3
Molecular biology
　in screening, I:2.7
　in therapy, I:2.7
Moraxella catarrhalis
　in acute bronchitis, III:4.2
　in pneumonia, III:4.3t, 4.4t
Morphine sulfate, for MI, II:11.4
Mortality rate, interventions affecting, and total deaths prevented, I:2.2, 2.2t
Motivational skills, I:1.2, 1.3t
MRI. *See* Magnetic resonance imaging
Mucous membranes
　color, I:3.10
　examination, I:3.4, 3.10
Multicenter Unsustained Tachycardia Trial (MUSTT), II:6.6
Multiple endocrine neoplasia
　type I, thyroid nodules in, IV:4.6
　type II, IV:7.1, 7.2
　　pheochromocytoma in, IV:7.1–7.2
　　thyroid nodules in, IV:4.6
Multiple lentigines, IV:11.8t
Multiple Risk Factor Intervention Trial, II:8.2, 8.2f, 8.5, IV:18.2, 18.2t
Multiple system organ failure, III:10.4–10.5
　causes, III:10.4–10.5
　criteria for, III:10.5t
　therapy for, III:10.5
Multisystem atrophy, IV:1.2
Mumps, orchitis, IV:11.7
Murmurs. *See* Heart murmur(s)
Mustard repair, II:23.2t, 23.4f, 23.5
MVP. *See* Mitral valve, prolapse
Mycobacterium tuberculosis, III:4.3t, 4.4, 4.4t
Mycoplasma pneumoniae
　in acute bronchitis, III:4.2
　in pneumonia, III:4.3, 4.3t, 4.4t
Myocardial biopsy, in heart failure, II:2.7
Myocardial contusion, II:27.1–27.7

complications, II:27.3, 27.3t
diagnostic criteria, II:27.1–27.7, 27.2t
ECG findings with, II:27.2
echocardiography, II:27.7
imaging, II:27.7
mechanism of injury, II:27.2, 27.2f, 27.2t
vs. myocardial infarction, II:27.2
outcome with, II:27.2–27.3, 27.3t
predictors for, II:27.3–27.6
probability, calculation using ISS and ECG, II:27.6, 27.6t
radionuclide angiography, II:27.7
transesophageal echocardiography, II:27.7
triage algorithm for, II:27.3–27.5
Myocardial infarct/infarction
 acute
  diagnosis, age and, II:32.5, 32.6t
  in elderly, II:32.6t
  onset, circadian variation in, II:11.1
  prevalence, age and, II:32.4
  signs and symptoms, II:11.1–11.2
  stroke risk with, II:30.2
  treatment, age and, II:32.5
 arrhythmic complications, II:11.3
 asymptomatic, II:1.3
 cardiac arrest with, II:6.1–6.2
 cardiogenic shock complicating, II:3.3, 3.3f
 conduction disturbances with, II:11.3
 with coronary trauma, II:27.8
 diagnosis, II:3.4t
 drug therapy for, II:11.4–11.5, 11.6t, 11.7t
 ECG findings with, II:1.5–1.6, 1.6f; 11.2, 11.2f, 11.3t
 echocardiography with, II:11.2–11.3
 emergency evaluation for, II:1.7
 expansion, II:11.4t
 extension, II:11.4t
 hemodynamic complications, II:11.3, 11.4t, 11.5t
 imaging, II:11.2–11.3
 laboratory findings with, II:11.2
 lipid-lowering therapy after, clinical intervention trial, II:8.6
 location, ECG leads indicating, II:11.2, 11.3t
 long-term management strategies, II:11.7, 11.8f
 mechanical complications, II:11.3, 11.4t
 mortality, in-hospital, II:3.1
 non-Q wave, II:10.1–10.6, 11.1
  cardiology consultation and, II:10.5
  coronary arteriography and intervention with, II:10.5, 10.5f
  creatine kinase with, II:10.4, 10.4t
  diagnosis, II:10.2
  diagnostic testing with, II:10.2–10.4
  ECG findings with, II:10.2–10.4, 10.3f
  emergency treatment, II:10.5
  history-taking with, II:10.2
  hospitalization for, II:10.5
  initial assessment for, II:10.2
  laboratory testing with, II:10.2
  pathophysiology, II:10.1, 10.2f
  physical examination with, II:10.2
  treatment, II:10.4f, 10.4–10.5
 pain, II:1.2
 pathophysiology, II:10.1, 10.2f
 pericarditis and, II:21.1
  management, II:21.3–21.4
 postinfarction evaluation, II:11.7, 11.8f
 in pregnancy, II:33.4
 prognostic factors in, II:11.7
 Q-wave, II:11.1–11.9
  diagnosis, II:11.1–11.3
  diagnostic criteria, II:11.1
  management, II:11.4–11.7
  physical findings with, II:11.1–11.2

 radionuclide scintigraphy with, II:11.3
 radionuclide ventriculography with, II:11.3
 secondary prevention, chronic drug therapy for, II:11.7t
 serum lipids after, II:8.4
 temporary pacing and, II:11.3
 thrombolytic therapy for, II:11.4, 11.5–11.6, 11.5t
  contraindications to, II:11.6–11.7
  early adjunctive therapy with, II:11.6
  recommendation for, II:11.6–11.7
 treatment
  angioplasty in, II:11.7
  early adjunctive therapy with thrombolysis, II:11.6
  long-term adjunctive therapy, II:11.7
Myocardial ischemia, II:9.1–9.7. See also Myocardial infarct/infarction
 asymptomatic, II:1.3
 clinical features, II:9.1–9.2
 ECG findings with, II:1.5–1.6, 1.6f
 emergency evaluation for, II:1.7
 vs. esophageal pain, II:1.1
 noninvasive tests for, II:1.7–1.8
 pain with, II:1.1–1.3
  characteristics, II:1.3f, 1.3–1.4
  duration, II:1.3
  inciting factors, II:1.3–1.4
  patterns of relief, II:1.4
 physical findings with, II:1.4–1.5
 with pulmonary edema, II:1.5
 silent, age and, II:32.4
 threshold for, II:9.2, 9.2f
Myocardial oxygen supply and demand
 β-adrenergic blockers and, II:9.3f
 calcium channel blockers and, II:9.3f
 determinants, II:9.1
 nitrates and, II:9.3f
Myocardial perfusion imaging, II:1.8. See also Dipyridamole-thallium imaging
 in heart failure, II:2.7
Myocarditis
 acute, II:19.4–19.5
  clinical spectrum, II:19.1
 asymptomatic, II:19.1
 bacterial, II:19.3t, 19.7
 catecholamine, IV:7.3
  with pheochromocytoma, IV:7.3
 of Chagas' disease, II:19.7–19.8
 chronic active, II:19.4–19.5
 chronic persistent, II:19.4–19.5
 clinicopathologic classification, II:19.4
 coxsackievirus, II:19.6
 definition, II:19.1
 diagnosis, II:3.4t
 diphtherial, II:19.7
 echovirus, II:19.6
 endomyocardial biopsy in, II:19.4–19.5, 19.6
 fulminant, II:19.4–19.5
 fungal, II:19.3t
 giant cell, II:19.6
 heart transplantation in, II:19.6
 helminthic, II:19.3t, 19.8
 histology, Dallas criteria for, II:19.4, 19.4t
 human immunodeficiency virus, II:19.6
 incidence, II:19.1
 infectious
  acute, autoimmune mechanism, II:19.2
  autoimmune mechanism, II:19.2
  chronic, autoimmune mechanism, II:19.2
  disease mechanism, II:19.1–19.2, 19.2f
  endomyocardial biopsy in, II:19.2
  etiologies, II:19.2, 19.3t
 influenza, II:19.6

 in Lyme disease, II:19.7
 metazoal, II:19.3t, 19.8
 in polymyositis and dermatomyositis, II:31.6
 protozoal, II:19.3t. See also Toxoplasmosis; Trypanosomiasis
 rickettsial, II:19.3t
 spirochetal, II:19.3t
 streptococcal, II:19.7
 in toxoplasmosis, II:19.8
 viral, II:2.2, 19.1–19.4
  antimyosin antibody imaging in, II:19.4
  clinical course, II:19.5–19.6
  diagnosis, II:19.2
  ECG findings with, II:19.2–19.3
  echocardiography in, II:19.3f, 19.3–19.4
  histology, II:19.4, 19.4t, 19.5f
  incidence, II:19.1
  signs and symptoms, II:19.2
  specific agents, II:19.6
  treatment, II:19.5–19.6
Myocardium
 in rheumatoid arthritis, II:31.5
 in scleroderma, II:31.5
 stunned, II:1.5
 in systemic lupus erythematosus, II:31.4
Myosin heavy chain, gene mutations, and hypertrophic cardiomyopathy, II:16.1
Myotonic dystrophy, IV:11.4
Myxedema coma, IV:3.3
 in elderly, IV:21.4
Myxoma(s), II:26.1–26.2
 atrial, II:30.3, 30.3f
 auscultatory features, II:26.2
 clinical manifestations, II:26.1, 26.2t
 conditions mimicked by, II:26.3t
 familial, II:26.2
 location, II:26.2t
 recurrence, II:26.6
 treatment, II:26.6

N

Nail beds, examination, I:3.4
Nails
 clubbing, I:3.4, 3.10–3.11
 color, I:3.10
 examination, I:3.10
National health expenditures, I:6.1–6.3, 6.2f, 7.3. See also Health care cost(s)
Near-syncope
 and congestive cardiomyopathy, II:17.9, 17.9f
 evaluation, II:2.5
 in hypertrophic cardiomyopathy, II:16.2
Negligence
 contributory, I:10.4
 medical
  claims for, standards for establishing, I:10.1–10.4
  definition, I:10.1–10.2
Nelson's syndrome, IV:5.9–5.10
Neoplasms, of lung, III:3.1–3.7
Nephropathy, diabetic. See Diabetic nephropathy
Neuroendocrinology, IV:1.1–1.8
Neurofibromatosis, pheochromocytoma and, IV:7.1
Neurological examination, of lower extremity, I:3.3, 3.4t
Neurologic ischemic events, with mitral valve prolapse, II:13.8
Neuromuscular disease(s)
 acute respiratory failure with, III:10.1, 10.4, 10.4t
 lung volumes in, III:1.3t

19

Neuropathy
  amyloid-induced, II:31.8
  diabetic. *See* Diabetic neuropathy
New York Heart Association, functional classification, II:2.8, 17.5–17.6, 17.7*t*
Niacin
  flushing with, II:8.8
  lipid-lowering therapy, II:8.8, 8.8*t*
    clinical intervention trial, II:8.6
Nicotine replacement, effects, on smoking cessation, III:2.6, 2.7*f*
Nicotinic acid, lipid-lowering therapy, II:8.8, 8.8*t*
Nifurtimox, for Chagas' disease, II:19.8
Nitrates
  for angina, II:9.4–9.5
  for congestive heart failure, II:17.8
  effects on myocardial oxygen supply and demand, II:9.3*f*
  mechanism of action, II:9.4
  for MI, II:11.4
Nitroglycerin
  for MI, II:11.6*t*
  for unstable angina, II:10.5
Nitroprusside
  for MI, II:11.6*t*
  for mitral regurgitation, II:12.5–12.6
Noninvasive cardiac testing, II:1.7–1.8, 9.2. *See also specific modality*
Nonsteroidal antiinflammatory drugs
  effects, on menstrual blood loss, IV:9.4, 9.5*t*
  for pleuritic pain, III:8.2
Norepinephrine
  indications for, II:3.6
  plasma, with pheochromocytoma, IV:7.2, 7.3*t*, 7.4, 7.4*t*
  for septic shock, III:10.6
  urinary, with pheochromocytoma, IV:7.3*t*, 7.3–7.4
Norethindrone, for anovulation, IV:9.4, 9.4*t*
Normal, definitions, I:4.1–4.2, 4.2*t*
  diagnostic, I:4.2, 4.2*t*
  therapeutic, I:4.2, 4.2*t*
Normetanephrine
  plasma, with pheochromocytoma, IV:7.2, 7.3*t*, 7.4
  urinary, with pheochromocytoma, IV:7.3*t*, 7.3–7.4
NQMI. *See* Myocardial infarct/infarction, non-Q wave
Nuclear cardiology. *See* Myocardial perfusion imaging
Nutrition, hypercholesterolemia and, IV:18.3–18.6

O

Obesity
  cardiovascular disease and, II:7.7, 8.2
  congestive cardiomyopathy and, II:17.2
  hyperandrogenemia and amenorrhea in, IV:10.4
  and hypercholesterolemia, IV:18.4
  lung volumes in, III:1.3*t*
  screening recommendations for, I:2.6*t*
  upper body, in females, IV:18.1
Obstructive lung disease, pulmonary hypertension in, II:24.6
Occidental cultural heritage, I:9.3, 9.5*t*
Occupational asthma, III:7.1–7.3
  allergic form, III:7.1
  characteristics, III:7.1
  diagnosis, III:7.2–7.3
  nonallergic irritant-induced, III:7.1
  prognosis in, III:7.3
  referral for, III:7.3
  treatment, III:7.3
Octreotide
  for acromegaly, IV:2.10*f*, 2.11
  in pheochromocytoma imaging, IV:7.5–7.6
OKT3, for viral myocarditis, II:19.5
Oligomenorrhea, IV:10.1
Oophoritis, autoimmune, IV:10.5
Open-lung biopsy, III:1.6
Oral cancer, screening recommendations for, I:2.6*t*
Oral contraceptives
  for anovulation, IV:9.4, 9.4*t*
  drug interactions, with glucocorticoids, IV:6.5*t*
  for hypoestrogenism, IV:10.6–10.7
Oral hypoglycemics
  for diabetes in elderly, IV:21.2–21.3
  drug interactions, with glucocorticoids, IV:6.5*t*
Orchiectomy
  plus nilutamide, for prostate cancer, IV:20.8–20.9, 20.9*t*
  for prostate cancer, IV:20.8–20.9, 20.9*t*
Orchitis, postpubertal, IV:11.7
Organ failure, hypoglycemia in, IV:14.6, 14.7*t*
Orthopnea, in pregnancy, II:33.3
Orthostatic hypotension, II:5.3
  with mitral valve prolapse, II:13.6
Ortner's syndrome, II:12.2
Osler's nodes, II:20.2
Oslo Dietary and Smoking Intervention Trials, II:8.4–8.5
Osmoreceptors
  high-set, IV:1.3, 1.3*t*
  hypothalamic, IV:1.2
Osmotic diuresis, IV:1.2*t*
Osteomalacia
  in elderly, laboratory findings in, IV:21.5*t*
  tumor-related, IV:19.5–19.6
Osteoporosis
  in elderly, laboratory findings in, IV:21.5*t*
  postmenopausal, IV:22.3
  screening recommendations for, I:2.6*t*
Ovarian cancer, and malignant pleural effusions, III:8.7*t*
Ovarian failure
  primary, IV:10.2, 10.5
  secondary, IV:10.2
Ovarian tumor(s), lipoid cell, IV:10.5
Ovulation, tests for, IV:22.2*t*
Oxygen, arterial partial pressure, III:1.2
  decreased, in hypoventilation, III:9.3
Oxygen therapy
  for acute severe asthma, III:10.4
  for central sleep apnea, III:9.7
  for COPD, III:2.9
  for hypoventilation, III:9.3
  for MI, II:11.4
  for pneumoconiosis, III:7.5
  for primary spontaneous pneumothorax, III:8.3
  for pulmonary hypertension, III:5.4
  transtracheal catheter delivery, III:2.9, 2.9*f*
Oxytocin
  hemodynamic effects, II:33.4
  SIADH caused by, IV:1.4, 1.5*t*

P

Pacemaker implantation
  indications for, II:3.7
  temporary, indications for, II:11.3
  in viral myocarditis, II:19.5
Pacemaker syndrome, II:4.3, 4.4*f*
Paget's disease, in elderly, laboratory findings in, IV:21.5*t*
Pain
  abdominal. *See* Abdominal pain
  hand, I:3.2–3.3
  knee, I:3.4–3.5, 3.5*t*
  low back, I:3.3–3.4
Palpitations, II:4.1–4.3
  with atrioventricular dissociation, II:4.3, 4.4*f*
  causes, II:4.1–4.3
  characteristics, II:4.3–4.4, 4.5*t*
  definition, II:4.1
  diagnostic evaluation, II:4.5, 4.6*t*, 4.7*f*
  drugs associated with, II:4.5*t*
  ECG findings with, II:4.2, 4.2*f*, 4.4
  history-taking with, II:4.3, 4.5*t*
  laboratory testing with, II:4.4–4.5
  mechanisms, II:4.1–4.3
  with mitral valve prolapse, II:13.6, 13.6*t*
  patient evaluation with, II:4.3–4.5
  physical examination of patient with, II:4.4
  with premature ventricular beats, II:4.3, 4.3*f*
  risk stratification with, II:4.5, 4.6*t*, 4.7*f*
Pamidronate, for hypercalcemia of malignancy, IV:19.2*t*
Pancoast's syndrome, management, III:3.6
Pancreatic cancer
  screening recommendations for, I:2.6*t*
  SIADH with, IV:1.4, 1.5*t*
Pancreatitis, clinical features, III:8.5*t*
Panic attacks, mitral valve prolapse and, II:13.6, 13.6*t*, 13.7*t*
Papanicolaou smear, effectiveness, I:2.2
Papaverine hydrochloride, intracavernosal injection, IV:12.6
Papillary fibroelastoma, cardiac
  clinical manifestations, II:26.3*t*
  treatment, II:26.6
Papillary muscle
  dysfunction, postinfarction, II:11.4*t*
  rupture, II:11.4*t*
Parasites, differential diagnosis, III:6.9*t*
Parathyroid adenoma(s), IV:13.2–13.3
Parathyroid hormone
  actions, IV:13.1
  circulating, measurement, IV:13.3
  immunoradiometric assay, IV:13.3
Parathyroid hormone–related peptide, IV:19.1
Parlodel. *See* Bromocriptine
Paroxysmal nocturnal dyspnea, in pregnancy, II:33.2, 33.3
Patches, intracardiac, II:23.2, 23.2*t*
Patent ductus arteriosus, II:22.5–22.7. *See also* Eisenmenger's syndrome
  in adult, II:22.2
  anatomy, II:22.5
  auscultatory findings with, II:22.6
  complications, II:22.7
  diagnosis, II:22.6
  echocardiography, II:22.6, 22.6*f*
  moderate-sized, physical findings with, II:22.5
  pathophysiology, II:22.5
  physical findings with, II:22.5–22.6
  with pulmonary hypertension, physical findings with, II:22.5–22.6
  repair, II:23.6
  small, physical findings with, II:22.5
  treatment, II:22.7
Patient(s)
  belief system, eliciting, I:1.4, 1.4*t*
  breaking bad news to, I:1.5, 1.5*t*
  difficult, coping with, I:1.5, 1.5*t*
PE. *See* Pulmonary embolism
Peak expiratory flow rate, in diagnosis of occupational asthma, III:7.2
Penicillamine, for collagen vascular disorders, III:6.8

Penile brachial blood pressure index, IV:12.5, 12.7*t*
Penile implants, IV:12.6–12.7
Penile vascular flow, evaluation, IV:12.5
Penis at 12 syndrome, IV:11.5
Pentamidine, precautions with, II:19.6
Percussion, in physical diagnosis, I:3.4*t*
Percutaneous transluminal coronary angioplasty, in elderly, results, II:32.4, 32.5*t*
Pergolide, for hyperprolactinemia, IV:10.7–10.8
Pericardial cyst, clinical manifestations, II:26.3*t*
Pericardial disease(s), II:21.1–21.8
    referrals for, II:21.7
Pericardial effusion(s), II:21.4–21.5
    in cardiac amyloidosis, II:31.8
    chest radiography with, II:21.4–21.5, 21.4*t*, 21.5*f*
    clinical features, II:21.4
    ECG findings with, II:21.4
    echocardiography, II:21.4–21.5
    laboratory findings with, II:21.4–21.5, 21.4*t*
    malignant, treatment, II:21.5
    management, II:21.5
    with metastatic disease, II:26.2–26.3
    pathogenesis, II:21.4
    in rheumatoid arthritis, II:31.5
    in scleroderma, II:31.5
Pericardial friction rubs, II:1.5, 21.2
Pericardial knock, II:21.6
Pericardiocentesis
    in cardiac tamponade, II:21.5
    diagnostic, in pericarditis, II:21.3
    echocardiographic evaluation for, II:21.7
    indications for, II:3.7
Pericarditis
    acute, II:21.1–21.4
        clinical features, II:21.2
        ECG findings with, II:21.2, 21.2*f*
        etiology, II:21.1, 21.2*t*
        management, II:21.3–21.4
        pathophysiology, II:21.1
    anticoagulation and, II:21.3–21.4
    bacterial, II:21.1, 21.2, 21.3
        management, II:21.3
    cardiac enzymes in, II:21.3
    chest pain in, II:21.2
    chest radiography in, II:21.3
    constrictive, II:21.5–21.7
    ECG findings with, II:1.6
    effusive-constrictive, II:21.6
    friction rub in, II:21.2
    in HIV-infected (AIDS) patient, II:21.1
    idiopathic, management, II:21.3
    laboratory findings in, II:21.2–21.3
    with metastatic disease, II:26.2
    myocardial infarction and, management, II:21.3–21.4
    postinfarction, II:11.4*t*
    in rheumatoid arthritis, II:31.5
    in scleroderma, II:31.5
    in systemic lupus erythematosus, II:31.3–31.4
    thrombolytic therapy and, II:21.3–21.4
    tuberculous, II:21.1, 21.3
        management, II:21.3
    uremic, management, II:21.3, 21.3*t*
    viral, management, II:21.3
Pericardium, functions, II:21.1
Perimenopause, IV:22.1–22.2
    contraception in, IV:22.2, 22.2*t*
    endometrial risk in, IV:22.2
    hormone replacement therapy in, IV:22.2
    tests for, IV:22.2*t*
Peripartum cardiomyopathy, II:33.4
Peripheral arterial aneurysm(s), II:29.6–29.7

Peripheral arterial disease, II:29.1–29.7
    occlusive, II:29.1–29.6
        acute, II:29.1–29.2
        causes, II:29.2
        chronic, II:29.1–29.2
        diagnosis, II:29.2–29.3
        differential diagnosis, II:29.3
        distribution, II:29.1–29.2
        Fontaine classification, II:29.2, 29.2*t*
        less common types, clinical features, II:29.3, 29.5*t*
        management, II:29.5–29.6
        prognosis for, II:29.5
        referrals for, II:29.6
Peripheral arterial occlusion. *See also* Peripheral arterial disease, occlusive
    acute, II:29.6
        management, II:29.6
        referral for, II:29.6
    embolic, II:29.6, 29.6*t*
    thrombotic, II:29.6, 29.6*t*
Peripheral neuropathy, and bronchogenic carcinoma, III:3.3*t*
Peripheral vascular disease, II:7.1, 29.1–29.10. *See also* Peripheral arterial disease
    blood lipids and, II:7.4–7.6
    in diabetes mellitus, IV:16.7–16.8
    incidence, age and, II:7.1, 7.2*f*
    screening recommendations for, I:2.6*t*
Permanent neonatal lupus, II:31.4
Permax. *See* Pergolide
Pesticide inhalation, effects, III:7.5–7.6
Phalen's sign, I:3.3
Pharmacohemodynamic testing, in heart failure, II:2.7
Pharynx, reconstruction, for obstructive sleep apnea, III:9.6
Phenobarbital, drug interactions, with glucocorticoids, IV:6.5*t*
Phenoxybenzamine
    dosage and administration, IV:7.6, 7.7*t*
    indications for, IV:7.6
    mechanism of action, IV:7.6
    for pheochromocytoma, IV:7.6–7.7, 7.7*t*
Phentolamine
    intracavernosal injection, IV:12.6
    intraoperative, with pheochromocytoma surgery, IV:7.7
    for pheochromocytoma, IV:7.6–7.7, 7.7*f*, 7.7*t*
Phenylephrine hydrochloride
    indications for, II:3.6
    for septic shock, III:10.6
Phenytoin, drug interactions, with glucocorticoids, IV:6.5*t*
Pheochromocytoma, IV:7.1–7.9
    acute respiratory distress syndrome with, IV:7.3
    associated disorders, IV:7.1–7.2
    associated neuroectodermal syndromes, IV:7.1
    biochemical assays with, IV:7.3–7.4, 7.3–7.4
    catecholamine and catecholamine metabolite levels with, IV:7.2, 7.3*t*
    clinical features, IV:7.1, 7.2*t*
    clonidine suppression test with, IV:7.4*f*, 7.4*t*, 7.4–7.5
    computed tomography, IV:7.5–7.6, 7.6*f*
    diagnosis, IV:7.1, 7.2*t*
    diagnostic tests for, IV:7.4, 7.4*t*
    distribution, IV:7.5, 7.5*f*
    epidemiology, IV:7.1
    familial, IV:7.1–7.2, 7.2*t*
    imaging, IV:7.4*t*, 7.5
    incidence, IV:7.1
    localization, IV:7.2, 7.5*f*, 7.5–7.6
    magnetic resonance imaging, IV:7.5–7.6

    malignant, treatment, IV:7.7, 7.7*t*
    medical control, IV:7.6–7.7, 7.7*t*
    myocardial sequelae, IV:7.3
    pharmacologic diagnosis, IV:7.5
    physical findings with, IV:7.2*t*, 7.3
    plasma catecholamines with, IV:7.4, 7.4*t*
    in pregnancy, IV:7.8
    scintigraphy, IV:7.5–7.6, 7.6*f*
    signs and symptoms, IV:7.1, 7.2–7.3, 7.2*t*
    survival rate with, IV:7.7
    treatment, IV:7.6–7.7
        medical, IV:7.6–7.7, 7.7*t*
        surgical, IV:7.6
    tumor localization, IV:7.5–7.6
    urinalysis with, IV:7.3–7.4, 7.3*t*
    urinary catecholamines with, IV:7.3*t*, 7.3–7.4
Phlegmasia cerulea dolens, II:29.7, 29.7*f*
Phosphodiesterase inhibitors, for congestive heart failure, II:17.8*t*, 17.9
Phrenic nerve stimulation, for hypoventilation, III:9.3
Physical activity, cardiovascular disease and, II:7.7
Physical diagnosis, I:3.1–3.5. *See also* Diagnostic tests
    of heart murmurs, I:3.2–3.3
    of pulmonary disorders, I:3.3–3.4, 3.4*t*
Physical examination
    with chest pain, II:1.4–1.5
    with congestive cardiomyopathy, II:17.2–17.3
    in heart failure, II:2.2–2.3
Physician(s)
    "compleat," attributes, I:9.4, 9.6*f*
    incomes and expenses, I:6.5, 7.3
    numbers of, in US, I:6.5, 6.5*f*, 7.3
    payments to, modalities for, I:6.6
    practice settings, trends in, I:6.5*f*, 6.5–6.6
    specialty mix, and Medicare funding of graduate medical education, I:7.3
Physician–patient relationship, I:10.2
Piperacillin, for nosocomial pneumonia, III:4.7*t*
Pirbuterol, for acute severe asthma, III:10.4
Pistol-shot systolic sound, with aortic regurgitation, II:14.7
Pituitary adenoma(s), IV:2.1
    cell origin, IV:2.6*t*
    clinical syndromes with, IV:2.6*t*
    diagnosis, IV:2.6
    hormone production by, IV:2.6*t*
    local neurologic effects, IV:2.5–2.6
    magnetic resonance imaging, IV:2.6, 2.6*f*
    prolactin-secreting, in males, IV:11.9, 11.9*t*
Pituitary disorder(s), diabetes insipidus in, IV:1.2
Pituitary gland. *See also* Hypothalamic-pituitary axis; Hypothalamic-pituitary-thyroid axis
    anterior, IV:2.1–2.12
        dysfunction, clinical syndromes with, IV:2.4–2.12
        function, testing, quadruple bolus method, IV:2.4*f*, 2.5*t*
    posterior, in anorexia nervosa, IV:1.7, 1.7*t*
Pituitary tumor(s), IV:2.5–2.6. *See also* Pituitary adenoma(s)
    corticotropin-dependent, IV:5.5–5.6
    diagnosis, IV:2.6
    gonadotropin-secreting, IV:2.6*t*, 2.9
    growth hormone-secreting, IV:2.6*t*, 2.6–2.8
    hormone production by, IV:2.6*t*
    local neurologic effects, IV:2.5–2.6
    prolactin-secreting, IV:2.6*t*, 2.8–2.9, 2.9*t*
        management, IV:2.10*f*, 2.11
    thyroid-stimulating hormone (thyrotropin)-secreting, IV:2.6*t*, 2.9
    transsphenoidal resection, IV:2.11, 2.11*f*
    treatment, IV:2.11, 5.9–5.10, 5.10*t*

Plaque, atherosclerotic, formation, II:8.1
Plasma aldosterone:plasma renin activity ratio, IV:8.2
Pleura
 costal parietal, injury to, III:8.2
 diaphragmatic
  central, inflammation, III:8.2
  peripheral, inflammation, III:8.2
 diseases, III:8.1–8.10
Pleural abrasion
 for malignant pleural effusions, III:8.9
 for primary spontaneous pneumothorax, III:8.3
 for secondary spontaneous pneumothorax, III:8.3
Pleural effusion(s), III:8.1–8.2
 asbestos, benign, clinical features, III:8.5t
 bloody, differential diagnosis, III:8.2
 conditions associated with, III:8.1
 vs. consolidation, I:3.10, 3.10t
 malignant, III:8.3–8.9
  causes, III:8.7t
  cytology in, III:8.8
  epidemiology, III:8.3
  significance, III:8.3
  survival with, III:8.8, 8.8f
  treatment, III:8.8–8.9, 8.9t
 paramalignant, III:8.3–8.6
  chest radiography in, III:8.6–8.7, 8.7f
  clinical features, III:8.6
  diagnosis, III:8.6–8.8
  etiology, III:8.7t
  treatment, III:8.9t
 physical diagnosis, I:3.3, 3.4, 3.4t
 physical findings with, I:3.11t
 uremic, clinical features, III:8.5t
Pleural fluid analysis
 in diagnosis of pleurisy, III:8.2
 in malignant pleural effusions, III:8.7–8.8
Pleural friction rub(s), II:1.5, III:8.2
Pleurectomy
 for malignant pleural effusions, III:8.9
 for primary spontaneous pneumothorax, III:8.3
Pleurisy, III:8.1–8.2
 clinical features, III:8.2
 differential diagnosis, III:8.2
 diseases that cause, clinical features, III:8.4t–8.5t
 treatment, III:8.2
 viral, clinical features, III:8.4t
Pleuritic pain, II:1.4
 with pulmonary embolism, II:25.2
Pleuroperitoneal shunt, III:8.9
Plicamycin, for hypercalcemia of malignancy, IV:19.2t
Pneumoconiosis(es), III:7.3–7.5
 coal-workers,' exposure settings for, III:7.4t
 diagnosis, III:7.4
 differential diagnosis, III:7.5t
 disease progression in, III:7.4f
 inorganic, III:6.1
 interstitial, differential diagnosis, III:6.3t
 occupational exposure causing, III:7.4t
 prognosis in, III:7.5
 treatment, III:7.5
Pneumocystis carinii pneumonia, III:4.3t, 4.4, 4.4t
 in heart transplant recipient, II:34.7
Pneumonia, III:4.1
 atypical
  physical diagnosis, I:3.4t
  physical findings with, I:3.11t
 bacterial
  clinical features, III:8.4t
  differential diagnosis, III:8.2
 as cause of death, III:2.2t

community-acquired, III:4.2–4.6
 clinical features, III:4.3
 diagnosis, III:4.4–4.5
 etiologic pathogens in, III:4.3–4.4
  in hospitalized patients, III:4.4t
  in outpatient therapy, III:4.3t
 hospitalization for, III:4.4
  indications for, III:4.4t
 prevention, III:4.5–4.6
 radiographic features, III:4.3, 4.3f
 severity, III:4.4
 therapy for, III:4.5, 4.5t
consolidating
 computed tomography scans, III:1.4f
 radiographs, III:1.4f
eosinophilic, III:6.10f
 chronic, differential diagnosis, III:6.9t
nosocomial, III:4.6–4.7
 diagnosis, III:4.6
 pathologic pathogens in, III:4.6
 prevention, III:4.7, 10.8
 risk factors for, III:4.6t
 therapy for, III:4.6–4.7
 in ventilated patients with respiratory failure, III:10.7–10.8
physical diagnosis, I:3.3, 3.4t
SIADH with, IV:1.4, 1.5t
typical
 physical diagnosis, I:3.4t
 physical findings with, I:3.11t
vaccination for, III:2.6–2.7
 indications for, III:4.5–4.6
Pneumothorax, III:8.2–8.3
 classification, III:8.2
 clinical features, III:8.5t
 differential diagnosis, III:8.2, 8.3
 iatrogenic, III:8.2
 in interstitial lung disease, III:6.4t
 physical diagnosis, I:3.3, 3.4t
 physical findings with, I:3.11t
 primary spontaneous, III:8.2–8.3
  causes, III:8.2
  clinical and physiologic features, III:8.2–8.3
  diagnosis, III:8.3
  prevention of recurrence, III:8.3
  treatment, III:8.3
 secondary spontaneous, III:8.2, 8.3
  causes, III:8.3, 8.6t
  clinical features, III:8.3
  diagnosis, III:8.3
  prevention of recurrence, III:8.3
  treatment, III:8.3
 spontaneous, III:8.6f
  in histiocytosis X, III:6.8, 6.10f
 traumatic, III:8.2
Point-of-service plans, I:6.4
Polyarteritis, cardiac involvement in, II:31.6
Polyarteritis nodosa, III:6.8
 cardiac involvement in, II:31.6
Polychondritis, cardiac involvement in, II:31.2t, 31.7
Polycystic ovary syndrome, IV:10.3f, 10.3–10.4
Polydipsia, primary, IV:1.2t, 1.3
Polymerase chain reaction, detection of viral genome, II:19.4
Polymyositis
 cardiac involvement in, II:31.2t, 31.6
 diagnosis, II:31.6
Polyp(s)
 endocervical, IV:9.3
  surgical therapy for, IV:9.5
 endometrial, IV:9.3
  surgical therapy for, IV:9.5
 uterine, IV:9.3, 9.4f

Polysomnogram, III:9.6f
Polyuria, hypotonic
 of diabetes insipidus, IV:1.2t
 differential diagnosis, IV:1.2t
Popliteal artery
 aneurysm, II:29.6
 entrapment, clinical features, II:29.3, 29.5t
POSCH. *See* Program on the Surgical Control of the Hyperlipidemias
Positive end-expiratory pressure, III:10.3
 mechanism, III:10.3f
Positron emission tomography, II:1.8
POS plans. *See* Point-of-service plans
Postcardiac injury syndrome
 clinical features, III:8.4t
 treatment, III:8.2
Posterior cruciate ligament, tear, I:3.4
Postmenopausal patient, IV:22.1–22.6. *See also* Menopause
 dyslipoproteinemia in, IV:22.5
 follow-up, IV:22.5–22.6
Postural hypotension, with pheochromocytoma, IV:7.3
Potassium balance, regulation, IV:8.1, 8.2f
PPOs. *See* Preferred provider organizations
Pravastatin, lipid-lowering therapy, II:8.8, 8.8t
Prazosin hydrochloride
 indications for, IV:7.6–7.7
 for pheochromocytoma, IV:7.6–7.7, 7.7t
Precipitin antibody, findings in interstitial lung disease, III:6.5t
Predictive value, of screening test, I:2.2f, 2.2–2.3
 prevalence and, I:2.3, 2.3t
Prednisolone, pharmacology, IV:6.2t
Prednisone
 for collagen vascular disorders, III:6.8
 pharmacology, IV:6.2t
 for sarcoidosis, III:6.5
Preferred provider organizations, I:6.4, 6.5, 6.5f, 7.4
Pregnancy
 acquired valvular heart disease in, II:33.2–33.4
 anticoagulation in, II:33.4
 autoimmune thyroid disease and, IV:3.6
 congenital heart disease and, II:33.4
 diabetes in. *See* Gestational diabetes
 diabetes insipidus in, IV:1.2
 glucocorticoid therapy in, IV:6.3
 heart disease in, II:33.1
 heart in, II:33.1–33.5
 hematologic effects, II:33.1–33.2, 33.2f
 hemodynamic effects, II:33.1, 33.2, 33.2f
 hyperthyroidism in, management, IV:3.5
 hypertrophic obstructive cardiomyopathy and, II:33.5
 and hypothyroidism, management, IV:3.3
 Marfan syndrome and, II:33.4–33.5
 myocardial infarction in, II:33.4
 pheochromocytoma in, IV:7.8
 prosthetic heart valves and, II:33.4
 pulmonary hypertension in, II:33.4
 virilization during, IV:10.4
Preload, II:3.2, 3.2f
Premature atrial beats, with acute MI, II:11.3
Premature ventricular beats, with acute MI, II:11.3
Prepatellar bursitis, I:3.4
Presyncope
 evaluation, II:6.5–6.6, 6.6f
 with mitral valve prolapse, II:13.6
 in pregnancy, II:33.2
Prevalence, effect on predictive value of screening test, I:2.3, 2.3t
Prevention. *See* Preventive medicine
Preventive medicine

future opportunities, I:2.7
interventions in
  effectiveness, I:2.2–2.3
  mortality benefit, I:2.2, 2.2t
  primary, I:2.1, 2.2f
  screening in, I:2.1–2.2
  secondary, I:2.1, 2.2f
  tertiary, I:2.1, 2.2f
Proarrhythmias, II:6.2
Probucol, lipid-lowering therapy, II:8.8
Progesterone, for hypoventilation, III:9.3
Progesterone in oil, for anovulation, IV:9.4, 9.4t
Progestin(s), therapy with, for menstrual irregularity, IV:10.8
Progestin-withdrawal test, measurement, IV:10.5
Program on the Surgical Control of the Hyperlipidemias, II:8.7
Progressive systemic sclerosis, interstitial, differential diagnosis, III:6.3t
Prolactin, IV:2.2f
  hypersecretion, testing for, IV:2.4
  reserve, testing for, IV:2.4
  secretion
    by pituitary tumors, IV:2.6t, 2.8–2.9, 2.9t
    in males, IV:11.9, 11.9f
    management, IV:2.10f, 2.11
    regulation, IV:2.3–2.4
  serum. *See also* Hyperprolactinemia
    normal, IV:2.9
Prolactinoma, management, IV:2.10f, 2.11
Propranolol
  dosage and administration, IV:7.7, 7.7t
  indications for, IV:7.7
  for pheochromocytoma, IV:7.7, 7.7t
Propylthiouracil, for hyperthyroidism, IV:3.4, 3.5f
Prostacyclin, for pulmonary hypertension, III:5.5
Prostaglandin E$_1$, intracavernosal injection, IV:12.6
Prostaglandin synthetase inhibitor, for diabetes insipidus, IV:1.4t
Prostate
  age-related changes and disorders, IV:20.1–20.11. *See also* Benign prostatic hyperplasia
  volume, age-related changes in, IV:20.2f
  weight, age-related changes in, IV:20.1, 20.2f
Prostate cancer, IV:20.6–20.9
  diagnosis, IV:20.7
  prevalence, IV:20.6
  screening, IV:20.6f, 20.7
    recommendations for, I:2.6t
  stage C, downstaging, with total androgen blockade, IV:20.9
  stage D$_2$, total androgen blockade for, IV:20.9, 20.10f
  staging, IV:20.7f, 20.7–20.8, 20.8f
  treatment, IV:20.7f, 20.8–20.9, 20.9t
    castration in, IV:20.8–20.9, 20.9f
    with megestrol acetate plus diethylstilbestrol or estradiol, IV:20.9, 20.11f
    and survival, IV:20.9, 20.10f
    total androgen blockade in, IV:20.8–20.9, 20.9f
Prostate-specific antigen, screening, for prostate cancer, effectiveness, I:2.2t, 2.2–2.3
Prostate-specific antigen test, IV:20.6f, 20.7
Prostate symptom score, IV:20.5t, 20.5–20.6
Prostatism. *See* Benign prostatic hyperplasia
Protozoal myocarditis, II:19.3t. *See also* Toxoplasmosis; Trypanosomiasis
Proximate cause, I:10.3–10.4
Pseudohermaphroditism, male, with androgen receptor defects, IV:11.6
Pseudohypoparathyroidism, IV:13.1, 13.5, 13.5t

Pseudomonas aeruginosa pneumonia, III:4.4, 4.4t
Pseudo-pseudohypoparathyroidism, IV:13.5
Public policy. *See* Health policy
Pulmonary alveolar proteinosis, III:6.8, 6.10f
Pulmonary angiography
  complications, II:25.5–25.6
  for pulmonary embolism, II:25.5–25.6, 25.6f
  in pulmonary hypertension, II:24.3
Pulmonary arteriography, in diagnosis of pulmonary thromboembolism, III:5.6
Pulmonary arteriovenous fistula
  anatomy, II:22.11
  angiocardiography with, II:22.11, 22.11f
  complications, II:22.11
  diagnosis, II:22.11
  pathophysiology, II:22.11
  physical findings with, II:22.11
  treatment, II:22.11
Pulmonary artery catheter/catheterization, II:3.3, 3.6t, 3.7t
Pulmonary artery insufficiency, auscultatory findings, II:20.5
Pulmonary atresia, in adult, II:22.2
Pulmonary circulation, disorders, III:5.1–5.8
Pulmonary diagnostic tests, III:1.1–1.6
Pulmonary disease, SIADH with, IV:1.4, 1.5t
Pulmonary edema
  flash, II:1.5, 2.2
  myocardial ischemia with, II:1.5
  in pregnancy, II:33.3
Pulmonary embolism, II:25.1–25.8
  chest radiographic findings with, II:25.4, 25.4t
  clinical features, III:8.5t
  and deep venous thrombosis, II:25.1
  diagnosis, II:3.5t, 25.2–25.4, 25.5t
    strategy for, II:25.6f, 25.6–25.7
  ECG findings with, II:1.6, 25.2–25.4, 25.4t
  hemodynamic parameters for, II:3.6t
  predisposing factors for, II:25.1, 25.2t
  probability, evaluation, II:25.5, 25.5f, 25.6f
  pulmonary angiography for, II:25.5–25.6, 25.6f
  residual impairment after, II:25.6
  signs and symptoms, II:25.2, 25.4t
  treatment, II:25.3t, 25.7, 25.7t
  ventilation-perfusion lung scan with, II:25.4f, 25.4–25.5, 25.5t
Pulmonary eosinophilic granuloma. *See* Histiocytosis X
Pulmonary fibrosis, idiopathic, III:6.10
  clinical features, III:6.1–6.2
  diagnosis, III:6.10
  interstitial, differential diagnosis, III:6.3t
Pulmonary function test(s)
  in heart failure, II:2.7
  in pulmonary hypertension, II:24.2f, 24.3
Pulmonary function testing, III:1.1–1.2
  in COPD, III:2.2
  in diagnosis of occupational asthma, III:7.2
  in diagnosis of pulmonary hypertension, III:5.3–5.4
Pulmonary hemosiderosis
  idiopathic, III:6.8
Pulmonary hypertension, II:24.1–24.6, III:5.1–5.6
  with atrial septal defect, II:22.2–22.3
  cardiac catheterization in, II:24.3
  causes, II:24.1, 24.2, 24.2t
  chest radiography in, II:24.2, 24.2f
  chronic thromboembolic
    differential diagnosis, III:5.4
    perfusion lung scan in, III:5.4, 5.4f
  classification, by etiology, III:5.2t
  in collagen vascular disease, II:24.6
  with congenital heart disease, II:24.6
  diagnosis, II:24.2–24.3, 24.2t, III:5.2

differential diagnosis, III:5.2–5.4
echocardiography in, II:24.3
with left ventricular diastolic dysfunction, II:24.6
with mitral stenosis, II:12.2, 24.6
natural history, III:5.6
in obstructive lung disease, II:24.6
patent ductus arteriosus with, physical findings with, II:22.5–22.6
pathophysiology, II:24.1
in pregnancy, II:33.4
primary, II:24.3–24.4
  electrocardiogram in, III:5.3, 5.3f
  radiography in, III:5.3, 5.3f
  survival rate, II:24.5, 24.5f
  treatment, II:24.5f, 24.5–24.6
prognosis in, III:5.6
pulmonary angiography in, II:24.3
pulmonary function testing in, II:24.2f, 24.3
referrals for, II:24.1–24.2, 24.5
role of the generalist in, II:24.1–24.2
treatment, II:24.3–24.5, III:5.4–5.6
  algorithm for, III:5.5f
  general measures for, II:24.6–24.7, 25.1t
unexplained, associated conditions, II:24.2, 24.2t
ventilation-perfusion lung scan in, II:24.2f, 24.3
Pulmonary infiltration with eosinophilia, III:6.8
  causes, III:6.9t
  differential diagnosis, III:6.9t
  drug-induced, differential diagnosis, III:6.9t
Pulmonary nodule, solitary, management, III:3.6
Pulmonary stenosis, valvular, II:15.4–15.5
  in adult, II:22.2
  anatomy, II:22.8
  complications, II:22.8
  congenital, intracardiac repair for, sequelae and residua after, II:23.4
  diagnosis, II:22.8
  ECG findings with, II:15.4, 15.5f
  grading, II:15.4–15.5, 15.5t
  management, II:15.5, 15.5t
  pathophysiology, II:22.8
  physical findings with, II:22.8
Pulmonary thromboembolism, III:5.6–5.7
  diagnosis, III:1.4f, 5.6
    algorithm for, III:5.7f
  prevention, III:5.7
  risk factors in, III:5.6
  sources, III:5.6
  therapy for, III:5.6–5.7
Pulmonary valve, regurgitation, postoperative, with intracardiac repair for congenital heart disease, II:23.2, 23.2t
Pulmonary varix, II:22.2
Pulmonary vascular disease
  differential diagnosis, III:5.2
  HIV-associated, differential diagnosis, III:5.2
Pulmonary vascular resistance, determinants, II:3.1
Pulmonary vasculitis, III:6.8
Pulmonary vasoconstriction, cocaine-induced, differential diagnosis, III:5.2
Pulmonic valve
  disease, II:15.4–15.5
    acquired, II:15.5
    congenital, II:15.4–15.5
  regurgitation, II:15.5
    diagnosis, II:15.5
    functional, II:15.5
    management, II:15.5
    organic, II:15.5
Pulse
  extremity, reduced or absent, II:29.2
  paradoxic, II:21.4, 21.4t

23

Pulsus paradoxus, II:21.4, 21.4t, 21.6
Pulsus parvus et tardus, I:3.2
Pus, with empyema, III:8.2
PVD. See Peripheral vascular disease
Pyrimethamine, for toxoplasmosis, II:19.8

Q

Quincke's pulse, II:14.7
Quinolone
    for acute bronchitis, III:4.2
    plus clindamycin, for community-acquired pneumonia, III:4.5t
    plus penicillin, for community-acquired pneumonia, III:4.5t

R

Radial nerve
    dysfunction, I:3.2, 3.3t
    screening examination, I:3.3t
Radiation exposure, thyroid cancer and, IV:4.6
Radioallergosorbent test, in diagnosis of occupational asthma, III:7.3
Radioiodine therapy, for hyperthyroidism, IV:3.4–3.5
Radionuclide angiography, of myocardial contusion, II:27.7
Radionuclide studies
    in deep venous thrombosis, II:25.1
    in heart failure, II:2.7
    indications for, II:4.6t
    with myocardial infarction, II:11.3
Radionuclide ventilation/perfusion scans, III:1.4f, 1.4–1.5
Radionuclide ventriculography, with myocardial infarction, II:11.3
Radiotherapy
    for bronchogenic carcinoma, III:3.6
    for sarcoidosis, III:6.5
Rales, I:3.4, 3.10
    end-inspiratory, III:6.1–6.2
Rapid corticotropin stimulation test, IV:5.13, 5.13t
Rastelli repair, II:23.2t, 23.5, 23.6f
Reactive airways dysfunction syndrome, III:7.1–7.2
Receiver operating characteristic curve, I:4.4, 4.4f
5α-Reductase deficiency, IV:11.5, 11.6f
Referral letter(s), I:5.3, 5.4f
    with problem list, I:5.3, 5.4f
    problem list in, I:5.3, 5.4f
Referrals, I:5.1–5.2, I:5.1–5.2. See also Consultant(s); Consultation
    for aortic regurgitation, II:14.9
    for aortic stenosis, II:14.5–14.6
    awkward issues in, I:5.3–5.4, I:5.3–5.4
    of cardiac arrest survivors, II:6.7
    for congestive cardiomyopathy, II:17.9
    for infectious endocarditis, II:20.7
    for mitral regurgitation, II:12.6
    for mitral stenosis, II:12.4
    for occlusive arterial disease, II:29.6
    for patient with syncope, II:5.4–5.5
    for pericardial disease, II:21.7
    problems in, I:5.2
    for pulmonary hypertension, II:24.1–24.2, 24.5
    reasons for, I:5.1, I:5.1–5.2, I:5.2t, I:5.2t
    steps in, I:5.2t, I:5.2t, I:5.2–5.3, I:5.2–5.3
    timing, I:5.2, I:5.2
    for varicose veins, II:29.7, 29.9
Regional blood flow, in pregnancy, II:33.2, 33.3f
Regional enteritis, cardiac involvement in, II:31.6–31.7

Reifenstein's syndrome, IV:11.6–11.7
Reiter's syndrome
    aortitis in, II:28.6
    cardiac involvement in, II:31.2t, 31.6–31.7
Relapsing polychondritis, cardiac involvement in, II:31.7
Renal failure
    in intensive care unit, causes, III:10.8
    with respiratory failure, III:10.8
Renin–angiotensin–aldosterone system, II:3.1–3.2
Renin-angiotensin system, IV:8.1, 8.2f
Renin secretion, by tumors, IV:19.6
Reperfusion therapy, for MI, II:11.4
Reproductive problems, male, IV:12.1–12.8
Residual volume, in normal and disease states, III:1.3t
Res ipsa loquitur, I:10.3
Respiration, normal, III:9.4f
    airflow and respiratory movement in, III:9.5f
Respiratory center, III:9.1
Respiratory distress syndrome. See Acute respiratory distress syndrome; Adult respiratory distress syndrome
Respiratory failure
    acute, III:10.1–10.4
    complications, III:10.7t
        gastrointestinal, III:10.7
        management, III:10.7–10.8
        related to airway management, III:10.7
        risk factors for, III:10.7
    due to neuromuscular disease, III:10.4
        diagnosis, III:10.4
        treatment, III:10.4
    etiology, III:10.2t
    classification, III:10.1, 10.2t
    hypercapnic, III:10.3
        causes, III:10.3
    hypoxemic, III:10.2–10.3
Respiratory musculature, III:9.1
Respiratory stimulant drugs, for hypoventilation, III:9.3
Respiratory tract viruses, in pneumonia, III:4.3t
Restrictive cardiomyopathy, II:18.1–18.8
    abnormal diastolic filling of ventricles in, II:18.1
    with amyloidosis, II:18.4f, 18.4–18.6, 18.5f
    angiography in, II:18.3
    with carcinoid heart disease, II:18.6
    clinical features, II:18.1–18.2
    computed tomography in, II:18.3
    vs. constrictive pericarditis, II:21.6, 21.7f
    diagnosis, II:18.2–18.3
    differential diagnosis, II:17.6, 17.7t, 18.1
    ECG findings in, II:18.2
    echocardiography in, II:18.2
    endomyocardial biopsy in, II:18.3
    with endomyocardial fibrosis, II:18.3
    with eosinophilic myocardial disease, II:18.3–18.4, 18.4f
    etiology, II:18.1
    with Fabry's disease, II:18.6
    geographic distribution, II:18.1
    with hemochromatosis, II:18.6–18.7
    hemodynamic parameters in, II:18.2f, 18.3
    idiopathic, II:18.1
    magnetic resonance imaging in, II:18.3
    pathophysiology, II:18.1
    primary, II:18.1
        causes, II:18.3–18.4
    prognosis for, II:18.3
    with sarcoidosis, II:18.6
    secondary, II:18.1
        causes, II:18.4–18.7
    signs and symptoms, II:18.1–18.2
    treatment, II:18.3

ultrasound in, II:18.2
Reticulum cell sarcoma, SIADH with, IV:1.4, 1.5t
Retinopathy, diabetic. See Diabetic retinopathy
Revascularization, in coronary artery disease, II:9.6
Reverse T_3, serum, and nonthyroidal illness, IV:3.6, 3.6f
Rhabdomyoma, cardiac
    clinical manifestations, II:26.3t
    treatment, II:26.6
Rheumatic disease(s)
    cardiac involvement in, II:31.1, 31.2t
    stroke risk with, II:30.2–30.3
Rheumatic fever
    acute, II:31.1–31.3
        antibiotic therapy, II:31.3, 31.3t
        cardiac involvement in, II:31.1–31.3, 31.2t
        diagnosis, II:31.1–31.3
        Jones criteria for, II:31.1, 31.3t
        secondary prophylaxis after, II:31.3, 31.3t
        treatment, II:31.3, 31.3t
    antibiotic prophylaxis for, II:12.3
    diagnosis, II:12.1, 12.2t
    mitral regurgitation with, II:12.4
    and mitral stenosis, II:12.1–12.2, 12.2t
Rheumatoid arthritis
    cardiac involvement in, II:31.2t, 31.4–31.5
    treatment, glucocorticoids in, IV:6.1–6.2
Rheumatoid pleurisy, clinical features, III:8.4t
Rhonchi, I:3.4, 3.10, 3.11t
Ribavirin therapy, for viral myocarditis, II:19.6
Rickettsial myocarditis, II:19.3t
Rifampin, drug interactions, with glucocorticoids, IV:6.5t
Right-to-left shunt(s)
    arterial, II:22.10t
    atrial, II:22.10t
    in congenital heart disease, II:22.9–22.12
    diagnosis, III:1.5
    intracardiac repair for, II:23.5
    venous, II:22.10t
    ventricular, II:22.10t
Right ventricle
    acute strain, ECG findings with, II:1.6
    function, assessment, after surgery for congenital heart disease, II:23.5
    infarction
        diagnosis, II:3.4t
        hemodynamic parameters for, II:3.6t
Right ventricular failure, differential diagnosis, III:5.3
Rivero-Carvallo maneuver, I:3.3, 3.7
ROC curve. See Receiver operating characteristic curve
Roentgenography, chest, III:1.3–1.4, 1.4f
Roger's disease, II:22.4
Romantilde's sign, II:19.7
Rotator cuff tears, I:3.6
Rothmund-Thomson syndrome, IV:11.8t
Roth spots, II:20.2
RU486, for adrenal tumor, IV:5.10t
Rud syndrome, IV:11.8t

S

SAECG. See Signal-averaged electrocardiograms
St. Thomas Atherosclerosis Regression Trial, II:8.5
Saline solution, for SIADH, IV:1.5, 1.6t
Salt-losing tendency, in elderly, IV:21.5
Sarcoidosis, II:18.6, III:6.4–6.5, 6.6f
    clinical features, III:6.2, 6.2f; 8.4t
    differential diagnosis, III:6.9t
    vs. hypersensitivity pneumonitis, III:6.7t

interstitial, differential diagnosis, III:6.3*t*
intrathoracic changes in, stages, III:6.5
multisystem involvement in, III:6.6*f*
thyroid involvement in, IV:4.5
Sarcoma. *See also* Angiosarcoma; Lymphosarcoma
   cardiac, II:26.2
      clinical manifestations, II:26.3*t*
      treatment, II:26.6
   reticulum cell, SIADH with, IV:1.4, 1.5*t*
Scalene maneuver, in occlusive arterial disease, II:29.4*f*
Scandinavian Simvastatin Study, II:8.7
Schmidt's syndrome, IV:5.12
Sciatica, I:3.3, 3.4*t*
Sciences
   ascendancy, I:9.2–9.3
   humanities and
      bidirectional relationship between, I:9.2–9.3
      dichotomy between, I:9.2
      metaphorical split between, I:9.3
Scintigraphy, of pheochromocytoma, IV:7.5–7.6, 7.6*f*
Sclerodactyly, I:3.2
Scleroderma
   cardiac involvement in, II:31.2*t*, 31.5
   diagnosis, II:31.5
   treatment, II:31.5
Screening, I:2.1–2.8. *See also* Diagnostic tests
   definition, I:2.1–2.2
   for diabetic nephropathy, IV:16.5
   for diabetic retinopathy, IV:16.3, 16.3*t*
   future opportunities, I:2.7
   general, I:2.2
   mass, I:2.2
   in preventive medicine, I:2.1–2.2
   for prostatic carcinoma, IV:20.6*f*, 20.7
   recommendations
      from American Cancer Society, I:2.5
      from American College of Physicians, I:2.5
      bias in, I:2.4, 2.5*f*
      from Canadian Task Force, I:2.5
      comparative, I:2.5
      criteria for, I:2.2–2.4
      evaluation, I:2.4–2.5
         quality of evidence and, I:2.4, 2.5*t*
      for metabolic diseases, I:2.6*t*
      for neoplastic diseases, I:2.6*t*
      sources, I:2.5
      for specific conditions, I:2.5
      from US Preventive Services Task Force, I:2.5
      for vascular diseases and risk factors, I:2.6*t*
   routine, I:2.2
   selective, I:2.2
   target, importance, I:2.2, 2.2*t*
   tests, effectiveness, I:2.2–2.4
   threshold for, I:2.4–2.5
   types, I:2.2
Sedimentation rate, findings in interstitial lung disease, III:6.5*t*
Semen, analysis, IV:12.3–12.4
Semimembranous bursitis, I:3.4
Sensitivity, of tests, I:2.2, 2.2*f*, 4.3*f*, 4.3–4.4
Sepsis
   etiology, III:10.5
   organisms causing, III:10.5–10.6
Sepsis syndrome, III:10.5, 10.5*f*
Septic shock, II:3.1, 3.2, III:10.5–10.6
   clinical presentation, III:10.6
   hemodynamic parameters in, II:3.6*t*
   treatment, III:10.6
Sertoli-cell-only syndrome, IV:11.5
Sex, cardiovascular disease risk and, II:7.1, 7.2*f*, 7.3*f*, 8.2

Sexual history, I:1.4, 1.4*t*
Sheehan's syndrome, IV:5.13
Shock. *See also* Cardiogenic shock; Septic shock
   treatment, III:10.5
Shock state, II:3.2, 3.2*f*
Shortness of breath. *See also* Dyspnea
   causes, I:3.10, 3.11*t*
   etiology, I:3.3
   physical examination with, I:3.10–3.11, 3.11*t*
   physical findings with, I:3.3*t*, 3.3–3.4, 3.4*t*
Shoulder, physical examination, I:3.5–3.6, 3.6*t*
Shy-Drager's disease, II:5.3
Shy-Drager syndrome, IV:1.2
SIAD. *See* Syndrome of inappropriate antidiuresis
SIADH. *See* Syndrome of inappropriate antidiuretic hormone secretion
Sick euthyroid patient, IV:3.6
Sickle cell disease, male hypogonadism in, IV:11.10
Signal-averaged electrocardiograms
   in heart failure, II:2.4
   indications for, II:4.6*t*, 5.4
Silicosis, III:7.3
   differential diagnosis, III:7.5*t*
   exposure settings for, III:7.4*t*
   prognosis in, III:7.5
   treatment, III:7.5
Simvastatin, lipid-lowering therapy, II:8.8, 8.8*t*
   clinical intervention trial, II:8.7
Sinus bradycardia, with acute MI, II:11.3
Sinus of Valsalva, aneurysms, repair, II:23.6
Sinus tachycardia, with acute MI, II:11.3
Sipple syndrome, IV:7.1
   pheochromocytoma in, IV:7.1
Situs inversus, II:22.2
Skin cancer, screening recommendations for, I:2.6*t*
Skin tests, in diagnosis of occupational asthma, III:7.3
SLE. *See* Systemic lupus erythematosus
Sleep apnea
   central, III:9.5, 9.7
      airflow and respiratory movement in, III:9.5*f*
      treatment, III:9.7
   cycle of events in, III:9.6*f*
   mixed, III:9.5
      airflow and respiratory movement in, III:9.5*f*
   obstructive, III:9.5–9.7
      airflow and respiratory movement in, III:9.5*f*
      clinical features, III:9.6, 9.6*f*
      definition, III:9.5
      diagnosis, III:9.6
      sleep polysomnogram in, III:9.6*f*
      treatment, III:9.6–9.7
Smoke inhalation, management, III:7.8
Smokers, identification, III:2.5
Smoking
   and bronchogenic carcinoma, III:3.1–3.2, 3.2*t*
   cessation, III:2.6
      for acute bronchitis, III:4.2
      behavioral stages, III:2.6*t*
      effects, on pulmonary function decline, III:2.5, 2.5*f*
      physician's 4 A's to, III:2.6*t*
   and interstitial lung disease, III:6.2
Sodium
   balance, regulation, IV:8.1
   excretion, diabetes insipidus with, IV:1.2
   serum. *See* Hyponatremia
Sodium chloride, supplements, indications for, II:13.9
Sodium ipodate, for hyperthyroidism, IV:3.4
Solitary thyroid nodules, IV:4.5–4.8
   adenoma, IV:4.5–4.6
   autonomous functioning, IV:4.5–4.6, 4.6*f*

   carcinoma, IV:4.6–4.7, 4.7*t*
   colloid nodule, IV:4.5
   cyst, IV:4.6, 4.6*f*
   cytopathology, IV:4.7
   differential diagnosis, IV:4.5*t*
   evaluation, IV:4.7*t*
   fine-needle aspiration biopsy, IV:4.7
   isotope scan, IV:4.7, 4.7*f*
   treatment, IV:4.7–4.8, 4.8*f*
Somatostatin, IV:2.2*f*
   actions, IV:2.3
SPAF. *See* Stroke Prevention in Atrial Fibrillation
Specific-agent-inhalation challenge, in diagnosis of occupational asthma, III:7.2
Specificity, of tests, I:2.2, 2.2*f*, 4.3–4.4
Speed's sign, I:3.6
Sperm antibodies, vasectomy and, IV:12.8
Sperm function tests, IV:12.4
Spirochetal myocarditis, II:19.3*t*
Spirometry, III:1.1, 1.2*f*
   with COPD, III:2.2, 2.3*f*
Spironolactone
   for adrenal tumor, IV:5.10*t*, 5.11
   for hirsutism, IV:10.8
Spondyloarthropathies, cardiac involvement in, II:31.2*t*, 31.6–31.7
Spondylolisthesis, I:3.3–3.4
Sputum cytology, in diagnosis of bronchogenic carcinoma, III:3.5
Sputum examination, III:1.5
   in interstitial lung disease, III:6.5*t*
   in physical diagnosis, I:3.4*t*
Sputum Gram stain, in diagnosis of acute bronchitis, III:4.2, 4.2*f*
Standard of care, appropriate, determining, I:10.2
Staphylococcus aureus pneumonia, III:4.3, 4.3*t*, 4.4*t*
Statute of limitations, I:10.4
Stein-Leventhal syndrome, IV:10.3
Steroid(s). *See also* Adrenal steroids; Glucocorticoid(s)
   biosynthesis, IV:5.1, 5.2*f*, 5.2*t*
Steroid sulfatase deficiency, IV:11.8*t*
Streptococcal infection, and acute rheumatic fever, II:31.1–31.3
Streptococcal myocarditis, II:19.7
Streptococcus pneumoniae
   in acute bronchitis, III:4.2
   in pneumonia, III:4.3, 4.3*t*, 4.4*t*
Streptokinase
   dosage and administration, II:11.5*t*
   for MI, II:11.5–11.6
   pharmacology, II:11.5*t*
   for pulmonary thromboembolism, III:5.7
   stroke risk with, II:11.6
Stress echocardiography, II:1.8
   in coronary artery disease, II:9.3
   in older patients, II:32.4
Stress imaging, in older patients, II:32.4
Stress testing. *See* Exercise (stress) testing
Stridor, I:3.4, 3.10
Stroke
   cardiac sources, II:30.1–30.4, 30.2*f*
   cardioembolic
      diagnosis, II:30.1–30.2
      high-risk groups, II:30.2–30.3, 30.2*t*, 30.3*f*
      medium-risk groups, II:30.3–30.4
      pathophysiology, II:30.1, 30.2*f*
      prevalence, II:30.1
      sources, II:30.1–30.2, 30.2*f*, 30.2*t*
   with coronary artery bypass grafting, II:30.5
   incidence, age and, II:7.1, 7.2*f*
   prevention, II:30.4–30.5, 30.4*t*
   risk, with cardiac disorders, II:30.1
   with thrombolytic therapy, II:11.6

Stroke Prevention in Atrial Fibrillation, II:30.2, 30.4
Sturge-Weber disease, pheochromocytoma and, IV:7.1
Subacromial bursitis, I:3.6
Subacute thyroiditis, IV:4.4–4.5
    clinical features, IV:4.4–4.5
    diagnosis, IV:4.4–4.5
    granulomatous, IV:3.6, 3.7t
    treatment, IV:4.5
Subphrenic abscess, clinical features, III:8.5t
Sudden (cardiac) death
    causes, II:6.1–6.2, 6.2t
    and congestive cardiomyopathy, II:17.9, 17.9f
    electrophysiologic abnormalities with, II:6.2, 6.4
    familial pattern, II:6.2
    and hypertrophic cardiomyopathy, II:16.1
    incidence, II:6.1
    with mitral valve prolapse, II:13.8
Sulfadiazine, for toxoplasmosis, II:19.8
Sulfonylureas
    for diabetes in elderly, IV:21.2–21.3
    for non-insulin-dependent diabetes mellitus (NIDDM), IV:14.5, 14.5t
Superior vena cava syndrome, management, III:3.6
Supraspinatus tendinitis, I:3.6
Surgery
    for bronchogenic carcinoma, III:3.5–3.6
    central arterial, II:23.6
    intraatrial, for congenital heart disease, II:23.4–23.5
    intraventricular, for congenital heart disease, II:23.5–23.6
Swan neck deformity, I:3.2
Sympathomimetics, for congestive heart failure, II:17.8t, 17.9
Syncope, II:5.1–5.5
    with aortic stenosis, II:14.2
    auscultatory findings with, II:5.3
    autonomic dysfunction and, II:5.3
    autonomic testing and, II:5.4
    cardiogenic, II:5.1
    carotid sinus massage and, II:5.4
    causes, II:5.3t, 6.2
    and congestive cardiomyopathy, II:17.9, 17.9f
    diagnostic approach to, II:5.2f
    ECG findings with, II:5.3–5.4
    echocardiography and, II:5.4
    evaluation, II:2.5, 6.5–6.6, 6.6f
    factitious, II:5.2
    history-taking with, II:5.1–5.3
    in hypertrophic cardiomyopathy, II:16.2
    hypotensive, II:5.4
    laboratory evaluation, II:5.3–5.4, 5.4t
    management, II:5.4–5.5
    with mitral valve prolapse, II:13.6
    multiple events, II:5.3
        management, II:5.4
    with myxoma, II:26.1
    neurogenic, II:5.1
    patient's memory, II:5.2–5.3
    physical findings with, II:5.3, 5.3t
    in pregnancy, II:33.2
    prevalence, II:5.1
    psychogenic, II:5.1
    in pulmonary hypertension, II:24.2
    referral for, II:5.4–5.5
    signal-averaged electrocardiograms and, II:5.4
    single event, management, II:5.4
    vasodepressor, II:5.3
    vasovagal, II:5.3
    witnessed vs. unwitnessed, II:5.2

Syndrome of apparent mineralocorticoid excess, IV:8.4, 8.4f
Syndrome of inappropriate antidiuresis
    diagnosis, IV:19.3, 19.3t
    drug-related, IV:19.3, 19.3t
    referral guidelines, IV:19.3
    signs and symptoms, IV:19.3t
    treatment, IV:19.3
Syndrome of inappropriate antidiuretic hormone secretion, IV:1.4–1.6
    and bronchogenic carcinoma, III:3.3t
    causes, IV:1.4, 1.5t
    diagnosis, IV:1.4–1.5
    treatment, IV:1.5–1.6, 1.6f
Syphilis, screening recommendations for, I:2.7t
Systemic lupus erythematosus
    cardiac involvement in, II:31.2t, 31.3–31.4
    interstitial, differential diagnosis, III:6.3t
    lung involvement in, III:6.7f
    myocardial involvement in, II:31.4
    permanent neonatal lupus and, II:31.4
Systemic sclerosis, cardiac involvement in, II:31.2t, 31.5
Systemic vascular resistance (SVR)
    calculation, II:3.7t
    normal value, II:3.7t
Systolic Hypertension in the Elderly Program, II:7.2–7.3, 32.6, 32.7f

T

T_3. *See* Triiodothyronine
T_4. *See* Thyroxine
Tachycardia, II:1.5
    in pregnancy, II:33.3
Tachypnea
    in pregnancy, II:33.3
    with pulmonary embolism, II:25.2
Tactile fremitus, in physical diagnosis, I:3.4t
Takayasu's arteritis
    clinical features, II:28.5
    diagnosis, II:28.5
    occlusive arterial disease and, II:29.3
    pathophysiology, II:28.5
    prognosis for, II:28.5
    treatment, II:28.5
Talc insufflation
    for malignant pleural effusions, III:8.9
    for secondary spontaneous pneumothorax, III:8.3
Talc poudrage, for primary spontaneous pneumothorax, III:8.3
Talc slurry
    for malignant pleural effusions, III:8.9
    for primary spontaneous pneumothorax, III:8.3
    for secondary spontaneous pneumothorax, III:8.3
TEE. *See* Transesophageal echocardiography
Temporal arteritis. *See* Giant cell arteritis
Tendinitis
    bicipital, I:3.6
    supraspinatus, I:3.6
Teratoma, clinical manifestations, II:26.3t
Terazosin
    for benign prostatic hyperplasia, IV:20.6, 20.6f
    indications for, IV:7.6–7.7
    for pheochromocytoma, IV:7.6–7.7, 7.7t
Terbutaline, for acute severe asthma, III:10.4
Testes
    chemotherapy and, IV:11.7
    undescended, IV:11.7
Testicular failure
    autoimmune, IV:11.7

    postpubertal, IV:11.1, 11.2t
    prepubertal, IV:11.1, 11.2t
    treatment, IV:11.3–11.4
Testicular feminization, IV:11.6
Testicular irradiation, IV:11.7
Testicular trauma, IV:11.7
Testosterone
    production, enzyme defects in, IV:11.5, 11.5t, 11.6f
    replacement, dosage and administration, IV:11.10
    serum, in Klinefelter's syndrome, IV:11.3, 11.4f
    supplementation, in older men, IV:21.6
Testosterone enanthate, for male contraception, IV:12.7
Test threshold, I:2.4–2.5, 4.6
Tetracycline(s)
    for acute bronchitis, III:4.2
    for community-acquired pneumonia, III:4.5t
    as sclerosing agent, for malignant pleural effusions, III:8.9
Tetrahydro-18-oxocortisol, urinary, IV:8.4, 8.4f
Tetralogy of Fallot, II:22.10–22.11
    in adult, II:22.2
    anatomy, II:22.10
    clinical features, II:22.10
    diagnosis, II:22.10–22.11
    intracardiac repair for, II:23.5f, 23.5–23.6, 23.6f
    sequelae and residua after, II:23.2, 23.3t
    pathophysiology, II:22.10
    physical findings with, II:22.10–22.11
    pink, II:22.4
    treatment, II:22.11
Thallium-201 stress testing, in coronary artery disease, II:9.3
Theophylline
    for COPD, III:2.7
    efficacy, III:2.8f
    toxicity, III:2.7
Therapeutic relationship, developing and maintaining, I:1.2, 1.2t
Thiazide diuretics, for diabetes insipidus, IV:1.4t
Thirst perception, IV:1.2
Thoracentesis, III:1.6, 1.6t
    in diagnosis of bronchogenic carcinoma, III:3.5
    in diagnosis of pleurisy, III:8.2
Thoracic aortic aneurysm(s), II:28.2–28.3
    clinical presentation, II:28.3
    diagnosis, II:28.2f, 28.3
    imaging, II:28.2f, 28.3
    pathophysiology, II:28.2–28.3
    prognosis for, II:28.3
    treatment, II:28.3
Thoracic outlet maneuver(s), in occlusive arterial disease, II:29.3, 29.4f
Thoracoscopy, III:1.6
Thromboangiitis obliterans
    clinical features, II:29.3, 29.5t
    occlusive arterial disease due to, II:29.2
    prognosis for, II:29.5
Thromboembolism. *See also* Embolism/emboli
    aortic, II:28.6
    in infectious endocarditis, II:20.2–20.3
Thromboendarterectomy, for chronic thrombotic pulmonary hypertension, III:5.4
Thrombolytic therapy
    age and, II:32.5
    cerebrovascular complications, II:30.5
    contraindications to, II:11.6–11.7
    for coronary artery trauma, II:27.8
    for deep venous thrombosis, II:25.3t, 29.7
    for MI, II:11.4, 11.5–11.6, 11.5t
        early adjunctive therapy with, II:11.6
        recommendation for, II:11.6–11.7

pericarditis and, II:21.3–21.4
for pulmonary embolism, II:3.6, 25.3t, 25.7, 25.7t
Thrombophlebitis, superficial
diagnosis, II:29.7
differential diagnosis, II:29.7
management, II:29.7
recurrence, II:29.7, 29.8t
Thymoma, SIADH with, IV:1.4, 1.5t
Thyroidectomy, for hyperthyroidism, IV:3.5
Thyroid function tests, IV:3.1–3.2
drugs affecting, IV:3.2t
Thyroid gland. See also Hypothalamic-pituitary-thyroid axis
carcinoma, IV:4.6–4.7, 4.7t
medullary, IV:7.1
disorders, IV:3.1–3.7. See also Graves' disease; Hyperthyroidism; Hypothyroidism
autoimmune, IV:3.6, 4.1–4.3
in elderly, IV:21.4–21.6
screening recommendations for, I:2.6t
examination, IV:4.1
function, and nonthyroidal illness, IV:3.6, 3.6f
masses, IV:4.1–4.9. See also Goiter; Solitary thyroid nodules
Thyroiditis
Hashimoto's lymphocytic, IV:3.2, 3.6
infectious, IV:4.5
lymphocytic, IV:3.6, 3.7t
postpartum, IV:3.6, 4.3
subacute, IV:4.4–4.5
subacute granulomatous, IV:3.6, 3.7t
Thyroid-stimulating hormone (thyrotropin), IV:2.2f
deficiency, IV:2.5
reserve, test for, IV:2.1
response to TRH, IV:2.1, 3.2
secretion, by pituitary tumors, IV:2.6t, 2.9
serum
measurement, IV:3.2
and nonthyroidal illness, IV:3.6, 3.6f
normal, IV:3.2
Thyroid storm, IV:3.5–3.6
treatment, IV:3.6t
Thyrotropin-releasing hormone, IV:2.2f
TSH response to, IV:3.2
D-Thyroxine, lipid-lowering therapy, clinical intervention trial, II:8.6
Thyroxine, serum
and nonthyroidal illness, IV:3.6, 3.6f
normal, IV:3.1
test, IV:3.1
Tilt-table testing, II:2.5
indications for, II:4.6t
Tinel's sign, I:3.3
Tinkles, I:3.8
Tissue plasminogen activator
dosage and administration, II:11.5t
for MI, II:11.5–11.6
pharmacology, II:11.5t
stroke risk with, II:11.6
Tobacco, chewing, and syndrome of apparent mineralocorticoid excess, IV:8.4
Toes
clubbing, with patent ductus arteriosus, II:22.6, 22.6f
Tolazamide, for non-insulin-dependent diabetes mellitus (NIDDM), IV:14.5, 14.5t
Tolbutamide, for non-insulin-dependent diabetes mellitus (NIDDM), IV:14.5, 14.5t
Toluene diisocyanate, III:7.2
Tomography, conventional, pulmonary, III:1.5
Torsade de pointes, II:6.2
ventricular proarrhythmia, II:6.2, 6.3f

Total lung capacity, III:1.2
Toxoplasmosis, myocarditis in, II:19.8
Tracheostomy
contraindications to, III:7.7
for obstructive sleep apnea, III:9.6–9.7
Transesophageal echocardiography
of aortic dissection, II:28.4–28.5
of cardiac sources for emboli, II:30.4
with cardiac tumors, II:26.4–26.5
in congenital heart disease, II:23.2–23.3
with mitral stenosis, II:12.2, 12.3f
of myocardial contusion, II:27.7
of ulcerated plaques in aortic arch, II:30.4
Transposition of the great arteries, intracardiac repair for
sequelae and residua after, II:23.3t, 23.4
surgical procedures, II:23.4f, 23.5
Transsphenoidal resection, of pituitary tumor, IV:2.11, 2.11f
Transthoracic needle aspiration biopsy, in diagnosis of bronchogenic carcinoma, III:3.5, 3.5f
Transurethral resection of prostate, for benign prostatic hyperplasia, IV:20.6
vs. finasteride therapy, IV:20.4, 20.4f
Trauma
cardiac, nonpenetrating, II:27.1–27.10. See also Coronary artery trauma; Myocardial contusion
complications, II:27.3, 27.3t
mechanism of injury, II:27.1, 27.2t
outcome with, II:27.2–27.3, 27.3t
occlusive arterial disease due to, II:29.2
Travel history, and interstitial lung disease, III:6.2
Triamcinolone, pharmacology, IV:6.2t
Trichinosis, myocarditis in, II:19.8
Tricuspid valve
atresia, II:14.9
intracardiac repair for, sequelae and residua after, II:23.3t
disease, II:15.1–15.4
acquired, II:15.2–15.4
congenital, II:15.1–15.2
incompetence, auscultatory findings, II:20.5
regurgitation, II:15.3–15.4
auscultatory features, II:15.4
ECG findings with, II:15.4
functional, II:15.3–15.4
intracardiac repair for, sequelae and residua after, II:23.4
organic, II:15.3–15.4, 15.4t
physical findings with, I:3.3
regurgitation (insufficiency), I:3.7t, 3.7–3.8
replacement, indications for, II:15.3, 15.4
stenosis, II:15.2–15.3, 15.2t, 15.3f, 15.3t
auscultatory features, II:15.3, 15.3t
Trigger finger, I:3.2
Triglyceride(s), serum
and cardiovascular disease, IV:18.2
coronary heart disease risk and, II:7.4–7.6
decision cutoffs with, II:8.3, 8.4t
measurement, II:8.2–8.4
Triiodothyronine
for hypothyroidism, IV:3.3
serum
and nonthyroidal illness, IV:3.6, 3.6f
normal, IV:3.1
test, IV:3.1
Triiodothyronine uptake test, IV:3.2
Trimethoprim/sulfamethoxazole
for acute bronchitis, III:4.2
for community-acquired pneumonia, III:4.5t
Troleandomycin, drug interactions, with glucocorticoids, IV:6.5t

Tropical eosinophilia, differential diagnosis, III:6.9t
Trypanosoma cruzi. See Chagas' disease
Trypanosomiasis, II:19.7–19.8
Tube drainage
with instillation of sclerosing agent
for malignant pleural effusions, III:8.9
technique for, III:8.9
for secondary spontaneous pneumothorax, III:8.3
Tuberculosis
differential diagnosis, III:6.9t
miliary, interstitial, differential diagnosis, III:6.3t
pericarditis in, II:21.1, 21.3
management, II:21.3
pleurisy in, clinical features, III:8.4t
screening recommendations for, I:2.7t
SIADH with, IV:1.4, 1.5t
Tuberculous pericarditis, II:21.1, 21.3
management, II:21.3
Tuberous sclerosis, pheochromocytoma and, IV:7.1
Tube thoracostomy
with instillation of sclerosing agent, for primary spontaneous pneumothorax, III:8.3
for primary spontaneous pneumothorax, III:8.3
for secondary spontaneous pneumothorax, III:8.3
Tumor(s). See also *specific tumor*
acromegaly caused by, IV:19.5, 19.5f
adrenal. See Adrenal tumor(s)
apical pulmonary, diagnosis, III:3.4
cardiac. See Cardiac tumors
chromaffin, IV:7.2, 7.3
ectopic Cushing's syndrome with, IV:19.3–19.4
human chorionic gonadotropin production by, IV:19.6
Hümle cell, IV:4.5
hypoglycemia caused by, IV:19.4t, 19.5
lung. See Lung(s), tumors
nonendocrine, hormone production by, IV:19.1, 19.2f, 19.2t
osteomalacia caused by, IV:19.5–19.6
ovarian, lipoid cell, IV:10.5
pituitary. See Pituitary tumor(s)
renin-secreting, IV:19.6
Tumor plop, II:26.2
Turner syndrome, IV:10.2
24-hour monitoring, II:1.8
indications for, II:4.6t
Typhoid fever, II:19.7

U

UAP. See Angina pectoris, unstable
Ulceration
ischemic, II:29.2, 29.2f, 29.2t
stress, therapy for, III:10.7
venous stasis, II:29.2t, 29.8, 29.9f
Ulcerative colitis, cardiac involvement in, II:31.6–31.7
Ulnar nerve, screening examination, I:3.3t
Ultrasound
B-mode, in deep venous thrombosis, II:25.1–25.2
in deep venous thrombosis, II:29.7
in diagnosis of pleurisy, III:8.2
in differential diagnosis of renal failure, III:10.8
of lungs, III:1.4
in restrictive cardiomyopathy, II:18.2
Univentricular heart, intracardiac repair for, II:23.2t, 23.6f, 23.7
sequelae and residua after, II:23.3t

University of California–San Francisco Familial Hypercholesterolemia trial, II:8.6–8.7
Uremia, pericarditis with, management, II:21.3
Urinalysis, with pheochromocytoma, IV:7.3–7.4, 7.3*t*
Urine, catecholamines in, with pheochromocytoma, IV:7.3*t*, 7.3–7.4
Urogenital atrophy, postmenopausal, IV:22.3
Urokinase
    for coronary artery trauma, II:27.8
    dosage and administration, II:11.5*t*
    pharmacology, II:11.5*t*
    for pulmonary thromboembolism, III:5.7
US Preventive Services Task Force, screening recommendations from, I:2.5
Uterine bleeding, abnormal (dysfunctional). *See* Abnormal uterine bleeding
Uterine fibroids, IV:9.2–9.3, 9.3*f*
    medical therapy for, IV:9.4–9.5
    surgical therapy for, IV:9.5
Uterine polyps, IV:9.3, 9.4*f*
Uterus, gravid, hemodynamic effects, II:33.2, 33.2*f*
Utilization review, I:6.4, 7.3
Uvulopalatopharyngoplasty, for obstructive sleep apnea, III:9.6–9.7

V

Vaccine(s), live attenuated viral, drug interactions, with glucocorticoids, IV:6.4*t*
Values
    analysis, I:9.2
    and ethics, I:8.2
Valvotomy, for congenital heart disease, sequelae and residua, II:23.3
Valvular heart disease
    acquired, in pregnancy, II:33.2–33.4
    congenital, in adult, II:22.7–22.9
    in elderly, II:32.8
        diagnosis, II:32.8
        prevalence, II:32.8
        treatment, II:32.8
    physical findings with, II:1.5
Vancomycin, for nosocomial pneumonia, III:4.7*t*
Vanillylmandelic acid, urinary, with pheochromocytoma, IV:7.3*t*, 7.3–7.4
Vanishing testis syndrome, IV:11.5
Varicocele, gonadotropin response to GnRH with, IV:11.1, 11.3*f*
Varicose vein(s), II:29.8–29.9
    pulmonary, II:22.2
    superficial phlebitis, II:29.7
Vasculitis
    cardiac involvement in, II:31.2*t*, 31.6
    in polymyositis and dermatomyositis, II:31.6
Vasectomy, IV:12.7–12.8, 12.8*t*
    acceptability, IV:12.8
    complications, IV:12.8
    reversal, IV:12.8
    sperm antibodies and, IV:12.8
Vasoactive intestinal (poly)peptide, IV:2.2*f*
Vasodilator therapy
    for congestive heart failure, II:17.8
    for pheochromocytoma, IV:7.7, 7.7*t*
    for pulmonary hypertension, III:5.4–5.5
Vasopressin, IV:1.2
    aqueous, for diabetes insipidus, IV:1.3–1.4, 1.4*t*
    deficiency, IV:2.5
    plasma, in SIADH, IV:1.5
    secretion, in elderly, IV:21.5–21.6
    urinary, in SIADH, IV:1.5
Venous disease, II:29.7–29.9. *See also* Chronic venous insufficiency; Deep venous thrombosis
Venous stasis ulceration, II:29.2*t*, 29.8, 29.9*f*
Venous thrombosis. *See also* Deep venous thrombosis
    diagnosis, II:29.7
    differential diagnosis, II:29.7
    management, II:29.7, 29.8*f*
    recurrence, II:29.7, 29.8*t*
    superficial, II:29.7
Ventilation-perfusion lung scan
    in diagnosis of pulmonary thromboembolism, III:5.6
    in differential diagnosis of pulmonary hypertension, III:5.4
    with pulmonary embolism, II:25.4*f*, 25.4–25.5, 25.5*t*
    in pulmonary hypertension, II:24.2*f*, 24.3
Ventilatory control disorders, III:9.1–9.8
Ventricle(s). *See also* Left ventricular; Right ventricle
    single. *See also* Univentricular heart
        intracardiac repair for, sequelae and residua after, II:23.3*t*
Ventricular dysfunction. *See also* Heart failure
    clinical features, II:2.1
    initial evaluation, II:2.1–2.7
    physical findings with, II:1.5
Ventricular fibrillation
    with acute MI, II:11.3
    sudden cardiac death due to, II:6.1–6.2
Ventricular septal defect, I:3.7*t*, 3.7–3.8. *See also* Interventricular septal defect
Ventricular septal rupture
    diagnosis, II:3.4*t*
    hemodynamic parameters for, II:3.6*t*
Ventricular tachycardia, II:6.2
    with acute MI, II:11.3
Verapamil. *See also* Calcium channel blockers
    for angina, II:9.5
    for hypertrophic cardiomyopathy, II:16.4
    precautions with, II:9.5
    in viral myocarditis, II:19.5
Vertebra, compression fracture, I:3.3
Viral infection
    congestive cardiomyopathy and, II:17.1–17.2, 17.3*t*
    myocarditis due to, II:19.1–19.4
Viral pericarditis, management, II:21.3
Virilization
    in congenital adrenal hyperplasia, IV:10.3, 10.3*t*
    during pregnancy, IV:10.4
    tumoral, IV:10.5
Visual acuity loss, screening recommendations for, I:2.7*t*
Vital capacity, in normal and disease states, III:1.3*t*
Vitruvian Man, I:9.1, 9.2*f*
Vitums' sign, I:3.3, 3.7
Volume, homeostasis, IV:8.1, 8.2*f*
Volume expansion
    in elderly, IV:21.5
    indications for, II:13.9
    with pheochromocytoma, IV:7.3
von Hippel-Lindau disease, pheochromocytoma and, IV:7.1–7.2, 7.1–7.2
VSD (ventricular septal defect). *See* Interventricular septal defect

W

Warfarin therapy
    in congestive heart failure, II:17.9
    for deep venous thrombosis, II:25.2
    for MI, for secondary prevention, II:11.7*t*
    for pulmonary thromboembolism, III:5.6
    in stroke prevention, II:30.4–30.5, 30.4*t*
    teratogenicity, II:33.4
Water balance
    disorders, IV:1.1–1.6
    regulation, IV:1.1–1.2
Water deprivation test, IV:1.3, 1.3*t*
Water intoxication, in elderly, IV:21.5–21.6
Water load test, oral, IV:1.5, 1.5*t*
Water restriction, for SIADH, IV:1.6, 1.6*t*
Weakness, lower extremity, I:3.4, 3.4*t*
Wegener's granulomatosis, III:6.8
    cardiac involvement in, II:31.6
    and polyarteritis, differential diagnosis, III:6.9*t*
Weight gain, in congestive cardiomyopathy, II:17.2
Weight loss, for obstructive sleep apnea, III:9.6
Wheezes, I:3.4, 3.10, 3.11*t*
White blood cell count, cardiovascular disease and, II:7.7
Wolff-Parkinson-White syndrome, II:6.6, 22.12, 23.4
    electrophysiologic abnormalities with, II:6.2
World War II, medical advances in, I:7.2
Wristdrop hand, I:3.3

X

Xanthomas, II:8.3, 9.2
XX karyotype, in males, IV:11.4
XXXY karyotype, IV:11.3
XXY karyotype, IV:11.2–11.3
XY/XO mixed gonadal dysgenesis, IV:11.4
XYY syndrome, IV:11.4

Y

Yergason's sign, I:3.6

Z

Zoladex, plus flutamide, for prostate cancer, IV:20.8–20.9, 20.9*t*

Color Plates
II. Cardiology

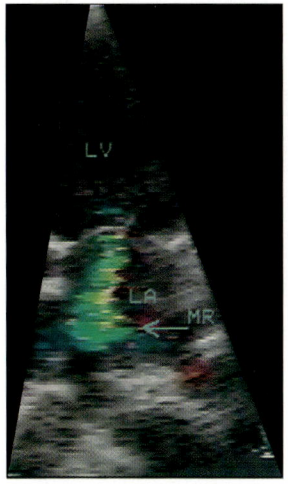
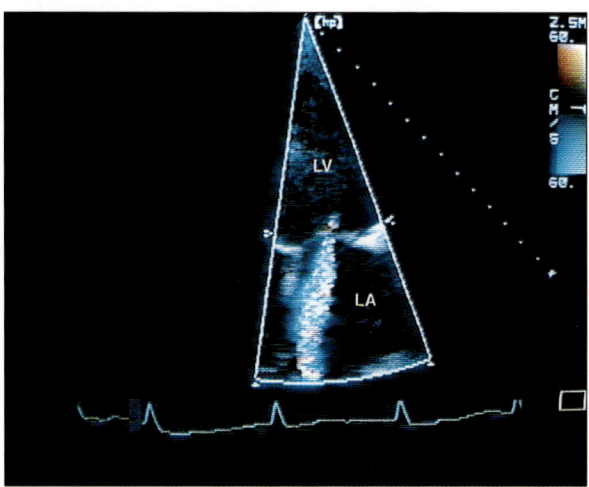

Chapter 2, Figure 3B, p. II:2.5   Chapter 12, Figure 3, p. II:12.5

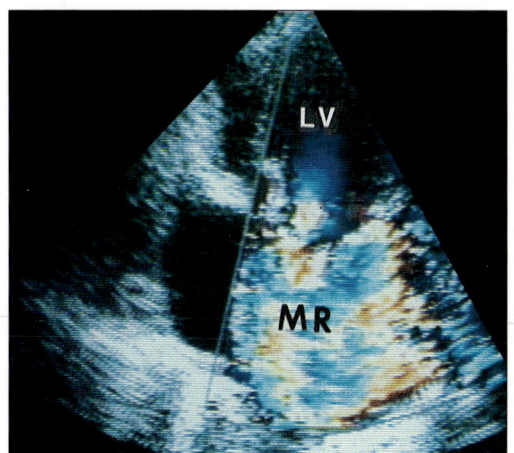 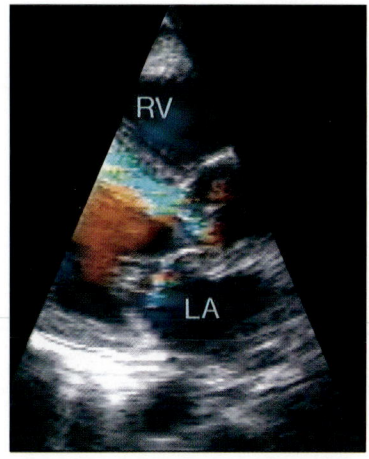 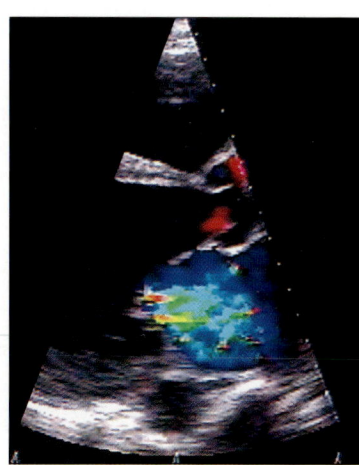

Chapter 13, Figure 12, p. II:13.7   Chapter 14, Figure 8B, p. II:14.8   Chapter 17, Figure 9C, p. II:17.6

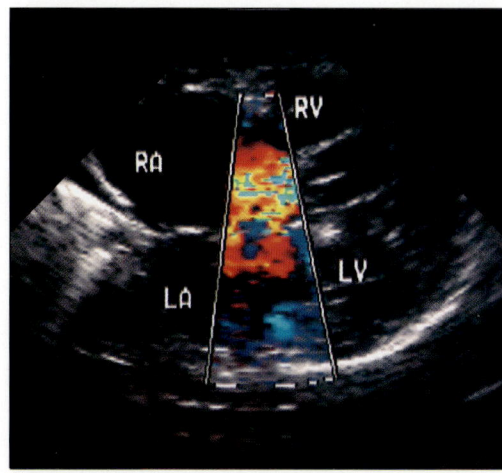 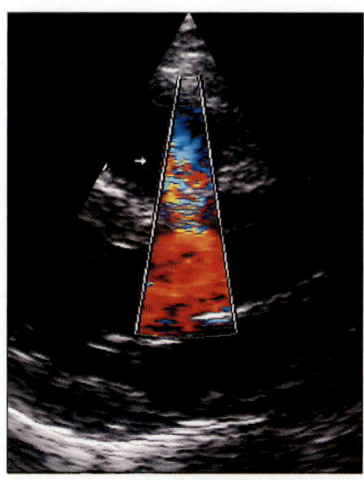

Chapter 22, Figure 2, p. II:22.3   Chapter 22, Figure 3, p. II:22.5

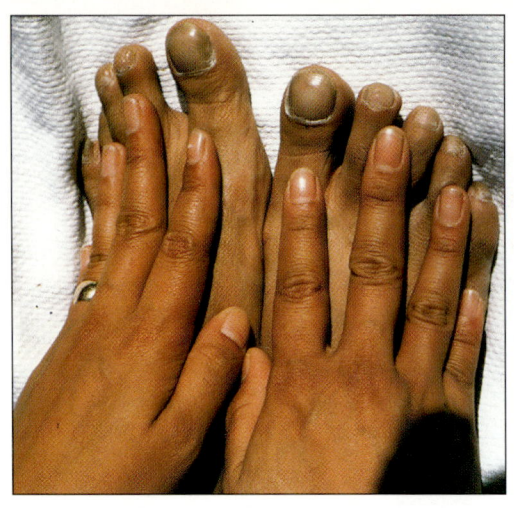

Chapter 22, Figure 4, p. II:22.6

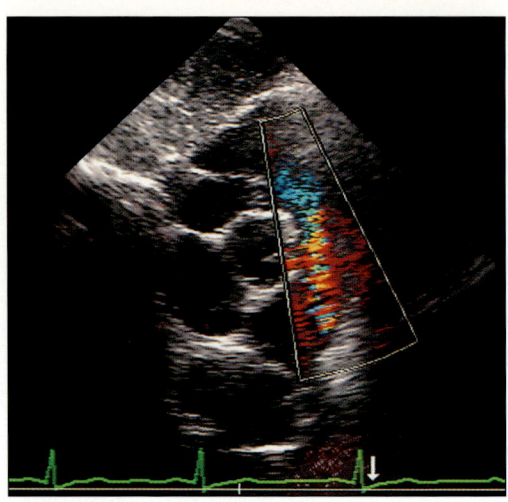

Chapter 22, Figure 5, p. II:22.6

III. PULMONARY AND CRITICAL CARE MEDICINE

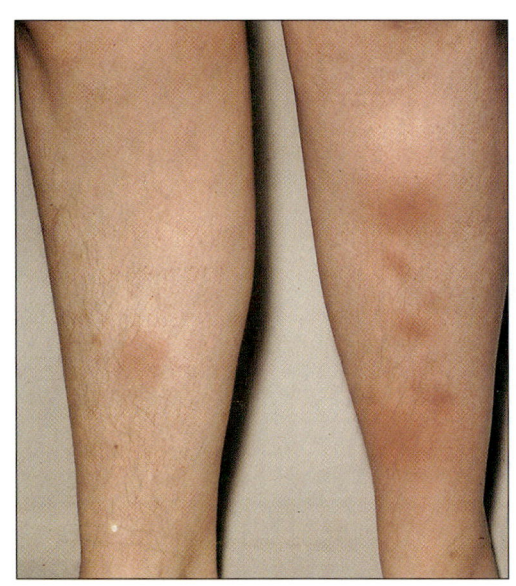

Chapter 6, Figure 2B, p. III:6.2

IV. ENDOCRINOLOGY AND METABOLIC DISEASE

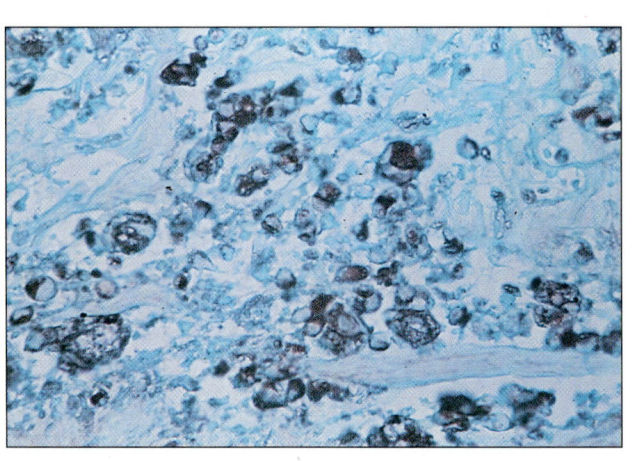

Chapter 19, Figure 1, p. IV:19.2